Seventh Edition

Handbook
of
Applied Therapeutics

Seventh Edition

Handbook
of
Applied Therapeutics

Mary Anne Koda-Kimble, PharmD
Professor and Dean, TJ Long Chair in Chain Pharmacy Practice
School of Pharmacy, University of California at San Francisco
San Francisco, California

Lloyd Yee Young, PharmD
Professor and Chair, Department of Clinical Pharmacy
TA Oliver Chair in Clinical Pharmacy
School of Pharmacy, University of California at San Francisco
San Francisco, California

Wayne A. Kradjan, PharmD
Dean and Professor
College of Pharmacy, Oregon State University
Corvallis, Oregon

B. Joseph Guglielmo, PharmD
Professor, Division of Clinical Pharmacy
School of Pharmacy, University of California at San Francisco
San Francisco, California

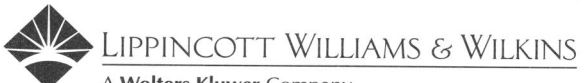

LIPPINCOTT WILLIAMS & WILKINS
A **Wolters Kluwer** Company
Philadelphia · Baltimore · New York · London
Buenos Aires · Hong Kong · Sydney · Tokyo

Editor: David Troy
Managing Editor: Matthew J. Hauber
Marketing Manager: Chris Kushner
Project Editor: Paula C. Williams
Designer: Armen Kojoyian
Compositor: Graphic World, Inc.
Printer: Vicks Lithograph & Printing

351 West Camden Street
Baltimore, Maryland 21201–2436 USA

530 Walnut Street
Philadelphia, Pennsylvania 19106–3621 USA

Printed in the United States of America

Library of Congress Cataloging-in-Publication Data

LOC data is available 0-7817-3484-3

To purchase additional copies of this book, call our customer service department at **(800) 638–3030** or fax orders to **(301) 824–7390**. International customers should call **(301) 714–2324**.

Visit Lippincott Williams & Wilkins on the Internet: http://www.LWW.com. Lippincott Williams & Wilkins customer service representatives are available from 8:30 am to 6:00 pm, EST.

02 03 04 05
1 2 3 4 5 6 7 8 9 10

Preface

The text, *Applied Therapeutics: The Clinical Use of Drugs,*[1] provides a unique blend of factual information and practical application for both the beginning student and the mature practitioner. The case study format brings alive clinical concepts that cannot be envisioned in a standard textbook. Nevertheless, in the day-to-day-management of patients, the clinician often needs quick access to the "clinical pearls" in order to formulate rapid therapeutic decisions. It is for this purpose that the first edition of *The Handbook of Applied Therapeutics* was published. Now, several editions and many years later, this newest edition has been prepared to reflect the substantial increase in drug knowledge since the 1996 publication of the 6th edition.

In these times of national attention on medical errors, escalating costs, and shortages of nurses and pharmacists, we hope that the ready accessibility of clinically important drug information will make the *Handbook of Applied Therapeutics* a valuable tool for assisting in the safe and efficient use of drugs. The authors have abstracted hundreds of valuable tables and other information from the 7th edition of *Applied Therapeutics: The Clinical Use of Drugs* and have supplemented it with dozens of new tables that represent the collective expertise of the editors and authors of the original text. To achieve portability of size, only the most essential data have been included. Therefore, the user is strongly encouraged to refer to the primary text for more detail and for literature documentation.

B. Joseph Guglielmo
Mary Anne Koda-Kimble
Wayne A. Kradjan
Lloyd Yee Young
November 2001

---

[1]*Applied Therapeutics: The Clinical Use of Drugs, 7th ed.*, 2001, edited by Mary Anne Koda-Kimble, Lloyd Yee Young, Wayne A. Kradjan, and B. Joseph Guglielmo (ISBN 0–7817–3137–2).

Acknowledgments

The editors of the *Handbook of Applied Therapeutics* have abstracted and compiled hundreds of valuable tables and other information based upon the work of contributing authors from the 7th edition of *Applied Therapeutics: The Clinical Use of Drugs*. We are indebted to each of the authors for their thoughtful work in preparing their original chapters for *Applied Therapeutics* and fully acknowledge that the Handbook is derived from their chapters. We appreciate the excellent coordination of editors, production staff, and other support personnel by Matt Hauber, Managing Editor of Lippincott Williams & Wilkins. Finally, a deeply appreciative thank you to our spouses, Deter Guglielmo, Donald Kimble, Carolyn Kradjan, and Linda Young for your long-standing patience and support as we worked on yet another edition.

Notice to Reader

Drug therapy information is constantly evolving. Our ever-changing knowledge and experience with drugs and the continual development of new drugs necessitates changes in treatment and drug therapy. The editors, authors, and publisher of this work have made every effort to ensure that the information provided herein was accurate at the time of publication. *It remains the responsibility of every practitioner to evaluate the appropriateness of a particular opinion or therapy in the context of the actual clinical situation and with due consideration of any new developments in the field.* Although the authors have been careful to recommend dosages that are in agreement with current standards and responsible literature, the student or practitioner should consult several appropriate information sources when dealing with new and unfamiliar drugs.

Table of Contents

VII. Nutrition Issues

VIII. Dermatological Disorders

IX. Arthritic Disorders

X. Women's Health

XI. Endocrine Disorders

XII. Eye Disorders

XIII. Neurological Disorders

XIV. Infectious Diseases

x

Chapter 1

Interpretation of Clinical Laboratory Tests

Principles

♦ The serum, urine, and other fluids of patients are analyzed routinely; however, lab tests should only be ordered if the results of the test will affect decisions about the therapeutic management of the patient.

♦ Clinicians should use the normal values listed by their own laboratory facility when interpreting laboratory tests results, rather than those published in reference texts, because laboratories may use different methods of assay.

Laboratory Error should always be considered when laboratory results do not correlate with clinical expectations. Common sources of laboratory error are as follows:

♦ Spoiled specimen (e.g., improper handling or delay in assay);
♦ Specimen taken at wrong time;
♦ Incomplete specimen collection (e.g., 24-hr urine);
♦ Faulty reagents;
♦ Technical errors (e.g., calibration of instrument, interchange of patient names);
♦ Diagnostic and therapeutic procedures (e.g., digital prostate exam before PSA assay);
♦ Medications (e.g., interference with testing procedure or altering values by virtue of pharmacological properties).

Units of Measure

♦ Most countries report clinical laboratory values in the metric system (SI units), except in the United States.
♦ Table 1.1 lists SI units and symbols.

Serum Chemistry Reference Values in SI and conventional units are listed in Table 1.2.

Hematologic Laboratory Values are listed in Table 1.3.

Coagulation Tests

♦ Control of bleeding depends on the formation of a platelet plug and the formation of a stable fibrin clot.

♦ The prothrombin time (PT), international normalized ratio (INR), and activated partial thromboplastin time (aPTT) are commonly used laboratory tests of coagulation to assist clinicians in localizing the specific factor responsible for a coagulation abnormality. Clinical applications of laboratory tests of coagulation are described in Chapter 13: Thrombosis.

Urinalysis

♦ Gross appearance should be clear and color should be slightly yellow depending on the degree of dilution. Urinalysis may reveal clouds of crystals, bilirubin, blood, porphyrins, proteins, food or drug colorings, or melanin.

♦ Specimen pH normally is acidic (pH 4.6 to 8).

♦ Specific gravity should be 1.020 to 1.025, and variances reflect renal concentrating mechanisms.

♦ Proteinuria often reflects renal injury, but a positive qualitative test for urine protein should be repeated after a few days because transient proteinuria can accompany various physiologic and pathologic states.

♦ Microscopic examination of urine sediment for RBCs, WBCs, casts, yeast, crystals, and epithelial cells provides clues to various conditions.

Urine Drug Screening

♦ Detection time in urine for commonly abused substances (e.g., cocaine) are listed in Table 1.4.

Table 1.1 • SI Units and Symbols

Physical Quantity Measured	Unit	Symbol
Length	Meter	m
Mass	Kilogram	kg
Time	Second	s
Amount of substance	Mole	mol
Temperature	Kelvin	K
Electric current	Ampere	A
Luminous intensity	Candela	Cd
Area	Square meter	m^2
Volume	Cubic meter	m^3
Force	Newton	N
Pressure	Pascal	Pa
Work energy	Joule	J
Density	Kilogram per cubic meter	kg/m^3
Frequency	Hertz	Hz

Notes:

Table 1.2 • Blood Chemistry Reference Values

Laboratory Test	Conventional Units (Normal Reference Values)	SI Units (Normal Reference Values)	Conversion Factor	Comments
Acid phosphatase	0–3 KA units	0–5.5 U/L	1	From prostate; different form in erythrocytes and platelets. ↑ in prostatic carcinoma or vigorous prostatic massage.
ALT	0–3.5 U/L	0–3.5 U/L[a]	1	From heart, liver, muscle, kidney, pancreas. ↑ negligible unless parenchymal liver disease. More liver-specific than AST.
Albumin	4–6 g/dL	40–60 g/dL	10	Produced in liver; important for intravascular osmotic pressure. ↓ in liver disease, malnutrition, ascites, hemorrhage, protein-wasting nephropathy.
Alk Phos	30–120 U/L	30–120 U/L	1	Large amounts in bile ducts, placenta, bone. ↑ in bile duct obstruction, obstructive liver disease, rapid bone growth (e.g., Paget's), pregnancy.
AST	0–35 U/L	0–35 U/L	1	Large amounts in heart and liver; moderate amounts in muscle, kidney, and pancreas. ↑ with myocardial infarction and liver injury.
Bilirubin				
Total	0.1–1 mg/dL	2–18 μmol/L	17.1	Breakdown product of hemoglobin, bound to albumin, conjugated (direct) in liver. ↑ with hemolysis, cholestasis, liver injury.
Direct	0–0.2 mg/dL	0–4 μmol/L	17.1	
BUN	8–18 mg/dL	3–6.5 mmol/L	0.357	End product of protein metabolism, produced by liver, transported in blood, excreted renally. ↑ in renal dysfunction, high protein intake, upper GI bleeding, volume contraction.
Calcium				
Total	8.8–10.2 mg/dL	2.20–2.56 mmol/L	0.250	Regulated by body skeleton redistribution, parathyroid hormone, vitamin D, calcitonin. Plasma level affected by changes in albumin concentration (40% bound to albumin).
	4.4–5.1 mEq/L	2.20–2.56 mmol/L	0.250	Physiologically active form. Unbound "free" calcium remains unchanged as albumin fluctuates.
Unbound	4–4.6 mg/dL	1.0–1.15 mmol/L	0.250	Total calcium ↓ when albumin ↓.
	2.0–2.3 mEq/L	1.0–1.15 mmol/L	0.250	
CO_2 content	22–28 mEq/L	22–28 mmol/L	1	Sum of HCO_3 and dissolved CO_2. Reflects acid-base balance and compensatory pulmonary (CO_2) and renal (HCO_3) mechanisms. Primarily reflects HCO_3.
Chloride	95–105 mEq/L	95–105 mmol/L	1	Important for acid-base balance. ↓ by GI loss of chloride-rich fluid (vomiting, diarrhea, GI suction, intestinal fistulas, overdiuresis).
Cholesterol				
Total	<200 mg/dL	<5.2 mmol/L	0.02586	Desirable = Total <200; LDL <130; HDL >50 mg/dL; ↑ LDL or ↓ HDL are risk factors for cardiovascular disease. High in hypothyroid, nephrotic syndrome, systemic lupus erythematosus, multiple myeloma, obstructive liver disease.
LDL	<130 mg/dL	<3.362 mmol/L	0.02586	
HDL	>50 mg/dL	>1.29 mmol/L	0.02586	

(continued)

Table 1.2 • Blood Chemistry Reference Values (continued)

Laboratory Test	Normal Reference Values		Conversion Factor	Comments
	Conventional Units	SI Units		
CK	0–150 U/L	0–150 U/L	1	In tissues that use high energy (skeletal muscle, myocardium, brain). ↑ by IM injections, myocardial infarction, acute psychotic episodes. Isoenzyme CK-MM in skeletal muscle; CK-MB in myocardium; CK-BB in brain. MB Fraction >5% in MI.
Creatinine	0.6–1.2 mg/dL	50–110 μmol/L	88.4	Major constituent of muscle; rate of formation constant; affected by muscle mass; excreted renally. ↑ in renal dysfunction. Cimetidine and trimethoprim interfere.
Cl$_{Cr}$	75–125 mL/min	1.24–2.08 mL/s	0.01667	Reflects glomerular filtration rate; ↓ in renal dysfunction.
GGT	0–30 U/L	0–30 U/L	1	Sensitive test reflecting hepatocellular injury; not helpful in differentiating liver disorders. Usually high in chronic alcoholics.
Globulin	2.3–3.5 g/dL	23–35 g/L	10	Active role in immunologic mechanisms. Immunoglobulins ↑ in chronic infection, rheumatoid arthritis, multiple myeloma.
Glucose	70–110 mg/dL	3.9–6.1 mmol/L	0.05551	↑ in diabetes or by adrenal corticosteroids.
Iron				Body stores ⅔ in hemoglobin; ⅓ in bone marrow, spleen, liver; only small amount present in plasma. Blood loss major cause of deficiency.
Male	80–180 μg/dL	14–32 μmol/L	0.1791	
Female	60–160 μg/dL	11–29 μmol/L	0.1791	↑ needs in pregnancy and lactation.
TIBC	250–460 μg/dL	45–82 μmol/L	0.1791	↑ capacity to bind iron with iron deficiency.
LD	50–150 U/L	50–150 U/L	1	High in heart, kidney, liver, and skeletal muscle. 5 isoenzymes—LD$_1$ mostly in heart, LD$_5$ mostly in liver and skeletal muscle. Pleural fluid to serum LD ratio >0.6 suggests exudative rather than transudative effusion.
Magnesium	1.6–2.4 mEq/L	0.8–1.20 mmol/L	0.5 1	Malabsorption, severe diarrhea, alcoholism, pancreatitis, diuretics, hyperaldosteronism causes for hypomagnesemia (symptoms of weakness, depression, agitation, seizures, hypokalemia, and arrhythmias). Renal failure can cause hypermagnesemia.
	1.8–3.0 mg/dL	0.8–1.20 mmol/L	0.5 1	

Test	Conventional units	SI units	Conversion factor	Comments
Phosphate[b]	2.5–5 mg/dL	8.8–1.60 mmol/L	0.3229	↑ with renal dysfunction, hypervitaminosis D, and hypoparathyroidism. ↓ with excess aluminum antacids, malabsorption, renal losses.
Potassium	3.5–5 mEq/L	3.5–5 mmol/L	1	↑ by renal dysfunction, acidosis, hemolysis, burns, crush injuries. ↓ by diuretics, alkalosis, protracted vomiting, severe diarrhea.
Sodium	135–147 mEq/L	135–147 mmol/L	1	Low sodium usually because of dilution with water (e.g., excess serum antidiuretic hormone) and treated with water restriction.
SGOT	See AST			
SGPT	See ALT			
Triglycerides	<160 mg/dL	<1.80 mmol/L	0.01129	↑ by alcohol, saturated fats, drugs (propranolol, diuretics, oral contraceptives).
Uric acid	2–7 mg/dL	120–420 μmol/L	59.48	↑ in gout, neoplastic or myeloproliferative disorders, and drugs (diuretics, niacin, low-dose salicylate, cyclosporine).

[a]Enzyme activity can be reported as U/L, where 1 unit equals the amount of enzyme generating 1 μmol of product per minute, or as a katal (kat) unit, which reports product formation in moles per second. The U/L will be used in this book rather than the katal.
[b]Phosphate as inorganic phosphorus.

Alk Phos, alkaline phosphatase; ALT, alanine aminotransferase; AST, aspartate aminotransferase; BUN, blood urea nitrogen; CO_2, carbon dioxide; CK, creatine kinase, formerly known as creatine phosphokinase (CPK); Cl_{Cr}, creatinine clearance; GGT, gamma-glutamyl transferase; HDL, high-density lipoprotein; KA units, King-Armstrong units; LD, lactate dehydrogenase, formerly known as LDH; LDL, low-density lipoprotein; MI, myocardial infarction; SGOT, serum glutamate oxaloacetic transaminase; SGPT, serum glutamate pyruvate transaminase; TIBC, total iron-binding capacity.

Table 1.3 • Hematologic Laboratory Values[a]

Laboratory Test	Normal Reference Values		Comments
	Conventional Units	SI Units	
ESR			Nonspecific; ↑ with inflammation, infection, neoplasms, connective tissue disorders, pregnancy, nephritis. Useful monitor of temporal arteritis and polymyalgia rheumatica.
Male	0–20 mm/hr	0–20 mm/hr	
Female	0–30 mm/hr	0–30 mm/hr	
Hct			↓ with anemias, bleeding, hemolysis. ↑ with polycythemia, chronic hypoxia.
Male	39–49%	0.39–0.49 I[a]	
Female	33–43%	0.33–0.43 I[a]	
Hgb			Similar to hematocrit.
Male	14–18 g/dL	140–180 g/L	
Female	11.5–15.5 g/dL	115–155 g/L	
MCH	27–33 pg	27–32 pg	Measures weight of Hgb in average RBC.
MCHC	33–37 g/dL	330–370 g/L	More reliable index of red cell hemoglobin than MCH. Measures concentration of Hgb in average RBC. Concentration will not change with weight or size of RBC.
MCV	76–100 μm³	76–100 fL[b]	Describes cell size (macrocytic and microcytic).
Platelets	130,000–400,000/mm³	$1.3–1.4 \times 10^{11}$/L	$<1.0 \times 10^{11}$/L = thrombocytopenia; $<0.2 \times 10^{11}$/L = ↑ risk for bleeding.
RBC count			
Male	$4.3–5.9 \times 10^{6}$/mm³	$4.3–5.9 \times 10^{12}$/L	
Female	$3.5–5 \times 10^{6}$/mm³	$3.5–5 \times 10^{12}$/L	
Reticulocyte count (adults)	0.1–2.4%	0.001–0.024 I[a]	An ↑ suggests ↑ number of immature erythrocytes released in response to stimulus (e.g., iron in iron deficiency anemia).
WBC count	3,200–9,800/mm³	$3.2–9.8 \times 10^{9}$/L	Consists of neutrophils, lymphocytes, monocytes, eosinophils, and basophils.
Bands	3–5%	0.03–0.05 I[a]	An ↑ in neutrophils suggests bacterial or fungal infection. ↑ in bands and immature neutrophils suggests bacterial infection. Absolute neutrophil count (% neutrophils × WBC count) <100 ↑ risk of bacteremia; >1,000 = low risk of infection.
Neutrophils	54–62%	0.54–0.62 I[a]	
Lymphocytes	25–33%	0.25–0.33 I[a]	
Monocytes	3–7%	0.03–0.07 I[a]	Eosinophils ↑ with allergies and parasitic infections.
Eosinophils	1–3%	0.01–0.03 I[a]	
Basophils	<1%	<0.01 I[a]	

[a]With the SI, the concept of number fraction replaces %. Thus, for mass fraction, volume fraction, and relative quantities, the unit "I" is used to replace former units.
[b]fL, femtoliter; femto, 10^{-15}; pico, 10^{-12}; nano, 10^{-9}; micro, 10^{-6}; milli, 10^{-3}.
ESR, erythrocyte sedimentation rate; MCH, mean corpuscular hemoglobin; MCHC, mean cell hemoglobin concentration; MCV, mean cell volume; RBC, red blood cell; WBC, white blood cell.

Table 1.4 • Detection Times in Urine with Enzyme-multiplied Immunoassay Technique (EMIT) Methods[53]

Drug	Detection Time in Urine
Amphetamines	Within 24–48 hr after ingestion. Oral decongestants (ephedrine, pseudoephedrine, or phenylpropanolamine) may give positive results.
Barbiturates	1 dose of 250 mg phenobarbital detectable for up to 9 days. Others detectable for up to 1–2 days.
Benzodiazepines	1 dose usually not detectable. Up to 5–7 days in chronic users.
Cocaine	Up to 48 hr after a single dose.
Codeine	1 dose of 120 mg detectable for up to 48 hr. Excreted and detected as morphine.
Heroin	1 dose of 10 mg detectable for up to 24 hr, 4–5 days for chronic users.
Marijuana	≤5 days after occasional use, 21–32 days after last dose in chronic users.
Methadone	≈3 days. Possible interference from high levels of chlorpromazine, promethazine, and dextromethorphan.
Methaqualone	Typical dose ≥5 days.
Morphine	1 dose of 10 mg detectable for 24–48 hr.
Phencyclidine	1 dose detectable for 7 days, up to 14 days in chronic users.
Propoxyphene	Up to 48 hr after a single dose.

Table 1.5 • Therapeutic Drug Concentrations[a]

Laboratory Test	Normal Reference Values Conventional Units	SI Units	Conversion Factor
Amitriptyline	50–200 ng/mL	180–820 nmol/L	3.61
Carbamazepine	4–12 µg/mL	17–51 µmol/L	4.23
Desipramine	50–200 ng/mL	170–200 nmol/L	3.75
Digoxin	0.5–2 ng/mL	0.6–2.6 nmol/L	1.28
Disopyramide	2–6 µg/L	6–18 µmol/L	2.946
Ethosuximide	40–110 µg/mL	280–780 µmol/L	7.084
Imipramine	50–200 ng/mL	180–710 nmol/L	3.566
Iron Male	80–180 µg/dL	14–32 µmol/L	0.179
Female	60–160 µg/dL	11–29 µmol/L	0.179
Lidocaine	1–5 µg/mL	4.5–21.5 µmol/L	4.267
Lithium	0.5–1.5 mEq/L	0.5–1.5 µmol/L	1
Phenobarbital	15–50 µg/mL	65–215 µmol/L	4.34
Phenytoin	5–20 µg/mL	20–80 µmol/L[b]	4
Procainamide	4–10 µg/mL	17–42 µmol/L	4.25
Quinidine	1.2–4 µg/mL	3.7–12.3 µmol/L	3.08
Salicylate	20–25 mg/dL	1.4–1.8 mmol/L	0.07
Theophylline	5–15 µg/mL	28–83 µmol/L	5.55
Valproic acid	50–100 µg/mL	350–700 µmol/L	7.0

[a]Drug concentrations of antibiotics are presented in the Infectious Disorders chapters.
[b]Unbound phenytoin = 0.5 – 2 mg/mL = 2–8 mmol/L.

The reader is referred to Chapter 2: Interpretation of Clinical Laboratory Tests, written by *Lloyd Y. Young, Pharm.D.,* and *Eileen G. Holland, Pharm.D.,* in the seventh edition of **Applied Therapeutics: The Clinical Use of Drugs** for a more in-depth discussion. The editors of this handbook express their thanks to Drs. Young and Holland and acknowledge that this chapter is based upon their work.

Notes:

Chapter 2

Herbs and Nutritional Supplements

General Information

♦ **German Commission E.** An expert panel assembled by the German Federal Health Agency to review the available information on herbs and to determine which ones achieved "reasonable certainty of efficacy and absolute safety." Monographs have recently been translated into English.

♦ **Dietary Supplement Health and Education Act (DSHEA).** An act passed in 1994 to regulate *dietary supplements,* defined as botanicals, vitamins, minerals, tissue extracts, and amino acids. Dietary supplements are regulated as foods, not pharmaceuticals. They cannot be removed from the market unless the Food and Drug Administration (FDA) proves that the product poses a serious or unreasonable risk to consumers.

♦ **Definitions.** In this chapter *"herbal remedy"* is used for botanicals and *"nutritional supplement"* is used for hormones, vitamins, minerals, cofactors, enzymes, amino acids, and others. Any product that alters the structure and function of the body or endogenous process for the treatment or prevention of disease is a *drug.*

♦ **Dietary Supplement Labeling Requirements**
  - Must include *"dietary supplement"* as part of the product name
  - Must include a *"supplement facts"* panel on as many as 14 ingredients when present in "significant amounts."
  - *Source.* Products derived from plants must designate the plant part and the Latin binomial. Nonherbal dietary supplements must indicate the source: animal, human, or synthetic
  - *High potency* is used if the ingredients exceed 100% of the dietary reference intake (DRI). DRI is the nutritional requirement for a population, while the recommended dietary allowance (RDA) is based on individual requirements. The *"% Daily Value"* or % RDA must be designated; however, these are outdated and often low. New RDAs are anticipated in 2005.

♦ **Claims.** Dietary supplements can make only "structure-function" claims, which may include the supplement's role in the person's well-being. They must also include the disclaimer: "This statement has not been evaluated by the Food and Drug Administration. This product is not intended to diagnose, treat, cure, or prevent any disease." Proposed indications, level of evidence, and doses for herbs and nutritional supplements addressed in this chapter are summarized in Table 2.1.

♦ **Product Formulations**
  - *Teas* are prepared by drying the herb, which is marketed in its course cut form or in tea bags. They can be prepared by *infusion* (steeping the herb in boiling or hot water for 10 minutes, then straining), *decoction* (placing the herb in cold water, which is heated to a boil and steeped for 10 minutes, or by *maceration* (allowing the herb to stand in water at room temperature for many hours before straining).
  - *Extracts* are concentrated formulations of fluids, powders, solids, and volatile oils.

Extraction of the dried herb with ethanol (tinctures), water, or both is used to make fluid extracts. Solid extracts are prepared by evaporating the solvent. Distillation or lipophilic extraction is used to prepare volatile oils.

- *Oil macerates* are prepared by allowing fresh or dried herbs to stand in oil at room temperature for many hours.
- *Fresh pressed juice* is prepared by macerating the herb in water and then squeezing the juice from it. If alcohol is used, the preparation becomes a *fresh herbal tincture.*

♦ **Good Manufacturing Processes (GMPs)** were designed to protect consumers from contamination and improper conditions during manufacturing of pharmaceuticals. Dietary supplements are considered foods and are therefore not subject to the same level of GMPs. Consequently, problems related to product purity, potency, and contamination have been documented.

♦ **Herbal Hazards**

- *Adulteration* with misidentified plant products, heavy metals, prescription medications, and other substances have been reported in cases of toxicity.
- *Adverse effects.* See Table 2.2.
- *Inappropriate consumer use* includes overuse, self-treatment of serious conditions such as cancer or infection, use during pregnancy or lactation, and use in children or other vulnerable populations. All of these practices can lead to adverse consequences.

♦ **Patient Recommendations.** See Table 2.3.

Garlic (*Allium sativum*)

♦ **Preparations**

- Allicin is responsible for garlic's odor, and many of its reported therapeutic effects. It is formed when an odorless precursor (alliin) is exposed to allinase, a very unstable enzyme.
- Powdered formulations are generally preferable to oil formulations because the activity of alliin and allinase activity can be preserved and concentrated. Enteric coating prevents allinase degradation in the stomach and releases allicin in the small intestine, minimizing the odor.
- Look for preparations standardized to 1.3% alliin or 0.5% allicin

♦ **Dose.** 600 to 900 mg of enteric-coated powdered garlic in two to three divided doses is typically recommended. This is equivalent to ½ to 1 clove of fresh garlic daily.

♦ **Effects and Uses**

- *Lipid-lowering Effects.* Based on meta-analyses of several small studies, 600- and 900-mg doses reduce total cholesterol 5 to 12% (conservatively, 5 to 8%) after 1 month, an effect that can last 6 months. TG levels may be reduced by 13%, but there seems to be no effect on HDL-C. May inhibit HMG-Co-A reductase.
- *Hypotensive Activity.* Meta-analysis indicates that 600 and 900 mg of garlic reduce the systolic and diastolic blood pressures by 7.7 and 5 mm Hg, respectively. Underlying mechanisms of action may include stimulation of nitric oxide synthesis, inhibition of angiotensin-converting enzyme, and reduction in intracellular calcium. Watch for potential interactions with antihypertensive medications.
- *Antiatherosclerotic Effects.* A few clinical trials and epidemiologic studies suggest that garlic may decrease plaque volume and aortic stiffness. This has been attributed to garlic's potential to reduce coronary risk factors: hyperlipidemia, hypertension, platelet aggregation, LDL-oxidation, and fibrin formation.
- *Antiplatelet and Thrombolytic Effects.* In a few studies using larger sample sizes (60 to 120 people), substantial reductions in spontaneous platelet aggregation and

plasma viscosity were observed. Doses of 800 mg per day of garlic powder for 4 to 12 weeks were used. Mechanisms of action may include inhibition of thromboxane formation and platelet aggregation, stimulation of nitrous oxide synthesis, and an increase in plasminogen activation. Watch for drug-drug interactions with warfarin.

• *Other Effects.* Reports include anticarcinogenic, anti-infective, and antidiabetic or hypoglycemic effects.

♦ **Adverse Drug Reactions and Interactions**

• *Adverse drug reactions* include nausea (6%), hypotension (1.3%), and allergy (1.1%). Odiferous effects occur in 20 to 40% of people taking 300 to 900 mg. Since antiplatelet effects might increase the risk of postoperative bleeding, advise patients to avoid garlic 7 to 10 days before and after surgery.

• *Drug Interactions.* None have been reported. However monitor patients taking antihypertensives and anticoagulants.

Gingko (Gingko biloba)

♦ **Preparations.** Gingko biloba extracts (GBEs) are prepared from the leaves of the gingko tree. The German E Commission recommends an herb:extract ratio of 50:1, which means that 50 parts of ginkgo leaves are used to generate one part extract. Extracts should be standardized to contain 22 to 27% flavone glycosides and 5 to 7% terpene lactones. Crude leaf teas are not likely to have sufficient potency. GBE is available in 40-, 60-, and 120-mg capsules or tablets.

♦ **Dose.** The recommended dose is 120 to 240 mg per day of GBE orally in two to three divided doses. Clinical benefits may not be observed for 4 to 6 weeks, but short-term memory benefits have been observed within 1 hour of a 600-mg dose.

♦ **Effects and Uses**

• *Neuroprotection.* The German Commission E developed criteria for nootropic or cognition-enhancing therapies. A meta-analysis of eight studies meeting these criteria showed positive effects on cognitive testing or symptoms. GBE was recommended for patients with Alzheimer's disease or vascular or mixed-type degenerative dementia. Potential mechanisms of action include improved cerebral blood flow, antioxidant effects, antagonism of platelet-activating factor, and alterations in neurotransmitter concentrations and binding sites.

• *Other Effects.* In animals, GBE may minimize stress response by minimizing the elevation in steroids; however, there are no human studies. GBE may improve pain at rest or pain-free walking distance (by 45%) in people with intermittent claudication. Subjects took 120 mg/day for 6 months. Data on improved short-term memory and many other proposed effects are inconclusive.

♦ **Adverse Drug Reactions and Interactions**

• Adverse effects are minimal and are found in only 1.69% of patients. Side effects occurring with a frequency of >0.5% include nausea, headache, stomach upset, diarrhea, allergy, anxiety, and insomnia.

• No drug-drug interactions have been reported but monitor for bleeding in patients taking antiplatelet agents or anticoagulants on the basis of case reports of intraocular and intracranial bleeding.

St. John's Wort (Hypericum perforatum)

♦ **Preparations.** Products are prepared from the dried above-ground parts of the plant and are typically standardized by the hypericin content, but this may not be the active ingredient. The alcoholic extracts have been used most often in clinical studies. They are formulated with an herb:extract ratio of 4:1 or 7:1 and should contain no less than 0.3% hypericin. Tea formulations are less concentrated and contain about 300 mg or 1/3 of the recommended antidepressant dose. Each tablet contains 300 mg hypericum with 0.3% hypericin or 900 mcg of hypericin. (Note: Although hyperforin, 2 to 4% of the crude herb, is considered the primary antidepressant constituent, most commercial preparations do not bear this standardized marker.)

♦ **Dose.** Hypericum extract 900 mg/day in three divided doses is the dose most commonly used. The onset of effect takes 2 to 4 weeks.

♦ **Effects and Uses**

- *Antidepressant.* Hypericum appears to be more effective than placebo in the treatment of mild-to-moderate depression and has a more tolerable side effect profile when compared to prescription antidepressants. Their use is not recommended in patients with severe depression, suicidal ideation, therapy resistance, or complicated depressive courses. Many mechanisms of action have been proposed, including inhibition of the reuptake of serotonin, dopamine, and norepinephrine.

- *Other Effects.* Hypericum has antiviral and antiproliferative effects in vitro, but insufficient evidence exists for its use in the treatment of AIDS or cancer at this time. Its use has also been studied for the treatment of seasonal affective disorder, depression with somatic symptoms, and reactive depression. Its topical use for wound healing is considered obsolete.

♦ **Adverse Drug Reactions and Interactions**

- Relatively few side effects have been reported in people taking 900 mg/day. These have included GI disturbances (8.5%), dizziness/confusion (4.5%), tiredness/sedation (4.3%), dry mouth (4%), restlessness (2.5%), and headache (1.7%). Photosensitization, serotonin syndrome, mania, and hypomania have appeared as case reports.

- Hypericum induces cytochrome P450, and there are case reports of reduced serum levels of drugs metabolized by this enzyme: digoxin, theophylline, cyclosporine, warfarin, indinavir, and ethinylestradiol/desogestrel. Avoid the combined use with agents that could enhance adrenergic or serotonergic neurotransmission: amphetamines, phenylephrine, phenylpropanolamine, antidepressants. Watch for serotonergic syndrome in patients taking this combination.

Echinacea (*Echinacea purpurea*)

♦ **Preparations**

- Products can vary markedly due to plant parts used, confusion among morphologically similar species, addition of non-Echinacea plant species, and method of extraction. The German Commission E approved the root of *E. pallida* (as a 1:5 water-alcohol extract) and the above-ground parts of *E. purpurea* (freshly pressed juice in 22% ethanol by volume as a preservative) for clinical use.

♦ **Dose**

- *E. Purpurea* (e.g., Echinaguard): 6 to 9 mL/day in divided doses (e.g., 15 to 30 drops of E. purpurea juice, equivalent to 0.75 to 1.5 mL, two to five times daily).

- *E. pallida* root: 900 mg/day in divided doses

- The German Commission E recommends that use not exceed 8 weeks because the mechanism for reported immune modulation is unclear.

- Topical preparations should contain at least 15% of the freshly pressed juice.

♦ **Effects and Uses**

- *Treatment of Cold and Upper Respiratory/Flu-like Syndromes.* Evidence to date suggests that cold symptoms and their duration may be reduced when echinacea is taken early in the course of the illness. The mechanism of action is unclear but is proposed to be immune modulation or stimulation. Enhanced phagocytic activity has been observed in humans.

- *Prophylaxis of Cold and Upper Respiratory/Flu-like Syndromes.* The prophylactic benefit has not been established. There are no differences in the frequency of URI infections, time to first occurrence, duration, and severity in people who take Echinacea prophylactically for 8 or more weeks.

- *Other uses* include adjuvant cancer treatment to minimize hematological toxicity or enhance recovery; supportive treatment of lower urinary tract infections, treatment of recurrent vaginal candidiasis, and wound healing (topical use).

♦ *Adverse Drug Reactions and Interactions*

- Few adverse effects have been reported: flu-like symptoms, unpleasant taste, and upset stomach have occurred. No drug interactions have been reported.

- Until the effects of Echinacea's immune modulating effects are more clearly defined, the German Commission E considers its use in people infected with HIV or with disorders that could be activated by immunostimulation (e.g., multiple sclerosis, rheumatoid arthritis, tuberculosis) to be contraindicated.

Saw Palmetto *(Serenoa repens)*

♦ *Preparations.* Saw palmetto berry is composed of many constituents, but the active ingredients are unknown. It is commercially formulated as a concentrated fat-soluble extract that is standardized to contain 85–95% fatty acids and sterols.

♦ *Dose.* 1 to 2 grams of the berry or 320 mg of the lipophilic extract per day, taken as 160 mg orally twice a day. The extract is available as 80- and 160-mg tablets. Onset of action is in 4 to 6 weeks.

♦ *Effects and Uses*

- *Benign Prostatic Hypertrophy (BPH).* Saw palmetto improves overall urinary tract symptoms by about 28% compared with placebo in men with mild-to-moderate BPH. Its efficacy was similar to finasteride at 6 months and slightly less than α-blockers at 1 and 3 months. The benefits beyond 6 months remain uncertain. The mechanism of action is unclear, but it does not alter PSA levels.

♦ *Adverse Drug Reactions and Interactions*

- *Side Effects* occur with an incidence of 1 to 3% and include hypertension, decreased libido, abdominal pain, erectile dysfunction, back pain, urinary retention, and headache. GI upset can be resolved if the herb is taken with food.

- *Drug Interactions.* None have been reported.

Ginseng *(Panax spp.)*

♦ *Preparations*

- There are a variety of species distinguished by their country of origin (Chinese or Korean, American, Japanese, Sanchi). All contain ginsenosides (28 types) that are thought to be responsible for the reported effects of ginseng. Other plants reported to have similar effects but are not of the Panax species include Siberian and Brazilian "ginseng." The German Commission E has approved both the Panax species and Siberian ginseng.

- The plant root is generally used for commercial manufacturing, and the time required for maturation and optimal ginsenoside levels is 5 to 6 years. Thus, commercial supply can be scarce, leading to high prices or plant substitution.

- Ginsenoside content in *P. ginseng* roots is assessed by Rg_1 content; 1.5% is considered standard. Ginseng extract should be standardized to contain at least 7% ginsenosides.

- The crude herb or extract formulations are preferred. Crude ginseng products are available as fresh (<4 years old), peeled and dried white (4 to 6 years of age), or steamed and dried red (>6 years). These products can be powdered, extracted, or made into teas.

♦ **Dose.** The Commission E recommends 1 to 2 g *P. ginseng* or its equivalent (200 to 400 mg of an extract such as Ginsana). For Siberian ginseng, the dose is 2 to 3 g of the crude root or its equivalent. Continuous use should be limited to 3 months.

♦ **Effects and Uses**

- *Ergogenic and Nootropic Effects.* The German Commission E has approved ginseng as "a tonic to counteract weakness and fatigue, as a restorative for declining stamina and impaired concentration, and as an aid to convalescence." The effects of ginseng on physical (ergogenic) and mental (nootropic) performance have been inconsistent.

- *Glucose Homeostasis.* There is some evidence that in people with type 2 diabetes ginseng may decrease fasting glucose levels and HbA_{1c} (200 mg, species unspecified) and postprandial glucose concentrations (3 g American ginseng 40 minutes before meals). Studies are small, and in some cases the species of ginseng is not specified.

- *Cardiovascular Effects and Lipid Homeostasis.* The hypotensive and antihyperlipidemic effects of ginseng have not been clearly demonstrated.

- *Immune Modulation.* Ginseng may enhance immune function in healthy patients. For example, fewer cases of influenza occurred in a group who received Ginsana 100 mg daily plus influenza vaccine versus those who received the vaccination alone.

- *Anticarcinogenic/Antitumor Effects.* Epidemiologic studies suggest that chronic use of ginseng extract or powder (once or more per month) may reduce the odds ratio for developing certain cancers.

- *Liver Function.* Improved hepatic function in people with alcohol or drug-induced chronic liver disease has not been clearly demonstrated.

- *Male Erectile Dysfunction and Fertility.* Ginseng may enhance fertility and erectile dysfunction in men (300 mg *P. ginseng* extract). Sperm numbers and motility were enhanced, and hormone levels (e.g., testosterone) were increased in one study.

♦ **Adverse Drug Reactions and Interactions**

- *CNS stimulation,* insomnia, hypertension and nervousness have been reported, as have Stevens-Johnson syndrome and cerebral arteritis.

- *Antiplatelet properties* might increase the bleeding risk in patients taking anticoagulant medicines. Pre- and postoperative patients should be advised to discontinue ginseng 7 to 10 days before and after surgery.

- *Estrogenic Effects.* Vaginal bleeding and mastalgia have occurred after the acute and chronic use of ginseng.

- *Drug Interactions.* Irritability, sleeplessness, and manic behavior have been reported in patients using psychiatric medicines (e.g., lithium, neuroleptics). Thus, such patients should be alert for mood changes if they choose to take ginseng. A few other cases of interactions with other drugs have been reported.

Dehydroepiandrosterone (DHEA) and Wild Yams (Dioscorea Extracts)

♦ **Physiology**

- DHEA is a precursor hormone secreted by the adrenal cortex and CNS. It rapidly converts to the sulfate ester (DHEAS) and ultimately to estrogen or testosterone. In men, DHEA is primarily converted to estrogen; in premenopausal women it is primarily converted to testosterone; in postmenopausal women it is converted to both. This model explains the rationale for its use and side effects. See Table 2.4.

* Although no specific function has been attributed to DHEAS, endogenous levels have correlated with a variety of disease states. Levels of DHEA and DHEAS decline with age, and levels in men exceed those of women.

◆ **Preparations**

* *DHEA.* Many doses and formulations of DHEA are available in the U.S., including tablets, capsules, sublingual tablets, and sublingual sprays. Doses available include but are not limited to 5, 10, 25, 30, 50, and 100 mg.

* *Wild (Mexican, Dioscorea floribunda) Yam Extract* has been marketed as a natural way to supplement endogenous female hormones. The yam with the most abundant source of steroids is a Mexican yam, which has been used to produce cortisone, estrogen, and progesterone derivatives commercially. However, DHEAS levels do not correspond with the hormonal activity of Dioscorea, and there are no long-term safety studies. Also, because the products are not standardized, it is difficult to assess the amount of hormones released. The dose has not been established.

◆ **Dose**

* *DHEA.* Pharmacologic doses are much higher than replacement doses: 1600 mg versus 25 to 100 mg/day, respectively.

◆ **Uses and Effects (See Table 2.5)**

* *Weight Loss.* The effect of DHEA on body fat and weight loss is uncertain. It cannot be recommended for this purpose.

* *Antioxidant Properties.* DHEA and Dioscorea extracts may have antioxidant effects, but the beneficial effects on health, well-being, or longevity are unknown.

* *Alzheimer's Disease (AD).* Research to date does not support a correlation between DHEA synthesis or metabolism and AD, and there is no evidence that DHEA improves symptoms or slows progression of AD.

* *Cardiovascular Risk.* DHEAS levels are a poor predictor of cardiovascular morbidity or mortality in both men and women, and no studies have evaluated the effect of exogenous DHEA supplementation on cardiovascular risk reduction.

* *Lipid Effects.* The effects of DHEA on cholesterol levels are modest and variable. Pharmacologic doses may decrease total cholesterol in postmenopausal women but decreases in HDL-C make it undesirable. DHEA does not seem to alter cholesterol regulation and synthesis in men.

* *HIV Infection.* Low or declining DHEA and DHEAS levels may be an independent predictor for the progression to AIDS. Large doses (750 mg three times daily) were associated with a slower decline in CD4+ cell count than lower doses (250 mg three times daily), but since viral loads were not measured it is difficult to assess the benefits. Replacement doses (50 mg daily) improved energy, cognitive and physical functioning, emotional well-being, and health perception. Interaction with protease inhibitors has not been studied.

* *Systemic Lupus Erythematosus.* DHEA (50 to 200 mg/day) may decrease dose requirements for corticosteroids and disease activity index. However, many patients discontinue therapy because of side effects or perceived lack of efficacy. DHEA is considered an orphan drug for SLE in the United States.

* *Glucose Homeostasis.* The effect of DHEA on glucose homeostasis is poorly defined, even though low levels are observed in insulin-resistant states (e.g., hypertension, obesity, and type 2 diabetes mellitus).

- ◆ **Adverse Effects and Drug Interactions**
  - *Benign Prostatic Hyperplasia.* There is some concern that DHEA may worsen BPH or prostate cancer, because both of these conditions are sensitive to testosterone and DHEA could increase adrenal testosterone production. Avoid use in these situations and watch for symptoms suggestive of prostatic hypertrophy.
  - *Cancer Risk.* The relationship between DHEA or DHEAS levels and cancer risk is under study. Because the effects of DHEA supplementation have not been fully studied, any one with cancer should avoid use of DHEA.
  - *Thyroid Function Tests.* In postmenopausal women, DHEA may decrease thyroid-binding globulin and slightly decrease TT_4. This was not observed in men.
  - *Mexican Yams.* Reported side effects (8 pills of high-dose extracts) include headache, xerostomia, nausea, vomiting, and sleep difficulties. Lower doses (2 to 4 pills/day) had no side effects.
  - *DHEA* in pharmacological doses produced nasal congestion, headache, fatigue, nausea, gynecomastia, breast tenderness, and insomnia in 25 to 40% of subjects.
  - *Drug interactions* have not been studied. None have been reported.

Glucosamine and Chondroitin

- ◆ **Physiology.** Glucosamine has been promoted for use alone and in combination with chondroitin to treat and prevent osteoarthritis (OA). Glucosamine is used to increase cartilage formation, and chondroitin is said to inhibit cartilage-destroying enzymes.
- ◆ **Preparations**
  - *Glucosamine* is derived from chitin, which is found in yeast, fungi, and marine invertebrates, but a synthetic product is preferred. Many salts are available, but the sulfate is preferred because it is required for cartilage synthesis and is the form best studied. Many products have added herbs, minerals, vitamins, and amino acids, but there is no evidence that these enhance the effect of glucosamine.
- ◆ **Dose**
  - *Glucosamine sulfate.* 500 mg (two 250-mg capsules) three times per day with meals (1500 mg/day) is the usual dose. Up to 3000 mg/day has been used in some studies.
  - *Chondroitin sulfate.* 400 mg three times daily has been used. Since it is likely to be broken down into individual glucosamine monomers before it is absorbed, patients should use one or the other.
- ◆ **Use in Osteoarthritis**
  - *Glucosamine* seems to improve symptoms (swelling, movement limitations) and alleviates pain associated with OA. Pain scores improve as early as 7 days; joint tenderness, swelling, and restriction of active movements improve in about 14 days; improved passive movements improve in 21 days. Ibuprofen has a faster onset of action, but after 8 weeks, pain scores were significantly improved over those treated with ibuprofen.
  - *Chondroitin.* In one study, 400 mg three times daily appeared to be as effective in relieving pain as diclofenac sodium (Voltaren), 50 mg three times daily.
- ◆ **Adverse Reactions and Drug Interactions**
  - *GI Effects.* The most common adverse effects of glucosamine include epigastric pain, tenderness, heartburn, diarrhea, constipation, and nausea. Overall, it is well tolerated and better tolerated than NSAIDs. Take with food.
  - *Glucose Homeostasis.* Glucosamine may increase insulin resistance and thereby

increase glucose concentrations, but this is not well documented. Monitor people with type 2 diabetes for deterioration in blood glucose control.

• *Drug Interactions.* None have been reported to date.

Shark Cartilage

♦ **Preparations.** Chondroitin-6-sulfate is the primary ingredient found in shark cartilage, but it is not known whether this is the active ingredient. There is no evidence that one formulation or source is superior to another, but the product should not have been exposed to excessive heat during the manufacturing process, because this could denature active proteins.

♦ **Dose.** The most commonly recommended oral dose is 1 g/kg per day in three divided doses. To avert enzymatic degradation, maximize absorption, and minimize GI irritation, shark cartilage has been administered as a retention enema for 25 minutes (20 g bulk powder diluted in 20 mL tepid water).

♦ **Uses and Effects**

• *Cancer.* Limited information suggests that shark cartilage is not effective in preventing or slowing the progression of cancer.

• *Other.* Shark cartilage has been advocated for many disorders, including cancer, psoriasis, diabetic retinopathy, neurovascular glaucoma, inflammation, Kaposi's sarcoma, and arthritic pain. It is also said to have antimicrobial properties and antioxidant effects. None of these uses has been well studied.

♦ **Adverse Reactions and Drug Interactions**

• *Gastrointestinal upset* is the most common dose-limiting effect. Since one case of hepatitis has been reported, patients should be warned against using a product that has a changed odor or color.

• *Contraindications* include any situation in which neovascularization is crucial for tissue growth and repair, such as pregnancy, wound healing, and normal growth.

• *Drug Interactions.* Avoid use with anticoagulants since shark cartilage contains proteins that resemble heparin and others that enhance the effects of tissue plasminogen activator.

Zinc Lozenges

♦ **Physiology and Mechanism of Action**

• Zinc is a trace element that is an enzymatic cofactor. Zinc ions protect cell membranes from lysis resulting from complement activation and toxin release.

• The mechanism of action is controversial, and many have been proposed. The rationale for the use of zinc lozenges in the symptomatic relief of the common cold is based on supraphysiologic concentrations of Zn^{2+} in the oral and nasal passage, which prevent rhinoviral binding and activation.

• Neutral and negatively charged zinc ions may worsen symptoms.

♦ **Preparations**

• Many salt forms of zinc are available, each of which vary in solubility, palatability, and zinc ion release characteristics. Zinc acetate (ZA), zinc gluconate (ZG), and zinc gluconate-glycine (ZGG) have been studied for treating the common cold.

• Product selection should be based on palatability.

♦ **Dose.** ZGG (13.3 mg), ZA (10 mg) and ZG (23 mg) lozenges dissolved completely in the mouth every 2 hours while awake for 5 to 10 days or until symptoms are resolved.

◆ Uses and Effects

- *Common Cold.* Meta-analyses indicate that adult patients with colds who used zinc lozenges were 50% less likely to have cold symptoms at 1 week, compared to placebo. Zinc appears to shorten the subjective duration of respiratory symptoms by 1 to 2 days. Improvements are most likely to be seen if zinc is started within 1 to 2 days from the start of symptoms. Effectiveness and doses in children are not well characterized.

- *Zinc Deficiency.* Because the systemic absorption of zinc from lozenges is not known, they should not be used to treat cases of deficiency. Instead therapeutic zinc supplementation at doses of 150 mg/day for 1 to 3 months should be used. The recommended daily allowance for males is 15 mg/day.

- *Allergic Rhinitis.* There is no clinical information on its use in this condition, but zinc does have antihistaminic properties and may inhibit inflammatory processes.

◆ Adverse Reactions

- Poor palatability results most often in discontinuation. Nausea, taste disturbances, and mouth irritation also are commonly reported. Use after a meal or food may minimize the nausea.

- Chronic use could lead to copper and other nutrient imbalances.

- Avoid in women who are pregnant or lactating.

Melatonin

- ◆ **Physiology.** Melatonin is an endogenous hormone secreted by the pineal gland in response to darkness. Secretion increases progressively after the onset of darkness, usually between 9 PM and 4 AM, and peaks between 2 and 4 AM.

- ◆ **Preparations.** Melatonin is available as 0.1-, 0.3-, 1-, 5-, and 10-mg oral tablets or capsules in immediate- and sustained-release (IR and SR) formulations. Synthetic formulations should be used exclusively, since animal- or human-derived products carry a risk for viral transmission, contamination, and variable potency.

◆ Dose

- *Jet lag.* 5 mg IR formulation on the evening of departure and then for the next 1 to 3 days after arrival at the destination.
- *Insomnia.* 5 mg IR formulation
- *Immune modulation.* 10 to 20 mg nightly
- *Anticancer.* 20 to 40 mg per day

◆ Uses and Effects

- *Jet Lag.* Melatonin has some hypnotic effects, which may help. However, improvement in jet lag symptoms seems to be more closely related to resynchronization by regular light-dark stimuli. Patients should be advised to maximize exposure to daylight, to go to bed at the same time each night, and to avoid caffeine and daytime naps.

- *Insomnia.* Many studies have documented the hypnotic effect of melatonin in improving sleep onset and quality in healthy volunteers. It is unlikely to improve total sleep time. Melatonin 5 mg orally caused peak hypnotic effects within 3 hours when taken at noon, compared to 1 hour when taken at 9 PM. The effect of patient age, dose, duration of therapy, and sleep disorder etiology on melatonin efficacy remains to be studied.

- *HIV.* The lay press has suggested that melatonin enhances the immune system in people with HIV and protects against AZT toxicity, as well as the AIDS-wasting syndrome. None of these claims is supported by clinical trials, but in vitro and animal studies indicate that melatonin may enhance the immune response.

- *Anticancer Effects.* The antitumor effects of melatonin have been studied in vitro and in small clinical trials involving patients with metastatic breast cancer, malignant melanoma, and glioblastoma. In all of these cancers, some beneficial effect has been observed, which may be related to melatonin's immune modulating or antioxidant effects. It may also lessen cytotoxicity associated with chemotherapy or radiation therapy. Melatonin should be used only in consultation with an oncologist.

◆ *Adverse Reactions and Drug Interactions*

- Drowsiness is a major effect.
- Melatonin in high doses (75 to 300 mg per day) can inhibit ovulation, and it may suppress prolactin secretion. Thus, it should not be used in women who are trying to conceive or in those who are lactating.

Notes:

Table 2.1 • Summary of Herbal Products and Nutritional Supplements Reviewed

Herbal/Nutritional Supplement	Proposed Indication(s)	Authors' Interpretation of Level of Evidence for Use in a Clinical Setting[a]	Dosing
Garlic *Allium sativum*	Hyperlipidemia Hypertension Antiplatelet Antiatherosclerotic Cancer prevention Antitumor/antiproliferative Antimicrobial Diabetes/hypoglycemia	Promising Promising Promising Promising Investigational Unknown Investigational Unknown	Standardized to contain 1.3% alliin or 0.6% allicin (600–900 mg powdered garlic/day in 2 to 3 divided doses) Equivalent to 1.8–2.7 g fresh garlic daily (one clove is approximately 3 g)
Ginkgo *Ginkgo biloba*	Dementia Peripheral vascular disease Stress/anxiety Short-term memory Tinnitus/hearing loss Sexual dysfunction	Promising Promising Unknown Unknown Unknown Investigational	Gingko biloba extract (GBE) standardized to contain 22–24% flavone glycosides and 5–7% terpene lactones (120–240 mg/day in 2 or 3 divided doses)
St. John's Wort *Hypericum perforatum*	Mild-to-moderate depression Antiviral Wound healing (topical)	Promising Investigational Unknown	Alcoholic extract standardized to contain at least 0.3% hypericin or 5% hyperforin (900 mg/day in 3 divided doses)
Echinacea *Echinacea purpurea* *Echinacea pallida*	Cold treatment Cold prophylaxis Urinary tract infection (supportive treatment) Wound healing	Promising Unknown Unknown Unknown	6–9 mL of *E. purpurea* fresh pressed juice or 900 mg/day of *E. pallida* root (1:5 tincture, 50% ethanol); administer in divided doses (e.g., 15–30 drops of *E. purpurea* juice equivalent to 0.75–1.5 mL, 2 to 5 times daily)
Saw palmetto *Serenoa repens*	Benign prostatic hyperplasia	Promising	Lipophilic extract standardized to contain 85–95% fatty acids and sterols; 160 mg 2 times daily
Panax ginseng	Adaptogen Ergogenic Immune modulation Anticancer/antitumor Diabetes/hypoglycemia	Unknown Unknown Investigational Investigational Unknown	*P. ginseng* extract standardized to contain at least 7% ginsenosides; 1–2 g of the crude root or its equivalent (1 g of crude root is equivalent to 200 mg of the extract)

Supplement	Indication	Status	Dosing
Panax ginseng (continued)	Hyperlipidemia	Unknown	
	Hypertension/cardiovascular	Unknown	
	Hepatoprotectant	Unknown	
	Erectile dysfunction/infertility	Investigational	
Dehydroepiandrosterone (DHEA)	Weight loss	Unknown	Replacement dosing: men 50–100 mg daily; women 25–50 mg daily
	Anticancer	Unknown	Systemic lupus erythematosus: 50–200 mg daily
	Antioxidant effects	Investigational	Hyperlipidemia: 1,600 mg daily in divided doses
	Hormone replacement therapy	Investigational	HIV: 750–2,250 mg in 3 divided doses
	Aging	Doubtful	
	Alzheimer's disease	Investigational	
	Cardiovascular protection	Investigational	
	Hyperlipidemia	Doubtful	
	HIV	Doubtful	
	Systemic lupus erythematosus	Promising	
	Diabetes	Doubtful	
Glucosamine	Osteoarthritis	Promising	500–1,000 mg 3 times daily
	Wound healing	Doubtful	
	Antioxidant	Investigational	
Shark cartilage	Anticancer	Doubtful	1 g/kg/day or 80–100 g/day given in 3 divided doses
	Antimicrobial	Doubtful	
Zinc	Common cold	Promising	ZGG: 13.3 mg Q 2 hr while awake
	Allergic rhinitis	Investigational	ZG: 23 mg Q 2 hr while awake
			ZA: 10 mg Q 2 hr while awake
Melatonin	Jet lag	Promising	Jet lag: 5–8 mg IR the evening of departure and for 3–5 days after
	Insomnia	Promising	Insomnia: 0.3–5 mg once nightly for sleep onset
	Reproduction	Investigational	Higher dosages may be required for sleep maintenance
	Antioxidant	Investigational	
	Immune modulation	Investigational	
	Anticancer	Investigational	
	Aging	Doubtful	
	Depression	Investigational	

aPromising: A sufficient number of double-blind, placebo-controlled studies have been conducted that indicate that an effect may exist.
Investigational: Studies have indicated promising results in animal models or in epidemiologic studies. Small trials in humans may currently be underway.
Unknown: There is an equivalent amount of scientific evidence, which shows both positive and negative results or studies that have been conducted and indicate positive findings but were generally of poor study design, or there is a relative lack of trials that have been performed for this indication.
Doubtful: Studies that have been conducted have generally shown no effect.

Table 2.2 • Hazards Associated with Some Nutritional Supplements

Supplement/Latin Binomial	References	Associated Clinical Use[a]	Toxicity	Recommendation
Comfrey rhizome, roots, leaves *Symphytum* spp.	4, 11, 19, 20	Internal digestive aid External wound healing	Pyrrolizidine alkaloids—hepatotoxicity	Avoid ingestion. External application only. Limit use to 4–6 wk. Do not use on unbroken skin.
Coltsfoot flower, leaves *Tussilago farfara*	4, 11, 19	Upper respiratory tract infections	Pyrrolizidine alkaloids—hepatotoxicity	Avoid herb, root, or flower products. Leaf can be used as an external anti-inflammatory agent. Limit use to 4–6 wk.
Germander leaves, tops *Teucrium chamaedrys*	11, 19, 21	Diet aid	Hepatotoxicity	Avoid.
Borage leaves, tops *Borago officinalis*	4, 11, 19	Anti-inflammatory, diuresis	Pyrrolizidine alkaloids —hepatotoxicity	Avoid.
Chaparral leaves, twigs *Larrea tridentata*	11, 19, 22	Anti-infective, antioxidant, anticancer	Hepatotoxicity	Avoid.
Sassafras root bark *Sassafras albidum*	19, 23	Tonic, blood thinner	Safrole oil—hepatocarcinogen in animal studies	Avoid.
Aconite (found in some Chinese herbal remedies) *Aconitum* spp.	24, 25	Analgesic	Alkaloids—cardiac and central nervous system toxicity	Avoid.
Pennyroyal Extract from *Mentha pulegium* or *Hedeoma pulegoides*	11, 26	Digestive aid, induction of menstrual flow, abortifacient	Pulegone and its metabolite—hepatic and renal failure	Avoid.

Life root, whole plant *Senecio aureus*	19	Induction of menstrual flow	Pyrrolizidine alkaloids—hepatotoxicity	Avoid.
Poke root, root of plant *Phytolacca americana*	19, 27	Antirheumatic	Hemorrhagic gastritis	Avoid.
Jin Bu Huan (a Chinese herbal remedy)	28	Analgesic, sedative	Hepatotoxicity—mechanism unknown, but levotetrahydropalmatine is structurally similar to pyrrolizidine alkaloids	Avoid.
Ephedra *Ma huang, Ephedra* spp.	18, 19	Weight loss, stimulant, bronchodilation	Extension of pharmacologic effects	Avoid use in patients in whom stimulant effects could be harmful (e.g., hypertension, diabetes, heart disease, anxiety, hyperthyroidism).
Royal jelly from the honeybee (*Apis mellifera*)	29	Tonic	IgE-mediated bronchospasm and anaphylaxis in patients with atopy or asthma	Avoid use in patients with history of asthma, atopy, or allergies.
Guar gum *Cyamopsis psorabides* or *tetragonolobus*	11, 30	Weight loss, diabetes, hypercholesterolemia	Esophageal, small-bowel obstruction	Avoid.

aAssociated clinical use is based on patient report at time of event or reported use in listed references.

Table 2.3 • Guidelines for Selecting or Recommending an Herbal Remedy or Dietary Supplement Product

- Read all labels carefully.
- Never share these products with others.
- Avoid using in children.
- Avoid if you are pregnant or trying to become pregnant or nursing.
- Never take more than the recommended amount listed on the label.
- Do not select a product that does not have dosing recommendations on the label.
- Avoid products that do not carry a lot number or expiration date.
- Discard products without an expiration 1 year from the date of purchase.
- Select products that list the manufacture's name, address, and telephone number.
- Avoid purchasing these products from mail-order companies; instead purchase from pharmacies and large outlet nutrition stores.
- Speak to your health care professional if you are trying to treat a life-threatening condition, such as cancer, HIV, and others.
- If you are taking a prescription medicine, do not take an herbal remedy or dietary supplement for the same condition.
- Avoid taking multiple-ingredient preparations; select single-ingredient products that list the strength per dose.
- Do not store these products in a medicine cabinet or glove compartment; store them in a dry environment out of direct sunlight and humidity.
- The term *natural* does not mean safe; be diligent and report any unusual experiences to your doctor or pharmacist.
- Store products away from young children and pets.
- Always inform your health care provider of the products you are taking; keep a list if necessary or bring them with you to your appointment.
- Do not take these products with alcohol until you know it is safe to do so or are familiar with the effects.
- Check with your health care provider if you are taking "blood-thinning" drugs; some products may interact.
- Never use these products in place of proper rest and nutrition; eat a balanced diet.
- Do not expect a cure or unrealistic results; these agents are not "cure-alls."
- If it sounds too good to be true, it probably is; use discretion when evaluating claims.

Notes:

Table 2.4 • Theoretical Basis of the Effects of DHEA[a,288]

Patients	Hormonal Environment		Effect of DHEA		Potential Outcome
	Estrogens	Androgens	Estrogenic	Androgenic	
Premenopausal women	High	Low	Decreases estradiol effect by binding competitively to estrogen receptor	Enhances androgenic effect on fat distribution and CVD, which are balanced by high estrogens	If DHEA is low, breast cancer risk is increased since estradiol effect is unopposed.
Postmenopausal women	Low	Low	Bind to unoccupied estrogen receptors and enhances estradiol effects	Enhanced androgenic effect on fat distribution and CVD, which are less well balanced by low estrogen levels	If DHEA is high, both pathways are active with androgenic predominance: 1. Androgenic effects (central obesity, insulin resistance, risk for CVD) 2. Estradiol-like effect (increased risk for breast cancer)
Men	Low	High	Binds to unoccupied estrogen receptors and enhances estradiol effects	Negligible additional androgenic effect	If DHEA is high, estrogenic effect may offer protection against CVD.

[a]CVD = Coronary vascular disease.
Reprinted with permission from Ebeling P, Koivisto VA. Physiological importance of dehydroepiandrosterone. Lancet 1994;343:1479. © The Lancet Ltd.

Table 2.5 • DHEA: General Recommendations

- Because DHEA is a precursor hormone, women should avoid using DHEA during pregnancy and lactation.
- Replacement doses are associated with few adverse effects but may depend on gender and menopausal status. If patients decide to replace low DHEA levels, they should start with the lowest tolerable DHEA dosage.
- Patients should be informed that the hormonal protective effects of DHEA have not been clearly defined and have not been compared to standard pharmaceuticals.
- The long-term safety and efficacy of DHEA has not been systematically studied; with long-term supplementation, endogenous regulation of DHEA may be adjusted to account for the excess hormone.
- DHEA is not released from wild yam extracts.

- The antioxidant properties of DHEA have not been applied in a clinical setting; it is unknown whether DHEA improves longevity or well-being.
- The role of DHEA in diabetes has not been defined. Patients should not use DHEA to help regulate their insulin or blood glucose levels.
- There is no evidence to prove DHEA supplementation reverses age-related diseases, including cancer, cardiovascular disease, and Alzheimer's disease.
- DHEA may have a role in improving the quality of life of patients with systemic lupus erythematosus, but side effects limit medication adherence.
- DHEA is not effective in preventing HIV disease progression.
- DHEA drug interactions have not been formally studied.

The reader is referred to Chapter 3: Herbs and Nutritional Supplements, written by *Catherine E. Dennehy, Pharm.D.,* and *Candy Tsourounis, Pharm.D.,* in the seventh edition of **Applied Therapeutics: The Clinical Use of Drugs** for an extensive analysis of the human studies, postulated mechanisms of action, pharmacokinetics, and "therapeutic use" of these agents. All notations to reference numbers are based on the reference list at the end of that chapter. The editors of this handbook express their thanks to Drs. Dennehy and Tsourounis and acknowledge that this chapter is based upon their work.

Notes:

Chapter 3

Anaphylaxis and Drug Allergies

Definition

Drug allergies or drug hypersensitivity reactions are defined in this chapter as unpredictable adverse drug reactions, often dose independent, that are immunologically mediated.

Predisposing Factors

The prevalence of allergic reactions can be affected by either drug idiosyncrasies or patient-related variables.

Age and Gender. Adults are more susceptible to drug allergies than children. Females are more prone to cutaneous reactions than males.

Genetic Factors. Patients with allergic rhinitis, allergic asthma, or atopic dermatitis tend to experience more severe drug reactions. Slow acetylators are more likely to develop antinuclear antibodies and symptoms of systemic lupus erythematosus when treated with procainamide or hydralazine.

Associated Illnesses. Maculopapular rashes are more common in ampicillin-treated patients with Epstein-Barr virus infections.

Acquired immunodeficiency syndrome (AIDS) patients with *Pneumocystis carinii* pneumonia experience a high prevalence of cutaneous reactions to sulfonamides.

Previous Drug Administration. Frequent intermittent drug exposure, route of administration (e.g., topical administration highest risk of sensitization), and occasionally high dose (e.g., penicillin-induced hemolytic anemia) can influence development of drug allergy.

Immunopathologic Classifications

Allergic drug reactions can be classified into 4 different immunological types (see Table 3.1).

Diagnosis

Allergic drug reactions can be differentiated from other types of adverse drug reactions by assessing common clinical features of the allergic drug reaction (see Table 3.2) and by a detailed drug history (see Table 3.3).

Skin testing and drug rechallenge are the most definitive methods of diagnosing drug allergy; however, skin test antigens currently are available only for penicillin (see Table 3.4).

Categories of Drug Allergies

Drug allergies can be grouped into 3 categories: *generalized reactions, organ-specific reactions, and pseudoallergic reactions.*

Generalized reactions involve multiple organ systems and have variable clinical manifestations

 ◆ **Anaphylactic reactions** usually begin soon after exposure and can cause significant respiratory and cardiovascular failure. For treatment see Table 3.5.
 ◆ **Serum Sickness Drug Reactions.** See Tables 3.6 and 3.10.
 ◆ **Drug-Induced Fever.** See Tables 3.7 and 3.10.
 ◆ **Drug-Induced Hypersensitivity Vasculitis.** See Tables 3.8 and 3.10.
 ◆ **Autoimmune Drug Reactions.** The clinical characteristics of autoimmune drug reactions can be found in Tables 3.9 and 3.10.

Organ-Specific Reactions. The drug allergies in this chapter are grouped into categories of generalized reactions, organ-specific reactions, and pseudoallergic reactions. The organ-specific hypersensitivity drug reactions affecting the blood can be found in Chapter 83, Drug-Induced Blood Disorders; those affecting the liver in Chapter 27, Adverse Effects of Drugs on the Liver; those affecting the lung in Chapter 23, Drug-Induced Pulmonary Disorders; those affecting the kidney in Chapter 28, Acute Renal Failure; and those affecting the skin in Chapter 35, Dermatotherapy.

Pseudoallergic reactions involve drug reactions that exhibit clinical signs and symptoms of an allergic response but are not immunologically mediated (see Table 3.11). These pseudoallergic reactions can be manifested as relatively benign symptoms or as severe life-threatening events indistinguishable from anaphylaxis. The specific drug-induced pseudoallergic reactions are described in Table 3.12.

Prevention and Management of Allergic Reactions

The first step in managing an allergic reaction is to determine its etiology. Secondly, a decision as to whether or not to discontinue the suspected drug should be made based upon the severity of the reaction, the condition being treated, and the availability of suitable alternatives. If a suitable alternative exists, the offending agent should be stopped and the reaction treated symptomatically. If it is inappropriate or not possible to change to an alternative therapy, desensitization can be considered.

 Desensitization protocols for β lactams and trimethoprim-sulfamethoxazole are provided in Tables 3.13, 3.14, and 3.15.

Notes:

Table 3.1 • Immunopathologic Classification of Allergic Drug Reactions

Immunologic Class	Antibody	Mechanism	Common Clinical Manifestations
Type I (anaphylactic)	IgE	Drug-hapten reacts with IgE antibody on the surface of mast cells and basophils, resulting in the release of mediators	Anaphylaxis
Type II (cytotoxic)	IgG IgM	*Hapten–Cell Reaction:* Drug interacts with cell surfaces resulting in the formation of an immunogenic complex and the production of antibodies *Immune Complex Reaction:* Drug reacts with antibody in circulation forming a complex, which with complement, binds to the cell, resulting in injury (hematologic reactions only) *Autoimmune Reaction:* Drug induces autoantibody production against red blood cells	Hemolytic anemia, granulocytopenia, thrombocytopenia
Type III (immune complex)	IgG	Same as type II immune complex reactions (nonhematologic reactions)	Serum sickness
Type IV (cell mediated)		Interaction of sensitized T lymphocytes with drug antigen	Contact dermatitis

Adapted from reference 6.

Table 3.2 • Clinical Features of Allergic Drug Reactions

- Have no correlation with known pharmacologic properties of the drug
- Require an induction period on primary exposure but not on readministration
- Can occur with doses far below therapeutic range
- Often include a rash, angioedema, serum sickness syndrome, anaphylaxis, and asthma
- Occur in a small proportion of the population
- Disappear on cessation of therapy and reappear after readministration of a small dose of the suspected drug(s) of similar chemical structure
- Desensitization may be possible

Reprinted from Assem E-S K. Drug allergy and tests for its detection. In: Davies DM, ed. Textbook of Adverse Drug Reactions. 3rd Ed. New York: Oxford University Press, 1985:689 by permission of Oxford University Press.

Table 3.3 • Detailed Drug History

- Prior allergic and medication encounters
- Nature and severity of reaction
- Temporal relationships between drugs and reaction (dose, date initiated, duration)
- Prior exposure to the same or structurally related medications subsequent to the reaction
- Effect of drug discontinuation
- Response to treatment
- Prior diagnostic testing or rechallenge
- Route of administration (e.g., preservatives in formulations)
- Other medical problems if any

From references 3 and 19.

Notes:

Table 3.4 • Penicillin Skin Testing Procedure

Agent	Procedure	Interpretation
Penicilloyl penicillin (Pre-Pen) major determinant	Scratch test 1 drop of full-strength solution $(6 \times 10^{-5}$ mol/L)[a]	*No wheal or erythema after 10 min:* Proceed with intradermal test. *Wheal or erythema within 10 min:* Choose alternative agent, desensitization if no other alternatives exist
Penicilloyl penicillin (Pre-Pen)	*Intradermal test:* 0.01–0.02 mL PPL (Pre-Pen)[a] *Saline:* negative control *Histamine:* positive control (optional; useful if it is suspected that patient may be anergic)	*Negative response:* Induration size similar or less than saline control *Positive response:* Induration 1–4 mm or more greater than saline control with or without erythema; choose alternative agent, desensitization if no other alternatives exist
Penicillin G potassium (<1 wk old) most important of the minor determinants	Scratch test 1 drop of 10,000 U/mL solution	Same as scratch test with PPL (see above)
Penicillin G potassium	*Intradermal test:* 0.002 mL 10,000 U/mL solution *Serial testing* with 10, 100, or 1,000 U/mL solutions can be performed in those with strong history/serious reactions	Same as intradermal test with PPL (see above)

[a]The penicilloyl derivative of penicillin conjugated to polylysine (PPL) is administered initially as a scratch test. If no wheal or erythema develops, then intradermal testing is performed. From Schwarz Pharma, Kremers Urban Company, Milwaukee, Wis.

Table 3.5 • Drug Therapy of Anaphylaxis

Drug	Indication	Adult Dosage	Complications
Initial Therapy			
Epinephrine	Hypotension, bronchospasm, laryngeal edema, urticaria, angioedema	0.3–0.5 mL of 1:1000 SC or IM Q 10–20 min PRN. 3–5 mL of 1:10,000 IV over 5 min Q 10–20 min PRN. 1 mL of 1:1,000 in 500 mL of dextrose 5% IV at a rate of 0.5–5 µg/min. 3–5 mL of 1:10,000 intratracheally Q 10–20 min PRN	Arrhythmias, hypertension, nervousness, tremor
Oxygen	Hypoxemia	40–100%	None
Metaproterenol	Bronchospasm	0.3 mL of 5% solution in 2.5 mL of saline via nebulizer	Arrhythmias, hypertension, nervousness, tremor
or			
Albuterol		0.5 mL of 0.5% solution in 2.5 mL of saline via nebulizer	
or			
Isoetharine		0.5 mL of 1% solution in 2 mL of saline via nebulizer	
IV fluids	Hypotension	1 L of crystalloid or colloid Q 20–30 min PRN	Pulmonary edema, CHF
Secondary Therapy[a]			
Antihistamines			
H_1-receptor antagonists	Hypotension, urticaria	Diphenhydramine or hydroxyzine 25–50 mg IV/IM/PO Q 6–8 hr PRN	Drowsiness, dry mouth, urinary retention; may obscure symptoms of continuing reaction
H_2-receptor antagonists		Cimetidine 300 mg IV over 3–5 min or PO Q 6–8 hr PRN *or* Ranitidine 50 mg IV over 3–5 min Q 8 hr PRN or 150 mg PO BID PRN	

Corticosteroids	Bronchospasm; patients undergoing prolonged resuscitation or severe reaction	Hydrocortisone sodium succinate 100 mg IM/IV Q 3–6 hr for 2–4 doses or Methylprednisolone sodium succinate 40–125 mg IV Q 6 hr for 2–4 doses	Hyperglycemia, fluid retention
Aminophylline	Bronchospasm	6 mg/kg loading dose (if necessary) IV over 30 min followed by 0.3–0.9 mg/kg/hr as a maintenance dose[b]	Arrhythmias, nausea, vomiting, nervousness, seizures
Norepinephrine	Hypotension	4 mg in 1 L dextrose 5% IV at a rate of 2–12 µg/min	Arrhythmias, hypertension, nervousness, tremor
Glucagon[c]	Refractory hypotension	1 mg in 1 L of dextrose 5% IV at a rate of 5–15 µg/min	

[a]Although not effective during acute anaphylaxis, these agents may reduce or prevent recurrent or prolonged reactions.
[b]Doses are for aminophylline; to convert to theophylline, multiply by 0.8. Lower rates may be required in elderly patients, those taking medications that reduce aminophylline metabolism, those with hepatic dysfunction, and those with CHF. Higher doses may be required in younger patients or cigarette smokers.
[c]Glucagon may be particularly useful in patients taking β-adrenergic blockers, because it can increase both cardiac rate and contractility regardless of β-adrenergic blockade.
Adapted from references 4, 5, and 6. Choice of agent and starting doses should be patient specific, weighing safety and efficacy.
CHF, congestive heart failure; IM, intramuscularly; IV, intravenously; PO, orally; PRN, as needed; SC, subcutaneously.

Table 3.6 • Hypersensitivity Reactions to Drugs: Serum Sickness

Clinical manifestations	Fever, cutaneous eruptions (95% of cases), lymphadenopathy, and joint systems (10–50%). Onset 1–2 weeks after exposure, 2–4 days in sensitized individuals. Laboratory data relatively nonspecific: elevated ESR and circulating immune complexes. Complements C3 and C4 are often low while activation products C3a and C3a des-arginine are elevated. RF sometimes present. UA may reveal proteinuria, hematuria, or an occasional cast.
Prognosis	Usually mild and self-limiting. Most resolve within a few days to weeks after withdrawal of inciting agent.
Treatment	Aspirin and antihistamines can relieve arthralgias and pruritus. Corticosteroids may be required for severe cases and tapered over 10–14 days.

From references 23–26.
ESR, erythrocyte sedimentation rate; RF, rheumatoid factor; UA, urinalysis.

Table 3.7 • Hypersensitivity Reactions to Drugs: Drug-induced Fever[48–55]

Frequency	True frequency is unknown because fever is a common manifestation and almost any drug may cause fever. However, it has been estimated that 3–5% of hospitalized patients experiencing adverse drug reaction suffer from drug fever alone or as part of multiple symptoms.
Clinical manifestations	Temperatures may be $\geq 38°C$ and do not follow a consistent pattern. Although patients may have high fevers with shaking chills, patients generally have few symptoms or serious systemic illness. Skin rash (18%), eosinophilia (22%), chills (53%), headache (16%), myalgias (25%), and bradycardia (11%) may occur in patients with drug fever. Onset of fever after exposure to the offending agent is highly variable, ranging from an average of 6 days for antineoplastics to 45 days for cardiovascular agents. Occurrence of fever independent of the dose of the offending agent.
Treatment	Although drug fever may be treated symptomatically (e.g., with antipyretics, cooling blankets), stopping the offending agent is the only therapy that will eliminate fevers completely. Patients generally experience defervescence within 48–72 hr of stopping the suspect drug.
Prognosis	Drug fever usually benign, although one review found a mean of increased length of hospitalization of 9 days per episode of drug fever. Rechallenge with the offending drug usually results in rapid return of the fever. Although re-exposure to the suspect drug was previously thought to be potentially hazardous, there is little risk of serious sequelae.

Table 3.8 • Hypersensitivity Reactions to Drugs: Clinical Manifestations of Drug-induced Vasculitis[33,51,140,141]

- Palpable purpura and maculopapular rash occurring symmetrically on the extremities
- Multiple organ systems may be involved:
  - *Renal*: microscopic hematuria to nephrotic syndrome and acute renal failure
  - *Liver*: enlarged liver, elevated enzymes, and arthralgias
- Laboratory data usually show nonspecific abnormalities of inflammation: elevated ESR and leukocytosis. Peripheral eosinophilia may be present and serum complement concentrations can be low. Histologic findings upon biopsy reveal granulocytes in venule or arteriole walls
- Onset typically 7–10 days after initiation therapy

From references 33, 51, 140, and 141.
ESR, erythrocyte sedimentation rate.

Table 3.9 • Hypersensitivity Reactions to Drugs: Autoimmune Drug-induced Lupus

Frequency	Less likely to affect females and Blacks than idiopathic SLE. Drug-induced lupus is more common in individuals with slow acetylator phenotype.
Clinical manifestations	Milder disease than idiopathic SLE. Arthralgias, myalgias, fever, malaise, pleurisy, and slight weight loss. Mild splenomegaly and lymphadenopathy. *Onset:* usually abrupt, occurring several months to years after continuous therapy with the offending drug. Classic butterfly malar rash, discoid lesions, oral mucosal ulcers, Raynaud's phenomenon, and alopecia are unusual features with DIL, as opposed to idiopathic SLE. *Laboratory studies:* positive ANA (predominantly single-stranded DNA and antihistone antibodies), anemia, and elevated ESR. Many patients demonstrate ANAs *without* development of lupus disease. It is, therefore, not necessary to discontinue therapy in asymptomatic patients with positive ANAs.
Treatment	Clinical features subside and disappear days to weeks after discontinuation of the offending drug. Serologic tests resolve more slowly. ANAs may persist for a year or longer.
Prognosis	DIL does not predispose to development of idiopathic SLE. Lupus-inducing drugs do not appear to ↑ the risk of exacerbation of idiopathic SLE. However, long-term treatment with interferon-γ may worsen pre-existing SLE.

From references 101, 102, 105–107, 127, 136, and 142–150.
ANA, antinuclear antibody; DIL, drug-induced lupus; ESR, erythrocyte sedimentation rate; SLE, systemic lupus erythematosus.

Table 3.10 • Allergic Reactions to Drugs

Serum Sickness

6-Mercaptopurine[27]	Furazolidone[28]	Minocycline[29]
Antithymocyte globulin[26,30–32]	Hemophilus B vaccine[33]	Pentoxifylline[34]
Carbamazepine[35]	Indomethacin[36]	Phenytoin[37–39]
Cefaclor[40]	Intravenous immune globulin[41]	Rabies vaccine[29]
Ciprofloxacin[42,43]	Iron dextran[44]	
Fluoxetine[45,46]	Itraconazole[47]	

Drug Fever[48–59]

Allopurinol	Digoxin	Nitrofurantoin
Aminoglycosides	Epinephrine	Oral contraceptives
Amphetamine	Folate	Para-aminosalicylate
Amphotericin B	Griseofulvin	Penicillins
Anesthetics, inhaled	Heparin	Phenytoin
Antacids	Hydralazine	Procainamide
Anticholinergics	Hydroxyurea	Propylthiouracil
Antihistamines	Ibuprofen	Quinidine
Antilymphocyte globulin	Imipenem	Quinine
Antineoplastics	Insulin	Ranitidine
Azathioprine	Interferon	Rifampin
Barbiturates	Iodides	Salicylates
Bleomycin	Isoniazid	Streptokinase
Carbamazepine	Iron dextran	Streptomycin
Cephalosporins	Macrolide antibiotics	Sulfonamides
Chloramphenicol	Mebendazole	Sulindac
Cimetidine	Metoclopramide	Tacrolimus
Clofibrate	Methyldopa	Tetracyclines
Cocaine	Monoamine oxidase inhibitors	Tolmetin
Corticosteroids	Muromonab-CD3	Triamterene
Cyclosporine	Neuroleptics	Trimethoprim
Diazoxide	Nifedipine	Vancomycin
		Vitamins

(continued)

Table 3.10 • Allergic Reactions to Drugs (continued)

Drug-induced Vasculitis

Allopurinol[60,61]	Mefloquine[62]	Ritodrine[63]
Azathioprine[64]	Methotrexate[65]	Sotalol[66]
Carbamazepine[67]	Naproxen[68]	Sulfadiazine[69]
Cephalosporins[70]	Nizatidine[71]	Terbutaline[72]
Cimetidine[73]	Ofloxacin[74,75]	Torasemide[76]
Ciprofloxacin[77–79]	Penicillin[80]	Trimethadione[67]
Clarithromycin[81]	Phenytoin[67]	Valproate[82]
Furosemide[83]	Phenylbutazone[84]	Vitamins[69]
Hydralazine[85]	Pneumococcal vaccine[86]	Warfarin[87]
Hydrochlorothiazide[72]	Procainamide[88]	Zidovudine[89]
L-Trypthophan[90]	Propylthiouracil[91–93]	

Autoimmune Drug Reactions

Anticonvulsants[67,94–100]	Interferon[101–104]	Procainamide[105–110]
β-Blockers[105,111]	Isoniazid[112–114]	Quinidine[115–118]
Chlorpromazine[119–122]	Methyldopa[123–126]	Sulfasalazine[127–132]
Estrogen[133]	Minocycline[134]	Terbinafine[135]
Hydralazine[105,136,137]	Penicillamine[138]	Zafirlukast[139]

Table 3.11 • Hypersensitivity Reactions to Drugs: Pseudoallergic Reactions

Frequency	Highly variable, depending on the agent involved. For example, up to 30% of patients taking aspirin develop a cutaneous pseudoallergic response. On the other hand, pseudoallergic reactions to other agents, such as phytonadione and thiamine, are rare.
Clinical manifestations	Range from benign reactions (e.g., pruritus and flushing) to a life-threatening clinical syndrome indistinguishable from anaphylaxis.
Treatment	Pseudoallergic reactions treated the same as true allergic reactions (i.e., according to the clinical presentations of the patient). Thus, some reactions simply may require removal of the suspect agent, while some anaphylactoid reactions may require aggressive therapy (e.g., epinephrine, antihistamines, corticosteroids).
Prognosis	As with true allergic reactions, patients who have experienced a pseudoallergic drug reaction may have a similar reaction upon re-exposure. However, the severity of response may lessen with repeated administration. Furthermore, for some drugs, the frequency and severity of the reaction also may be influenced by the dose and/or rate of IV administration. Pretreatment regimens to reduce the frequency and the severity of responses have been developed for some drugs well known to cause pseudoallergic reactions (e.g., radiocontrast media).

From references 5, 9, and 151–163.

Table 3.12 • Pseudoallergic Reactions

Pseudoallergic Reactions

Acetylcysteine[160]	Immune globulin[151]	Phytonadione[151]
ACE inhibitors[155]	Methotrexate[175]	Polyoxyethylated castor oil (Cremophor EL—a solubilizing agent used in parenteral drugs, e.g., cyclosporine, paclitaxel)[181,182]
Angiontensin II-receptor blocking agents[164–174]	Minocycline[176]	Protamine[9]
Aspirin[156,159]	Narcotic analgesics[151]	Pyrethrin with piperonyl butoxide[152]
β-Adrenergic blockers[151]	NSAIDs[156,164]	Quaternary ammonium muscle relaxants[5,151]
Ciprofloacin[5,157,161,162]	Ondansetron[158,163]	Radiocontrast media[154]
Cisplatin[178]	Paclitaxel[177]	Reserpine[151]
Corticosteroids[179,180]	Pentamidine[151]	Thiamine[164]
Deferoxamine[151]		Vancomycin[9,153]

Table 3.13 • β-Lactam Oral Desensitization Protocol

Stock Drug Concentration (mg/mL)[a]	Dose No.	Amount (mL)	Drug Dose (mg)	Cumulative Drug (mg)
0.5	1[b]	0.05	0.025	0.025
	2	0.10	0.05	0.075
	3	0.20	0.10	0.175
	4	0.40	0.20	0.375
	5	0.80	0.40	0.775
5.0	6	0.15	0.75	1.525
	7	0.30	1.50	3.025
	8	0.60	3.00	6.025
	9	1.20	6.00	12.025
	10	2.40	12.00	24.025
50	11	0.50	25.00	49.025
	12	1.20	60.00	109.025
	13	2.50	125.00	234.025
	14	5.00	250.00	484.025

[a]Dilutions using 250 mg/5 mL of pediatric suspension.
[b]Oral dose doubled approximately every 15–30 minutes.
Adapted from references 192 and 194. Dosing for the oral protocol is arbitrary and should be adjusted for individual patients based on the clinical sensitivity and the desired drug dose end point.

Table 3.14 • β-Lactam Desensitization Protocol

Stock Drug Concentration (mg/mL)[a]	Dose No.[b]	Amount per 50 mL (mg/mL)[c]	Cumulative Drug (mg)
0.005	1[a]	0.0001	0.005
0.025	2	0.0005	0.030
0.125	3	0.0025	0.155
0.625	4	0.0125	0.780
3.125	5	0.0625	3.905
15.625	6[a]	0.3125	19.530
31.25	7	0.625	50.780
62.50	8	1.25	113.280
125.00	9	2.5	238.280
250.00	10[d]	5.0	488.280

[a]Stock drug solutions are prepared using serial dilutions of the desired goal (e.g., 500 mg of β-lactam). Doses 1–5 represent fivefold dilutions; doses 6–10 represent twofold dilutions.
[b]Interval between doses is 15–30 minutes. If desensitization is interrupted for >2 half-lives of the β-lactam, desensitization should be repeated.
[c]Mix 1 mL of stock drug solution in 50 mL 5% dextrose/0.225 normal saline or other compatible solution. Infuse each dose over 20–45 minutes. Dilution volume may vary with patient age and weight.
[d]If all 10 doses are administered and tolerated, the remaider of a full therapeutic dose of the β-lactam should be administered.
Adapted from reference 231. Dosing for the IV protocol is arbitrary and should be adjusted for individual patients based on the clinical sensitivity and the desired drug dose end point.

Table 3.15 • Oral Trimethoprim-Sulfamethoxazole Desensitization Protocol

Hour	Trimethoprim Component (Concentration or Tablet)	Volume	Dose of TMP-SMZ
0	0.0008 mg/mL	5 mL	0.004/0.02 mg
1	0.008 mg/mL	5 mL	0.04/0.2 mg
2	0.08 mg/mL	5 mL	0.4/2 mg
3	0.8 mg/mL	5 mL	4/20 mg
4	8 mg/mL	5 mL	40/200 mg
5	160 mg	1 tablet	160/800 mg

ᵃStock solution of trimethoprim-sulfamethoxazole may be prepared by appropriate dilutions of the commercially available suspension (8 mg trimethoprim/40 mg sulfamethoxazole per mL) with simple syrup or distilled water. Adapted with permission from Gluckstein D, Ruskin J. Rapid oral desensitization to trimethoprim-sulfamethoxazole (TMP-SMZ) use in prophylaxis for *Pneumocystis carinii* in patients with AIDS who were previously intolerant to TMP-SMZ. Clin Infect Dis 1995; 20:849. This protocol should serve as a guide only. Obtaining informed consent from the patient before initiating desensitization is advisable.

The reader is referred to Chapter 4: Anaphylaxis and Drug Allergies, written by *Paul M. Beringer, Pharm.D.*, and *Robert K. Middleton, Pharm.D.*, in the seventh edition of **Applied Therapeutics: The Clinical Use of Drugs** for a more in-depth discussion. All notations to reference numbers are based on the reference list at the end of that chapter. The editors of this handbook express their thanks to Drs. Beringer and Middleton and acknowledge that this chapter is based upon their work.

Notes:

Chapter 4

Managing Acute Drug Toxicity

Policies and Procedures

Practice sites can lessen stress and anxiety provoked by drug or other chemical exposures (accidental or purposeful) by establishing policies and procedures for effective communication. Among the most important principles are:

♦ Calm the caller by reassuring him that telephoning for assistance was appropriate

♦ Determine the identity of the patient (the caller or someone else) and age (if a child)

♦ Determine if the patient is conscious, breathing, and has a pulse. Obtain the phone number and address if it is determined that emergency personnel should be summoned. Call 911.

♦ Provide the telephone number and address of the nearest accredited poison control center. Educate all personnel as to how to quickly access this information.

General Principles

♦ In most situations, it is best to help the patient contact a poison center rather than trying to care for the patient yourself. They are better prepared to obtain the necessary information, make assessments, and recommend specific treatment.

♦ Basic support of airways, breathing, and circulation (the "ABC's") is paramount. Help the patient summon emergency personnel and provide CPR guidance to administer while waiting for help to arrive.

♦ In less life-threatening situations, management often centers around symptomatic and supportive care until the substance is cleared from the body.

Information Resources

♦ Medical Toxicology: Diagnosis and Treatment of Human Poisonings

♦ Goldfrank's Toxicologic Emergencies

♦ Poisoning and Drug Overdose (pocket-sized)

♦ Posindex (quarterly CD ROM database)

♦ Toxicologic, Occupational Medicine and Environmental Series (TOMES) database

Gather History of Exposure

If referral to a poison center is not available, try to determine:

♦ Why the individual believes an accidental ingestion or overdose occurred.

♦ Probable intoxicant(s).

♦ Maximum amount of substance(s) ingested.

- ♦ Dosage form(s).
- ♦ When the ingestion or exposure occurred.
- ♦ The state of consciousness of the patient.
- ♦ Current symptoms. Are they consistent with alleged substance(s) ingested?
- ♦ Prior medical problems and likely medications for treatment of medical problems.
- ♦ Allergies.

Interpret Laboratory Data

- ♦ *Qualitative urine drug screen* may be useful in patients with coma of unknown etiology or when history is inconsistent with clinical findings.
- ♦ *Quantitative tests of drugs* in serum can be useful:
  - • If concentration of the substance correlates with toxic effects;
  - • If turnaround time for results is rapid;
  - • If treatment can be guided by the serum concentration of the drug.
- ♦ *Pharmacodynamic and pharmacokinetic behavior* of drugs can be substantially altered by large drug overdoses, especially with drugs associated with dose-dependent pharmacokinetics.
  - • Rate of drug absorption is generally slowed by large oral overdoses.
  - • Time to reach peak serum drug concentrations can be prolonged with large oral overdoses.
  - • Volume of distribution of a drug can be increased.
  - • Usual metabolic pathways can become saturated, and secondary pathways can be important.

Most Common Reported Toxic Substances. See Table 4.1.

Decontamination

After the airway and cardiopulmonary systems are supported, efforts should be directed toward removing the toxic substance from the patient. Consider one of the following if the ingestion is large enough to produce clinically significant toxicity.

- ♦ *Activated Charcoal*
  - • Adsorption of substances to activated charcoal is usually the preferred method of GI decontamination.
  - • A 50-gm dose should be mixed into a slurry with water and sorbitol.
  - • Sorbitol is usually administered concurrently to remove the charcoal-drug complex from the GI tract before possible disassociation of toxic drug from charcoal.
  - • Effectiveness varies with location of toxic substance and amount present in GI tract.
- ♦ *Syrup of Ipecac-induced Emesis*
  - • Removes substances from the stomach and possibly from the proximal small bowel.
  - • Not effective for removal of substances from more distal bowel.
  - • Contraindications to emesis are described in Table 4.2.
  - • Administration of 15 mL to children <10 yr old and 30 mL to older children and adults induces emesis in about 80%-90%. Repeat dose in 30–45 minutes if no emesis.
  - • Vomiting begins in about 20 minutes after administration of syrup of ipecac. May be less effective if patient is lying down; encourage ambulation if possible.

♦ **Gastric Lavage**
♦ **Whole Body Irrigation**
- A *polyethylene glycol-balanced electrolyte solution* (Colyte, GoLYTELY) can remove substances from the entire GI tract. Simple cathartics and laxatives are ineffective.
- Slower than ipecac or gastric lavage
- Useful for removal of sustained-release dosage forms

Antidotes
♦ Specific antidotes exist for only a small fraction of ingested substances
- *Naloxone* can displace opioids from receptor sites.
- *Flumazenil* can displace benzodiazepines from receptor sites.
- *Acetylcysteine* can inhibit the formation of toxic acetaminophen metabolites. (See below.)
- *Alcohol or 4-methyl pyrazole* for methanol
- *Antidigoxin FAB fragment* can bind digoxin and prevent binding to the receptor. (See Chapter 16: Heart Failure)
- *Deferoxamine* can chelate iron and form ferrioxamine, which is eliminated in the urine. See below for dosing of deferoxamine.

Management of Specific Drug Overdoses
♦ Acute and chronic *salicylate* toxicity
- Possible causes: aspirin or topical methylsalicylate (oil of wintergreen) in liniments.
- The potential symptoms and severity of *acute salicylism* can be predicted both by the dose ingested (see Table 4.3) and serum levels (see Figure 4.1). Other common signs are respiratory alkalosis or metabolic acidosis (especially in children), hypokalemia, hypernatremia, hyperthermia, and tinnitus.
- *Chronic salicylate intoxication* usually is associated with ingestion of >100 mg/kg/day for >2 to 3 days.
- Treatment of acute toxicity:
  Activated charcoal and/or gastric lavage to minimize further absorption.
  Hypotonic (1/4 to 1/2 normal) saline and 20–40 mEq/L potassium as needed for hypernatremia and hypokalemia.
  Sodium bicarbonate (50 mEq IV bolus or 1–2 mEq/kg to each liter of IV fluid) as needed for metabolic acidosis.
  Vitamin K if prothrombin time is prolonged.
  Hemodialysis if seizures occur.
♦ *Acetaminophen* ingestion
- The risk of hepatotoxicity can be estimated by serum levels drawn 4–24 hours after acute ingestion (see Figure 4.2)
- Treatment:
  Activated charcoal 50 g with sorbitol if <4 hours since ingestion. Remove charcoal by lavage or wait 4 hours before starting acetylcysteine.
  Acetylcysteine (Mucomyst) 140 mg/kg orally as first dose, diluted to a concentration of <5 per cent using a carbonated beverage or fruit juice to mask the sulfur odor. Then 70 mg/kg Q 4 hours for 72 hours. If vomiting occurs within first hour, repeat

the loading dose. Consider antiemetic drugs or a duodenal feeding tube if vomiting continues.

- Monitor AST and ALT levels and prothrombin time daily for 72 hours.
- ◆ *Iron* ingestion
  - The symptoms, toxic serum concentrations, and stages of acute iron toxicity are found in Table 4.4
  - Treatment:

  Syrup of ipecac more effective than activated charcoal or lavage for iron removal (see above for ipecac dosing).

  Chelation: If serum concentration >500 µg/dL or ingestion >60 mg/kg, start *deferoxamine (Desferal)* 20 mg/kg (1 gm in adults) IM or slow IV followed by 10 mg/kg (500 mg in adults) Q 4 hr × 2 doses. May give further doses at 4- to 12-hour intervals, not to exceed 120 mg/kg (6 g in adults) in 24 hours. To avoid histamine-related side effects (flushing, generalized erythema, urticaria, hypotension, shock, seizures), do not exceed 4–15 mg/hr infusion rate.

Table 4.1 • Substances Most Commonly Reported in Toxic Exposures

Cases	Deaths
Poison Centers	726 *Total*
2,155,592 Total	Analgesics
Cleaning substances	Antidepressants
Analgesics	Stimulants and street drugs
Cosmetics	Cardiovascular drugs
Plants	Alcohols
Cough/cold preparations	
Emergency Departments	**Medical Examiner**
531,800 Total	*9,216 Total*
Alcohol with other drugs	Cocaine
Cocaine	Heroin/morphine, opiates not specified
Heroin/morphine	Alcohol with other drugs
Marijuana/hashish	Codeine
Acetaminophen	Marijuana/hashish

Notes:

Table 4.2 • Contraindications to Emesis

CNS Depression
Patients who are lethargic or unresponsive, lack a gag reflex, or are otherwise unable to adequately protect their airway are at risk of pulmonary aspiration

Caustic Ingestions
Esophageal and oropharyngeal mucous membranes can be further damaged when re-exposed to caustic solids or liquids upon emesis. Emesis also can cause gastric or esophageal perforation of the weakened visceral wall. Pulmonary aspiration of the caustic substance is a risk as well

Seizure Activity
The postictal patient is at risk of aspirating gastric contents should another seizure develop

Petroleum Distillates
Systemic toxicity from low viscosity agents (e.g., mineral seal oil) is low, but the risk of aspiration is high when vomiting is induced. Emesis also is not indicated when compounds of very high viscosity (e.g., motor oil, mineral oil) have been ingested because these agents also have low systemic toxicity. In contrast, emesis may be induced when the following are ingested: halogenated hydrocarbons (e.g., carbon tetrachloride); large volumes (>1 mL/kg) of compounds with potent CNS activity (e.g., gasoline, paint thinner); or petroleum distillates serving as a base for a toxic chemical or pesticide. For these agents, emesis carries a lower risk of aspiration than gastric lavage

Foreign Body Ingestion
Can cause further damage to esophageal tissue or mucous membranes

---

Table 4.3 • Signs and Symptoms of Acute Salicylate Intoxication

Dose Ingested (mg/kg)	Severity	Anticipated Symptoms
<150	Asymptomatic	None
150–300	Mild-to-moderate	*Mild*: mild-to-moderate hyperpnea, occasional lethargy *Moderate*: severe hyperpnea, lethargy, agitation
300–500	Severe	Severe hyperpnea, coma, occasional convulsions
>500	Potentially lethal	Coma, convulsions, cardiovascular collapse

---

Table 4.4 • Stages of Iron Toxicity

Stage	Time after Ingestion	Symptoms
I	Within 6 hours	Nausea, vomiting, diarrhea, abdominal pain common if ingestion >20 mg/kg. Blood in vomitus or stool possible. If severe (ingestion of >60 mg/kg elemental iron, serum iron >500 µg/dL) may see lethargy, seizures, tachycardia, hypotension.[a]
II	12–24 hours	Asymptomatic or decreasing symptoms. May mark recovery if ingestion was small but may be misleading if a large dose is ingested.
III	12–48 hours	CNS (lethargy, coma, seizures) and/or cardiovascular toxicity (hypotension, pulmonary edema). Metabolic acidosis, hypoglycemia, hepatic necrosis, renal damage, coagulopathy also possible.
IV	4–6 weeks	Late GI tract sequalae: gastric scarring, pyloric strictures, and permanent functional abnormalities.

[a]Peak serum concentrations (2–6 hours postingestion) >300–350 µg/dL are usually associated with toxicity. Concentrations >500 µg/dL predict severe toxicity.

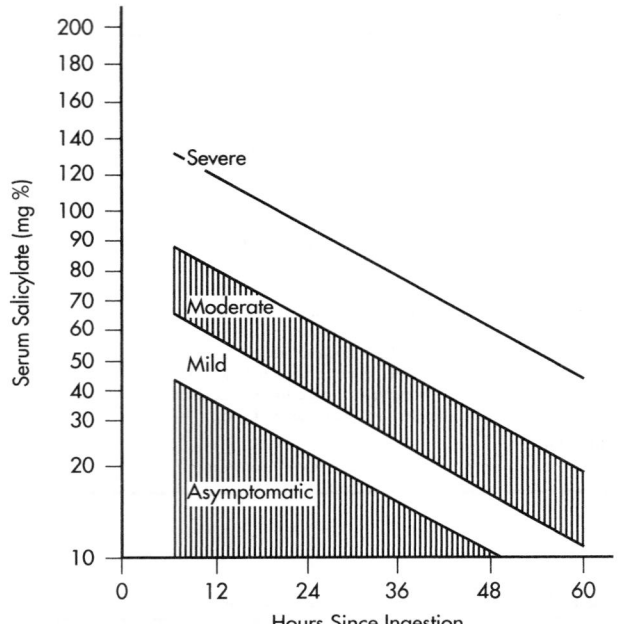

Fig. 4.1 Done Nomogram for Interpretation of Severity of Acute Salicylate Poisoning.
(Reproduced by permission of Pediatrics 1960; 26:800–807).

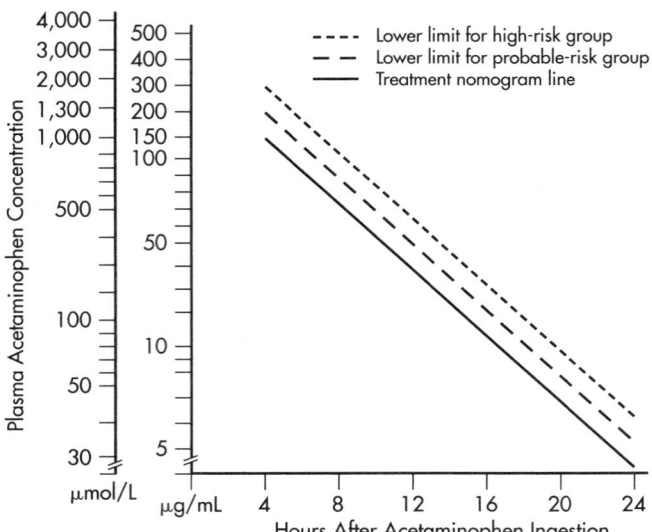

Fig. 4.2 Nomogram for Interpretation of Severity of Acetaminophen Poisoning. (Copyright 2001 Massachusetts Medical Society. All rights reserved.)

The reader is referred to Chapter 5: Managing Acute Drug Toxicity, written by *William A. Watson, Pharm.D.,* and *Frank Paloucek, Pharm.D.,* in the seventh edition of **Applied Therapeutics: The Clinical Use of Drugs** for a more in-depth discussion. All notations to reference numbers are based on the reference list at the end of that chapter. The editors of this handbook express their thanks to Drs. Watson and Paloucek and acknowledge that this chapter is based upon their work.

Notes:

Notes:

Chapter 5

Nausea and Vomiting

General Principles

♦ Nausea and vomiting (N/V) are usually self-limiting events without serious sequelae. Protracted vomiting may result in dehydration, malnutrition, metabolic alkalosis, hyponatremia, hypokalemia, and hypochloremia. Infants and children are at greatest risk.

♦ Repeated retching may result in tears and bleeding at the gastroesophageal junction (Mallory-Weiss syndrome). Aspiration of gastric acid may produce a chemical pneumonitis.

Etiology

Viral gastroenteritis is the most common cause of N/V. Bacterial infections, drugs, motion sickness, cancer chemotherapy, and pregnancy also are frequently encountered etiologies. Chronic N/V may signify a serious underlying problem and warrants medical attention. Table 5.1 lists these and other causes of N/V.

Management Principles

Nondrug therapies include removal or treatment of the underlying cause.

Antiemetic drugs should be used cautiously if pregnancy is suspected.

♦ *Available products* are listed in Table 5.2 along with their primary indication and recommended doses.

♦ *Adverse Effects.* See Table 5.3.

♦ *References to key National and International Antiemetic Guidelines for specific types of nausea and vomiting.* See Table 5.4.

Motion Sickness

Motion sickness occurs when perceptions of motion by visual, vestibular, and sensory proprioceptors provide conflicting information.

General measures for prevention of motion sickness are found in Table 5.5.

♦ The belladonna alkaloids (scopolamine) and antihistamines are the most effective agents against motion sickness. Transdermal scopolamine provides a constant delivery of drug over a prolonged period. After delivering a priming dose of 140 μg over the first few hours, 5 μg/hr is released over 72 hr. For severe symptoms, a combination of amphetamine plus either an antihistamine or scopolamine may be necessary. Phenothiazines are less effective.

♦ Recommendations for traveler's and drug therapy of motion sickness are summarized in Tables 5.6 and 5.7, respectively.

Postoperative Nausea and Vomiting (PONV)

The incidence of PONV ranges from 1 to 43% of surgeries and varies by the type of anesthetic used, anatomical location of the surgery, age, and gender of the patient.

♦ Antiemetic drugs can be given both prophylactically and for treatment. See Table 5.8. Also see Chapter 7: Perioperative Care.

Chemotherapy-associated Nausea and Vomiting (CANV)

The emetogenic potential of various single agents is listed in Table 5.9. Cisplatin is the most frequently implicated. Combination chemotherapy is at least as emetogenic as the most emetogenic single agent it contains.

Acute nausea and vomiting occur 1–2 hr after administration and is usually controlled within 24 hr. However, some experience persistent or delayed N/V that can last for days to weeks. The potential to cause N/V varies among agents, dose, route, patients, and treatment courses in the same patient.

Anticipatory emesis is N/V that starts before administration of chemotherapy and is a problem in patients who have been inadequately treated previously or in those receiving highly emetogenic regimens. The hospital or clinic environment or other treatment-related associations (e.g., smells) can trigger emesis.

Management

♦ *Premedication (prophylaxis),* given as a single dose 15–60 minutes prior to chemo-therapy, reduces the incidence of acute CANV. A combination of a $5HT_3$ receptor antagonist plus dexamethasone is recommended for high-to-moderate risk regimens. (See Table 5.10 for recommended doses in both adults and children.) Lorazepam may be added to reduce anxiety and anticipatory nausea. Monotherapy is adequate for intermediate risk regimens. No premedication is necessary for low-risk regimens.

♦ *Delayed CANV* may begin as late as 16–24 hr after chemotherapy, and emesis may last up to 96 hours. Dexamethasone and other agents may be used as monotherapy for delayed CANV or breakthrough emesis (see Table 5.11). A combination of dexameth-asone 4–8 mg BID plus metoclopramide 0.5 mg/kg QID is common but may have a higher risk of extrapyramidal side effects in children. Refractory emesis may require combination therapy.

Diabetic Gastroparesis

See Chapter 47: Diabetes Mellitus.

Nausea and Vomiting in Pregnancy

See Chapter 43: Obstetrics.

Pediatric Nausea and Vomiting

See Chapter 89: Pediatric Considerations.

Notes:

Table 5.1 • Causes of Nausea and Vomiting

Acute Symptoms

Anxiety

Drugs
  Antibiotics (erythromycin, quinolones, flucytosine, nitrofurantoin)
  Anticholinergics
  Cancer chemotherapy
  Digoxin
  Opioids
  Theophylline

Fluid and Electrolyte Abnormalities
  Hypercalcemia
  Volume Depletion
  Water intoxication

Migraine Headache

Peritonitis

Radiation Therapy

Tube Feeding

Vestibular Disorders
  Meniere's syndrome
  Motion sickness
  Otitis interna

Viral Hepatitis

Chronic Symptoms

Mechanical Obstruction
  Peptic or gastric ulcer
  Gastric or pancreatic carcinoma
  Pancreatic pseudocyst

Metabolic and Endocrine Disturbances
  Adrenal insufficiency
  Diabetic ketoacidosis
  Hyperparathyroidism
  Uremia

Metastasis
  Brain
  Hepatic
  Meninges ($\uparrow$ intracranial pressure)

Pregnancy

Psychogenic
  Anorexia nervosa
  Bulimia
  Rumination

Notes:

Table 5.2 • Available Antiemetic Agents[a]

Drug	Type of Emesis Used For	Available Dosage Forms	Recommended Dosage Regimen
Antihistamines			
Buclizine (Bucladin-S)	Motion sickness	*Tab:* 50 mg	*Adults:* 50 mg PO 30 min before exposure and Q 4–6 hr
Cyclizine (Marezine)	Motion sickness	*Tab:* 50 mg *Inj:* 50 mg/mL	*Adults:* 50 mg PO or IM 30 min before exposure and Q 4–6 hr (*max:* 200 mg/day) *Children:* 25 mg PO 30 min before exposure and Q 4–6 hr (*max:* 75 mg/day)
Dimenhydrinate (Dramamine)	Motion sickness	*Tab:* 50 mg *Oral solution:* 15 mg/mL *Inj:* 50 mg/mL	*Adults:* 50–100 mg PO, IM, or IV 30 min before exposure and Q 4 hr *Children:* 1.25 mg/kg PO or IM Q 4–6 hr (*max:* 300 mg/day)
Meclizine (Antivert, Bonine)	Motion sickness	*Tab:* 12.5, 25, 50 mg	*Adults:* 25–50 mg PO 1 hr before exposure and Q 4–6 hr
Anticholinergics			
Scopolamine (Transderm–Scop)	Motion sickness, postoperative	*Transdermal system:* 0.5 mg/72 hr *Inj:* 0.3, 0.4, 1 mg/mL	*Adults:* Apply 4 hr before exposure and Q 72 hr; preoperative 0.2–1 mg IM, IV, or SQ
Butyrophenones			
Haloperidol (Haldol)	Chemotherapy, postoperative	*Tab:* 0.5, 1, 2, 5, 10, 25 mg *Oral solution:* 2 mg/mL *Inj:* 5 mg/mL	*Adults:* 1–2 mg PO or IM Q 8 hr
Droperidol (Inapsine)	Chemotherapy, postoperative	*Inj:* 2.5 mg/mL	*Adults:* 0.5–1 mg IV Q 4 hr
Dopamine Antagonist			
Metoclopramide (Reglan)	Chemotherapy, gastric stasis	*Tab:* 10 mg; oral solution 5 mg/mL *Inj:* 5 mg/mL	*Adults:* Chemotherapy: 1–2 mg/kg IV or PO 30–60 min before exposure and Q 2–3 hr (*max:* 12 mg/kg) *Stasis:* 10 mg PO, IM, or IV 30 min before meals and HS
Cannabinoid			
Dronabinol (Marinol)	Chemotherapy	*Cap:* 2.5, 5, 10 mg	*Adults:* 5 mg/m^2 1–3 hr before and Q 2–4 hr. May ↑ dose by 2.5 mg/m^2 to max of 15 mg/m^2/dose
Nabilone (Cesamet)	Chemotherapy	*Cap:* 1 mg	*Adults:* 1 or 2 mg PO Q 8 and 12 hr. Give 1st dose before chemotherapy

Drug	Indication	Formulations	Dosage
Corticosteroids Dexamethasone (Decadron, Hexadrol, Dexone)	Chemotherapy	*Tab:* 0.25, 0.5, 0.75, 1, 1.5, 2, 4, 6 mg *Inj:* 4, 10, 20, 24 mg/mL	*Adults:* 10–20 mg PO or IV before chemotherapy
Phenothiazines Prochlorperazine (Compazine)	Chemotherapy, postoperative, general	*Tab:* 5, 10, 25 mg *Rectal suppository:* 2.5, 5, 25 mg *Oral solution:* 5 mg/5 mL *Inj:* 5 mg/mL; extended release *Cap:* 10, 15, 30 mg	*Adults:* 5–10 mg PO, IM, or IV Q 6–8 hr
Promethazine (Phenergan, Anergan)	Postoperative, motion sickness	*Tab:* 12.5, 25, 50 mg *Oral solution:* 6.25, 25 mg/5 mL *Inj:* 25, 50 mg/mL *Rectal suppository:* 12.55, 25, 50 mg	*Adults:* 25 mg PO or IM 30–60 min before exposure and Q 8–12 hr *Children:* 0.5 mg/kg PO 30–60 min before exposure and Q 8–12 hr
Thiethylperazine (Torecan)	Chemotherapy, postoperative, general	*Tab:* 10 mg *Rectal suppository:* 10 mg *Inj:* 5 mg/mL	*Adults:* 10 mg PO, IM, or PR Q 8 hr
Chlorpromazine (Thorazine)	Postoperative	*Tab:* 10, 25, 50 mg *Oral solution:* 10 mg/5 mL, 30, 100 mg/mL *Inj:* 25 mg/mL	*Adults:* 12.5–25 mg PO or IM Q 4–6 hr *Children:* 0.275–0.55 mg PO or IM Q 4–6 hr
Serotonin (5-HT₃) Antagonists Dolasetron (Anzemet)	Chemotherapy	*Inj:* 20 mg/mL *Tab:* 50, 100 mg	*Adults and Children >2 yr:* 1.8 mg/kg up to 100 mg 30 min before chemotherapy
	Postoperative	*Inj:* 20 mg/mL *Tab:* 50, 100 mg	*Adults and Children >2 yr:* 0.35 mg/kg up to 12.5 mg 15 min before anesthesia *Adults:* 100 mg PO 2 hr before surgery *Children:* 1.2 mg/kg PO up to 100 mg 2 hr before surgery
Granisetron (Kytril)	Chemotherapy	*Inj:* 1 mg/mL *Tab:* 1 mg	*Adults and Children >2 yr:* 10 μg/kg 30 min before chemotherapy *Adults:* 1 mg Q 12 hr × 2 doses

(continued)

Table 5.2 • Available Antiemetic Agents[a] (continued)

Drug	Type of Emesis Used For	Available Dosage Forms	Recommended Dosage Regimen
Ondansetron (Zofran)	Chemotherapy	Inj: 2 mg/mL	Adults and Children >4 yr: 0.15 mg/kg 30 min before chemotherapy and then 4 and 8 hr
		Tab: 4, 8 mg	Adults: 32 mg before chemotherapy
			Adults and Children >12 yr: 8 mg TID
			Children 4–14 yr: 4 mg TID
	Postoperative	Inj: 2 mg/mL	Adults: 4 mg IV immediately before induction or postoperatively if symptoms occur
	Radiation	Tab: 4, 8 mg	Adults: 8 mg TID
Miscellaneous			
Benzquinamide (Emete–Con)	Postoperative	Inj: 25 mg/mL	Adults: 0.5–1 mg/kg IM Q 3–4 hr
Diphenidol (Vontrol)	Postoperative, chemotherapy, labyrinthine disturbances	Tab: 25 mg	Adults: 25–50 mg PO Q 4 hr
			Children: >6 months, 0.88 mg/kg Q 4 hr
Trimethobenzamide (Tigan)	General	Cap: 100, 250 mg	Adults: 250 mg PO Q 6–8 hr or 200 mg PR or IM Q 6–8 hr
		Inj: 100 mg/mL	
		Rectal suppository: 100, 200 mg	

[a]Cap = Capsule; HS = At bedtime; IM = Intramuscular; Inj = Injection; IV = Intravenous; PO = Oral; PR = Per rectum; Tab = Tablet.

Notes:

Table 5.3 • Antiemetic Side Effects

Drug	Side Effects
Phenothiazines, butyrophenones	Drowsiness, dry mouth, constipation, blurred vision, hypotension, dystonias[a]
Metoclopramide	Dystonias,[a] diarrhea
Ondansetron	Headache, sedation, transient LFT elevations[c]
Antihistamines	Drowsiness, dry mouth, confusion
Scopolamine[b]	Drowsiness, dry mouth, blurred vision, confusion, tachycardia, hypotension
Corticosteroids (short course, high dose)	Euphoria, insomnia, psychosis, mild fluid retention, hyperglycemia, GI bleeding
Cannabinoids	Orthostatic hypotension, altered mental perceptions ("high"), especially in elderly

[a]Dystonias and other extrapyramidal effects are infrequent, even with high doses. Combined treatment with antihistamines may ↓ this side effect.
[b]Side effects of scopolamine are ↓ when transdermal patches are used.
[c]LFT, liver function test.

Table 5.4 • National and International Antiemetic Guidelines

American Society of Clinical Oncology[18]	Acute and delayed CIE Anticipatory emesis Emesis in pediatric oncology High-dose chemotherapy Breakthrough emesis Radiation-induced emesis
American Society of Health-Systems Pharmacists[17]	Adult acute and delayed CIE Radiation-induced emesis Postoperative nausea and vomiting Pediatric CIE, radiation-induced emesis, PONV
Multinational Association of Supportive Care in Cancer[19]	Adult acute and delayed CIE Radiation-induced emesis High-dose chemotherapy Pediatric CIE Multiple day and rescue
National Comprehensive Cancer Center Network[20]	Acute and delayed CIE Radiation-induced emesis Anticipatory emesis Breakthrough emesis

CIE, chemotherapy–induced emesis; PONV, postoperative nausea and vomiting.

Notes:

Table 5.5 • General Measures for Prevention of Motion Sickness

1. Minimize exposure.
   - Be located in the middle of the plane or boat, where movement is least.
   - Be in a semirecumbent position.
   - Minimize head and body movements.
2. Restrict visual activity.
   - Fix vision on the horizon or some other stable external object.
   - Avoid fixation on a moving object.
   - Avoid reading
   - Close eyes if below deck or in an enclosed cabin.
3. Improve ventilation and remove noxious stimuli.
4. Reduce the magnitude of the motion stimulus.
   - Avoid or minimize acceleration and deceleration and turning or moving of the vehicle.
5. Engage in distracting activity.
   - Be in control of the vehicle.
   - Perform mental activity.

Table 5.6 • Recommendations for Travelers

I. Short-term exposure (≤6 hr)
   A. Mild to moderate
      1. Recommended
         a. Dimenhydrinate
      2. Alternatives
         a. Meclizine
         b. Promethazine
   B. Intensive
      1. Recommended
         a. Promethazine plus amphetamine
      2. Alternatives
         a. Dimenhydrinate
         b. Scopolamine patch

II. Long-term exposure (>6 hr)
   A. Mild
      1. Recommended
         a. Dimenhydrinate as needed
      2. Alternatives
         a. Scopolamine patch
         b. Meclizine as needed
         c. Promethazine as needed
   B. Moderate to severe
      1. Recommended
         a. Scopolamine patch
      2. Alternatives
         a. Repeated doses of dimenhydrinate
         b. Repeated doses of promethazine
         c. Repeated doses of meclizine

Adapted from reference 16.

Table 5.7 • Recommendations for Prevention of Motion Sickness

Drug	Oral Dose (mg)	Time to Efficacy (hr)	Dose Frequency (hr)	Use in Pregnancy	Use in Children
Amphetamine	5–10	1–2	Q 4–6	No	Not <3 yr
Cyclizine	50	1–2	Q 4–6	? No	Yes
Dimenhydrinate	50–100	1–2	Q 4–6	? No	Not <2 yr
Meclizine	25–50	2	Q 6–24	? No	Yes
Promethazine	25	1.5–2	Q 4–6	Yes	Not <2 yr
Scopolamine patch	Patch	8	Q 72	No	No

Adapted from reference 16.

Table 5.8 • Antiemetics for Management of Postoperative Nausea and Vomiting in Adults and Pediatrics

Agents	Regimen	Route
Prophylaxis—Adults		
Droperidol	0.625–0.125 mg 5 min before terminating anesthesia	IV
Ondansetron	4 mg immediately before induction of anesthesia	IV
	8 mg 1 hr before induction of anesthesia	PO
Dolasetron	12.5 mg intraoperatively	IV
	100 mg PO 1 hr before induction of anesthesia	PO
Metoclopramide	10 mg given near end of procedure (20 mg may be used)	IV
Promethazine	25 mg 1 hr before induction of anesthesia	PO
	12.5–25 mg immediately before induction of anesthesia	
Prochlorperazine	5–15 mg 1 hr before induction of anesthesia	PO
	5–10 mg 1–2 hr before induction of anesthesia; may repeat once in 30 minutes if needed	IM
	5–10 mg 15–30 min before induction of anesthesia; may repeat once as needed	IV
Treatment—Adults		
Ondansetron	1–4 mg postoperatively	IV
Metoclopramide	10 mg may be given Q 4–6 hr as needed postoperatively	IV
Promethazine	10–25 mg Q 4–6 hr as needed postoperatively	PO
	12.5–25 mg Q 4 hr as needed postoperatively	IM/IV
Prochlorperazine	5–15 mg postoperatively	PO
	5–10 mg; may repeat once in 30 min as needed	IM
	5–10 mg; may repeat once as needed	IV
Droperidol	0.625–0.125 mg as needed	IV
Dolasetron	12.5 mg postoperatively	IV
Prophylaxis—Pediatrics		
Dolasetron	>2 yr old; 1.8 mg/kg immediately before induction	IV
Ondansetron	0.05 mg/kg (range of 0.05–0.15 mg/kg)	IV
Droperidol	0.015–0.075 mg/kg/dose	IV
Treatment—Pediatrics		
Chlorpromazine	0.55 mg/kg	PO/IM
Droperidol	0.1 mg/kg/dose	IV
Ondansetron	0.05 mg/kg/dose	IV

Adapted from reference 17.

Notes:

Table 5.9 • Emetogenic Potential of Single Chemotherapy Agents

Hesketh[a]	ASCO[b]	MASCC[c]
Level 5 Carmustine (>250 mg/m^2) Cisplatin (>50 mg/m^2) Cyclophosphamide Dacarbazine (>500 mg/m^2) Mechlorethamine Streptozocin	**High** Actinomycin Carboplatin Carmustine (>250 mg/m^2) Cisplatin (>50 mg/m^2) Cyclophosphamide (>1,500 mg/m^2) Cytarabine (>1 g/m^2) Dacarbazine Daunorubicin Doxorubine Epirubicin Idarubicin Ifosfamide Lomustine Mechlorethamine	**High** Carmustine Cisplatin Cyclophosphamide Dacarbazine Mechlorethamine Streptozocin
Level 4 Carboplatin Carmustine (<250 mg/m^2) Cisplatin (<50 mg/m^2) Cyclophosphamide (>750–1,500 mg/m^2) Cytarabine (>1 g/m^2) Doxorubicin Methotrexate (>1,000 mg/m^2) Procarbazine (oral)		**Moderate to High** Anthracyclines Carboplatin Carmustine Cisplatin Cyclophosphamide Cyclophosphamide (oral) Cytarabine Hexamethylmelamine Ifosfamide Irinotecan Methotrexate Mitoxantrone Procarbazine Topotecan
Level 3 Cyclophosphamide (≤750 mg/m^2) Cyclophosphamide (oral) Doxorubicin (20–60 mg/m^2) Epirubicin (≤90 mg/m^2) Hexamethylmelamine (oral) Idarubicin Ifosfamide Methotrexate (250–1,000 mg/m^2) Mitoxantrone (<15 mg/m^2)	**Intermediate** Docetaxel Etoposide Gemcitabine Irinotecan Mitomycin Mitoxantrone Paclitaxel Teniposide Topotecan	**Low to Moderate** Etoposide Fluorouracil Gemcitabine Methotrexate Mitomycin Taxoids
Level 2 Docetaxel Etoposide 5–Fluorouracil Gemcitabine Methotrexate (50 mg/m^2; 250 mg/m^2) Mitomycin Paclitaxel	**Low** Bleomycin Busulfan Cladribine Fludarabine Fluorouracil Methotrexate (≤50 mg/m^2) Vinblastine Vincristine Vinorelbine	**Low** Bleomycin Busulfan Chlorambucil (oral) 2–Chlorodeoxyadenosine Fludarabine Hydroxyurea Methotrexate L–phenylalanine mustard 6–Thioguanine (oral) Vinblastine Vincristine Vinorelbine
Level 1 Bleomycin Busulfan (<4 mg/kg/day) Chlorambucil (oral) 2–Chlorodeoxyadenosine Fludarabine Hydroxyurea Methotrexate (≤50 mg/m^2) L–phenylalanine mustard (oral) Thioguanine (oral) Vinblastine Vincristine Vinorelbine		

[a]From Hesketh P et al. J Clin Oncol 1997;15:103. Level 5 = vomiting within 24 hours in >90% of patients. Level 4 = 60–90% of patients. Level 3 = 30–60% of patients. Level 2 = 10–30% of patients. Level 1 = <10% of patients.
[b]ASCO = American Society of Clinical Oncology
[c]MASCC = Multination Association of Supportive Care in Cancer.

Notes:

Table 5.10 • Recommendations for Prevention of Acute Chemotherapy-induced Emesis

Agent	Dose	Schedule[a]	Route
Adults			
Level 3–5 or Moderate, Moderately High, or High Risk			
Ondansetron	8 mg	Single dose	IV
	24 mg		PO
or			
Granisetron	10 µg/kg	Single dose	IV
	2 mg	Single dose	PO
or			
Dolasetron	1.8 mg/kg or	Single dose	IV
	100 mg	Single dose	IV
plus			
Dexamethasone	20 mg	Single dose	PO or IV
Level 2 or Intermediate, Low-to-Moderate Risk			
Ondansetron	8 mg	BID	PO
or			
Granisetron	2 mg	QD	PO
or			
Dolasetron	100 mg	QD	PO
or			
Dexamethasone	8 mg	BID	PO
Pediatrics			
Level 3–5			
Ondansetron	0.15 mg/kg/dose	4 hr × 3	IV
or			
Granisetron	20–40 µg/kg	Single dose	IV
or			
Dolasetron	1.8 mg/kg	Single dose	IV
plus			
Dexamethasone	5–10 mg/m^2	Single dose	PO or IV

[a]Single dose administered once 15–60 minutes before chemotherapy administration.
Adapted from references 17–20 and product information.

Notes:

Table 5.11 • Standard Doses of Non–5HT$_3$–Receptor Antagonist Antiemetics for Prevention and Management of Chemotherapy–induced Emesis

Agents	Dose/Schedule[a]	Route
Phenothiazines		
Prochlorperazine	10–40 mg Q 6–8 hr	PO, IV, IM
	25 mg Q 6–8 hr	PR
Thiethylperazine	10 mg Q 8 hr	PO, IM, IV, PR
Perphenazine	4–5 mg Q 6 hr	PO, IV, IM
Butyrophenones		
Haloperidol	1–3 mg Q 2–8 hr	PO, IM, IV
Droperidol	5–15 mg × 1; 2–7.5 mg Q 2 hr	IV
Cannabinoids		
Marinol	5–10 mg/m^2 Q 3–4 hr	PO
Corticosteroids		
Dexamethasone	20 mg before chemotherapy	PO, IV
	4–8 mg Q 12 hr (delayed)	PO
Methylprednisolone	0.5–1 mg/kg before chemotherapy or Q 12 hr IV (maximum total 4 mg/kg/24 hr)	IM, PO
Substituted benzamides		
Metoclopramide	1–3 mg/kg Q 2 hr × 2–5 doses (maximum total, 12 mg/kg/24 hr)	IV
	0.5 mg/kg Q 2–6 hr (delayed)	PO
Benzodiazepines		
Lorazepam	1–2 mg before chemotherapy	IV, SL
	1 mg Q 6–12 hr	PO
Miscellaneous		
ACTH	1 mg Q 12 hr × 3	IM
Scopolamine	1 patch Q 72 hr	TD

[a]Dose and schedule pertain to use as antiemetics with chemotherapy only.
ACTH, adrenocorticotropin hormone; IM, intramuscularly; IV, intravenously; PO, orally; SL, sublingually; TD, transdermally; PR, per rectum.
Adapted from references 17–20 and product information.

The reader is referred to Chapter 5: Nausea and Vomiting written by *Celeste Lindley, Pharm. D.* in the seventh edition of **Applied Therapeutics: The Clinical Use of Drugs** for a more in-depth discussion. All notations to reference numbers are based on the reference list at the end of that chapter. The editors of this handbook express their thanks to Dr. Lindley and acknowledge that this chapter is based upon her work.

Notes:

Chapter 6

Pain

Description

♦ Pain is an unpleasant situation disturbing a patient's comfort, thought, sleep, emotion, or normal daily activity. It serves a useful purpose by alerting an individual to an injury, but persistent or chronic pain serves no useful purpose. Anxiety, fatigue, prior experience, emotional status, as well as the extent of tissue injury, can influence the perception of pain. Since pain is a subjective experience, it is the patient, not the caregiver who can best describe the intensity of pain and the benefit of therapy. See Figures 6.1–6.3 for examples of pain assessment tools.

♦ *Somatic pain* is caused by nociceptor stimulation of skin, muscle, tendons, joints, or periosteum of bone. Also includes headache, dental pain, and menstrual cramps. It is usually well localized and responsive to nonsteroidal anti-inflammatory drugs (NSAIDs) or acetaminophen. Can combine NSAIDs with opiods if indicated. Opioids alone often are less effective.

♦ *Visceral pain* is caused by stretching of the omentum of the gastrointestinal (GI) tract and pericardium, organ damage, or bone pain. It is often diffuse and difficult to localize. Most responsive pain to opioids but also may respond to NSAIDs.

♦ *Neuropathic (deafferentation) pain* is caused by nerve involvement: diabetic neuropathy, herpes zoster (shingles), trigeminal neuralgia, phantom limb, post-thalamic CVA, or vincristine neuropathy. It is often described as burning, lancinating, piercing, and numbness. Neuropathic pain responds poorly to opioids. Antidepressants and anticonvulsants often are effective.

Treatment

♦ *General Principle.* Pain often is undertreated. The goal of both acute and chronic pain is to reduce pain to the lowest tolerable intensity and prevent it from recurring. This may require high, frequent doses. Fear of habituation or addiction is not an appropriate reason for using low doses of opioids, especially if maximal pain relief has not been achieved.

♦ *Nonmalignant Pain.* When approaching pain therapy, one must differentiate between *acute* and *chronic* nonmalignant pain. (See Table 6.1.)

♦ *Cancer Pain.* The principles of cancer pain management are discussed in Table 6.2.

♦ *Nonnarcotic analgesics* are indicated for either acute or chronic pain and often are equally as effective as opioids for somatic pain (e.g., dental pain). NSAIDs are the analgesics of choice for the management of mild-to-moderate pain involving musculoskeletal tissues and are effective for inflammation, peripheral tissue injury, menstrual pain, and painful bone metastases. Acetaminophen lacks anti-inflammatory effects.

• *Dosing.* See Table 6.3.

• *Adverse Effects.* See Table 6.4.

♦ **Opioid Analgesics.** Morphine is the gold standard against which other opioids are compared. Table 6.5 and Table 6.6 may be used as a starting point in determining dose requirements and equivalencies between various opioids. These tables, however, should be used cautiously since individual patient needs vary considerably. Before using Tables 6.5 and 6.6, the following points also should be considered:

Dose equivalencies are for single dose only. Methadone has a long half-life (24 hr); thus, dose equivalency may be different with chronic dosing. *Caution:* Possible accumulation and overdose may occur with methadone 2–3 days after starting therapy.

Dose equivalency between intramuscular and oral may be dose dependent. Morphine undergoes extensive first-pass metabolism, but its relative bioavailability and accumulation of active metabolite (morphine 6-glucuronide) may increase with larger doses or with chronic dosing.

Actual dose given must be adjusted for each patient. Doses given are average starting doses. Start with small doses in the elderly or those with chronic obstructive airways disease or small body size. Patients with severe pain may need larger doses to start. Note the relative "ceiling effect" with codeine, meperidine, and pentazocine: each increment of additional pain relief is accompanied by a larger increment of adverse effects when doses exceed the "ceiling"'(e.g., seizures from meperidine metabolites).

Tolerance occurs with chronic dosing. Much larger doses may be required in cancer patients (e.g., several hundred mg/day of morphine or equivalent). *Caution:* cross-tolerance is not complete; reduce dose by 50% when interchanging drugs.

Duration of action of meperidine is always short. Duration of methadone is the longest. Duration of morphine is dose dependent. Sustained-release morphine tablets are available for every 8–12 hr dosing. Transdermal fentanyl is administered every 72 hours.

Alternative-to-frequent parenteral injection. Continuous infusions (either intravenous or subcutaneous), patient-controlled analgesic devices, or epidural administration may be considered in patients requiring frequent intermittent parenteral injection. (See Table 6.6.)

Mixed agonist/antagonists may precipitate withdrawal if given to a patient dependent upon other opioids. (See Table 6.5.)

♦ **Combination Products.** Combination therapy of an opioid with either acetaminophen or an NSAID provides superior pain relief to either drug given alone. Claims of either superior effect or decreased side effects from different products are unfounded.

Available Combination Products. See Table 6.7.

♦ **Adverse Effects.** See Table 6.8.

♦ **Adjunctive Therapy**

Antihistamines. Hydroxyzine (Vistaril, Atarax) and promethazine (Phenergan) are used in conjunction with narcotics to decrease histamine-induced itching, decrease anxiety, prevent narcotic-induced nausea, and impart a sedative effect. Hydroxyzine, but not promethazine, also may have mild analgesic properties, but documentation of enhanced analgesia is not well supported. Usual doses of hydroxyzine are 25–50 mg Q 6–8 hr.

Antidepressants are commonly used in treatment of neuropathic pain and pain associated with insomnia or depression (see description: Neuropathic pain). It is unclear whether these drugs have intrinsic analgesic properties or if they only alter the psychological response to pain. The onset of effect may be rapid, an indication of true analgesic effect. Amitriptyline (Elavil), imipramine (Tofranil), and doxepin (Sinequan) have all been recommended. Fluoxetine (Prozac) and sertraline (Zoloft) are less sedating, but there are less data on effectiveness.

Anticonvulsants. Carbamazepine (Tegretol) and gabapentin (Neurontin) are used in the management of diabetic neuropathy, trigeminal neuralgia, and other neuropathic pain syndromes with varying degrees of success. Phenytoin probably is not effective.

Corticosteroids. Dexamethasone (Decadron) can reduce pain associated with cerebral and spinal cord edema and is also used for neuropathic and bone pain refractory to other agents. Mood elevation, antiemetic activity, and appetite stimulation are other beneficial effects.

Topical. Capsaicin (Zostrix) 0.75% for diabetic neuropathy and post-herpetic neuralgia depeletes substance P at receptor. It also causes increased burning initially. Relief takes 2–3 weeks.

Other modalities include mexiletine, transcutaneous nerve stimulators (TENS), acupuncture, hypnosis, biofeedback, local anesthetics (nerve blocks), and alcohol injections (nerve ablation).

Table 6.1 • Principles of Acute versus Chronic Nonmalignant Pain Treatment[a]

Acute Pain	Chronic Pain
Cause easy to identify (e.g., tissue damage)	Original source of pain often healed. Degree of pain often out of proportion to amount of tissue damage. Influenced by anxiety, depression, prior pain experience, social factors
Goal: ↓ suffering	Goal: functional patient. Total pain relief not always a realistic goal
High-dose, frequent PRN[a] dosing often indicated	PRN[a] dosing not acceptable; use fixed dose and time interval (e.g., sustained-release formulations)
Avoid underdosing; little risk of addiction or respiratory depression	Greater risk of tolerance and dependence, but this should not prevent aggressive pain management.
Aspirin, NSAIDS,[a] opioids all may be acceptable, depending on cause (see description of somatic and visceral pain on page 6.1)	Avoid opioids unless NSAIDs fail. Add antidepressants or anticonvulsants for neuropathic pain.
	Consider cognitive interventions (relaxation, self-hypnosis, psychotherapy); physical manipulation (heat, cold, massage, electrical nerve stimulation, physical therapy); regional anesthesia; spinal analgesia; and surgery if drug treatment fails.

[a]NSAIDs = Nonsteroidal anti-inflammatory drugs; PRN = As needed.

Notes:

Table 6.2 • Principles of Cancer Pain Management

1) A unique form of chronic pain that has elements of acute pain due to existence of a known organic cause
2) Avoid "as needed" treatment plans that ↑ anxiety by delaying onset of pain relief
3) Avoid underdosing the patient. Use the dose necessary to control pain, regardless of total amount administered
4) Continue using acetaminophen or NSAIDs in the management of chronic pain. Add narcotics to these agents. Consider all sources of acetaminophen to keep total dose <4 gm/day.
5) Psychological dependence is uncommon when narcotics are used to treat chronic pain. Not a valid reason to justify use of low doses
6) Sustained-release dosage forms or methadone on a fixed time schedule are preferred dosing for narcotics. Use rapid release preparations for breakthrough pain
7) Use dose equivalency tables to interchange analgesics. (See Table 6.5.)
8) After pain control has been stabilized, gradual dosage reduction can be attempted. If pain reappears, titrate up to optimal dose
9) Meperidine and agonist-antagonist agents (e.g., pentazocine) are undesirable. Meperidine has a short duration of action. Normeperidine, the major metabolite, lowers the seizure threshold (risk in patient with brain metastases) and accumulates in renal failure. Agonist-antagonists may precipitate withdrawal in patients receiving potent narcotics
10) In patients with renal or hepatic dysfunction, avoid analgesics with a long biological $t_{1/2}$ such as methadone or levorphanol or those which are metabolized to toxic metabolites (e.g., meperidine metabolized to normeperidine)
11) Use psychotropic drugs in patients with anxiety, depression, or insomnia
12) Give patients concurrent laxatives and stool softeners

Notes:

Table 6.3 • Nonnarcotic Analgesics[a]

Drug	Indicated for Mild Pain (Rating 1–3 on Pain Intensity Scale) Usual Starting Dose	Usual Maximum Dose (mg/day)[b]
Acetylated Salicylates[c]		
Aspirin (ASA)	650 mg Q 4–6 hr	6000
Nonacetylated Salicylates[c]		
Choline salicylate (Arthropan)	870 mg = 648 mg (ASA)	
Choline magnesium salicylate (Trilisate)	500 mg = 218 mg (ASA)	
Diflunisal (Dolobid)	50 mg Q 12 hr	
Salsalate (Disalcid)	500 mg = 648 mg (ASA)	
Nonsteroidal Anti-inflammatory Drugs (NSAIDs)[d]		
Celecoxib (Celebrex)[g]	200 mg QD or 100 mg BID	200 mg BID
Diclofenac		
Na⁺ (Voltaren)	25–50 mg Q 6–8 hr	300
K⁺ (Cataflam)	25–50 mg Q 6–8 hr	200
Etodolac (Lodine)	200–400 mg Q 6–8 hr	1200
Fenoprofen (Nalfon)	200 mg Q 4–6 hr	3200
Flurbiprofen (Ansaid)	50 mg Q 6 hr	300
Ibuprofen (Advil, Motrin, OTCs)[e]	400 mg Q 6 hr	3200
Indomethacin (Indocin)	25 mg Q 6 hr	200
Ketoprofen (Orudis)[e]	50 mg Q 6 hr	300
Ketoprofen SR (Oruvail)	200 mg QD	200
Ketorolac (Toradol)-only NSAID with parenteral dosage form	15–30 mg IM Q 6 hr 10 mg PO 4–6 hr	120 40
Meclofenamate (Meclomen)	50 mg Q 4 hr	400
Mefenamic acid (Ponstel)	250 mg Q 6 hr	1000
Nabumetone (Relafen)	500 mg QD-BID	2000
Naproxen		
(Naprosyn)	250 mg Q 8–12 hr	1250
Na⁺ (Anaprox, Alleve)[e]	275 mg Q 12 hr	1375
Oxaprozin (Daypro)	600 mg QD	1200
Piroxicam (Feldene)	20 mg QD	20
Rofecoxib (Vioxx)[g]	12.5 mg QD	50 mg QD
Sulindac (Clinoril)	150 mg Q 12 hr	400
Tolmetin (Tolectin)	400 mg Q 8 hr	1800
Other (Not Antiinflammatory)		
Acetaminophen (Tylenol)[f]	650 mg Q 4 hr	4000[f]

[a] SR = Sustained release; OTC's = Over-the-counter.

[b] These agents exhibit a "ceiling," or maximum dose, effect. Higher doses increase side effect risk without further pain reduction.

[c] Enteric-coated (EC) ASA tablets are slowly (6–8 hr) but completely absorbed; therefore, only indicated for chronic pain management with continuous dosing. EC ASA causes less gastric irritation, compared to buffered ASA. Nonacetylated salicylates cause less gastric irritation than ASA. Diflunisal is longer acting but no more effective.

[d] All NSAIDs have analgesic properties, but not all are approved for use as analgesics. All NSAIDs are equally effective. Can be used for minor trauma, dental pain, dysmenorrhea, metastatic bone pain, arthritis. Nabumetone, naproxen, oxaprozin, sulindac, and piroxicam have longer half-lives. Naproxen Na is absorbed faster than naproxen. Nabumetone and sulindac are prodrugs converted to an active metabolite.

[e] Ibuprofen available as liquid (100 mg/5 mL) and OTC (200 mg). Naproxen sodium available as liquid (125 mg/ 5 mL) and OTC (220 mg). Ketoprofen available OTC (12.5 mg).

[f] Caution: Patients often unknowingly obtain acetaminophen from multiple products. Total doses exceeding 4 gm QD, especially combined with alcohol or malnutrition, increase risk for hepatotoxicity.

[g] Celecoxib and rofecoxib are relatively Cox-2 inhibitors.

Table 6.4 • Side Effects of Nonnarcotic Drugs[a]

Side Effect	Comment
GI[a] irritation and bleeding	Most with ASA, indomethacin, and ketorolac. Less, but not absent with other NSAIDs. Least with Cox-2 inhibitors (celecoxib and rofecoxib) and possibly nabumetone. Acetaminophen = 0. Risk factors include age >60, male gender, alcohol use, smoking, corticosteroids or anticoagulant therapy, and history of gastric ulcer or bleed.
↓ platelet aggregation	Irreversible with ASA (platelet function returns to normal in 5–7 days). Reversible with other NSAIDs (1–3 days to regain normal platelet function). Acetaminophen = 0.
Na[a] retention	Renal prostaglandin inhibition. Edema, hypertension. ↓ diuretic effects. Not with acetaminophen.
Renal insufficiency	↑ risk in elderly or if volume depleted. Especially use low dose of ketorolac in these populations. May be less with sulindac or nabumetone since no active drug excreted by kidney. Can occur with acetaminophen with very large doses used chronically
Hepatotoxicity	Acetaminophen overdose (>10 gm) or chronic high dose (>4 gm). Risk factors include alcohol use and malnutrition. Rare hypersensitivity with NSAIDs (e.g., ibuprofen).
Asthma	ASA and all NSAIDs due to prostaglandin inhibition, ↑ leukotrienes in lung. Risk ↑ in patients with nasal polyps and allergy history. Not with acetaminophen.
Hyperuricemia	Low-dose ASA. Other NSAIDs used to treat acute gout
Reye's syndrome	Possibly associated with aspirin in children and teenagers with viral illnesses
Tinnitus	ASA toxicity (see Chapter 4: Managing Acute Drug Toxicity)

[a]ASA = Acetylsalicylic acid; GI = Gastrointestinal; Na = Sodium; NSAIDs = Nonsteroidal antiinflammatory drugs.

Notes:

Table 6.5 • Single Dose Equivalences of Opioids[a]

Drug	Equivalent Dose (mg) Parenteral	PO
Narcotic Agonists		
Morphine (MSIR, MS Contin, Oramorph SR)	5	30 (15) (30 rectal)
Alfentanil (Alfenta)	0.2–0.4	—
Codeine	30–60	90 (60 rectal)
Fenatyl (Sublimaze, Duragesic transdermal)	0.05–0.1	—
Hydrocodone (Lorcet, Lortab, Vicodin)	10	10–15
Hydromorphone (Dilaudid)	0.6–0.7	3–4 (3 rectal)
Levorphanol (Levo-Dromaran)	1	2
Meperidine (Demerol)	25–50	100–150
Methadone (Dolophine)	5 (1.25–2.5)	5–10 (1.25–2.5)
Oxycodone (Oxycontin, Roxicodone)	—	10–15
Sufentanil (Sufenta)	0.1–0.2	—
Mixed Agonist/Antagonists		
Buprenorphine (Buprenex)	0.2	—
Butorphanol (Stadol)	1.5	—
Dezocine (Dalgan)	25	4 (3–8)
Nalbuphine (Nubain)	10	4 (3–8)
Pentazocine (Talwin)	30	100
Other		
Propoxyphene (Darvon)	—	65–130[b]
Tramadol (Ultram)[c]	50	75–150

[a]Single-dose equivalent doses provided only as a guide; individual patient variation exists. With repeated administration, the equivalent dose may be lower (in parentheses).
[b]Propoxyphene napsylate (Darvon-N) 100–200 mg.
[c]Tramadol is a centrally acting analgesic with only weak opioid agonist properties. Also affects serotonin receptors. Only available in U.S. as 50 mg tablets. May cause sedation, dizziness, nausea, dry mouth, sweating. May cause seizures with overdose.

Table 6.6 • Recommended Starting Opioid Analgesic Doses[a,b]

Drug	Dose Based on Weight	Average Adult Dose
Phenanthrene Analogs		
Codeine		
IV	0.2–0.4 mg/kg Q 2 hr	15–30 mg Q 2 hr
IM	0.4–0.8 mg/kg Q 3 hr	30–60 mg Q 3 hr
PO	0.8–1.5 mg/kg Q 3 hr	60–120 mg Q 3 hr
PR	0.8–1.5 mg/kg Q 3 hr	60–120 mg Q 3 hr
Morphine Sulfate[d]		
IV	0.05–0.07 mg/kg Q 2 hr	3–5 mg Q 2 hr
IM	0.14–0.17 mg/kg Q 3 hr	10–12 mg Q 3 hr
PO	0.4 mg/kg Q 3 hr	30 mg Q 3 hr; 30–60 mg SR Q 8–12 hr
PR	0.4–0.6 mg/kg Q 3 hr	30–40 mg Q 3 hr
PCA		
Concentration	1.0 mg/mL	1.0 mg/mL
Basal	0–0.014 mg/kg/hr	0–1.0 mg/hr
Bolus	0.014 mg/kg/6 min	1.0 mg/6 min

(continued)

Table 6.6 • Recommended Starting Opioid Analgesic Doses[a,b] (continued)

Drug	Dose Based on Weight	Average Adult Dose
Phenanthrene Analogs (continued)		
Hydromorphone[e]		
IV	0.01–0.014 mg/kg Q 1 hr	0.75–1.0 mg Q 2 hr
IM	0.02–0.03 mg/kg Q 3 hr	1.5–2.0 mg Q 3 hr
PO	0.05–0.09 mg/kg Q 3 hr	4.0–6.0 mg Q 3 hr
PR	0.04–0.09 mg/kg Q 3 hr	3.0–6.0 mg Q 3 hr
PCA		
Concentration	0.2 mg/mL	0.2 mg/mL
Basal	0–0.003 mg/kg/hr	0–0.2 mg/hr
Bolus	0.003 mg/kg/6 min	0.2 mg/6 min
Levorphanol[c]		
IV	0.014 mg/kg Q 2 hr (Q 3 hr)	1.0 mg Q 2 hr (Q 3 hr)
IM	0.02–0.03 mg/kg Q 4 hr (Q 6 hr)	1.5–2.0 mg Q 4 hr (Q 6 hr)
PO	0.03–0.06 mg/kg Q 4 hr (Q 6 hr)	2.0–4.0 mg Q 4 hr (Q 6 hr)
Oxymorphone		
IV	0.01–0.014 mg/kg Q 2 hr	0.75–1.0 mg Q 2 hr
IM	0.014–0.02 mg/kg Q 3 hr	1.0–1.5 mg Q 3 hr
PR	0.07–0.14 mg/kg Q 3 hr	5–10 mg Q 3 hr
Phenylpiperidine Analogs		
Meperidine		
IV	0.35–0.7 mg/kg Q 2 hr	25–50 mg Q 2 hr
IM	1.0–1.4 mg/kg Q 3 hr	75–100 mg Q 3 hr
PO	1.4–2.0 mg/kg Q 3 hr	100–150 mg Q 3 hr
PCA		
Concentration	10 mg/mL	10 mg/mL
Basal	0–0.14 mg/kg/hr	0–10 mg/hr
Bolus	0.14 mg/kg/6 min	10 mg/6 min
Fentanyl[f,g]		
IV	0.5 µg/kg Q 2 hr	25–50 µg Q 2 hr
IM	1.0 µg/kg Q 3 hr	75–100 µg Q 3 hr
Transdermal		25–50 µg/hr Q 3 days
PCA		
Concentration	10 µg/mL	10 µg/mL
Basal	0–0.14 µg/kg/hr	0–10 µg/hr
Bolus	0.14 µg/kg/6 min	10 µg/6 min
Phenylheptanone Analog		
Methadone[c]		
IV	0.03 mg/kg Q 2 hr (Q 3 hr)	2.5 mg Q 2 hr (Q 3 hr)
IM	0.03–0.07 mg/kg Q 4 hr (Q 6 hr)	2.5–5.0 mg Q 4 hr (Q 6 hr)
PO	0.07–0.14 mg/kg Q 4 hr (Q 6 hr)	5–10 mg Q 4 hr (Q 6 hr)

[a]IM = Intramuscular; IV = Intravenous; PO = Oral; PCA = Patient-controlled analgesia; PR = Rectal; SC = Subcutaneous.
[b]Recommended starting dose for patients without prior opioid exposure. The actual dose must be titrated to the patient's need.
[c]The dosing interval should be ↑ with repeated dosages to avoid drug accumulation and toxicity.
[d]Oral morphine comes as solution (10 mg/2.5 mL; 10, 20, or 100 mg/5 mL). Soluble tablets (10, 15, 30 mg); rapid release tablets (15, 30 mg) and SR tablets (15, 30, 60, 100 mg). Suppositories = 5, 10, 20, 30 mg. Injectable as 0.5, 1, 2, 3, 4, 5, 8, 10, 15 mg/mL. Be careful of different morphine strengths when using for PCA pumps. Keep volume <1 mL/hr for SC PCA. Intrathecal dose = 0.2–1 mg Q 24 hr (keep volume <2 mL). Epidural dose = 2–10 mg Q 12–24 hr. Respiratory depression, facial and generalized pruritus may occur 1–3 hr after epidural dose. Rapidly reversed by continuous SC naloxone infusion without affecting analgesia.
[e]Hydromorphone injection as 1, 2, 3, 4, 10 mg/mL. High concentration for SC PCA (max: 1 mL/hr) or continuous SC infusion (max: 2 mL/hr).
[f]Fentanyl also available as lozenges (100, 200, 300, 400, 600, 800, 1200 µg) and transdermal patch (25, 50, 75, 100 µg/hr). Replace patch Q 3 days. Onset delayed 24–36 hr at initial application. Supplement with short-acting opioids as needed. Morphine 60 mg/day or 360 mg/day oral about equal to fentanyl 100 µg/hr patch. Epidural dose = 50 µg.
[g]Alfentanil (Alfenta) and Sufentanil (Sufenta) sometimes given as continuous IV infusion as anesthetic adjunct to fentanyl.

Table 6.7 • Combination Analgesic Products

Acetaminophen[a] plus	Codeine (Tylenol #3, #4)[b]
	Codeine and caffeine[c] (Anacin #3, Phenaphen #3)[b]
	Hydrocodone (Lorcet, Lortabs, Vicodin, Vicodin ES)[d]
	Oxycodone (Percocet, Tylox)[e]
	Propoxyphene napsylate (Darvocet)
Aspirin plus	Codeine (Empirin #3, #4)[b]
	Codeine, caffeine, butalbital (Fiorinal #3)[b,c]
	Dihydrocodeine and caffeine (Synalgos DC)[c]
	Hydrocodone and caffeine (Damason)[c]
	Oxycodone (Percodan)
Ibuprofen plus	Hydrocodone (Vicoprofen)[f]

[a] Caution: Although combinations of acetaminophen plus opioids are very effective, excessive use may lead to inadvertent acetaminophen toxicity and risk of hepatic or renal injury.
[b] #3, #4 designate 30 or 60 mg of codeine, respectively.
[c] Benefit from caffeine is debated. May have mild analgesic effect, but dose is generally subtherapeutic. Vasodilator properties may help migraine.
[d] Lorcet = 5/500, 7.5/650, or 10/650 (hydrocodone/acetaminophen); Lortab = 2.5/500, 5/500, or 7.5/500, 10/500; Vicodin = 5/500, ES = 7.5/500, HP = 10/660.
[e] Percocet = 5/325 (oxycodone/acetaminophen); Tylox = 5/500.
[f] Vicoprofen 7.5/200 (hydrocodone/ibuprofen).

Table 6.8 • Opioid Side Effects[a,b]

Side Effect	Comment
Nausea	Less if taken lying down
Drowsiness	Caution about driving, alcohol
Dysphoria, hallucinations	Especially pentazocine
Constipation	Frequent complaint with chronic use. Daily stool softener or laxative often necessary.
Itching	Due to histamine release; may be ↓ with antihistamines
Skin rash	True allergy. Differentiate from above. Codeine, morphine may cross-react. Meperidine, methadone different chemical structure
Respiratory depression	Rare except in overdose, including propoxyphene. Caution in COPD[b]
Miosis	Pinpoint pupils. Caution in head trauma
Biliary colic	Spasm of sphincter of Oddi
Fetal CNS[b] depression	Caution in pregnancy at delivery.
Anxiety, restlessness, tremor and seizures	Toxic meperidine, propoxyphene, and tramadol metabolites in chronic high dose, acute overdose, elderly patients, or renal impairment. Also, accumulation of morphine 6 glucuronide if renal impairment.
Tolerance	↑ dose requirements
Dependence[c] (see Table 6.9)	Withdrawal includes agitation, sweating, goosebumps, abdominal pain

[a] CNS = Central nervous system; COPD = Chronic obstructive pulmonary disease.
[b] If overdose is suspected, give naloxone (Narcan 0.2–0.4 mg IM). May need to repeat Q 60–90 min until drug is cleared from system.
[c] Withdrawal symptoms may be suppressed by clonidine in doses up to 1.2 mg/day. If using transdermal patch, supplement with clonidine tablets for first 24 hr.

Notes:

Table 6.9 • Signs and Symptoms of Physical Dependence Due to Opioid Withdrawal

Body aches	Insomnia
Diarrhea	Irritability
Loss of appetite	Runny nose
Nausea/vomiting	Sneezing
Stomach cramps	Tachycardia
Goosebumps	Uncontrolable yawning
Shivering	Weakness/fatigue
Sweating	Fever

Table 6.10 • Opioid Drug Interactions

Target Drugs	Interactions
Cytochrome P450 2D6 Substrates Codeine Hydrocodone Oxycodone Propoxyphene Tramadol	Codeine metabolized to morphine in liver during absorption. Genetic slow metabolizers (females > males) may not obtain analgesia with codeine. Inhibitors of 2D6 (e.g., amiodarone, citalopram, fluoxetine, fluvoxamine, paroxetine, ritonavir, quinidine, terbinafine) may reduce conversion to active drug. Possible serotonin syndrome with tramadol. Significance of these interaction risks needs further evaluation.
Cytochrome P450 3A4 Substrates Alfentanil Fentanyl Methadone Sufentanil	Inhibitors of 3A4 (e.g., clarithromycin, cyclosporine, delaviridine, diltiazem, erythromycin, fluvoxamine, indinavir, itraconazole, ketoconazole, nefazadone, nelfinavir, ritonavir, saquinavir, verapamil, zafirlukast) may slow metabolism and increase toxicity. Inducers of 3A4 (e.g., barbiturates, carbamazepine, efavirenz, rifabutin) may decrease analgesic response. Phenytoin reported to induce metabolism of methadone and precipitate withdrawal. Cimetidine reported to decrease methadone metabolism and induce opioid toxicity.

Notes:

Date_____
Patient's name_____Age_____Room_____
Diagnosis_____Physician_____
Evaluator_____

1. LOCATION: Patient or clinician marks drawing.

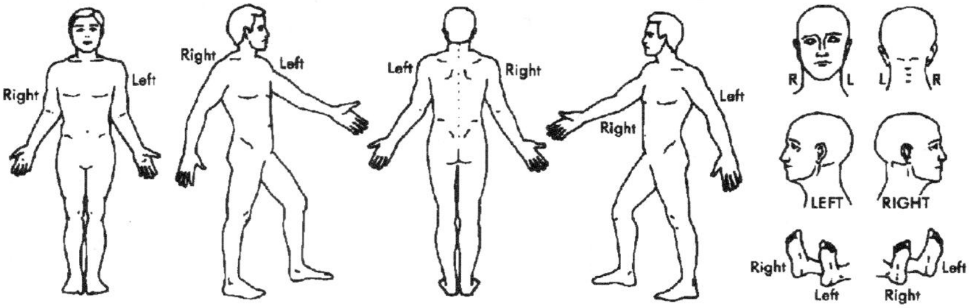

2. INTENSITY: Patient rates the pain. Scale used _____
    Present: _____
    Worst pain gets: _____
    Best pain gets: _____
    Acceptable level of pain: _____
3. QUALITY: (Use patient's own words, e.g., prick, ache, burn, throb, pull, sharp) _____

4. ONSET, DURATION, VARIATIONS, RHYTHMS: _____

5. MANNER OF EXPRESSING PAIN: _____

6. WHAT RELIEVES THE PAIN? _____

7. WHAT CAUSES OR INCREASES THE PAIN? _____

8. EFFECTS OF PAIN: (Note decreased function, decreased quality of life.)
    Accompanying symptoms (e.g., nausea) _____
    Sleep _____
    Appetite _____
    Physical activity: _____
    Relationship with others (e.g., irritability) _____
    Emotions (e.g., anger, suicidal, crying) _____
    Concentration _____
    Other _____
9. OTHER COMMENTS: _____

10. PLAN: _____

Fig. 6.1 Initial Pain Assessment Tool. (Modified from McCaffery M, Pasero C. Pain: Clinical Manual. St. Louis: Mosby, 1999:60.)

Notes:

Date: ___/___/___   Time: _____

Name: _____ _____ ___
         Last   First   MI

1) Throughout our lives, most of us have had pain from time to time (such as minor headaches, sprains, and toothaches). Have you had pain other than these everyday kinds of pain today?

   1. Yes   2. No

2) On the diagram, shade in the areas where you feel pain. Put an X on the area that hurts the most.

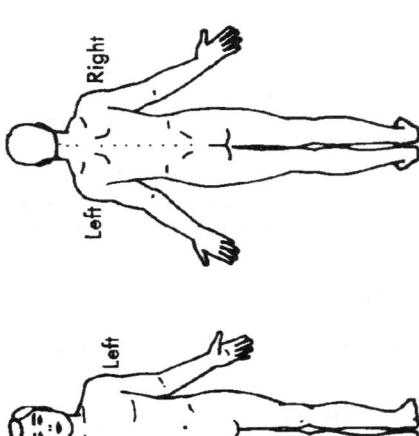

Left   Right   Right   Left

7) What treatments or medications are you receiving for your pain?

_____

8) In the past 24 hours, how much relief have pain treatments or medications provided? Please circle the one number that most shows how much relief you have received?

   0   1   2   3   4   5   6   7   8   9   10
   No   Complete
   relief   relief

9) Circle the one number that describes how, during the past 24 hours, pain has **interfered** with your:

   A. General activity

   0   1   2   3   4   5   6   7   8   9   10
   Does not   Completely
   interfere   interferes

   B. Mood

   0   1   2   3   4   5   6   7   8   9   10
   Does not   Completely
   interfere   interferes

C. Walking ability

0 1 2 3 4 5 6 7 8 9 10
Does not   Completely
interfere   interferes

D. Normal work (includes both work outside the home and housework)

0 1 2 3 4 5 6 7 8 9 10
Does not   Completely
interfere   interferes

E. Relations with other people

0 1 2 3 4 5 6 7 8 9 10
Does not   Completely
interfere   interferes

F. Sleep

0 1 2 3 4 5 6 7 8 9 10
Does not   Completely
interfere   interferes

G. Enjoyment of life

0 1 2 3 4 5 6 7 8 9 10
Does not   Completely
interfere   interferes

3) Please rate your pain by circling the one number that best describes you pain at its **worst** in the past 24 hours.

0 1 2 3 4 5 6 7 8 9 10
No   Pain as bad as
pain   you can imagine

4) Please rate your pain by circling the one number that best describes your pain at its **least** in the past 24 hours.

0 1 2 3 4 5 6 7 8 9 10
No   Pain as bad as
pain   you can imagine

5) Please rate your pain by circling the one number that best describes your pain on the **average.**

0 1 2 3 4 5 6 7 8 9 10
No   Pain as bad as
pain   you can imagine

6) Please rate your pain by circling the one number that tells how much pain you have **right now.**

0 1 2 3 4 5 6 7 8 9 10
No   Pain as bad as
pain   you can imagine

Fig. 6.2 Brief Pain Inventory (Short Form). (From Pain Research Group, Department of Neurology, University of Wisconsin-Madison.)

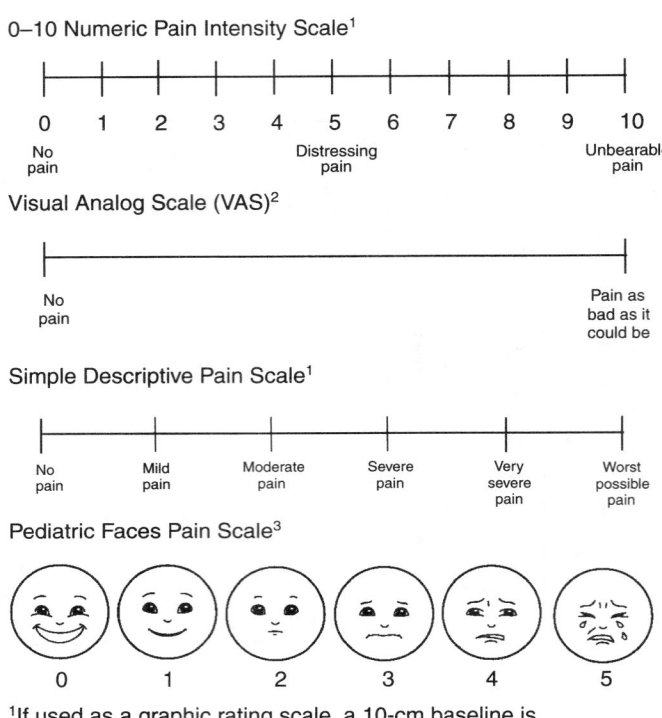

0–10 Numeric Pain Intensity Scale[1]

| 0 | 1 | 2 | 3 | 4 | 5 | 6 | 7 | 8 | 9 | 10 |

No pain   Distressing pain   Unbearable pain

Visual Analog Scale (VAS)[2]

No pain   Pain as bad as it could be

Simple Descriptive Pain Scale[1]

No pain   Mild pain   Moderate pain   Severe pain   Very severe pain   Worst possible pain

Pediatric Faces Pain Scale[3]

| 0 | 1 | 2 | 3 | 4 | 5 |

[1]If used as a graphic rating scale, a 10-cm baseline is recommended.

[2]A 10-cm baseline is recommended for VAS scales.

[3]Recommended for persons age 3 years and older. Explain to the person that each face is for a person who feels happy because he has no pain (hurt) or sad because he has some or a lot of pain. Face 0 is very happy because he/she does not hurt at all. Face 1 hurts just a little bit. Face 2 hurts a little more. Face 3 hurts even more. Face 4 hurts a whole lot. Face 5 hurts as much as you can imagine, although you don't have to be crying to feel this bad. Ask the person to choose the face that best describes how he/she is feeling.

Fig. 6.3 Pain Intensity Scales. (Adapted from Patt RB. Cancer Pain. Philadelphia: JB Lippincott, 1993; and Wong DL. Whaley and Wong's Essentials of Pediatric Nursing. St. Louis: Mosby, 1997.)

The reader is referred to Chapter 7: Pain, written by *Elaine Taylor, Pharm.D.* and *Peter J.S. Koo, Pharm.D.*, in the seventh edition of **Applied Therapeutics: The Clinical Use of Drugs** for a more in-depth discussion. Other topics included in their chapter include patient-controlled analgesia; pain management in opioid-dependent patients; obstetrical pain; spinal analgesia; topical anesthetics; and management of pain in head injury, myocardial infarction, liver disease, elderly patients, children, dysmenorrhea, and headaches. The editors of this handbook express their thanks to Drs. Taylor and Koo and acknowledge that this chapter is based upon their work.

Chapter 7

Perioperative Care

Perioperative Care covers the following three surgical periods:
- *Preoperative*
- *Intraoperative*
- *Postoperative*

These activities can occur both as inpatients and as outpatients. A variety of different medications may be given during each of these three periods.

PREOPERATIVE MEDICATIONS

Table 7.1 lists indications for giving premedicants. Patients should be individually assessed for their specific requirements considering the factors in Table 7.2. Not all patients require premedicants.

Table 7.3 lists medications commonly used preoperatively, their major indications, routes of administration, and dosages. Midazolam is the most common sedative premedicant, followed by diazepam and lorazepam for adults and ketamine and transmucosal fentanyl for children.

Aspiration Pneumonitis Prophylaxis

Regurgitation or aspiration of undigested or semidigested gastric contents into the respiratory tract can cause inflammation (chemical pneumonitis) and possible obstruction.

The primary risk factors for aspiration pneumonitis are gastric pH <2.5 to 3.5 and a gastric volume >25 to 50 mL.

Table 7.4 lists other risk factors and clinical situations that may require pneumonitis prophylaxis.

Medications to reduce pneumonitis risk (see Table 7.3 for specific drugs and doses)
- Antacids. 30 mL 15–30 minutes before anesthesia to raise gastric pH >2.5.
  - Nonparticulate formulations preferred since suspension particles act as foci for inflammation if aspirated.
  - Pros: rapid-acting and effective on fluid already in the stomach.
  - Cons: Short duration (<1 hour), incomplete mixing with stomach fluids, addition of gastric volume.
- Gastric motility stimulants. PO 60 minutes before or IV 15–30 minutes before anesthesia induction.
  - Reduce gastric volume (speed emptying) but do not affect pH.
  - Metoclopramide also antiemetic and lowers esophageal sphincter pressure.
  - Atropine or anticholinergics may offset effects on upper GI tract.
- H_2 receptor antagonists. PO 1–3 hours before or IV 30–60 minutes before anesthesia induction.
  - Pros: longer duration (4–6 hours cimetidine or ranitidine; 10–12 hours famotidine) extends through maintenance and emergence from anesthesia.

- Cons: slower onset in emergency surgery, possible aspiration of particulate matter from tablets.
- Proton pump inhibitors. No evidence for cost effectiveness over H_2 antagonists for this indication.

INTRAOPERATIVE MEDICATIONS DURING SURGERY

- *Intravenous general anesthetic induction agents* induce unconsciousness, amnesia, analgesia, muscle relaxation, immobility, and attenuation of reflexes to noxious stimuli.

  Table 7.5 lists the most common induction agents and their clinical uses besides induction. Drugs commonly used for IV induction include ultrashort-acting barbiturates (thiopental, methohexital), etomidate, propofol, and ketamine. Synthetic opioids (fentanyl, sufentanil, alfentanil) and benzodiazepines (midazolam) are less frequently used. Induction agents that do not accumulate during repeat or continuous dosing may also be used for anesthesia maintenance. Some agents may be used at lower doses for pre- or postoperative sedation and analgesia.

  Pharmacokinetics (see Table 7.6). The onset and duration of effect are the most important pharmacokinetic properties of IV anesthetic induction agents. Most have a rapid onset and short duration due to redistribution of drug from the brain to other tissues.

  Adverse effects and costs of induction agents are compared in Table 7.7. Most worrisome are cardiovascular effects (that may be exaggerated during endotracheal intubation). Etomidate and opioids have the most stable cardiovascular profile. Postoperative nausea and vomiting (PONV) and hangover may delay recovery or discharge from day surgery. CNS effects include hiccups, myoclonus, seizures, euphoria, hallucinations, and emergence delirium. Because of cost, propofol is often limited to anesthesia induction in outpatient procedures lasting <2 hours and in patients known to be sensitive to PONV. Ketamine may be advantageous in pediatrics because it can be given IM and has analgesic properties and little respiratory depression. Delirium, hallucinations, and psychiatric emergence reactions in 5–30% of cases offset this benefit.

- *Volatile inhalation agents* produce similar clinical effects as the IV drugs described above but are more useful for *anesthesia maintenance* because their effects can be titrated through the lungs via a face mask or endotracheal tube and anesthesia machine. Desflurane and sevoflurane have low blood solubility, making them ideal for ambulatory surgery or inpatients when rapid wakeup is desired (e.g., neurosurgery).

  Combinations of small doses of more than one inhalation agent plus a low-dose IV general anesthetic and a neuromuscular blocking agent are titrated to achieve a desired balance of sedation, amnesia, rapid loss of consciousness, muscle relaxation (to facilitate endotracheal intubation), and reduced side effects.

  Table 7.8 lists the pharmacologic and pharmacokinetic properties of the volatile anesthetic agents. Potency is compared by the *minimum alveolar concentration (MAC)* that prevents movement in 50% of subjects in response to a painful stimulus. The lower the agent's MAC, the greater the anesthetic potency. Factors that influence the uptake and distribution of volatile inhalation agents include the inspired concentration, solubility in blood (blood/gas partition coefficient), lung blood flow, organ distribution, tissue solubility, and tissue mass. Low-solubility agents have faster onset and more rapid CNS removal.

- *Neuromuscular blocking agents* are adjuncts to general anesthesia to facilitate endotracheal intubation and relax skeletal muscle during surgery. Also used in the ICU to paralyze mechanically ventilated patients.

The classification, cardiovascular adverse effects, pharmacokinetic/pharmacodynamic parameters, and elimination pathways of the commonly used neuromuscular blocking agents are found in Tables 7.9, 7.10, 7.11, and 7.12, respectively.
Caution: Neuromuscular blocking agents do not affect consciousness or pain threshold. An anesthetic agent, sedative, and/or analgesia must be administered simultaneously.

Succinylcholine advantages include rapid onset, ultrashort duration of action, relatively low cost, and ability to be used intramuscularly in children. Adverse effects include hyperkalemia; arrhythmias; fasciculations; muscle pain; myoglobinuria; trismus; phase II block; and increased intraocular, intragastric, and intracranial pressures.

Succinylcholine is contraindicated in patients with skeletal muscle myopathies, acute burns, multiple trauma, extensive denervation of skeletal muscle, upper motor neuron injury, or known risk for malignant hyperthermia. Rapid-onset nondepolarizing agents (rocuronium or rapacuronium) are preferred in these patients.

Cisatracurium, vecuronium, pipecuronium, and doxacurium are preferred for patients with unstable cardiovascular profiles.

Patients' renal and hepatic function must be considered when choosing a neuromuscular blocking agent (see Table 7.12). Renally eliminated agents (doxacurium, metocurine, pancuronium, pipecuronium, and tubocurarine) have prolonged duration in patients with renal failure. Metabolism may be via plasma cholinesterase (pseudocholinesterase), Hoffman elimination (a pH and temperature dependent nonbiologic process that does not require renal, hepatic, or enzymatic function), nonspecific esterases, or via hepatic enzymes.

Table 7.13 lists drugs that can potentiate or antagonize neuromuscular blocking agents.

♦ *Local Anesthetics and Regional Anesthesia.* Selective anesthesia for a specific surgical site is preferred to general (total body) anesthesia in some high-risk patients to shorten surgical duration; reduce cardiovascular or pulmonary stress; and avoid postoperative nausea, vomiting, and laryngeal irritation.

Types of regional anesthesia include:

• Epidural
• Spinal (intrathecal)
• Intravenous regional
• Peripheral nerve block
• Topical
• Local infiltration

Table 7.14 lists the currently available local anesthetics and the forms of regional anesthesia they may be used for. The physiochemical and pharmacokinetic properties of local anesthetics are found in Table 7.15. They may be given in combination with sodium bicarbonate (to increase speed of onset and reduce pain), epinephrine (to prolong duration of action and slow vascular absorption), hyaluronidase, or opioids.

CNS side effects (confusion, tremor, seizures) and cardiac toxicity (hypotension, prolonged QT interval, re-entrant arrhythmias) occur from systemic absorption of high doses or accidental IV injection. Ester-type local anesthetics (benzocaine, procaine, and tetracaine) produce allergic reactions via conversion to the metabolite para-aminobenzoic acid (PABA). True allergy to amide-type anesthetics is rare, but reactions may be due to preservatives (e.g., methylparabens) or accidental intravascular injection of an epinephrine-containing products.

Lidocaine is metabolized by cytochrome P450 (CYP) 3A4, which may be inhibited by cimetidine. Levobupivicaine is affected by CYP 3A4 and 1A2 inhibitors and inducers.

Cocaine produces intense and prolonged vasoconstriction in addition to analgesia. It is indicated only for topical anesthesia of the nose, throat, and oral cavity. Application to mucosal surfaces results in systemic absorption, with plasma levels persisting up to 6 hours and a risk of hypertension, tachycardia, myocardial infarction, and CNS stimulation. Alternatives include topical mixtures of another local anesthetic (lidocaine or tetracaine) with a vasoconstricting sympathomimetic (phenylephrine or oxymetazoline).

♦ *Cardioplegia solution* is administered via a cardiopulmonary-bypass pump into the coronary vasculature during cardiac surgery to produce an elective cardiac arrest (cardioplegia), providing the surgeon with a bloodless operative field and a flaccid heart on which to work.

Contents of cardioplegia solutions vary during the induction of arrest and maintenance of the arrest. A separate reperfusion solution is used. Cardioplegia solution prevents myocardial ischemic damage during induction and maintenance of arrest, whereas reperfusion solution minimizes reperfusion injury at the end of surgery before aortic unclamping.

The characteristics of cardioplegia solution vehicles and additives are found in Tables 7.16 and 7.17, respectively. Blood is the preferred vehicle over crystalloid because of fewer ECG changes, improved recovery rates, and better preservation of high-energy phosphates. Premixed ratios of blood to crystalloid composition range from 1:1 to 8:1, with 4:1 being the most common.

Hyperkalemic solutions induce a rapid diastolic arrest. Hyperosmolar solutions minimize myocardial edema during arrest and sodium bicarbonate counteracts ischemia-induced metabolic acidosis.

Traditionally, cardioplegia solutions have been chilled to 4 to 8°C (hypothermic) during all phases of cardioplegia to decelerate the metabolic activity of the heart, reduce ischemia, and maintain cardiac arrest. Newer techniques use intermittent normothermia (37°C) during induction and reperfusion or tepid (29°C) cardioplegia during all phases.

Investigational additives include oxygen-free radical scavengers (e.g., catalase, superoxide dismutase, and glutathione), adenosine, and L-arginine.

Postoperative Medications

♦ *Antiemetic agents for postoperative nausea and vomiting (PONV)*

Table 7.18 identifies the risk factors for PONV. Complications can include dehydration, electrolyte imbalance, pulmonary aspiration (especially if airway reflexes are blunted by anesthesia), and tension on suture lines.

Commonly used antiemetic agents, usual doses, and side effects are listed in Table 7.19. The reader is also referred to Chapter 5, Nausea and Vomiting, for further information on antiemetic drugs.

♦ Analgesic agents and postoperative pain management

One or more of the following techniques can be used to manage postoperative pain:

• Systemic administration of opioids, NSAIDs, and acetaminophen. See Chapter 6, Pain.

• Patient-controlled analgesia (PCA) (on-demand IV administration of opioids). Morphine is most commonly used, but hydromorphone is preferred in patients with renal impairment. See Table 7.20 and also Chapter 6, Pain.

• Epidural analgesia (continuous infusion or on-demand, usually with an opioid/local anesthetic mixture).

Table 7.21 lists the drugs, concentrations, and typical infusion rates for epidural administration. Bupivicaine produces analgesia without significant motor blockade or tachyphylaxis. Single doses of lipophilic opioids (fentanyl and sufentanil) have a rapid onset of action, short duration, less dermatomal spread, and greater systemic absorption. However, after continued infusion, fentanyl's dermatomal (regional) specificity is lost, and analgesia is achieved via systemic blood levels. Morphine (relatively hydrophilic) has a slower-onset, longer duration of effect, more dermatomal spread and migration to the brain, and less systemic absorption. It retains a spinal mechanism with continued infusion. Hydromorphone acts in a manner similar to that of morphine. Meperidine has significant systemic absorption. See Table 7.22 for pharmacokinetic comparisons of the epidural opioid analgesics.

Adverse effects: Pruritus is more common with epidural infusion than by IV administration. Also monitor for nausea, vomiting, sedation, confusion, constipation, ileus, urinary retention, and respiratory retention. Local anesthetics are associated with hypotension, urinary retention, lower limb paresthesias and numbness, and lower limb motor block. Epidural and spinal hematoma may occur in anticoagulated patients.

- Local nerve block
- Cognitive-behavioral interventions (e.g., relaxation, imagery)
- Massage or application of heat or cold
- Transcutaneous electrical nerve stimulation

Table 7.1 • Indications for Preoperative Medications

Relieve fear and anxiety

Produce sedation

Provide analgesia

Produce amnesia

Facilitate smooth anesthetic induction

Reduce anesthetic requirements

Prevent autonomic responses/reduce hemodynamic instability during surgery

Decrease salivation and secretions

Reduce risk factors for aspiration pneumonia (reduce gastric fluid volume/raise gastric pH)

Prevent or minimize allergic reactions.

Table 7.2 • Assessing Patient Need for Premedications

Preexisting medical conditions and overall health status that may affect risk of complications or predict likelihood of survival.
- Diabetes
- Coronary artery disease

Age
- Elderly more sensitive to opioids, CNS depressants, anticholinergics

Degree of anxiety

Duration and type of surgery.
- Inpatient or outpatient. Avoid long-acting sedatives or anesthetics for short-duration outpatient surgery.

Drug allergies

Previous experience with drugs

Concurrent drug therapy.
- Possible drug interactions or additive responses

Table 7.3 • Indications, Routes of Administration, and Doses of Preoperative Agents [a,b]

Agent	Indications	Routes of Administration	Doses [c]
Benzodiazepines			
Diazepam (Valium)	Anxiolysis, amnesia, sedation	PO IV PR	*Adults:* 5–20 mg; *pediatrics:* 0.1–0.5 mg/kg *Adults:* 2–20 mg (titrate dose); *pediatrics:* 0.1–0.2 mg/kg *Pediatrics:* 0.1–0.75 mg/kg (max, 20 mg)
Lorazepam (Ativan)	Anxiolysis, amnesia, sedation	PO IV	0.025–0.05 mg/kg (range, 1–4 mg for adults) *Adults:* 0.025–0.04 mg/kg; *pediatrics:* 0.03–0.05 mg/kg
Midazolam (Versed)	Anxiolysis, amnesia, sedation	PO IM IV PR IN SL	*Adults:* 15 mg; *pediatrics:* 0.25–1 mg/kg (max, 20 mg) *Adults:* 0.05–0.1 mg/kg; *pediatrics:* 0.08–0.3 mg/kg *Adults:* 1–2.5 mg (titrate dose); *pediatrics:* 0.1–0.15 mg/kg (titrate dose) *Pediatrics:* 0.3–1 mg/kg *Pediatrics:* 0.2–0.3 mg/kg *Pediatrics:* 0.2–0.4 mg/kg
Opioids			
Morphine	Analgesia, sedation	IM IV	*Adults:* 5–10 mg; *pediatrics:* 0.1–0.2 mg/kg Titrate dose
Meperidine (Demerol)	Analgesia, sedation	IM IV	*Adults:* 50–150 mg; *pediatrics:* 1–2 mg/kg Titrate dose
Fentanyl (Sublimaze)	Analgesia, sedation	IV OTM[d]	*Adults:* 1–2 μg/kg (titrate dose) *Adults:* 5 μg/kg (max, 400 μg); 2.5–5 μg/kg (>65 years old; max, 400 μg); *pediatrics:* 5–15 μg/kg (max, 400 μg)
Anticholinergics			
Atropine (A)	Antisialagogue (S > G > A), sedation (S > A)	PO IM/IV	*Pediatrics:* 0.02 mg/kg *Adults:* 0.3–1 mg; *pediatrics:* 0.02 mg/kg IM, 0.01 mg/kg IV
Scopolamine (S)	Sedation, amnesia, antisialagogue	IM/IV	*Adults:* 0.2–0.3 mg; *pediatrics:* 0.02 mg/kg IM, 0.01 mg/kg IV
Glycopyrrolate (G) (Robinul)	Antisialagogue	IM/IV	*Adults:* 0.1–0.3 mg; *pediatrics:* 0.01 mg/kg

Drug	Action	Route	Dosages
Dissociative Anesthetics			
Ketamine (Ketalar)[e]	Sedation, amnesia, analgesia	PO	*Pediatrics: 6 mg/kg*
		IM	*Adults: 2–5 mg/kg; pediatrics: 2–5 mg/kg*
		IV	*Adults: 0.5–1 mg/kg*
		PR	*Pediatrics: 3 mg/kg*
		IN	*Pediatrics: 3 mg/kg*
Gastric Motility Stimulants			
Metoclopramide (Reglan)	Reduce gastric volume, antiemetic	PO	*Adults: 10 mg; pediatrics: 0.1 mg/kg*
		IV	*Adults: 0.1–0.2 mg/kg (10–20 mg); pediatrics: 0.1 mg/kg*
H$_2$-Receptor Antagonists			
Cimetidine (Tagamet)	↑ gastric pH	PO	*Adults: 300 mg; pediatrics: 7.5 mg/kg*
		IV	*Adults: 300 mg; pediatrics: 7.5 mg/kg*
Ranitidine (Zantac)	↑ gastric pH	PO	*Adults: 150 mg; pediatrics: 2 mg/kg*
		IV	*Adults: 50 mg; pediatrics: 0.5–1 mg/kg*
Famotidine (Pepcid)	↑ gastric pH	PO	*Adults: 40 mg; pediatrics: 0.5–0.6 mg/kg*
		IV	*Adults: 20 mg; pediatrics: 0.3–0.4 mg/kg*
Nizatidine (Axid)	↑ gastric pH	PO	*Adults: 150 mg*
Nonparticulate Antacids			
Sodium citrate (Citra pH)	↑ gastric pH	PO	*Adults: 30 mL*
Sodium citrate/citric acid (Bicitra)	↑ gastric pH	PO	*Adults: 30 mL*
Sodium bicarbonate/citric acid/ potassium bicarbonate (Alka-Seltzer Gold)	↑ gastric pH	PO	*Adults: 2 tabs dissolved in minimal fluid*
α$_2$-Agonists			
Clonidine (Catapres)	Anxiolysis, potentiate action of anesthetic agents, sedation, analgesia	PO	*Adults: 0.005 mg/kg*

[a] IM = Intramuscular; IN = Intranasal; IV = Intravenous; OTM = Oral transmucosal; PO = Oral; PR = Rectal; SL = Sublingual.
[b] General dosage guidelines; doses must be individualized based on patient-specific parameters.
[c] Doses listed are for agents when used as sole premedicant; doses may need to be reduced if premedicants are administered in combination (e.g., opioids, benzodiazepines).
[d] Risk of hypoventilation with its use; anesthesia care provider should be present and resuscitative/suction equipment available, indicated when an opioid analgesic effect beyond sedation is indicated.
[e] The duration and depth of sedation from ketamine is determined by the dose and route of administration. Low dosages (0.025 to 0.075 mg/kg IV or 2 to 3 mg/kg IM) should produce light sedation for a short period of time. Higher dosages will produce deep sedation to the point of general anesthesia. In addition, airway reflexes are depressed, increasing the patient's risk for aspiration. An anesthesia care provider should be present and resuscitative/suction equipment should be readily available.

Table 7.4 • Risk Factors for Aspiration Pneumonitis

Nonfasted patients having emergency surgery (e.g., trauma)
• Use nonparticulate antacids (see Table 7.3)

Abnormal airways (e.g., intubated, history of COPD)

Increased abdominal pressure (e.g., obesity or pregnancy)

Incompetent lower esophageal sphincter
• Hiatal hernia
• Gastroesophageal reflux disease (GERD)
• Older age
• Medication-induced (anticholinergics, benzodiazepines, calcium channel blockers, halothane, opioids, thiopental

Delayed gastric emptying
• History of diabetes (diabetic gastroparesis)
• Obesity
• Opioids
• Peptic ulcer disease or hyperchlorhydria
• Pregnancy (hormonal changes)
• Pain or stress

History of previous upper GI surgery

Table 7.5 • Common Clinical Uses of Intravenous Anesthetic Agents[a]

Etomidate (Amidate)
IV induction

Ketamine (Ketalar)
Analgesia
Sedation
IV induction
IM induction

Methohexital (Brevital)
IV induction
PR induction
Sedation

Midazolam (Versed)
Anxiolysis
Amnesia
Sedation

Propofol (Diprivan)
Sedation
IV induction
Maintenance of general anesthesia

Thiopental
IV induction
PR induction

[a]IM = Intramuscular; IV = Intravenous; PR = Rectal.

Table 7.6 • Pharmacokinetic Comparison of Common Intravenous Anesthetic Agents

Drug	Half-Life (hr)	Onset (sec)	Clinical Duration (min)[a]	Hangover Effect[b]
Etomidate (Amidate)	2–5	≤30	3–12	+
Ketamine (Ketalar)	1–3	30–40	10–15	++ – +++
Methohexital (Brevital)	4	≤30	4–8	+
Midazolam (Versed)	1–4	30–60	17–20	+++[c]
Propofol (Diprivan)	0.5–7	≤30	4–10	0–+
Thiopental (Pentothal)	11	≤30	5–8	++

[a]Time from injection of agent to return to conscious state.
[b]Residual psychomotor impairment after awakening.
[c]When midazolam is administered as the induction agent (e.g., 0.15 mg/kg).

Table 7.7 • Adverse Effects and Costs of IV Induction Agents[a]

Adverse Effect	Etomidate (Amidate)	Ketamine (Ketalar)	Methohexital (Brevital)	Midazolam (Versed)	Propofol (Diprivan)	Thiopental (Pentothal)
Adreno-corticoid suppression	+[b]	−	−	−	−	−
Cerebral protection	+	−	+	+	+	+
Cardiovascular depression	−	−	++	+	++	++
Emergence delirium or euphoria	−	++	−	−	+	−
Myoclonus	+++	+	++	−	+	+
Nausea/ vomiting	+++	++	++	+	−	++
Pain on injection	++	−	+	−	++	+
Respiratory depression	++	−	++	+/++	++	++
Relative cost	++++	++	++	+++++	+++	+

[a]+ to +++++ = likelihood of adverse effect relative to other agents (or increasing cost for cost comparison); − = no effect; IV = intravenous.
[b]Not shown to be clinically significant in single dose.

Table 7.8 • Pharmacologic and Pharmacokinetic Properties of the Volatile Inhalation Agents

Property/Effect	Desflurane	Sevoflurane	Isoflurane	Halothane	Enflurane
MAC in O_2 (adults)	6.0	1.71	1.15	0.77	1.7
Blood/gas partition coefficient[a]	0.42	0.69	1.46	2.54	1.91
Brain:blood partition coefficient[b]	1.29	1.7	1.6	1.9	1.4
Muscle:blood partition coefficient[c]	2.02	3.13	2.9	3.4	1.7
Fat:blood partition coefficient[d]	27.2	47.5	45	51	36
Metabolism	0.02%	3%	0.2%	15–20%	2%
Molecular weight (g)	168	201	184.5	197.4	184.5
Liquid density[e]	1.45	1.505	1.496	1.87	1.517

MAC = Minimum alveolar concentration to prevent movement in 50% of subjects.
[a]The greater the blood:gas partition coefficient, the greater the blood solubility.
[b]The greater the brain:blood partition coefficient, the greater the brain solubility.
[c]The greater the muscle:blood partition coefficient, the greater the muscle solubility.
[d]The greater the fat:blood partition coefficient, the greater the fat solubility.
[e]Density determined at 25°C for desflurane, isoflurane, and enflurane and at 20°C for sevoflurane and halothane.

Table 7.9 • Classification of Neuromuscular Blocking Agents

Agent	Type of Block[a]	Clinical Duration of Action[b]	Structure
Atracurium (Tracrium)	−	Intermediate	Benzylisoquinolinium
Cisatracurium (Nimbex)	−	Intermediate	Benzylisoquinolinium
Doxacurium (Nuromax)	−	Long	Benzylisoquinolinium
Metocurine (Metubine)	−	Long	Benzylisoquinolinium
Mivacurium (Mivacron)	−	Short	Benzylisoquinolinium
Pancuronium (Pavulon)	−	Long	Steroidal
Pipecuronium (Arduan)	−	Long	Steroidal
Rapacuronium (Raplon)	−	Short[c]	Steroidal
Rocuronium (Zemuron)	−	Intermediate	Steroidal
Succinylcholine (Anectine, Quelicin)	+	Ultrashort	Acetylcholine-like
Tubocurarine	−	Long	Benzylisoquinolinium
Vecuronium (Norcuron)	−	Intermediate	Steroidal

[a]+ = depolarizing; − = nondepolarizing.
[b]Time from injection of agent to return to twitch height to 25% of control (time at which another dose of agent will need to be administered to maintain paralysis); in general, clinical duration of a standard intubating dose of ultrashort agents ranges from 3 to 5 minutes, short agents from 15 to 30 minutes, intermediate agents from 30 to 40 minutes, and long agents from 60 to 120 minutes.
[c]From a single intubation dose.

Table 7.10 • Causes of Cardiovascular Adverse Effects of Neuromuscular Blocking Agents[a]

Agent	Histamine Release[b]	Autonomic Ganglia	Vagolytic Activity	Sympathetic Stimulation
Atracurium[b] (Tracrium)	+	−	−	−
Cisatracurium (Nimbex)	−	−	−	−
Doxacurium (Nuromax)	−	−	−	−
Metocurine (Metubine)	++	Weak block	−	−
Mivacurium (Mivacron)	+	−	−	−
Pancuronium (Pavulon)	−	−	++	+
Pipecuronium (Arduan)	−	−	−	−
Rapacuronium (Raplon)	+	−	+	−
Rocuronium[c] (Zemuron)	−	−	−/+	−
Succinylcholine (Anectine, Quelicin)	+	Stimulates	−	−
Tubocurarine	+++	Blocks	−	−
Vecuronium (Norcuron)	−	−	−	−

[a]+ − +++ = Likelihood of developing the cardiovascular adverse effect relative to the other agents; − = No effect.
[b]Histamine release is dose and rate related; cardiovascular changes can be lessened by minimizing dose and injecting agent slowly.
[c]Produces an increase in heart rate of approximately 18% with intubating dose of 0.6 mg/kg; effect usually transient and resolves spontaneously.

Notes:

Table 7.11 • Pharmacokinetic and Pharmacodynamic Parameters of Action of Neuromuscular Blocking Agents[a]

Agent	Cl (mL/kg/min)	Vd$_{ss}$ (L/kg)	Half-Life (min)	ED95 (mg/kg)	Initial Dose[b,c] (mg/kg)	Onset (min)	Clinical Duration of Action of Initial Dose (min)
Atracurium[d] (Tracrium)	5–7	0.2	20	0.2	0.4–0.5	2–3	20–45
Cisatracurium (Nimbex)	4.6	0.15	22	0.05	0.15–0.2	1.5–3	40–75
Doxacurium (Nuromax)	1–2.5	0.2	100–120	0.025	0.05–0.08	4–6	100–160
Metocurine (Metubine)	1–2	0.4	80–120	0.28	0.2–0.5	3–5	60–100
Mivacurium[c] (Mivacron)	50–100[e]	0.2	2[e]	0.07	0.15–0.25	1.5–3	12–20
Pancuronium (Pavulon)	1–2	0.3	80–120	0.07	0.04–0.1	3–5	60–100
Pipecuronium (Arduan)	2.4	0.3	80–120	0.05	0.07–0.085	3–5	60–120
Rapacuronium (Raplon)	6.6	0.3	141	1.15[f]	1.5	1–1.5	12–17
Rocuronium[d] (Zemuron)	4.0	0.3	60–70	0.25–0.3	0.5–1.0	1–1.5	20–40
Succinylcholine[d] (Anectine, Quelicin)	Unknown	Unknown	Unknown	0.2	1.0–1.5	0.5–1	4–6
Tubocurarine	1–2	0.3–0.6	80–120	0.5	0.5–0.6	3–5	60–90
Vecuronium[d] (Norcuron)	4.5	0.4	50–70	0.05	0.08–0.1	2–3	20–35

[a] Cl = Clearance; ED95 = Effective dose causing 95% muscle paralysis; Vd$_{ss}$ = Steady-state volume of distribution.
[b] Dose when nitrous oxide-opioid technique is used.
[c] Intermittent maintenance doses to maintain paralysis, as a general rule, will be approximately 20 to 25% of the initial dose.
[d] Also can be administered as a continuous infusion to maintain paralysis; suggested infusion ranges under balanced anesthesia are as follows: atracurium, 4 to 12 μg/kg per minute; cisatracurium, 1 to 2 μg/kg per minute; mivacurium, 3 to 12 μg/kg per minute (higher in children); rocuronium, 6 to 14 μg/kg per minute; succinylcholine, 50 to 100 μg/kg per minute; vecuronium, 0.8 to 2 μg/kg per minute.
[e] Values reflect contribution of trans-trans and cis-trans isomers only.
[f] Value represents ED90.

Table 7.12 • Elimination of Neuromuscular Blocking Agents

Agent	Renal	Hepatic	Biliary	Plasma
Atracurium (Tracrium)	<5%	—	—	Hofmann elimination, ester hydrolysis
Cisatracurium (Nimbex)	16%	—	7%	Hofmann elimination
Doxacurium (Nuromax)	60–90%	—	Yes	—
Metocurine (Metubine)	80–100%	—	<2%	—
Mivacurium (Mivacron)	<10%	—	Minor	Plasma cholinesterase
Pancuronium (Pavulon)	60–80%	15–40%	5–10%	—
Pipecuronium (Arduan)	60–90%	—	20–25%	—
Rapacuronium (Raplon)	10–20%	Yes	28%	—
Rocuronium (Zemuron)	Up to 30%	Yes	Yes	—
Succinylcholine (Anectine, Quelicin)	—	—	—	Plasma cholinesterase
Tubocurarine	40–60%	<1%	10–20%	—
Vecuronium (Norcuron)	20–30%	20–30%	30–50%	—

Table 7.13 • Drugs That Potentiate and Antagonize Neuromuscular Blocking Agents

Potentiate
- Aminoglycosides
- Amphotericin B
- Clindamycin
- Dantrolene
- Furosemide
- Lidocaine
- Magnesium
- Quinidine

Antagonize
- Adrenocorticosteroids (chronic administration)
- Carbamazepine
- Phenytoin
- Theophylline

Notes:

Table 7.14 • Clinical Uses of Local Anesthetic Agents

Agent	Primary Clinical Use
Esters	
Chloroprocaine (Nesacaine)	Local infiltration, nerve block, epidural
Cocaine	Topical
Procaine (Novocain)	Local infiltration, nerve block, spinal
Tetracaine (Pontocaine)	Topical, spinal
Amides	
Bupivacaine (Marcaine, Sensorcaine)	Local infiltration, nerve block, epidural, spinal
Etidocaine (Duranest)	Local infiltration, nerve block, epidural
Levobupivacaine (Chirocaine)	Nerve block, epidural
Lidocaine (Xylocaine)	Local infiltration, nerve block, spinal, epidural, topical, IV regional
Mepivacaine (Carbocaine, Polocaine)	Local infiltration, nerve block, epidural
Ropivacaine (Naropin)	Local infiltration, nerve block, epidural

IV = Intravenous.

Notes:

Table 7.15 • Physicochemical and Pharmacokinetic Properties of Local Anesthetic Agents

Agent	pK$_a$	Partition Coefficient[a]	% Protein Binding	Onset	Duration[b]	Maximum Recommended Dose[c] Plain (mg)	With Epi (mg)
Esters							
Cocaine[d]	—	—	—	—	—	100–200	—
Chloroprocaine (Nesacaine)	9.1	720	—	Fast	Short	600–800	1,000
Procaine (Novocain)	8.9	81	6	Fast	Short	400–500	600
Tetracaine (Pontocaine)	8.4	3,615	76	Slow	Long	100 (topical)	—
Amides							
Bupivacaine (Marcaine, Sensorcaine)	8.1	1,565[e]	95	Moderate	Long	175	225
Etidocaine (Duranest)	7.9	4,900	94	Fast	Long	300	—
Levobupivacaine (Chirocaine)	8.1	1,624[e]	>97	Moderate	Long	—	—
Lidocaine (Xylocaine)	7.8	30	70	Fast	Moderate	300	7 mg/kg
Mepivacaine (Carbocaine, Polocaine)	7.7	90	77	Moderate	Moderate	300	500
Ropivacaine (Naropin)	8.1	775	94	Moderate	Long	200	500

EPI = Epinephrine.
[a] Octanol/buffer partition coefficient (25°C).
[b] Depends on injection site, dose, addition of epinephrine, and so on. In general, a short duration is <1 hour, a moderate duration is 1 to 3 hours, and a long duration of action is 3 to 12 hours when the local anesthetic is administered without epinephrine.
[c] Maximum recommended single dose for infiltration or peripheral nerve block in 70-kg adults.
[d] Topical use only; concentrations >4% are not recommended due to increased risk for systemic adverse effects.
[e] Oleyl alcohol/water partition coefficient.

Table 7.16 • Advantages and Disadvantages of Cardioplegia Solution Vehicles[a]

Vehicle	Advantages	Disadvantages
Blood	Oxygen-carrying capacity Active resuscitation Reduction in systemic hemodilution Avoidance of reperfusion damage Provision of inherent buffering, oncotic, and rheologic effects Provision of physiologic calcium concentration Presence of endogenous oxygen-free radical scavengers	Possible sludging at low temperatures Possible unfavorable shift in oxyhemoglobin association curve Potential for poor distribution of solution beyond coronary stenoses Possible RBC crenation
Crystalloid	History of effectiveness Ease of solution preparation Low cost Minimal potential for capillary obstruction	Minimal oxygen-carrying capacity Possible damage of coronary endothelium Reduced efficacy (compared with blood) in preserving left ventricular function postoperatively Systemic hemodilution Possible role in production of late myocardial fibrosis

[a]RBC = Red blood cell.

Notes:

Table 7.17 • Commonly Used Cardioplegia Solution Additives

Additive	Frequently Used Concentration[b]	Function
Amino acid substrates (glutamate/aspartate[c])	11–12 mL/L[d]	Improves myocardial metabolism; improves metabolic and functional recovery in energy-depleted hearts
Calcium	At least trace amounts (0.1 mEq/L)	Maintains integrity of myocardial cell membrane; prevents "calcium paradox"[e]
Chloride	90–110 mEq/L	Establishes a solution similar in composition to extracellular fluid
CPD solution[a]	12 mL/L[f] 45 mL/L[d]	Chelates calcium in blood-based cardioplegia solution to produce safe levels of hypocalcemia for rapid diastolic arrest; limits postischemic calcium accumulation and improves postischemic performance
Glucose	5–10 g/L safely used	Helps achieve desired osmolarity of solution; serves as a metabolic substrate for the heart
Magnesium	32 mEq/L	Reduces magnesium loss during ischemia; reduces calcium influx and potassium efflux during ischemia; has a weak arresting action on heart
Potassium	15–30 mEq/L[g]	Induces rapid diastolic arrest
Sodium	120–140 mEq/L	Necessary for protective action of potassium; establishes a solution similar in composition to extracellular fluid
Sodium bicarbonate or THAM[a]	Variable; added until desired pH is obtained	Provides buffering capacity; helps maintain physiologically normal pH range; counters acidosis produced by ischemia

[a] CPD = Citrate-phosphate-dextrose; THAM = Trihydroxymethylaminomethane.
[b] Concentration delivered to patient; concentration dependent on other cardioplegia solution additives (concentration of any one additive may be changed by inclusion of other additives).
[c] Not commercially available in parenteral formulation; each mL of solution contains 178.4 mg monosodium L-glutamate and 163.4 mg monosodium L-aspartate (for preparation directions, see reference 184).
[d] Warm, blood-based induction and reperfusion solutions.
[e] Calcium paradox is a condition that results in rapid consumption of high-energy phosphates, extensive ultrastructural damage of myocardial cells, and myocardial contracture; it results from an influx of calcium into the myocardial cells, resulting from the introduction of a calcium-containing perfusate (i.e., blood) into the system during reperfusion after the use of a cardioplegia solution completely lacking in calcium.
[f] Cold, blood-based induction and maintenance solutions.
[g] Lower concentrations (5 to 10 mEq/L) used during maintenance phase.

Notes:

Table 7.18 • Risk Factors for Developing Postoperative Nausea and Vomiting

Patient	Procedure Type	Anesthesia and Analgesia	Postoperative
• Female gender • History of motion sickness • History of PONV[a] • *Nonsmoker* • *Younger age (<50 years old)* • *Anxiety*	• ENT,[a] *strabismus,*[b] or dental surgery • Breast surgery[c] • Gynecologic surgery[c] • Orthopedic surgery, especially shoulder[d] • Plastic surgery, especially breast augmentation[c] • Laparoscopic surgery • Thyroid surgery • Long duration of surgery[e]	• General anesthesia • Intraoperative use of opioids, especially higher dosages • Use of inhalation anesthetic agents • Long duration of anesthesia[e]	• Pain • Ambulation or movement • Administration of opioids, especially higher dosages

[a]ENT = Ear, nose, and throat; PONV = Postoperative nausea and vomiting.
[b]Incidence most likely depends on the age of the patient, with a higher incidence in children than in adults.
[c]The high incidence of PONV found in most studies is most likely because the studies were performed in patients at high risk for PONV (e.g., young female patients undergoing general anesthesia with inhalation anesthetic agents) rather than due to the surgical procedure itself.
[d]The high incidence of PONV after shoulder surgery may be due to postoperative pain and administration of opioids.
[e]60 to 180 minutes; the risk of PONV does not further increase with surgical duration >180 minutes.

Table 7.19 • Classification, Proposed Site(s) of Action, Usual Dose, and Adverse Effects of Select Antiemetic Drugs[a]

Antiemetic Drug	Proposed Site(s) of Action	Usual Adult Dose	Adverse Effects
Butyrophenones Droperidol (Inapsine)	Blocks dopaminergic stimulation of the CTZ	0.625–1.25 mg IV[b]	Sedation, hypotension, tachycardia, restlessness, EP reactions[c]
Serotonin Antagonists Dolasetron (Anzemet)	Blocks 5HT3 receptors of vagal afferent nerves in the GI tract and the CTZ	12.5 mg IV[b]	Headache, dizziness, mild drowsiness, transient elevation of liver enzymes, rare cases of ECG alterations
Ondansetron (Zofran)	Blocks 5HT3 receptors of vagal afferent nerves in the GI tract and the CTZ	4 mg IV[b]	Headache, dizziness, mild drowsiness, transient elevation of liver enzymes, rare cases of ECG alterations
Benzamides Metoclopramide (Reglan)	Blocks dopaminergic, serotonin, and some H_1-receptors in the CTZ; increases lower esophageal sphincter tone and enhances gastric emptying and small bowel motility	0.1–0.2 mg/kg (10–20 mg) IV or IM Q 4–6 hr	Sedation, restlessness, diarrhea, agitation, anxiety, fatigue, EP reactions[c,d]

(continued)

Table 7.19 • Classification, Proposed Site(s) of Action, Usual Dose, and Adverse Effects of Select Antiemetic Drugs^a (continued)

Antiemetic Drug	Proposed Site(s) of Action	Usual Adult Dose	Adverse Effects
Phenothiazines Prochlorperazine (Compazine)	Blocks dopaminergic receptors in the CTZ	5–10 mg PO, IM, or IV Q 3–4 hr (maximum of 40 mg/24 hr); 25 mg PR BID	Sedation, restlessness, skin sensitization, hypersensitivity reactions, hypotension (with IV use), EP reactions^c; lowers seizure threshold
Antimuscarinics Dimenhydrinate (Dramamine)	Blocks acetylcholine receptors in the vestibular apparatus	50–100 mg PO, IM, or IV Q 4–6 hr (maximum of 400 mg/24 hr)	Sedation, dry mouth, blurred vision, urinary retention, confusion
Promethazine (Phenergan)	Competes with histamine for H_1-receptor and blocks dopaminergic receptors in the CTZ; has affinity for muscarinic cholinergic receptors in the VC and CTZ	12.5–25 mg PO, IV, or IM, or PR Q 4 hr	Sedation, lethargy, skin sensitization, hypersensitivity reactions, hypotension (with IV use), EP reactions^c

^{a}5HT3 = Serotonin type 3 receptor; CTZ = Chemoreceptor trigger zone; ECG = Electrocardiogram; EP = Extrapyramidal; GI = Gastrointestinal; H_1 = Histamine type 1; VC = Vomiting center.
^{b}Single dose only for prevention or treatment of postoperative nausea and vomiting.
^{c}EP reactions may be more common than expected, with elderly patients (droperidol, prochlorperazine), young adults (<30 years old) (metoclopramide, prochlorperazine), and children (prochlorperazine) at the greatest risk. The most common EP reaction is akathisia (motor restlessness).
^{d}When metoclopramide is administered to patients taking a selective serotonin reuptake inhibitor, the risk of EP reaction may be increased.

Table 7.20 • Adult Analgesic Dosing Recommendations for IV Patient-Controlled Analgesia^{a,b}

Drug	Usual Concentration	Demand Dose (mg)		Lock-Out Interval (min)	4-Hour Limit (mg)
		Usual	Range		
Fentanyl (as citrate) (Sublimaze)	10 µg/mL	0.01–0.015	0.01–0.05	5–10	0.2–0.4
Hydromorphone HCl (Dilaudid)	0.2 mg/mL	0.1–0.2	0.05–0.5	5–15	4–6
Meperidine HCl (Demerol)	10 mg/mL	10–20	5–30	5–15	200–300^c
Morphine Sulfate	1 mg/mL	1–1.5	0.5–2.5	5–15	20–30

^{a}HCL = Hydrochloride; IV = Intravenous.
^{b}Analgesic doses are based on those required by a healthy 55- to 70-kg, opioid-naive adult. Analgesic requirements vary widely between patients. Doses may need to be adjusted because of age, condition of the patient, and prior opioid use.
^{c}Limit of 600 mg/24 hours and duration of 48 hours.

Notes:

Table 7.21 • Adult Analgesic Dosing Recommendations for Epidural Infusion[a]

Agent[b]	Bolus Dose	Infusion Concentration	Infusion Rate	Demand Dose	Lock-Out Interval (min)
Bupivacaine HCl (Sensorcaine, Marcaine)	Not applicable	0.625–1.25 mg/mL	2–20 mg/hr	0.625–2 mg	10–30
Fentanyl (as citrate) (Sublimaze)	100 μg	3–10 μg/mL	20–100 μg/hr	10–20 μg	10–15
Hydromorphone HCl (Dilaudid)	1–1.5 mg	0.05–0.075 mg/mL	0.04–0.4 mg/hr	0.15 mg	30
Meperidine HCl (Demerol)	30–100 mg	1–2 mg/mL	5–20 mg/hr	10–20 mg	12–20
Morphine sulfate	5 mg	0.05–0.1 mg/mL	0.1–0.3 mg/hr	0.5–1 mg	20–30
Sufentanil (as citrate) (Sufenta)	10–50 μg	1 μg/mL	5–10 μg/hr	5 μg	10

[a]HCl = Hydrochloride.
[b]Usually administered in combination (e.g., bupivacaine with an opioid). In general, lower concentrations of bupivacaine (e.g., 0.0625%) are administered in thoracic epidurals and lower concentrations of fentanyl (e.g., 3 μg/mL) and possibly, bupivacaine, are administered to elderly patients. Bolus and demand doses, as well as infusion rates, should be reduced in elderly patients, and patients with severe underlying systemic disease or pre-existing respiratory or cardiovascular compromise.

Table 7.22 • Pharamacokinetic Comparison of Common Epidural Opioid Analgesics

Agent	Partition Coefficient[a]	Onset of Action of Bolus (min)	Duration of Action of Bolus (hr)	Dermatomal Spread
Fentanyl (Sublimaze)	813	5	3–6	Narrow
Hydromorphone (Dilaudid)	1.4	15	6–17	Intermediate–wide
Meperidine (Demerol)	39	5–10	4–6	Intermediate
Morphine Sulfate	1.4	30	12–24	Wide
Sufentanil (Sufenta)	1,778	5	4–7	Narrow

[a]Octanol pH buffer.

Notes:

The reader is referred to Chapter 8: Perioperative Care, written by *Andrew J. Donnelly, Pharm.D., M.B.A.,* and *Julie Golembiewski, Pharm.D.,* in the seventh edition of **Applied Therapeutics: The Clinical Use of Drugs.** Other topics included in their chapter include drug interactions with perioperative drugs (especially opioids and general anesthetics) and effects of herbal medicines on perioperative procedures. The editors of this handbook express their thanks to Drs. Donnelly and Golembiewski and acknowledge that this chapter is based on their work.

Notes:

Chapter 8

Acid-Base Disorders

Acid-Base Disorders

Acid-base disturbances can be induced both by underlying medical conditions and drugs. Responses to drugs may also be altered by acid-base disturbances.

Arterial Blood Gas Measurements

Arterial blood gas measurements (ABGs) are the key to assessing acid-base balance, reported as *arterial pH, partial pressure of carbon dioxide (PaCO$_2$)*, and serum *bicarbonate (HCO$_3^-$)* concentration. Table 8.1 on page 8.5 lists the normal values for these laboratory parameters.

Several important principles must be understood to properly assess blood gas measurements.

♦ *Arterial pH* is determined primarily by the ratio of base to acid in the blood as described by the *Henderson-Hasselbalch equation,* with HCO$_3^-$ as the primary base and *carbonic acid (H$_2$CO$_3$)* as the major acid.

$$pH = pKa + \log \frac{base}{acid} = pKa + \log \frac{HCO_3^-}{H_2CO_3} = 6.1 + \log \frac{HCO_3^-}{H_2CO_3}$$

♦ Because most carbonic acid is present in the blood as *CO$_2$ gas,* its concentration is reflected by PaCO$_2$. Thus, CO$_2$ gas is considered to be an acid, and the Henderson-Hasselbalch equation can be reduced to the following simplified form:

$$pH = pKa + \log \frac{HCO_3^-}{CO_2\ gas} \cong \frac{HCO_3^-}{PaCO_2}$$

♦ CO$_2$ gas is measured by PaCO$_2$ *not* serum total CO$_2$.

♦ The "CO$_2$" value reported by the laboratory on a general electrolyte screen from a *venous blood* sample ("total CO$_2$") is essentially a measure of plasma HCO$_3^-$ as explained below:

Total CO$_2$ in the *venous blood* is made up of approximately 20 parts of HCO$_3^-$ (a base) and 1 part CO$_2$ gas (an acid via conversion to H$_2$CO$_3$).

The small amount of CO$_2$ gas in the blood is best measured via *arterial blood gas* determinations, reported as PaCO$_2$.

Example:

Venous Blood			Arterial Blood Gas	
HCO$_3^-$	24.0 mEq/L			
Dissolved CO$_2$ gas	1.2 mEq/L	yields →	PaCO$_2$	40 mm Hg
Total CO$_2$ content	25.2 mEq/L			

◆ The body attempts to maintain a constant 20:1 ratio of HCO_3^- to CO_2 gas, again illustrated by a simplified version of the Henderson-Hasselbalch equation:

$$pH \cong \frac{HCO_3^-}{CO_2 \text{ gas}} \cong \frac{20}{1}$$

HCO_3^- is regulated primarily by the kidneys via secretion of H^+ and reabsorption of HCO_3^-.

$PaCO_2$ is controlled by pulmonary ventilation as CO_2 gas is retained or exhaled by the lungs.

◆ Chloride provides valuable clues for metabolic disorders, especially metabolic alkalosis. If chloride is lost in the urine, another anion (e.g., HCO_3^-) must be retained in its place to maintain electroneutrality of the blood (see Table 8.2).

◆ Consider the patient's clinical status when assessing blood gas results. Presence of a respiratory illness, diabetes, renal failure, or toxic ingestion provide clues as to what form of acid-base disorder is likely to be present.

◆ Be aware that mixed acid-base imbalances may occur in the same patient.

Respiratory vs Metabolic Disorders

Common laboratory findings for the four basic acid-base disorders are summarized in Table 8.2.

◆ *Primary changes:*

Metabolic disorders primarily affect the HCO_3^- portion of the ratio.

Respiratory disorders primarily alter the CO_2 gas portion of the ratio (i.e., $PaCO_2$).

◆ Changes that occur to *correct (compensate)* the primary disorder as the body attempts to restore the 20:1 ratio of HCO_3^- to CO_2 gas.

Lungs compensate for metabolic disorders and kidneys compensate for respiratory disorders (see Table 8.3). Renal compensation is sluggish and requires 36–72 hr to reach maximum effect.

When $PaCO_2$ and HCO_3^- are outside normal compensatory ranges (see Table 8.3), suspect *mixed-acid base disorders,* inadequate extent of compensation, or inadequate time for compensation.

In long-standing acid-base disorders, the pH may be nearly normal, but the value of the primary defect will always be more abnormal than that of the compensatory value.

Metabolic Acidosis

Metabolic acidosis is associated with HCO_3^- loss (e.g., diarrhea), decreased acid excretion by the kidney (e.g., renal tubular acidosis), or increased endogenous acid production (e.g., diabetic ketoacidosis). Table 8.4 lists the common causes of metabolic acidosis sorted by the presence or absence of an *anion gap.* (See Table 8.1 for formula to calculate the anion gap and the normal value.)

Lactic Acidosis

◆ Lactic acidosis represents a metabolic acidosis with an anion gap. Common causes of lactic acidosis are listed in Table 8.5. It is important to correct the underlying cause and to administer IV bicarbonate to maintain a pH >7.20 to 7.25.

◆ The bicarbonate dose may be estimated as follows:

$$\text{HCO}_3^- \text{ Dose (in mEq)} = (0.5 \text{ L/kg})\left(\begin{array}{c} \text{Body wt} \\ \text{in kg} \end{array}\right)\left(\begin{array}{c} \text{Desired HCO}_3^- \\ \text{Increment} \\ \text{in mEq/L} \end{array}\right)$$

Replace 50% over 3–4 hours; remainder over 24 hours.

◆ Once the pH is 7.20–7.25, the serum [HCO]$_3^-$ should not be increased by more than 4–6 mEq/L over 6–12 hr to avoid the risks of overalkalinization [paradoxical central nervous system (CNS) acidosis; decreased affinity of hemoglobin for oxygen leading to tissue hypoxia and lactic acid production; sodium overload; and hypokalemia].

◆ See Table 8.6 for dosage forms to replace HCO$_3^-$.

◆ Risk of long-term HCO$_3^-$ administration:

  • Excess HCO$_3^-$ converted to $H_2CO_3^-$, then to CO_2 gas causing paradoxical metabolic acidosis with rapid penetration of CO_2 gas into CNS.

  • Decreased O_2 release from hemoglobin, arrhythmogenic, increased serum osmolality.

Metabolic Alkalosis

Often associated with chloride loss

◆ KCl loss via diuresis or diarrhea

◆ HCl loss via vomiting or NG suction

Metabolic alkalosis can be categorized according to saline responsiveness (see Table 8.7).

Treatment

◆ Calculate chloride deficit in mEq = 0.2 L/kg (wt in kg) × (103 − observed Cl⁻)

◆ Treat underlying cause. Replace potassium and chloride with KCl. NaCl may be used if hyperkalemic. Sodium overload may occur in patients with liver disease, renal failure, or congestive heart failure.

◆ If rapid correction is desired, administer 0.1–0.2 N HCl in D$_5$W or normal saline (NS) into a central venous line. First make a 1 N stock solution of 95 mL 37.5% HCl qs to 1 L with sterile water. Then make the 0.1 N injection solution (100 mEq Cl⁻/L) using 100 mL of the 1 N stock solution filtered via acid-resistant filter qs to 1 L with D$_5$W or NS. Use glass only; no rubber, metal, or membrane filters. Administer at an initial rate of 100–125 mL/hr (10–12.5 mEq/hr) and monitor arterial blood gases every 4 hr.

Respiratory Acidosis

◆ Respiratory acidosis occurs when pulmonary ventilation is inadequate. Common causes of respiratory acidosis are listed in Table 8.8.

◆ Dyspnea, headache, drowsiness, disorientation, confusion, flushing, peripheral dilation, tachycardia, and arrhythmias are common symptoms.

Treatment

◆ Treatment involves correction of the underlying disorder and giving supplemental oxygen. IV NaHCO$_3$ is not recommended unless the respiratory acidosis is severe and the patient is hemodynamically unstable or exhibiting CNS symptoms.

◆ *Doxapram* is reserved for patients unresponsive to NaHCO$_3$ and mechanical ventilation.

♦ **Medroxyprogesterone acetate** (Provera) 20 mg TID may improve chronic respiratory acidosis caused by CNS-mediated hypoventilation.

Respiratory Alkalosis

♦ Excessive rate or depth of respiration increases CO_2 excretion. Common causes of respiratory alkalosis are summarized in Table 8.9.

♦ **Symptoms** of respiratory alkalosis include peripheral and perioral paresthesias, light-headedness, confusion, and tachycardia.

♦ **Treatment.** Respiratory alkalosis is usually not a severe disorder; treatment involves correcting the underlying disease. In cases of acute anxiety, the patient should rebreathe expired air from a paper bag.

Mixed Acid-Base Disorders

A normal pH, despite obvious defects in $PaCO_2$, HCO_3^-, or chloride, should raise suspicion of mixed acidosis and alkalosis.

♦ Calculate excess ion gap (i.e., total anion gap minus the normal anion gap of 12)

This step is only done if an anion gap is present. The presence of an increased anion gap always indicates a metabolic acidosis. This second correction helps to detect whether a second acid-base abnormality is also present.

Add the calculated excess anion gap value to the measured HCO_3^- concentration. If the sum is greater than a normal serum HCO_3^-, there is a co-existent metabolic alkalosis. If the sum is less than a normal HCO_3^-, there is a co-existent nonanion gap metabolic acidosis.

♦ A decreased anion gap may be present in alkalosis with HCO_3^- excess.

Notes:

Table 8.1 • Normal Values for Laboratory Tests

Test	Normal Range
Arterial Blood Gases (ABGs)	
pH	7.36–7.44
PaO_2	90–100 mm Hg
$PaCO_2$	35–45 mm Hg
Total CO_2 Content[a]	24–30 mEq/L
Anion Gap[b] **(AG)**	7–14 mEq/L

[a]Primarily $[HCO_3]$ and some CO_2. Ratio = 20:1. Used to estimate $[HCO_3]$.
[b]Anion Gap = $(Na^+ + K^+) - (Cl^- + HCO_3^-)$. An ↑ anion gap generally indicates presence of an organic acid (e.g., ketones or lactic acid).

Table 8.2 • Laboratory Values in the Four Basic Acid-Base Disorders

Disorder	Arterial pH	Primary Change	Compensatory Change
Metabolic acidosis	↓	↓ HCO_3^-	↓$PaCO_2$
Respiratory acidosis	↓	↑ $PaCO_2$	↑ HCO_3^-
Metabolic alkalosis	↑	↑ HCO_3^-	↑ $PaCO_2$
Respiratory alkalosis	↑	↓ $PaCO_2$	↓ HCO_3^-

Table 8.3 • Normal Compensation in Simple Acid-Base Disorders[a]

Disorder	Compensation[b]
Metabolic Acidosis	↓ $PaCO_2$ (mm Hg) = (1.0 to 1.4) × ↓ HCO_3^- (mEq/L)
Metabolic Alkalosis	↑ $PaCO_2$ (mm Hg) = (0.5 to 1.0) × ↑ HCO_3^- (mEq/L)
Respiratory Acidosis	
Acute	↑ HCO_3^- (mEq/L) = 0.1 × ↑ $PaCO_2$ (mm Hg)
Chronic	↑ HCO_3^- (mEq/L) = 0.4 × ↑ $PaCO_2$ (mm Hg)
Respiratory Alkalosis	
Acute	↓ HCO_3^- (mEq/L) = 0.2 × ↓ $PaCO_2$ (mm Hg)
Chronic	↓ HCO_3^- (mEq/L) = (0.4 to 0.5) × ↓ $PaCO_2$ (mm Hg)

[a]For example, a patient who has metabolic acidosis with a total CO_2 content of 14 mEq/L (↓ of 10 mEq/L from normal) would be expected to have respiratory compensation resulting in a ↓ in $PaCO_2$ of 10–14 mm Hg (from a normal of 40 mm Hg to a new value of 26–30 mm Hg). This degree of respiratory compensation results in an arterial pH between 7.29 and 7.35. If no respiratory compensation has occurred, arterial pH would fall to 7.17.

$$pH = 6.1 + \log \frac{HCO_3^-}{(0.03)(PaCO_2)}$$

[b]Based upon change from normal $HCO_3^- = 24$ mEq/L and $PaCO_2 = 40$ mm Hg.

Notes:

Table 8.4 • Common Causes of Metabolic Acidosis

Normal Anion Gap[a] (Loss of HCO_3^- with CL^- Retention)	Elevated Anion Gap (Retention of Fixed Acid)

Hypokalemic
    Diarrhea
    Carbonic anhydrase inhibitors
    Renal tubular acidosis (RTA)[b]
        Proximal
        Distal
 	
Hyperkalemic
    Hypoaldosteronism
    Hydrochloric acid or precursor ingestion
    Potassium-sparing diuretics
        Amiloride
        Spironolactone
        Triamterene
	Renal Failure (uremic acidosis)
	
	Lactic Acidosis (see Table 8.5)
	
	Ketoacidosis
	    Starvation
	    Ethanol
	    Diabetes mellitus
	
	Drug Intoxications[c]
	    Ethylene glycol
	    Methanol
	    Salicylates (aspirin)

[a]Patients are generally hyperchloremic.
[b]Drugs associated with RTA include acetazolamide, lithium, heavy metal ingestion (lead, cadmium, copper, mercury), amphotericin B, toluene.
[c]Calculate osmolality gap. See Chapter 9: Fluid and Electrolyte Disorders. If >10 mOsm/kg, one of these unmeasured, osmotically active substances should be considered.

Table 8.5 • Common Causes of Lactic Acidosis[a]

Type A[b]	Type B
Anemia	**Diabetes Mellitus**
Carbon Monoxide Poisoning	**Liver Failure**
CHF	**Renal Failure**
Shock	**Seizure Disorder**
Sepsis	**Leukemia**

	Drugs
	    Biguanides (metformin)
	    Didanoside
	    Ethanol
	    Isoniazid
	    Methanol
	    Salicylates
	    Zidovudine

[a]CHF = Congestive heart failure.
[b]Associated with tissue hypoxia.

Table 8.6 • Dosage Forms for Replacement of HCO_3^-

Dosage Form	Amount of HCO_3^- Provided
$NaHCO_3$ Injection (7.7%)	44.6 mEq/HCO_3^-/50 mL
$NaHCO_3$ Tabs 300 mg, 600 mg	1.8–4.8 gm/day = 24–64 mEq HCO_3^-
Shohl's solution: 90 gm Na citrate + 140 gm citric acid/L	1 mEq HCO_3^-/mL 30–60 mL/day

Table 8.7 • Classification of Metabolic Alkalosis

Saline-Responsive	Saline-Unresponsive
Diuretic Therapy	**Normotensive**
Extracellular Volume Contraction	Potassium depletion
	Hypercalcemia
Gastric Acid Loss	**Hypertensive**
Vomiting	Mineralocorticoids
Nasogastric suction	Hyperaldosteronism
Exogenous Alkali Administration	Hyperreninism
	Licorice
Blood Transfusions	

Table 8.8 • Common Causes of Respiratory Acidosis[a]

Airway Obstruction	**Cardiopulmonary**
Foreign body aspiration	Cardiac arrest
Asthma	Pulmonary edema or infiltration
COPD	Pulmonary embolism
Beta-adrenergic blockers	Pulmonary fibrosis
CNS Disturbances	**Neuromuscular**
Cerebral vascular accident	Amyotrophic lateral sclerosis
Sleep apnea	Guillain-Barré syndrome
Tumor	Myasthenia gravis
CNS depressant drugs	Hypokalemia
Barbiturates	Hypophosphatemia
Benzodiazepines	Drugs
Opioids	Aminoglycosides
	Antiarrhythmics
	Lithium
	Phenytoin

[a]CNS = Central nervous system; COAD = Chronic obstructive airways disease.

Table 8.9 • Common Causes of Respiratory Alkalosis[a]

CNS Disturbances	**Pulmonary**
Bacterial septicemia	Pneumonia
Cerebrovascular accident	Pulmonary edema
Fever	Pulmonary embolus
Hepatic cirrhosis	**Tissue Hypoxia**
Hyperventilation	High altitude
Anxiety–induced	Hypotension
Voluntary	CHF
Meningitis	**Other**
Pregnancy	Excessive mechanical ventilation
Trauma	Rapid correction of metabolic acidosis
Drugs	
Progesterone derivatives	
Respiratory stimulants	
Salicylate overdose	

[a]CNS = Central nervous system; CHF = Congestive heart failure.

Notes:

The reader is referred to Chapter 9: Acid-Base Disorders, written by *S. Troy McMullin, Pharm.D., Thomas G. Hall, Pharm.D.,* and *Rachel L. Kleiman-Wexler, Pharm.D.,* in the seventh edition of **Applied Therapeutics: The Clinical Use of Drugs** for a more in-depth discussion. The editors of this handbook express their thanks to Drs. McMullin, Hall, and Kleiman-Wexler and acknowledge that this chapter is based upon their work.

Notes:

Chapter 9

Fluid and Electrolyte Disorders

Basic Principles

Body Fluid Compartments

Body water distributes into intracellular fluid (ICF) and extracellular fluid (ECF) compartments as shown in Table 9.1.

> **Total body water (TBW)** = 0.5 L/kg × body weight,
> where 0.5 L/kg is the volume of distribution of water in the body.

Estimation of Osmolality

+ **Normal plasma osmolality** (280–295 mOsm/kg) is determined by the number of particles in solution per kg H_2O, not size or valence; for example, NaCl liberates 2 particles (ions) in solution, producing 2 mOsm/mmol of salt. Nondissociable solutes (glucose, albumin) generate 1 mOsm/mmol of particles. Plasma osmolality reflects the osmolality of total body water because all body fluid compartments are iso-osmotic.

+ **Effective osmolality (E_{osm})** is the number of osmoles acting to hold fluid in the ECF. It does not include urea, ethanol, and methanol because these readily penetrate the cell.

$$E_{osm} = (2)(Na \text{ in mEq/L}) + \frac{Glucose \text{ in mg/dL}}{18}$$

+ **Osmol gap.** An osmol gap exists when the difference between the measured (by freezing point depression) and calculated osmolality is >15 mOsm/kg. An osmol gap is encountered when an unknown solute (e.g., ethyl alcohol, ethylene glycol, isopropanol, paraldehyde, methanol) has accumulated or when the serum sodium has been artifactually decreased (e.g., hyperlipidemia).

Common Intravenous (IV) Solutions

+ Electrolyte concentrations and other characteristics of common IV solutions are provided in Table 9.2.

Assessing Fluid and Electrolyte Balance

+ To determine daily fluid and electrolyte needs, first determine basal needs (see Table 9.3).
+ Then, correct for existing diseases or imbalances by identifying, measuring, and replacing unusual fluid and electrolyte loss through diuresis, vomiting, burns, fever, diarrhea, GI drainage, and "third-spacing" (e.g., ascites, intestinal obstruction, blisters). (See Table 9.4.)

Sodium

♦ Important principles

- Laboratory results for serum sodium *[Na+]* indicate the *concentration* of sodium in the vascular space and reflect *water balance,* not absolute amount of sodium in the body.
- For example, *dilutional* hyponatremia: [Na+] <130 mEq/L caused by excess vascular free water. Total body sodium may be normal, depleted, or excessive.
- For example, hypernatremia: [Na+] >150 mEq/L due to hemoconcentration of sodium in the vasculature. Total body sodium may be normal, depleted, or excessive.
- *Volume depletion (dehydration)* indicates loss of both sodium and water from the body. If this loss is isotonic, serum sodium concentration will be unchanged ("normal"), even when total body sodium stores are markedly depleted.

Hyponatremia

♦ Most cases of hyponatremia reflect an increase of total body water (impaired free water clearance by the kidneys via an ADH defect or excess water ingestion).

♦ Hyponatremia can be associated with normal, increased, or decreased total body sodium or extracellular volume (see Table 9.6).

♦ Drugs that induce hyponatremia are listed in Table 9.5 based upon their primary mechanism of action.

♦ *Interpretation of Serum Sodium*

Factitious Hyponatremia. Watch for factitious hyponatremia (low sodium with normal osmolality): It occurs when plasma water is displaced by lipids or protein.

True hyponatremia can occur in the presence of *hyperglycemia,* which draws water from intracellular to extracellular space. Plasma Na+ falls 1.3 to 1.6 mEq/L for each 100 mg/dL increment of plasma glucose above normal.

♦ *Symptoms* occur when the [Na+] is <120 mEq/L and include anorexia, nausea, vomiting, weakness, muscle cramps, twitching, lethargy, confusion, and seizures.

♦ The **clinical presentation,** calculation of saline deficits, and **treatment** of hyponatremia are described in Table 9.6.

Hypernatremia

♦ Three primary causes of hypernatremia are:

- Pure *water loss* from inability of the kidney to conserve free H_2O (e.g., ADH deficiency from diabetes insipidus).
- *Hypotonic fluid loss* (dehydration) from osmotic or loop diuretics, diarrhea, vomiting, or excessive sweating. Accompanying decreased sensorium, physical inability to drink, or blunted thirst reflex worsen the condition.
- Pure *salt gain* from infusion of hypertonic saline (rare).

♦ *Symptoms.* When the [Na+] approaches 160–170 mEq/L, patients experience fatigue, muscle weakness, cramps, lethargy, and irritability.

♦ *Treatment*

$$\text{Calculate water deficit} = \text{Normal TBW} - \text{Present TBW}$$

$$= (0.5 \times \text{lean body weight}) \times \frac{(1 - \text{Normal Na concentration})}{(\text{Observed Na concentration})}$$

Replace half of calculated deficit with a hypotonic solution over 12–24 hours, remainder over 24–48 hours. Do not exceed a 0.5 mEq/L serum Na increase per hour.

Use D_5W if pure water loss. Use ½ or ¼ normal saline if Na deficit is also present. Correct other electrolytes as indicated.

Instruct the patient to drink more water regardless of thirst.

Clinical Use of Diuretics

♦ *Classification.* Diuretics reduce the reabsorption of sodium and chloride in the kidney tubules, thereby enhancing solute and fluid excretion. Individual diuretic agents can be categorized according to their sites of action within renal tubules (see Figure 9.1).

♦ *Potency.* Loop diuretics (i.e., furosemide, bumetanide, torsemide, and ethacrynic acid) are more potent than thiazide diuretics (e.g., hydrochlorothiazide, chlorthalidone), and both loop and thiazide diuretics are more potent than the potassium-sparing diuretics (e.g., amiloride, spironolactone, triamterene). Metolazone is characterized as a thiazide diuretic but has a potency intermediate between those of the other thiazides and loop diuretics.

♦ *Indications.* Diuretics are indicated for the treatment of hypertension and for volume expansion disorders. The goal of diuretic therapy when used for volume expansion disorders (e.g., CHF) is the provision of symptomatic relief without causing intravascular depletion. See Chapter 11: Essential Hypertension and Chapter 16: Heart Failure for a more detailed discussion of the indications, dosing, side effects, and clinical monitoring of diuretics.

Potassium

♦ Total body stores approximate 45–55 mEq/kg; plasma concentration is 3.5 to 5 mEq/L.

♦ Since 98% is located intracellularly, small shifts in potassium from the intracellular to the extracellular space can cause large changes in plasma concentrations.

♦ The dietary intake of potassium (50–100 mEq/day) primarily is excreted renally.

♦ Pathologic conditions that alter [K^+] are summarized in Table 9.7.

Hypokalemia

♦ Three main causes of hypokalemia are:

• Decreased dietary potassium.

• Shift of potassium from the extracellular to the intracellular space (alkalosis, stress, insulin)

• Increased urinary or GI losses.

♦ Drugs that induce hypokalemia are listed in Table 9.8.

Clinical Presentation. May be asymptomatic until [K^+] <3.0 mEq/L.

♦ *Neuromuscular manifestations* include weakness, myalgias, fasciculations, cramps, and areflexia (e.g., difficulty climbing stairs or lifting objects—proximal muscle weakness).

♦ *Electrocardiogram (ECG) changes* include ST depression, flattened T waves, U waves, a prolonged PR interval, QRS widening, and arrhythmia.

♦ *Renal manifestations* include polyuria, chloride wasting, metabolic alkalosis, and sodium retention.

Treatment

♦ *Estimate Total Body Deficit.* There is a 100–200 mEq per 1 mEq/L decrement if the [K^+] is >3 mEq/L. When [K^+] <3 mEq/L, each additional 1 mEq/L decrement represents a 200–400 mEq/L deficit. Use estimates cautiously when hypokalemia is due to intracellular K+ shifts. Measure electrolyte content of body fluid losses.

♦ **Oral Potassium.** The chloride salt of potassium (13.4 mEq K+/gm) is preferred, except in the presence of renal tubular acidosis or chronic HCO_3^- wasting diarrhea, when an alkalinizing salt may be preferred. Wax matrix and microencapsulated formulations are preferred. There are no major differences between these products. Select the product on the basis of cost and patient preference. Maintenance doses usually are 40–100 mEq/day. (See Table 9.9.)

♦ **K-sparing diuretics** [spironolactone (Aldactone); triamterene (Dyazide); and amiloride (Midamor)] or salt substitutes also may be used to maintain K+ balance.

♦ **Parenteral Potassium.** If [K+] is 72.5 mEq/L, replace with IV KCl in concentrations of 30-40 mEq/L. Do not exceed a rate of 10 mEq/hr, unless [K+] is <2 mEq/L or the patient has life-threatening symptoms. Concentrated solutions may be infused (usual maximum concentration is 60–80 mEq/L, although higher concentrations have been used in extreme emergencies) at a rate not >40 mEq/hr and with ECG monitoring. Avoid glucose solutions that promote intracellular uptake of K+. The chloride salt of K+ is preferred in the setting of alkalosis; use acetate in the setting of acidosis; use PO_4^- salt in the setting of hypophosphatemia.

Hyperkalemia

♦ Three primary causes of hyperkalemia are:
- Decreased renal excretion.
- Redistribution of K+ from the intracellular to the extracellular space (acidosis).
- Increased exogenous intake in the presence of renal failure.

♦ Caution: There could be spurious hyperkalemia in hemolyzed blood sample, WBC >500,000 or Platelets >750,000

♦ Drugs that induce hyperkalemia are listed in Table 9.10.

Clinical Presentation

♦ **Neuromuscular manifestations** include lower extremity paresthesias and weakness; can progress to upper extremities and pulmonary musculature.

♦ **ECG changes** include peaked T waves (>6 mEq/L); widening of QRS and P waves (>7 mEq/L); arrhythmias; and cardiac arrest (>8 mEq/L).

♦ **Moderate to Severe.** Hyperkalemia is considered moderate to severe if serum potassium concentrations are 6.5–8.0 mEq/L with only peaked T waves.

♦ **Severe.** Hyperkalemia is considered severe if the serum potassium is >8 mEq/L with QRS widening, atrioventricular block, and dysrhythmias.

Treatment of hyperkalemia is presented in Table 9.11.

Magnesium

♦ Magnesium is primarily located intracellularly (65% bone, 20% muscle).

♦ Normal serum Mg concentration = 1.4 to 1.75 mEq/L (20% protein bound).

♦ Dietary intake usually is 20–30 mEq/day in the U.S. Normally 30–40% absorbed, ↑ to 80% in deficiency states.

♦ Most magnesium is excreted renally and a small amount from the GI tract.

♦ Patients with renal insufficiency can accumulate magnesium if exogenous intake is not restricted.

Hypomagnesemia

Hypomagnesemia generally is caused by:
♦ Decreased intake or absorption (e.g., malnutrition, alcoholism, malabsorption).

♦ Increased GI or urinary losses (e.g., vomiting, diarrhea, NG suction, and drugs such as diuretics, laxatives, aminoglycosides, cisplatin, cyclosporine, amphotericin B).

Clinical Presentation

♦ **Central nervous system (CNS) manifestations** include personality changes, agitation, confusion, delirium, seizures, depression, apathy, nausea, and vomiting.

♦ **Neurological manifestations** include positive Chvostek's and Trousseau's sign, hypocalcemic tetany, tremors, and weakness.

♦ **ECG changes** are similar to hypokalemia, and include prolonged PR and QT intervals, flattened and widened T waves, and ventricular arrhythmias.

Treatment

♦ **Duration.** Since 50% of the dose administered by any route is lost renally, magnesium should be replenished over several days.

♦ **Parenteral MgSO$_4$.** 1 mEq/kg on day 1 as 10% solution (1/2 in first 3 hr, rest over 24 hr); then 0.5 mEq/kg IV QD on days 3–5. More aggressive replacement (16–32 mEq MgSO$_4$ IV over 4 min) may be needed in patients with arrhythmias or seizures.

♦ **Oral replacement.** Choose one of the following if patient is not symptomatic. Diarrhea is a limiting factor.
  • Liquid antacids, 30–60 mL QID (magnesium content varies).
  • Milk of magnesia, 5 mL QID (1 mL = 36 mg or 3 mEq magnesium).
  • Magnesium oxide tablets, 250–500 mg (12.5–25 mEq) QID.
  • Decreased deep tendon reflexes (DTRs) reflect excessive magnesium replacement (serum Mg >4 mEq/L). Patients in renal failure are at highest risk.

Hypermagnesemia

♦ **Causes** include renal failure in association with an exogenous Mg^{++} load (e.g., antacids), toxemia treated with MgSO$_4$, hypothyroidism, Addison's disease, and lithium.

♦ **Clinical presentation** varies by serum magnesium concentration:
  • 2–4 mEq/L: nausea, vomiting, anorexia, drowsiness, lethargy, diaphoresis.
  • 4–6 mEq/L: decreased DTRs.
  • >6 mEq/L: absent DTRs, altered consciousness.
  • >8–10 mEq/L: flaccid paralysis, hypotension, difficulty talking or swallowing. Prolonged PR interval, widened QRS, ventricular arrhythmias.
  • 15 mEq/L: complete heart block, asystole.

♦ **Treatment**
  Prevention is the best treatment: therefore, exogenous intake should be limited.
  IV calcium, 5–10 mEq repeated PRN, may be used to antagonize toxicity.
  IV furosemide plus 0.45 NaCl may help accelerate renal clearance if fluids are not contraindicated.
  Dialysis can be helpful.

Phosphorus

♦ Phosphorus (P) is found primarily in bone (85%) and soft tissue (14%); there is <1% in ECF.

♦ Dietary intake typically is 800–1500 mg/day (milk, meat, vegetables).

♦ Phosphorus is excreted into the GI tract and renally.

♦ 1 mmol of phosphate (PO_4^- + $PO_4^=$) contains 1 mmol of elemental P, but 1 mmol phosphate is 3× the weight of P (1 gm P = 32 mmol). Thus it is preferred to express doses of either as mmol equivalents, not mg equivalents.

♦ Normal serum P levels are 2.7–4.5 mg/dL (0.9–1.5 mmol/L) in adults.

Hypophosphatemia

Causes

♦ Impaired absorption (e.g., malabsorption, NG suction, vomiting, $A1OH_2$ antacids, sucralfate).

♦ Increased renal elimination (e.g., hyperglycemic diuresis, renal tubular acidosis, hyperparathyroidism, hypokalemia, hypomagnesemia, and volume overload).

♦ Intracellular shift (e.g., glucose and insulin, alkalosis).

♦ Hypophosphatemia commonly is associated with diabetic ketoacidosis, chronic alcoholism, recovery from malnutrition (total parenteral nutrition therapy), and burns.

Clinical Presentation

♦ Most symptoms are related to impaired cellular energy stores and tissue hypoxia.

♦ Muscle weakness, respiratory failure, decreased cardiac contractility, paresthesias, seizures, coma, and hemolysis also have been observed.

♦ **Chronic hypophosphatemia** can be associated with rickets, osteomalacia, bone pain, diabetes, hypercalciuria, and hypermagnesemia.

Treatment

♦ **Parenteral replacement** is used in severe symptomatic cases (serum P <1 mg/dL) or when the patient is NPO. Empiric regimens range from 0.08–0.5 mmol P/kg over 4–12 hr to 0.32 mmol P/kg in 0.45% saline Q 12 hr until the serum phosphorus is >2 mg/dL. Measure concentrations before each dose and switch to oral therapy when serum phosphorus ≥2 mg/dL. Watch for K+ or Na+ overload.

♦ **Oral Replacement.** Use when serum phosphorus levels are ≥2 mg/dL. An oral dose of 30–60 mmol/day (e.g., 5 mL Fleets or Neutra-Phos BID = 40 mmol) can be administered. Dilute and titrate dose slowly to minimize diarrhea.

♦ Replacement preparations are listed in Table 9.12.

Hyperphosphatemia

Causes

♦ Impaired excretion (e.g., renal failure, volume depletion).

♦ Increased endogenous or exogenous phosphorus loads (e.g., excess supplements, hemolysis, cytotoxic therapy).

♦ A shift from intracellular to extracellular space (e.g., acidosis).

♦ **Drugs** including disodium etidronate, vitamin D intoxication, diuretics (volume depletion), and phosphate-containing laxatives and enemas.

Clinical Presentation

♦ Hyperphosphatemia is associated with hypocalcemia (tetany, convulsions, arrhythmias, hypotension).

♦ $CaPO_4$ can precipitate in the cornea, lung, kidney, blood vessels, and cardiac conduction system, especially when the product of the serum [Ca^{++}] × the serum [P] exceeds 60–75 mg/dL in uremic patients.

♦ CHF, renal failure, ileus, nausea, and vomiting also may occur.

Treatment

♦ Eliminate exogenous phosphorus.

♦ Excretion of phosphorus can be aided by PO_4^- binding antacids: $A1OH_3^-$ 30–40 mL with meals and HS or $CaCO_3$ if calcium is low. If the P is >6 mg/dL, use $AlOH_3$ *before* $CaCO_3$ to avoid soft tissue precipitation.

♦ P also can be dialyzed.

Calcium

♦ Most calcium (99%) is found in bone, but calcium that is found in ECF and ICF plays a critical physiologic role.

♦ Normal serum concentrations are 8.5–10.5 mg/dL; 47% (4–5 mg/dL) is ionized (free).

♦ Since 40% of calcium is bound to albumin in plasma, albumin concentrations can alter measured $[Ca^{++}]$ without altering the free or active form. Each 1 gm/dL change in albumin causes a 0.8 mg/dL change in $[Ca^{++}]$ in the same direction.

$$\frac{Corrected}{Calcium} = \frac{Observed}{Calcium} + 0.8 \left(\frac{Normal}{Albumin} - \frac{Observed}{Albumin} \right)$$

Hypercalcemia
Causes

♦ **Malignancy** (breast, lung, renal cell, multiple myeloma, and bone metastases) and hyperparathyroidism are the most common causes.

♦ **Secondary hyperparathyroidism** commonly is associated with acute or chronic renal failure.

♦ **Other causes** include granulomatous disorders and drugs (e.g., vitamin A and D intoxication, thiazides, estrogens, tamoxifen, lithium, and excessive calcium ingestion).

Clinical presentation often is nonspecific.

♦ **Neurological manifestations** include lethargy, confusion, headaches, seizures, and ataxia.

♦ **Neuromuscular manifestations** include weakness, myalgia, hyporeflexia, and arthralgias.

♦ **Chronic renal manifestations** include polyuria, nocturia, and polydipsia.

♦ **Metabolic complications** include hypermagnesuria and alkalosis.

♦ **Cardiovascular effects** include hypertension, arrhythmias, and a shortened QT interval.

♦ **GI symptoms** include constipation, nausea and vomiting, anorexia, dyspepsia, weight loss, peptic ulcer disease, and pancreatitis.

Treatment of hypercalcemia is described in Table 9.13. Aggressiveness depends upon acuteness of onset and symptoms. Treat vigorously if serum calcium is ≥13 mg/dL.

Notes:

Table 9.1 • Body Fluid Compartments

Body Fluid	% Total Body Weight	Comments
Total Body Water (TBW)^a	Infants: 75–85% Adult male: 50–60% Adult female: 45–50%	Gender differences can be attributed to greater proportion of adipose tissue
Intracellular fluid (ICF)	30–40% (2/3 of TBW)	K^+, Mg^{++}, PO_4^- primary electrolytes
Extracellular fluid (ECF)	15–20% (1/3 of TBW)	Na^+, Cl^-, HCO_3^- primary electrolytes
Intravascular (plasma)	5%	Normal saline (NS) acutely $\uparrow$ ECF, but not ICF. D_5W distributes equally between ICF and ECF because insulin promotes uptake of glucose in ICF. NS best to replace intravascular volume
Interstitial/lymph	12%	
Connective tissue, bone, transcellular components	2%	

^{a}TBW = 0.5 L/kg × body weight in kg, where 0.5 L/kg = volume of distribution of water.

Table 9.2 • Common IV Solutions^a

Solution	Glucose (gm/L)	NaCl (mEq/L)	Osmolality (mOsm/L)	Energy (cal/L)
0.45% NaCl	0	77	154	0
0.9% NaCl	0	154	308	0
3.0% NaCl	0	513	1026	0
5.0% NaCl	0	855	1710	0
5.0% DW	50	0	252	170
10% DW	100	0	505	340
5% DW/0.45% NaCl	50	77	406	170
5% DW/0.9% NaCl	50	154	560	170

^{a}D = Dextrose; IV = Intravenous; W = Water; NaCl = Sodium Chloride.

Table 9.3 • Basic Fluid and Electrolyte Requirements

Basic Fluid Requirements
Sensible (measurable) losses (replace with 0.45% or 0.9% saline)

Stool	200 mL/day
Urine	500–1500 mL/day
Sweat	Varies with humidity and body and environmental temperatures

Insensible Losses (Replace with D_5W)

Skin	500 mL/day
Lungs	400 mL/day
Total	2600 mL/day

Basic Electrolyte Requirements

Potassium	40–60 mEq/day
Sodium	50–90 mEq/day

Table 9.4 • Body Fluid Volumes and Electrolyte Content[a]

Source	Volume (L/day)	Na⁺ (mEq/L)	K⁺ (mEq/L)	Cl⁻ (mEq/L)	HCO₃⁻ (mEq/L)
Salivary glands	1.5 (0.5–2)	10 (2–10)	26 (20–30)	10 (8–18)	30
Stomach	1.5 (0.1–4)	60 (9–116)	10 (0–32)	130 (8–54)	—
Duodenum	(0.1–2)	140	5	80	—
Ileum	3 (0.1–9)	140 (80–150)	5 (2–8)	104 (43–137)	30
Colon	—	60	30	40	—
Pancreas	(0.1–0.8)	140 (113–185)	5 (3–7)	75 (54–95)	115
Bile	(0.05–0.8)	145 (131–164)	5 (3–12)	100 (89–180)	35

[a]Mean value (range in parentheses).

Table 9.5 • Common Etiologies of Syndrome of Inappropriate Antidiuretic Hormone

Tumors
Small-cell lung carcinoma (most common), pancreas, duodenum, ureter, nasopharynx, leukemia, Hodgkin's disease, thymoma

CNS Disorders
Mass lesions (tumor, brain abscess, hematoma)
Inflammatory disease (encephalitis, meningitis, lupus)
Degenerative diseases (Guillain-Barré syndrome, spinal cord lesion)
Miscellaneous (psychosis, head trauma, subarachnoid hemorrhage, delirium tremens)

Pulmonary Disorders
Pneumonia, tuberculosis, acute respiratory failure, chronic obstructive pulmonary disease

Endocrine Disorders
Hypothyroidism, glucocorticoid deficiency

Drug-Induced
Antidiuretic hormones: desmopressin, oxytocin
Psychotropic agents: antipsychotics, carbamazepine[a], MAOIs, tricyclic antidepressants
Antineoplastic agents: adenosine arabinoside, cyclophosphamide[a,b], vinblastine, vincristine[a]
Diabetic agents: chlorpropamide[a,b], tolbutamide
Miscellaneous: bromocriptine[a], clofibrate[a], clonidine, morphine[a], nicotine[a], NSAIDs[b], thiazide diuretics[c]

Postoperative State (Surgery)
Hypoxia, nausea, pain, narcotics, hypotension

Others
AIDS, senile atrophy, idiopathic

ADH = Antidiuretic hormone, AIDS = Acquired immunodeficiency disorder, MAOIs = Monoamine oxidase inhibitors, NSAIDs = Nonsteroidal antiinflammatory drugs.
[a]Exerts exogenous ADH-like effect
[b]Increases renal responsiveness to endogenous ADH.
[c]Alters renal diluting capacity.

Notes:

Table 9.6 • Clinical Presentation and Treatment of Hyponatremia[a]

Na+ and H$_2$O Status	Clinical Presentation/Cause	Treatment
Edematous, Fluid Overload (Hypervolemic, Hypotonic) ↑ Total Body Na+ ↑↑ Total Body H$_2$O	*Cirrhosis/CHF/nephrotic syndrome:* A ↓ in renal blood flow activates renin angiotensin system. ↑ aldosterone leads to ↑ Na+, and ↑ ADH leads to free H$_2$O retention. Urine Na+ is low (0–20 mEq/L) and urine osmolality ↓. Diuretics can induce paradoxical effects on urine Na+ and osmolality. This form also can occur in patients with renal failure who drink excessive amounts of water. Patients have symptoms of fluid overload (ascites, distended neck veins, edema).	Fluid and Na restriction. Correct underlying disorder (e.g., paracentesis for ascites). Diurese cautiously; avoid ↓ ECF and accompanying ↓ tissue perfusion. ↑ BUN may indicate overly rapid diuresis.
Nonedematous Hypovolemic (Hypotonic with ECF Depletion) ↓↓ Total Body Na+ ↓ Total Body H$_2$O	Occurs in: *GI fluid loss (e.g., diarrhea) with hypotonic electrolyte-poor fluid replacement, overdiuresis, "third spacing," Addison's disease, renal tubular acidosis, osmotic diuresis.* Replacement of fluid losses with solute-free fluid predisposes these patients to hyponatremia. Kidneys concentrate urine to conserve fluid (urine Na+ <10 mEq/L). *Symptoms:* nonedematous; ECF depletion (collapsed neck veins, dehydration, orthostasis). *Neurologic symptoms:* (See Hyponatremia: Symptoms in text).	Discontinue diuretics. Replace fluid and electrolyte (especially K+) losses. 0.9% saline preferred unless Na+ deficit severe, then use 3%–5% saline. See footnote *b* for method of estimating Na+ deficit.
Nonedematous, Normovolemic (Normovolemic, Hypotonic) ↓ Total Body Sodium ↑ Total Body H$_2$O	*SIADH[a]:* Hyponatremia, hypo-osmolality, renal Na+ wasting (>40 mEq/L), absence of fluid depletion, U$_{osm}$ >P$_{osm}$, normal renal and adrenal function. Free H$_2$O retained while Na+ lost. *Causes:* a) ADH production (infectious disease, vascular disease, cerebral neoplasm, cancer of lung, pancreas, duodenum); b) exogenous ADH administration; c) drugs (see Table 9.5); d) psychogenic polydipsia.	*Chronic treatment:* Restrict fluids to less than urine loss. *Demeclocycline* (300–600 mg BID) induces reversible diabetes insipidus. *Emergency Treatment* for unresponsive patients includes *furosemide* diuresis to achieve negative H$_2$O balance with careful replacement of Na+ and K+ using hypertonic saline solutions.[c] See footnote *c* for method of calculating TBW excess and type of solutions to use.

[a]ADH = Antidiuretic hormone; BUN = Blood urea nitrogen; CHF = Congestive heart failure; ECF = Extracellular fluid; GI = Gastrointestinal; NS = Normal saline (0.9% Na); SIADH = Syndrome of Inappropriate ADH.
[b]Estimate Na deficit: (mEq) = (0.5 L/kg × wt in kg) (Na desired − Na observed), where 0.5 L/kg is volume of distribution (Vd) of Na in the body. Rate of Na and fluid repletion used depends on severity. Mild: Replace with NS. 1st third over 6–12 hours at a rate of <0.5 mEq/L per hour, remaining 2/3 over 24–48 hr. *Severe* (e.g., seizures): Use 3%–5% saline, rate gauged by patient's ability to tolerate Na and volume load. Monitor CNS function, skin turgor, BP, urine Na, signs of Na/H$_2$O overload, especially in patients with cardiovascular, renal, and pulmonary disease.
[c]Total body water (TBW) = 0.5 L/kg × wt in kg.

$$\text{TBW excess} = \text{TBW} - \text{TBW} \frac{\text{(Observed serum Na)}}{\text{(Desired serum Na)}}$$

Remove estimated excess free water with IV furosemide (1 mg/kg). Repeat as necessary. Since furosemide generates a urine that resembles 0.45% NaCl, urine losses of Na and K must be carefully measured and replaced hourly with hypertonic salt solutions. *Correction Rate:* 1–2 mEq Na/hr in symptomatic patients; 0.5 mEq/hr in asymptomatic patients.

Table 9.7 • Factors Which Alter Serum Potassium

Factor	Comment
Drugs	See Tables 9.8 and 9.10.
Acid/base imbalances	Metabolic acidosis $\uparrow$ [K^+] by 0.2–1.7 mEq/L for each 0.1 unit $\downarrow$ in pH. Respiratory acid/base disorders not routinely associated with K^+ shifts. Metabolic alkalosis shifts K^+ intracellularly by 0.3 mEq/L for each 0.1 unit pH $\uparrow$.
Dietary intake and IV fluids	May be either excessive or insufficient.
Hyperosmolarity	$\uparrow$ [K^+] by 0.3–0.6 mEq/L per each 10 mOsm increment.
Cell lysis or destruction (e.g., hemolysis, trauma, rhabdomyolysis)	Liberates intracellular potassium, thereby $\uparrow$ [K^+], particularly if renal function poor.
Rapid cell synthesis (e.g., treatment of megaloblastic anemia)	K^+ utilization exceeds stores leading to hypokalemia.
Renal failure	[K^+] $\uparrow$ in acute renal failure, especially if exogenous potassium given.
$\downarrow$ exogenous intake	Obligatory renal and intestinal losses in the face of $\downarrow$ intake (including K^+-free parenteral fluids) precipitate hypokalemia.
$\uparrow$ renal or GI[a] losses	Hypokalemia can be secondary to $\uparrow$ GI[a] or renal losses of K^+. *GI[a]:* vomiting, diarrhea, fistular drainage, NG[a] suction. *Renal:* hyperaldosteronism induced by hypovolemia or $\downarrow$ urine flow, diuresis, renal tubular acidosis, large Na^+ loads, hypercalcemia, hypomagnesemia.

[a]GI = Gastrointestinal; NG = Nasogastric.

Table 9.8 • Drugs That Most Commonly Induce Hypokalemia[a]

Drug	Mechanism	Predisposing Factors
Acetazolamide	Marked $\uparrow$ in renal K^+ loss	Most profound with short-term therapy
Amphotericin	Renal K^+ loss (renal tubular acidosis)	Concurrent piperacillin, ticarcillin
β_2-agonists	Intracellular shift of K^+	—
Cisplatin	Renal K^+ loss secondary to renal tubular damage	May be dose-related but can occur after a single 50 mg/m^2 dose
Corticosteroids	Renal K^+ loss. Enhanced Na^+ reabsorption at distal tubule and collecting ducts in exchange for K^+ and H^+	Supraphysiologic doses of agents with moderate-to-strong mineralocorticoid activity (e.g., prednisone, hydrocortisone)
Insulin with glucose	Intracellular shift of K^+	Predictable effect when insulin administered to patients with diabetic ketoacidosis. Combination used to treat hyperkalemia
Penicillins piperacillin ticarcillin	High Na^+ load and nonreabsorbable anions can $\uparrow$ K^+ loss	Was more common with carbenicillin when it was available. Newer penicillins are used in lower doses. Less likely to produce hypokalemia
Thiazide and loop diuretics	Renal K^+ loss. $\uparrow$ Na^+ delivery to the late distal tubule, resulting in Na^+ resorption in exchange for K^+	Patients with hyperaldosteronism (e.g., cirrhosis, CHF) predisposed. May be dose-related

[a]CHF = Congestive heart failure.

Table 9.9 • Potassium Supplements

KCl Liquids (Various)
    10% = 20 mEq/15 mL
    20% = 40 mEq/15 mL

Controlled-Release Tablets or Capsules

Kaon Cl-10	10 mEq/tab
Klotrix	10 mEq/tab
K-Tab	10 mEq/tab
K-Dur 10	10 mEq/tab
K-Dur 20	20 mEq/tab
Micro-K Extencaps	8 mEq/cap
Micro-K-10 Extencaps	10 mEq/cap
Slow-K	8 mEq/tab

Table 9.10 • Drugs That Induce Hyperkalemia[a]

Drug	Mechanism	Predisposing Factors
ACE inhibitors	Hypoaldosteronism, impaired excretion	Renal compromise
Nonspecific β-adrenergic blockers	Impaired β_2-mediated cellular uptake	Exercise, tissue damage
Cyclosporine	Impaired excretion	Renal/cardiac transplant
Digitalis	Impaired Na^+/K^+ pump	Renal compromise; intoxication
K^+ supplements	Exogenous K^+ load	Renal compromise
Heparin	Impairs aldosterone synthesis	—
Lithium	Impairs aldosterone synthesis	—
K^+ penicillins	Exogenous K^+ load	Renal compromise
K^+-sparing diuretics	Impaired K^+ secretion	Renal compromise, K^+ supplements
NSAIDs	Impaired K^+ secretion, hypoaldosteronism	—
Pentamidine	Impaired excretion, cellular shift	Renal impairment
Salt substitutes (K^+-containing)	Exogenous K^+ load	Renal compromise
Succinylcholine	Impaired cellular distribution	Head trauma, neuromuscular disease

[a]ACE = Angiotension-converting enzyme; NSAIDs = Nonsteroidal anti-inflammatory drugs.

Notes:

Table 9.11 • Treatment of Hyperkalemia

Drug	Mechanism	Dose	Comment
$CaCl_2$	Reverse cardiotoxicity caused by K^+	10–20 mL 10% $CaCl_2$ IV over 1–3 min. May repeat once.	*Onset:* 1–3 min. *Duration:* 30–60 min. [K^+] remains unchanged
Insulin and glucose	Redistribution of K^+ intracellularly	5–10 U regular insulin with 50 ml 50% dextrose, then $D_{10}W$ infused at 50 mL/hr[a]	*Onset:* 15–30 min *Duration:* several hr. Watch for hypoglycemia and hypokalemia. Does not ↓ total body K^+
β_2-agonists (e.g., Albuterol)	Redistribution of K^+ intracellularly	2 or 4 mg PO TID-QID. Inhalation: 20 mg in 4 mL saline via nebulizer	*Onset:* 30–60 min. *Duration:* 2 hr.
Sodium polystyrene sulfonate (Kayexalate)	Cationic binding resin. 1 gm of resin binds 0.5–1 mEq K^+ in exchange for Na^+	*Oral:* 15–20 gm with 20–100 mL 70% sorbitol Q 4–6 hr. PRN preferred *Retention enema:* 50 gm in 50 mL (70% sorbitol and 150 mL H_2O). Retain 30 min and follow with nonsaline irrigation	*Onset:* Slow; 50 gm will lower [K^+] by 0.5–1 mEq/L over 4–6 hr. Watch for Na^+ overload (100 mg Na^+/1 gm Kayexalate)
$NaHCO_3$	Redistribution of K^+ intracellularly	50 mEq IV over 5 min. Repeat PRN	*Onset:* variable, ≈30 min. May work best in acidosis. Watch for Na^+ overload and hyperosmolar state. No change in total body K^+
Dialysis	Removal of K^+	—	Use as last resort

[a]Glucose unnecessary in patients with high glucose concentrations.

Notes:

Table 9.12 • Phosphorus Replacement Preparations

Product	Potassium (mmol)	Sodium (mmol)	Phosphorus (mmol)[c]
K-Phos Neutral tablets	1.15	12.6	8
Uro-KP-Neutral tablets	1.27	10.9	8
Neutra-Phos			
capsules[a]	7.13	7.13	8
powder[b]	7.13	7.13	8
Neutra-Phos K			
capsules[a]	14.25	0	8
powder[b]	14.25	0	8
Fleets Phospho-Soda (per mL)	0	4.8	4.1
K Phosphate IV (per mL)	4.4	0	3
Na Phosphate IV (per mL)	0	4	3
Milk			
whole (per cup)	9	5.3	7.3
skim (per cup)	9.1	5.5	7.5

[a]Phosphorus content after reconstituting 1 capsule in 75 mL water. Capsules must be reconstituted and not swallowed.
[b]Phosphorus content after reconstituting 1 packet in 75 mL water.
[c]1 gm P = 32 mmol of P.

Table 9.13 • Treatment of Hypercalcemia[a]

Intervention	Dose	Comment
Saline and furosemide	1–2 L NS. Then furosemide 80–100 mg Q 2–4 hr. Establish and maintain normovolemia. Other electrolytes as needed.	Saline diuresis and volume expansion depresses Ca^{++} reabsorption in tubules. Lowers $[Ca^{++}]$ within 24 hr. Treatment of choice in patients without CHF or renal failure.
Calcitonin	4 IU/kg SC or IM Q 12 hr. ↑ dose or use another therapy if unresponsive after 24 hr. (Max: 8 IU/kg Q 6 hr). Human calcitonin = 0.5 mg if allergic or resistant to salmon.	Inhibits osteoclast resorption and renal reabsorption of calcium. Calcimar (salmon-derived) is preferred over human-derived calcitonin because it is more potent and longer acting. Preferred 2nd-line agent because it has a rapid onset (6 hr) and is nontoxic. It can be used safely in CHF and renal failure. Nausea is the major adverse effect. Tolerance occurs in 24–72 hr. Concomitant plicamycin can lead to hypocalcemia.
Plicamycin	25 μg/kg/day IV over 4–6 hr. Repeat PRN in 48 hr. Renal failure: 12.5 μg/kg.	Inhibits osteoclast bone resorption. Onset 24–48 hr; duration 3–14 days. Common side effects: N/V, minimized by slow IV. Since the dose is 10% of an antineoplastic dose, cytotoxic effects less severe. Obtain baseline renal and hepatic function, platelet counts.
Biphosphonates (Etidronate) (Pamidronate)	Etidronate: 7.5 mg/kg IV QD × 3 days over at least 2 hr. Maintenance: 20 mg/kg/day PO. Pamidronate: 60–90 mg IV over 4 hr × 1. Repeat in 7 days PRN.	Inhibits osteoclast reabsorption in malignancy state. Efficacy 75%–100%. Onset 48 hr. Duration, days. Concomitant hydration is imperative. Do not use in renal failure. Adverse effects: ↑ P, ↑ SrCr, N/V (oral).

(continued)

Table 9.13 • Treatment of Hypercalcemia*ᵃ* *(continued)*

Intervention	Dose	Comment
Gallium Nitrate	100–200 mg/M^2/day continued IV infusion × 5 days.	Potent inhibitor of osteoclast-mediated bone resorption. Onset 5–6 days, duration 7 days. Nephrotoxic at high doses (1,400 mg/M^2/day).
Phosphate	IV PO$_4^-$ not recommended. PO PO$_4^-$: gradually titrate to 30–60 mmol/day (1–3 gm/day in divided doses)	Inhibits bone resorption; soft tissue calcification. IV onset 24 hr, but not drug of choice. Oral agents used for chronic therapy. (See Table 9.12.) Contraindicated in renal failure.
Corticosteroids	Prednisone 60–80 mg/day. Hydrocortisone 5 mg/kg/day IV × 2–3 days.	Impair GI absorption and bone resorption. Onset several days. Best in patients with multiple myeloma, vitamin D intoxication, granulomatous conditions. Can be used in CHF, renal failure.
Indomethacin	75–150 mg/day.	Reports of efficacy are mixed.

*ᵃ*CHF = Congestive heart failure; GI = Gastrointestinal; IM = Intramuscular; IV = Intravenous; NS = Normal saline; N/V = Nausea and vomiting; SrCr = Serum creatinine.

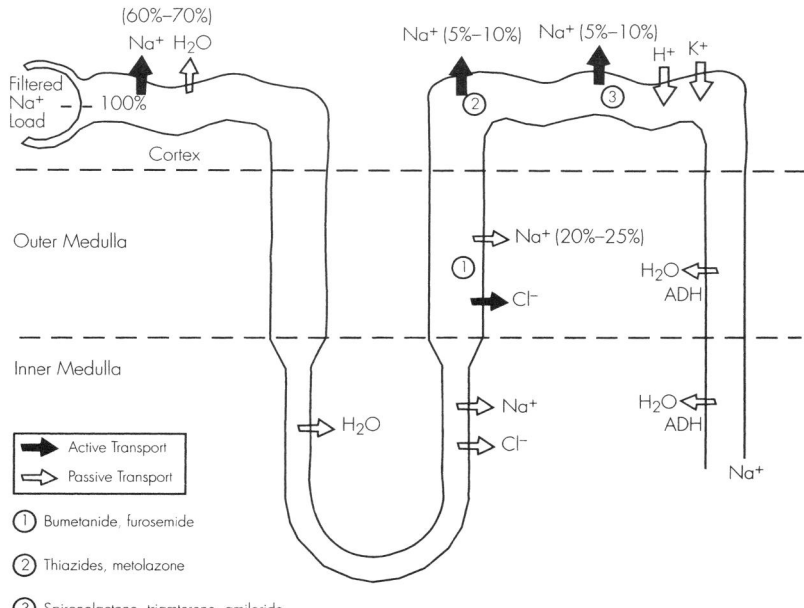

Fig. 9.1 Probable Sites of Sodium Reabsorption and Diuretic Action in the Nephron. Note: To produce diuresis, the drug must first be actively secreted tubularly into the nephron. If tubular secretion is impaired, the diuretic response will be less. The loop diuretics are most effective, resulting in an excretion of 15%–25% of the sodium filtered through the glomerulus. Thiazide only results in excretion of 5%–10% of filtered sodium.

The reader is referred to Chapter 10, written by *Allan Lau, Pharm.D.,* in the seventh edition of **Applied Therapeutics: The Clinical Use of Drugs** for a more in-depth discussion. Another topic included in his chapter relates to nephrotic syndrome. The editors of this handbook express their thanks to Dr. Lau and acknowledge that this chapter is based upon his work.

Notes:

Chapter 10

Dyslipidemias

Definitions

- ◆ **Fats (lipids)** are combinations (esters) of fatty acids plus an alcohol. The 2 main fats in the body are:
  - *Triglycerides* (glycerol esterified with 3 fatty acids). *Normal:* <150 mg/dL (1.69 mmol/L).
  - *Cholesterol esters* (cholesterol alcohol esterified with fatty acids). *Normal total cholesterol:* <200 mg/dL (5.17 mmol/L).
- ◆ **Lipoproteins** are complexes that solubilize and transport hydrophobic fats in the blood. They are composed of an oily inner lipid core of triglyceride and/or cholesterol esters. This core is surrounded by a hydrophilic outer coat of protein (apoproteins), phospholipids, and soluble (unesterified) cholesterol alcohol. Lipoproteins are classified by their density (separation via ultracentrifuge) or electrophoretic mobility. (See Table 10.1.)

Lipoprotein Profiling

- ◆ National Cholesterol Education Program (NCEP) Adult Treatment Panel III (ATP-III) guidelines, updated in 2001, recommend a full lipid panel every 5 years in adults over age 20 years. Low density lipoprotein cholesterol (LDL-C) is a better predictor of coronary heart disease than total cholesterol (TC).
- ◆ See Table 10.2 for assessment of normal and abnormal lipid values.

Categorization of Lipid Disorders

Based upon lipoprotein profiling, physical examination for the presence of tendon or palmar xanthomas, family history for CHD, and the age of onset of coronary symptoms (if any) in the patient, a presumptive diagnosis of type of lipid disorder can be made. (See Table 10.3.)

Risk Factor Assessment for Hypercholesterolemia

- ◆ NCEP guidelines (see table 10.4) have identified risk factors for CHD in patients with increased LDL-C.
- ◆ Presence of diabetes or noncoronary vascular disease (e.g., peripheral vascular disease, intermittent claudication) are considered *"coronary heart disease equivalents,"* placing patients in the highest risk category for intensive therapeutic interventions.

Goals of Therapy

- ♦ Based upon these risk factors and the presence or absence of CHD (or CHD equivalents) in the patient, NCEP recommends the LDL treatment goals listed in Table 10.5.
- ♦ The long-term goal is to prevent cardiac events and premature death.

Treatment

- ♦ **Primary Prevention.** In patients with increased LDL, but no history of CHD (or CHD equivalents), there is increasing evidence of reduced incidence of angina, heart attacks, and strokes as well as reduction of mortality risk. Use of drug therapy is controversial because of high cost, but it may be cost effective in high-risk patients (e.g., strong family history or coexistent diabetes) when nondrug therapies fail.

- ♦ **Secondary Prevention.** In patients with increased LDL and a history of CHD (or CHD equivalents), there is strong evidence of fewer heart attacks and strokes and prolonged survival. Use of drug therapies definitely indicated when nondrug therapies fail.

- ♦ **Therapeutic Lifestyle Changes (TLC)** always are considered initial intervention for both primary and secondary prevention. It includes:
  - Smoking cessation (may include nicotine gum, transdermal therapy or bupropion [Zyban]).
  - Exercise
  - *Antioxidant vitamins (A, C, E).* Long-term, high doses may slow atherogenesis. Assessments of value await further data.
  - Diet modification. (See Table 10.6.)

- ♦ **Other Interventions.** Remove or reduce dose of possible drugs affecting plasma lipids. (See Table 10.7.)
  Treat other possible causes of dyslipidemia:
  - Hypothyroidism. Thyroid supplements (L-thyroxine) may normalize LDL levels.
  - Metabolic syndrome. Note increased CHD risk in patients with combined obesity, diabetes, hypertension, low HDL, and high triglyceride (TG). Diabetes also is a possible contraindication to niacin.
  - Nephrotic syndrome.
  - Obstructive liver disease.

Drug Therapy

- ♦ Drug therapy is indicated if 3–6 months of lifestyle modification fails to achieve LDL goals. May initiate sooner in high-risk patients.
- ♦ Initial drug of choice guided by type of disorder present and cost/compliance considerations (see Tables 10.8 and 10.9).
  - Statins produce the most effective LDL lowering and have highest patient acceptance, but cost of drug and laboratory monitoring is high.
  - Niacin is the least expensive drug and has the most desirable lipid-lowering potential (decreased LDL, decreased TG, increased HDL), but acute reactions (flushing, itching) and the risk of hepatotoxicity at high doses limit patient and physician acceptance. Also relatively contraindicated in diabetes.
  - Bile acid resins are free of systemic side effects (not absorbed), but compliance is limited by taste and inconvenience of preparation. May increase TG in mixed hyperlipidemia.

- Consider estrogens in postmenopausal females.
- Gemfibrozil (Lopid) primarily is indicated for lowering TG or raising HDL; reserve for mixed hyperlipidemia. Not recommended for LDL lowering only.
- Probucol (Lorelco) is limited by poor bioavailability and a tendency to decrease HDL. However, it may slow atherogenesis by inhibiting oxidation of LDL.
- Combinations are acceptable if single drug fails to achieve LDL goal in 6–12 months.
- The relative efficacy of lipid-lowering drugs is both drug and dose dependent. Especially note dosage differences between various statins (see Tables 10.10 and 10.11). Table 10.12 lists monitoring parameters, adverse effects, and drug interactions with major cholesterol-lowering drugs.

HYPERTRIGLYCERIDEMIA
Clinical Presentation

- *Normal:* <150 mg/dL (1.69 mmol/L). Little risk unless >500 mg/dL (see Table 10.2).
- Increased VLDL or chylomicrons.
- The primary symptom of hypertriglyceridemia is pancreatitis (abdominal pain) and eruptive xanthomas. Hypertriglyceridemia alone is a small risk factor for CHD. Hypertriglyceridemia associated with any of the following is a definite risk factor for CHD: Strong family history of CHD, elevated LDL, low HDL, smoking history, diabetes, or chronic renal failure.

Treatment Principles

- **Step One.** Dietary restriction (decrease carbohydrates, restrict alcohol, and restrict saturated fats). (See Table 10.6.)
- **Step Two.** Remove offending drugs (see Table 10.7).
- **Optimize insulin therapy** in patients with diabetes to enhance lipoprotein lipase activity.
- **Drugs of Choice.** Statins, fibrates (gemfibrozil or fenofibrate), and niacin are all effective triglyceride-lowering agents. Avoid bile acids since they may increase triglyceride.
  - Patients with hypertriglyceridemia and normal cholesterol: Fibrates may be drug of choice here. Niacin most effective and least expensive, but most side effects; avoid in diabetes. Combinations may be required if severe. Caution regarding increased myositis risk with combined statin plus fibrate.
  - Patients with combined hypertriglyceridemia and elevated LDL-C: Both statins and niacin lower both LDL-C and TG, but statins better tolerated. Atorvastatin was first statin approved for TG lowering, but all are effective with varying dose-response relationships. Effects of fibrates on LDL-C are complex. They may lower LDL-C 10–25% in patients with normal TG, but have less effect or even paradoxically raise LDL-C in patients with combined disease.

Fish Oils

Fish oils are rich in omega-3 polyunsaturated fatty acids (linolenic acid). They decrease the synthesis and enhance clearance of VLDL. The effects on LDL are varied: synthesis of LDL is reduced, but LDL may paradoxically increase as VLDL metabolism is enhanced. The effects on HDL are variable. Fish oil supplements are of little value unless combined with a proper diet containing several fish meals per week. They appear to be equally as effective as vegetable oils (omega-6 fatty acids) in controlling lipids. Omega-3 fatty acids are metabolized to eichsopentanoeic acid and docosahexaenoic acid that compete with arachidonic acid for the cyclooxygenase enzyme. Thromboxane A_3 that is produced then competes with thromboxane A_2; inhibition of platelet aggregation and increased bleeding time may result. Although this may protect against coronary events and transient ischemic attacks, it also can increase the risk for intracranial bleeds. PGI_3, a prostacyclin analog that also is produced, has potent vasodilator activity and inhibits platelet aggregation.

Notes:

Table 10.1 • Classification and Properties of Plasma Lipoproteins[a]

	Chylomicron[b]	VLDL[c]	LDL[d]	HDL[e]
Density (gm/mL)	<0.94	0.94–1.006	1.006–1.063	1.063–1.210
Composition (%)				
Protein (PR)	1–2	6–10	18–22	45–55
Triglyceride	85–95	50–65	4–8	2–7
Cholesterol	3–7	20–30	51–58	18–25
Phospholipid (PL)	3–6	15–20	18–24	26–32
Physiologic origin	Intestine (dietary)	Intestine (dietary) and liver	End product of VLDL catabolism	Liver and intestine
Physiologic function	Transports dietary TG to liver	Transports endogenous TG and CH	Transports CH to extrahepatic cells	Transports CH from extrahepatic cells to liver
Plasma appearance	Cream layer	Turbid	Clear	Clear
Electrophoretic mobility	Origin	Prebeta	Beta	Alpha
Apolipoproteins	A-IV, B-48, C-I, C-II, C-III	B-100, C-I, C-II, C-III, E	B-100, (a)	A-I, A-II, A-IV

[a]CH = Cholesterol; HDL = High-density lipoprotein; LDL = Low-density lipoprotein; TG = Triglyceride; VLDL = Very low-density lipoprotein.
[b]Chylomicrons (exogenous triglycerides) are very, very low-density triglyceride-rich particles obtained from the diet. They are rapidly metabolized via hepatic lipase and lipoprotein lipase (LPL) enzymes.
[c]VLDL are triglyceride-rich particles derived primarily from hepatic synthesis (endogenous triglyceride). They contain nearly 100% of the total blood TG measured in fasting patients and 15–20% of total blood cholesterol.
[d]LDL carry two-thirds of body cholesterol ester. Transports cholesterol to tissues; associated with CHD. Most LDL is derived from metabolism of VLDL by LPL to a "cholesterol-rich remnant." LDL is associated with atherosclerosis only after it is oxidized in vascular cell walls to foam cells. Small dense LDL is most atherogenic.
[e]HDL also is called α-lipoprotein; carries 15% of total body cholesterol. Picks up (scavenges) cholesterol from tissues and returns it to the liver for metabolism; high levels of HDL cholesterol protect against CHD. ↑ by aerobic exercise and estrogen (especially premenopause). HDL$_2$ is most protective.

Notes:

Table 10.2 • Classification of Lipid Values for Selecting Adults at Risk[a]

Risk	TC	LDL-C[b]	HDL-C	TG
Optimal (especially high risk patients)	<150 mg/dL (<3.88 mmol/L)	<100 mg/dL (<2.58 mmol/L)	>60 mg/dL[c] (>1.58 mmol/L)	
Normal (above optimal for high risk patients)	150–200 mg/dL (3.88–5.17 mmol/L)	100–129 mg/dL (2.58–3.33 mmol/L)	40–60 mg/dL (1.05–1.58 mmol/L)	<150 mg/dL
Borderline high risk	200–239 mg/dL[c] (5.18–6.19 mmol/L)	130–159 mg/dL (3.36–4.11 mmol/L)	<40 mg/dL (<1.05 mmol/L)	150–199 mg/dL
High risk	>240 mg/dL (>6.20 mmol/L)	160–189 mg/dL (4.14–4.88 mmol/L)	<35 mg/dL (<0.92 mmol/L)	200–499 mg/dL
Very high risk		>190 mg/dL (>4.91 mmol/L)	<30 mg/dL (<0.78 mmol/L)	>500 mg/dL[d]

[a]CHD = Coronary heart disease; HDL-C = High density lipoprotein cholesterol; LDL-C = Low density lipoprotein cholesterol; TG = Triglyceride; TC = Total cholesterol.
[b]LDL-C = TC − (TG/5 + HDL-C). Desirable LDL-C:HDL-C ratio = <2.
[c]HDL-C >60 mg/dL may be cardioprotective. Premenopausal women may have TC >200 mg/dL, but may actually have low risk because of a high HDL-C (>100 mg/dL) and a low LDL-C.
[d] ↑ TG alone is a smaller contributor to CHD than LDL-C. Combined ↑ LDL-C and/or ↓ HDL-C with an ↑ TG is an additive and significant risk factor, especially if diabetes also present. TG >1000 mg/dL may cause acute pancreatitis.

Table 10.3 • Characteristics of Common Lipid Disorders[a]

Disorder	Metabolic Defect	Lipid Effect	Main Lipid Parameter	Diagnostic Features
Familial hyper-cholesterolemia (heterozygous)[b]	Dysfunctional or absent LDL receptors	↑ LDL-C	LDL-C: 250–450 mg/dL	Fam Hx, CHD, tendon xanthomas, arcus senilus
Familial defective apoB-100	Defective apoB on LDL and VLDL	↑ LDL-C	LDL-C: 250–450 mg/dL	Fam Hx, CHD, tendon xanthomas
Dysbetalipopro-teinemia (Type III hyperlipidemia)	ApoE2:E2 pheno-type, ↓ VLDL remnant clearance	↑ remnant VLDL, ↑ IDL	LDL-C: 300–600 mg/dL TG: 400–800 mg/dL	Palmar xanthomas, tuberoeruptive xanthomas
Polygenic hyper-cholesterolemia[c]	↓ LDL clearance	↑ LDL-C	LDL-C: 160–250 mg/dL	None distinctive
Familial combined hyperlipidemia[d]	↑ apoB and VLDL production	↑ CH, TG, or both	LDL-C: 250–350 mg/dL TG: 200–800 mg/dL	Fam Hx, CHD Fam Hx, hyperlipidemia
Familial hyperapo-betalipoproteinemia	↑ apoB production	↑ apoB	ApoB: >125 mg/dL	None distinctive
Hypoalphalipopro-teinemia	↑ HDL catabolism	↓ HDL-C	HDL-C: <35 mg/dL	None distinctive

[a]ApoB = Apolipoprotein B; ApoE = Apolipoprotein E; CH = Cholesterol; CHD = Coronary heart disease; Fam Hx = Family history; HDL = High-density lipoprotein; HDL-C = High-density lipoprotein cholesterol; IDL = Intermediate-density lipoprotein; LDL = Low-density lipoprotein; LDL-C = Low-density lipoprotein cholesterol; TG = Triglyceride; VLDL = Very low-density lipoprotein.
[b]0.2% of U.S. population have heterozygous pattern of 50% reduction in LDL receptor. Very rare = total absence of LDL receptors with LDL-C >450 mg/dL, and premature death. Arcus senilus = cholesterol deposits in iris of eye.
[c]25%–36% of U.S. population. Most prevalent disorder.
[d]1%–2% of U.S. population.

Table 10.4 • Coronary Heart Disease Risk Factors[a]

Positive Risk Factors (↑ Risk)
- Age: Male ≥45 yr
  Female ≥55 yr or premature menopause without estrogen replacement therapy

- Family history of premature CHD (definite MI), or sudden death before 55 yr in father or other male 1st-degree relative or before 65 yr in mother or other female 1st-degree relative

- Current cigarette smoking

- Hypertension (≥140/90 mm Hg or on antihypertensive drugs)

- Low HDL cholesterol (<35 mg/dL)

  Negative Risk Factor (↓ Risk, Protective)
- High HDL cholesterol (≥60 mg/dL)

[a]CHD = Coronary heart disease; HDL = High density lipoprotein; LDL = Low density lipoprotein; MI = Myocardial infarction. In the guidelines released in 2001, presence of diabetes is considered a CHD risk equivalent and thus is *not counted* when conducting a risk assessment for the purpose of identifying the LDL-C goal (see Table 10.5). Obesity is not counted as a risk factor, but may contribute to insulin resistance, hypertension, and other risk factors.

Table 10.5 • Treatment Decisions Based on LDL-C

Goal	Therapeutic Lifestyle Intervention Indicated	Consider Drug Therapy	Primary Goal LDL-C Treatment Goal	Secondary Goal Non–HDL-C[a] Treatment Goal
No CHD with 0–1 risk factors	≥130 mg/dL	≥190 mg/dL	<160 mg/dL	<190 mg/dL
No CHD with ≥2 risk factors[b]				
a. 10 yr CHD risk 10–20%	≥130 mg/dL	≥130 mg/dL	<130 mg/dL	<160 mg/dL
b. 10 yr CHD risk <10%	≥130 mg/dL	≥160 mg/dL	<130 mg/dL	<160 mg/dL
With CHD or CHD equivalent or 10 yr CHD risk >20%[c]	>100 mg/dL	≥130 mg/dL	≤100 mg/dL	<130 mg/dL

[a]Non-HDL-C = Total Cholesterol – HDL cholesterol. The secondary treatment goal is triggered when a fasting triglyceride level of >200 mg/dL or an HDL-C <40 mg/dL is encountered.
[b]Patients with two or more risk factors (see Table 10.4) should receive a global risk assessment. Patients with a 10–20% risk of a CHD event in 10 years via global risk assessment have a lower LDL-C goal than those with <10% risk. Those with a >20% 10 year risk move to the CHD equivalent category (see footnote c).
[c]CHD equivalent includes primary prevention patients who have diabetes, peripheral vascular disease or a >20% risk of a CHD event in 10 years via global assessment.
CHD = Coronary heart disease; HDL-C = High density lipoprotein cholesterol; LDL-C = Low density lipoprotein cholesterol.

Notes:

Table 10.6 • Diet Therapy for High Blood Cholesterol[a]

Nutrient	Recommended Intake
Total Fat	25–30% of total daily calories
Saturated fats[b]	<7% of total daily calories
Polyunsaturated fats[c]	Up to 10% of total daily calories
Monounsaturated fats[d]	Up to 20% of total daily calories
Carbohydrates[e]	55–60% of total daily calories
Carbohydrate fiber	20–30 g/day
Protein	~15% of total daily calories
Cholesterol[f]	<200 mg/day
Total calories	Adjust to maintain normal body weight
Physical activity	Expend 200 calories/day

[a]Allow 6 weeks to adapt to diet and physical activity. A total of 12 weeks is generally required to fully implement and assess diet changes. LDL-C may reduce by 5–14% with diet and exercise.
[b]Saturated fats primarily from animal sources. Fish, veal, poultry without skin lower in saturated fat. Coconut and palm oils are low in cholesterol, but high in saturated fats.
[c]Polyunsaturated fats from vegetable sources. Trans fatty acids (e.g., hard margarines) should be avoided: high in calories and raise LDL-C.
[d]Monounsaturated fats: olive oil, canola oil, and fish products. Also rich in omega-3 fatty acids.
[e]Preferred carbohydrates sources: whole grains, fruit, and vegetables. Avoid high sugar, high calorie "fast foods." May reduce carbohydrates to 40–50% and raise monounsaturated fats to 20% in patients with diabetes.
[f]200 mg cholesterol = 1 egg (but low in saturated fat). Also high in organ meats.

Table 10.7 • Drug-Induced Hyperlipidemia[a]

Drug	Effect on Plasma Lipids Cholesterol	Triglycerides	HDL-C	Comments
Diuretics Thiazides	↑ 5%–7%, initially, ↑ 0%–3% later	↑ 30%–50%	↑ 1%	Effects transient. Monitor for long-term effects.
Loop	No change	No change	↓ to 15%	
Indapamide	No change	No change	No change	
Metolazone	No change	No change	No change	
Potassium sparing	No change	No change	No change	
β-Blockers Nonselective	No change	↑ 20%–50%	↓ 10%–15%	Nonselective β-blockers have greater effects than selective. β-blockers with ISA or α-blocking effects are lipid neutral.
Selective	No change	↑ 15%–30%	↓ 5%–10%	
α-Blocking	No change or ↓	No change	No change	
α-Agonists and antagonists (e.g., prazosin and clonidine)	↓ 0%–10%	↓ 0%–20%	↓ 0%–15%	In general, drugs which affect α receptors ↓ cholesterol and ↑ HDL-C.
ACE[a] Inhibitors	No change	No change	No change	
Calcium Channel Blockers	No change	No change	No change	

(continued)

Table 10.7 • Drug-Induced Hyperlipidemia[a] (continued)

Drug	Effect on Plasma Lipids Cholesterol	Triglycerides	HDL-C	Comments
Oral Contraceptives				
Monophasics	↑ 5%–20%	↑ 10%–45%	↑ 15% to ↓ 15%	Effects due to reduced lipolytic activity and/ or ↑ VLDL synthesis. Mainly due to progestin component.
Triphasics	↑ 10%–15%	↑ 10%–15%	↑ 5%–10%	
Glucocorticoids	↑ 5%–10%	↑ 15%–20%	—	
Ethanol	No change	↑ up to 50%	—	Marked elevations can occur in hypertriglyceridemic patients.
Isotretinoin	↑ 5%–20%	↑ 50%–60%	↓ 10%–15%	Chances may reverse 8 weeks after drug is DC.
Cyclosporine	↑ 15%–20%	No change	No change	

[a]ACE = Angiotensin-converting enzyme; DC = Discontinued; HDL-C = High-density lipoprotein cholesterol; ISA = Intrinsic sympathomimetic activity.

Table 10.8 • Drugs of Choice for Dyslipidemia[a]

Lipid Disorder	Single Drugs of Choice	Combination Drugs of Choice
Polygenic hypercholesterolemia with desirable TGs and HDL-C	Statin or bile acid resin or niacin	Statin + resin or statin + niacin or resin + niacin
Familial hypercholesterolemia with desirable TGs and HDL-C	Statin or bile acid resin or niacin	Statin + resin or statin + niacin or resin + niacin
Mixed hyperlipidemia in nondiabetic patients (↑ LDL-C and ↑ TGs)	Statin or niacin or fibrate[b]	Statin + niacin or statin + fibrate[c] or niacin + resin or niacin + fibrate
Mixed hyperlipidemia in diabetic patients (↑ LDL-C and ↑ TGs)	Statin or fibrate	Statin + fibrate[c] or statin + resin or fibrate + resin
Polygenic hypercholesterolemia with isolated low HDL	Statin or niacin or estrogen (postmenopausal women)	Statin + niacin

[a]HDL = High-density lipoprotein; HDL-C = High-density lipoprotein cholesterol; LDL-C = Low-density lipoprotein cholesterol; TGs = Triglyceride.
[b]Effects of fibrates on LDL-C are complex. They may lower LDL-C 10–25% in patient with normal TG, but have less effect or even paradoxically raise LDL-C in patients with combined disease.
[c]Use statin + fibrate combination cautiously as there is an increased risk of myopathy. Fibrates relatively ineffective in lowering LDL except in combination with other drugs.

Notes:

Table 10.9 • Dosages of Selected Lipid-Modulating Drugs

Drug	Initial Dosage	Usual Dosage	Maximum Dosage[a]	Comment
Cholestyramine	4 g before main meal	4 g BID before heaviest meals	8 g BID before heaviest meals	May prescribe 24 g/day, but few patients can tolerate.
Colestipol	5 g powder or 2 g tabs QD before main meal	5 g of powder or 4 g of tabs BID before heaviest meals	10 g powder or 8 g of tabs BID before heaviest meals	May prescribe 30 g of powder per day, but few patients can tolerate.
Colesevelam	6 × 0.63 g tablets per day	Same	7 × 0.63 g tablets per day	Less bulk is associated with less gastrointestinal intolerance.
Niacin	100–125 mg BID with food	750–1,000 mg BID	1,500 mg BID	Dosages up to 6 g/day have been used, but few can tolerate. Dosages may be increased 200–250 mg/day every 3–7 days until desired dosage has been obtained.
Atorvastatin	10 mg QD	10–20 mg QD	80 mg QD	Administer any time of day.
Cerivastatin	0.4 mg Q PM	0.4 mg Q PM	0.8 mg Q PM	Removed from market by FDA
Fluvastatin	20–40 mg QHS	20–40 mg QHS	40 mg BID	Modified-release form with similar efficacy and less bioavailability (and less risk of adverse effects) is currently under development for delivering the top dose.
Lovastatin	20 mg with dinner	20–40 mg with dinner	40 mg BID	Administration with food increases bioavailability.
Pravastatin	10–20 mg HS	10–20 mg HS	40 mg HS	Administer with food to reduce dyspepsia.
Simvastatin	20 mg Q PM	20–40 mg Q PM	80 mg Q PM	Administer with food to reduce dyspepsia.
Gemfibrozil	600 mg BID	Same	Same	
Fenofibrate	67–201 mg QD	Same	Same	

[a]The relative efficacy of lipid-lowering drugs is both drug and dose dependent (see Tables 10.10 and 10.11). Especially note dosage differences between various statins.

Table 10.10 • Average Effects of Selected Drugs on Lipoprotein Cholesterol and Triglycerides[a]

Drug	LDL	HDL	TG
Bile acid resins	−15%–30%	±3%	+3%–10%
Niacin	−15%–30%	+20%–35%	−30%–60%
Statin	−25%–60%	+5%–15%	−10%–45%
Estrogens[b]	−10%–25%	+10%–20%	+10%–50%
Fibrates[c]	±10%	+10%–30%	−20%–50%

[a] HDL = High-density lipoprotein; LDL = Low-density lipoprotein; TG = Triglyceride.
[b] Caution: recent evidence indicates lack of cardiovascular protection and possibly increased risk when used for secondary prevention.
[c] Fibrates = gemfibrozil (Lopid) and fenofibrate (TriCor).

Table 10.11 • Dose-Related LDL-C Lowering of Major Drugs

Drug	Daily Dosage	LDL-C Lowering
Bile acid resins (colestipol)	5 g	−15%
	10 g	−23%
	15 g	−27%
Niacin (crystalline)	1,000 mg	−6%
	1,500 mg	−13%
	2,000 mg	−16%
	3,000 mg	−22%
Atorvastatin	10 mg	−39%
	20 mg	−43%
	40 mg	−50%
	80 mg	−60%
Cerivastatin[a]	0.2 mg	−25%
	0.3 mg	−31%
	0.4 mg	−34%
	0.8 mg	−44%
Fluvastatin	20 mg	−22%
	40 mg	−24%
	80 mg	−34%
Lovastatin	20 mg	−24%
	40 mg	−34%
	80 mg	−40%
Pravastatin	10 mg	−22%
	20 mg	−32%
	40 mg	−34%
Simvastatin	5 mg	−26%
	10 mg	−30%
	20 mg	−38%
	40 mg	−41%
	80 mg	−47%

[a] Removed from market by FDA following deaths associated with rhabdomyolysis.

Notes:

Table 10.12 • Monitoring Parameters, Adverse Effects, and Drug Interactions with Major Cholesterol-Lowering Drugs[a]

Drug	Adverse Effects	Drug Interactions	Monitoring Parameters
Bile acid resin	Indigestion, bloating, nausea, constipation, abdominal pain, flatulence. May ↑ TG	GI binding and reduced absorption of anionic drugs, including fat-soluble vitamins, warfarin, beta blockers, digitoxin, thyroxine, thiazide diuretics. (Administer drugs 1–2 hr before or 4 hr after bile acid resin)[b]	Lipid profile Q 4–8 wk until control; then TC Q 6–12 months long-term. Check TG level after stable dose achieved, then PRN.
Niacin[c]	Flushing, itching, tingling, headache, nausea, gas, heartburn, fatigue, rash, worsening of peptic ulcer, elevation in serum glucose and uric acid, hepatitis and elevation in hepatic transaminase levels	Hypotension with BP-lowering drugs, such as alpha blockers, possible. Diabetics on insulin or oral agents may require dose adjustment because of ↑ in serum glucose levels	Lipid profile after 1000–1500 mg/day and then after stable dosage achieved; then TC Q 6–12 months long-term. LFTs at baseline and Q 6–8 wk for 1st yr, then PRN symptoms. Uric acid and glucose at baseline and again after stable dose reached (or symptoms produced), more frequently in diabetics. Monitor sitting and standing BP in hypertensive and elderly patients.
Statins	Headache, dyspepsia, myositis (myalgia + CPK >10 × normal), elevation in hepatic transaminase levels	Increased myositis risk with concurrent use of drugs that inhibit or compete for P450 3A4 system (e.g., cyclosporine, erythromycin, calcium blockers, fibrates, nefazodone, niacin, ketoconazole); risk greater with lovastatin and simvastatin; caution with concurrent fibrate or niacin use; lovastatin increases the protime with concurrent warfarin	Lipid profile Q 4–8 wk after dose change, then TC Q 6–12 months long-term. LFTs at baseline and Q 6–8 wk for 1st yr, then PRN symptoms. Measure CPK if patient has symptoms of myalgia.

[a]BP = Blood pressure; CPK = Creatine phosphokinase; GI = Gastrointestinal; LFTs = Liver function tests; TC = Total cholesterol; TG = Triglyceride.
[b]Binding of other drugs and vitamins less with colesevelam than with cholestyramine and colestipol.
[c]Niacin–related flushing, itching may be reduced by taking each dose with 325 mg aspirin. Liver toxicity greatest with SR preparation, especially if dose >1500 mg/day.

Notes:

The reader is referred to Chapter 11: Dyslipidemias, written by *Jam...* in the seventh edition of **Applied Therapeutics: The Clinical U**... in-depth discussion. Other topics included in his chapter include effect... insulin resistance syndrome, hypertension management in patients with a... other complex mixed disorders. The editors of this handbook express their... McKenney and acknowledge that this chapter is based upon his work.

Notes:

Chapter 11

Essential Hypertension

Blood Pressure (BP): Classification and Measurement

♦ **Classification.** Table 11.1 lists the classification scheme for hypertension advocated by the 6th report of the Joint National Committee on Detection, Evaluation and Treatment of High Blood Pressure (JNC VI). A systolic pressure (SBP) >140 mm Hg or a diastolic pressure (DBP) >90 mm Hg is a cause for concern.

♦ Most treatment guidelines are based upon the diastolic reading, but some patients (especially the elderly or those with aortic valve dysfunction) have isolated systolic hypertension (SBP ≥140 mm Hg) with a normal diastolic pressure (<90 mm Hg)

♦ Mean arterial pressure (MAP) $= \dfrac{(SBP - DBP)}{3} + DBP$

♦ **Measurement.** Table 11.4 and Figure 11.1 detail the proper technique for measuring blood pressure and the types of sounds heard when deflating the BP cuff.

♦ **Primary versus Secondary Hypertension.** There is no identifiable cause in the majority of hypertensive cases (primary hypertension). However, in some instances, a causative factor, including drug-induced hypertension, is present. These secondary causes of hypertension should be treated or removed, if possible, before beginning other therapies. (See Table 11.3.)

Treatment

♦ **Goals of Therapy.** The treatment goals of hypertension are to normalize pressure (<140/90), avoid hypotension or other adverse drug effects, and prevent or retard end-organ damage (heart, kidney, brain, eyes). The goal value is more aggressive (<130/85) in patients with diabetes and other high-risk populations (Table 11.2).

Caution: Hypertension often is asymptomatic; headaches and nose bleeds are not reliable signs of hypertension.

♦ **The JNC VI algorithm** for selecting hypertension therapy is found in Figure 11.2. Lifestyle modification (nondrug therapy) should be initiated before starting drug therapy in low-risk patients. (See Table 11.5). Drug therapy is started sooner in **higher-risk patients.** (See Tables 11.6 to 11.8.) Any of the drugs listed may be used as monotherapy, although diuretics or beta blockers generally are recommended first. Direct vasodilators (e.g., hydralazine) and α_2–agonists (e.g., clonidine) are not recommended as monotherapy because their effect is limited by salt and water retention or adverse effects. They require coadministration of a diuretic for optimal effect.

◆ ***Individualization of Drug Therapy.*** A modification of the stepped-care approach individualizes drug therapy to patient characteristics and/or coexisting disease. Some of the variables to consider are:

Age. Younger patients may respond better to beta blockers than the elderly. Older patients may respond better to diuretics, angiotensin-converting enzyme (ACE) inhibitors, or calcium blockers than to beta blockers. The elderly exhibit more side effects and should be started on lower doses (e.g., 12.5 mg hydrochlorothiazide, 6.25 mg captopril).

Race. Blacks have a higher incidence of hypertension, often at an earlier age, and it is more severe. They may respond better to diuretics or calcium blockers than to beta blockers or ACE inhibitors. Beta blockers may be added as part of combination therapy or if other diseases indicate a need. Whites may respond best to beta blockers and ACE inhibitors.

Concurrent Diseases. Various disease states either may be improved by the proper choice of drug therapy or worsened by improper choice. (See Table 11.9.) Whenever possible, an agent that benefits more than one condition should be chosen. (See Figure 11.2.)

Lipid Status. Diuretics may increase serum cholesterol and triglyceride levels. Beta blockers may increase triglycerides and lower high-density lipoprotein cholesterol. These changes are dose related and often transient. The clinical significance of these biochemical changes is unknown.

◆ ***Antihypertensive Drugs***

Diuretics remain a first-line choice of therapy. They are effective as single drug therapy for diastolic pressure <100 mm Hg. Diuretics also are used as adjuvant therapy for those drugs that cause fluid retention. Despite the large number of different thiazide diuretics, none are superior in efficacy or less expensive than hydrochlorothiazide. Potassium-sparing diuretics have a minimal BP lowering effect, but are used in combination with thiazides to minimize potassium loss. (See Tables 11.10 and 11.18.)

Beta blockers are especially useful in younger patients, those with concurrent angina, vascular headaches, or postmyocardial infarction. The availability of a large number of different beta blockers with varying pharmacokinetic and pharmacodynamic variables can be confusing. However, they all appear to be equal in their antihypertensive efficacy. Propranolol remains the gold standard because of the availability of inexpensive generic products. The longer-acting products (atenolol, nadolol) and those with relative β_1 selectivity (atenolol, metoprolol) are widely used. (See Tables 11.11, 11.12, and 11.18.)

ACE inhibitors, angiotensin II receptor antagonists, and calcium channel blockers (CCBs) are equally effective as diuretics and beta blockers as first-line drugs. Their primary drawback is higher cost. (See Tables 11.13 to 11.16.) Recent epidemiologic evidence suggests that high-dose, immediate-release CCBs may be associated with an increased incidence of angina or myocardial infarction. Until this risk is better defined, avoid doses >30 mg of immediate-release nifedipine (or equivalent doses of other CCBs). Sustained release dosage forms appear to be safer.

Other Drugs. A variety of other drugs are available for either single-drug therapy or adjuvant therapy of hypertension. Table 11.17 summarizes the mechanism of action of available products, and usual doses for these drugs. Table 11.18 lists the common side effects and contraindications.

◆ ***Discontinuing Drug Therapy.*** After several months or years of continuous good hypertension control in patients with mild hypertension, cautious step-down or discontinuation of therapy may be considered. Even then, nondrug treatment should continue. Rapid discontinuation of therapy can result in a gradual or abrupt return of blood pressure to pretreatment levels. Rarely, a rebound hypertensive crisis may occur after withdrawal from high-dose clonidine (>0.6 mg/day) or beta blockers.

Patient Education

Noncompliance is a major cause of poor response to antihypertensive therapy. Appropriate counseling and patient follow-up are needed to understand the risks of untreated hypertension and to minimize the side effects of drugs. (See Table 11.19 for Patient Education principles.)

Table 11.1 • Classification of Blood Pressure for Adults Aged 18 Years and Older[a]

Category	Systolic (mm Hg)		Diastolic (mm Hg)
Optimal[b]	<120	and	<80
Normal	<130	and	<85
High-normal	130–139	or	85–89
Hypertension[c]			
Stage 1	140–159	or	90–99
Stage 2	160–179	or	100–109
Stage 3	>180	or	≥110

[a]Not taking antihypertensive drugs and not acutely ill. When systolic and diastolic pressures fall into different categories, the higher category should be selected to classify the patient's blood pressure status. For instance, 160/92 mm Hg should be classified as stage 2 hypertension, and 174/120 mm Hg should be classified as stage 3. Isolated systolic hypertension is defined as a systolic blood pressure of ≥140 mm Hg and diastolic blood pressure of <90 mm Hg and staged appropriately (e.g., 170/82 mm Hg is defined as stage 2 isolated systolic hypertension). In addition to classifying stages of hypertension on the basis of average blood pressure levels, clinicians should specify presence or absence of target-organ disease and additional risk factors. This specificity is important for risk classification and management.
[b]Optimal blood pressure with respect to cardiovascular risk is below 120/80 mm Hg. However, unusually low readings should be evaluated for clinical significance.
[c]Based on the average of two or more readings taken at each of two or more visits after an initial screening.

Table 11.2 • Goal BP Values for Patients with Hypertension

Subclassification/ Comorbid Conditions	Goal Blood Pressure Value
Uncomplicated hypertension	<140/90 mm Hg
Diabetes or congestive heart[a]	<130/85 mm Hg
Renal insufficiency/failure[a]	<130/85 mm Hg, or <125/75 mm Hg if proteinuria >1 g/day
Isolated systolic hypertension	Interim goal systolic pressure <160 mm Hg, long-term goal systolic pressure <140 mm Hg

[a]The JNC VI recommends drug therapy for patients with heart failure, renal insufficiency, or diabetes if blood pressure is in the high-normal range (≥130/85 mm Hg).

Notes:

Table 11.3 • Secondary Causes of Hypertension

Renal Disease
Renoparenchymal disease
Renovascular disease

Coarctation of the Aorta

Primary Aldosteronism

Cushing's Syndrome (Hyperadrenalism)

Pheochromocytoma (Adrenal Tumor)

Pregnancy

Increased Intracranial Pressure

Drug-induced
Adrenalcorticosteroids
Alcohol
Amphetamines/anorexiants (e.g., phentermine, sibutramine)
Appetite suppressants (including some herbal products containing ephedra, caffeine, and MaHuang)
Cyclosporine
Estrogens
Licorice
MAOIs
NSAIDs
Oral contraceptives
Oral decongestants (e.g., phenylpropanolamine, pseudoephedrine)
Thyroid hormone excess
TCAs
Venlafaxine

MAOIs = Monoamine oxidase inhibitors; NSAIDs = Nonsteroidal anti-inflammatory drugs; TCAs = Tricyclic antidepressants.

Table 11.4 • Recommended Technique for Blood Pressure Measurement

1. Patient should be seated for 5 minutes with arm bared, unrestricted by clothing, and supported at heart level. Smoking or food ingestion should not have occurred within 30 minutes before the BP measurement.
2. Choose the appropriate blood pressure cuff size for the patient. The bladder width should be at least 40% and the bladder length at least 80% of the upper arm circumference. Wrap the cuff snugly around the arm, with the bladder centered over the brachial artery.
3. Take measurements with a mercury sphygmomanometer, a recently calibrated aneroid manometer, or a validated electronic device.
4. Inflate the cuff to determine the SBP by observing the point at which the radial pulse is no longer palpable. Deflate the cuff and wait 15 to 30 seconds before reinflating.
5. Position the stethoscope over the brachial artery and rapidly inflate the cuff to 20 to 30 mm Hg above the point determined in Step 4. Deflate the cuff at a rate of 2 mm Hg per second, listening for phase I and phase V (phase IV for children) Korotkoff sounds. Phase V, at the disappearance of sound, is the DBP in adults. Listen for 10 to 20 mm Hg below phase V for any further sound, then deflate the cuff completely.
6. Record the BP in even numbers and document the patient's position, arm used, and cuff size.
7. Obtain two BP readings in the same arm and average them. Allow 1 to 2 minutes to elapse before repeating the BP measurement. If the readings differ by >5 mm Hg, obtain additional measurements. The BP should be taken in both arms at the initial visit, with the BP taken in the arm with the higher reading at subsequent visits.

BP = Blood pressure; DBP = Diastolic blood pressure; SBP = Systolic blood pressure.

Notes:

Table 11.5 • Lifestyle Modifications for Hypertension Treatment or Prevention

Weight loss if overweight

Limiting alcohol intake (ethanol: ≤1 oz/day for men; <0.5 oz/day 1 for women and lower weight people)

Increasing aerobic exercise/activity (30 to 45 minutes most days of the week)

Reducing sodium intake (sodium: ≤2.4 g/day)

Maintaining an adequate intake of dietary potassium, calcium, and magnesium

Reducing daily intake of dietary saturated fat and cholesterol

Smoking cessation

Table 11.6 • Hypertension Risk Evaluation

Major Risk Factors	TOD/CCD
Family history of cardiovascular disease (women <65 years, men <55 years)	Heart disease (left ventricular hypertrophy, angina/prior myocardial infarction, prior coronary revascularization, heart failure)
Smoking	Stroke or transient ischemic attack
Dyslipidemia	Nephropathy
Diabetes mellitus	
Age >60 years	Peripheral arterial disease
Sex (men and postmenopausal women)	Retinopathy

CCD = Clinical cardiovascular disease; TOD = Target organ disease.

Table 11.7 • JNC VI Hypertension Risk Classification

Risk Group A	No major risk factors and no TOD/CCD
Risk Group B	At least one major risk factor other than diabetes and no TOD/CCD
Risk Group C	Diabetes and/or TOD/CCD (patients may have additional major risk factors)

CCD = Clinical cardiovascular disease; TOD = Target organ disease.

Table 11.8 • Hypertension Risk Stratification and Initial Treatment[a]

Blood Pressure Stages (mm Hg)	Risk Group A	Risk Group B	Risk Group C
High-normal (130–139/85–89)	Lifestyle modification	Lifestyle modification	Drug therapy[c]
Stage 1 (140–159/90–99)	Lifestyle modification (up to 12 months)	Lifestyle modification (up to 6 months)[b]	Drug therapy
Stages 2 and 3 (≥160/≥100)	Drug therapy	Drug therapy	Drug therapy

[a]Lifestyle modification is adjunctive therapy for all patients recommended for drug therapy.
[b]For patients with multiple risk factors, initial drug therapy with lifestyle modification should be considered.
[c]For patients with diabetes, heart failure, or renal insufficiency.

Table 11.9 • Individualized Drug Therapy Based Upon Special Patient Characteristics

Clinical Situation	Preferred Agent(s)	Requires Special Monitoring	Relatively or Absolutely Contraindicated
Angina pectoris	Beta blockers, calcium antagonists	High-dose, immediate-release nifedipine[d]	Direct vasodilators
Cardiac failure	Diuretics, ACE inhibitors	Beta blockers	Calcium antagonists, labetalol
Post-MI[a]	Beta blocker without ISA[a]	High-dose, immediate-release nifedipine[d]	Direct vasodilators
Renal artery stenosis[b]			ACE[a] inhibitors
Renal insufficiency			
Early renal insufficiency	ACE[a] inhibitors?[c]; calcium antagonists?[c]		Potassium supplements; potassium-sparing agents
Advanced renal insufficiency	Loop diuretics	ACE[a] inhibitors	Potassium supplements; potassium-sparing agents
Prostatic hypertrophy	α_1-antagonists	α_2-agonist, diuretic	
Sexual dysfunction		Diuretics, beta blocker	Guanethidine
Asthma, COPD[a]			Beta blockers, labetalol
Diabetes mellitus Type I		Beta blockers, diuretic	
Hyperlipidemia		Diuretics, beta blockers	
Vascular headaches	Beta blockers		Direct vasodilators
Depression, confusion		Beta blockers, α_2-agonists, reserpine	
Intention tremor	Beta blocker		

[a]ACE inhibitor = Angiotension-converting enzyme inhibitor; COPD = Chronic obstructive pulmonary disease; ISA = Intrinsic sympathomimetic activity; MI = Myocardial infarction.
[b]Either bilateral renal arterial disease or severe stenosis in artery to a solitary kidney.
[c]Encouraging data are emerging for these agents, but it is not known if they are superior to other antihypertensives.
[d]See statement regarding epidemiologic finding with nifedipine in Antihypertensive Drugs: Calcium Channel Blockers and ACE inhibitors.

Table 11.10 • Diuretics

Category	Selected Products	Usual Dosage Range (mg/day)[a]	Dosing Frequency
Thiazide	Chlorthalidone (Hygroton)	12.5–50	QD
	Hydrochlorothiazide (Esidrix, Hydrodiuril, Microzide)	12.5–50	QD
	Indapamide (Lozol)[b]	1.25–5	QD
	Metolazone (Zaroxolyn)	2.5–10	QD
Loop[b]	Bumetanide (Bumex)	0.5–4	QD to BID
	Ethacrynic acid (Edecrin)	25–100	BID to TID
	Furosemide (Lasix)	40–240	QD to BID
	Torsemide (Demadex)	5–100	QD to BID
Potassium-sparing	Amiloride (Midamor)	5–10	QD
	Spironolactone (Aldactone)	25–100	QD
	Triamterene (Dyrenium)	25–100	QD
Diuretic combinations	Triamterene/Hydrochlorothiazide (Maxide, Dyazide)	37.5–75/25–50	QD
	Spironolactone/Hydrochlorothiazide (Aldactazide)	25–50/25–50	QD
	Amiloride/Hydrochlorothiazide (Moduretic)	5/50	QD

[a]Geriatric patients may be more sensitive and require lower doses.
[b]Metolazone and loop diuretics are no more effective than thiazides, except in patients with renal insufficiency.

Table 11.11 • Pharmacodynamic Properties of β-Blocking Agents and Dosage Schedules[a]

Drug	Usual Dosage Range (mg/day)[b]	Daily Dosing Frequency[c]	Relative Selectivity[d]	Intrinsic Sympathomimetic Activity[e]	Lipid Solubility[f]
Atenolol (Tenormin)	25–100	1	++	0	Low
Acebutolol (Sectral)	200–1,200	2	++	+	Moderate[g]
Bisoprolol (Zebeta)	25–200	1	++	0	Low
Betaxolol (Kerlone)	5–20	1	++	0	Low
Carteolol (Cartrol)	2.5–10	1	0	++	Low
Carvedilol (Coreg)	12.5–50	2	0	0	High
Labetalol (Trandate, Normodyne)[h]	200–800	2	0	0	Moderate
Metoprolol (Lopressor)	50–200	1 or 2	+	0	Moderate to high
Nadolol (Corgard)	20–240	1	0	0	Low
Penbutolol (Levatol)	20–80	1	0	+	High
Pindolol (Visken)	10–60	2	0	+++	Moderate
Propranolol (Inderal)	40–240	2	0	0	High
Timolol (Blocadren)	20–40	2	0	0	Low to moderate

[a]All drugs listed are equally effective despite different pharmacodynamic properties.
[b]These dosage ranges are suggested. Higher doses have been used.
[c]All these drugs (even those with short t1/2) can be given once or twice daily for treatment of hypertension. There is no reason to use SR propranolol for treatment of hypertension.
[d]None are entirely β1 specific. Use cautiously in patients with asthma, COPD, or peripheral vascular insufficiency (e.g., Reynauds). Atenolol may be slightly more β1 specific at usual doses than are either acebutolol or metoprolol.
[e]ISA = Intrinsic sympathomimetic activity. Whether ISA has a protective effect in patients predisposed to bradycardia, CHF, or vasospasm is controversial. ISA also may protect against adverse lipid effects.
[f]Lipid solubility may predict other drug characteristics. Highly lipid-soluble agents have shortest t1/2, a greater percentage of hepatic metabolism, more variability in dose due to high presystemic (1st-pass) metabolism, and possibly more CNS side effects. Low lipid solubility drugs have longer t1/2, ↑ renal clearance, narrower dosage ranges, and possible ↓ CNS penetration.
[g]Acebutolol has an active metabolite of moderate lipid solubility.
[h]Concurrent alpha-blocking property of labetalol adds to antihypertensive effect since it counteracts vasoconstriction from beta blockade. Clinical relevance of this is not well documented. Alpha blockade also may be protective in peripheral vascular disease, asthma, or adverse disorders.

Table 11.12 • Pharmacokinetic Properties of β-Adrenoceptor Blockers

Drug	Absorption[a] (%)	Bioavailability[a] (%)	Metabolism/ Excretion	Protein Binding (%)	Half-Life[b] (hr)
Acebutolol	90	40	Hepatic/renal/ biliary	30–36	3–4
Atenolol	50	40	Renal	6–16	6–7
Betaxolol	100	89	Hepatic/renal	50	14–22
Bisoprolol	90	80	Hepatic/renal	30	9–12
Carteolol	80	85	Hepatic/renal	23–30	6
Carvedilol	90	25–35	Hepatic	95–98	6–10
Labetalol	100	30–40	Hepatic/renal	50	6–8
Metoprolol	95	50	Hepatic/renal	12	3–7
Nadolol	30	30	Renal	30	20–24
Penbutolol	100	100	Hepatic/renal	80–98	5
Pindolol	>95	87–90	Hepatic/renal	40	3–4
Propranolol	90	40	Hepatic	90	4
Timolol	90	61	Hepatic/renal	<10	4

[a]High absorption drug with low bioavailability indicates high presystemic (first-pass) hepatic metabolism, which roughly correlates with a more lipid-soluble drug. Conversely, less lipid-soluble drugs may have poor intrinsic absorption but little presystemic metabolism.
[b]The duration of antihypertensive effect exceeds the drug half-life and no more than twice-daily dosing is necessary.

Notes:

Table 11.13 • Angiotensin-Converting Enzyme (ACE) Inhibitors in Hypertension[a]

Drug	Starting Dose[b] (mg/day)	Usual Maintenance Dose Range (mg/day)	Dosing Frequency[c]	Onset (hr)	Duration (hr)	Elimination[d]
Benazepril (Lotensin)[e]	10	20–40	QD	1	24	Renal
Captopril (Capoten)	25	50–150	BID	0.25–0.5	2–12	50% hepatic
Enalapril (Vasotec)	5	10–40	QD	1	24	Renal
Fosinopril (Monopril)	10	20–40	QD	1	24	Hepatic/renal
Lisinopril (Prinivil, Zestril)	10	20–40	QD	1	24	100% renal
Moexipril (Univasc)	7.5	7.5–30	QD	1.5	24	Hepatic
Perindopril (Aceon)	4	4–8	QD	1.5	24	Hepatic/renal
Quinapril (Accupril)	10	20–80	QD	1	>30	Renal
Ramipril (Altace)	2.5	2.5–20	QD	1–2	24	Renal
Trandolapril (Mavik)	1	2–4	QD	4	24	Hepatic/renal

[a]All ACE inhibitors are equally effective. Also see Chapter 16: Heart Failure for further details on ACE inhibitors.
[b]Starting dose should be decreased 50% if patient is on a diuretic, has heart failure, or is being aggressively diuresed.
[c]When the higher doses are used, BID dosing for QD products and TID dosing for captopril may be needed.
[d]Only captopril and lisinopril active as parent drug. Benazepril, enalapril, fosinopril, moexipril, perindopril, quinapril, ramipril, and trandolapril are hepatically metabolized to active metabolites (benazeprilat, enalaprilat, fosinoprilat, moexiprilat, quinaprilat, ramiprilat) that are eliminated primarily renally. Fosinoprilat 50% via biliary excretion.
[e]Also available as combination with amlodipine (Lotrel) as 2.5/10, 5/10, 5/20 (amlodipine/benazepril).

Table 11.14 • Angiotensin II–Receptor Antagonists

Drug	Usual Dosage Range (mg/day)	Starting Dose (mg/day)	Dosing Frequency
Candesartan (Atacand)	4–32	16	QD
Irbesartan (Avapro)	75–300	75–150	QD
Losartan potassium (Cozaar)	25–100	25–50	QD to BID
Temisartan (Micardis)	20–80	40	QD
Valsartan (Diovan)	80–320	80	QD

Table 11.15 • Pharmacologic Actions of Calcium Channel Blockers

	Verapamil	Diltiazem	Dihydropyridines
Peripheral vasodilation	↑	↑	↑↑
Heart rate	↓↓	↓	↑
Cardiac contractility	↓↓	↓	0/↓[a]
SA/AV nodal conduction	↓	↓	0
Coronary blood flow	↑	↑	↑↑

[a]No significant decreases are seen with amlodipine,[217] and possibly felodipine.
↑ = increase, ↑↑ = marked increase, ↓ = decrease, ↓↓ = marked decrease, 0 = no change.

Table 11.16 • Calcium Channel Blockers

Drug	Usual Dosage Range (mg/day)	Dosing Frequency
Nondihydropyridines		
Diltiazem, immediate-release tablet (Cardizem, generic)	90–360	TID
Diltiazem, sustained-release capsule (Cardizem SR, Tiamate)	120–360	BID
Diltiazem, sustained-release capsule (Dilacor XR)[b]	120–480	QD
Diltiazem, sustained-release capsule (Cardizem CR, Tiazac)[b]	120–360	QD
Verapamil, immediate-release tablet (Calan, Isoptin, generic)	80–480	BID
Verapamil, sustained-release tablet (Calan SR, Isoptin SR, generic)[b]	120–480	QD to BID
Verapamil, sustained-release capsule (Verelan)[b]	120–480	QD to BID
Verapamil, controlled-onset extended-release tablet (Covera HS)[c]	180–480	QHS
Verapamil, chronotherapeutic oral drug absorption system (Verelan HS)[c]	100–400	QHS

(continued)

Notes:

Table 11.16 • Calcium Channel Blockers (continued)

Drug	Usual Dosage Range (mg/day)	Dosing Frequency
Dihydropyridines		
Amlodipine, immediate-release tablet (Norvasc)[d]	2.5–10	QD
Felodipine, extended-release tablet (Plendil)	2.5–10	QD
Isradipine, immediate-release capsule (DynaCirc)	5–10	BID
Isradipine, controlled-release tablet (DynaCirc CR)	5–10	QD
Nicardipine, immediate-release capsule (Cardene)	60–120	TID
Nicardipine, sustained-release capsule (Cardene SR)	60–120	BID
Nifedipine, sustained-release[e] tablet (Procardia XL, Adalat CC)	30–120	QD
Nisoldipine, extended-release tablet (Sular)	10–40	QD

Also see Tables 14.5 and 14.6 in Chapter 14: Ischemic Heart Disease.
[a]All calcium channel blockers (CCBs) are equally effective; they also have a mild diuretic effect. Note: immediate release (IR) diltiazem, nifedipine, and verapamil should be avoided in hypertension (HTN). Nimodipine also not indicated for HTN.
[b]Because of short t½ most of these drugs are given TID in immediate release forms. Many sustained release (SR) products exist but vary in release characteristics. Thus, they are not directly interchangeable. Diltiazem SR capsules and verapamil SR tabs still require BID dosing. Absorption of verapamil SR is more rapid and duration of action is shorter if taken on an empty stomach, further reducing its SR characteristics; generally must be given Q 12 hr with food to maintain SR release, even though total bioavailability is reduced. Diltiazem CD caps (copolymer-coated SR beads) release 40% of dose in first 12 hours and 60% over the next 12 hours, allowing QD dosing. Dilacor XR, made as SR tablets contained within a capsule, can be given QD. Procardia XL uses "GITs" technology and effectively releases drug over 24 hr. Adalat CC also releases over 24 hours but uses a core-coat release mechanism.
[c]Covera HS (a "GITs" formulation) and Verelan HS (a beaded capsule) are "chronotherapeutic" agents. An outer coating delays initial release for 4–5 hours with both, followed by sustained release. They are taken at bedtime but offer a peak response in the early AM when BP is often highest. Because they use different delivery systems, they are not interchangeable.
[d]Also available in combination with benazepril (Lotrel) as 2.5/5, 2.5/10, 5/10, and 5/20 mg (amlodipine/benazepril).
[e]Only sustained-release nifedipine is approved for hypertension. Immediate release should be avoided.

Table 11.17 • Other Drugs Used in Hypertension

Drugs/Mechanism of Action	Usual Dose
α₁-Blockers[a]	
Doxazosin (Cardura)	1–8 mg QD-BID
Prazosin (Minipress)	1–5 mg BID-TID
Terazosin (Hytrin)	1–5 mg QD-BID
α₂-Agonists (Central)	
Clonidine (Catapres)	0.1–0.6 mg QD-BID
Clonidine Transdermal (Catapres TTS)[b]	0.1–0.3 mg/24 hr Q wk
Guanabenz (Wytensin)	4–16 mg BID
Methyldopa (Aldomet)	250–500 mg BID-TID
Vasodilators[b]	
Hydralazine (Apresoline)	12.5–50 mg BID-TID
Minoxidil (Loniten)	2.5–10 mg BID-TID
Adrenergic Neuron Blockers	
Reserpine (Serpasil)	0.1–0.25 mg QD
Guanethidine (Ismelin)	10–50 mg QD
Guanadrel (Hylorel)	5–25 mg BID-TID

[a]Vasodilators may cause fluid retention and reflex tachycardia. May need concurrent diuretic and/or beta blocker therapy.
[b]Transdermal clonidine patch may ↓ incidence of side effects and ↑ compliance. Acceptability limited by skin rash.

Table 11.18 • Side Effects and Contraindications of Antihypertensive Agents

	Side Effects		
	Innocuous but Sometimes Annoying	Harmful or Potentially Harmful	Contraindications
Oral Diuretics Thiazide type	↑ urination (onset of therapy), weakness, muscle cramps (onset of therapy), hyperuricemia (sometimes with gout), GI disturbances	Hypokalemia,[a] hyponatremia,[b] hyperglycemia, hypercalcemia,[b] hypovolemia, azotemia,[b] (↑ BUN), skin rash[b] (cross-reacts with sulfa drugs), photosensitivity,[b] purpura,[b] marrow depression,[b] lithium toxicity[b] (patients on lithium therapy), pancreatitis, hypercholesterolemia, hypertriglyceridemia	Persistent anuria/ oliguria, advanced renal failure
Loop diuretics	↑ urination (onset of therapy), weakness, muscle cramps (onset of therapy), hyperuricemia (sometimes with gout), GI disturbances	Hypokalemia,[a] hyponatremia,[b] hyperglycemia, hypocalcemia,[b] hypovolemia, azotemia[b] (↑ BUN), skin rash[b] (cross-reacts with sulfa drugs), photosensitivity,[b] lithium toxicity[b] (patients on lithium therapy), pancreatitis, hypercholesterolemia, hypertriglyceridemia. Hearing loss with large IV doses	Not contraindicated in renal failure
Spironolactone	Hirsutism, menstrual irregularities, gynecomastia, GI disturbances	Hyperkalemia,[b] hyponatremia[b]	Renal failure, hyperkalemia, hyponatremia
Beta Blockers	Bradycardia, weakness, lethargy, GI disturbances	CHF (carvedolol, metoprolol approved for CHF), bronchospasm[b] (in patients with asthmatic propensity), hypoglycemia (nonselectives can mask the warning symptoms of or potentiate hypoglycemia), hyperglycemia (nonselectives can ↓ insulin secretion in Type II diabetes patients), aggravation of arterial insufficiency[b] (in patients with peripheral occlusive arterial disease), nightmares, insomnia,[b] impotence, hypertriglyceridemia, ↓ HDL	Asthma, 2nd or 3rd degree heart block, CHF (unless due to an arrhythmia amenable to therapy with propranolol or diastolic CHF), "brittle" diabetes mellitus
ACE Inhibitors (all)	Dizziness, faintness, lightheadedness (check orthostatic BP), palpitation, taste changes,[d] cough	Hypotension (more frequent in elderly), skin rash (disappears or discontinuation), proteinuria,[d] leukopenia[d]	Renal artery stenosis, volume depletion, pregnancy

(continued)

Table 11.18 • Side Effects and Contraindications of Antihypertensive Agents *(continued)*

| | Side Effects | | |
	Innocuous, but Sometimes Annoying	Harmful or Potentially Harmful	Contraindications
Angiotensin II Receptor Antagonist	Same as ACE inhibitors, except without cough	Same as ACE inhibitors	Same as ACE inhibitors
Calcium Channel Blockers			
Nifedipine, nicardipine, isradipine, felodipine	Dizziness, lightheadedness, headache, weakness, nausea	Peripheral edema, hypotension, tachycardia. Possibly angina or MI with high-dose, immediate-release nifedipine	Severe hypotension
Verapamil and diltiazem	Dizziness, lightheadedness, headache, weakness, nausea, constipation	AV block, bradycardia (may lead to CHF), digoxin interaction[f]	Severe CHF, 2nd or 3rd degree AV block, sick sinus syndrome, severe hypotension
α_1-Blockers	Headache, palpitation, dizziness	Sudden collapse and loss of consciousness related to orthostatic hypotension (usually after initial dose of prazosin; minimize by always using low 1st dose at bedtime)	None
α_2-Agonists	Dry mouth, drowsiness/lethargy, constipation, skin rash with transderm	"Rebound hypertension,"[g] parotid pain[a]	
Methyldopa	Drowsiness, lethargy, dry mouth, sexual difficulty, direct Coombs' test, nasal congestion	Abnormal liver function tests, hepatitis,[b] drug fever,[b] hemolytic anemia,[b] retroperitoneal fibrosis,[b] skin rash,[b] orthostatic hypotension, depression[b]	Coombs' positive hemolytic anemia, hepatic disease
Hydralazine	Tachycardia,[h] palpitation,[h] headache,[h] flushing,[h] nasal congestion, GI disturbances	Aggravation of angina,[b,h] lupus-like syndrome,[b] drug fever,[b] skin rash[b]	Symptomatic angina (unless used with propranolol)
Minoxidil	Tachycardia,[h] hypertrichosis, initial rise in plasma renin activity	Na and water retention (can lead to CHF or pulmonary edema), pericardial effusion	Advanced renal disease, limited to patients unresponsive to usual high BP therapy, pheochromocytoma
Reserpine	Bradycardia, lethargy, lassitude, nasal congestion	Depression,[b] activation of peptic ulcer,[b] parkinsonian state[b]	Depression (past or present), parkinsonism

(continued)

Notes:

Table 11.18 • Side Effects and Contraindications of Antihypertensive Agents *(continued)*

	Side Effects		
	Innocuous, but Sometimes Annoying	Harmful or Potentially Harmful	Contraindications
Guanethidine	Bradycardia, exercise hypotension (especially following meals), weakness, retrograde ejaculation or impotence, nasal congestion	Orthostatic hypotension, potentially harmful in patients with cerebral or myocardial ischemia and advanced renal insufficiency, drug sensitivity (rare)[b]	Interacts with TCAs, sympathomimetic amines

[a]Incidence of hypokalemia is 20%–30%. Routine use of potassium supplements and/or concurrent potassium-sparing diuretics should be discouraged unless hypokalemia is documented or the patient is taking digitalis glycoside.
[b]Usually requires cessation of therapy, at least temporarily.
[c]See text for predicting side effects and choice of beta blocker.
[d]Skin rash, proteinuria, leukopenia, and taste change are minimized by using low doses of captopril or any of the other ACE inhibitors. Also see Table 11.9 for use of ACE inhibitors in renal failure.
[e]Adverse reactions may be less frequent with diltiazem. Also see Chapter 14: Ischemic Heart Disease for further characterization of calcium channel blockers.
[f]Verapamil may ↑ digoxin levels. Also see Chapter 16: Congestive Heart Failure.
[g]Rebound hypertension worse after doses >0.6 mg/day.
[h]These side effects are minimized or prevented by coadministration of a beta blocker.

Table 11.19 • Patient Education[a]

Patient/Clinician Discussions
• Establish a BP goal

• High BP cannot be cured, only controlled

• Treatment should not be discontinued without medical consultation, and chronic treatment is usually necessary to control BP

• BP levels cannot be determined by the way a patient feels

• Potential adverse consequences of poor adherence to antihypertensive therapy and uncontrolled BP

• Patients should verbalize understanding of their diagnosis

• Encourage patients to openly discuss their medications and any problems or side effects

Clinical Responsibilities to Enhance Patient Education and Improve Patient Compliance
• Involve patients' families or caregivers in the treatment process

• Encourage patients to self-monitor BP

• Ask open-ended questions and provide encouragement for achieving goals

• Tailor treatment regimens to maximize compliance (i.e., QD or BID medications, dosage forms)

• Provide oral and written instructions and information on drug regimens and goals

• Provide alternative treatments and be willing to modify the patient's regimen

• Minimize cost of therapy

• Provide assistance to noncompliant patients (i.e., pillboxes, frequent follow-up visits, mail and/or telephone refill reminders)

• Contact patients who fail to attend follow-up appointments

• Collaborate with other health care providers (i.e., pharmacists, physicians, nutritionists, nurses)

[a]BP = Blood pressure.

Notes:

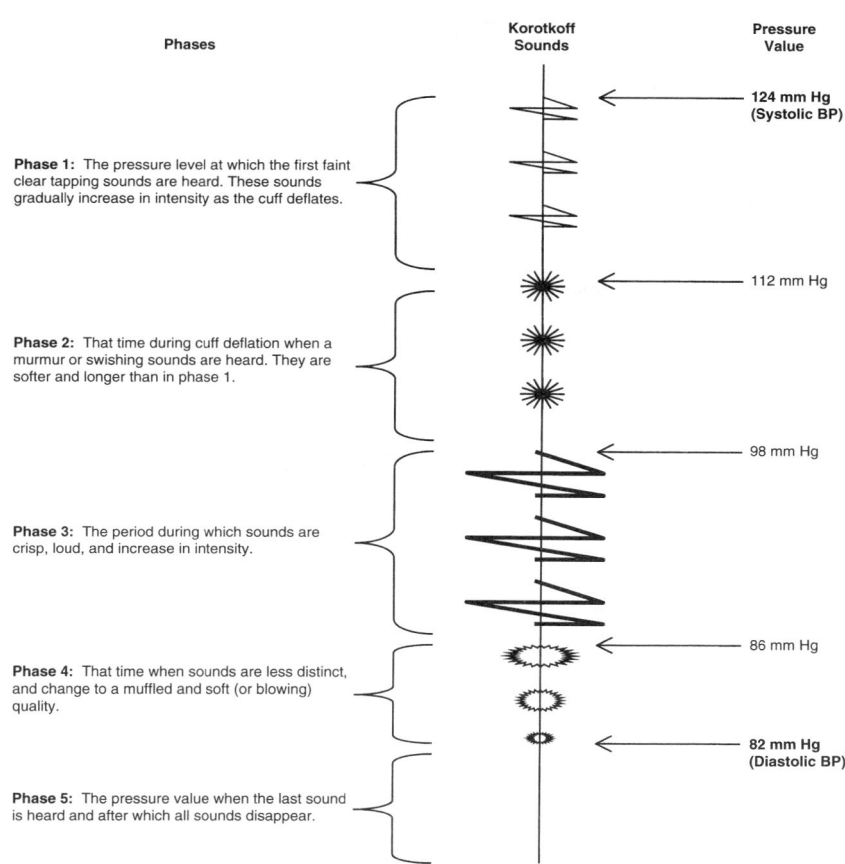

Fig. 11.1 Phases of the Korotkoff Sounds Heard When Indirectly Measuring Blood Pressure.

Notes:

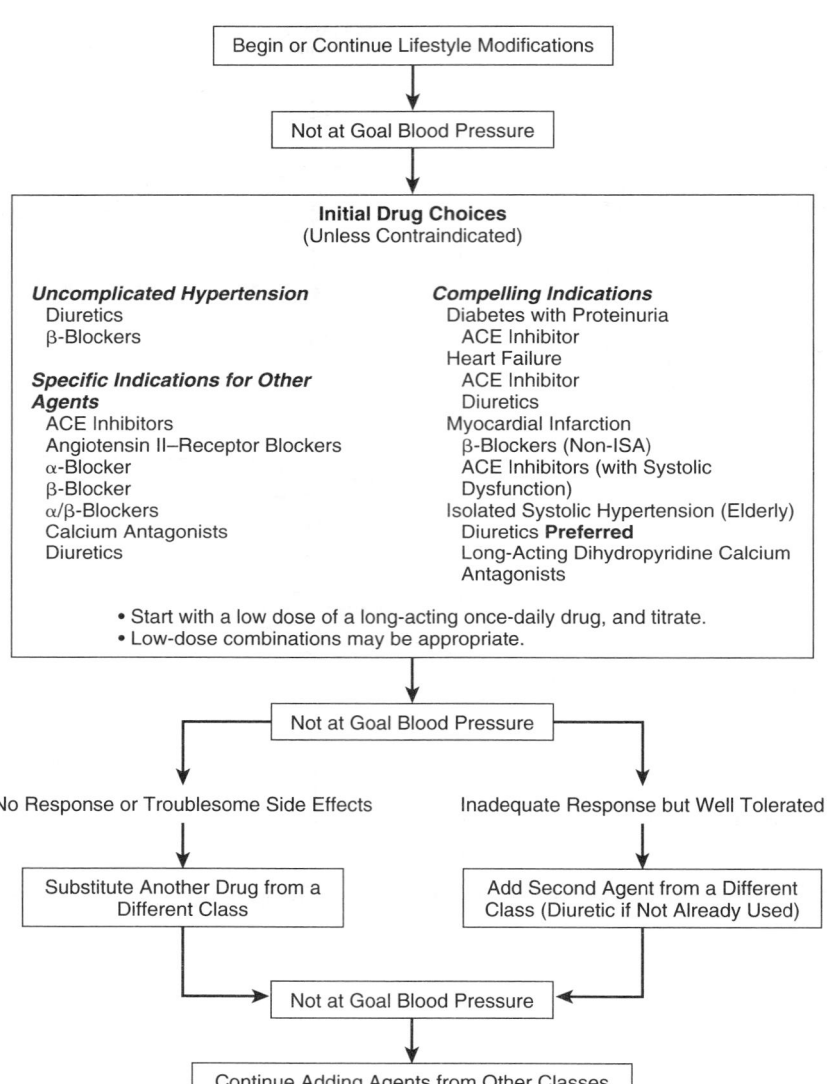

Begin or Continue Lifestyle Modifications

↓

Not at Goal Blood Pressure

↓

Initial Drug Choices
(Unless Contraindicated)

Uncomplicated Hypertension
Diuretics
β-Blockers

Specific Indications for Other Agents
ACE Inhibitors
Angiotensin II–Receptor Blockers
α-Blocker
β-Blocker
α/β-Blockers
Calcium Antagonists
Diuretics

Compelling Indications
Diabetes with Proteinuria
  ACE Inhibitor
Heart Failure
  ACE Inhibitor
  Diuretics
Myocardial Infarction
  β-Blockers (Non-ISA)
  ACE Inhibitors (with Systolic Dysfunction)
Isolated Systolic Hypertension (Elderly)
  Diuretics **Preferred**
  Long-Acting Dihydropyridine Calcium Antagonists

• Start with a low dose of a long-acting once-daily drug, and titrate.
• Low-dose combinations may be appropriate.

↓

Not at Goal Blood Pressure

No Response or Troublesome Side Effects

Inadequate Response but Well Tolerated

Substitute Another Drug from a Different Class

Add Second Agent from a Different Class (Diuretic if Not Already Used)

Not at Goal Blood Pressure

↓

Continue Adding Agents from Other Classes
Consider Referral to a Specialist

Fig. 11.2 JNC VI Treatment Algorithm for the Management of Hypertension.

Notes:

The reader is referred to Chapter 12: Essential Hypertension, written by *Joseph J. Saseen* and *Barry L. Carter, Pharm.D.*, in the seventh edition of **Applied Therapeutics: The Clinical Use of Drugs** for a more in-depth discussion. All notations to reference numbers are based on the reference list at the end of that chapter. The editors of this handbook express their thanks to Drs. Saseen and Carter and acknowledge that this chapter is based upon their work.

Notes:

Notes:

Chapter 12

Peripheral Vascular Disorders

PERIPHERAL VASCULAR DISORDERS

Peripheral vascular disorders are divided into two major categories:
- ♦ **Arterial** diseases (see Table 12.1).
- ♦ **Venous** disorders (see Table 12.2).

Arterial Diseases

- ♦ Arterial diseases are characterized by *poor perfusion of the extremities,* in particular the lower extremities. These are subdivided further when due to either:
- • Vascular occlusion or
- • Vasospasm.

Vascular Occlusion: Intermittent Claudication (IC)
Sites of Atherosclerosis and Correlation to Symptoms
- ♦ **Iliac or ilioaortic artery** involvement correlate to buttock pain and impotence.
- ♦ **Femoropopliteal artery** involvement correlate to calf and thigh pain.
- ♦ **Tibial artery** involvement correlate to foot pain.

Treatment
- ♦ Goals of treatment are prevention of further pain, arresting progression of underlying disease, and decreasing risk of cardiovascular events.
- ♦ Prevention and nondrug therapies (see Table 12.1)
- ♦ **Pentoxifylline** (Trental) is the only FDA-approved drug for IC.
- ♦ **Proposed Mechanisms of Action**
  - • Improved hemorrheology: Increased red blood cell (RBC) deformability, decreased blood viscosity, improved blood flow to impaired microcirculation.
  - • Inhibition of platelet and red cell aggregation, ↓ plasma fibrinogen.
- ♦ **Dose.** 300 mg sustained-release (SR) tablet TID. Reduce to BID if gastrointestinal (GI) distress, hypotension, flushing, or headache occurs.
- ♦ May increase pain-free walking distance.
  - • Onset: 2–3 weeks; 6–8 weeks to full benefit.
  - • It is difficult to separate value of supervised exercise programs and smoking cessation from effect of pentoxifylline.
  - • "Statistically significant" increase in walking distance may not be "clinically significant."
  - • Side effects: dyspepsia, nausea, vomiting, headache, dizziness
- ♦ **Vasodilator therapy** generally is of little value because:
  - • Occluded vessels are maximally dilated from hypoxia-induced release of adenosine, CO_2, and potassium.

- Preferential dilation of healthy vessels leads to shunting of blood away from occluded vessels ("steal phenomenon").

Verapamil (80–240 mg QD) improved walking distance in one small, but well-controlled trial.

Consider niacin if lipid lowering is indicated and the patient is not diabetic.

Consider nitrates or a calcium channel blocker if the patient has coexistent angina or congenital heart disease.

Papaverine (150–300 mg SR BID) and nifedipine (30–60 mg TID) may improve walking distance; clinical trials are small and poorly controlled.

No evidence of benefit with cyclandelate (Cyclospasmol) or isoxuprine (Vasodilan).

Monitor for vasodilator side effects, including facial warmth and flushing, itching, hypotension, dizziness, tachycardia, palpitations, and headache. Watch for hepatotoxicity with niacin and papaverine and atrioventricular block with papaverine or calcium channel blockers.

♦ **Other Therapeutic Considerations**

- Aspirin: 80–325 mg/day, especially if there is evidence of coronary artery disease (CAD) or cerebrovascular disease (CVD).

- Ticlodipine (Ticlid) 250 mg BID and clopidogrel (Plavix) 75 mg BID are expensive alternatives to aspirin as antiplatelet drugs. Caution re neutropenia with ticlopidine and diarrhea and thrombotic thrombocytopenic purpura (TTP) with clopidogrel. (Also see Table 13.3 in Chapter 13: Thrombosis.)

- Cilostazol (Pletal) 100 mg BID, a phosphodiesterase III inhibitor with vasodilating and antiplatelet effects, has labeled indication for use in IC (based on improved walking distance). It is a P450 3A4 substrate; reduce dose to 50 mg BID if taking concurrent 3A4 inhibitors. Use is contraindicated in heart failure. Other side effects are headache, diarrhea, and dizziness.

- Ginko bilboa (120 mg QD) shown to improve walking distance is one study, possibly due to antiplatelet effects.

- Vitamin E. 400–800 units QD. No controlled studies available.

- Angioplasty of iliac or superficial femoral arteries with stent placements.

- Arterial bypass grafting or endarterectomy.

- Amputation

Vasospasm: Drug Therapy for Raynaud's Phenomenon

♦ **Calcium Channel Blockers.** Nifedipine immediate-release 10–30 mg TID is the best documented and is beneficial in two-thirds of patients.

The benefits of SR nifedipine, diltiazem, and other vasoselective calcium blockers are inconclusive.

♦ α_1-**Adrenergic Antagonists.** Prazosin (1 mg TID) yields moderate benefit in two-thirds of patients.

There are limited data regarding terazosin and none for doxazosin.

Thymoxamine is investigational.

♦ **Other Vasodilators.** Nitroglycerin ointment applied TID to affected areas may reduce symptoms, but is limited by systemic absorption and side effects (headache, flushing).

Niacin may be used if the patient has concurrent atherosclerosis and is not diabetic.

ACE inhibitors (via inhibition of bradykinin) have not been shown to be of benefit.

Kentaserin (an investigational serotonin receptor antagonist) 40 mg BID-TID decreases the frequency, but not the duration, of attacks. Side effects include headache, weakness, dizziness, sedation, edema, dry mouth, and a prolonged QT interval.

Venous Disorders

Venous disorders (see Table 12.2) include *deep vein thrombophlebitis* (see Chapter 13: Thrombosis) and functional failure of the valves in the veins of the lower extremities. The latter results in *chronic venous insufficiency* and/or venous distention *(varicose veins).*

MUSCULOSKELETAL DISORDERS
Nocturnal Leg Muscle Cramps

- ♦ **Definition.** Idiopathic involuntary contractions occurring at rest and causing intense pain and a visible or palpable knot in the affected muscles.

- ♦ **Clinical Presentation.** Nocturnal leg muscle cramps usually occur in the early hours of sleeping with the calf and small muscle of foot most often affected. Muscles that are already in a shortened position are most vulnerable (e.g., tight bed sheets pushing toes downward when calf and foot muscles already are partially contracted.)

- ♦ **Incidence.** Rare and episodic to several times per night. More prevalent in middle to older age.

- ♦ **Prevention** includes:
  - *Nondrug Therapy.* Muscle stretching exercises and dorsiflexion of foot several times a day. Dorsiflexion is grasping the toes and pulling them upward in the opposite direction of the cramp.
  - Loosening bed sheets. Patients may use a canopy to raise sheets at the end of the bed.
  - Sleeping on stomach with toes extended downward over the end of bed.
  - *Drug Therapy.* Quinine (200–325 mg at dinner and/or HS) is widely used, but highly controversial. It has been discontinued as an over-the-counter medication and may be withdrawn from the market completely.

    Mechanism. Increased refractory period of skeletal muscle and decreased excitability of motor end plate.

    Efficacy. Contradictory results on reduction in frequency, duration, and severity. Higher doses (BID) possibly more effective, but increased side effects.

    Side effects include GI intolerance; cinchonism, which is dose related and characterized by tinnitus; headache; nausea; and vertigo. Rarer side effects include thrombocytopenia (cross-reacts with quinidine; also quinine in tonic water); hemolysis if patient is G6PD deficient; optic atrophy; delirium; and arrhythmias.
  - Supplementing electrolyte (sodium, potassium, calcium, magnesium) if deficient.
  - Verapamil (120 mg at HS) decreased cramping after 6 days in one open-labeled study with only 8 subjects.
  - Vitamin E, 800 units/day. Little evidence of benefit.

- ♦ **Treatment** includes:
  - Dorsiflexion of foot at first sign of cramp.
  - Identify and treat other causes of cramping (see Table 12.3).

Notes:

Table 12.1 • Arterial Vascular Diseases

	Intermittent Claudication	Raynaud's
Synonyms	Arteriosclerosis obliterans, angina of the extremities	*Raynaud's disease* = Idiopathic or primary disorder (genetic?) *Raynaud's phenomenon* = Secondary to other causes
Clinical presentation	Aching, cramping, tightness, or weakness of buttocks, thigh, calf, or feet during exertion. Relieved by rest. Loss of leg and foot hair, ↓ pulse in feet, cold feet, absence of leg sweating. Numbness, rest pain, ischemia, ulceration, or necrosis indicate severe disease. Often concomitant CAD[a] or CVD,[a] high incidence of MI[a] and stroke	Sudden onset of pain and cyanosis (white, blue, patchy color) of fingertips upon exposure to cold or emotional stress. Feet affected less often. Digits are normal or cool and moist between attacks. *Severe cases:* atrophy of skin, nail loss, ulceration of fingertips
Cause/pathophysiology	Atherosclerotic plaque occluding vessel (see Figure 12.1). *Endothelial dysfunction:* ↓ vasodilatory response to thromboxane, serotonin, nitric oxide,[a] ↑ secretion of vasoconstrictive substances (e.g., endothelin), ↑ platelet aggregation. *Abnormal hemorrheology:* ↓ erythrocyte deformability; ↑ blood viscosity	Vasospasm causing ischemia of peripheral arteries. Exaggerated sympathetic response to precipitating stimuli. ↑ platelet aggregation
Precipitating/risk factors	Diabetes, hypertension, cigarette smoking, ↑ LDL, ↑ TG, ↓HDL[a] (metabolic syndrome)	Cold exposure, cigarette smoking (nicotine-induced vasoconstriction), RA,[a] scleroderma, SLE,[a] trauma (e.g., use of vibrating machinery). *Drugs:* ergots, beta blockers,[c] alpha agonists (decongestants), imipramine, clonidine
Prevention/general management (see text for drug therapies)	Stop smoking, exercise, diabetes control (diet, insulin, oral agents), lipid-lowering diet and drugs[b] (use caution with niacin if diabetes), hypertension treatment (ACE inhibitors,[a] calcium blockers, or α_1-antagonists preferred).[c] *Foot care:* Keep feet warm, dry; properly fitted shoes. Immediate treatment of abrasions, infection, or ulcers	Stop smoking, cold avoidance, warm water soaks, mittens and other hand protection, avoidance of precipitating drugs and occupations, treatment of associated diseases

[a]ACE inhibitor = Angiotensin-converting enzyme inhibitor; CAD = Coronary artery disease; CVD = Cerebral vascular disease; HDL = High-density lipoprotein; IC = Intermittent claudication; LDL = Low-density lipoprotein; MI = Myocardial infarction; RA = Rheumatoid arthritis; SLE = Systemic lupus erythematosus; TG = Triglyceride.
[b]Cholesterol reduction may slow or reverse atherosclerotic process and also may restore endothelial responsiveness to nitric oxide.
[c]Risk of beta blockers: May ↓ blood flow via unopposed α activity. Cold feet and worsening of Raynaud's well documented. Evidence for potentiating IC is conflicting; meta-analysis indicates lack of effect. If beta blockers indicated for concurrent disease, begin with low dose.

Notes:

Table 12.2 • Peripheral Venous Disorders

	Thrombophlebitis	Venous Insufficiency	Varicose Veins
Clinical findings	Calf tenderness, pain, and swelling in the involved extremity	Progressive edema of lower leg with varicosites, stasis pigmentation (brown discoloration of ankle or foot) due to vascular leakage	Dilated elongated superficial veins in the thigh or lower leg that are most visible when standing
Complications	Pulmonary embolism	Stasis dermatitis (acute or chronic eczematous eruptions) and ulcerations at or above the ankle	Ulceration if trauma or irritation of the thin atrophic pigmented skin of the lower leg or ankle region. May become chronic lesion and painful
Treatment	Heparin, warfarin	Wound care. Avoid antibiotics unless culture proven infection	Compression stockings, leg elevation, flexing. *Sclerotherapy:* Sodium tetradecyl (Sotradecol) or ethanolamine oleate (Ethamolin). Surgical vein stripping

Table 12.3 • Other Possible Causes of Muscle Cramps

Drug-induced Cramps	Biochemical Causes
Alcohol	Hyponatremia
Antipsychotics (dystonia)	Dehydration
Beta agonists (e.g., albuterol, terbutaline, salbutamol)	Calcium deficiency
Cimetidine	Magnesium deficiency
Clofibrate	Hemodialysis
Diuretics	
Lithium	
Narcotic analgesics	
Nicotinic acid	
Nifedipine	
Penicillamine	

Notes:

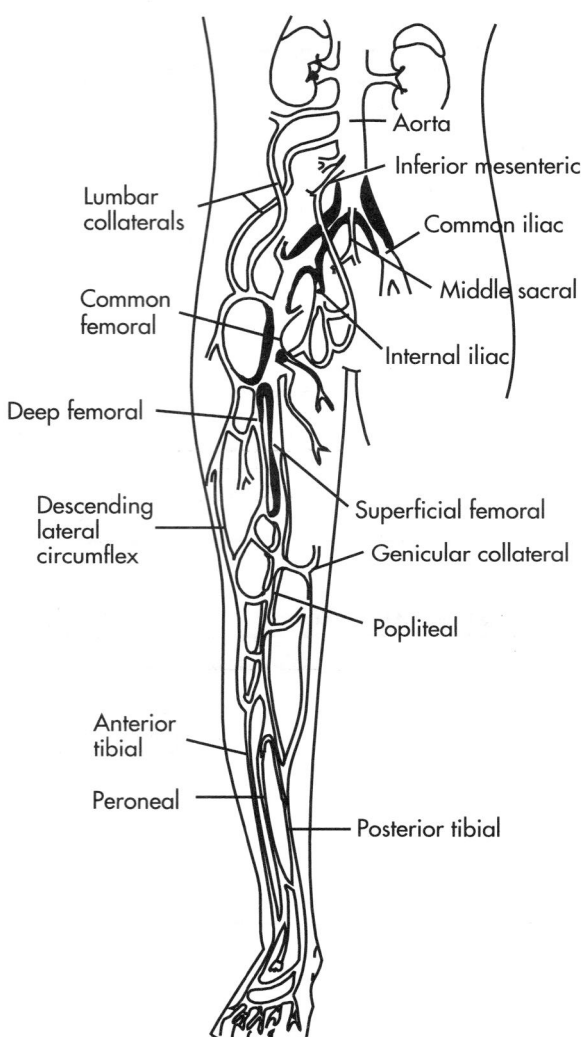

Fig. 12.1 Common Sites of Atherosclerosis (Shown in Black) in the Aorta and Lower Extremities. (Reproduced with permission from Peripheral Vascular Disease. St. Louis: Mosby Yearbook; 1996: 208.)

The reader is referred to Chapter 13: Peripheral Vascular Disorders, written by *Anne P. Spencer, Pharm.D.* and *C. Wayne Weart, Pharm.D.,* in the seventh edition of **Applied Therapeutics: The Clinical Use of Drugs** for a more in-depth discussion. The editors of this handbook express their thanks to Drs. Spencer and Weart and acknowledge that this chapter is based upon their work.

Chapter 13

Thrombosis

Definitions

+ ***Thrombosis*** is the process of abnormal fibrin blood clot formation. Small *superficial veins* or the larger, *deep venous* system may be affected.

+ ***Embolus*** is a small part of a clot that breaks off and travels to another site in the body. Emboli that become trapped in small capillaries (e.g., pulmonary tree) cause ischemia or infarction of the surrounding tissue.

+ ***Embolic events*** include pulmonary embolism (PE), myocardial infarction (MI), cerebrovascular accident (CVA; "strokes"), and transient ischemic attacks (TIAs), as summarized in Table 13.1.

+ ***Endothelialization*** is adherence of a thrombus to the vessel wall and usually takes 7–10 days. Clot resolution (i.e., thrombolysis) may take considerably longer.

Predisposing Factors for Thromboembolism

Predisposing factors include: immobilization, obesity, trauma, surgery, estrogen use, pregnancy, peripheral vascular and coronary artery disease, atrial fibrillation, left ventricular dysfunction (CHF, PostMI), venous occlusion by tumors, and foreign material within the vasculature (e.g., artificial heart valves and venous catheters).

Signs and Symptoms

+ ***Deep Venous Thrombosis (DVT).*** Unilateral leg or arm swelling, local tenderness or pain, erythema, warmth, venous "cord," weak or absent pulse below the thrombosis.

+ ***Pulmonary Embolism (PE).*** Dyspnea, pleuritic chest pain, anxiety, cough, tachypnea, tachycardia, rales, hemoptysis, hypoxia, VQ mismatch. Prior history of DVT in 80% of patients.

Treatment

+ ***Heparin.*** The action of heparin is facilitated by binding to the naturally circulating anticoagulant, antithrombin III (AT III, also called heparin co-factor). The heparin AT III complex attaches to and irreversibly inactivates thrombin (factor IIa) as well as activated factors IX, X, XI, and XII. Only about one third of the molecules in standard (unfractionated) heparin bind to AT III, leading to large variability in response. In cases of acute DVT or PE, thrombin must be inactivated directly, a process that may require relatively large doses of heparin. Due to the multiplier effect of the clotting cascade, inactivation of relatively small amounts of factor Xa (*before* clot has formed) prevents the production of large quantities of thrombin and serves as the basis for low-dose heparin prophylaxis after surgery or during immobilization. Other properties of heparin are listed in Table 13.2.

Low molecular weight heparins [e.g., enoxaparin (Lovenox), dalteparin (Fragmin), and tinzaparin (Innohep)] selectively inactivate factor Xa with minimal effect on thrombin. Initial indications were for prophylaxis only (e.g., orthopedic surgery), but they are now used as initial treatment of uncomplicated DVT as subcutaneous (SC) injections given at home. The prophylactic dose of enoxaparin is a fixed dose of 30 mg Q 12 hr, and dalteparin is given as a fixed dose of 2500 units Q 24 hr. Treatment doses are enoxaparin 1 mg/kg SC Q 12 hr, dalteparin 200 IU SC Q 24 hr, and tinzaparin 175 units/kg SC Q 24 hr. None of these drugs require laboratory monitoring at any of these doses. The incidence of bleeding and thrombocytopenia is less than with standard heparins.

Dosing of heparin is summarized in Tables 13.3 (prophylaxis), 13.4 (acute treatment), and 13.5 (adjusted dose subcutaneous administration).

♦ **Warfarin.** Warfarin interferes with the hepatic production and activation of vitamin K-dependent clotting factors II, VII, IX, and X. Commercially available warfarin (Coumadin) is a racemic mixture containing equal parts of the highly active S(−) isomer and the less potent R(+) warfarin.

Pharmacokinetics. (See Table 13.2.) The pharmacodynamic response of warfarin is a composite of both its long elimination half-life and the pharmacokinetics of the inhibited clotting factors. Although warfarin may rapidly inhibit the production of new clotting factors, the full anticoagulant effect is not seen until the pre-existing stores of the factors are reduced to a new steady state, a process that takes 7–10 days (e.g., 3–5 half-lives of factor II). Paradoxical thromboembolism may occur early in the course of treatment in patients with protein C or S deficiencies.

Therapeutic range and duration of therapy for warfarin are dependent on the type of thromboembolic event (see Table 13.6). The *prothrombin time (PT),* normalized to the *International Normalized Ratio (INR),* is used to monitor warfarin. *Intensity* of anticoagulation is classified as low (INR 2–3) or high (INR 2.5–3.5).

Initiating and Adjusting Warfarin Doses. A recommended protocol for initiating and early monitoring/adjustment of warfarin is found in Table 13.7. Typically 10 mg is given for the first 2–3 days, but as indicated in Table 13.7, some highly sensitive patients require early dosage reduction. The INR on day 4 is used to predict chronic daily dosing. Single doses of warfarin produce some effect on the prothrombin time in 24 hours, but the maximal effect is not seen until 36 hours. When assessing a patient's response after several days of dosing, one must consider the cumulative effect of each dose. For example, if a patient has received a 10-mg dose each evening for 3 days and the PT is drawn on the fourth morning, the measured PT reflects residual effects of the first dose, maximal effects of the second dose, and initial effects of the third dose. Ideally, doses should be changed as infrequently as possible, taking into account the pharmacokinetics of coagulation factors. Patients who show a rapid change in INR (i.e., >1.8 after the first 10-mg dose) are sensitive to the drug and may require small maintenance doses (=2.5 mg/day). If only minimal changes are seen in the INR after 3–4 days of 10-mg dosing, a maintenance dose of =10 mg/day may be needed. On average, patients will show some response by 48 hr and will need a final maintenance dose of 4–5 mg/day to achieve an INR of 2–3.

Atrial Fibrillation. See Table 13.8 for stroke prevention dosing in patients with atrial fibrillation.

Treatment During Pregnancy. See Table 13.9.

Outpatient Monitoring. Once the final maintenance dose has been determined, large dosage changes are rarely indicated. Giving the same dose every day (e.g., 6 mg QD) provides more predictable responses than alternating doses (e.g., 5 mg alternating with 7.5 mg QOD). Usually, outpatient dosage increments do not exceed addition or deletion of 2.5–5 mg/week. Algorithms for dosage adjustment based on target INRs are found in Figures 13.1 and 13.2.

Drug Interactions and Patient Counseling. See Tables 13.10, 13.11, and 13.12, respectively.

♦ **Newer Drugs**

- **Bivalirudin (Angiomax).** Direct reversible thrombin inhibitor. Alternative to heparin (in combination with aspirin) during percutaneous angioplasty. 1 mg/kg IV bolus, then 2.5 mg/kg/hr IV infusion × 4 hours.

- **Danaparoid (Orgaran).** A heparanoid compound that inactivates factor X and IIa via AT-III. 750 units SC BID pre and post hip replacement surgery.

- **Argatroban (Novastan).** A synthetic direct thrombin inhibitor. 2 µg/kg/min continuous infusion.

- **Lepirudin (Refludan).** A recombinant form of the direct thrombin inhibitor hirudin. 0.4 mg/kg IV bolus, then 0.15 mg/kg/hr infusion.

Acute Treatment (at Onset of Symptoms)

- ♦ **Goal of Therapy.** Symptomatic relief and prevention of clot extension.
- ♦ **Superficial or Calf DVT.** Local heat and NSAIDs.
- ♦ **Ileo-femoral DVT or PE.** IV heparin load and continuous IV infusion (see Table 13.4). Begin warfarin days 1–3 (see Table 13.7). Continue heparin for 4–7 days until warfarin reaches therapeutic levels (i.e., target INR achieved).
- ♦ **If Severe and Within First 24 Hours.** Thrombolytic agents may be indicated. See Chapter 15: Myocardial Infarction (MI) for dosing of thrombolytic agents.

Prophylaxis

- ♦ Anticoagulation and/or mechanical interventions (elastic stockings, leg elevation, pneumatic compression) may be given to prevent thrombosis in high-risk situations including prolonged bedrest, post-MI or surgical procedures. Prophylaxis is most effective for GI, gynecological, and some orthopedic surgery. Success after hip surgery is improved by using larger heparin doses or low molecular weight heparin.

- ♦ Adjusted dose subcutaneous heparin may be indicated in patients with poor IV access, following hip surgery, or for outpatients with warfarin intolerance (e.g., allergy or pregnant females).

Antiplatelet Drugs

Aspirin, dipyridamole, clopidogrel (Plavix), and ticlopidine (Ticlid) all act to slow or prevent platelet aggregation. They are used in a variety of disorders including general cardiovascular prophylaxis, unstable angina, postmyocardial infarction, and cerebrovascular disorders. The general properties of these drugs are listed in Table 13.13. Also see Table 14.7 in Chapter 14: Ischemic Heart Disease for indications and dosing of glycoprotein II_b/III_c receptor antagonists.

Fibrinolytic Agents

Fibrinolytic agents have the advantage over other anticoagulants in that they directly dissolve thrombi rather than just prevent their extension. However, they are extremely expensive and are only associated with improved patient outcome when compared to heparin if they are started within the first 3–6 hr of severe PE. Dosing of fibrinolytic agents is outlined in Chapter 15: Myocardial Infarction (MI).

Table 13.1 • Examples of Embolic Events[a]

Type of Event	Source of Embolus	Site of Damage
PE	DVT of thigh or ileofemoral vein[c]	Capillaries of lung
MI (See Chapter 15: Myocardial Infarction)	May be primary thrombosis of an atherosclerotic coronary artery or an embolism dislodged from a clot in the atrium or ventricle of the heart (mural thrombi)	Coronary arteries
CVA (stroke) (See Chapter 52: Cerebrovascular Disorders)	May be primary thrombosis of an atherosclerotic cerebral capillary or an embolism from a mural thrombi (e.g., following cardioversion of atrial fibrillation)	Cerebral venous system
TIA[b]	Platelet emboli	Cerebral arterioles or capillaries

[a]CVA = Cerebrovascular accident; DVT = Deep venous thrombosis; MI = Myocardial infarction; PE = Pulmonary embolus; TIA = Transient ischemic attack.
[b]Symptoms of a CVA and a TIA are similar, but the duration of a TIA is <24 hr. CVA is caused by a fibrin clot in the venous system. TIA is caused by a platelet clot in the arteriolar system.
[c]Superficial vein thrombosis and DVT of the calf have a lower risk of PE than DVT of the thigh or ileofemoral region.

Table 13.2 • Clinical Pharmacokinetics and Monitoring of Anticoagulants[a]

Parameter	Unfractionated Heparin	Warfarin
Absorption	Parenteral only	Oral 100% (not given parenterally)
Vd	Plasma volume (~0.07 L/kg)	≈7.6–13.9 L
Metabolism/Cl	Hepatic metabolism and uptake by reticuloendothelial system. Also uptake (consumption) by thrombin and other clotting factors	Hepatic
Elimination t½	30–150 min[b]	36–42 hr
Protein binding	Bound to antithrombin III and other serine proteases	99.4% bound to albumin
Cp (therapeutic)	0.2–0.4 U/mL	1.5 mg/L
Side effects	Bleeding,[c] thrombocytopenia,[d] osteoporosis	Bleeding,[c] skin necrosis, drug interactions
Treatment of bleeding	*Mild:* Slow or stop infusion *Severe:* Protamine 1 mg/100 U of estimated heparin remaining in body	*Mild:* Hold 1–2 doses, observe and restart at lower dose *Severe:* Vitamin K or fresh-frozen plasma

[a]Cl = Clearance; Cp = Plasma concentration; t½ = Half-life; Vd = Volume of distribution.
[b]Clearance of heparin is faster (t½ shorter) with large thrombosis and before endothelialization. Therefore, dose requirements may be higher during the early stages of DVT or PE.
[c]Monitor hemoccult of stool; observe for bleeding from injection sites, hematuria, nose bleeds, gum bleeding, ↑ menstrual flow, and bruising of subcutaneous sites. Monitor platelets with prolonged heparin therapy. Significant GI bleeding or hematuria may indicate an underlying lesion (e.g., ulcer or tumor). Rare = Intracranial bleed with mental status changes, headache.
[d]Two forms of heparin-induced thrombocytopenia. Type I = Direct (reversible, common) effect to cause platelet sequestration and clumping. Onset = Rapid; platelets above 100,000/mm³. Type II = Immune-mediated binding of heparin to IgG. Complex binds to platelet to cause aggregation. Onset = delayed; rare. Platelet count below 100,000/mm³; possible arterial thrombosis (white clot syndrome). Both occur with low molecular weight heparin (LMWH), but at lower incidence than unfractionated. LMWH contraindicated in patients with a history of type II thrombocytopenia. Consider argatroban or lepirudin.

Table 13.3 • Prevention of Venous Thromboembolism

Clinical Setting	Prophylaxis
General Surgery	
Low-risk patients (age <40 yr; no other risk factors)	Early ambulation
Moderate risk patients (age >40 yr; no other risk factors)	Elastic stockings (ES) or intermittent pneumatic compression (IPC) or low-dose unfractionated heparin (UFH)[a]
High-risk patients (age >40 yr, and other risk factors)	IPC or UFH[a] or enoxaparin[b] or dalteparin[c]
Very high-risk patients (multiple risk factors)	IPC or UFH[a] or enoxaparin[b] or dalteparin[c]
Total Hip Replacement/Hip Fracture Surgery	Enoxaparin[b] or dalteparin[c] or low-intensity warfarin[d] or danaparoid[e]
Total Knee Replacement	IPC or enoxaparin[b] or dalteparin[c] or low-density warfarin[d]
Intracranial Neurosurgery	IPC with or without ES; or [either IPC or ES] *plus* either [UFH[a] or enoxaparin[b] or dalteparin[c]]
Spinal Cord Injury	Enoxaparin[b] or dalteparin[c]
Multiple Trauma	IPC or enoxaparin[b] or dalteparin[c]
Prolonged Bedrest/Immobility	ES or IPC or UFH[a] or low-intensity warfarin[d]

[a] Low-dose unfractionated heparin (UFH) = 500 U SC 2–12 hr before surgery and then Q 12 hr postoperative until ambulatory. aPTT monitoring not required. May add or substitute aspirin 80–325 mg Q day.
[b] Enoxaparin = Low molecular weight heparin. Usual dose 30 mg SC Q 12 hr (mg SC Q 12 hr).
[c] Dalteparin = Low molecular weight heparin. Usual dose 2500 units SC Q 24 hr.
[d] Low-intensity warfarin = INR 2–3.
[e] Danaparoid 75 units SC BID

Table 13.4 • Heparin Protocol for Acute Thromboembolic Event[a]

1. Suggested loading dose:	Treatment: 80 U/kg (rounded to nearest 500 U)
	Prevention: 70 U/kg (rounded to nearest 500 U)
2. Suggested initial infusion:[b]	Treatment: 18 U/kg/hr (rounded to nearest 100 U)
	Prevention 15 U/kg/hr (rounded to nearest 100 U)
3. First aPTT check:	6 hr after initiating therapy
4. Dosing adjustments:[d]	Per chart below (rounded to nearest 100 U)

aPTT[c] (sec)	Heparin Bolus	Infusion Hold Time	Infusion Rate Adjustment	Next aPTT
<40–49	4,000 U	0	↑ 200 U/hr	In 6 hr
50–59	2,000 U	0	↑ 100 U/hr	In 6 hr
60–100	0	0	None	Q AM
101–110	0	0	↓ 100 U/hr	In 6 hr
111–120	0	0	↓ 200 U/hr	In 6 hr
>120	0	30 min	↓ 200 U/hr	In 6 hr

[a] University of Washington Medical Center. Consider argatroban or lepirudin if history of heparin induced thrombocytopenia.
[b] For home treatment, substitute subcutaneous low molecular weight heparin for IV unfractionated heparin. Use enoxaparin 1 mg/kg SC Q 12 hr or dalteparin 200 IU/kg SC Q 24 hr. No need to monitor aPTT. Continue 5 days or until warfarin is therapeutic.
[c] aPTT = Activated partial thromboplastin time. Based on aPTT reagent-specific therapeutic range of 60–100 sec corresponding to in vitro heparin concentrations of 0.2–0.4 U/mL. Caution: Immediately after a loading dose, the aPTT will be immeasurable (i.e., the blood will not clot). Even after 6 hr, some residual effect from the loading dose may remain. Waiting for 8 hr will generally overcome this complication.
[d] As clot endothelializes over 7–10 days, dose requirement may decrease.

Table 13.5 • Heparin Protocol for Adjusted-Dose Subcutaneous Administration[a]

Initial Dosage
A. Initial therapy with adjusted-dose SC heparin
   1. Give SC heparin 240 U/kg × 1.
   2. Check first aPTT 6 hr after first dose.
   3. Adjust dosing per chart below.
B. Conversion from continuous infusion heparin to adjusted-dose SC heparin
   1. Calculate total 24-hr heparin requirement necessary to maintain therapeutic aPTT.
   2. Divide 24-hr heparin requirement by 2 to determine initial Q 12 hr SC dosing requirement.
   3. Discontinue IV heparin and administer initial Q 12 hr SC dose within 1 hr.
   4. Check first aPTT 6 hr after first dose.
   5. Adjust dosing per chart below.
C. Conversion from warfarin to adjusted-dose SC heparin
   1. Discontinue warfarin.
   2. Give 240 U/kg SC heparin within 24 hr.
   3. Check first aPTT 6 hr after first dose.
   4. Adjust dosing per chart below.

Dosing Adjustments

aPTT[b] (sec)	Dosing Adjustment[c]	Next aPTT
<40	↑ by 48 U/kg Q 12 hr	6 hr after dose
40–59	↑ by 24 U/kg Q 12 hr	6 hr after dose
60–100	No change	Q AM
101–120	↓ by 12 U/kg Q 12 hr	6 hr after dose
121–140	↓ by 24 U/kg Q 12 hr	6 hr after dose
>140	↓ by 36 U/kg Q 12 hr	6 hr after dose

[a]University of Washington Medical Center. aPTT = activated partial thromboplastin time; IV = intravenous; SC = subcutaneous.
[b]Based on aPTT reagent-specific therapeutic range of 60–100 sec corresponding to in vitro heparin concentrations of 0.2–0.4 U/mL.
[c]Rounded to nearest 500 U.

Table 13.6 • Optimal Therapeutic Range and Duration of Warfarin Therapy[a]

Indication	Target INR Range (Duration)
Atrial Fibrillation (AF)	
Age <65 and no risk factors	None (aspirin 325 mg QD)
Age 65–75 and no risk factors	2.0–3.0 (long term)[d]
Age <75 with moderate risk factors (diabetes, coronary artery disease, thyrotoxicosis)	2.0–3.0 (long term)[d]
Age <75 with high-risk factors for stroke (history of TIA/stroke/TE; hypertension, CHF, decreased LV function; rheumatic mitral valve disease; valve replacement)	2.0–3.0 (long term)
Age >75	2.0–3.0 (long term)
Precardioversion (AF or flutter >48 hr)	2.0–3.0 (3 wk)
Postcardioversion (in NSR)	2.0–3.0 (4 wk)
Cardioembolic Stroke	
With risk factors for stroke (AF, CHF, LV dysfunction; mural thrombus, history of TIA/stroke/TE)	2.0–3.0 (long term)
Following embolic event despite anticoagulation	2.0–3.0 (long term)[e]
Left Ventricular Dysfunction	
Ejection fraction <30%	2.0–3.0 (long term)
Transient, following myocardial infarction	2.0–3.0 (3 mo)
Following embolic event despite anticoagulation	2.0–3.0 (long term)[e]

(continued)

Table 13.6 • Optimal Therapeutic Range and Duration of Warfarin Therapy [a] (continued)

Indication	Target INR Range (Duration)
Myocardial Infarction (MI)	
Following anterior MI	2.0–3.0 (3 mo)
Following inferior MI with transient risk(s) (AF, CHF, LV dysfunction, mural thrombus, history of TE)	2.0–3.0 (3 mo)
Following initial treatment with persistent risks	2.0–3.0 (long term)
Thromboembolism (DVT, PE)	
Treatment/prevention of recurrence	
• Transient risk factors	2.0–3.0 (3–6 mo)
• Idiopathic	2.0–3.0 (6 mo)
• Persistent risk factors (AT-III, protein C, protein S deficiencies; factor V Leiden; malignancy)	2.0–3.0 (long term)
• Antiphospholipid antibody syndrome	2.5–3.5 (long term)
Following recurrent DVT/PE	2.0–3.0 (long term)
Valvular Disease	
Aortic valve disease with mitral valve disease, AF, or history of systemic embolization	2.0–3.0 (long term)
Mitral annular calcification with AF or history of systemic embolization	2.0–3.0 (long term)
Mitral valve prolapse:	
• With AF or history of systemic embolization	2.0–3.0 (long term)
• With history of TIA despite ASA therapy	2.0–3.0 (long term)
• s/p embolic event despite anticoagulation	2.0–3.0 (long term) [e]
Rheumatic mitral valve disease:	
• With AF, history of systemic embolization, LA >5.5 cm	2.0–3.0 (long term)
• s/p embolic event despite anticoagulation	2.0–3.0 (long term) [e]
Valve Replacement—Bioprosthetic	
Aortic or mitral	2.0–3.0 (3 mo) [e]
• With LA thrombus	2.0–3.0 (>3 mo) [e]
• With history of systemic embolism	2.0–3.0 (3–12 mo) [e]
• With AF	2.0–3.0 (long term) [e]
Following systemic embolism	2.0–3.0 (long term) [e]
Valve Replacement—Mechanical	
Aortic	
Bileaflet	
In NSR, normal ejection fraction, normal LA size	2.0–3.0 (long term)
All others	2.5–3.5 (long term) [f]
Tilting disk	2.5–3.5 (long term) [f]
Ball and cage	2.5–3.5 (long term) [f]
Mitral	
Bileaflet	2.5–3.5 (long term) [f]
Tilting disk	2.5–3.5 (long term) [f]
Ball and cage	2.5–3.5 (long term) [f]
With additional risk factors or following TE	2.5–3.5 (long term) [f]

[a]ASA = Acetylsalicylic acid; AT-III = Antithrombin III; CHF = Congestive heart failure; LA = Left atrial; LV = Left ventricular; NSR = Normal sinus rhythm; s/p = Status post; TE = Thromboembolism; TIA = Transient ischemic attack.
[b]INR = International normalized ratio. Standardizes prothrombin time (PT) by correcting for variations in different batches of thromboplastin.

$$INR = \left(\frac{Patient's\ PT}{Control\ Valve} \right)^{c}$$

where c = International Sensitivity Index value assigned to the current batch of thromboplastin (usually between 2 and 3).
[c]Use aspirin 325 mg QD alone
[d]May *substitute* aspirin 325 mg QD for warfarin
[e]*Add* aspirin 325 mg QD (clopidogrel or ticlopidine if aspirin contraindicated) to warfarin.
[f]May lower INR to 2–3 *and add* aspirin 81 mg QD

Table 13.7 • Flexible Initiation Dosing Protocol for Warfarin Therapy[a]

Day	a.m. PT INR	p.m. Warfarin Dose (mg)
1 (baseline)	<1.4	10
2	<1.8	10
	1.8	1
	>1.8	0.5
3	<2	10
	2–2.1	5
	2.2–2.3	4.5
	2.4–2.5	4
	2.6–2.7	3.5
	2.8–2.9	3
	3–3.1	2.5
	3.2–3.3	2
	3.4	1.5
	3.5	1
	3.6–4	0.5
	>4	None
		Maintenance Dose
4	<1.4	>8
	1.4	8
	1.5	7.5
	1.6–1.7	7
	1.8	6.5
	1.9	6
	2–2.1	5.5
	2.2–2.3	5
	2.4–2.6	4.5
	2.7–3	4
	3.1–3.5	3.5
	3.6–4	3
	4.1–4.5	Omit 1 dose, then 2
	>4.5	Omit 2 doses, then 1

[a]Algorithm for initiating warfarin dosing to obtain target INR of 2–3. Start with 10 mg on day 1. Final doses will be higher if target INR = 2.5–3.5.

Table 13.8 • Stroke Risk Stratification of Patients with Atrial Fibrillation

Risk Category	Characteristics	Strategy for Stroke Prevention
High risk	Age >75 Age <75 with high-risk factors: • Previous transient ischemic attack, stroke, or systemic embolism • Poor left ventricular function • Hypertension • Rheumatic mitral valve disease • Prosthetic heart valve	Warfarin to INR 2.0–3.0[a]
Moderate risk	Age 65–75 with no other risk factors Age <75 with moderate-risk factors: • Diabetes • Coronary artery disease • Thyrotoxicosis	Warfarin to INR 2.0–3.0 or aspirin 325 mg[a]
Low risk	Age <65 with no other risk factors	Aspirin 325 mg

[a]See Table 13.6 for duration of treatment.

Table 13.9 • Recommendations for Anticoagulation in Pregnancy

Clinical Condition	Peripartum	Alternative Strategy	Postpartum
DVT/PE before pregnancy; not currently anticoagulated	UFH 5,000 U SC Q 12 hr	LMWH/prevention doses	Warfarin to INR 2–3 for 4–6 wk
DVT/PE before pregnancy; currently anticoagulated	SC UFH/treatment doses	LMWH/treatment doses	Warfarin to INR 2–3 until full course completed (minimum, 4–6 wk)
New DVT/PE during pregnancy	IV UFH/treatment doses for 5–10 days, followed by SC UFH/treatment doses	LMWH/treatment doses	Warfarin to INR 2–3 until full course completed (minimum, 4–6 wk)
Currently anticoagulated for other reasons (e.g., atrial fibrillation, valve replacement)	SC UFH/treatment doses		Warfarin to appropriate INR intensity

DVT = Deep venous thrombosis; LMWH = Low-molecular-weight heparin; PE = Pulmonary embolism; SC = Subcutaneous; UFH = Unfractionated heparin.

Table 13.10 • Clinically Significant Warfarin Drug Interactions

Mechanism	Effect on Prothrombin Time	Drugs/Drug Classes
Increased synthesis of clotting factors	Decreased	Estrogens, vitamin K
Reduced catabolism of clotting factors	Decreased	Methimazole, propylthiouracil
Induction of warfarin metabolism	Decreased	Barbiturates, carbamazepine, chronic alcohol use, dicloxacillin, griseofulvin, nafcillin, phenytoin, primidone, rifampin
Reduced absorption of warfarin	Decreased	Cholestyramine, colestipol, sucralfate
Unexplained mechanisms	Decreased	Azathioprine, cyclophosphamide, cyclosporine, mesalamine
Increased catabolism of clotting factors	Increased	Thyroid hormones
Decreased synthesis of clotting factors	Increased	Cefamandole, cefmetazole, cefoperazone, cefotetan, moxalactam, vitamin E
Impaired vitamin K production by gastrointestinal flora	Increased	Broad-spectrum antibiotics
Inhibition of warfarin metabolism	Increased	Acute alcohol use, allopurinol, amiodarone,[b] azithromycin, cimetidine,[c] ciprofloxacin,[c] clarithromycin,[a] disulfiram,[b] erythromycin,[b,c] fluconazole,[a,b] fluorouracil, fluoxetine,[a] fluvoxamine,[b] grapefruit juice,[a] isoniazid,[a] itraconazole,[a] ketoconazole, metronidazole,[b] miconazole,[a,b] norfloxacin,[c] ofloxacin, omeprazole,[a] phenytoin, propafenone, quinidine,[a] sulfamethoxazole,[b] sulfasoxazole

(continued)

Table 13.10 • Clinically Significant Warfarin Drug Interactions (continued)

Mechanism	Effect on Prothrombin Time	Drugs/Drug Classes
Unexplained mechanisms	Increased	Acetaminophen, androgens, ascorbic acid, clofibrate, corticosteroids, gemfibrozil, statins
Increased bleeding risk	No effect	Aspirin/acetylated salicylates, clopidogrel, nonsteroidal anti-inflammatory drugs, selective serotonin reuptake inhibitors, ticlopidine

[a]Inhibition of CYP3A4, primary metabolic pathway for (R)-warfarin.
[b]Inhibition of CYP2C9, primary metabolic pathway for (S)-warfarin.
[c]Inhibition of CYP1A2, primary metabolic pathway for (R)-warfarin.

Table 13.11 • Potential Warfarin Interactions with Dietary Supplements

Presumed Mechanism	Possible Effect	Case Reports	Potential Interactions
Inhibition of platelet aggregation	↑ risk of bleeding	Garlic,[a] ginkgo[a]	Cassio, clove, feverfew, ginger
Contains salicylate derivatives	↑ risk of bleeding		Liquorice, meadowsweet, poplar, willow
Enhanced fibrinolysis	↑ risk of bleeding		Dehydroepiandrosterone (DHEA)
Procoagulant activity	↑ risk of thromboembolism		Agrimony, yarrow
Contains Coumarin constituents	↑ PT/INR	Dan shen (Salvia)	Alfalfa, aniseed, arnica, artemesia, celery seed, chamomile, dong quai (Angelica), fenugreek horse chestnut, melilot, prickly ash, quassia, red clover, sweet woodruff, tonka beans
Unknown	↑ PT/INR	Ginseng	

[a]Case reports of bleeding when used alone.

Table 13.12 • Key Elements of Patient Education Regarding Warfarin

Identification of generic and brand names
Purpose of therapy
Expected duration of therapy
Dosing and administration
Visual recognition of drug and tablet strength
What to do in case a dose is missed
Importance of prothrombin time monitoring
Recognition of signs and symptoms of bleeding
Recognition of signs and symptoms of thromboembolism
What to do in case bleeding or thromboembolism occurs
Recognition of signs and symptoms of disease states that influence warfarin dosing requirements
Potential for interactions with prescription and over-the-counter medications
Dietary considerations and use of alcohol
Avoidance of pregnancy
Significance of informing other health care providers that warfarin has been prescribed
When, where, and with whom follow-up will be provided

Table 13.13 • Mechanism, Indications, and Dosage of Antiplatelet Drugs

	Aspirin (acetylsalicylic acid)	Clopidogrel (Plavix)	Ticlopidine (Ticlid)
Mechanism	Acetyl group binds to and inactivates platelet cyclo-oxygenase. ↓ thromboxane A_2 production causes ↓ platelet aggregation[a]	Inhibits ADP-induced platelet aggregation and thus binding of fibrinogen to gp IIb/IIIa receptor[b]	Same as clopidogrel[c]
Possible Indication[d]			
Unstable angina	Doses from 325 mg QD-QID have been shown to ↓ nonfatal MI and mortality. 325 mg QD recommended	Not indicated.[e] Used in combination with aspirin following coronary stent placement.	Not indicated[e]
MI prophylaxis with or without prior history of CAD or MI	Doses from 64–325 mg QD have been shown to ↓ incidence of MI[d]	75 mg QD in patients with recent MI or established peripheral artery disease	Not indicated[e]
Post coronary artery bypass surgery	↑ graft patency with doses of 325 mg QD-TID starting 48 hr post-op	Not indicated[e]	Not indicated[e]
Thrombotic stroke prevention	325 mg BID in patients with history of TIAs. May combine with dipyridamole.[d]	75 mg QD in patients with history of TIAs or recent thrombotic stroke[f]	250 mg BID with food in patients with history of TIAs or completed thrombotic stroke[f]
Mechanical heart valve placement[g]	Fewer thrombotic events at a dose of 1000 mg QD taken in combination with dipyridamole 100 mg QD. ASA alone is ineffective	Not indicated[e]	Not indicated[e]
Artificial grafts (e.g., dialysis)	↑ patency with dose of 325 mg QD. May combine with dipyridamole.[h]	Not indicated[e]	Not indicated[e]
Side Effects	GI irritation, bleeding (see Chapter 6: Pain)	Diarrhea, nausea, dyspepsia, GI bleeding, rare TTP	Diarrhea, nausea, dyspepsia, GI bleeding, rash, ↑ serum cholesterol, neutropenia[j]

Also see Table 14.7 in Chapter 14: Ischemic Heart Disease for Indications and Dosing of Glycoprotein IIb/IIIc Receptor Antagonists

[a]The effects of ASA on platelet cyclo-oxygenase are irreversible over the 8-day life span of the platelet. ASA also inhibits vessel wall cyclo-oxygenase to inhibit prostacyclin production. This latter effect may not be desirable. Apparently, low doses of ASA (300 mg/day) selectively inhibit platelet cyclo-oxygenase. Very small doses of ASA (60 mg/day) may also preferentially inactivate platelet cyclo-oxygenase during the "first pass" through the portal vein after oral absorption, followed by rapid metabolism to inactive salicyclic acid.

[b]Effect of clopidogrel irreversible for the life of the platelet. Maximal effect (40–60% inhibition) at 3–7 days. Return to baseline 5 days after discontinuation. Metabolized to active and inactive metabolites; kinetics poorly characterized.

[c]Effect of ticlopidine is irreversible for the life of the platelet. 50% effect in 4 days; maximal effect in 8–11 days. Primarily hepatic metabolism. Dose-dependent pharmacokinetics; $t^{1/2} = 12.6$ hr single dose, 4–5 days multiple dose. Clearance ↓ with age.

[d]For unexplained reasons, most of aspirin's beneficial effects on the heart and in stroke prevention have been limited to men only. Aggrenox = 200 mg extended release dipyridamole with 25 mg aspirin. One capsule BID for patients with history of stroke or TIA.

[e]Not indicated means not FDA-approved indication. Consider use in patients unable to tolerate aspirin.

[f]Clopidogrel and ticlopidine equally effective in men and women.

[g]Anticoagulation with warfarin recommended.

[h]Dipyridamole (Persantine) 75 mg TID prolongs graft patency. Mechanism: inhibits phosphodiesterase thus ↑ platelet cyclic AMP and platelet prostacyclin. Inhibits adenosine uptake into platelets.

[i]TTP = Thrombotic thrombocytopenic purpura.

[j]Neutropenia = 2.4%. CBC must be monitored every 2 weeks for 1st 3 months. Reserve for use in patients with aspirin failure or intolerance, or in women.

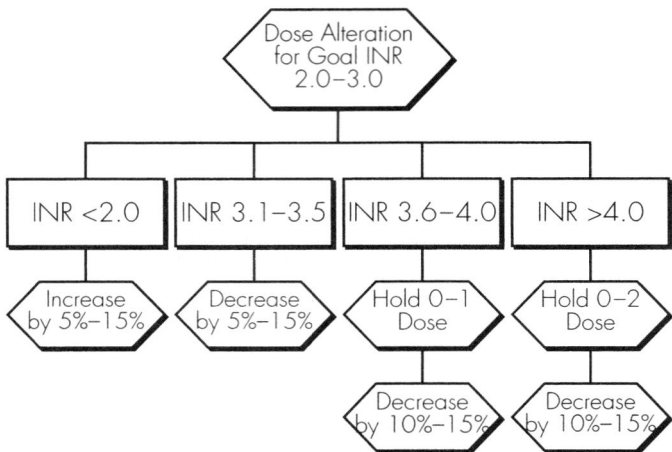

Fig. 13.1 Warfarin Maintenance Dosing Protocol for Goal INR 2.0–3.0

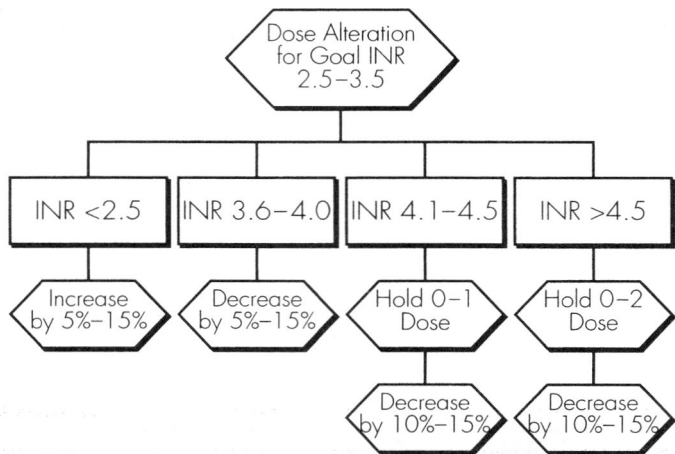

Fig. 13.2 Warfarin Maintenance Dosing Protocol for Goal INR 2.5–3.5

The reader is referred to Chapter 14: Thrombosis, written by *Ann K. Wittowsky, Pharm.D.*, in the seventh edition of **Applied Therapeutics: The Clinical Use of Drugs** for a more in-depth discussion. Other topics covered in this chapter include management of overcoagulation and disseminated intravascular coagulation (DIC). The editors of this handbook express their thanks to Dr. Wittowsky and acknowledge that this chapter is based upon her work.

Notes:

Chapter 14

Ischemic Heart Disease: Anginal Syndromes

Angina Pectoris

- ♦ **Definition.** Angina pectoris is a symptom of myocardial ischemia in the absence of infarction. Angina typically implies severe chest pain or discomfort during strenuous exercise, but it may develop unexpectedly with little or no exertion. Some patients describe a pressure sensation or heaviness instead of pain.
- ♦ **Characteristics.** The characteristics of angina are listed in Table 14.1.
- ♦ **Coronary Blood Flow.** Figure 14.1 illustrates the anatomy and distribution of the major coronary arteries. The anterior and lateral portions of the left ventricle receive blood flow from the *left coronary artery (LCA)*. This artery divides into two major branches, the *left anterior descending (LAD)* and the *circumflex*. The *right coronary artery (RCA)* supplies blood to most of the right ventricle, as well as the posterior part of the left ventricle.
- ♦ **Classification and Clinical Presentation.** Table 14.2 classifies angina into five categories based upon the patient's presenting symptoms.

General Management

- ♦ *Goals of therapy* are to relieve or prevent symptoms and to prevent myocardial infarction and death.
- ♦ *Lifestyle Alterations.* In chronic stable angina, alterations of lifestyle, including avoidance of stresses known to precipitate an attack, may suffice. Supervised exercise and smoking cessation programs are encouraged, and patients should be discouraged from leading a totally inactive lifestyle.
- ♦ *Dietary and drug therapy of dyslipidemias and hypertension* may slow progression and possibly cause regression of coronary plaque. (See Chapter 10: Dyslipidemias and Chapter 11: Essential Hypertension.)
- ♦ *SL Nitroglycerin.* Prophylactic sublingual nitroglycerin taken 5–10 minutes before known inciting events (e.g., exercise, coitus) helps minimize the number of symptomatic episodes. SL nitroglycerin also reduces the duration and intensity of anginal pain when taken at the onset of an acute attack. (See Table 14.3.)
- ♦ *Aspirin.* Antiplatelet therapy with aspirin, 75–125 mg QD, should be given to all patients for general cardiovascular protection, unless contraindicated by GI or other intolerance. Aspirin also is given for acute unstable angina. Clopidogrel (Plavix), 75 mg QD, or ticlopidine (Ticlid), 250 mg BID, may be substituted for patients intolerant of aspirin and in women. (See Chapter 13: Thrombosis for details on aspirin, clopidogrel, and ticlopidine dosing and side effects.)
- ♦ *Frequent or recurrent angina* is best treated with chronic scheduled drug therapy using either a beta-adreneric blocker, a long-acting nitrate, or a long-acting calcium channel

blocker (CCB). Unless contraindicated, a beta blocker is usually given first because of greater efficacy in comparative trials to the other drugs; superiority for preventing silent myocardial ischemia; and lower morbidity and mortality in patients with hypertension, acute MI, and heart failure. Otherwise, the choice of drug is based on the presence of concurrent diseases and side effect profile. For example, nitrates are preferred to CCBs in patients with heart failure while CCBs are preferred in supraventricular arrhythmia. Combination therapy with two or three drugs may be required in more advanced disease.

♦ *Unstable angina* may require temporary hospitalization, bed rest, platelet inhibitor therapy (aspirin), or anticoagulation. Invasive measures may be required including percutaneous transluminal angioplasty (balloon angioplasty) or coronary artery bypass graft surgery.

Nitrates

♦ *Mechanisms.* Nitrates work by two mechanisms: 1) dilating epicardial coronary arteries and 2) venodilation to decrease preload and ventricular filling pressure.

♦ *Short-acting nitrates* (e.g., SL nitroglycerin and translingual spray) are primarily used for immediate prophylaxis or to abort an acute attack.

♦ *Longer-acting nitrates* are used either alone or in combination with other drugs to decrease the incidence of attacks.

♦ *Commonly prescribed organic nitrates* are listed in Table 14.3.

♦ *Transdermal Nitroglycerin.* Transdermal patches come in a variety of delivery systems (see Table 14.4), but they are equally effective in releasing the drug in a reliable manner over a 24-hr period. Patients may prefer one system over another based upon comfort, aesthetics, and adhesiveness. Contact dermatitis has been reported with transdermal patches.

Duration of Effects. With the first few applications, exercise tolerance and anti-anginal protection may last for 24 hr after a single morning application, but continued use is associated with the development of tachyphylaxis resulting in only a 4–18 hr duration of effect. Dosage regimens should maintain a nitrate-free interval (e.g., bedtime).

Beta-adrenergic blockers reduce myocardial oxygen demand by decreasing catecholamine-mediated increases in heart rate, contractility, and blood pressure. They also may have mild platelet inhibitory effects. A detailed listing of the available beta blockers and their classifications as to beta$_1$ specificity, metabolism, half-life, dose recommendations, and side effects is found in Chapter 11: Essential Hypertension.

♦ *Indications.* This drug class is especially indicated in patients following MI or with concurrent hypertension, arrhythmias, or vascular headaches that are also responsive to beta blockade. However, they should be used with caution in patients with chronic obstructive pulmonary disease (COPD), asthma, or peripheral vascular disorders. Recent evidence indicates that benefit outweighs risk in patients with diabetes or heart failure (bisoprolol, carvedilol, or metoprolol preferred), but each patient should be assessed individually.

♦ *Cautions.* Patients should be cautioned that abrupt withdrawal may lead to a rebound increase in underlying cardiac disease and possibly an increased risk of MI or sudden death.

Calcium channel blockers, such as amlodipine, bepridil, diltiazem, nicardipine, nifedipine, and verapamil, are all approved for this use and are equally effective. They are safe for use in asthma and COPD. However, CCBs should be used with caution in patients with CHF; verapamil has the most negative inotropic effect. Amlodipine and felodipine are preferred in patients with CHF.

♦ *Mechanisms of Action* (see Table 14.5), CCBs inhibit calcium entry and/or release in the cell. The net result of this inhibition is insufficient intracellular calcium, which limits myocardial and smooth muscle contraction. Dilation of large coronary arteries and relief of vasospasm is the basis for their use in vasospastic angina. Calcium channel blockers also produce peripheral arterial vasodilation and decrease workload (afterload) on the heart. In addition some possess negative inotropic properties (especially verapamil) similar to those of the beta blockers. Bepridil also blocks fast sodium channels in the heart, but is reserved for refractory cases because of the risk of torsade de pointes and agranulocytosis.

♦ *Additive Benefit.* Calcium channel blockers have an additive benefit in patients with: hypertension (see Chapter 11: Hypertension); supraventricular arrhythmias [verapamil and diltiazem slow AV node conduction (see Chapter 17: Cardiac Arrhythmias)]; peripheral vasospastic disorders (e.g., Raynauds); and possibly chronic migraine.

♦ *Dosing.* See Table 14.6 and Table 11.16 in Chapter 11: Essential Hypertension. Sustained release dosage forms of diltiazem, felodipine, nicardipine, nifedipine, and verapamil or intrinsically long-acting drugs (e.g., amlodipine and isradipine) are preferred. Avoid immediate release diltiazem, nifedipine, or verapamil to minimize hypotension and reflex tachycardia.

♦ *Adverse Effects.* See Table 14.5 and also Table 11.8 in Chapter 11: Essential Hypertension.

Angiotensin-Converting Enzyme (ACE) inhibitors do not have direct anti-ischemic properties, but reduce morbidity and mortality in patients with CHF, acute MI, and diabetes. Ramipril (Altace) decreased incidence of death, MI, stroke, and angina in one trial of patients with coronary artery disease (CAD) without heart failure. The future role of ACE inhibitors in treating CAD is being investigated further.

Variant Angina (Coronary Artery Spasm, Prinzmetal's Angina)

♦ Because of their antispasmodic effects and low side effects, CCBs are generally selected over nitrates or beta blockers.

♦ Nitrates are acceptable alternatives to CCBs, but beta blockers may worsen vasospastic angina by allowing unopposed alpha-mediated vasoconstriction.

Acute Coronary Syndrome (Unstable Angina and Non-Q Wave Myocardial Infarction)

♦ *Medical Therapy.* These conditions are a medical emergency falling between chronic stable angina and MI. Aggressive therapy, including hospitalization and combined therapy with up to 5 drugs, is indicated: aspirin (325 mg chewable), intravenous (IV) NTG infusion, IV or oral beta blockers, heparin (either IV unfractionated or SC fixed-dose low molecular weight), and calcium channel blockers.

♦ *Angioplasty.* Failure of aggressive drug therapy necessitates many invasive procedures. Percutaneous transluminal coronary angioplasty (PCTA) is a nonsurgical method of mechanically dilating a coronary artery obstruction through arterial intimal disruption, plaque fissuring, and stretching of the arterial wall. A balloon dilating catheter is advanced through the afflicted coronary artery to the obstruction site. Balloon inflations are repeated until the plaque is compressed and coronary blood flow resumes. Angioplasty generally is performed in patients with single-vessel disease and symptomatic ischemia, although it can be beneficial in some patients with multivessel disease. The lesion must be accessible by the catheter and is usually in the proximal portion of the vessel. Clinical improvement may be marked, but reocclusion is common and is an indication for coronary artery bypass graft surgery.

- **Glycoprotein (Gp) IIb/IIIc receptor antagonists** administered IV during PCTA and for 12–24 hours afterward decrease the risk of death, acute MI, or the need for repeat PCTA. Abciximab (ReoPro), eptifibatide (Integrilin), and tirofiban (Aggrastat) are all available in the U.S. Major adverse effects are bleeding and thrombocytopenia. See Table 14.7 for indications and dosing.

- **Intraluminal stents** are "metal scaffolding" devices placed into the vessel walls after balloon inflation during angioplasty. They provide a physical barrier to reoccurrence of stenosis at the site. Combined aspirin and clopidogrel are given for 2–4 weeks after stent placement, followed by aspirin continued for life.

- **Coronary artery bypass graft (CABG) surgery** uses either the patient's saphenous vein (from the leg), internal mammary artery, or a vein from a pig to create a "bypass graft" to allow blood to flow past the obstruction in the diseased artery. Candidates for CABG include patients with left main coronary disease, patients with three vessel disease with coexistent left ventricular dysfunction, survivors of sudden cardiac death, and those refractory to medical management and PCTA.

Table 14.1 • Characteristics of Angina Pectoris[a]

Symptoms
- Sensation of pressure or heavy weight on chest alone or with pain
- Pain described variably as feeling of tightness, burning, crushing, squeezing, vice-like, aching, or "deep"
- Gradual ↑ in intensity followed by gradual fading away (distinguished from esophageal spasm)[a]
- SOB[b] with feeling constriction about the larynx of upper trachea

Location of Pain or Discomfort
- Over the sternum or very near to it
- Anywhere between epigastrium and pharynx
- Occasionally limited to left shoulder and left arm
- Rarely limited to right arm
- Lower cervical or upper thoracic spine
- Left interscapular or suprascapular area

Radiation of Pain
- Medial aspect of left arm
- Left shoulder
- Jaw
- Occasionally, right arm

Duration of Symptoms
- 0.5–30 min

ECG
- ST segment depression ≥2 mm
- T wave inversion

Precipitating Factors
- Mild, moderate, or heavy exercise, depending on patient
- Effort that involves use of arms above the head
- Cold environment
- Walking against the wind
- Walking after a large meal
- Emotions: fright, anger, or anxiety
- Coitus

Nitroglycerin Relief[a]
- Relief of pain occurring within 45 sec to 5 min of taking nitroglycerin

[a]Esophageal spasm and other GI disorders occasionally mimic anginal pain and also can be relieved by nitroglycerin.
[b]SOB = Shortness of breath.

Notes:

Table 14.2 • Classification of Angina: Presenting Signs[a]

Chronic Stable Angina (Exercise-induced Angina)
Angina that is reproducible with a certain level of physical activity: usually due to atherosclerosis, platelet aggregation, and thrombi that all contribute to narrowing of coronary arteries.[b] Pain is relieved by rest or nitroglycerin

Unstable Angina (Crescendo Angina, Preinfarction Angina)
Change in angina characterized by ↑ intensity. frequency, or duration of symptoms. This may be premonitory of impending infarction

Prinzmetal Variant (Vasospastic) Angina
Due to spasm of coronary artery; may occur at rest. May be detected by ergonovine maleate provocation test

Mixed Angina
With both atherosclerosis and vasospasm

Silent Myocardial Ischemia
Transient change in myocardial perfusion that is detectable on ECG but does not result in pain or discomfort

[a]Discomfort arises when the O_2 supply to coronary arteries is unable to meet O_2 requirements (demand) for myocardial function.
[b]Ischemia develops when stenosis exceeds narrowing of lumen. >50% to 75% obstruction = Risk for Angina. >80% obstruction = High grade lesion. >95% obstruction = Functional absence of flow; risk of infarction.

Notes:

Table 14.3 • Commonly Prescribed Organic Nitrates

Nitrates	Dosage Form	Duration	Onset (min)	Usual Dosage
Short-acting				
NTG	SL	10–30 min	1–3	0.4–0.6 mg[a,b]
NTG	Translingual spray	10–30 min	2–4	0.4 mg/metered spray[a,b]
NTG	IV	3–5 min[c]	1–2	Initially 5 µg/min. ↑ Q 3–5 min until pain is relieved or hypotension occurs
Long-acting[d]				
NTG	SR capsule	4–8 hr	30	6.5–9 mg Q 8 hr
NTG	Topical ointment[e]	4–8 hr	30	½"–2" Q 4–6 hr[f] (Table 14.4)
NTG	Transdermal patch	4–8 hr	30	0.2–0.4 mg/hr[f]
NTG	Transmucosal	3–6 hr	2–5	1–3 mg Q 3–5 hr[f]
ISDN[g]	SL	2–4 hr	2–5	2.5–10 mg Q 2–4 hr[f]
	Chewable	2–4 hr	2–5	5–10 mg Q 2–4 hr[f]
	Oral	2–6 hr	15–40	10–60 mg Q 4–6 hr[f]
	SR	4–8 hr	15–40	40–80 mg Q 6–8 hr[f]
ISMN[h]	Tab (ISMO, Monoket)	7–8 hr	30–60	10–20 mg BID (a.m. and midday) to start. Titrate to 20–40 mg BID[f]
	SR tab (Imdur)	8–12 hr	30–60	60 mg QD to start. Titrate to 30–120 mg QD

[a]When using sublingual or translingual spray forms of nitroglycerin, patients should administer the dose while sitting to minimize tachycardia, hypotension, dizziness, headache, and flushing. The optimal dose relieves symptoms with ≤10–15 mm Hg drop in systolic BP or ≤10 beat/min rise in pulse. Pain relief is rapid (onset 1–2 min; relief in 3–5 min), but up to 3 doses at 5-min intervals may be given. After this, medical assistance should be summoned.
[b]Sublingual NTG tablets are degraded rapidly by heat, moisture, and light. They should be stored in a cool, dry place; do not leave the lid open or refrigerate. Tablets should be stored in the original manufacturer's container or a glass vial since the tablets volatilize and bind to many plastic vials and cotton. Previously, stinging of the tongue was an indicator of fresh tablets, but newer formulations only cause stinging in ~75% of patients.
[c]Duration after infusion discontinued.
[d]Longer-acting forms of nitrates are effective drugs, but one must understand their limitations to optimize effectiveness. Sublingual ISDN tablets display an onset and duration intermediate between that of sublingual NTG and oral ISDN. Because of high presystemic (1st-pass) metabolism of the oral forms of both NTG and ISDN, very large doses may be required compared to sublingual or chewable dosage forms. Small oral doses (2.5 mg NTG, 5 mg ISDN) are probably not effective; doses as large as 9 mg NTG and 60 mg ISDN are not uncommon. Despite claims for longer activity, ointments and oral forms are often only effective for 4–8 hr, even when given as SR preparations. Also, continued daily use leads to rapid development of tolerance (see f).
[e]Squeeze ½"–2" of ointment onto the calibrated paper enclosed in the package with tube. Carefully spread the ointment on chest in a thin layer ≈2" × 2" in size. Keep area covered with applicator paper. Wipe off previous dose before adding new dose or if hypotensive. If another person applies the ointment, avoid contact with fingers or eyes to prevent headache or hypotension.
[f]Dosage regimens should maintain a nitrate-free interval (e.g., bedtime) to ↓ tolerance development. Give last oral dose or remove ointment or transdermal patch at 7 p.m. Give last dose of SR ISDN in early afternoon.
[g]ISDN = Isosorbide dinitrate.
[h]ISMN = Isosorbide monohydrate = Major active metabolite of ISDN. 100% bioavailable; no first-pass metabolism, but tolerance may still occur. Rapid release (ISMO, Monoket) as 10- and 20-mg tablets. SR form (Imdur) as 60-mg tablets. OK to cut Imdur in half, do not crush or chew.

Notes:

Table 14.4 • Transdermal Nitroglycerin Systems[a]

Distributor/Product	Surface Area (cm²)	Total NTG Content (mg)
Schwarz Pharma		
Deponit 0.2 mg/hr (5 mg/24 hr)	16	16
Deponit 0.4 mg/hr (10 mg/24 hr)	32	32
Roberts		
Nitrodisc 0.2 mg/hr (5 mg/24 hr)	8	16
Nitrodisc 0.3 mg/hr (7.5 mg/24 hr)	12	24
Nitrodisc 0.4 mg/hr (10 mg/24 hr)	16	32
Key Pharmaceuticals		
Nitro Dur 0.1 mg/hr (2.5 mg/24 hr)	5	20
Nitro Dur 0.2 mg/hr (5 mg/24 hr)	10	40
Nitro-Dur 0.3 mg/hr (7.5 mg/24 hr)	15	60
Nitro-Dur 0.4 mg/hr (10 mg/24 hr)	20	80
Nitro-Dur 0.6 mg/hr (15 mg/24 hr)	30	120
Nitro-Dur 0.8 mg/hr (20 mg/24 hr)	40	160
Summit		
Transderm-Nitro 2.5 (0.1 mg/hr)	5	12.5
Transderm-Nitro 5 (0.2 mg/hr)	10	25
Transderm-Nitro 10 (0.4 mg/hr)	20	50
Transderm-Nitro 15 (0.6 mg/hr)	30	75
Transderm-Nitro 20 (0.4 mg/hr)	40	100
3M Pharm		
Minitran 0.1 mg/hr (2.5 mg/24 hr)	3.3	9
Minitran 0.2 mg/hr (5 mg/24 hr)	6.7	18
Minitran 0.4 mg/hr (10 mg/24 hr)	13.3	36
Minitran 0.6 mg/hr (15 mg/24 hr)	20	54

[a]Also generic in 0.2, 0.4, and 0.6 mg/hr.

Notes:

Table 14.5 • Calcium Channel Blockers

	Dihydropyridine Derivatives[a]	Diltiazem	Verapamil	Bepridil
Peripheral vasodilation[b]	+++	++	++	++
Coronary vasodilation[b]	+++	+++	++	+++
Negative inotrope[c]	+/−	++	+++	++[f]
AV node suppression[c]	+/−	+	++	+[f]
Heart rate	↑ (reflex)	↓	↓	↓[f]
Pharmacokinetics[d]				
Dosing[e]				
Side Effects				
Nausea, vomiting	+ (most)	+/−	+/−	+/−
Constipation	Not observed	+/−	+	Not observed
Hypotension, dizziness[g]	++	+	+	+
Flushing, headache	++	+	+	+
Bradycardia, CHF symptoms	+/−	+	++	+/−
Reflex tachycardia, angina	+[g]	Not observed	Not observed	++
Peripheral edema	+	+/−	+/−	Not observed
Drug Interactions[h]				Unknown

Also see Tables 11.15 and 11.16 in Chapter 11: Essential Hypertension.
[a]Dihydropyridine derivatives FDA approved for angina: Amlodipine (Norvasc), nicardipine (Cardene), and nifedipine (Adalat, Procardia). See Table 14.6 for others that are approved for hypertension but have been used clinically for angina. Investigational: nitrendipine (Baypress)
[b]Peripheral and coronary vasodilation helpful for angina, hypertension, and possibly CHF, but peripheral dilation is the basis for side effects of flushing, headache, and hypotension.
[c]AV node suppression is helpful for controlling supraventricular arrhythmias, but this property plus the negative inotropic effect may worsen CHF. Nifedipine has less negative inotropic effect than verapamil and diltiazem, but still may worsen CHF. Amlodipine may have the least negative inotropic effect.
[d]All have poor bioavailability due to high 1st-pass metabolism and all are eliminated primarily by hepatic metabolism; intra- and interindividual variability in bioavailability and metabolism is extensive. Diltiazem, nifedipine, nicardipine, and verapamil have short t½ (<5 hr) requiring frequent dosing or use of SR products. Amlodipine, isradipine (8 hr), felodipine (10–20 hr), and bepridil (42 hr) have longer t½. The long t½ of bepridil makes dosage titration difficult.
[e]See Table 14.6 in this chapter and Table 11.16 in Chapter 11: Essential Hypertension.
[f]Bepridil affects both sodium channels and calcium channels. Ventricular conduction can be depressed with prolonged QT interval on ECG. Ventricular toxicity including torsades de pointes has been reported. Hypokalemia and 2 cases of agranulocytosis also have been reported.
[g]Hypotension and reflex tachycardia most with immediate release nifedipine, occasional with immediate-release diltiazem and verapamil, minimal with sustained release products or intrinsically long-acting agents.
[h]Diltiazem and verapamil = weak CYP 3A4 inhibitors and strong p-glycoprotein inhibitors. ↑ cyclosporine and digoxin bioavailability via increased GI transport and possibly less gut metabolism. Case reports of cyclosporine renal toxicity with diltiazem. Bradycardia and heart failure risk with combined verapamil and digoxin via additive AV block and negative inotropic effects. Risk of interaction with drugs metabolized by CYP 3A4 not known.

Notes:

Table 14.6 • Calcium Channel Blockers in Anginal Syndromes[a]

	FDA Approved[b]	Usual Dose for Chronic Stable Angina[c]	Product Availability[d]
Dihydropyridines			
Amlodipine (Norvasc)	Angina	2.5–10 mg QD	2.5, 5, 10 mg tab
	Hypertension		
Felodipine (Plendil)	Hypertension	5–20 mg QD	5, 10 mg ER tab
Isradipine	Hypertension		
(DynaCirc)		2.5–10 mg BID	2.5, 5 mg IR cap
(DynaCirc CR)		5–10 mg QD	5, 10 mg CR tab
Nicardipine	Angina (IR only)		
(Cardene)	Hypertension	20–40 mg TID	20, 30 mg IR cap
(Cardene SR)		30–60 mg BID	30, 45, 60 mg SR cap
Nifedipine	Angina (not Adalat CC)		
(Adalat, Procardia, generic)	Hypertension (CC and XL only)	10–30 mg TID	10, 20 mg IR cap
(Adalat CC)		30–180 mg QD	30, 60, 90 mg ER tab
(Procardia XL)		30–180 mg QD	30, 60, 90 mg ER tab
Nisoldipine (Sular)	Hypertension	20–60 mg QD	10, 20, 30, 40 mg ER tab
Diphenylalkylamines			
Verapamil	Angina (IR and Covera HS only)	30–120 mg TID/QID	40, 80, 120 mg IR tab
(Calan, Isoptin, generic)	Hypertension	120–240 mg BID	120, 180, 240 mg SR tab
(Calan SR, Isoptin SR, generic)	SVT	120–480 mg Q HS	180, 240 mg DR, ER tab
(Covera HS)		120–480 mg QD	120, 180, 240, 360 mg ER cap
(Verelan)		200–400 mg Q HS	100, 200, 300 mg DR, ER tab
(Verelan HS)			

(continued)

Table 14.6 • Calcium Channel Blockers in Anginal Syndromes[a] (continued)

	FDA Approved[b]	Usual Dose for Chronic Stable Angina[c]	Product Availability[d]
Benzothiazepines			
Diltiazem	Angina	30–120 mg TID/QID	30, 60, 90, 120 mg IR tab
(Cardizem, generic)	Hypertension	60–180 mg BID	60, 90, 120, 180 mg SR cap
(Cardizem SR and generic)		120–360 mg QD	120, 180, 240, 300, 360 mg cap
(Cardizem CD and generic)		120–480 mg QD	120, 180, 240 mg ER cap
(Dilacor XR)		120–480 mg QD	120, 180, 240 mg ER cap
Tiamate ER		120–480 mg QD	120, 180, 240, 300, 360, 420 mg ER cap
Tiazac ER			
Bepridil (Vascor)	Refractory angina	200–400 mg QD	200, 300, 400 mg tab

Also see Tables 11.15 and 11.16 in Chapter 11: Essential Hypertension.

[a]Cap = capsules. CD = controlled diffusion. CR = controlled release. DR = delayed release. ER = extended release. FDA = Food and Drug Administration. HS = bedtime. IR = immediate release. SR = sustained release. SVT = supraventricular including atrial fibrillation, atrial flutter, and reentry. Tab = tablets. XL and XR = extended release.

[b]FDA approved indications vary among IR and ER products. However, most all have been used clinically for both angina and hypertension. Avoid IR release products in hypertension.

[c]Because of short half lives, most of these drugs are given TID if using IR tabs or caps. Amlodipine and bepridil have a long half-life and are given QD.

[d]Caution: Substituting one long-acting dosage form with another, even for the same drug, is not recommended. Cardizem SR capsules and verapamil SR tabs (Calan SR, Isoptin SR) still require BID dosing. Absorption of verapamil SR is more rapid and duration of action is shorter if taken on an empty stomach, generally it must be given Q 12 hours with food to maintain SR release, even though total bioavailability is reduced. Release characteristics of Verelan-beaded capsules have more reliable sustained-release characteristics allowing QD dosing, with or without food. Covera HS and Verelan HS are taken at bedtime to optimize AM release when blood pressure is often highest, but these two products are not interchangeable. Cardizem CD (copolymer-coated sustained-release beads) release 40% of the dose in the first 12 hours and 60% over the next 12 hours allowing QD dosing. Dilacor XR and Tiazac ER caps also given QD. Procardia XL uses the "GITS" technology and effectively releases the drug over 24 hours. Adalat CC also given QD but not GITS formulation. Some formularies allow therapeutic substitution of these two dosage forms.

Table 14.7 • Indications and Dosing of Glycoprotein II$_b$/III$_c$ Receptor Antagonists

Indication	Abciximab (ReoPro)	Eptifibatide (Integrilin)	Tirofiban (Aggrestat)
Percutaneous transluminal coronary angioplasty (PCTA)	0.25 mg/kg IV bolus, then 10 μg/min IV infusion × 12 hr	135 μg/kg IV bolus, then 0.5 μg/kg/min IV infusion × 20–24 hr	Not approved use
Coronary stent placement	0.25 mg/kg IV bolus, then 10 μg/min IV infusion × 12 hr	Not approved use	Not approved use
Acute coronary syndrome (unstable angina and non-Q-wave MI)	Not approved use	180 μg/kg IV bolus, then 2.0 μg/kg/min IV infusion × 72–96 hr	0.4 μg/kg/min IV load × 30 minutes, then 0.1 μg/kg/min IV infusion × 48–102 hr Reduce dose by 50% if CrCl <30 mL/min

CrCl = Creatinine clearance; IV = Intravenous.

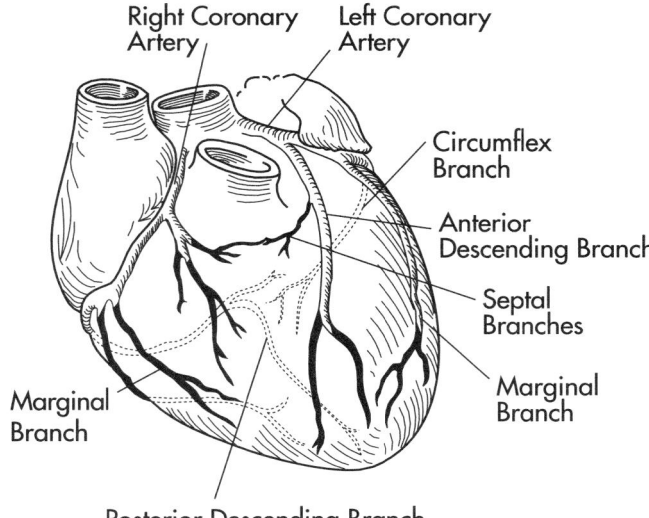

Fig. 14.1 Coronary Artery Distribution and Major Branches. (Reprinted with permission from Essentials of Human Physiology. Chicago: Yearbook Medical Publishers, Inc; 1978.)

The reader is referred to Chapter 15: Ischemic Heart Disease, written by *Toby Trujillo, Pharm.D.*, and *Paul E. Nolan, Pharm.D.*, in the seventh edition of **Applied Therapeutics: The Clinical Use of Drugs** for a more in-depth discussion. Other topics included in this chapter include microvascular ischemia and silent ischemia. The editors of this handbook express their thanks to Drs. Trujillo and Nolan and acknowledge that this chapter is based upon their work.

Notes:

Chapter 15

Myocardial Infarction (MI)

Definitions

+ ***Myocardial Infarction.*** Cellular death or necrosis of cardiac muscle and surrounding tissue secondary to severe or prolonged ischemia.
+ ***Myocardial Remodeling.*** Increased wall stress within the left ventricle causes thinning and stretching of the infarcted segment of the myocardial muscle leading to progressive left ventricular *dilation* and *hypertrophy.* This process, also known as infarct expansion, occurs over days to weeks after the MI.

Etiology

+ The most common is acute thrombus (clot) formation following fissuring or rupture of lipid-rich atheromatous plaque and platelet activation in an already stenotic vessel.
+ A rare or coexisting cause is coronary artery spasm.

Clinical Presentation

+ One or more of the following may be present:
  • Prolonged substernal chest pain or pressure (exaggerated angina).
  • Shortness of breath.
  • Diaphoresis.
  • Nausea with or without vomiting (may be interpreted as indigestion).
  • Hypotension or hypertension.
  • New heart murmurs, tachycardia or bradycardia, PVCs, or other arrhythmias.
+ Twenty percent of infarctions are "silent" (without pain). These "silent" infarctions:
  • Are more common in the elderly or patients with diabetes or hypertension.
  • May present with hypotension, weakness, or confusion (cerebrovascular symptoms)

Classification of MI and Prognosis

+ MI is classified by the region of the heart affected. It can be:
  • Anterior (these MIs have the poorest prognosis).
  • Lateral.
  • Inferior.
+ MI also is classified by electrocardiogram (ECG) changes:
  • **Q waves.** The presence of new Q waves may indicate more extensive necrosis and higher immediate mortality. *Non-Q wave infarcts* (25%–35% of events; also called

"acute coronary syndrome") often have more postinfarction angina (possibly signifying infarct extension) and earlier reinfarction; however, the prognostic distinction between Q wave and non-Q wave infarcts is still debated.

- **ST segment elevation** is seen in 90% of Q wave infarcts and 40% of non-Q wave infarcts. Also helps to define region of heart affected.
- ◆ **Early mortality.** Up to 10%–15%. Reduced to 5–10% with thrombolytic therapy.
- ◆ Increased risk of **sudden death** for 1–2 years postinfarction.

Cardiac Enzyme Monitoring

- ◆ *Creatinine kinase MB isoenzyme (CK-MB)* increases 3–6 hr post-MI, peaks in 12–24 hr, and returns to normal in 36–48 hr. This cycle is delayed if vessel reperfusion is slowed.
- ◆ *Lactate Dehydrogenase (LDH).* A ratio of $LDH_1:LDH_2 >1$ indicates myocardial damage. Onset is in 24–48 hr, and it peaks in 3–6 days.
- ◆ *Troponins.* More sensitive as late markers of MI than is LDH.

Management

- ◆ Goals of therapy:
  - Limit extension of myocardial necrosis.
  - Prevent reinfarction.
  - Control complications [pain, hypertension or hypotension, ventricular irritability, congestive heart failure (CHF)].
- ◆ Unless contraindicated, 4 classes of drugs are used in nearly all MI patients: a thrombolytic, a beta blocker, nitroglycerin (NTG), and aspirin. Morphine, lidocaine, heparin, warfarin, and stool softeners also are widely used. The role for angiotensin-converting enzyme (ACE) inhibitors and calcium channel blockers still is being defined. Cardiac complications such as arrhythmias and CHF are treated as presented in other chapters.

Thrombolysis

- ◆ *Goal.* Open and restore blood flow to the occluded artery as soon as possible to prevent further tissue necrosis.
- ◆ Table 15.1 lists the pharmacologic properties and dosing of the 6 thrombolytics currently available in the U.S. Urokinase is rarely used for MI. Unless contraindications are present (see Table 15.2) or administration is delayed beyond 12 hr, all patients should receive a thrombolytic. There is also a trend toward fewer MI complications with more fibrin-specific thrombolytics administered 12–24 hours post onset of MI symptoms.
- ◆ *Reperfusion* rates range from 60%–70%; *reocclusion* may occur in 10%–20%. tPA may be slightly faster and have higher reperfusion rates than streptokinase, but intracranial bleeding and cost are higher with tPA.
- ◆ *Side Effects.* Bleeding, especially intracranial bleeding, is a possible complication of all thrombolytics. Allergic reactions occur only with streptokinase and anistreplase. The incidence of post-MI thrombotic strokes has been reduced by thrombolytics, but hemorrhagic strokes are increased. It is suggested that patients over age 75 have a lower incidence of stroke with streptokinase than with tPA or reteplase.

Percutaneous Transluminal Coronary Angioplasty (PTCA)

- ◆ Alternative to thrombolytic therapy when thrombolytics are contraindicated or fail.

♦ Occluded vessels achieve patency faster with PCTA than with thrombolytics. PCTA may be associated with lower 5-year mortality, recurrent ischemia, or rehospitalization.

♦ Optimal results if performed within 12 hours of onset of pain.

Antiplatelet Therapy. (See Chapter 13: Thrombosis.)

♦ Aspirin 160–325 mg (chewed) given concurrently with thrombolytics increases the rate of vessel patency and is recommended for all patients.

♦ Aspirin 160–325 mg QD is recommended for lifetime prophylaxis against reinfarction unless contraindicated by gastrointestinal bleeding or intolerance.

♦ Clopidogrel (Plavix) 75 mg QD or ticlopidine (Ticlid) 250 mg BID are recommended if patient has an aspirin intolerance or aspirin is contraindicated.

♦ Aspirin and clopidogrel combined post stent placement.

Glycoprotein (GP) II$_b$/III$_c$ Receptor Antagonists

See Table 14.7 in Chapter 14: Ischemic Heart Disease for indications and dosing of abciximab, eptifibatide, and tirofiban.

Heparin

♦ Heparin should be given to all patients not receiving thrombolytics. Give 60 units/kg IV heparin bolus, then begin heparin infusion at 12 units/kg/hr to achieve aPTT 1.5–2 times control. (See Chapter 10: Thrombosis for further details of heparin dosing.)

♦ Heparin may also enhance efficacy rates (patency) when used as an adjunct to tPA (alteplase, reteplase, or tenecteplase). An initial 60 unit/kg IV bolus is given soon after the first bolus of tPA and the maintenance infusion should run concurrently with the tPA infusion and after.

♦ There is no evidence of additional benefit (reduced rate of reinfarction or stroke) when heparin is given to patients receiving streptokinase or anistreplase. Heparin may increase incidence of bleeding complications in these patients.

♦ **Subcutaneous low molecular weight heparin** (e.g., enoxaparin 1 mg/kg) should be given to patients with non-ST-segment elevation MI.

Warfarin

♦ Warfarin is recommended for stroke reduction and prevention of re-infarction in all patients with:
  • Atrial fibrillation.
  • A dilated left ventricle.
  • Postinfarct CHF.
  • Ventricular aneurysm.
  • Evidence of a mural thrombus in the left ventricle.

♦ Titrate dose to an INR of 2–3 for 1–3 months. (See Chapter 13: Thrombosis for details on warfarin pharmacology and dosing.)

♦ Some clinicians use warfarin in all patients without a contraindication.

Beta Blockers

♦ *Rationale.* Beta blockers decrease myocardial oxygen consumption, limit amount of myocardial damage, provide pain relief, decrease incidence of myocardial rupture, and prevent occurrence of life-threatening arrhythmias. There is evidence of decreased mortality, both immediately postinfarction and long term, with atenolol, metoprolol, propranolol, and timolol.

♦ Immediate IV administration is recommended for all patients unless evidence of cardiac decompensation [left ventricular hypertrophy, decreased ejection fraction (EF)] is present. Use with caution in patients with a past history of systolic CHF, asthma. chronic obstructive pulmonary disease, or diabetes.

♦ β_1-selective agents (atenolol or metoprolol) generally are preferred. For IV adminis- tration give metoprolol 5 mg IV Q 5 min for 3 doses.

♦ Titrate dose to a resting heart rate between 50–60 beats/minute and an exercise heart rate of <120 beats/minute and a resting systolic BP of 100–120 mm Hg.

♦ Once stabilized (including those with early cardiac decompensation), begin oral therapy. Continue for at least 2 years. (See Chapter 11: Essential Hypertension for details on beta blocker pharmacology and dosing.)

Nitrates

♦ Use SL and IV nitroglycerin as indicated for pain relief.

♦ Vasodilator effect of IV nitroglycerin also may reduce left ventricular filling pressure (preload) and systemic vascular resistance (afterload) to prevent left ventricular hypertrophy and CHF.

♦ IV routinely given for 24–48 hr, in a 15 µg bolus dose, then 5–10 µg/minute. Titrate dose up to maximum of 200 µg/minute to achieve pain relief and either a 10% decrease in mean arterial pressure or a 10%–30% decrease in pulmonary capillary wedge pressure. Keep systolic BP >90 mm Hg. Tolerance may develop requiring larger doses if the infusion is continued for prolonged periods. (See Chapter 14: Ischemic Heart Disease: Anginal Syndromes for nitrate dosing information.)

ACE Inhibitors

♦ Vasodilators reduce afterload and preload, thereby reducing oxygen demand and myocardial wall stress, which may slow "myocardial remodeling" (see Definitions).

♦ ACE inhibitors provide the most benefit in patients with large anterior MIs, evidence of left ventricular hypertrophy, EF <40%, or clinical evidence of CHF.

♦ Early IV administration is not recommended; excessive hypotension may offset any potential benefit.

♦ Begin oral therapy 2–3 days postinfarct and continue for at least 3 years. Begin with a captopril test dose of 6.25 mg, then 12.5–50 mg TID. If BP, renal function, and potassium level are stable, switch to a longer-acting agent (e.g., enalapril, lisinopril, benazepril, ramipril, or others). See Chapter 11: Essential Hypotension for ACE inhibitor pharmacology and dosing.

Calcium Channel Blockers

♦ *Positive attributes* include coronary and peripheral vasodilation and reduction of coronary vasospasm to reduce coronary ischemia, provide pain relief, and reduce CHF.

♦ Use diltiazem or verapamil for patients who either do not tolerate beta blockers or have continued chest pain despite beta blockers and nitrates. Avoid use in patients who are in heart failure or who have pulmonary congestion. Best results with diltiazem PO starting 24–72 hr post-MI in patients with non-Q wave infarcts.

♦ Avoid nifedipine or other dihydropyridines secondary to reflex tachycardia. These drugs may be indicated if angina persists.

♦ Use caution with verapamil and nifedipine secondary to negative inotropic effect.

♦ See Chapter 14: Ischemic Heart Disease and Chapter 11: Essential Hypertension for pharmacology and dosing.

Antiarrhythmics

♦ Ventricular irritability is common during the immediate post-MI period. If ectopy develops, lidocaine (1–1.5 mg/kg IV load, then 1–4 mg/kg/minute constant infusion) is generally the drug of choice for life-threatening ventricular arrhythmias, but specific treatment is individualized, depending upon the type of arrhythmia present. Alternatives include procainamide and amiodarone. (See Chapter 17: Cardiac Arrhythmias for principles of lidocaine, procainamide, and amiodarone dosing and treatment of arrhythmias in general.)

♦ Routine use of prophylactic lidocaine to prevent ventricular tachycardia and fibrillation in patients without ectopy is controversial. Patients under age 65, seen within 6 hr of onset of symptoms, and showing evidence of a new Q wave MI and ST segment elevation may benefit the most.

♦ Suppression of asymptomatic or mildly symptomatic ventricular ectopy with chronic oral therapy is not recommended due to increased risk of mortality from proarrhythmic effect of the drugs. Avoid flecainide, encainide, and moricizine.

Other Therapies

♦ *Morphine* 2–5 mg IV Q3–5 min PRN is the drug of choice for chest pain unrelieved by nitrates and thrombolytics. It also helps to relieve anxiety and reduce afterload and preload with minimal reflex tachycardia.

♦ *Oxygen* via nasal cannula to all patients until ischemic pain is relieved. Continue only if hypoxia persists by blood gases.

♦ *Docusate* or other stool softeners are used to prevent cardiac stress related to straining.

Notes:

Table 15.1 • Thrombolytic Agents[a]

	tPA[b] Alteplase (Activase) Reteplase (Retavase) Tenecteplase (TNKase)	Anistreplase (APSAC)[c] (Eminase)[c]	Streptokinase[d] (Streptase)	Urokinase[e] (Abbokinase)
Source	See footnote b	β-hemolytic streptococci	β-hemolytic streptococci	Human fetal culture or urine
Clot selectivity/fibrin specificity[f]	Modest to high	Low	Low	Modest
Antigenicity[g]	None	Yes, streptococci derived	Yes, streptococci derived	None
Half-life[h] (min)	alteplase: 3–9 α, 72 β; reteplase: 13–20 α, 98–135 β; TNKase: 11–24 α, 41–138 β	90–110 min	23 min	11–16 min
Dosing[i-k]	Alteplase: 1.25 mg/kg IV (*max*: 100 mg) over 90 min given as 15-mg bolus, then 0.75 mg/kg (*max*: 50 mg) over 30 min, then 0.5 mg/kg (*max*: 35 mg) over 60 min. *DVT/PE[a]*: 100 mg IV over 2 hr. Reteplase: 10 unit IV bolus; repeat 30 min later TNKase: 30 mg (if <60 kg) to 50 mg max. (if >90 kg) as single IV bolus	30 units IV over 2–5 min	*IV*: 1.5 million units infusion over 1 hr (investigational over 30 min) *Intra-arterial*: 20,000 units STAT, then 200 units/min for 1 hr *DVT/PE[a]*: 250,000 units IV over 30 min, then 100,000 units/hr infusion for 24–72 hr	*Intra-arterial*: 6,000 units/min until lysis (up to 2 hr). Average dose = 500,000 units *DVT/PE[a]*: 4400 units/kg IV over 10 min, then 4400 units/kg/hr infusion for 12 hr
Cost	High	Moderate	Lowest	Highest

[a]DVT = Deep venous thrombosis; PE = Pulmonary embolism; tPA = Recombinant tissue-type plasminogen activator.

[b]Alteplase = Direct-acting tissue plasminogen activator (PA) produced by recombinant DNA technology (rt-PA). PA binds to fibrin in a thrombus, then catalyzes cleavage of endogenous plasminogen peptide bonds to form plasmin. Plasmin in turn enzymatically dissolves the fibrin matrix of the thrombus. Reteplase (r-PA) and TNKase are genetically modified further to have greater fibrin specificity, longer half-lives, and more convenient dosing regimens.

[c]APSAC = Anisoylated plasminogen streptokinase activator complex. A complex of streptokinase and human blood-bound plasminogen to which a P-anisoyl group has been added to mask the catalytic center of the complex. In solution, gradual hydrolysis of the anisoyl group exposes the catalytic center and causes activation of plasminogen into plasmin. Essentially a "slow-release form" of streptokinase.

[d]Streptokinase binds to plasminogen to form on active plasminogen-streptokinase complex. The complex then cleaves other molecules of plasminogen to form plasmin, an active fibrinolytic enzyme that enhances dissolution of fibrin clots.

[e]Urokinase is a plasminogen activator that cleaves plasminogen and converts it to its active form, plasmin.

[f]Systemic administration of both streptokinase and urokinase has the potential disadvantage of plasmin activation not only at the site of thrombosis but also in the systemic circulation. tPA directly and more selectively binds to the fibrin-plasminogen complex in the clot, possibly ↓ the risk of systemic bleeding.

[g]Antigenicity caused by formation of neutralizing antibodies to streptococci-derived products. Titers measurable within a few days following administration and persist in 50% of patients at 4 yr. Allergic reactions, fever, and hypotension may occur in 15%–30%. Repeat administration of streptokinase or APSAC if reocclusion occurs soon after initial dose or later during a subsequent MI may be ineffective or associated with allergic reactions. tPA is indicated for repeat treatment in these patients.

[h]α = distribution half-life in minutes; β = terminal half-life in minutes.

[i]Effectiveness is time dependent. When treatment is started within 3 hr of anterior MI, streptokinase and tPA are equally effective (↑ coronary artery reperfusion, preservation of left ventricular function, ↓ mortality). From 6–12 hr, tPA may be more effective than streptokinase. Some evidence of value even if treatment delayed for 24 hr.

[j]Efficacy enhanced by concurrent aspirin 325 mg. Following clot lysis, there is a paradoxical increase in local thrombin generation and enhanced platelet aggregability.

[k]Repeat infusions within 24–48 hr with tPA if initial dose fails are safe, but efficacy is unreliable. Angioplasty or bypass graft surgery probably indicated if facilities available.

Table 15.2 • Risk Factors Associated with Bleeding Complications Secondary to Thrombolytic Use

Major
Thrombolytics contraindicated

Intracranial tumor or recent head trauma
Known or suspected aortic dissection
Previous hemorrhagic stroke at any time
Nonhemorrhagic stroke or cerebrovascular events within 1 yr
Active internal bleeding (excluding menses)
Major surgery within 2 wk

Important
Relative contraindication

Uncontrolled hypertension ≥180 mm Hg systolic, ≥110 mm Hg diastolic)
Remote thrombotic stroke
Recent transient ischemic attacks
Puncture of a noncompressible vessel
Cardiopulmonary resuscitation for >10 min
Recent trauma or major surgery (>2 but <4 wk)
Recent internal bleeding within 2–4 wk
Active peptic ulcer
Known bleeding diathesis or current use of anticoagulants (INR >2)
Pregnancy
History of chronic severe hypertension
For streptokinase or anistreplase: prior exposure (especially within 2–5 days) or prior allergic reaction
Diabetic retinopathy or other hemorrhagic ophthalmic conditions

Minor
Increased risk of bleeding

Older age
Female
Small body size
CPR[a] for <10 min

INR = International normalized ratio.
From references 6 and 11.

The reader is referred to Chapter 16: Myocardial Infarction, written by *Jean M. Nappi, Pharm.D.*, in the seventh edition of **Applied Therapeutics: The Clinical Use of Drugs** for a more in-depth discussion. All notations to reference numbers are based on the reference list at the end of that chapter. The editors of this handbook express their thanks to Dr. Nappi and acknowledge that this chapter is based upon her work.

Notes:

Chapter 16

Heart Failure

Definitions

♦ *Heart failure (HF)* results when the heart fails to pump sufficient blood to meet the body's needs.

♦ *Congestive heart failure (CHF).* A specific subset of HF characterized by left ventricular (LV) systolic dysfunction and a classic array of symptoms. (See Table 16.1.)

♦ *Afterload.* Forces acting on the *arterial* circulation to affect the impedance or resistance against which the left ventricle must pump during ejection; analogous to arterial resistance or pressure. Arterial dilators (e.g., hydralazine) decrease afterload to allow increased cardiac output.

♦ *Preload.* Forces acting on the *venous* circulation to affect myocardial wall function. Elevated preload aggravates congestive failure. Venous dilators (e.g., nitrates) decrease venous return, thus decreasing preload and relieving ventricular congestion.

♦ *Contractility.* The inherent ability of the myocardium (cardiac muscle) to develop force (contract) independent of preload or afterload. Contractility is synonymous with inotropism.

♦ *Ejection Fraction (EF).* Percent of LV volume expelled during systole. Normal: 60%–70%; <40% is usually symptomatic.

Classification

Heart failure can be classified as either low or high output failure. Low output failure is further subdivided into *systolic dysfunction* (classical congestive failure) and *diastolic dysfunction.* (See Table 16.2.)

Signs and Symptoms

♦ Systolic and diastolic failure present with similar symptoms, except for a normal EF in diastolic dysfunction.

♦ The symptoms of CHF can be divided into those that primarily reflect LV failure and those that denote right ventricular (RV) failure. (See Table 16.1.)

♦ Left-side failure usually occurs first. As volume accumulates in the LV, blood backs up into the pulmonary vasculature, causing increased pressure and pulmonary congestion. Elevated left side pressure and high pulmonary pressure force the RV to work harder until it eventually fails as well.

♦ Isolated right-sided failure is usually associated with stenosis or spasm of the pulmonary artery. For example:

  • Idiopathic primary pulmonary hypertension

- Drug-induced pulmonary hypertension (heroin, methylphenidate, fenfluramine, dexfenfluramine)
- Chronic obstructive pulmonary disease (COPD)

Treatment

♦ **Helpful nondrug interventions** include: correction of aggravating diseases (e.g., hypertension, anemia, and hyperthyroidism); elimination of precipitating factors such as drugs with high sodium contents (see Table 16.3) and drugs that may induce CHF (see Table 16.4); institution of a low sodium diet containing no more than 1–2 gm Na^+ and 2.5–5 gm NaCl (1 mEq Na^+ = 23 mg; 1 gm NaCl = 17 mEq Na^+); bed rest during acute episodes; and light exercise when patient is stable. Patients should avoid cooking with salt and using canned or packaged foods high in sodium.

Drug Treatment

♦ The immediate goals of drug therapy are to provide symptomatic relief and reversal of the signs and symptoms found in Table 16.1.

♦ Long-range goals are to increase quality of life, increase tolerance of activities of daily life, avoid hospitalizations, minimize adverse drug effects, and increase time of survival.

♦ The treatment algorithm (Figure 16.1) developed by the Agency for Health Care Policy and Research (AHCPR) recommends diuretics and ACE inhibitors as first-line therapy, supplemented with digoxin, nitrates, and other vasodilators as clinically indicated. Revised guidelines in 1999 recommend addition of a β-blocker as either first-line therapy combined with an ACE inhibitor or as an early add on with or without digoxin.

♦ Combination therapy of 2–4 drugs is common in advance disease, e.g., diuretic + ACE inhibitor (or nitrate plus hydralazine) + beta blocker and/or digoxin.

♦ *Diuretics* are indicated in both systolic and diastolic dysfunction when sodium restriction fails to control volume expansion. The goal is symptomatic relief of CHF without causing intravascular depletion. Dosing of diuretics may be daily in patients with edema or pulmonary congestion. Intermittent or PRN regimens may be preferred in asymptomatic patients or titrated to changes in weight. Diuretics should be withheld if hypotension or prerenal azotemia develops.

- **Dosing and Adverse Effects of Diuretics.** See Chapter 11: Essential Hypertension, Tables 11.10 and 11.18

- **Renal Failure.** Use of diuretics in patients with renal insufficiency (Cl_{Cr} <30 mL/min), the loop diuretics (furosemide, bumetanide, torsemide) or metolazone are preferred. Metolazone is characterized as a thiazide diuretic but has a potency intermediate between that of the other thiazides and loop diuretics.

- **Monitoring Diuretic Response and Side Effects.** See Table 16.5.

- **Diuretic Sites of Action.** See Figure 9.1 in Chapter 9: Fluids and Electrolyte Disorders.

- **Diuretic Resistance.** The *bioavailability* of oral furosemide is approximately 50%–60% in both normals and those with CHF. Despite this poor bioavailability, the 24-hour diuresis after IV and oral drug is almost equivalent. However, the time of onset (5–10 min IV; 20–30 min PO) and the diuresis during the first 2–4 hr is greatest with IV therapy. Some patients with severe CHF may have further reduced oral bioavailability of furosemide (as low as 34%) requiring use of parenteral therapy. Bioavailability is more complete and predictable with bumetanide and torsemide, but clinical responses are equal. As CHF worsens, a relative *refractoriness* to diuretics may occur necessitating large doses of loop diuretics. Using furosemide as an example, initial doses may be 20–40 mg/day. The dose is increased in 40- to 80-mg increments to a maximum of 320–600 mg/day. Equivalent doses: 40 mg furosemide = 1 mg bumetanide = 10 mg torsemide.

• **Continuous IV infusions** of furosemide (2.5–4 mg/hr), bumetanide (1 mg/hr), and torsemide (3 mg/hr) may be more efficacious than intermittent bolus in severe CHF or renal insufficiency. Others recommend higher doses: furosemide (0.25 to 1 mg/kg/hr), bumetanide (0.1 mg/kg/hr), or torsemide (5–10 mg/hr).

• **Combination Diuretic Therapy.** Combinations of a loop diuretic and metolazone (5–10 mg) or a thiazide may be necessary in patients who do not diurese after large doses of furosemide. These two drugs work on different parts of the tubule and have an additive diuretic effect. Since the duration of action of metolazone exceeds that of furosemide, some patients may require a decrease in furosemide dose after starting metolazone.

♦ **Spironolactone.** Doses of 25 to 50 mg/day, combined with a loop diuretic, an ACE inhibitor, and digoxin, may impart a cardioprotective effect and improve survival in patients with severe HF (EF <35%) independent of diuresis or potassium retention.

♦ **Treatment of Hypokalemia.** Potassium supplementation or potassium-sparing diuretics are not needed unless serum potassium is <3.5 mEq/L (30%-50% of patients) or the patient is taking digoxin. The average replacement dose is 20–60 mEq/day of potassium, but some patients may require >100 mEq/day. Only the chloride salt of potassium should be used.

♦ **Angiotensin-Converting Enzyme Inhibitors (ACEIs).** This family of vasodilator drugs has mixed preload- and afterload-reducing properties plus a mild diuretic effect (via aldosterone inhibition). They are preferred over other vasodilators and digoxin because of proven symptom reduction, documented reduction in mortality rates, convenience of dosing, and fewer side effects. Also see Chapter 11: Essential Hypertension for other ACEI's and dosing summary.

• *Choice of drug and dosing.* Table 16.6 lists the ACEIs approved for use in systolic HF and their usual doses. Initiate therapy with captopril because its short half-life allows easier dosage titration. Switch to a longer-acting drug for maintenance and titrate to listed target dose or maximum tolerated dose. All of the agents appear to be equally effective. Efficacy in diastolic HF is less clear.

• *Adverse effects.* Monitor patient for hypotension, nonproductive cough, and hyperkalemia. Angioedema, presenting as facial and neck swelling and severe airflow obstruction, is a rare complication; ACEIs are contraindicated in patients with familial angioedema or prior ACEI-induced angioedema. Contraindicated in pregnancy; skull, facial, and kidney abnormalities documented with use in 2nd and 3rd trimester of pregnancy.

• *Effects on renal function. (See Figure 16.2.)* ACEIs may improve renal function if cardiac output is increased. However, ACEIs may induce prerenal azotemia and renal failure if patient becomes hypotensive or volume depleted. Monitor BP, BUN, and creatinine daily when starting therapy or if patient is on a diuretic.

♦ **Angiotensin Receptor Antagonists.** Although not FDA-approved for HF treatment, clinical trials with losartan (Cozaar), 12.5 to 50 mg/day, and candesartan (Atecand), up to 16 mg/day, show equal symptomatic efficacy to ACEIs with less cough. Mortality benefits are still to be determined. These drugs offer no benefit over ACEIs relative to hypotension, hyperkalemia, renal function changes, or angioedema. Reserve for use in patients intolerant of ACEIs. See Chapter 11: Essential Hypertension, Table 11.14 for other angiotensin receptor antagonists and dosing summary.

♦ **Other Vasodilators (see Table 16.7 for drugs and dosing).** Hydralazine is a potent arterial dilator that provides symptomatic relief of HF by decreasing LV afterload. Nitrates are venous dilators that decrease LV congestion by reducing preload. Nitrate monotherapy is especially beneficial in patients with pulmonary congestion. Used in combination, these two drugs can reduce HF-associated mortality, but to a lesser degree than ACEIs. They are reserved for use either as an alternative to ACEIs in patients who do not tolerate ACEIs or as adjuncts to ACEIs in patients with continuing symptoms.

◆ **Beta Adrenergic Blockers.** Counteract many of the adverse hemodynamic changes that occur with heart failure (e.g., autonomic overactivity). Current guidelines recommend starting both an ACEI and a beta blocker in all patients with mild-to-moderate systolic HF unless contraindicated or a past history of intolerance is present. Their role in severe (NYHA class IV) heart failure is still to be determined. Because these recommendations are new, many clinicians start an ACEI first and then add either a beta blocker and/or digoxin as secondary therapy. Beta blockers are first-line therapy for HF caused by diastolic dysfunction.

- *Carvedilol (Coreg).* First beta blocker to obtain FDA approval for HF. Mixed alpha blocker and non-selective beta blocker. May also have antioxidant properties.

  —*Dosage.* Start with 3.125 mg BID. Double dose Q 2 weeks up to 25 mg BID in patients weighing <85 kg or 50 mg BID in larger patients. Take with food to slow absorption rate and reduce hypotension.

  —*Adverse effects.* Reduce or hold dose if hypotension, bradycardia, fluid retention, or worsening heart failure symptoms occur.

  —*Metabolism and drug interactions.* Metabolized by cytochrome P450 2D6, causing stereospecific variability in metabolism. Rifampin induces 2D6 metabolism and reduces carvedilol serum concentrations. Cimetidine inhibits carvedilol metabolism. Effect of other 2D6 inhibitors (quinidine, fluoxetine, paroxetine, and propafenone) on carvedilol metabolism unknown. Carvedilol reported to increase digoxin serum levels by 15% via unknown mechanism.

- *Metoprolol (Lopressor, Toprol XL).* Start at 5 to 6.25 mg BID of rapid release or 12.5 mg QD of extended release, titrate up to 150–200 mg/day of extended release. Lower cost than carvedilol and documented efficacy.

- *Bisoprolol (Zebeta).* Titrate to 5–10 mg maximum dose.

◆ **Digitalis Glycosides.** Digoxin reduces symptoms of heart failure through a combination of positive inotropic effects (increased myocardial contractility) and other neurohumoral actions. Improvement in survival has not been shown with these drugs. Digoxin should be started in patients with moderate-to-severe systolic dysfunction not responding to ACEIs (with or without a beta blocker) or other vasodilators. Benefit may be greatest in patients with S_3 gallop rhythm or atrial fibrillation. Digoxin is contraindicated in diastolic dysfunction. Document an EF <40% before initiating therapy.

- *Pharmacokinetics and dosing.* See Table 16.8.

- *Interactions.* See Table 16.9.

- *Adverse Effects.* See Table 16.10.

- *Management of Toxicity.* See Table 16.11.

◆ **Calcium channel blockers.**

- *Systolic HF.* All are relatively contraindicated due to negative inotropic effects. Diltiazem and verapamil can increase serum digoxin levels and have additive AV blocking effect. Amlodipine and felodipine appear to be safest in heart failure patients with concurrent angina. See Table 16.7.

- *Diastolic HF.* Verapamil is an alternative drug of choice to beta blockers. Prolongs duration of diastole to allow more complete ventricular filling.

Table 16.1 • Signs and Symptoms of CHF[a]

	Left Ventricular Failure	Right Ventricular Failure[b]
Subjective	SOB DOE Orthopnea (2–3 pillows) PND, cough Weakness, fatigue, confusion	Peripheral edema Weakness, fatigue
Objective	LVH $\downarrow$ BP EF <40%[c] Rales, S_3 gallop rhythm Reflex tachycardia $\uparrow$ BUN (poor renal perfusion)	Weight gain (fluid retention) Neck vein distension Hepatomegaly Hepatojugular reflex

[a]BP = Blood pressure; BUN = Blood urea nitrogen; DOE = Dyspnea on exertion; EF = Ejection fraction; LVH = Left ventricular hypertrophy; PND = Paroxysmal nocturnal dyspnea; SOB = Shortness of breath.
[b]Isolated right-sided failure occurs with long-standing pulmonary disease (cor pulmonale) or after pulmonary hypertension.
[c]Ejection fraction normal in patients with diastolic dysfunction.

Table 16.2 • Classification and Etiology of Left Ventricular Dysfunction[a]

Type of Failure	Characteristics	Contributing Factors	Etiology
Low output, systolic dysfunction (dilated cardiomyopathy)[b] (60%–70% of cases)	Hypofunctioning left ventricle; enlarged heart (dilated left ventricle); $\uparrow$ left ventricular end-diastolic volume; EF <40%; $\downarrow$ stroke volume; $\downarrow$ CO; S_3 heart sound present	1. $\downarrow$ contractility (cardiomyopathy) 2. $\uparrow$ afterload (elevated SVR)	1. Coronary ischemia,[c] MI, mitral valve stenosis or regurgitation, alcoholism, viral syndromes, nutritional deficiency, calcium and K depletion, drug-induced, idiopathic 2. Hypertension, aortic stenosis, volume overload
Low output, diastolic dysfunction (30%–40% of cases)	Normal LV contractility; normal size heart; stiff left ventricle; impaired left ventricular relaxation; impaired left ventricular filling; $\downarrow$ left ventricular end-diastolic volume; normal EF; $\downarrow$ SV; $\downarrow$ CO; exaggerated S_4 heart sound	1. Thickened left ventricle (hypertrophic cardiomyopathy) 2. Stiff left ventricle (restrictive cardiomyopathy) 3. $\uparrow$ preload	1. Coronary ischemia,[c] hypertension, aortic stenosis and regurgitation, pericarditis, enlarged left ventricular septum (idiopathic hypertrophic subaortic stenosis) 2. Amyloidosis, sarcoidosis 3. Sodium and water retention
High-output failure (uncommon)	Normal or $\uparrow$ contractility; normal size heart; normal left ventricular end-diastolic volume; normal or $\uparrow$ EF; normal or increased stroke volume; $\uparrow$ CO	$\uparrow$ metabolic and oxygen demands	Anemia and hyperthyroidism

[a]CO = Cardiac output; EF = Ejection fraction; K = Potassium; MI = Myocardial infarction; SV = Stroke volume; SVR = Systemic vascular resistance.
[b]Same as congestive heart failure if symptoms also present.
[c]Heart failure caused by coronary artery ischemia or myocardial infarction classified as "ischemic" etiology. All other types combined as "nonischemic."

Table 16.3 • Sodium Content of Medicinals: Selected Adult Medications with an Extraordinarily High Sodium Content (100 mg/dose)[a]

Drug	Unit	mg Na$^+$/unit[b]	mEq Na$^+$/unit
Parenteral Products			
Ticarcillin	1 g	120–150	5.2–6.5
Oral Liquids			
Cerose-DM	15 mL	157	6.8
Phenergan Expectorant (Plain/VC)	15 mL	150	6.5
Phospho-Soda	5 mL	554	2.4
Tussar	15 mL	105	4.6
Vicks Cough Syrup	15 mL	162	7.0
Vicks Formula 44 Syrup	15 mL	202	8.8
Oral Solid Dosage Forms			
Alka Seltzer	1 tablet	295	12.8
Alka Seltzer Pain Relief	1 tablet	551	24.0
Bisodol Powder	1 tsp	156	6.8
Bromo Seltzer	80 mg capful	760	33.0
Eno	1 tsp	818	35.6
Goody's Headache Powder	1 pack	812	35.3
Kayexalate Powder (Suspension)	15 g (60 mL)	1,500	65.2
Soda Mint	1 tablet	90	3.9
Sodium Salicylate	10-gr tablet	97	4.2
Food Supplements			
Ensure	1 L	844	36.7
Isocal	1 L	530	23.0
Meritene	1 L	880–1,078	38.3–46.9
Osmolite	1 L	549	23.9
Sustacal	1 L	924–940	40.2–40.9
Vivonex	1 L	468–529	20.3–23.0
Miscellaneous			
Fleets Enema	120 mL	4,439	193.0

[a] 23 mg Na = 1 mEq.
[b] Average absorption = 275–400 mg/enema (12.0 –176.9 mEq).

Notes:

Table 16.4 • Drugs That May Induce CHF

Negative Inotropic Agents

Beta blockers[a]	Most evident with propranolol or other non-selective agents. May be less with agents with intrinsic sympathomimetic activity (acebutolol, carteolol, pindolol). Also may be caused by use of timolol eyedrops
Calcium channel blockers[a]	Verapamil has most negative inotropic and AV blocking effects; amlodipine has the least
Antiarrhythmic drugs	Most with disopyramide (Norpace). Also quinidine

Direct Cardiotoxins

Cocaine, amphetamines	Overdoses and long-term myopathy
Anthracycline cancer chemotherapeutic drugs	Daunomycin and daunorubicin (Adriamycin). Dose-related. Keep total cumulative dose <600 mg/m^2

Expansion of Plasma Volume

NSAIDs	Prostaglandin inhibition; Na$^+$ retention
Corticosteriods, androgens, estrogens	Mineralocorticoid effect; Na$^+$ retention
Licorice	Aldosterone-like effect; Na$^+$ retention
Antihypertensive vasodilators (hydralazine, methyldopa, prazosin, minoxidil)	↓ renal blood flow; activation of renin-angiotensin system
Drugs high in Na$^+$	See Table 16.3

[a]Beta blockers and verapamil may be beneficial in diastolic CHF. Some β blockers (bucindolol, carvedilol, metopralol) approved for treatment of systolic dysfunction by counteracting autonomic hyperactivity.

Table 16.5 • Monitoring Parameters with Diuretics

↓ CHF symptoms (see Table 16.1)
1–2 lb weight loss/day until "ideal weight achieved"[a]
Signs of volume depletion
   weakness
   hypotension, dizziness
   orthostatic changes in blood pressure[b]
   ↓ urine output
   ↑ BUN[c]
↓ Serum K, Mg
↑ Uric acid, glucose

[a]Weight loss may be greater during 1st few days when significant edema is present.
[b]↓ in systolic BP of 10-15 mm Hg or ↓ diastolic BP of 5-10 mm Hg.
[c]A rising BUN can be caused by either volume depletion from diuretics or poor renal flow from poorly controlled CHF. Small boluses of 0.9% saline may be given cautiously to differentiate a rising BUN from volume depletion versus poor cardiac output. If volume depletion is present, saline will cause ↑ urine output and ↓ BUN. However, if the patient has severe CHF, the saline could cause pulmonary edema.

Notes:

Table 16.6 • ACE Inhibitor Use in Systolic Dysfunction[a]

Drug	Dosage Form	Starting Dose[b]	Target Dose[c]	Maximum Dose
Captopril[d] (Capoten, generic)	12.5, 25, 50, 100 mg tablets	6.25–12.5 mg TID	50 mg TID	100 mg TID
Enalapril (Vasotec)	2.5, 5, 10, 20 mg tablets	2.5–5 mg QD	10 mg BID	20 mg BID
Fosinopril (Monopril)	10, 20, 40 mg tablets	5–10 mg QD	20 mg QD	40 mg QD
Lisinopril (Prinivil, Zestril)	2.5, 5, 10, 20, 40 mg tablets	2.5–5 mg QD	10–20 mg QD	40 mg QD
Quinapril (Accupril)	5, 10, 20, 40 mg tablets	5–10 mg QD	20 mg BID	20 mg BID
Ramipril (Altace)	1.25, 2.5, 5, 10 mg capsules	1.25–2.5 mg QD	5 mg BID	10 mg BID

[a]Benazepril, cilazapril, moexipril, and trandolapril not labeled for use in HF.
[b]Start with lowest dose if hypotensive or renal dysfunction. All but captopril given QD in AM at starting doses. Increase dose slowly at 2- to 4-week intervals to assess full effect and tolerance.
[c]Enalapril, quinapril, and ramipril could possibly be given QD instead of BID based on half-life.
[d]Captopril is short acting. Start with a 6.25- or 12.5-mg test dose, then 6.25 to 12.5 mg TID.
Adapted from reference 31.

Table 16.7 • Comparative Pharmacology of Non-ACE Inhibitor Unloading Agents[a,b]

Drug	Dose	Comments
Predominantly Afterload Reduction (Arterial Dilators)		$\downarrow$ SVR; $\uparrow$ CO
Direct Vasodilators (Oral)		
Hydralazine	*Start:* 12.5–25 mg *Maintenance:* 25–100 mg Q 6–8 hr	Concurrent diuretics to block Na^+ retention; less reflex tachycardia than when treating hypertension
Minoxidil	*Start:* 2.5–5 mg *Maintenance:* 5–20 mg Q 8–12 hr	Same as hydralazine
Calcium Channel Blockers (Oral)[c]		
Amlodipine	2.5–10 mg Q 24 hr	
Diltiazem[d]	30–90 mg Q 6–8 hr; 60–180 mg SR Q 12–24 hr	All relatively contraindicated due to concern about negative inotropic effect (V>D>N>A,F)[a]
Felodipine	5–20 mg Q 12–24 hr (*max:* 20 mg/day)	May $\uparrow$ digoxin levels (V>D>N)[a]
Verapamil[d]	40–60 mg Q 6–8 hr; 120–240 mg SR Q 12–24 hr	
Predominantly Preload Reduction (Venous Dilators)		$\downarrow$ PCWP and left ventricular filling pressure
Nitrates (NTG)		
IV[e]	5 µg/min; titrate to effect (*max:* 200 µg/min)	
SR	6.5–9 mg Q 8–12 hr PO	6–8 hr duration
Ointment	½ inch–2 inch Q 4–8 hr	3–6 hr duration
Transdermal	5–40 mg/day (remove at night)	Concern about tolerance with SR and transdermal
Isosorbide		
SL	5–20 mg Q 3–6 hr	Short-acting (1–3 hr)
Tablets PO	10–80 mg Q 4–6 hr	4–6 hr duration
SR	20–120 mg Q 6–8 hr	6–8 hr duration

(continued)

Table 16.7 • Comparative Pharmacology of Non-ACE Inhibitor Unloading Agents [a,b] (continued)

Drug	Dose	Comments
Mixed Afterload and Preload Reduction		
Nitroprusside	*Start:* 5–20 μg/min	Parenteral only
	Titrate: 300–800 μg/min	

[a]A = Amlodipine; D = Diltiazem; F = Felodipine; N = Nifedipine; V = Verapamil. ACE = Angiotensin-converting enzyme; CO = Cardiac output; IV = Intravenous; Na = Sodium; NTG = Nitrogen; PCWP = Pulmonary capillary wedge pressure; PO = Oral; SL = Sublingual; SR = Sustained release; SVR = Systemic vascular resistance.
[b]See Chapters 11: Essential Hypertension and 14: Ischemic Heart Disease for side effects. On balance, the benefits of afterload reduction exceed those of preload reduction.
[c]Calcium blockers not listed (e.g., nifedipine, nicardipine) are not recommended in HF.
[d]Diltiazem and verapamil are only for use in patients with supraventricular arrhythmias or primarily diastolic CHF.
[e]May bind to plastic IV bags and many plastic tubing sets.

Table 16.8 • Pharmacokinetic Dosing of Digoxin

Bioavailability (F)	
Tablets	0.75 (0.5–0.9)[a]
Elixir	0.80 (0.65–0.9)
Liquid-filled capsules	0.95 (0.8–1.0)
Half-Life ($t_{1/2}$)	
Normal	1.6–2 days
Renal failure	≥4.4 days
Children	0.7–1.5 days
Volume of Distribution (Vd)[b]	
Normal	6.7 (4–9) L/kg
Renal failure	Smaller: 4.7 (1.5–8.5 L/kg)
Clearance	
Normal	1.02 Cl_{Cr} + 57 mL/min or 2.7 mL/min/kg
Severe CHF	0.88 Cl_{Cr} + 23 mL/min
% Renally Cleared Unchanged	*PO:* 50%–60%
	IV: 70%–75%
% Nonrenal Elimination	40% (20%–55%)
% Eliminated/Day	14% + Cl_{Cr}/5
% Enterohepatic Recycling	6.8%
Protein Binding	20%–30%
Therapeutic Serum Concentration[c]	0.8–2 ng/mL (1.2–2.6 mmol/L)
Usual Digitalizing Dose[d]	0.5–1 mg or 0.01–0.02 mg/kg
Usual Maintenance Dose[e]	0.125–0.5 mg/day
Pediatric Dosing	
Neonate loading	0.01–0.03 mg/kg IV
Infant loading	0.01–0.05 mg/kg PO
>2 yr loading	0.05 mg/kg PO
Premature maintenance	0.001–0.009 mg/kg/day
Neonate maintenance	0.01 mg/kg/day
Infant maintenance	0.015–0.025 mg/kg/day
>2 yr maintenance	0.01–0.015 mg/kg/day

[a]Mean value with range in parentheses.
[b]Vd ↓ in renal failure, possibly because of change in protein binding.
[c]There is a poor correlation between digoxin serum concentrations and effect. Levels drawn <6 hr after a dose may be falsely elevated. Spironolactone and endogenous digoxin-like substances in the blood of neonates and renal failure patients may result in falsely elevated levels. Resting concentrations may be higher than those taken after exercise.
[d]In patients in acute distress, loading doses of digoxin are indicated since it takes several days (5 × $t_{1/2}$) to reach steady state with maintenance doses. A more specific loading dose can be calculated by multiplying the desired steady-state concentration by the volume of distribution.
[e]Dosages may be higher for supraventricular arrhythmias than for heart failure. The dosage should be adjusted lower in the elderly or those with renal insufficiency by first estimating Cl_{Cr} to calculate an estimated digoxin clearance. The dosage is estimated by multiplying the target serum concentration times the estimated clearance.

Table 16.9 • Digoxin Drug Interactions

Drug	Effect
Drugs Affecting Absorption	
Antacids	↓ bioavailability via adsorption
Cancer chemotherapy	Possible ↓ bioavailability (especially combination of cyclophosphamide and vincristine)
Cholestyramine (Questran)	↓ bioavailability via adsorption
Colestipol (Colestid)	↓ bioavailability via adsorption
Erythromycin	↑ bioavailability in persons who normally metabolize digoxin in intestinal tract, possibly by inhibiting p glycoprotein.
Laxatives	↓ bioavailability via hypermotility
Metoclopramide (Reglan)	↓ bioavailability via enhanced gastric emptying (slow-release digoxin only)
Neomycin	Malabsorption of digoxin
Omeprazole	↑ bioavailability (slight) due to altered gut metabolism
Propantheline (Pro-Banthine)	↑ bioavailability via slowed gastric emptying (slow-release digoxin only)
Psyllium hydrophilic mucilloid (Metamucil) and dietary bran fiber	Possible ↓ bioavailability
Sulfasalazine (Azulfidine)	Malabsorption of digoxin
Drugs Affecting Distribution and Excretion	
Alprazolam	↑ serum digoxin levels
Amiodarone (Cordarone)	↑ serum digoxin levels
Calcium channel blockers	↑ serum digoxin levels (especially diltiazem and verapamil), possibly by inhibiting p glycoprotein
Captopril	↑ serum digoxin levels
Propafenone	↑ serum digoxin levels; dose-related
Quinidine	↑ serum digoxin levels, complex interactions
Tiaconazole	↑ serum digoxin levels

Table 16.10 • Digoxin Side Effects[a]

Cardiac[b]
  Bradycardia (AV block) (pulse <50 BPM) (Prolonged PR interval)
  ↑ irritability [premature atrial tachycardia (PAT), premature ventricular contractions (PVCs), others]

GI (anorexia, nausea)

Visual (altered color perceptions, halos)

CNS (nightmares, psychosis, hallucinations)

Fatigue, weakness

Hyperkalemia (tall, peaked T waves on ECG)

Gynecomastia (long-term)

[a]Toxicity most prevalent when serum concentration ≥2 μg/L or if serum potassium <3.0 mEq/L or if serum magnesium ↓.
[b]Cardiac side effects may occur without other patient complaints.

Table 16.11 • Treatment of Digitalis Toxicity

Withhold digitalis

Potassium replacement (10–40 mEq/hr) unless hyperkalemia present

Magnesium replaced unless hypermagnesemia present

Atropine 0.5–1 mg for bradycardia

Lidocaine or phenytoin for ventricular ectopy

Antidote if above fails or if life-threatening: digoxin-specific antibody fragments (digoxin immune Fab)[a]

[a]Digoxin immune Fab: Each 38-mg vial will bind approximately 0.5 mg digoxin. Formula to estimate body load of digoxin (in mg) = 5.0 (serum digoxin concentration) (wt in kg)/1000, where 5.0 is the Vd of digoxin in L/kg. Empiric dose = 380 mg (10 vials)

Notes:

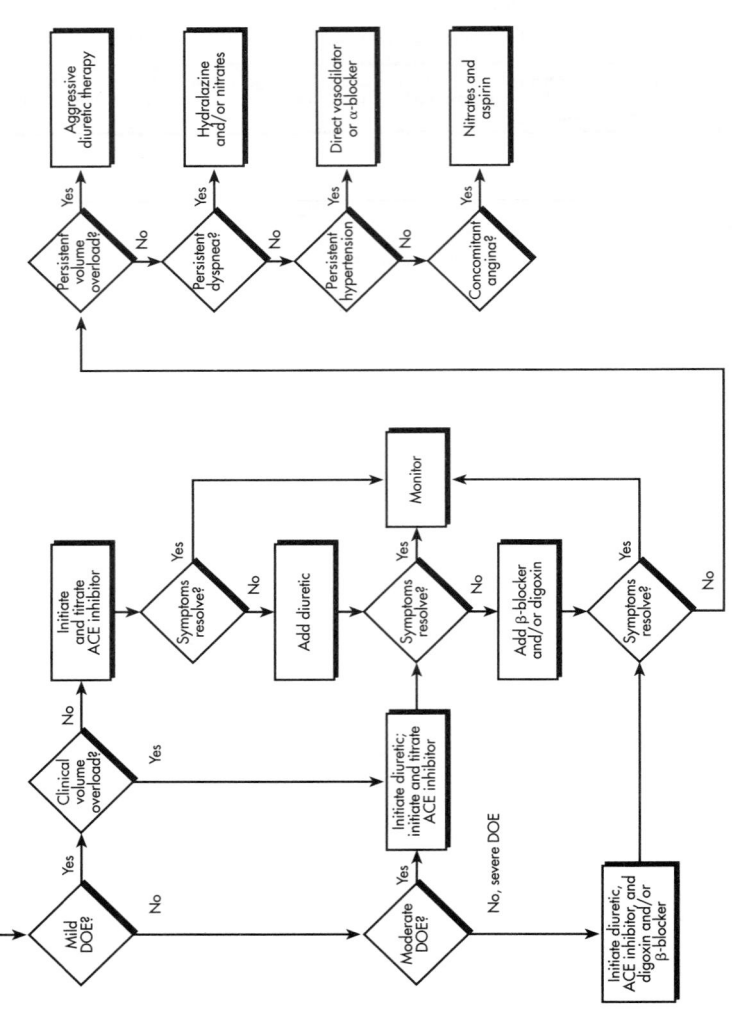

Fig. 16.1 Pharmacologic Management of Patients with Heart Failure. Reprinted with permission from Agency for Public Health Care Policy and Research. Heart Failure: Evaluation and Care of Patients with Left-Ventricular Systolic Dysfunction and adapted to integrate the role of β blockers.

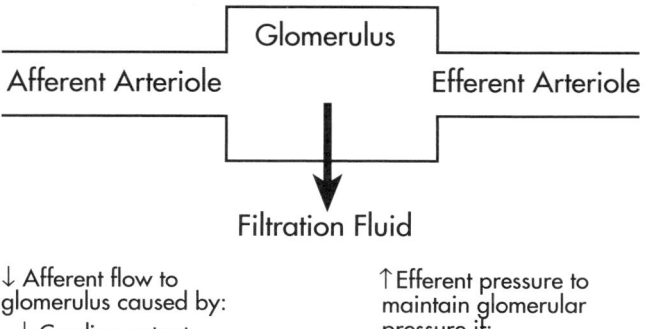

Filtration Fluid

↓ Afferent flow to
glomerulus caused by:

  ↓ Cardiac output
  Systemic hypotension
  Blood loss
  Overdiuresis, dehydration
  Renal artery stenosis
  (obstruction)
  Inhibition of PGE from NSAIDs

↑ Afferent flow to
glomerulus caused by:

  Systemic hypertension

↑ Efferent pressure to
maintain glomerular
pressure if:

  ↑ Production of
  angiotensin II via
  activation of renin-
  angiotensin system

↓ Efferent pressure to
protect glomerular
pressure if:

  ACE inhibitors block
  angiotensin II production

Fig. 16.2 Factors Affecting Renal Blood Flow. Normal glomerular filtration is dependent upon maintaining normal glomerular capillary pressure by regulating the balance of afferent and efferent arteriole. NSAID = Nonsteroidal anti-inflammatory drug; PGE = Prostaglandin E.

The reader is referred to Chapter 17: Heart Failure, written by *Wayne A. Kradjan, Pharm.D.*, in the seventh edition of **Applied Therapeutics: The Clinical Use of Drugs** for a more in-depth discussion. All notations to reference numbers are based on the reference list at the end of that chapter. The editors of this handbook express their thanks to Dr. Kradjan and acknowledge that this chapter is based upon his work.

Notes:

Notes:

Chapter 17

Cardiac Arrhythmias

Conduction Pathways: Electrocardiogram (ECG)

♦ **Conduction Scheme.** Electrical impulses normally begin in the SA node, the tissue with the greatest automaticity (ability to spontaneously depolarize). Each impulse spreads like a wave through the "working cells" of the atrium (causing the atrium to contract) until it reaches the AV node. The AV node acts as a "gate" to prevent excessive impulses from being conducted into the ventricles during certain arrhythmias. Alternatively, the AV node can spontaneously depolarize (function as the "pacemaker") if the SA node is damaged. From the AV node, the impulse travels through a specialized portion of the AV node called the bundle of HIS and then to the left and right ventricles via the left and right bundle branches. Finally the impulse reaches the terminal portions of the electrical system in the Purkinje fibers of the ventricles. From here, the current spreads like a wave through the working cells of the ventricles to cause ventricular contractions that translate into a heart beat or pulse wave.

♦ **Anatomy of Conduction System.** See Figure 17.1.

♦ **Relationship of Conduction System to ECG.** The relationship of this conduction scheme to the ECG is also illustrated in Figure 17.1.

Pathophysiology of Arrhythmias

Arrhythmias may be separated into those due to *abnormal impulse formation,* those due to *abnormal impulse conduction,* or a combination of both.

Abnormal Impulse Formation

Definition. Abnormal impulses can arise from either normal pacemaker sites (e.g., SA or AV node) or from outside the normal pacemaker system (e.g., an ectopic site). Those arising from the normal pacemakers generally are not pathologic and do not require treatment.

Abnormal Impulse Conduction

♦ **Definition.** Abnormal impulse conduction arrhythmias occur when normal conduction pathways are blocked causing impulses arriving from above to travel a more circuitous route to depolarize an area of myocardium.

♦ **Examples.** The simplest examples are left or right bundle branch blocks. If the left bundle branch is blocked, impulses travel first to the right ventricle by normal pathways and then eventually reach the left ventricle via wave-like conduction through ventricular muscle "worker cells."

♦ **Re-entry** (see Figure 17.2) is a more complex form of conduction defect caused by a transient or unidirectional disruption (block) of impulse conduction through one portion of a conduction pathway. An impulse reaching the blocked tissue conducts around it via an alternate pathway. If the conduction through the alternate pathway is slow, the impulse may return to the previously blocked tissue when it is no longer refractory and propagate a retrograde impulse through that tissue (i.e., the impulse "re-enters" the tissue that was originally blocked). This process then may repeat itself and perpetuate the arrhythmia.

- *Paroxysmal supraventricular tachycardia (PSVT) and Wolff-Parkinson-White (WPW) syndrome* are examples of re-entry arrhythmias through the AV node.
- Re-entry phenomenon also can occur in the ventricles at the level of the Purkinje fibers.
- Drugs may help break the re-entry cycle by increasing the effective refractory period of the tissue. (See Table 17.4.)

Classification of Arrhythmias
See Table 17.1.

Conduction Blocks
- **Definition.** Conduction blocks are interruptions in the normal electrical conduction pathways that have varying degrees of complications. These blocks can occur in the AV node, the bundle of HIS, or the left and right bundle branches.
- **Classification of AV Node Conduction Blocks.** See Table 17.2.

Clinical Features of Arrhythmias
- Arrhythmias can occur spontaneously or in conjunction with other cardiac disorders. Heart muscle damage following an MI is a frequent precipitating event.
- Subjectively, rhythm disturbances may be asymptomatic or they may be associated with a "fluttering sensation," "thumping," or "palpitation" in the chest.
- Unless the arrhythmia is accompanied by loss of consciousness, hypotension, reduced exercise tolerance, CHF, or dizziness (signifying inadequate cerebral or tissue perfusion), it is best to withhold drug therapy.
- Arrhythmias that result in a loss of cardiac output (e.g., ventricular fibrillation) can cause sudden loss of consciousness (syncope) and death.
- See Table 17.3 for risk factors of torsade de pointes including known precipitant drugs.

Antiarrhythmic Drugs
Vaughn-Williams Classification
- Table 17.4 classifies antiarrhythmic drugs according to their electrophysiologic effects (i.e., Vaughn-Williams classification).
- **Pharmacology.** Pharmacologically, drugs from within each Vaughn-Williams class are interchangeable, but individual responsiveness to each drug and side effects vary.

Arrhythmia Types and Drugs of Choice
The pathophysiology of arrhythmias and the pharmacology, pharmacokinetics, and side effect profiles of the available drugs are complex issues. Table 17.5 integrates the knowledge of each of these factors into the safest and most cost-effective recommendations for treatment of common arrhythmic processes.

Cardiopulmonary Resuscitation Drugs
See Table 17.6. The most frequently used drugs during cardiopulmonary resuscitation are epinephrine, lidocaine, and atropine. Calcium and bicarbonate frequently were used in the past, but their use now is controversial.

Table 17.1 • Classification of Arrhythmias[a]

Supraventricular (Arrhythmias That Arise from Above the Ventricle)
Those Arising from SA Node
Sinus tachycardia (e.g., pulse >100 with exercise or stress)
Sinus bradycardia (e.g., <60 in athlete)

Those Arising from Ectopic Sites in Atrium
Premature atrial contractions (isolated abnormal beats)
Atrial tachycardia [may be unifocal or multifocal (MAT)]
Atrial flutter
Atrial fibrillation (characterized by irregular ventricular activation)

Re-Entrant Rhythms (Involve AV Node, HIS Bundle)
Paroxysmal atrial tachycardia (PAT)
Paroxysmal supraventricular tachycardia (PSVT) (See Figure 17.2.)

Ventricular (Arise from Ectopic Sites in Purkinje System)
Premature Ventricular Contractions (PVCs)
Characterized on ECG by a broad QRS complex with an ↑ amplitude. (See Figure 17.3.)
  Subcategories include:
  Unifocal: from 1 site
  Couplets: 2 PVCs in a row. Triplets: 3 PVCs in a row
  Bigeminy: every other beat is a PVC. (See Figure 17.3A.) Trigeminy: every 3rd beat is a PVC
  V tach, nonsustained (NSVT): 3 or more consecutive PVCs lasting <30 seconds and terminating
    spontaneously. See Figure 17.3B.
  V tach, sustained (SuVT): Consecutive PVCs lasting >30 seconds, usual rate of 150-200 beats/min.
    See Figure 17.3C
  V fib: a totally disorganized rhythm; a medical emergency

Complex Ventricular Arrhythmias
Torsade de pointes (TdP): a complex ventricular arrhythmia that literally translated means "twisting
of the points." On a rhythm strip, one sees a prolonged QT interval and cycles of alternating electrical
polarity such that the QRS complex appears to be twisting around the isoelectric line of the recording.
It may either spontaneously terminate or degenerate into ventricular fibrillation. Symptoms: unexplained
syncope, seizures, sudden death. See Table 17.3 for predisposing factors for TdP, including drug
induced.

Idioventricular rhythms: seen during episodes of complete AV block. With no beats coming from above,
a new pacemaker arises from the ventricles at a very slow rate (40 beats/min)

Ventricular escape

[a]AV = Atrioventricular; ECG = Electrocardiogram; SA = Sino-atrial; V fib = Ventricular fibrillation; V tach = Ventricular tachycardial.

Table 17.2 • AV Node Conduction Blocks[a]

1st Degree AV Block
A partial block of conduction. ECG shows widened PR interval, but all impulses are conducted from
atrium to ventricles. May be result of digoxin therapy.

2nd Degree AV Block
Some, but not all, impulses conducted from atrium to ventricle. Subcategories include:
  Mobitz Type I (Wenckebach). PR interval progressively lengthens with each beat until an impulse
  fails to be conducted; the pattern continuously repeats itself. Usually every 2nd or 3rd beat fails to be
  conducted.
  Mobitz Type II. PR interval with fixed duration, but only a certain fraction of atrial impulses are conducted to ventricles (e.g., 2:1 Block = Every other beat is blocked; 3:1 Block = Every 3rd beat is
  blocked).

3rd Degree Block
Synonymous with complete AV block. No atrial beats are conducted to ventricles. Either HIS bundle or
a ventricular pacemaker takes over to maintain cardiac activity at a very slow rate (<40 beats/min).
This also may allow ectopic beats (PVCs) to arise.

[a]AV = Atrioventricular; ECG = Electrocardiogram; PVC = Premature ventricular contraction.

Table 17.3 • Torsade de Pointes Risk Factors

Prolonged QT interval
• Hereditary and idiopathic
• Drug induced (see below)

Hypokalemia

Hypomagnesemia

Hypothyroidism

Associated Drugs
• Antiarrhythmics	Class IA: quinidine
	Class IC: encainide, flecainide, propafenone, moricizine
	Class III: dofetilide, ibutilide, sotalol
• Antihistamines	Astemizole,[a] terfenadine[a]
• Dopaminergic agents	Amantadine
• Antidepressants	Maprotiline, tricyclics
• Antipsychotics	Haloperidol, thioridazine
• Antibiotics	Erythromycin, isoethionate, pentamidine, trimethoprim-sulfa
• Antimalarial	Quinine
• Miscellaneous	Arsenic, cisapride,[a] organophosphates

[a]Predominately as a drug interaction with a CYP 3A4 inhibitor (e.g., erythromycin) leading to accumulation of active drug (cisapride) or active metabolite (astemizole, terfenadine).

Notes:

Table 17.4 • Vaughn-Williams Classification and Pharmacology of Antiarrhythmic Drugs[a]

Drug	Pharmacokinetics	Indications	Route of Elimination	ECG Changes	Side Effects
Class I					
Drugs with local anesthetic effects and membrane-stabilizing properties. Affect upstroke velocity of phase 0. These are subdivided based on the magnitude of effects on phase 0, APD, and ERP					
Type IA. Moderate Slowing of Phase 0 Upstroke, Moderate Effects on ERP and APD. ↑ QRS and QT Interval					
Quinidine sulfate (83% quinidine; SR = Quinidex) Quinidine gluconate (62% quinidine; SR = Quinaglute)	$t\frac{1}{2} = 6.2 \pm 1.8$ hr (affected by age, cirrhosis) $Vd = 2.7$ L/kg (↑ in CHF, cirrhosis) $Cp = 2-6$ µg/mL	Atrial fibrillation (conversion or prophylaxis), PSVT, WPW, V tach, PVCs	Liver metabolism 80%; renal 20%. Also a P450 2D6 inhibitor	↑ PR, QRS, QT. Low doses speed AV conduction via vagolytic effect. High doses slow AV conduction	Diarrhea (most common), hypotension, N/V, cinchonism,[b] fever, thrombocytopenia, proarrhythmia
Procainamide (Pronestyl, Pronestyl SR, Procan SR)	$t\frac{1}{2} = 3 \pm 0.6$ hr $Vd = 1.9 \pm 0.3$ L/kg $Cp = 4-10$ µg/mL (Also consider NAPA concentration)[c]	Atrial fibrillation (conversion or prophylaxis), PSVT, WPW, V tach, PVCs	Liver metabolism 40%; renal 40%–60% NAPA (active metabolite) 100% renal	↑ PR, QRS, QT. Low doses speed AV conduction via vagolytic effect. High doses slow AV conduction	Hypotension, fever, SLE (joint pain, muscle pain, rash, pericarditis), headache, mood change, proarrhythmia
Disopyramide (Norpace, Norpace CR)[d]	$t\frac{1}{2} = 6 \pm 1$ hr $Vd = 0.59 \pm 0.15$ L/kg $Cp = 3-6$ µg/mL	Atrial fibrillation (conversion or prophylaxis), PSVT, WPW, V tach, PVCs	Liver metabolism 30%; renal 70%	↑ PR, QRS, QT. Low doses speed AV conduction via vagolytic effect. High doses slow AV conduction	Anticholinergic: dry mouth, blurred vision, urinary retention (especially older males), CHF, proarrhythmia
Type IB. Minimal Effects on Phase 0, Little Effect on ERP, ↓ APD. No Changes in QRS or QT Interval[e]					
Lidocaine (Xylocaine)	$t\frac{1}{2}\beta = 1.8 \pm 0.4$ hr $Vd = 1.1 \pm 0.4$ L/kg $Cp = 1.5-6$ µg/mL	Ventricular arrhythmias only (PVCs, V tach, V fib)	Liver metabolism 100%	—	CNS: Drowsiness, agitation, muscle twitching, seizures, paresthesias.
Mexiletine (Mexitil)	$t\frac{1}{2} = 10.4 \pm 2.8$ hr $Vd = 9.5 \pm 3.4$ L/kg $Cp = 0.5-2$ µg/mL	Ventricular arrhythmias only (PVCs, V tach, V fib)	Liver metabolism 80%–85%	None	CNS: Drowsiness, agitation, muscle twitching, paresthesias, seizures; N/V, diarrhea, proarrhythmia

(continued)

Table 17.4 • Vaughn-Williams Classification and Pharmacology of Antiarrhythmic Drugs[a] (continued)

Drug	Pharmacokinetics	Indications	Route of Elimination	ECG Changes	Side Effects
Class I (continued)					
Type 1B. Minimal Effects on Phase 0, Little Effect on ERP, ↓ APD. No Changes in QRS or QT Interval[e] (continued)					
Tocainide (Tonocard)	$t/2 = 13.5 \pm 2.3$ hr $Vd = 3 \pm 0.2$ L/kg $Cp = 6–15$ µg/mL	Ventricular arrhythmias only (PVCs, V tach, V fib)	Liver metabolism 60%–65%	None	CNS: Drowsiness, agitation, muscle twitching, paresthesias, seizures; N/V, diarrhea, proarrhythmia, agranulocytosis
Type IC. Marked Slowing of Phase 0 Upstroke, Minimal Effects on ERP or APD. ↑ QRS Width, No Change in QT Interval					
Encainide (Enkaid)[f]	$t/2 = 1.5 \pm 2$ hr chronic 6 hr	Severe ventricular arrhythmias only[f]	Liver metabolism; via P450-2D6, active metabolites	↑ PR, QRS	Mild negative inotropic effects. N/V, dizziness, tinnitus, proarrhythmia
Flecainide (Tambocor)[f]	$t/2 = 12–27$ hr $Vd = ?$ $Cp = 0.4–1$ µg/mL	A fib, PSVT, severe ventricular arrhythmias	Liver metabolism 75%; renal 25%	↑ PR, QRS	Dizziness, tremor, lightheadedness, flush, blurred vision, metallic taste, proarrhythmia
Propafenone (Rythmol)	$t/2 = 2$ hr (extensive metabolizers); 10 hr (poor metabolizers[h]) $Vd = 2.5–4$ L/kg $Cp = 0.06–1$ µg/mL	A fib, PSVT, WPW, severe ventricular arrhythmia	Liver metabolism via P450-2D6; active metabolites[g]	None	Mild negative inotropic effects. N/V, dizziness, tinnitus, blurred vision, taste changes, asthma, proarrhythmia
Type I, Mixed. Characteristics of Groups IA, B, and C					
Moricizine (Ethmozine)[f]	$t/2 = 1.3–3.5$ hr $Vd = >300$ L $Cp = $ undefined	Severe ventricular arrhythmias only[f]	Liver metabolism	None	Mild negative inotropic effects. N/V, dizziness, tinnitus, proarrhythmia
Class II					

β-adrenergic blocking agents. General myocardial depressants for both supraventricular and ventricular rhythm disturbances. See Chapter 11: Essential Hypertension for pharmacokinetic properties. Acebutolol (Sectral), atenolol (Tenormin), esmolol (Brevibloc), metoprolol (Lopressor), propranolol (Inderal) approved for arrhythmias

Class III
No membrane stabilizing effects, selectively ↑ APD

Drug	Pharmacokinetics	Indications	Metabolism/Elimination	ECG	Adverse effects
Amiodarone (Cordarone)	$t\frac{1}{2} = 40–60$ days $Vd = 60–100$ L/kg $Cp = 0.5–2.5$ μg/mL Erratic absorption (22%–86%)	Life-threatening V tach or V fib resistant to other drugs. Also SVT, A fib	Liver metabolism 100%. Inhibits CYP 1A2, 2C9, 2C19, ↑ digoxin and warfarin levels	↑ PR, ↑ QRS, ↑ QT, sinus bradycardia	Corneal microdeposits (80%), blurred vision, photophobia, skin discoloration, constipation; ↑ serum transaminases, hepatotoxicity, pulmonary fibrosis, ataxia, headache, thyroid abnormalities (hyper and hypo)
Bretylium (Bretylol)	$t\frac{1}{2} = 8.9 \pm 1.8$ hr $Vd = 5.9 \pm 0.8$ L/kg $Cp = $ undefined	V tach, V fib	Renal 80%–90%	None	Hypotension, N/V, lightheadedness, dizziness, transitory hypertension, and tachycardia
Dofetilide (Tikosyn)	$t\frac{1}{2} = 10$ hr $Vd = 3$ L/kg $Cp = $ undefined	Conversion A fib or A flutter to NSR. Also maintenance of NSR (restricted due to TdP risk)	80% renal via GFR and tubular secretion (cation transport system), 20% hepatic by CYP 3A4 (↑ levels with cimetidine, ketoconazole, trimethroprim, verapamil)	↑ QT	Headache, chest pain, dizziness, torsade de pointes (TdP)
Ibutilide (Corvert)	$t\frac{1}{2} = 6\ (2–12)$ hr $Vd = 11$ L/kg $Cp = $ undefined	Conversion A fib or A flutter to NSR	80% hepatic 7% renal unchanged 19% feces	↑ QT	Headache, nausea, dizziness, torsade de pointes (TdP)
Sotalol[h] (Betapace)	$t\frac{1}{2} = 10–20$ hr $Vd = 1.2–2.4$ L/kg $Cp = $ undefined	Life-threatening ventricular arrhythmias, A fib, PSVT	Renal 100%	None	Fatigue, dizziness, dyspnea, bradycardia, proarrhythmia

(continued)

Table 17.4 • Vaughn-Williams Classification and Pharmacology of Antiarrhythmic Drugs^a (continued)

Drug	Pharmacokinetics	Indications	Route of Elimination	ECG Changes	Side Effects
Class IV					
Calcium channel blockers. (See Table 14.4 and Chapter 14: Ischemic Heart Disease Anginal Syndromes for dosing information)^i					
Verapamil (Calan)	$t_{1/2}$ = 2–5 hr; Vd = 4.0 ± 0.9 L/kg; Cp = 100 ng/mL	PSVT; rate control of atrial fibrillation and flutter	Liver metabolism 90%–95%	↑ PR	Constipation, hypotension, bradycardia, dizziness, nausea

Unclassified

Digoxin. ↓ AV node conduction to control ventricular response to atrial fibrillation. Digoxin not a true antiarrhythmic since it ↑ irritability and automaticity of ectopic sites in atrium and ventricles. (See Chapter 16: Heart Failure for pharmacokinetics.)

Adenosine (Adenocard). An endogenous nucleoside. ↓ AV node conduction and interrupts AV re-entry pathways. Given as IV bolus to slow ventricular response in A Fib or to convert PSVT to NSR. *Side effects:* Facial flushing, SOB, dizziness, nausea, worsening of asthma

^{a}A fib = Atrial fibrillation; APD = Action potential duration; AV = Atrioventricular; CHF = Congestive heart failure; CNS = Central nervous system; Cp = Plasma concentration; CR = Controlled release; CYP = cytochrome P450; ECG = Electrocardiogram; ERP = Effective refractory period; GFR = Glomerular filtration; LFT = Liver function tests; NAPA = n-acetylprocainamide; NSR = Normal sinus rhythm; PSVT = Paroxysmal supraventricular tachycardia; PVC = Premature ventricular contraction; SLE = Systemic lupus erythematosus; SOB = Shortness of breath; SR = Sustained release; SVT = Supraventricular tachycardia; $t_{1/2}$ = Half-life; TdP = torsade de pointes; Vd = Volume of distribution; V fib = Ventricular fibrillation; V tach = Ventricular tachycardia; WPW = Wolf-Parkinson-White.
^{b}Cinchonism = Symptom complex seen if Cp >5 µg/mL with disturbed hearing, visual changes, ringing in the ears, headache, and confusion.
^{c}Procainamide metabolized to active metabolite n-acetylprocainamide (NAPA). NAPA is 100% renally cleared unchanged.
^{d}Not FDA-approved for atrial arrhythmias.
^{e}Phenytoin also classified as type IB agent.
^{f}Only indicated for treatment of life-threatening arrhythmias, such as sustained ventricular tachycardia. Encainide, flecainide, and moricizine were removed from the market except for persons previously using the drug because of mortality in CAST trials when used to treat asymptomatic PVCs.
^{g}10% of patients are genetically slow metabolizers (predicted by P450-2D6 metabolism).
^{h}Possesses both Class II (beta-blocker) and III activity.
^{i}Diltiazem may be substituted for verapamil.

Table 17.5 • Arrhythmia Types and Drugs of Choice[a]

Sinus Bradycardia

Step 1
Remove precipitating causes, such as vagal stimulation due to vomiting or bowel straining, digitalis, beta blockers, or calcium blockers

Step 2
Atropine 0.5–1 mg, repeat to 2 mg total

Step 3
Isoproterenol 100–200 µg bolus, 2–10 µg/min drip and/or pacemaker

1st Degree AV Block
No therapy needed. May be due to digitalis, class IA antiarrhythmics

2nd and 3rd Degree Heart Blocks
Same as for sinus bradycardia. Pacemaker usually required for 3rd degree block

Atrial Fibrillation (A fib)[b,c,d]
Goal: Relieve symptoms, control ventricular response, ↓ risk of stroke
    Conversion to NSR unlikely if onset >24–48 hr

Recent Onset (<48 hr)
Step 1. Rapid conversion or ventricular rate control[d]
If angina, hypotension, symptomatic: Electrical cardioversion

If hemodynamically stable: Control ventricular rate with one or more of following (some patients may spontaneously cardiovert during this maneuver):

Diltiazem IV[d,e,f]	20 mg (0.25 mg/kg) over 2 min, may repeat in 15 min; then 5–15 mg/hr IV infusion.
Verapamil IV[d,e,f]	5–10 mg (0.075–0.15 mg/kg) slow IV, may repeat in 30 min; then 5–10 mg/hr IV infusion.
Digoxin IV or PO[d,e,g]	0.5–1.5 mg load over 24 hr; then 0.125–0.5 mg QD; Adjust dose for renal function. See Chapter 16: Heart Failure

Beta blockers	
Esmolol IV	0.5 mg/kg over 1 min, then 30–50 µg/kg/min infusion
Metoprolol IV	5 mg at 1 mg/min, then 25–50 mg PO BID
Propranolol IV	0.5–1 mg. May repeat Q 2–5 min to max of 0.1–0.15 mg/kg, Then 0.04 mg/kg/min infusion or 10–120 mg PO TID.

Step 2. Slow conversion.
If convert to NSR: Discharge without medications.

If ventricular rate slowed, but still in A fib: Full dose IV unfractionated heparin or SC LMWH (See Chapter 13: Thrombosis). Then one or more of the following to attempt cardioversion:

Amiodarone IV[h]	1200 mg over 24 hours
Dofetilide PO[i,j,k]	0.5 mg Q 12 hr
Disopyramide PO[l]	200 mg Q 4 hr to max 800 mg in 24 hours
Flecainide PO	300 mg × 1
Ibutilide IV[j,m]	1 mg over 10 min (0.1 mg/kg if <60 mg). May repeat × 1.
Procainamide IV	100 mg Q 5 min to 1000 mg max
Propafenone PO	600 mg × 1
Quinidine SO$_4$ PO[n]	200 mg × 1, then 400 mg 1–2 hr later

Step 3. Maintenance
If convert to NSR: Discharge without medications
If fail to cardiovert: Start warfarin. Consider electrical cardioversion. Choose from the following:

Ventricular rate controller	
Digoxin PO[g]	0.125 to 0.5 mg QD.
Diltiazem PO[e,o]	180–360 mg/day (SR or CD preferred for fewer daily doses)
Verapamil PO[e,o]	120–480 mg/day (SR preferred for fewer daily doses)

(continued)

Table 17.5 • Arrhythmia Types and Drugs of Choice[a] (continued)

Antiarrhythmic

Amiodarone PO[h]	600 mg QD × 2 weeks, then 200–400 mg QD
Disopyramide PO[d,l,m]	100–150 mg QID or 200–300 mg BID SR
Dofetilide PO[i,j,k]	0.5 µg BID. Reduce dose if renal insufficiency.
Flecainide PO[m]	50–150 mg BID
Procainamide PO[d,i,m,p]	500–1000 mg QID as SR
Propafenone PO[m,q]	150–300 mg TID
Quinidine PO[d,n]	200–400 mg QID SO_4; 324–648 mg TID gluconate
Sotalol PO[i,j]	120–160 mg BID

Late onset (>48 hr), unknown time of onset, high risk for stroke
Step 1. Emergency electric cardioversion or rate control as in early onset.

Step 2. (Still in A fib.) Heparinize as above, then *warfarin × 3 weeks* followed by electrical cardioversion with or without ventricular rate controller and antiarrhythmic drugs.

Step 3. If sinus rhythm restored: Warfarin × 6–12 weeks, no antiarrhythmics
Failure of cardioversion or recurrence of A fib: Continue warfarin indefinitely.
Add drugs as in step 3 above (recent onset).

Step 4. Continued A fib with cardiac instability: Consider AV node ablation.

Paroxysmal Supraventricular Tachycardia (PSVT) or Atrial Flutter
Step 1. ↑ vagal tone via carotid sinus massage

Step 2. Break the re-entry circuit (Choose one)

Adenosine	6 mg IV bolus. Repeat up to 12 mg × 2 at 5–10 min intervals
Verapamil/diltiazem[f]	Same dose as A fib

Step 3. Failure of above
Digoxin or beta blocker *or* Class IA antiarrhythmics. Same dose as A fib

Premature Atrial Contractions and Other Ectopic Foci
Class IA antiarrhythmics

Ventricular Arrhythmias

Asymptomatic PVCs, no CAD: No treatment indicated[r]
Short course low-dose PO beta blocker (atenolol, metoprolol, propranolol) if palpitations are bothersome.

PVCs, Post-MI (<10 PVC/min): Beta blocker (metoprolol or propranolol) to reduce risk of reinfarction and cardiac arrest. Does not alter arrhythmia risk. (See Chapter 15: Myocardial Infarction)

PVCs, Post-MI (>10 PVC/min or Symptomatic)

Esmolol IV	0.5 mg/kg over 1 min, then 50–300 µg/kg/min infusion
Metoprolol IV	5 mg Q 5 min × 3. Then 50–200 mg PO BID
Propranolol IV	0.5–1 mg. May repeat Q 2–5 min to max of 0.1–0.15 mg/kg, then 0.04 mg/kg/min infusion or 10–120 mg PO TID

If beta blocker contraindicated (asthma, heart failure)

Amiodarone	600–800 mg QD (or 300–400 mg BID) × 7–14 days, then 300–400 mg QD

Nonsustained Ventricular Tachycardia (NSVT) Post-MI
No symptoms, EF >40%: No treatment indicated. Avoid Class IC drugs (proarrhythmic)
Symptomatic: Beta blocker or amiodarone as above

Sustained Ventricular Tachycardia (SVT)
If unstable: emergency cardioversion
If stable blood pressure:

Step 1. Loading dose, rapid conversion

Lidocaine[m]	1 mg/kg load, no faster than 50 mg/min. May repeat 0.5 mg/kg Q 8–10 min to 3 mg/kg total. Then 1–4 mg/min continued infusion. Lower dose if CHF or liver failure.
Procainamide[i,m]	12 mg/kg load @ 25–50 mg/min or 100 mg Q 5–10 min to max 1000 mg. Then 1–4 mg/min infusion. Lower dose if renal insufficiency.

(continued)

Table 17.5 • Arrhythmia Types and Drugs of Choice[a] *(continued)*

Step 2. Maintenance

Amiodarone[h]	200–500 mg QID × 1 week load, then 100–800 mg/day (300–400 mg usual)
Quinidine[i,n]	200–400 mg QID SO₄; 324–648 mg TID gluconate
Sotalol[i,j]	80–160 mg BID; 640 mg/day maximum

Step 3. Failure of above. May use EPS stimulation to identify preferred drug. Can choose from:

Encainide[m,s]	25–50 mg TID
Flecainide[m,s]	100–200 mg BID
Mexilitene[i,s]	200–400 mg TID
Moricizine[s,t]	200–300 mg TID
Propafenone[m,q,s]	150–300 mg TID
Tocainide[m,s]	400–600 mg TID

Torsade de Pointes

Discontinue proarrhythmic drugs (see Table 17.3)

Magnesium SO₄ IV	2-gm load, then 3–20 mg/min infusion up to 48 hr
Mexilitene	200–400 mg TID
Isoproterenol cardioacceleration @ 1–4 μg/min infusion	
Cardiac pacing	

[a]A fib = Atrial fibrillation; AV = Atrioventricular; CAD = Coronary artery disease; CD = Controlled diffusion; CHF = Congestive heart failure; EPS = Electrophysiologic stimulation; IV = Intravenous; LMWH = Low molecular weight heparin; MI = Myocardial infarction; NSR = Normal sinus rhythm; PO = Orally; PVC = Premature ventricular contraction; SC = Subcutaneous; SR = Sustained release; V tach = Ventricular fibrillation.

[b]Chronic A fib without symptoms or with a ventricular response <100 may not require treatment with antiarrhythmic drugs, but chronic anticoagulation with warfarin is recommended. Recent-onset A fib or patients with symptoms (lightheaded, dizzy, palpitations) require treatment. Electrical cardioversion may be used for recent-onset A fib instead of drugs.

[c]Conversion of chronic A fib to NSR may result in strokes due to dislodging of mural thrombi from the atrium. Anticoagulation may be required before cardioversion (with drugs or electrical shock), especially if A fib is long-standing or if patient has underlying mitral stenosis, hypertrophic cardiomyopathy, or ischemic heart disease. Ideally, anticoagulation should begin 3 weeks before cardioversion and continue for 4 weeks after achieving NSR.

[d]*Important Principle:* In many patients, ventricular rate control may be all that is required. Digoxin achieves this by slowing AV node conduction. However, digoxin will only convert A fib to NSR if underlying cause of the A fib is CHF. In some cases, digoxin may actually ↑ with digoxin due to ↑ automaticity of the atrial ectopic foci. Even when the atrial rate is sped up, ventricular response ↓. If a type IA drug (quinidine, procainamide, or disopyramide) is started without prior digitalization or treatment with a calcium blocker, the ventricular rate may paradoxically rise even though the atrial rate is slowed. This effect is caused by ↑ AV conduction due to antivagal properties of type IA drugs at low doses. At high doses, the type IA drugs will slow AV conduction and add to the digitalis effect. Since one cannot predict whether type IA drugs will speed or slow AV conduction, pretreatment with digoxin or calcium blockers is recommended.

[e]Calcium channel blockers may be preferred to digoxin since they maintain rate control better during exercise than digoxin. Digoxin is most effective at rest. Verapamil has greater AV blocking effects and more negative inotropic properties than diltiazem. Nifedipine has little AV blocking or negative inotropic effect.

[f]In PSVT, calcium blockers lead to NSR in up to 90% of cases. In A fib, they primarily act to control ventricular rate, similar to digoxin.

[g]Digoxin doses require adjustment in renal failure (see Chapter 16: Heart Failure).

[h]Very long half-life of amiodarone requires prolonged loading regimens. For maintenance, may be drug of choice for patients with heart disease. Must monitor liver function, pulmonary function, visual changes, thyroid function.

[i]Adjust dose in renal disease. See Table 14.3 for desired plasma level.

[j]Causes QT prolongation, risk of torsade de pointes. Avoid if bradycardia, hypokalemia, hypomagnesemia, history of QT prolongation, other drugs known to prolong QT (see Table 17.3). Observe for unexplained syncope, seizures, sudden death.

[k]Blood levels may be increased by concurrent cimetidine, verapamil, ketoconazole, or trimethoprim-sulfa.

[l]Avoid if prostate hypertrophy.

[m]Adjust dose in hepatic disease. See Table 14.3 for desired plasma level.

[n]Quinidine sulfate comes in SR and rapid-release and SR forms. Rapid-release is given QID; SR is given BID-TID. Quinidine gluconate comes in SR form given BID-TID. *Caution:* When converting from sulfate to gluconate salt, dosage adjustment may be required since sulfate is 83% quinidine and gluconate is only 62% quinidine. Quinidine may need dose adjustments in hepatic disease or in CHF. Keep levels of 2–5 μg/mL using double extraction assay or 1–4 μg/mL with TLC or HPLC.

[o]Diltiazem and verapamil are available in a variety of SR forms given QD or BID.

[p]Procainamide comes in both SR and rapid-release forms. Due to the very short t½ of procainamide, SR is given Q 6 hr and rapid-release is given Q 4 hr. Adjust dose in both renal and hepatic impairment. Keep levels at 3–14 μg/mL.

[q]Propofenone reported to ↑ digoxin and warfarin concentrations.

[r]Occasional to frequent PVCs are benign and may occur in both healthy persons and those with heart disease. No treatment indicated if asymptomatic. Use beta blockers to slow rate if palpitations or lightheadedness are uncomfortable. More aggressive therapy indicated if sustained V tach, V fib or if cardiac function compromised (hypotension, CHF, angina).

[s]↑ death with encainide, flecainide, and moricizine in CAST trial; possibly due to proarrhythmic effect.

[t]Moricizine induces cytochrome P450. Cimetidine inhibits moricizine metabolism.

Table 17.6 • Commonly Used Cardiopulmonary Resuscitation Drugs[a]

Drug	Dose	Rationale/Indications	Comments
Atropine	*Adult:* 0.5–1 mg IV push over 20–30 sec. Repeat at 3–5 min intervals up to total of 2 mg *Pediatric:* 0.02 mg/kg	Blocks parasympathetic activity due to excessive vagal activity. Useful in: sinus bradycardia, heart block, asystole, idioventricular or slow junctional rhythms	Must be given rapidly to avoid paradoxical vagal activity. Do not give when heart rate >60 beats/min.
Bretylium	*Initial:* 5–10 mg/kg IV push for V fib. Dilute in 50 mL D_5W and infuse 10 min for V tach in conscious patients. May repeat in 10 min up to a total of 30 mg/kg *Continuous infusion:* 1–2 mg/min *Intermittent infusion:* 5–10 mg/kg Q 6–8 hr	V tach and V fib unresponsive to lidocaine. Works best just before defibrillation	Questionable use in digitalis toxicity. Catecholamine release initially followed by hypotension.
Calcium	2–4 mg/kg IV over 2–4 min, repeat PRN up to 500 mg max. Flush lines before and after administration. Do not mix with bicarbonate	Reverses direct effects of K^+ on myocardial tissue	Use only for calcium blocker toxicity, hyperkalemia, or hypocalcemia. Use of calcium not recommended in cardiac arrest. Avoid in digitalis toxicity.
Epinephrine	0.02 mg/kg (0.5–1 mg) IV push (10 mL of 1:10,000 dilution). May be repeated in 3–5 min *Infusion:* 1–5 µg/min or titrate to desired effect *Endotracheal:* 2 mg (20 mL of 1:10,000)	Cardiac stimulant. Inotropic and chronotropic response. ↑ peripheral vascular resistance. Useful in asystole, electromechanical dissociation, V fib	*Infusion:* Give in central line if possible; also intracardiac. *Investigational:* 3–7 mg Q 5 min *or* 0.2–0.6 mg/min IV infusion (high dose)
Isoproterenol	2–10 µg/min by IV infusion may begin with 100–300 µg	Inotropic and chronotropic support. Useful in bradydysrhythmias	*Caution:* hypotension, tachyarrhythmias
Lidocaine	1 mg/kg IV bolus over 30–60 sec. Repeat 0.5 mg/kg if needed *Infusion:* 1–4 mg/min	Suppression of ventricular arrhythmias: V fib, V tach, digitalis toxicity	↓ loading dose by ½ in heart failure and/or liver failure. No infusion indicated during CPR.
Procainamide	100 mg IV push over 1–5 min up to 1 gm *Infusion:* 1–4 mg/min	Ventricular arrhythmias unresponsive to lidocaine, PVCs	Limit loading dose to 0.5 gm in heart failure. ↓ maintenance infusion by ½ in renal failure. *Caution:* hypotension; avoid if TCA or phenothiazine overdose.
Sodium bicarbonate	*Adult:* 1 mEq/kg IV push over 30–60 sec. 0.5 mEq/kg Q 10 min of continued arrest depending on arterial blood gases *Pediatric:* 1–2 mEq/kg initially followed by 1 mEq/kg Q 10 min	Reverses metabolic acidosis in shock, DKA, severe hypotension, and cardiac arrest. Restores responsiveness to catecholamines and may improve response to defibrillation	Use of bicarbonate generally not recommended in cardiopulmonary arrest. Manipulation of pH by hyperventilation should be attempted before use of bicarbonate. Use cautiously in presence of hypokalemia. Flush lines before and after use.

[a]DKA = Diabetic ketoacidosis; IV = Intravenous; TCA = Tricyclic antidepressant; V fib = Ventricular fibrillation; V tach = Ventricular tachycardia.

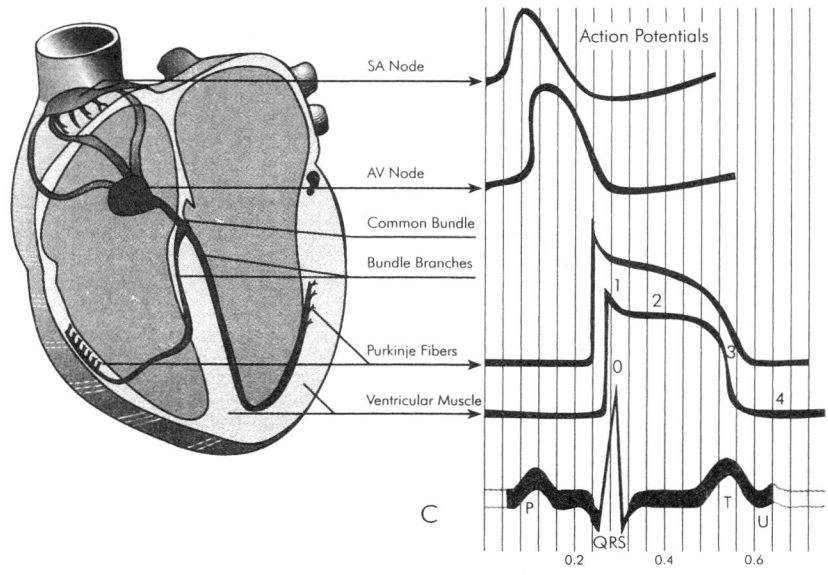

P wave = Atrial depolarization.
PR =   Rate of conduction through atria, AV node, and HIS bundle
QRS =   Ventricular depolarization, rate of conduction through bundle branches and
            ventricular muscle
T wave = Ventricular repolarization
QR =   Reflects duration of depolarization and repolarization of the ventricular myocardium

Fig. 17.1 The Cardiac Conduction System. A: Cardiac conduction system anatomy; B: Action potentials of specific cardiac cells; C: Relationship of surface electrocardiogram to the action potential.

Notes:

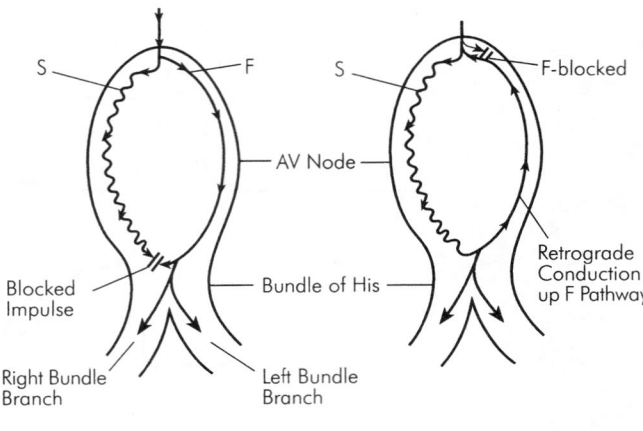

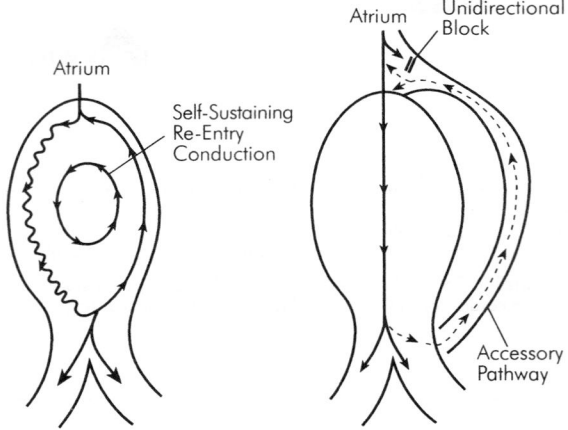

Fig. 17.2 Diagrammatic Representation of the AV Node in PSVT and WPW Syndrome.
F = Fast, S = Slow.

Notes:

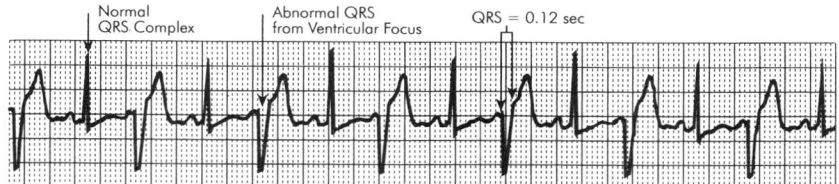

Fig. 17.3A Premature Ventricular Contractions Bigeminy. Every other beat is a premature ventricular (ectopic) contraction.

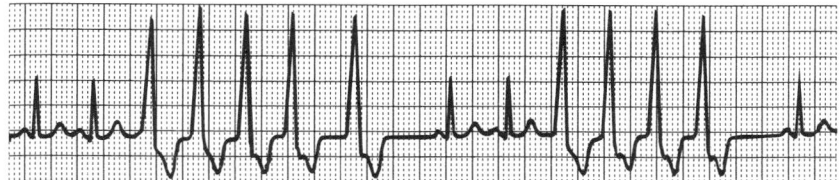

Fig. 17.3B Nonsustained Ventricular Tachycardia

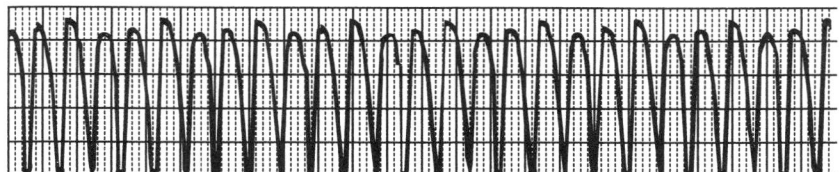

Fig. 17.3C Sustained Ventricular Tachycardia

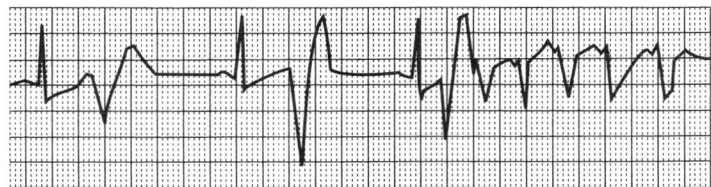

Fig. 17.3D R on T. R on T is used to describe the situation when the R wave of a PVC falls on the T-wave of the preceding beat. This is the vulnerable period during which depolarization (from a PVC) can result in re-entry and initiate ventricular tachycardia or fibrillation.

The reader is referred to Chapter 18: Cardiac Arrhythmias, written by *Moses S.S. Chow, Pharm.D.*, and *C. Michael White, Pharm.D.*, in the seventh edition of **Applied Therapeutics: The Clinical Use of Drugs** for a more in-depth discussion. Other topics covered in their chapter include an approach to reading ECGs, holter monitor, EPS principles, naturopathic therapies, and CPR guidelines. The editors of this handbook express their thanks to Drs. Chow and White and acknowledge that this chapter is based upon their work.

Notes:

Chapter 18

Hypertensive Emergencies

Hypertensive Emergencies Versus Hypertensive Urgencies

Acute hypertensive disorders are divided into two general categories: hypertensive emergencies and hypertensive urgencies. (See Table 18.1.) Signs and symptoms for these disorders are nonspecific and may overlap. Noncompliance and rebound hypertension following withdrawal of therapy should always be considered as an etiologic factor.

Treatment

* ◆ *Principles.* The rate of blood pressure lowering must be individualized. Ischemic damage to the heart and brain can be provoked by a precipitous fall in blood pressure, especially in the elderly, those with autonomic dysfunction, or with stenosis of cerebral or neck arteries. Patients with chronically elevated blood pressure are less likely to tolerate abrupt pressure reductions. Avoid reductions >20–30% if encephalopathy is present. In emergencies, reduce pressure no more than 20% (minutes to hours), then toward 160/100 mm Hg in 2–6 hours.
* ◆ *Hypertensive Emergencies.* See Table 18.2 for a discussion of drugs commonly used in hypertensive emergencies.
* ◆ *Hypertensive Urgencies.* See Table 18.3 for a discussion of drugs commonly used in hypertensive urgencies.

Notes:

Table 18.1 • Hypertensive Emergencies vs. Urgencies[a]

Emergencies	Urgencies
Stage 3 hypertension (Diastolic >120 mm Hg)[b]	Stage 3 hypertension (Diastolic >120 mm Hg)[b]
Potentially life-threatening	Not life-threatening

End organ damage present or high risk:
  CNS (dizziness, N/V, encephalopathy, confusion, weakness, intracranial or subarachnoid hemorrhage, stroke)
  Eyes (ocular hemorrhage or fundoscopic changes, blurred vision, loss of sight)
  Heart (left ventricular failure, pulmonary edema, MI, angina, aortic dissection)
  Renal failure/insufficiency
	Minimal end organ damage with no pending complications
	  Accelerated malignant hypertension
	  Optic disc edema
	  Coronary artery disease
	  Post- or perioperative hypertension
	  Pre- or post-kidney transplant

Pheochromocytoma crisis	

Drug-induced hypertensive crisis
  MAOI-tyramine interactions
  Overdose with PCP, cocaine, or LSD	

Eclampsia (complicated pregnancy)	
Requires immediate pressure reduction	Treated over several hours to days
Requires IV therapy (See Table 18.2)	Oral therapy or slower-acting parenteral drugs preferred. (See Table 18.3.)

[a]LSD = Lysergic acid diethlyamide; MAOI = Monoamine oxidase inhibitor; N/V = Nausea and vomiting; PCP = Phencyclidine.
[b]Degree of blood pressure elevation less diagnostic than rate of pressure rise and presence of concurrent diseases or end organ damage. See Chapter 11: Essential Hypertension for staging of hypertension.

Notes:

Table 18.2 • Parenteral Drugs Commonly Used in the Treatment of Hypertensive Emergencies[a]

Drug (Brand Name)	Dose/Route	Onset of Action	Duration of Action	Major Side Effects (All Can Cause Hypotension)	Mechanism of Action	Avoid or Use Cautiously in Patients with These Conditions
Nitroprusside[b] (Nitropress) 50 mg/2 mL (Most commonly used)	IV infusion[b]: Start: 0.5 μg/kg/min Usual: 2–5 μg/kg/min Max: 8 μg/kg/min	Seconds	3–5 min after D/C infusion	Nausea, vomiting, diaphoresis, weakness, thiocyanate toxicity,[c] cyanate toxicity (rare)[d]	Arterial and venous vasodilator	Renal failure (thiocyanate accumulation), pregnancy, increased intracranial pressure
Diazoxide (Hyperstat IV) 300 mg/20 mL	50–150 mg IV Q 5 min or as infusion of 7.5–30 mg/min[e]	1–5 min	4–12 hr	Hyperglycemia, Na retention,[e] tachycardia, painful extravasation	Arterial vasodilator	Angina pectoris, MI, aortic dissection, pulmonary edema, intracranial hemorrhage
Enalaprilat[f] (Vasotec IV) 1.25 mg/mL 2.5 mg/2 mL	0.625–1.25 mg IV Q 6 hr	15 min (max, 1–4 hr)	6–12 hr	Hyperkalemia	ACE inhibitor	Hyperkalemia. Renal failure in patients with dehydration or bilateral renal artery stenosis. Pregnancy (teratogenic)
Esmolol[g] (Brevibloc) 100 mg/10 mL 2,500 mg/10 mL concentrate	250–500 μg/kg × 1 min 50–100 μg/kg/min × 4 min may repeat	1–2 min	10–20 min	Nausea; thrombophlebitis; painful extravasation	β-Adrenergic blocker	Asthma, bradycardia, decompensated CHF; advanced heart block
Fenoldopam (Corlopam) 10 mg/mL 20 mg/2 mL 50 mg/5 mL	0.1–0.3 μg/kg/min	<5 min	30 min	Tachycardia, headache, nausea, flushing	Dopamine-1 agonist	Glaucoma
Hydralazine[h] (generic) 20 mg/mL	10–20 mg IV 10–50 mg IM	10–30 min (IV) 20–40 min (IM)	2–6 hr	Tachycardia, headache, angina	Arterial vasodilator	Angina pectoris, MI, aortic dissection
Labetalol[i] (Normodyne) 20 mg/4 mL 40 mg/8 mL 100 mg/20 mL 200 mg/20 mL	2 mg/min IV or 20–80 mg Q 10 min up to 300 mg total dose	≤5 min	3–6 hr	Abdominal pain, nausea, vomiting, diarrhea	α- and β-adrenergic blocker	Asthma, bradycardia, decompensated CHF

(continued)

Table 18.2 • Parenteral Drugs Commonly Used in the Treatment of Hypertensive Emergencies[a] (continued)

Drug (Brand Name)	Dose/Route	Onset of Action	Duration of Action	Major Side Effects (All Can Cause Hypotension)	Mechanism of Action	Avoid or Use Cautiously in Patients with These Conditions
Nicardipine[j] (Cardene IV) 25 mg/10 mL	IV loading dose 5 mg/hr increased by 2.5 mg/hr Q 5 min to desired BP or a max of 15 mg/hr × 15 minutes, followed by maintenance infusion of 3 mg/hr	2–10 min maximum 8–12 hr	40–60 min after D/C infusion	Headache, flushing, nausea, vomiting, dizziness, tachycardia; local thrombophlebitis change: infusion site after 12 hr	Arterial vasodilator (Ca channel blocker)	Angina, decompensated CHF; increased intracranial pressure
Nitroglycerin[k] (Tridil, Nitro-Bid IV, Nitro-Stat IV) 5 mg/mL 5 mg/10 mL 25 mg/5 mL 50 mg/10 mL 100 mg/20 mL	IV infusion pump 5–100 μg/min	2–5 min	5–10 min after D/C infusion	Methemoglobinemia, headache, tachycardia, nausea, vomiting, flushing, tolerance with prolonged use	Arterial and venous vasodilator	Pericardial tamponade, constrictive pericarditis, or increased intracranial pressure
Trimethaphan (Arfonad) 500 mg/10 mL	IV infusion pump 0.5–5 mg/min	1–5 min	10 min after D/C infusion	Tachyphylaxis, ileus, constipation, urinary retention, pupillary dilation	Ganglionic blocker	Postoperative glaucoma

[a]ACE = Angiotensin-converting-enzyme; CHF = Congestive heart failure; D_5W = 5% Dextrose in water; D/C = Discontinued; MI = Myocardial infarction; Na=sodium.

[b]Nitroprusside is drug of choice for acute hypertensive emergencies. Supplied as 50 mg of lyophilized powder that is reconstituted with 2–3 mL of D_5W yielding a red-brown solution. The contents of the vial are added to 250, 500, or 1000 mL of D_5W to produce a solution for IV administration at a concentration of 200, 100, or 50 µg/mL, respectively. The container should be wrapped with metal foil to prevent light-induced decompensation. Under these conditions, the solution is stable for 4–24 hours. A rising blood pressure may indicate loss of potency. A change in color to yellow does not ↓ effectiveness. The appearance of a drak brown, green, or blue color indicates loss in activity. The drug is more effective if the head of the bed is slightly raised. When changing to a new bag, the administration rate may require adjustment.

[c]Thiocyanate levels rise gradually in proportion to the dose and duration of administration. The $t_{1/2}$ of thiocyanate is 2.7 days with normal renal function and 9 days in patients with renal failure. Toxicity occurs after 7–14 days in patients with normal renal function and 3–6 days in renal failure patients. Thiocyanate serum levels should be measured after 3–4 days of therapy, and the drug should be discontinued if levels exceed 10–12 mg/dL. Thiocyanate toxicity causes a neurotoxic syndrome of toxic psychosis, hyperreflexia, confusion, weakness, tinnitus, seizures, and coma.

[d]Signs of cyanide toxicity include lactic acidosis, hypoxemia, tachycardia, altered consciousness, seizures, and the smell of almonds on the breath. Concurrent administration of sodium thiosulfate or hydroxycobalamin may reduce the risk of cyanide toxicity in high-risk patients.

[e]Diazoxide is administered as a bolus dose (13 mg/kg Q 5 minutes to a max of 150 mg/injection) or as a slow infusion (15–20 mg/min) until a diastolic pressure of 100 mm Hg is reached. Significant fluid retention following diazoxide can cause CHF and pulmonary edema. Concurrent loop diuretics are recommended (e.g., furosemide 40 mg IV) if diazoxide is given by rapid IV bolus. Reflex ↑ in heart rate and stroke volume are potentially dangerous in patients with angina or MI. Concurrent beta blockers may be protective.

[f]Not approved by the Food and Drug Administration for treatment of acute hypertension.

[g]Approved for intraoperative and postoperative treatment of hypertension.

[h]Parenteral hydralazine is an intermediate treatment between oral agents and more aggressive therapies such as nitroprusside or diazoxide. It can be given IV or IM, but there is no appreciable difference in onset of action (20–40 min) between the two routes. This slow onset minimizes hypotension.

[i]Labetalol is contraindicated in CHF due to its beta-blocking properties. A solution for continuous infusion is prepared by adding two 100-mg ampules to 160 mL of IV fluid to give a final concentration of 1 mg/mL. Infusions start at 2 mg/min and are titrated until a satisfactory response is achieved or a cumulative dose of 300 mg.

[j]Indicated for short-term treatment of hypertension when the oral route is not feasible or desirable.

[k]Requires special delivery system due to drug binding to PVC tubing. Also see Chapter 14: Ischemic Heart Disease and Chapter 15: Myocardial Infarction for further information regarding nitroglycerin.

Table 18.3 • Oral Drugs Commonly Used in the Treatment of Hypertensive Urgencies

Drug (Brand Name)	Dose/Route	Onset of Action	Duration of Action	Major Side Effects[a]	Mechanism of Action	Avoid or Use Cautiously in Patients with These Conditions
Captopril[b] (Capoten) 12.5-, 25-, 50-, 100-mg tablets	6.5–50 mg PO	15 min	4–6 hr	Hyperkalemia, angioedema, ↑ BUN if dehydrated, rash, pruritus, proteinuria, loss of taste	ACE inhibitor	Renal artery stenosis, hyperkalemia, dehydration, renal failure, pregnancy
Clonidine (Catapres) 0.1-, 0.2-, 0.3-mg tablets	0.1–0.2 mg PO initially, then 0.1 mg/hr up to 0.8 mg total	0.5–2 hr	6–8 hr	Sedation, dry mouth, constipation	Central α-2 agonist	Altered mental status, severe carotid artery stenosis
Labetalol (Normodyne, Trandate) 100-, 200-, 300-mg tablets	200–400 mg PO repeated Q 2–3 hr	30 min–2 hr	4 hr	Orthostatic hypotension, nausea, vomiting	α- and β-adrenergic blocker	Congestive heart failure, asthma, bradycardia
Minoxidil (Loniten) 2.5-, 10-mg tablets	5–20 mg PO	30–60 min Max response 2–4 hr	12–16 hr	Tachycardia, fluid retention	Arterial and venous vasodilator	Angina, congestive heart failure
Nifedipine[c] 10-, 20-mg capsules	10–20 mg PO May repeat in 20–60 min. Avoid bite and chew.	60 min PO. 15–30 min bite and chew	3–5 hr	Burning paresthesia, flushing, headaches, palpitations, edema	Calcium entry blocker	Severe aortic stenosis, coronary artery disease, cerebrovascular disease

[a]All may cause hypotension, dizziness, and flushing.
[b]Other oral ACE inhibitors too slow in onset to be useful but can be used for maintenance.
[c]Nifedipine not recommended for acute treatment because of serious side effects (angina, MI, stroke) associated with rapid-onset calcium blockers. Biting and chewing a perforated capsule and then swallowing the liquid contents may hasten the hypertensive effect (also risk of serious side effects) by ↓ the dissolution time of the gelatin outer coating. Nifedipine is not well absorbed buccally or sublingually.

The reader is referred to Chapter 19: Hypertensive Emergencies, written by *Robert J. Michocki, Pharm.D.*, in the seventh edition of **Applied Therapeutics: The Clinical Use of Drugs** for more in-depth discussion. The editors of this handbook express their thanks to Dr. Michocki and acknowledge that this chapter is based upon his work.

Notes:

Notes:

Chapter 19

Shock

Systemic Inflammatory Response Syndrome (SIRS)

- ♦ Umbrella term describing acute inflammatory responses manifest by two or more of the following:
  - Temperature >38°C or <36°C
  - Heart rate >96 beats/min
  - Respiratory rate >20 breaths/min or partial pressure of CO_2 ($PaCO_2$) <32 mm/Hg
  - White blood cell (WBC) count >12,000 cells/mm^2, <4,000 cells/mm^2, or >10 immature (band) forms
- ♦ Possible causes
  - Septic shock (infection)
  - Hemorrhagic shock
  - Trauma/tissue injury
  - Ischemia
  - Pancreatitis
  - Immune-mediated organ injury

Multiple Organ Dysfunction Syndrome (MODS)

- ♦ Progressive physiologic dysfunction in two or more organ systems in critically ill patients.
  - Possible consequence of SIRS including infection, septic shock, and other shock forms
  - Also caused by excessive host inflammatory responses following direct organ injury (trauma, surgery)

Hemodynamic Monitoring

- ♦ Monitoring the hemodynamic parameters of critically ill patients is important in the assessment of shock and the therapeutic interventions which affect blood volume, blood pressure, and blood flow. Such assessment has been made easier by the Swan-Ganz catheter.
- ♦ ***Parameters measured directly by the Swan-Ganz catheter*** are:
  - *Right Atrial Pressure (RAP).* The RAP is essentially equivalent to the central venous pressure (CVP) and reflects the filling pressure of the right heart.
  - *Right Ventricular Pressure (RVP).*
  - *Pulmonory Artery Pressure (PAP).*
  - *Pulmonary Capillary Wedge Pressure (PCWP).* The PCWP is a useful measure of left ventricular end diastolic pressure (i.e., preload).

♦ **Thermodilution Techniques.** Cardiac output (CO) is measured through thermodilation techniques.

♦ **Normal Hemodynamic Values and Derived Indices.** See Table 19.1.

Shock

♦ **Definition and Diagnosis.** See Table 19.2.

♦ **Classification and Precipitating Events.** See Table 19.3.

♦ **General Treatment Goals and Interventions.** The primary goals in treating shock and other medical emergencies are to maintain blood pressure and CO and to preserve cardiac, renal, and cerebral perfusion. It is important to maintain patient oxygenation (O_2 therapy, intubation if needed). Specific interventions include fluid challenges, fluid replacement, and treatment with either vasoactive drugs or inotropic agents. The exact role for each therapy must be individualized to the hemodynamic findings of the patient and the underlying etiology of the problem.

♦ **Fluid replacement (crystalloids, colloids, blood)** is the most important initial therapy in hypovolemic shock due to blood loss or in septic shock with significant "third spacing" of body fluids. Table 19.4 lists available fluid replacement products.

  • *Estimating Fluid Requirements.* Table 19.5 provides guidelines for estimating extent of volume loss, required replacement doses, and preferred type of fluid.

♦ **Vasoactive drugs and inotropic agents** play a greater role in cardiogenic shock than in hypovolemic shock. However, they are also important adjuncts to fluid replacement in hypovolemic shock, septic shock, and other forms of distributive shock if more conservative therapies are not effective. The pharmacologic properties of commonly prescribed inotropic agents and vasoconstricters are listed in Table 19.6. Tables 19.7 and 19.8 present guidelines for initiation of vasopressor therapy in cardiogenic and septic shock, respectively. Also see Table 19.9 for investigational agents for treatment of septic shock. The roles of arterial and venous vasodilator drugs (hydralazine, nitrates, nitroprusside) are discussed in Chapters 18: Hypertensive Emergencies and 16: Heart Failure.

Notes:

Table 19.1 • Normal Hemodynamic Values and Derived Indices

Indices	Equation	Normal Value	Units
Directly Measurable			
Blood pressure (BP) (systolic/diastolic)		120–140/80–90	mm Hg
Cardiac output (CO)	$CO = SV \times HR$	4–7	L/min
Central venous pressure (CVP)[a]		2–6	mm Hg[b]
Heart rate (HR) (pulse)		60–80	beats/min (BPM)
Mean pulmonary artery pressure (MPAP)		12–15	mm Hg
Pulmonary artery pressure (PAP) (systolic/diastolic)		20–30/8–12	mm Hg
Pulmonary capillary wedge pressure (PCWP)		5–12[c]	mm Hg
Derived Indices			
Cardiac index (CI)	$CI = \dfrac{CO}{BSA^d}$	2.5–4.2	L/min/m²
Left ventricular stroke work index (LVSWI)	$LVSWI = (MAP - PCWP)\,(SVI)\,(0.0136)$	35–85	gm/m²/beat
Mean arterial pressure (MAP)	$MAP = \dfrac{2\ (\text{diastolic BP}) + \text{systolic BP}}{3}$	80–100	mm Hg
Perfusion pressure (PP)	$PP = MAP - PCWP$	≥50	mm Hg
Pulmonary vascular resistance (PVR)	$PVR = \dfrac{(MAP - PCWP)}{CO}(80)$	20–120	dynes • sec/cm⁻⁵
Stroke volume (SV)	$SV = \dfrac{CO}{HR}$	60–130	mL/beat
Stroke volume index (SVI)	$SVI = \dfrac{SV}{BSA^d}$	30–75	mL/beat/m²
Systemic vascular resistance (SVR)[e]	$SVR = \dfrac{(MAP - CVP)}{CO}(80)$	800–1440	dynes • sec • cm⁻⁵

(continued)

Table 19.1 • Normal Hemodynamic Values and Derived Indices (continued)

Indices	Equation	Normal Value	Units
Derived Indices (continued)			
Systemic vascular resistance index (SVRI)	$SVRI = SVR \times BSA^d$	1680–2580	dynes $\cdot$ sec $\cdot$ cm^{-5} $\cdot$ m^2
Oxygen Delivery (Do$_2$)	$Do_2 = CO \times Cao_2$ where $Cao_2 = Hgb \times Sao_2 \times 13.9$	700–1200	mL/min
Oxygen Consumption (Vo$_2$)	$Vo_2 = CO \times Hgb \times 13.9 \times Sao_2 \times SVo_2)$	200–400	mL/min

[a]CVP is essentially synonymous with Right atrial pressure (RAP).
[b]2–6 mm Hg = 3–6 cm H$_2$O (conversion: 1 mm Hg = 1.34 cm H$_2$O).
[c]May optimally ↑ PCWP to 16-18 mm Hg in critically ill patients. PCWP <16 mm Hg is indication for fluid replacement. PCWP >20 mm Hg indicates onset of mild pulmonary congestion. PCWP >30 mm Hg associated with acute pulmonary edema; an indication for diuretic therapy.
[d]BSA = Body surface area = 1.7 m^2 (average male).
[e]SVR is synonymous with total peripheral resistance (TPR).

Notes:

Table 19.2 • Definition and Diagnosis of Shock

Definition
Syndrome of impaired tissue perfusion with inadequate oxygen delivery to skin, muscle, brain, kidneys, heart, and other vital organs. Usually, but not always, accompanied by hypotension.

Clinical Diagnostic Criteria. One or more of the following may be present:
Systolic BP <90 mm Hg or reduction of >40 mm Hg from baseline

Tachycardia (heart rate >90 beats/min)

Hyperventilation (respiratory rate >20 breaths/min or $PaCO_2$ <32 mm/Hg)

Oliguria ($\uparrow$ BUN, $\uparrow$ Cr, urine output <20 mL/hr)

Metabolic acidosis (lactic acidosis via anaerobic glycolysis), respiratory alkalosis

Cutaneous vasoconstriction (cold clammy skin, mental confusion)

White blood cell changes consistent with SIRS (see page 19.1)

Table 19.3 • Classification of Shock and Precipitating Events

Hypovolemic Shock. (Reduction in intravascular volume $\rightarrow$ reduced venous return $\rightarrow$ $\downarrow$ CO)
Compensatory changes = $\uparrow$ heart rate, $\uparrow$ myocardial contractility, $\uparrow$ SVR

Hemorrhagic
Gastrointestinal bleeding
Trauma, surgery
Internal bleeding: ruptured aortic aneurysm, retroperitoneal bleeding

Nonhemorrhagic
Dehydration: vomiting, diarrhea, diabetes mellitus, diabetes insipidus, overuse of diuretics
Sequestration: ascites, third-space accumulation
Cutaneous: burns, nonreplaced perspiration, and insensible water losses

Cardiogenic Shock. (Abnormality of cardiac function)
Nonmechanical Causes
Acute myocardial infarction with left ventricular dysfunction
Low cardiac output syndrome
End-stage cardiomyopathy

Mechanical Causes
Rupture of intraventricular septum
Mitral or aortic valve insufficiency
Papillary muscle rupture or dysfunction
Critical aortic stenosis
Pericardial tamponade
Arrhythmias
Pulmonary embolism

Distributive Shock. (Loss of vascular tone causing tissue hypoperfusion)
Septic Shock

Anaphylaxis

Neurogenic
Spinal injury, cerebral damage, severe dysautonomia

Drug-Induced
Anesthesia, ganglionic and adrenergic blockers, and overdoses of barbiturates, narcotics

Acute Adrenal Insufficiency

Notes:

Table 19.4 • Fluid Replacement Products[a]

Type of Fluid	Comment

Crystalloids[b,c,d]
Normal saline
  (0.9% NaCl)
Lactated Ringer's (LR)
  (simulated plasma electrolyte
  solution) (28 mEq/L lactate)
	Crystalloids distribute to both vascular and interstitial fluid compartments in a ratio of $1:3$.[d] The two products are interchangeable, but Ringer's considered drug of choice since it provides electrolytes and $\downarrow$ risk of hyperchloremic acidosis via conversion of lacate to HCO_3^-

Colloids[d,e]
Albumin
  250 mL 5% solution
  50 mL 25% solution
Hetastarch (hydroxy ethyl starch)
  250 mL 6% solution
	Colloids distribute primarily to vascular spaces.[d] They maintain oncotic pressure and keep volume in vascular compartments. The 2 products are interchangeable; hetastarch is less expensive and does not transmit hepatitis or AIDs virus. Dose related $\downarrow$ platelets and $\uparrow$ prothrombin time with hetastarch.

Blood Products Whole blood Packed red blood cells	To maintain Hct >25%–30%

[a]Crystalloids equally effective to colloids at much lower cost. Reserve colloids for patients who remain hemodynamically unstable after crystalloids. Colloids expand vascular volume at lower dose than crystalloids and with less salt load, but do not replace interstitial losses.
[b]In hypovolemic patients or septic shock (with "third spacing" of body fluids), give 250–500 mL Q 10–15 min to start; may require up to 5–10 L/day as 150–200 mL/hr continuous infusion or as 250–500 mL boluses. Titrate to urine output of >50 mL/hr and/or PCWP 18–20 mm Hg, CI >2.5 L/min/m² and MAP 65–75 mm Hg.
[c]In cardiogenic shock, a 100-mL challenge dose may be given to assess fluid status. This may $\uparrow$ preload and improve cardiac output in some patients. If PCWP >20 mm Hg, acute pulmonary edema or CHF may develop. If this occurs, give 40–80 mg IV furosemide.
[d]For each liter of crystalloid fluid infused, 750 mL passes into interstitium and 250 mL remains in plasma. All 250 mL of colloid stays in plasma.
[e]5% albumin and 6% hetastarch are isotonic. Required replacement volumes are 25%–50% of those recommended for crystalloids in footnote B. Use 25% (hypertonic) albumin if need to replace protein in a patient unable to tolerate large volumes.

Notes:

Table 19.5 • Estimated Fluid and Blood Losses on Patient's Initial Presentation[a,b]

	Class I	Class II	Class III	Class IV
Blood loss (mL)	Up to 750	750–1500	1500–2000	>2000
Blood loss (% BV)	Up to 15%	15%–30%	30%–40%	>40%
Pulse rate (BPM)	<100	>100	>120	>140
Blood pressure	Normal	Normal	↓	↓
Pulse pressure (mm Hg)	Normal or ↑	↓	↓	↓
Respiratory rate (breaths/min)	14–20	20–30	30–40	>35
Urine output (mL/hr)	>30	20–30	5–15	Negligible
CNS/mental status	Slightly anxious	Mildly anxious	Anxious and confused	Confused and lethargic
Fluid replacement (3:1 rule)[c]	Crystalloid	Crystalloid	Crystalloid and blood	Crystalloid and blood

[a] For a 70-kg male. BV = Blood volume; BPM = Beats per minute.
[b] Reprinted with permission from Advanced Trauma Life Support Program for Physicians, Student Manual. Chicago: American College of Surgeons; 1993:75.
[c] These guidelines are based upon the "three-for-one" rule. This derives from the empiric observation that most patients in hemorrhagic shock require as much as 300 mL of electrolyte solution for each 100 mL of blood loss. Applied blindly, these guidelines can result in excessive or inadequate fluid administration. For example, a patient with a crush injury to the extremity may have hypotension out of proportion to his blood loss and require fluids in excess of the 3:1 guideline. In contrast, a patient whose ongoing blood loss is being replaced requires less than 3:1. The use of bolus therapy with careful monitoring of the patient's response can moderate these extremes.

Table 19.6 • Inotropic Agents and Vasopressors[a]

Drug	Usual Dose (IV Infusion)	Receptor Specificity			Pharmacological Effect				Usual Infusion Concentration
		α	β$_1$	β$_2$	VD	VC	INT	CHT	
Amrinone[b]	0.75 mg/kg bolus, then 5–20 µg/kg/min	−	−	−	+	−	++	−	1000–2000 µg/mL
Dobutamine[b]	2.5–15 µg/kg/min	+	+++	++	++	−	+++	+	800–1600 µg/mL
Dopamine	0.5–2 µg/kg/min[c] (renal)	−	−	−	−[c]	+	−	−	
	2–5 µg/kg/min	+	+	−	−[c]	+	+	+	
	5–10 µg/kg/min	+	++	−	−[c]	++	++	++	
	15–20 µg/kg/min	+++	++	−	−[c]	+++	++	++	
Epinephrine[d]	0.01–0.1 µg/kg/min	+	+++	++	+	−	+++	++	4–8 µg/mL
	>0.1 µg/kg/min	+++	++	++	−	+++	+++	++	
Isoproterenol	0.01–0.1 mg/kg/min	−	++++	+++	+++	−	+++	+++	4–8 mg/mL
Milrinone	50 µg/kg bolus, then 0.375–0.75 µg/kg/min	−	−	−	++	−	++	−	
Norepinephrine[d]	0.5–1 µg/kg/min Highly variable; titrate to SBP 90–100 mm Hg	+++	++	−	−	++++	+[e]	+	16–32 µg/mL
Phenylephrine	0.5–5 µg/kg/min Highly variable; titrate to effect	+++	−	−	−	+++	−	−	40–80 µg/mL

[a] CHT = Chronotropic; INT = Inotropic; SBP = Systolic blood pressure; VC = Peripheral vascular vasoconstriction; VD = Peripheral vascular vasodilation. Amrinone onset 3–10 min, duration 1 hr. Prolonged amrinone t½ in heart failure. 2–3% incidence of thrombocytopenia with amrinone.

[b] Dobutamine and amrinone have more inotropic effect than dopamine.

[c] Dopamine at 0.5–2 µg/kg/min stimulates dopaminergic receptors causing vasodilation in the splanchnic and renal vasculature.

[d] Epinephrine has predominant inotropic effects; norepinephrine has predominant vasoconstrictive effect. Epinephrine may vasodilate at low dose, vasoconstrict at high doses.

[e] Cardiac output unchanged or may decline due to reflex vagal responses that slow the heart.

Table 19.7 • Guidelines for Initiation of Vasopressor Therapy in Septic Shock[a]

1) *Maximize arterial* and tissue oxygenation by providing supplemental oxygen with ventilatory support PRN; correct any existing anemia.
2) *Expand intravascular volume* with crystalloids to a PCWP of 16–18 mm Hg as tolerated. Supplement with colloids if albumin level <2 gm/dL or if patients has ARDS.
3) If volume expansion fails to maintain a MAP of ≥65 mm Hg, a CI >4.5 L/min/m^2, Do$_2$ >550 mL/min/m^2, and Vo$_2$ <150 mL/min/m^2 begin:
   a. Dopamine[b] if MAP and CI are low
   b. Norepinephrine[c] if MAP low, but CI adequate
4) If MAP does not ↑,
   a. Add dobutamine,[b] if CI falls below 3.5 L/min/m^2
   b. Add norepinephrine,[c] if SVRI falls below predefined range (see 5)
   c. Supplement with dopamine PRN to attain desired endpoints
5) *Titrate norepinephrine* to lowest effective dose which will maintain a MAP of 65 mm Hg; keep SVRI <800–1100 dynes • sec • cm^{-5} • m^2 to avoid excessive vasoconstriction.[c]

[a]Eradication of the source of infection with appropriate antibiotic therapy and surgical drainage is a primary treatment of septic shock. ARDS = Acute respiratory distress syndrome.
[b]Dobutamine may ↑ PCWP and SVR with ↑ doses, while dobutamine may ↓ PCWP and SVR with ↑ doses. Dobutamine may cause more arterial dilation and worsen hypotension. Thus dobutamine may be preferred in patients with ↓ CI, ↑ PCWP, and ↑ SVR with mild hypotension while dopamine may be preferred in patients with ↓ CI, normal or markedly ↑ PCWP and moderate to severe hypertension. Dobutamine has equal or greater inotropic effect; dopamine has more chronotropic effect (tachycardia). Net effect with dobutamine is ↑ CI due to a combination of inotropic effect (↑ stroke volume) and ↓ SVR (↓ afterload). At the same time, ↓ PWCP leads to ↓ LV filling pressure, ↓ myocardial O$_2$ consumption, and improved coronary blood flow. Dopamine increases urine output due to ↑ CI and ↑ renal blood flow (low dose only).
[c]When fluid therapy and inotropic support fail to maintain satisfactory MAP despite a high CI, vasopressor (norepinephrine and/or high-dose dopamine) is indicated. Excessive vasoconstriction may cause reflex decrease in CI and hypoperfusion of kidney and other vital organs.

Table 19.8 • Hemodynamic Subsets of Cardiogenic Shock[a]

Subset Type	PCWP (mm Hg)	CI (L/min/m^2)	SAP (mm Hg)	Treatment
1	Elevated (>18)	Reduced (<2.2)	<100	Vasodilator and/or dobutamine. May substitute amrinone for dobutamine
2	Elevated (>18)	Reduced (<2.2)	<90	Dopamine if severe hypotension. Add norepinephrine if still hypotensive after dopamine. May add dobutamine + intra-aortic balloon pump
3	Elevated (>18) with: Elevated RAP (>10) Elevated RVDP (>10)	Reduced (<2.2)	<100	Avoid diuretics. Use fluid resuscitation ± dobutamine

[a]CI = Cardiac index; PCWP = Pulmonary capillary wedge pressure; RAP = Right atrial pressure; RVDP = Right ventricular diastolic pressure; SAP = Systolic arterial pressure.

Notes:

Table 19.9 • Investigational Therapies for Septic Shock

Inflammatory Mediator (Target of Therapy)[a]	Potential Modulator
Bacterial endotoxin	Monoclonal antibodies HA-1-A (human-derived) E-5 (murine-derived) Bactericidal permeability-increasing protein (BPI)
Tumor necrosis factor (TNF)	Monoclonal antibodies (TNF-Mab) Soluble TNF receptors Soluble TNF receptor immunoglobulin
Interleukins (IL-1 and IL-6)	IL 1 receptor antagonists (IL-1 ra) Soluble IL 1 receptors IL-1 and IL-6 antibodies
Arachidonic acid metabolites	Cyclooxygenase inhibitors (e.g., ibuprofen) Thromboxane A2 receptor antagonists Leukotriene receptor antagonists, leukotriene inhibitors
Platelet-activating factor (PAF)	PAF receptor antagonists
Macrophages/neutrophils	Pentoxifylline
Modulators of coagulation disorders	Antithrombin III
Endothelium-derived factors/adhesion molecules	Nitric oxide (NO) synthase inhibitors Adhesion molecule monoclonal antibodies
Complement	Monoclonal antibodies to C5a fragment C1 inhibitor
Beta endorphin	Naloxone

[a]Also continuous hemofiltration to remove TNF, IL-1, IL-6, IL-8, and endotoxin.

The reader is referred to Chapter 20: Shock, written by *Chris Chalmers, Pharm.D., Andrew Barnes, Pharm.D.,* and *Laura Arrigoni, Pharm.D.,* in the seventh edition of **Applied Therapeutics: The Clinical Use of Drugs** for a more in-depth discussion. All notations to reference numbers are based on the reference list at the end of that chapter. The editors of this handbook express their thanks to Drs. Chalmers, Barnes, and Arrigoni and acknowledge that this chapter is based upon their work.

Notes:

Chapter 20

Asthma

PATHOPHYSIOLOGY AND CLINICAL FEATURES
Definitions and Clinical Presentation

Asthma is a chronic *inflammatory disease* of the airways.

♦ In susceptible individuals, this inflammation causes symptoms of *wheezing, breathlessness, chest tightness, mucous plugging, airway edema, and cough,* particularly at night, early in the morning, or *associated with exercise.*

♦ These episodes are generally associated with widespread, but variable, *airflow obstruction (hyperreactivity and bronchospasm)* that often is *reversible* either spontaneously or after treatment with bronchodilator drugs.

Hyperreactivity is defined as an exaggerated response of bronchial smooth muscle (bronchospasm) to *trigger stimuli* (see Table 20.1) that generally do not cause bronchospasm in a person without asthma.

• Onset often in childhood.

• Children more likely to have allergic component than adult onset.

Severity of asthma is divided into four categories: Mild intermittent, mild persistent, moderate persistent, and severe persistent. (See Table 20.2.)

Pulmonary Function Tests (PFTs)

Spirometry measures lung volumes and air flow dynamics. It is useful as an index of the degree of obstruction and the amount of reversibility. (See Figures 20.1, 20.2, and 20.3)

Forced Vital Capacity (FVC) and Forced Expiratory Volume in One Second (FEV$_1$)

The patient takes a deep breath (maximal inspiration) and then rapidly and forcefully blows out to maximal expiration (to residual volume). The total *volume* of air expired is the FVC; the amount expired during the first second is the FEV$_1$. (See Figures 20.2 and 20.3.)

• Normal FVC for average-sized, young adult male is 4-5 L (age, gender, body size dependent). Results may be reported as absolute volume (e.g., 3 L) or as a percentage of predicted normal (e.g., 3 L = 75% of a predicted normal of 4 L).

• Normal FEV$_1$ for average-sized, young adult male is 3.2–4 L, or about 80% of FVC. Results may be reported as an absolute volume (e.g., 2.4 L) or as a percentage of predicted normal (e.g., 2.4 L = 75% of predicted normal of 3.2 L). (See Figures 20.2 and 20.3.)

Peak expiratory flow rate (PEFR) is the *maximal flow rate* that can be produced during forced expiration following a deep breath to full inspiration. Patients can test PEFR at home with a hand-held *peak flow meter.* Normal PEFR is 550-700 L/min for an adult and as low as 150–200 L/min in children. Analogous to a traffic light, green, yellow, and red zones can be established for monitoring of patients with persistent asthma. (See Table 20.3 and Figure 20.4.)

"Reversible" Pulmonary Function

♦ Reversible pulmonary function is a 15% or greater increase in FVC, FEV_1, or PEFR after inhaling a bronchodilator. One also should look at the absolute volume change because a 15% change in severely obstructed patients can be small in absolute terms and provide little subjective benefit to the patient.

Example 1. A 20-year-old may have an FVC of 4.8 and an FEV_1 of 4 L when not experiencing asthma symptoms. During an acute asthma exacerbation, the FEV_1 in the same patient falls to 3 L. After bronchodilator therapy, the FEV_1 rises to 3.5 L, a change of 0.5 L or 17%.

Example 2. A 65-year-old smoker has a predicted normal FEV_1 of 3.8 L, but because of chronic bronchitis and asthma, his FEV_1 chronically runs at 0.8 L. Bronchodilators raise his FEV_1 to 1 L. Although his FEV_1 has increased by 0.2 L (a 25% change), this patient remains severely obstructed and continues to be short of breath.

♦ A *clinically significant* improvement is considered either an increase of >0.2 L in FEV_1 and/or subjective improvement in symptoms.

♦ Reversibility generally is assessed using a short-acting beta-agonist. Some patients without reversibility from a beta-agonist show reversibility with an inhaled anticholinergic (e.g., ipratropium).

Bronchoprovocation Testing. Bronchoprovocation testing is conducted by having the patient inhale increasingly larger challenge doses of methacholine, histamine, allergen, or cold air.

- PC_{20} = Lowest dose (provocative concentration) to cause a 20% decrease in FEV_1.
- Bronchoprovocation testing is an indicator of airway hyperresponsiveness. The smaller the dose of drug to cause reduced air flow, the more hyperresponsiveness that is present.
- Improvement in disease control (protection) is measured as at least a twofold increase in the dose of challenge drug to cause a 20% fall in FEV_1.
- Anti-inflammatory drugs improve hyperresponsiveness to a greater degree than bronchodilators. Several weeks of anti-inflammatory therapy may be necessary before improvement is seen.

Important Clinical Principle. Patients who show good reversibility of PEFR or FEV_1 after bronchodilators, but who continue to show a high degree of hyperresponsiveness are at risk of acute asthma attacks upon exposure to their personal trigger factors.

Hypoxemia and Oxygen Dissociation. See Figure 20.5.

GENERAL MANAGEMENT

General management of asthma includes:

♦ Patient Education

- Symptoms, especially nocturnal episodes and morning cough.
- Triggers: recognition and avoidance. (See Table 20.1.)
- PEFR monitoring: establish green, yellow, and red zones. (See Table 20.3.)
- Drug use; especially distinction between "relievers" (bronchodilators) and "controllers" (anti-inflammatories).
- MDI and nebulizer technique (technique and compliance should be checked at every visit).
- Prevention of exercise-induced symptoms.
- When to seek medical help. Develop rescue action plans for acute exacerbations.

♦ Environmental control.
  • Home
  • Occupational
♦ Pneumococcal and influenza vaccination.

Acute Disease Management

See Table 20.4 for emergency department and hospital treatment of asthma exacerbations and Table 20.5 for more detailed dosing information.

Chronic Disease Management: Asthma Treatment Algorithms and Goals

♦ See Figures 20.6 and 20.7 for a stepwise approach for managing children <5 years of age and adults, respectively.

Goals of asthma treatment
  • Prevent or minimize symptoms
  • Maintain normal or near normal pulmonary function
  • Maintain normal activity (including exercise)
  • Prevent exacerbations; minimize need for emergency visits or hospitalizations
  • Provide optimal pharmacotherapy with minimal or no adverse effects
  • Meet patients' and families' expectations of and satisfaction with asthma care

Important Principle. Bronchodilators provide symptom relief only ("relievers") while anti-inflammatory drugs are disease modifiers ("controllers").

♦ If symptoms of asthma occur greater than 3 times per week, including nocturnal asthma and exercise-induced asthma, an inhaled anti-inflammatory should be started.

Bronchodilators (Symptom "Relievers")

♦ *Beta-Adrenergic Agonists*
  • *Comparison of agents.* See Table 20.6.
  • *Dosing.* See Table 20.7.
  • *Adverse effects.* See Table 20.8.

Aerosol Therapy: Metered-Dose Inhaler (MDI) vs. Nebulization vs. Dry Powder Inhaler.
See Figures 20.8 and 20.9.

♦ Advantage over systemic therapy: Drug is administered directly into the lung in very small doses, which minimizes side effects and speeds time of onset.

♦ A *nebulizer* may be more effective in emergency therapy because more drug is delivered to the lung. For chronic therapy there is no difference in efficacy between MDI and the nebulizer if correct technique is used.

♦ *MDI* is limited by the patient's ability to use it correctly (see Table 20.9). *An extender device* (see Table 20.10) acts as a reservoir to hold the drug between MDI actuation and inhalation. These devices increase the efficiency of drug penetration into the lung in patients with poor technique, but do not improve efficiency in patients with good technique. Even with the very best technique, only 10% of the drug released from the MDI penetrates into the lung. Some patients cannot use MDIs because of throat irritation and bronchospasm from the propellant or the drug itself.

♦ *Dry powder inhalers (DPI)* are an alternative to MDIs (see Table 20.10). For some products (e.g., salmeterol, budesonide, and fluticasone), a single inhalation from a DPI is clinically similar to two puffs from the MDI. Patients should be instructed to inhale using a fast deep breath with a DPI, compared to a slow inhalation with an MDI. Throat irritation from the inhaled powder may cause coughing or paradoxical bronchospasm.

♦ Air jet nebulizers require an air source such as an oxygen tank, a wall-mounted air outlet, or a small compressor pump. (See Figures 20.8 and 20.9). A 3- to 4-mL solution of the drug is placed in the nebulizer, and the air source is turned on. It takes about 5–10 min to completely nebulize all of the drug from the nebulizer. Most forms of nebulization are highly inefficient; considerable drug may be left in the nebulizer at the end of therapy, and much of the drug is lost to the atmosphere. Mist production is continuous, but the patient only breathes intermittently. Efficiency is increased by nebulizers that only produce mist when the patient breathes.

♦ **Anticholinergic Bronchodilators**
- Anticholinergics generally are less effective than β_2-agonists in children with asthma, but equivalent to, or possibly more effective than, beta-agonists in patients with chronic bronchitis or emphysema. Compared to β_2-agonists, onset of effect after inhaled anticholinergics (5–10 min) and peak effects are delayed (30–60 min) (but near maximal effects by 10–20 min). Duration of action is 4-6 hr or longer. Tachyphylaxis has not been demonstrated.
- *Available products, dosing, and side effects.* See Tables 20.7 and 20.11.

LONG-TERM CONTROL MEDICATIONS

Anti-inflammatory agents (corticosteroids, cromolyn, and nedocromil) are the primary long-term control medications. Leukotriene modifiers (montelukast, zafirlukast, and zileuton) are secondary antiinflammatory agents. Long-acting beta agonists and theophylline are used as adjuncts to anti-inflammatory agents. While beta agonists and theophylline provide good symptom relief, underlying inflammation may not be controlled, leaving the patient susceptible to acute exacerbations.

Corticosteroids

General Principles. Corticosteroids have anti-inflammatory and mast cell stabilization properties that decrease airway hyperresponsiveness. Although they have no direct bronchodilator effect, corticosteroids enhance beta-agonist response and increase the number and density of beta receptors. In addition, corticosteroids are vasoconstrictors and decrease airway edema.

♦ **Inhaled Steroids**
- Inhalation is the preferred route of administration for ambulatory therapy and inhaled steroids are first-line therapy when asthma symptoms increase despite frequent PRN beta-agonist use. Wait 2–4 weeks to assess benefit and up to 6 months for full benefit.
- *Seasonal Asthma.* Scheduled, daily inhaled steroid use starting several weeks before and continuing throughout the known seasonal risk period is the preferred therapy. Year-round use is indicated for continuous symptoms.
- *Available Products, Starting Doses, and Dose Equivalencies.* See Tables 20.12 and 20.13.
- *Adverse Effects and Precautions.* See Table 20.12.

♦ **Systemic Steroids: Ambulatory Patient**
- Short course "burst therapy" with rapid taper is indicated if inhaled steroids are not effective or following emergency room therapy or recent hospitalization. Example

dose: 60–120 mg methylprednisolone IV or 40–60 mg prednisone PO for 1–4 doses. Discharge with prednisone 40–60 mg/day for 3–10 days. Not necessary to taper dose, but is frequently done.

- Continuous systemic therapy only if all other treatment options have been exhausted.
- *Adverse effects with short- and long-term systemic use.* See Table 20.12.
♦ **Systemic Steroids: Acute Exacerbations.** Systemic steroids are indicated to protect against late-phase reaction but have little effect on early-phase reaction. Either parenteral or oral dosing is acceptable, and the first dose should be given as early as possible because of their delayed onset (6–8 hr). Single-dose therapy is associated with recurrent symptoms; follow up with tapering doses.

IV Dosing. Hydrocortisone (100–200 mg Q 4–6 hr) or methylprednisolone (0.25–1 mg/kg Q 6 hr). May continue 24–72 hr if hospitalized. May rapidly reduce to 60–80 mg oral prednisone, then taper slowly over 1–3 weeks. Example dosage regimen: 60 mg for 2–3 days, 40 mg for 2–3 days, 30 mg for 2–3 days, 20 mg for 2–3 days, 15 mg for 2–3 days, 10 mg for 5–7 days, 5 mg for 5–7 days, 5 mg QOD for 2 weeks; then stop. If symptoms occur at any time, return to at least 20 mg/day. To minimize HPA axis suppression, the doses are given once daily in the morning.

Noncorticosteroid Anti-inflammatory Drugs

♦ **Cromolyn and Nedocromil**
These drugs stabilize mast cells and prevent the release of chemical mediators of inflammation, possibly by inhibiting calcium influx into the cell. They are the only drugs that inhibit both early- and late-phase bronchospastic responses. The major indication for cromolyn and nedocromil is continuous prophylaxis, and they are used primarily for allergic asthma. They also may benefit nonspecific bronchial hyperreactivity. Neither cromolyn nor nedocromil has any systemic side effects.

- *Caution.* Cromolyn and nedocromil are not bronchodilators and will not abort an acute attack.
- *Available Products, Dosing, and Side Effects.* See Table 20.12.

♦ *Leukotriene-modifying Drugs*

- *Leukotriene Receptor Antagonists:*
  (selectively inhibit LTD4 and LTE4 receptors)
  Montelukast (Singulair)
  Zafirlukast (Accolate)

- *5 Lipooxygenase Inhibitor:*
  Zileuton (Zyflo)

- Oral dosing is an advantage over inhaled drugs, but is less effective than inhaled steroids.

- Available products, dosing, side effects, and drug interactions. See Table 20.12.

Xanthine Derivatives: Theophylline, Aminophylline, and Oxtriphylline

Theophylline is a weak bronchodilator and may have mild anti-inflammatory properties. Its use is discouraged because of slow onset, variable response rates, side effect profile, and drug interaction risk. Reserve for difficult-to-control patients who fail other regimens. Also see Chapter 21: Chronic Obstructive Pulmonary Disease for expanded indications.

♦ **Converting from One Derivative to Another.** When converting a patient from one xanthine derivative to another, the differences in percent of active theophylline must be taken into account. Table 20.14 lists the percentage of anhydrous theophylline in various salts.

♦ **Pharmacokinetics.** See Table 20.15.

♦ **Intravenous Maintenance Dose.** *Caution:* Guidelines in Table 20.16 are only approximations and must be adjusted by careful monitoring of serum levels. There is a wide range of variability within each of the patient groups, and clearance often changes in the same patient during the early stages of an acute exacerbation. Doses may range from 100–200 mg/day in patients with severe liver failure to >2000 mg/day in adult smokers.

♦ **Dosage Adjustment: Chiou Method.** Obtaining a single serum concentration at 6–12 hr after the loading dose is of little value, because it is difficult to separate out the simultaneous influences of declining levels from the loading dose and accumulation from the infusion dose. The Chiou equation is a simple method for estimating the clearance of theophylline using two serum concentrations (C_1 and C_2) drawn at t_1 and t_2 separated by about 4–8 hr:

$$Cl = \frac{2Ri}{C_1 + C_2} + \frac{2Vd(C_1 - C_2)}{(C_1 + C_2)(T_1 - T_2)}$$

where Cl is clearance (L/kg/hr), Ri is the infusion rate (mg/kg/hr), and Vd is the volume of distribution (0.5 L/kg). The calculated clearance then is used to predict the correct infusion rate to achieve the desired serum theophylline concentration according to the following:

$$Ri = (Cp)(Cl)(Wt)$$

For the Chiou method to be correct, the following conditions must be met: 1) There is no dosage change; 2) Clearance is not changing and is linear; and 3) Vd is not changing.

♦ **Oral Dosing.** The total daily doses of oral theophylline are the same as for IV infusion. For patients on an infusion, the current hourly rate is multiplied by the desired dosing interval (usually 8 or 12 hr for time-released preparations) to ascertain the daily oral dose and the most appropriate tablet or capsule dosage strength. For patients not on an infusion, the information in Table 20.17 can be used as a starting point. When switching from IV aminophylline to oral theophylline, the dose must be reduced by 20%. Tables 20.18 and 20.19 provide other practical suggestions for starting and adjusting oral therapy.

- *Choice of Oral Dosage Form.* Rapid-release tablets and liquids are used when a more rapid response is desired or in patients who have difficulty swallowing. Sustained-release (SR) products allow longer dosing intervals and minimize peak-trough fluctuations. The bioavailability of most SR products is 100%. Significant differences exist in the *rate* of absorption between SR products. TheoDur, SloBid, and Theochron have the most desirable release characteristics and are given either Q 8 hr or Q 12 hr, depending upon both the rate of absorption of the product and the patient's metabolic clearance rate (see Table 20.20). Liquid preparations and rapid-release tablets must be given Q 4 hr to rapid metabolizers (children and smokers) and Q 6 hr to slower metabolizers (adult nonsmokers). See Table 20.21 for oral preparations with absorption abnormalities.

- *Monitoring Serum Concentrations.* Serum concentration monitoring with oral theophylline is complex. When the number of samples that can be drawn is limited, peak concentrations should be obtained: Rapid release products = 1–2 hr after dose; most SR products = 4–6 hr after morning dose; Theo 24, Uniphyl = 8–12 hr after dose. *Caution:* There is diurnal variation in absorption of SR products (absorption is faster in the morning and slower at night). With Q 12 hr dosing, samples should be drawn at *trough* (0–3 hr after evening dose) and early morning predose level (midway between peak and trough).

♦ **Adverse Effects of Theophylline.** See Table 20.22.

Table 20.1 • Trigger Stimuli of Asthma^a

Allergens: More Prevalent in Childhood Onset
Seasonal: grasses, pollens, molds
Perennial: house dust mites, animal dander or saliva, mildew, molds
More prevalent in childhood onset

Nonallergic: May Occur at All Ages
Chemical irritants and fumes (e.g., cigarette smoke, household cleaners, occupational exposure)
Dust
Upper respiratory viral infections
Rhinitis and sinusitis with postnasal drip
Exercise. Seen in 70%–90% of asthmatics and may be the only symptom for some. Symptoms develop 10–20 min after discontinuing exercise and last for 90–120 min
Cold, dry air; especially in exercise-induced asthma
GERD may be exacerbated by theophylline
Drugs (e.g., aspirin. NSAIDs, beta blockers). (See also Chapter 23: Drug-Induced Pulmonary Disorders)
Foods (e.g., sulfites)
Extreme emotions

^aGERD = Gastroesophageal reflux disease; NSAIDs = Nonsteroidal anti-inflammatory drugs.

Notes:

Table 20.2 • Classifying Severity of Asthma Clinical Features Before Treatment[a]

Severity	Symptoms[b]	Nighttime Symptoms	Lung Function[c]
Mild Intermittent	• Symptoms <2×/week • Asymptomatic and normal PEF between exacerbations • Exacerbations brief (hours to days); intensity varies	<2×/month	• FEV_1 or PEF >80% predicted • PEF variability <20%
Mild Persistent	• Symptoms ≥2×/week but less than 1×/day • Exacerbations may affect activity	≥2×/month	• FEV_1 or PEF ≥80% predicted • PEF variability 20-30%
Moderate Persistent	• Daily symptoms • Daily use of inhaled short acting beta agonist • Exacerbations affect activity • Exacerbations ≥2×/week; may last days	≥1×/week	• FEV_1 or PEF >60%–<80% predicted • PEF variability >30%
Severe Persistent	• Continual symptoms • Limited physical activity • Frequent exacerbations	Frequent	• FEV_1 or PEF <60% predicted • PEF variability >30%

[a] The presence of one feature of severity is sufficient to place a patient in that category. Individuals should be assigned to the most severe grade in which any feature occurs. Characteristics noted are general and may overlap due to variability. An individual's classification may change over time.
[b] Patients at any level of severity can have mild, moderate, or severe exacerbations. Some patients with intermittent asthma experience severe and life-threatening exacerbations separated by long periods of normal lung function and no symptoms.
[c] FEV_1 = Forced expiratory flow volume in one second; PEF = Peak expirator flow.

Table 20.3 • Pulmonary Function Target Zones

Indicators of Disease Control Using PEFR or FEV_1

Green zone	80%–100% of normal or of the individual's personal best with <20% variability between tests
Yellow zone	50%–80% of normal or personal best with 20%–30% variability. Indicates need to reevaluate therapy
Red zone	<50% of target. Seek treatment immediately

FEV_1 = Forced expiratory flow volume in one second; PEF = Peak expirator flow.

Notes:

Table 20.4 • Hospital Treatment of Acute Asthma Exacerbations

Stage 1: Emergency Department Therapy. Goal is to abort bronchospasm and prevent hospitalization

Beta-agonists (See Table 20.5 for child and adult doses)

Albuterol or equivalent by nebulization Q 20 min × 3 doses, then Q 1–4 hr (or continuous nebulization).

MDI[a] with extender as effective as nebulized therapy at lower cost if patient able to coordinate inhalation maneuver. See dose equivalencies to nebulizer in Table 20.5.

Use systemic (subcutaneous) only if unable to comply with nebulized

Corticosteroids (See Table 20.5 for child and adults doses)

Must use if on home steroids. Most others also receive 1–2 mg/kg (max 60 mg) as a single or in 2 divided IV or oral "burst" doses to prevent late phase response and potentiate beta agonists.

Inhaled steroids may be discontinued temporarily during acute episodes, but must be restarted after discharge

If not hospitalized, discharge with 40–60 mg prednisone QD for 3–10 days.

Anticholinergics (See Table 20.5 for child and adults doses)

Ipratropium less effective than beta agonists as monotherapy, but combination therapy may add to beta-agonist effect.

Theophylline

Not recommended due to lack of demonstrated benefit

Inferior response to beta-agonists in first 1–2 hr

Oxygen

2–4 L/min if PaO_2 <50 mm Hg

Cromolyn/nedocromil

No role in acute treatment, but continue if taking at home

Stage 2: Hospitalize if Stage 1 treatment fails to abort attack

Beta agonists

Continue using high, frequent doses PRN (up to Q 1–2 hr)

Use nebulizer if unable to use MDI with extender

Corticosteroids

Methylprednisolone IV 0.5 mg/kg Q 6 hr × 48–72 hr (or equivalent)

Convert to oral prednisone. Rapid taper at first, then slow taper as outpatient after down to 40 mg/day

Anticholinergics

Add ipratropium MDI 2 puffs Q 4–6 hr

Theophylline

Minimal benefit, additional cardiac side effects to beta agonists. Use only if all else fails.

Loading dose of 5 mg/kg IV or PO (6.5 mg/kg if aminophylline) to achieve 10 mg/L. ↑ dose if goal is 15 mg/L

Continuous IV aminophylline or PO theophylline (see Table 17.13 for dose recommendations)

Oxygen

Continue PRN for PaO_2 <50 mm Hg

Intubation, Ventilation

Only if severe hypoxia or distress

[a]MDI = Metered-dose inhaler. Frequent high doses of beta agonists are well tolerated with little or no side effects. Subcutaneous beta agonists may cause tremor or tachycardia. However, the pulse rate may ↓ in patients with anxiety-induced tachycardia associated with acute asthma.

Notes:

Table 20.5 • Dosages of Drugs for Asthma Exacerbations

Medications	Dosages	
	Adult Dose	Child Dose
Inhaled Short-Acting β₂-Agonists		
Albuterol		
Nebulizer solution (5 mg/mL) (0.5–1 mL of 0.5% solution in 4 mL saline)[a]	2.5–5 mg Q 20 min for 3 doses, then 2.5–10 mg Q 1–4 hr as needed or 10–15 mg/hr continuously	0.15 mg/kg (minimum dose, 2.5 mg) Q 20 min for 3 doses, then 0.15–0.3 mg/kg up to 10 mg Q 1–4 hr as needed or 0.5 mg/kg/hr by continuous nebulization
Metered-dose inhaler (MDI) (90 μg/puff)	4–8 puffs Q 20 min up to 4 hr, then every 1–4 hr as needed	4–8 puffs Q 20 min for 3 doses, then every 1–4 hr as needed
Systemic (Injected) β₂-Agonists		
Epinephrine		
1:1,000 (1 mg/mL)	0.3–0.5 mg Q 20 min for 3 doses SC	0.01 mg/kg up to 0.3–0.5 mg Q 20 min for 3 doses SC
Terbutaline (1 mg/mL)	0.25 mg Q 20 min for 3 doses SC	0.01 mg/kg Q 20 min for 3 doses, then every 2–6 hr as needed SC
Anticholinergics		
Ipratropium bromide		
Nebulizer solution (0.25 mg/mL)[a]	0.5 mg in 4 mL saline Q 30 min for 3 doses, then Q 2–4 hr as needed	0.25 mg Q 20 min for 3 doses, then every 2–4 hr
MDI (18 μg/puff)	4–8 puffs as needed	4–8 puffs as needed
Corticosteroids[b]		
Prednisone Methylprednisolone Prednisolone	120–180 mg/day in 3 or 4 divided doses for 48 hr, then 60–80 mg/day until PEF reaches 70% of predicted or personal best	1 mg/kg Q 6 hr for 48 hr, then 1–2 mg/kg/day (maximum, 60 mg/day) in 2 divided doses until PEF 70% of predicted or personal best

[a]For optimal delivery, dilute aerosols to minimum of 4 mL at gas flow rate of 6–8 L/min.
[b]No advantage has been found for higher-dose corticosteroids in severe asthma exacerbations, nor is there any advantage for intravenous administration over oral therapy, provided gastrointestinal transit time or absorption is not impaired. The usual regimen is to continue the frequent multiple daily dosing until the patient achieves an FEV₁ or PEF of 50% of predicted or personal best and then lower the dosage to twice daily. This usually occurs within 48 hours. Therapy following a hospitalization or emergency department visit may last from 3 to 10 days. If patients are then started on inhaled corticosteroids, studies indicate there is no need to taper the systemic corticosteroid dosage. If the follow-up systemic corticosteroid therapy is to be given once daily, one study indicates that it may be more clinically effective to give the dose in the afternoon at 3:00 PM with no increase in adrenal suppression.

Table 20.6 • Comparison of Selected β-Agonist Bronchodilators

Agent	Dosage Forms[a]	Receptor Selectivity		β₂ Potency[b]	Duration of Action (hr)[c]
		β_1	β_2		
Epinephrine[d]	Inj, AS, MDI	+++	+++	2	0.5–2
Isoproterenol (Isuprel)	Inj, AS, MDI, SL	++++	++++	1	0.5–2
Isoetharine (Bronkosol)	AS, MDI	++	+++	6	0.5–2
Metaproterenol (Alupent)	AS, MDI, PO	++	++	10	3–4
Terbutaline (Brethine)	Inj, MDI, PO	+	++++	4	4–8
Albuterol (Ventolin, Proventil)	AS, DPI, MDI, PO	+	++++	2	4–8
Levalbuterol (Xoprenex)	AS	+	++++	2	4–8
Bitolterol (Tornalate)	AS, MDI	+	++++	4	4–8
Pirbuterol (Maxair)	MDI	+	++++	4	4–8
Formoterol (Foradil)	DPI	+	++++	0.24	12
Salmeterol (Serevent)	DPI, MDI	+	++++	0.5	12

[a]AS = Aerosol solutions; DPI = Dry powder inhaler; Inj = Injectable; MDI = Metered-dose inhaler (also may be termed metered-dose aerosol); PO = Oral; SL = Sublingual. Not all dosage forms are currently available in the U.S.
[b]Relative molar potency at the β₂-receptor with 1 the most potent. This gives the amount of drug to achieve the same therapeutic effect.
[c]Onset and duration data apply to aerosol therapy only. Duration of bronchodilation only applies to otherwise stable asthmatics and is not applicable to acute severe asthma or protection from significant provocation (e.g., allergen, exercise, ozone). Duration may be shorter during acute exacerbation or with chronic therapy due to downregulation of β-receptors (tolerance). Oral tablets and syrups are slower in onset but may be slightly longer-acting than aerosols (especially if using sustained-release tablets).
[d]Epinephrine also has alpha (vasoconstrictor) effects. This may help decrease edema in the airways. Found in all OTC inhalers.

Notes:

Table 20.7 • Selected Bronchodilator Dosages^a

Preparations	For Chronic Maintenance Therapy^a		For Acute Severe Asthma	
	Pediatric	Adult	Pediatric	Adult
Albuterol (Proventil, Ventolin, Generic)				
Oral^d 2, 4 mg tab; 4, 8 mg ER: 2 mg/5 mL syrup	0.1–0.2 mg/kg Q 6–8 hr (not ER)	2–4 mg Q 6–8 hr; 4 mg ER Q 12 hr	NR	NR
Nebulizer Solution 0.5% (5 mg/mL) or 0.83% (2.5 mg/3 mL UD)	0.05–0.15 mg/kg Q 4–8 hr^c	2.5–5 mg Q 4–8 hr^c	0.15 mg/kg (*max:* 5 mg); then 0.05 mg/kg Q 20 min until improvement^c	5–10 mg; then 2–5 mg Q 20 min until improvement^c
Dry Powder Inhaler (Rotacaps) 200 µg/cap	1 cap Q 4–8 hr	1–2 caps Q 4–8 hr	NR	NR
MDI 0.09 mg/puff, 200 puffs and also as CFC free (Proventil HFA)^e	1–2 puffs Q 6 hr	2–3 puffs Q 4–8 hr	2 puffs Q 20 min ×3; then 2 puffs Q 1–2 hr	3–4 puffs Q 20 min ×3; then Q 1–2 hr
Bitolterol (Tornalate)				
Nebulizer Solution 0.2% (2 mg/1.0 mL)	NR	NR	NR	2–4 mg; then 1–2 mg Q 20 min until improved^c
MDI 0.37 mg/spray	1–2 puffs Q 6 hr	2–3 puffs Q 6 hr	1–2 puffs Q 1–2 hr	3–4 puffs Q 1–2 hr
Epinephrine HCl^b				
Injection 1:1000 (1 mg/mL)^c	NR	NR	0.01 mg/kg (*max:* 0.5 mg) SC Q 20 min ×3 doses	0.3–0.5 mg SC Q 20 min ×3 doses
Sustained Action Sus–Phrine 1:200 (5 mg/mL)	NR	NR	0.005–0.01 mg/kg (*max:* 0.75 mg) SC Q 6–10 hr	0.5–0.75 mg SC Q 6–10 hr
Fenoterol (Berotec)^f				
Oral 2.5, 5 mg tab	0.1–0.2 mg/kg Q 6–8 hr	2.5–5 mg Q 6–8 hr	NR	NR
Nebulizer Solution 0.5% (5 mg/mL)	0.025–0.075 mg/kg Q 6–8 hr	2.5–5 mg Q 6–8 hr	0.075 mg/kg Q 2 hr	2.5–5 mg Q 2 hr

MDI 0.16 mg/puff	1 puff Q 6 hr	1–2 puffs Q 6 hr	2 puffs Q 20 min × 3 then Q 1–2 hr	3 puffs Q 20 min × 3 then Q 1–2 hr
Formoterol (Foradil) *Dry Powder Inhaler* 12 μg/cap for DPI[a,g]	NR	1 DPI cap Q 12 hr	NR	NR
Isoetharine (generic) *Nebulizer Solution* 10 mg/mL	NR[a]	NR[a]	0.1–0.2 mg/kg Q 1–2 hr[c]	5–10 mg Q 1–2 hr[c]
Isoproterenol (Isuprel, generic) *Nebulizer Solution* 1:200 (5 mg/mL)	NR	NR	0.05–0.1 mg/kg Q 2 hr	3.5–7 mg Q 2 hr
MDI Various 45–131 μg/spray	NR	NR	NR	NR
Levalbuterol (Xopenex) *Nebulizer Solution* 0.63 and 1.25 mg/3 mL UD	NR	NR	0.63–1.25 mg; then 0.63 mg Q 20 min until improved	1.25–2.5 mg; then 1.25 mg Q20 min until improved
Metaproterenol (Alupent, generic) *Oral[d]* 10, 20 mg tab; 10 mg/5 mL syrup	0.3–0.5 mg/kg Q 4–6 hr ↑ by 0.25 mg/kg as tolerated	10–20 mg Q 4-6 hr	NR	NR
Nebulizer Solution[c] 5% (15 mg/0.3 mL) or 15 mg/2.5 mL unit dose	0.25–0.5 mg/kg (*max:* 15 mg) Q 4–6 hr[c]	15 mg Q 4 hr[c]	0.5 mg/kg Q 1–2 hr[c]	15 mg Q 1–2 hr[c]
MDI 0.65 mg/puff, 100, 200 puffs	1–2 puffs Q 4 hr	2 puffs Q 4 hr	2 puffs Q 1–2 hr	2–4 puffs Q 1–2 hr
Pirbuterol (Maxair, Autohaler) *MDI[a]* 0.20 mg/puff, 300, 400 puffs	1–2 puffs Q 4–6 hr	2 puffs Q 4-6 hr	2 puffs Q 20 min × 3; then Q 1 hr	3 puffs Q 20 min × 3; then Q 1 hr

(continued)

Table 20.7 • Selected Bronchodilator Dosages^a (continued)

Preparations	For Chronic Maintenance Therapy^a		For Acute Severe Asthma	
	Pediatric	Adult	Pediatric	Adult
Terbutaline (Brethine, Bricanyl)				
Injection 1 mg/mL	NR	NR	10 µg/kg (*max:* 0.25 mg SC) Q 2-6 hr PRN *or* 10-20 µg/kg IV over 10 min; then 0.2-0.4 µg/kg/min: ↑ in 0.1 µg/kg steps Q 15 min as necessary	0.25-0.5 mg SC Q 2-6 hr PRN *or* 10 µg/kg IV over 1 min, then 0.1 µg/kg/min. ↑ by 0.1 µg/kg/min Q 15 min to max of 0.4 µg/kg/min
Oral^d 2.5, 5 mg tab	0.075-0.2 mg/kg Q 6-8 hr	2.5-5 mg Q 6-8 hr	NR	NR
Aerosol (use injection)	0.2-0.4 mg/kg Q 6 hr	5-10 mg Q 6 hr	0.3 mg/kg; then 0.2 mg/kg Q 20 min until improvement	10 mg; then 5 mg Q 20 min until improvement
MDI 0.2 mg/puff, 300 puffs	1-2 puffs Q 6 hr	2 puffs Q 6 hr	2 puffs Q 20 min × 3; then Q 1 hr	3 puffs Q 20 min × 3, then Q 1 hr
Salmeterol (Serevent)				
MDI 25 µg/puff, 60, 120 puffs	1-2 puff Q 12 hr	2 puffs Q 12 hr	NR	NR
Dry powder inhaler^h 50 µg/actuation, 28 dose Diskus	1 puff Q 12 hr	1 puff Q 12 hr	NR	NR
Ipratropium Bromide (Atrovent)				
Aerosol 0.025% (0.25 mg/mL)	0.25 mg Q 6 hr	0.25-0.5 mg Q 6 hr	0.25 mg Q 4-6 hr	0.25-0.5 mg Q 4-6 hr
MDI 18 µg/puff	1-2 puffs Q 6 hr	2-3 puffs Q 6 hr	1-2 puffs Q 4 hr	2-3 puffs Q 4 hr

^a CFC = Chlorofluorocarbons; DPI = Dry powder inhaler; ER = extended release tablets; NR = Not recommended; MDI = Metered-dose inhaler; SC = Subcutaneous; UD = Unit dose.
^b Epinephrine also found in various OTC MDIs.
^c All aerosol doses should be diluted to a total volume of 3-5 mL. Note that although these doses are large compared to MDI, part will not be nebulized and part will be lost to the atmosphere. Total drug delivery to lung with MDI and aerosol at recommended doses are equivalent.
^d Oral beta agonists have unpredictable absorption due to high first-pass metabolism. Onset is slow (30-60 min) and incidence of side effects is higher.
^e NEW: Proventil HFA is a nonfluorocarbon containing MDI. It delivers the same amount of drug as the conventional MDI but with a warmer and less forceful spray.
^f Not available in the U.S.
^g Formoterol fumarate supplied as a powder-filled capsule that is placed in an "Aerolizer" for dry powder inhalation.
^h Salmeterol DPI also available as a combination product (Advair Diskus) containing 50 µg salmeterol with 100, 250 and 500 µg fluticasone.

Table 20.8 • Beta-Agonist Side Effects

Beta₁-mediated
  Tachycardia*ᵃ*
  Arrhythmia (rare)

Beta₂-mediated
  Nervousness
  Tremor
  Wakefulness
  Hypotension
  Flushing
  Hypokalemia–high dose only or fenoterol

Alpha–mediated
  Urine retention
  Hypertension

Other
  Red sputum from isoetharine
  Bronchospasm from MDI
  Cough from MDI
  Bisulfite allergy (nebulizer solutions)

*ᵃ*All more pronounced with oral therapy, compared to inhalation. However, some sensitive patients have CNS and cardiac intolerance even with low-dose MDI. Epinephrine, ephedrine, and high-dose oral "beta₂-selective agents" have residual beta₁-effect. *Note:* Pulse rate may slow as asthma improves.

Table 20.9 • Steps for Correct Use of Metered Dose Inhalers*ᵃ*

1. Shake the inhaler well and remove the dust cap.

2. Exhale *slowly* through pursed lips.*ᵇ*

3. If using the "closed-mouth" technique, hold the inhaler upright and place the mouthpiece between your lips. Be careful to not block the opening with your tongue or teeth.
   If using the "open-mouth" technique, open your mouth wide and hold the inhaler upright 1–2 inches from your mouth, making sure the inhaler is properly aimed.

4. Press down on the inhaler *once* as you start a *slow*, deep inhalation.*ᶜ*

5. Continue to inhale slowly and deeply through your mouth. Try to inhale over at least 5 sec.

6. Hold your breath for 10 sec (use your fingers to count to 10 slowly). If 10 sec makes you feel uncomfortable, try to hold your breath for at least 4 sec.

7. Exhale *slowly.*ᵈ*

8. Wait at least 30–60 sec before inhaling the next puff of medicine.

*ᵃ*If using a spacer, see manufacturer's instructions. Same basic principles of slow, deep inhalation with adequate breath hold apply. With spacers, put mouthpiece on top of your tongue to ensure tongue does not block aerosol.
*ᵇ*As long as exhalation is slow, can exhale over several seconds. Some experts insist on exhaling only a tidal volume, but the key is to exhale *slowly.*
*ᶜ*For dry powder inhaler, use rapid deep breath.
*ᵈ*If patient has concomitant rhinitis, exhaling through the *nose* may be of benefit when using corticosteroids, cromolyn, or ipratropium (i.e., some medication may deposit in nose).

Notes:

Table 20.10 • Examples of Spacer Devices and Dry Powder Inhalers

Spacer Devices

ACE (Aerosol Cloud Enhancer) (DHD)	150-mL conical holding chamber with one-way valve at mouthpiece; flow indicator whistle
AeroChamber (Monaghan Medical)	Holding chamber; cylinder with one-way valve that releases aerosol when subject inhales; flow indicator whistle
InspirEase (Schering)	Holding chamber consisting of a collapsible bag with a flow indicator whistle
Optihaler (Health Scan)	Holding chamber; cylinder; aerosol particles are directed away from mouth initially

Breath-activated Dry Powder Inhalers

Diskus	Holds 60 doses of salmeterol; has dose counter; lactose for taste with dose
Rotadisk	Disk with 4 doses of flutcasone inserted into dishaler; lactose for taste with dose
Rotahaler	Each dose of albuterol must be loaded; lactose for taste
Turbuhaler	Holds 200 doses of budesonide; red indicator when 20 doses are left; no taste

Table 20.11 • Anticholinergic Bronchodilators

Drug	Comment	Side Effects
Atropine	A tertiary amine: May be absorbed in a small percentage of patients after high doses	Dry mouth, bitter taste, blurred vision (if nebulized into the eye). Tachycardia, urine retention, constipation, and mental confusion occur only if the drug is absorbed
Ipratropium[a] (Atrovent)	A quaternary amine; not absorbed	Dry mouth and metallic taste

[a]See Tables 20.5 and 20.7 for available dosage forms and recommended doses.

Notes:

Table 20.12 • Long-Term-Control Medications

Name/Products	Indications	Potential Adverse Effects	Therapeutic Issues
Corticosteroids (Glucocorticoids) *Inhaled:* Beclomethasone (Beclovent, Vanceril) Budesonide (Pulmicort) Flunisolide (Aerobid) Fluticasone (Flovent, Advair') Triamcinolone (Azmacort)	• Long-term prevention of symptoms; suppression, control, and reversal of inflammation. • Reduce need for oral corticosteroid.	• Cough, dysphonia, oral thrush (candidiasis-sore throat, white plaques in mouth). • In high doses, systemic effects (e.g., adrenal suppression, osteoporosis, growth suppression, skin thinning, and easy bruising) may occur, although clinical significance of these effects has not been established.	• Spacer/holding chamber devices and mouth washing after inhalation recommended to decrease local side effects and systemic absorption. • Preparations are not absolutely interchangeable on a mcg or per puff basis (see Table 20.13). New delivery devices may provide greater delivery to airways, which may affect dose. • The risks of uncontrolled asthma should be weighed against the limited risks of inhaled corticosteroids. The potential but small risk of adverse events is well balanced by their efficacy.
Systemic: Methylprednisolone (Medrol) Prednisolone Prednisone	• For short-term (3–10 days) "burst": to gain prompt control of inadequately controlled persistent asthma. • For long-term prevention of symptoms in severe persistent asthma: suppression, control, and reversal of inflammation.	• Short-term use: reversible hyperglycemia, elevated WBC count (demargination), hypokalemia, increased appetite, fluid retention, weight gain, hypertension, jitteriness, euphoria, toxic psychoses, peptic ulcer, and rarely, aseptic necrosis of femur. • Long-term use: adrenal axis suppression, growth suppression, osteoporosis, dermal thinning, hypertension, diabetes, Cushing's syndrome (facial swelling, back hump), cataracts, muscle weakness, and—in rare instances—impaired immune function. • Consideration should be given to coexisting conditions that could be worsened by systemic corticosteroids, such as herpesvirus infections, *Varicella*, tuberculosis, hypertension, peptic ulcer, and *Strongyloides*.	• Use at lowest effective dose. For long-term use, AM or alternate-day dosing produces least toxicity. If daily doses are required, one study shows improved efficacy with no increase in adrenal suppression when administered at 3 PM rather than in the morning. • 7–14 days required for HPA axis suppression. May take months to restore activity once suppressed.

(continued)

Table 20.12 • Long-Term-Control Medications (continued)

Name/Products	Indications	Potential Adverse Effects	Therapeutic Issues
Cromolyn Sodium and Nedocromil Cromolyn (Intal) MDI: 800 µg/puff DPI (Spinhaler): 20 mg powder-filled capsule for inhalation Nebulizer soln: 1% (20 mg/2 mL) Nedocromil (Tilade) MDI: 2 mg/puff	• Long-term prevention of symptoms; may modify inflammation. • Preventive treatment prior to exposure to exercise or known allergen.	• Transient cough, bronchial irritation, nasal congestion, or bronchospasm with DPI use. May be decreased by drinking water before dose. • 15–20% of patients complain of an unpleasant or bitter taste from nedocromil MDI.	• Therapeutic response to cromolyn and nedocromil often occurs within 2 weeks, but a 4- to 6-week trial may be needed to determine maximum benefit. • Dose of cromolyn MDI (800 µg/puff) may be inadequate. • Usual nedocromil dose is 2 puffs (4 mg) BID to QID • Cromolyn nebulizer useful in infants unable to use MDI. • Albuterol and cromolyn may be nebulized together. Use face mask for patients with both asthma and rhinitis. • Safety is the primary advantage of these agents.
Long-Acting β₂-Agonists *Inhaled:* Salmeterol MDI: 25 µg/puff DPI (Diskus): 50 µg/puff Formoterol (Foradil) DPI: 12 µg/puff	• Long-term prevention of symptoms, especially nocturnal symptoms, *added to anti-inflammatory therapy.* • Prevention of exercise-induced bronchospasm. • *Not to be used to treat acute symptoms or exacerbations.* • Compared to short-acting inhaled beta₂-agonist, salmeterol (but not formoterol) has slower onset of action (15 to 30 minutes) but both have longer duration (>12 hours).	• Tachycardia, skeletal muscle tremor, hypokalemia, prolongation of QT_c interval in overdose. • A diminished bronchoprotective effect may occur within 1 week of chronic therapy. Clinical significance has not been established.	• *Not to be used to treat acute symptoms or exacerbations.* • Clinical significance of potentially developing tolerance is uncertain because studies show symptom control and bronchodilation are maintained. • Should not be used in place of anti-inflammatory therapy. • May provide more effective symptom control when added to standard doses of inhaled corticosteroid compared to increasing the corticosteroid dosage.

Methylxanthines

Theophylline, sustained-release tablets and capsules (See Tables 20.14 through 20.21 for more detailed product and dosing information.)

- Long-term control and prevention of symptoms, especially nocturnal symptoms.

- Dose-related acute toxicities include tachycardia, nausea and vomiting, tachyarrhythmias (SVT), central nervous system stimulation, headache, seizures, hematemesis, hyperglycemia, and hypokalemia.
- Adverse effects at usual therapeutic doses include insomnia, gastric upset, aggravation of ulcer or reflux, increase in hyperactivity in some children, difficulty in urination in elderly males with prostatism.

- Maintain steady-state serum concentrations between 5 and 15 mcg/mL. Routine serum concentration monitoring is essential due to significant toxicities, narrow therapeutic range, and individual differences in metabolic clearance. Absorption and metabolism may be affected by numerous factors, which can produce significant changes in steady-state serum theophylline concentrations.

Leukotriene Modifiers

Montelukast (Singulair)
10 mg tabs Q HS for adults
5 mg chew tabs Q HS for children age 6–12

Zafirlukast tablets*
Accolate 20 mg tab BID

- Long-term control and prevention of symptoms in mild persistent asthma for patients >12 years of age (>6 years of age with montelukast).

- Headache, dyspepsia, diarrhea, abdominal pain reported with all three agents.

- Montelukast: Single daily dosing, lower age indication, lack of food effects on absorption, and lower drug interaction potential are all potential advantages.
- Zafirlukast: BID dosing improves compliance compared to zileuton. Administration with meals decreases bioavailability; take at least 1 hour before or 2 hours after meals.
- Zafirlukast inhibits the metabolism of warfarin and increases prothrombin time; it is a competitive inhibitor of the CYP2C9 hepatic microsomal isozymes. (It has not affected elimination of terfenadine, theophylline, or ethinyl estradiol drugs metabolized by the CYP3A4 isozymes.)

(continued)

Table 20.12 • Long-Term-Control Medications (continued)

Name/Products	Indications	Potential Adverse Effects	Therapeutic Issues
Zileuton tablets Zyflo 600 mg tab QID		• Elevation of liver enzymes has been reported. Limited case reports of reversible hepatitis and hyperbilirubinemia. Zileuton > zafirlukast and montelukast.	• QID dosing of zileuton is a potential problem. • Zileuton is microsomal CYP3A4 enzyme inhibitor that can inhibit the metabolism of terfenadine, propranolol, warfarin, and theophylline. Doses of these drugs should be monitored accordingly. • Zileuton: Monitor hepatic enzymes (ALT) Q month × 3 months, then Q 1–3 months.

*Fluticasone DPI also available as a combination product (Advair Diskus) containing 100, 250, and 500 µg fluticasone with 50 µg salmeterol.

Notes:

Table 20.13 • Estimated Comparative Daily Dosages for Inhaled Corticosteroids

Drug	Low Dose	Adults Medium Dose	High Dose
Beclomethasone dipropionate	168–504 mcg	504–840 mcg	>840 mcg
MDI: 42 mcg/puff	(4–12 puffs—42 mcg)	(12–20 puffs—42 mcg)	(>20 puffs—42 mcg)
MDI: 84 mcg/puff	(2–6 puffs—84 mcg)	(6–10 puffs—84 mcg)	(>10 puffs—84 mcg)
Budesonide	200–400 mcg	400–600 mcg	>600 mcg
DPI: 200 mcg/dose	(1–2 inhalations)	(2–3 inhalations)	(>3 inhalations)
Neb: 0.25 and 0.5 mg/2 mL (Respules)	0.25 mg	0.5 mg	0.75 mg
Flunisolide	500–1,000 mcg	1,000–2,000 mcg	>2,000 mcg
MDI: 250 mcg/puff	(2–4 puffs)	(4–6 puffs)	(>8 puffs)
Fluticasone	88–264 mcg	264–660 mcg	>660 mcg
MDI: 44, 110, 220 mcg/puff	(2–6 puffs—44 mcg) OR	(2–6 puffs—110 mcg)	(>6 puffs—110 mcg) OR
	(2 puffs—110 mcg)	(1–3 puffs—220 mcg)	(>3 puffs—220 mcg)
DPI: 50, 100, 250 mcg/dose	(2–6 inhalations—50 mcg)	(3–6 inhalations—100 mcg)	(>6 inhalations—100 mcg) OR
	(1–3 inhalations—100 mcg)	(1–3 inhalations—250 mcg)	(>2 inhalations—250 mcg)
Triamcinolone acetonide	400–1,000 mcg	1,000–2,000 mcg	>2,000 mcg
MDI: 100 mcg/puff	(4–10 puffs)	(10–20 puffs)	(>20 puffs)

(continued)

Table 20.13 • Estimated Comparative Daily Dosages for Inhaled Corticosteroids (continued)

Drug	Children		
	Low Dose	Medium Dose	High Dose
Beclomethasone dipropionate	84–336 mcg	336–672 mcg	>672 mcg
MDI: 42 mcg/puff	(2–8 puffs—42 mcg)	(8–16 puffs—42 mcg)	(>16 puffs—42 mcg)
MDI: 84 mcg/puff	(1–4 puffs—84 mcg)	(4–8 puffs—84 mcg)	(>8 puffs—84 mcg)
Budesonide	100–200 mcg	200–400 mcg	>400 mcg
DPI: 200 mcg/dose (Turbuhaler)		(1–2 inhalations—200 mcg)	(>2 inhalations—200 mcg)
Neb: 0.25 and 0.5 mg/2 mL (Respules)	0.25 mg	0.5 mg	0.75 mg
Flunisolide	500–750 mcg	1,000–1,250 mcg	>1,250 mcg
MDI: 250 mcg/puff	(2–3 puffs)	(4–5 puffs)	(>5 puffs)
Fluticasone	88–176 mcg	176–440 mcg	>440 mcg
MDI: 44, 110, 220 mcg/puff	(2–4 puffs—44 mcg) OR	(4–10 puffs—44 mcg) OR	(>4 puffs—110 mcg) OR
	(1–2 puffs—110 mcg)	(2–4 puffs—110 mcg) OR	(>2 puffs—220 mcg)
		(1–2 puffs—220 mcg)	
DPI: 50, 100, 250 mcg/dose	(2–4 inhalations—50 mcg)	(2–4 inhalations—100 mcg)	(>4 inhalations—100 mcg) OR
	(1–3 inhalations—100 mcg)	(1–2 inhalations—250 mcg)	(>2 inhalations—250 mcg)
MDI: Triamcinolone acetonide 100 mcg/puff	400–800 mcg	800–1,200 mcg	>1,200 mcg
	(4–8 puffs)	(8–12 puffs)	(>12 puffs)

NOTES:

- **The most important determinant of appropriate dosing is the clinician's judgment of the patient's response to therapy.** The clinician must monitor the patient's response using several clinical parameters and adjust the dose accordingly. The stepwise approach to therapy emphasizes that once control of asthma is achieved, the dose of medication should be carefully titrated to the minimum dose required to maintain control, thus reducing the potential for adverse effect.
- The reference point for the range in the dosages for children is data on the safety of inhaled corticosteroids in children, which, in general, suggest that the dose ranges are equivalent to beclomethasone dipropionate 200–400 mcg/day (low dose), 400–800 mcg/day (medium dose), and >800 mcg/day (high dose).
- Some dosages may be outside package labeling.
- Metered-dose inhaler (MDI) dosages are expressed as the actuator dose (the amount of drug leaving the actuator and delivered to the patient), which is the labeling required in the United States. This is different from the dosage expressed as the valve dose (the amount of drug leaving the valve, all of which is not available to the patient), which is used in many European countries and in some of the scientific literature. Dry powder inhaler (DPI) doses (e.g., Turbuhaler) are expressed as the amount of drug in the inhaler following activation.

Table 20.14 • Percentage of Anhydrous Theophylline and the Equivalent Dose of Various Theophylline Salts

Salt	% Theophylline	Equivalent Dosage (mg)
Theophylline anhydrous	100	100
Theophylline monohydrate	91	100
Aminophylline anhydrous	86	116
Aminophylline dihydrate	79	127
Theophylline monoethanolamine	75	133
Oxtriphylline (choline theophylline)	64	156
Theophylline sodium glycinate	49	200
Theophylline calcium salicylate	48	208

Table 20.15 • Theophylline Kinetics and Loading Dose

Desired plasma concentration (Cp)	5–20 mg/L^a (5–20 μg/mL)
Vd	0.5 L/kg (0.3–0.7 L/kg)
Metabolism	90% hepatic via CYP1A2
Renal excretion unchanged	10%
t½	Highly variable (see Table 20.16)
Loading dose^b	5 mg/kg theophylline 6.5 mg/kg aminophylline

^{a}Aim for 8–12 mg/L for stable patient; 10–15 mg/L for acute exacerbation.
^{b}Loading doses may be given over 20–30 min IV or by rapid–release oral tablets or solution. Guidelines are for a 10 mg/L target concentration; ↑ by 50% for 15 mg/L. ↓ by 50% or more if patient was taking theophylline previously or use the equation:

$$LD = (Cp - Cp_{initial})(Vd)$$

where Cp is any desired concentration and $Cp_{initial}$ is existing drug concentration before the dose.

Notes:

Table 20.16 • Initial IV Maintenance Theophylline Infusion Rates

Patient Population	Average $t_{1/2}$ (hr)	Theophylline Infusion Rate (mg/kg/hr)[a]
Neonates (up to 24 days)[b,c]	20–30	0.08
Neonates (>24 days)[b,c]		0.12
Infants (6–52 wk)		0.008 (age in wk) + 0.21 mg/kg/hr
Young children (1–9 yr)[c]	3–4	0.8
Older children (9–12 yr)[c]		0.7
Adolescents (12–16 yr)		0.5
Adolescent (smoker)		0.7
Adult (>16 yr, nonsmoker)	7–8 (Range: 3–16)	0.4
Adult (smoker)	3–4	0.7[h]
Elderly (nonsmoker)[c]	10	0.3
CHF,[d] liver dysfunction, cor pulmonale, pneumonia, viral illness, high fever[e]		0.2 mg/kg/hr or ↓ above dose by 50%[e]
Cimetidine, ciprofloxacin, erythromycin, other enzyme inhibitors[f]		↓ above dose by 50%[f]
Carbamazepine, phenytoin, phenobarbital, rifampin, smoker[g]		↑ above dose by 50%[g]

[a]Doses to achieve 10 mg/L. Divide by 0.8 for aminophylline dose. Use lean body weight for obese patients.
[b]To achieve a target concentration of 7.5 mg/L for neonatal apnea.
[c]Clearance is slow in neonates due to immature hepatic function. During early childhood, clearance is most rapid. Clearance is slower in adults than in children. Clearance is further reduced with aging (>65 yr).
[d]CHF = Congestive heart failure.
[e]The influence of these variables is difficult to predict. Theophylline clearance may change several times in the same patient during fluctuations in various disease processes. In particular, acute respiratory failure may ↓ theophylline clearance. Therefore, as respiratory status changes, theophylline dosage adjustments may be required. Do not exceed 400 mg/day starting dose unless serum levels indicate the need for larger doses.
[f]As a general rule, enzyme inhibition effects are rapid (24–48 hr), except with erythromycin. However, the magnitude of change may be both time and dose dependent. Patients with theophylline serum concentrations >13 mg/L are at greatest risk of developing side effects with combination therapy.
[g]As a general rule, enzyme induction effects are slow (5 days–2 weeks). Conversely, after stopping the drug inducer or smoking, it may take several days for the inducing effect to significantly abate.
[h]Do not exceed 900 mg/day starting dose unless indicated by serum levels.

Table 20.17 • Theophylline Dosing Guide for Chronic Use[a,b]

Starting dose for children 1–15 years <45 kg: 12–14 mg/kg/day up to maximum of 300 mg/day

Starting dose for adults and children 1–15 years >45 kg: 300 mg/day

Titrate dose upward after 3 days if necessary and if tolerated to:
- 16 mg/kg/day up to maximum of 400 mg /day in children 1–15 years <45 kg
- 400 mg/day in adults and in children >45 kg

Titrate dose upward after 3 more days if necessary and if tolerated to:
- 20 mg/kg/day up to a maximum of 600 mg/day in children 1–15 years <45 kg
- 600 mg/day in adults and in children >45 kg

[a]Dose using ideal body weight or actual body weight, whichever is less. These dosages do not apply if liver disease, heart failure, or other factors documented to affect theophylline clearance are present. Doses must be guided by monitoring serum concentrations to ensure optimal safety and efficacy.
[b]Dosing schedule dependent on product selected; sustained-release products are much preferred if at all possible.

Table 20.18 • Adjusting Doses of Theophylline Based Upon Serum Concentrations

Peak Theophylline Concentration (mg/L)[a]	Approximate Adjustment in Daily Dose	Comment
<5.0	↑ by 25%	Recheck serum theophylline concentration
5–10	↑ by 25% if clinically indicated	Recheck serum concentration; ↑ dose only if poor response to therapy
10–12	Cautious 10% ↑ if clinically indicated	If asymptomatic, no ↑ needed. Recheck serum theophylline concentration before further dose changes
12–15	Occasional intolerance requires a 10% ↓	If asymptomatic, no dose change needed unless side effects present
16–20	↓ by 10–25%	Even if asymptomatic and side effects absent, a dose ↓ is prudent
20–24.9	↓ by 50%	Omit one dose even if asymptomatic and side effects absent; a dose ↓ is indicated
25–29.9	↓ by ≥50%	Omit next doses even if asymptomatic and side effects absent; a dose ↓ indicated; repeat serum theophylline concentration after dose adjustment
≥30	Omit next doses; ↓ by 60–75%	Seek medical attention and consult regional poison center even if not symptomatic; if ≥60 years of age, anticipate need for treatment of seizures

[a]It is important that levels are obtained at steady state. If laboratory results appear questionable, suggest repeat measurements.

Table 20.19 • FDA Guidelines for Theophylline Dosing in Infants[a]

Premature Neonates
  <24 days postnatal age: 1.0 mg/kg Q 12 hr
  ≥24 days postnatal age: 1.5 mg/kg Q 12 hr

Term Infants and Infants Up to 52 Weeks of Age
Total daily dose (mg) = [(0.2 × age in weeks) + 5.0] × (kg body wt)
• Up to age 26 weeks; divide dose into 3 equal amounts administered at 8-hr intervals
• >26 weeks of age; divide dose into 4 equal amounts administered at 6-hr intervals

[a]Final doses adjusted to a peak steady-state serum theophylline concentration of 5–10 mg/L in neonates and 10–15 mg/L in older infants.

Table 20.20 • Rules for Dosing Intervals with Sustained Release (SR) Theophylline[a,b]

1) Rapid excreters (e.g., dose >1200 mg/day in adults): TheoDur and Slo-Bid Q 8 hr; other SR Q 6 hr

2) Children, adult smokers, and 25% of nonsmokers (e.g., doses of 900–1200 mg/day in adults): TheoDur and Slo–Bid Q 12 hr, other SR Q 8 hr

3) Average nonsmoking adult (e.g., doses of 600–900 mg/day): All SR Q 12 hr

4) Very slow metabolizers (e.g., doses of 200–600 mg/day in adults): TheoDur, Slo–Bid Q 24 hr, other SR Q 12 hr

[a]Because of absorption rate differences, SR theophylline products should never be therapeutically interchanged without informing the prescriber.
[b]For patients with nocturnal asthma, larger doses may be given QD at bedtime.

Table 20.21 • Oral Theophylline Preparations with Absorption Abnormalities

Theo–24	Very slow absorption. <100% bioavailable when fasting. ↑ rate and extent of absorption with large fatty meal
Uniphyl	Same as Theo-24
TheoDur Sprinkle	↓ bioavailability with food

Notes:

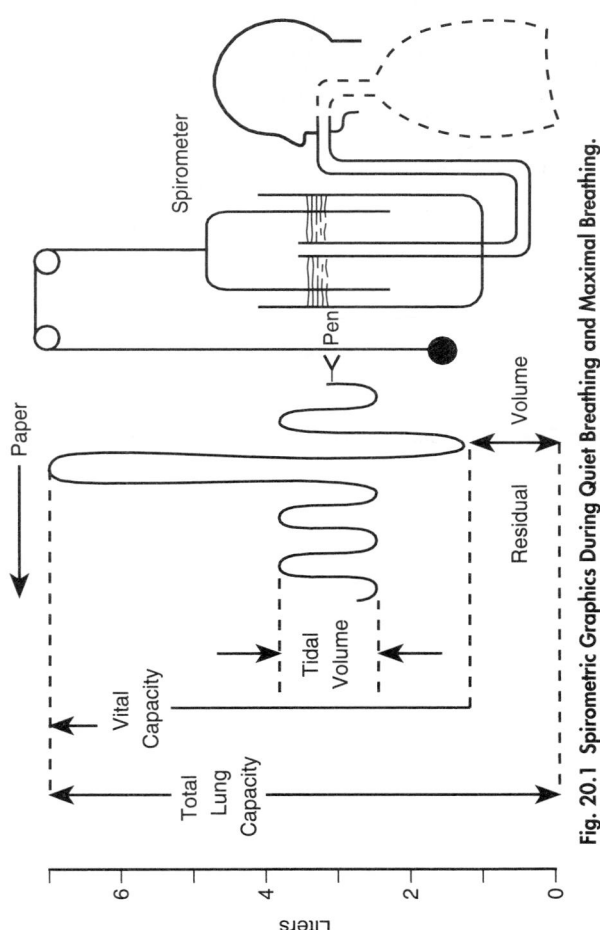

Fig. 20.1 Spirometric Graphics During Quiet Breathing and Maximal Breathing.

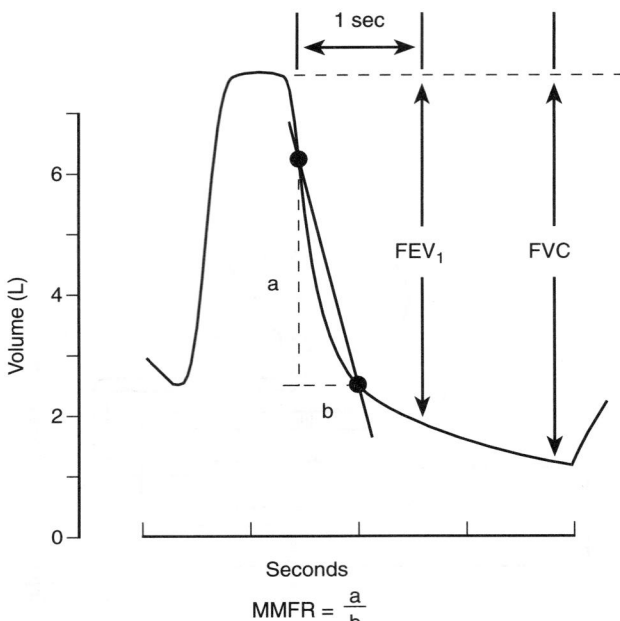

Fig. 20.2 Volume-Time Curve from a Forced Expiratory Maneuver.

Notes:

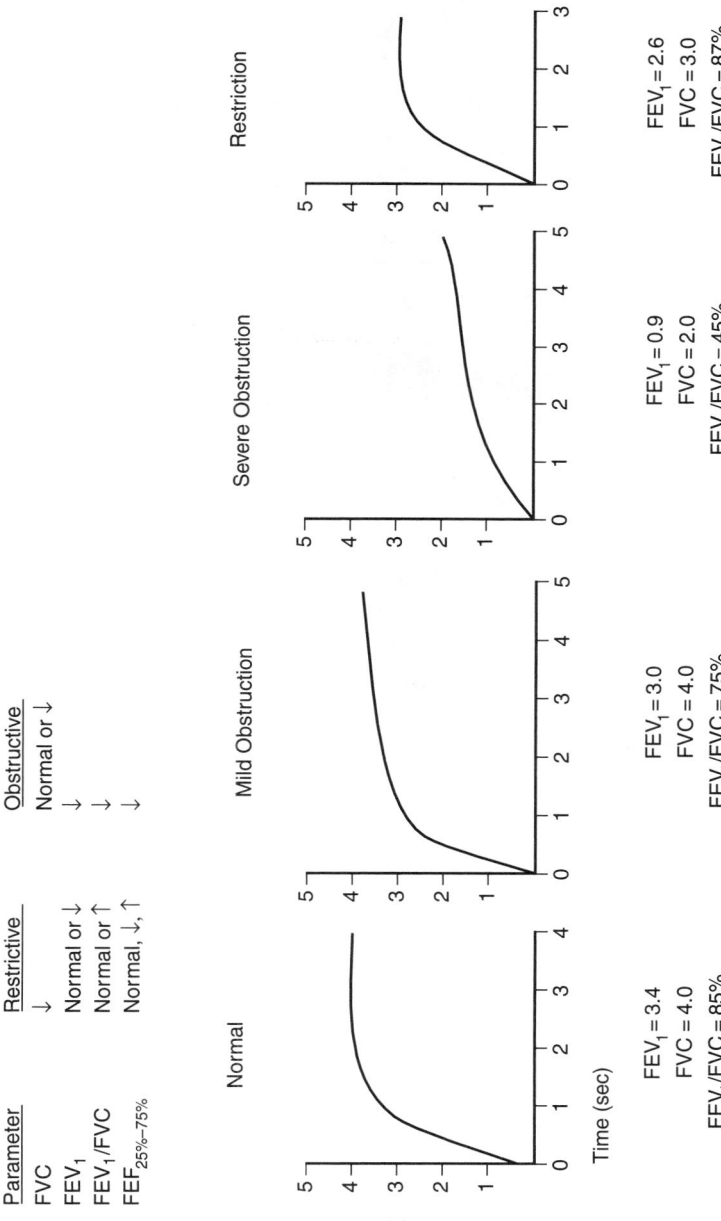

Fig. 20.3 Interpretation of Results of Spirometry. The graphs depicted are for illustration only. The interpretation of flow rates may vary with the age of the patient. (Reprinted with permission from National Institutes of Health. Guidelines for the Diagnosis and Management of Asthma. National Asthma Education Program Expert Panel Report, 1991; NIH Publication No. 91-3042.)

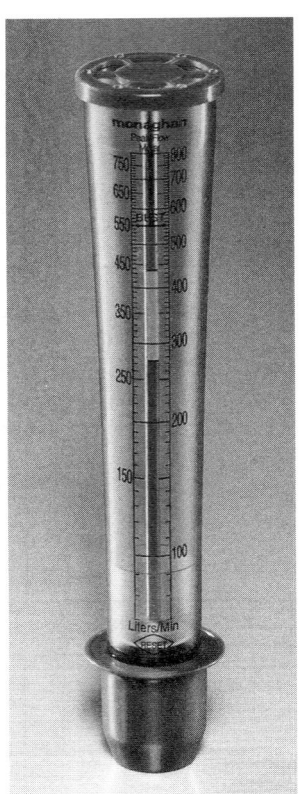

Fig. 20.4 Peak Flow Meter.

Notes:

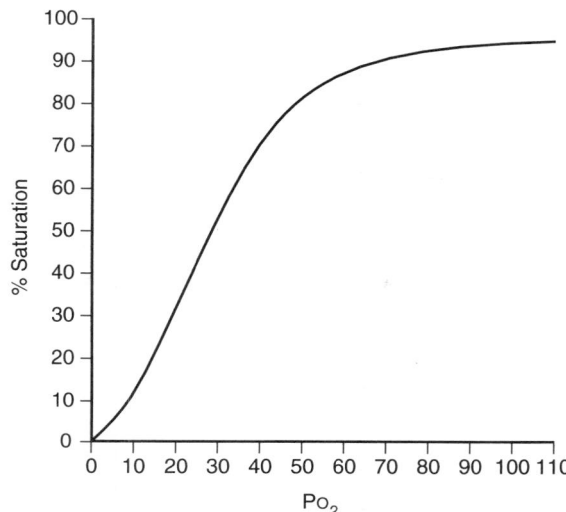

Fig. 20.5 The Oxygen Dissociation Curve Reveals that the Percent Saturation of Hemoglobin Increases Almost Linearly with Increases in the Arterial O_2 Tension Until a PaO_2 of 55 to 65 mm Hg is Reached. At PaO_2 values above this, the increase in hemoglobin saturation becomes proportionately less and relatively little additional oxygen is added to the hemoglobin despite large increases in PaO_2. (Reproduced with permission from Guenther CA, Welch MH. Pulmonary Medicine, 2nd Ed. Philadelphia; JB Lippincott, 1982.)

Notes:

Long-Term Control	Quick Relief
STEP 4 **Severe** **Persistent** ■ Daily anti-inflammatory medicine— High-dose budesonide nebulizer or other inhaled corticosteroid with spacer/holding chamber and face mask If needed, add systemic corticosteroids 2 mg/kg/day and reduce to lowest daily or alternate-day dose that stabilizes symptoms	■ Bronchodilator as needed for symptoms (see step 1) up to 3 times a day
STEP 3 **Moderate** **Persistent** ■ Daily anti-inflammatory medication. Either: Medium-dose budesonide nebulizer or other inhaled corticosteroid with spacer/holding chamber and face mask OR, once control is established: Medium-dose inhaled corticosteroid and nedocromil OR Medium-dose inhaled corticosteroid and long-acting bronchodilator (theophylline)	■ Bronchodilator as needed for symptoms (see step 1) up to 3 times a day
STEP 2 **Mild** **Persistent** ■ Daily anti-inflammatory medicine. Either: Cromolyn (nebulizer is preferred; or MDI) or nedocromil (MDI only) TID–QID Infants and young children usually begin with a trial of cromolyn or nedocromil OR Low-dose budesonide nebulizer or other inhaled corticosteroid with spacer/holding chamber and face mask	■ Bronchodilator as needed for symptoms (see step 1)

| STEP 1
Mild
Intermittent | ■ No daily medication needed. | ■ Bronchodilator as needed for symptoms <2 times a week.
Intensity of treatment will depend upon severity of exacer-
bation. Either:
  Inhaled short-acting beta₂-agonist by nebulizer or face
    mask and spacer/holding chamber
  OR
  Oral beta₂-agonist for symptoms
■ With viral respiratory infection:
  Bronchodilator Q 4–6 hours up to 24 hours (longer with
    physician consult) but, in general, repeat no more than
    once every 6 weeks
  Consider systemic corticosteroid if
    Current exacerbation is severe
    OR
    Patient has history of previous severe exacerbations |

Step down
Review treatment every 1 to 6 months. If control is sustained for at least 3 months, a gradual stepwise reduction in treatment may be possible.

Step up
If control is not achieved, consider step up. But first, review patient medication technique, adherence, and environmental control (avoidance of allergens or other precipitant factors).

NOTES:
■ **The stepwise approach presents guidelines to assist clinical decision making. Asthma is highly variable; clinicians should tailor specific medication plans to the needs and circumstances of individual patients.**
■ Gain control as quickly as possible; then decrease treatment to the least medication necessary to maintain control. Gaining control may be accomplished by either starting treatment at the step most appropriate to the initial severity of their condition or by starting at a higher level of therapy (e.g., a course of systemic corticosteroids or higher dose of inhaled corticosteroids).
■ A rescue course of systemic corticosteroid (prednisolone) may be needed at any time and step.
■ In general, use of short-acting beta₂-agonist on a daily basis indicates the need for additional long-term-control therapy.
■ It is important to remember that there are very few studies on asthma therapy for infants.
■ Consultation with an asthma specialist is *recommended* for patients with moderate or severe persistent asthma in this age group. Consultation should be *considered* for all patients with mild persistent asthma.

Fig. 20.6 Stepwise Approach for Managing Infants and Young Children (5 Years of Age and Younger) with Acute or Chronic Asthma Symptoms. (Reproduced with permission from National Institutes of Health. Expert Panel Report 2. Guidelines for the Diagnosis and Management of Asthma, 1997; NIH Publication No. 97-4051.)

| Treatment | Preferred treatments are in bold print. |
Long-Term Control	Quick Relief
STEP 4 **Severe** **Persistent**	Daily medications: ■ **Anti-inflammatory: inhaled cortico-steroid (high dose)** AND ■ Long-acting bronchodilator: either **long-acting inhaled beta$_2$-agonist,** sustained-release theophylline, or long-acting beta$_2$-agonist tablets AND ■ Corticosteroid tablets or syrup long term (2 mg/kg/day, generally do not exceed 60 mg per day).	Same as Step 1

STEP 3
Moderate
Persistent
	Daily medication:
	■ Either
	    Anti-inflammatory: inhaled cortico-steroid (medium dose)
	    OR
	    Inhaled corticosteroid (low-medium dose) and add a long-acting bronchodilator, especially for nighttime symptoms: either **long-acting inhaled beta$_2$-agonist,** sustained-release theophylline, or long-acting beta$_2$-agonist tablets.
	■ If needed
	    Anti-inflammatory: **inhaled cortico-steroids (medium-high dose)**
	    AND
	    Long-acting bronchodilator, especially for nighttime symptoms; either **long-acting inhaled beta$_2$-agonist,** sustained-release theophylline, or long-acting beta$_2$-agonist tablets.
		Same as Step 1

STEP 2 **Mild** **Persistent**	One daily medication: ■ **Anti-inflammatory:** either **inhaled corticosteroid** (low doses) or **cromolyn or nedocromil** (children usually begin with a trial of cromolyn or nedocromil). ■ Sustained-release theophylline to serum concentration of 5–15 mcg/mL is an alternative, but not preferred, therapy. Montelukast, zafirlukast or zileuton may also be considered for patients ≥12 years of age, although their position in therapy is not fully established.	Same as Step 1

Fig. 20.7 Stepwise Approach for Managing Asthma in Adults and Children Older than 5 Years of Age. (Reproduced with permission from National Institutes of Health. Expert Panel Report 2. Guidelines for the Diagnosis and Management of Asthma, 1997; NIH Publication No. 97-4051.)

	Treatment	Preferred treatments are in bold print.
	Long-Term Control	**Quick Relief**
STEP 1 **Mild** **Intermittent**	■ No daily medication needed.	■ Short-acting bronchodilator: **inhaled beta$_2$-agonists as** needed for symptoms. ■ Use of short-acting inhaled beta$_2$-agonists more than 2 times a week may indicate the need to initiate long- term-control therapy.

↓ **Step down**
Review treatment every 1 to 6 months; a gradual stepwise reduction in treatment may be possible.

↑ **Step up**
If control is not maintained, consider step up. First, review patient medication technique, adherence, and environmental control (avoidance of allergens or other factors that contribute to asthma severity).

NOTES:
■ **The stepwise approach presents general guidelines to assist clinical decision making; it is not intended to be a specific prescription. Asthma is highly variable; clinicians should tailor specific medication plans to the needs and circumstances of individual patients.**
■ Gain control as quickly as possible; then decrease treatment to the least medication necessary to maintain control. Gaining control may be accomplished by either starting treatment at the step most appropriate to the initial severity of the condition or starting at a higher level of therapy (e.g., a course of systemic corticosteroids or higher dose of inhaled corticosteroids).
■ A rescue course of systemic corticosteroid may be needed at any time and at any step.
■ Some patients with intermittent asthma experience severe and life-threatening exacerbations separated by long periods of normal lung function and no symptoms. This may be especially common with exacerbations provoked by respiratory infections. A short course of systemic corticosteroids is recommended.
■ At each step, patients should control their environment to avoid or control factors that make their asthma worse (e.g., allergens, irritants); this requires specific diagnosis and education.
■ Referral to an asthma specialist for consultation or comanagement is *recommended* if there are difficulties achieving or maintaining control of asthma or if the patient requires step 4 care. Referral may be *considered* if the patient requires step 3 care.

Fig. 20.7 *(continued)*

Notes:

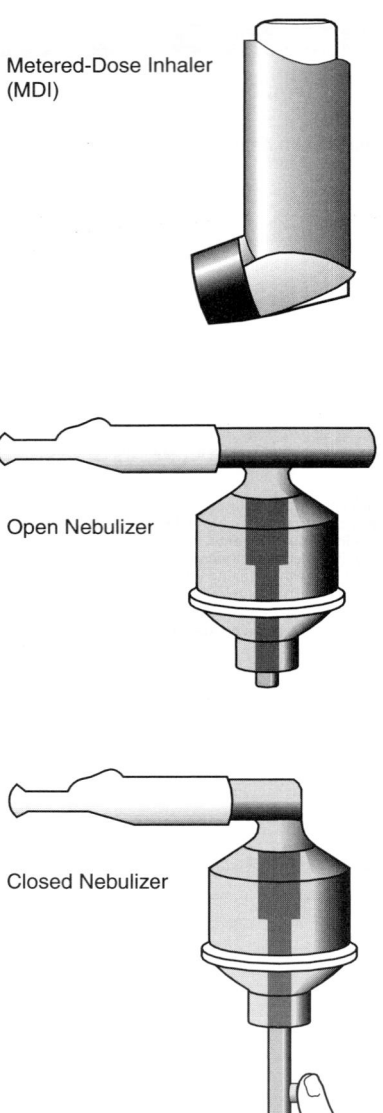

Metered-Dose Inhaler
(MDI)

Open Nebulizer

Closed Nebulizer

Fig. 20.8 Metered-Dose Inhaler and Nebulizer.

Notes:

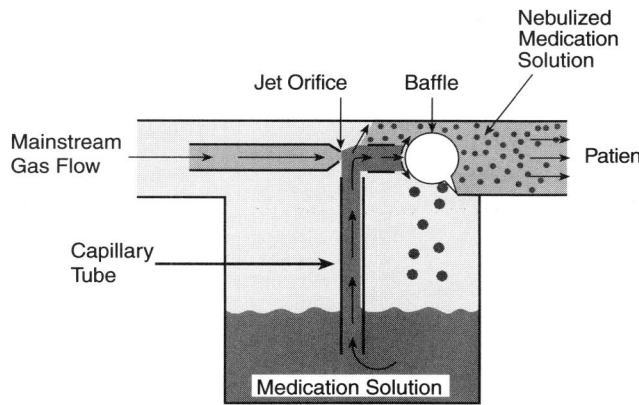

Fig. 20.9 Air Jet Nebulizer.

The reader is referred to Chapter 21: Asthma, written by *Timothy H. Self, Pharm.D.*, in the seventh edition of **Applied Therapeutics: The Clinical Use of Drugs** for a more in-depth discussion. The editors of this handbook express their thanks to Dr. Self and acknowledge that this chapter is based upon his work.

Notes:

Notes:

Chapter 21

Chronic Obstructive Pulmonary Disease

Pathophysiology and Clinical Features
Definitions and Clinical Presentation

- **Obstructive airways diseases** are disorders that obstruct the volume and/or rate of airflow into the lungs. Examples include asthma, chronic bronchitis, and emphysema. See Table 21.1 for a clinical comparison of these three disorders.

- **Chronic Obstructive Pulmonary Disease (COPD)** is defined as "a disease state characterized by the presence of airflow obstruction due to *chronic bronchitis* (and/or) *emphysema;* the airflow obstruction is generally progressive, may be accompanied by airway hyperreactivity, and may be partially reversible.

  - Asthma is specifically excluded from the definition of COPD, but a component of asthma may be present in some patients with COPD.

  - Cigarette smoking is the primary risk factor for development of COPD

- ***Bronchitis*** is defined as inflammation of the bronchioles.

- ***Chronic bronchitis*** is defined clinically as "the presence of chronic productive cough for 3 months in each of 2 consecutive years in a patient in whom other causes of chronic cough (e.g., heart failure) have been excluded."

- ***Emphysema*** is an anatomic pathology with "abnormal permanent enlargement of the airspaces distal to the terminal bronchioles, accompanied by destruction of their walls and without obvious fibrosis."

Restrictive lung diseases, in contrast to obstructive airways disease, are characterized by normal airways and alveoli but a decreased ability of the lung to expand due to loss of elasticity or anatomical destruction, e.g., pulmonary fibrosis, silicosis, scoliosis.

Staging Severity

Pulmonary function measurements of forced expiratory volume in one second (FEV_1) and the ratio of FEV_1 to forced vital capacity (FVC) are used to estimate the severity, prognosis, and reversibility of obstruction in COPD, as summarized in Table 21.2. See Chapter 20: Asthma for further interpretation of pulmonary function tests.

General Management Goals

The goals of treatment of COPD are similar to those of asthma but must be realistic. A return to normal functional ability and pulmonary function is generally not attainable. The disease is usually progressive, even with maximal treatment.

- Slow disease progression
- Minimize symptoms
- Maximize functional ability

♦ Prevent acute exacerbations
♦ Prolong survival

General Treatment Principles

♦ Educate patient with emphasis on understanding disease process and rationale for various components of care.
♦ Help patient develop *realistic* goals and expectations
♦ Annual influenza vaccination
♦ Pneumococcal vaccine (Pneumovax). Repeat Q 6 years or as indicated by titers
♦ Minimize unnecessary fear or anxiety
♦ Optimize strategies to improve functional ability
  • Pulmonary rehabilitation: breathing exercises, general physical conditioning, exercise training
♦ Coughing techniques, postural drainage, chest percussion for secretion mobilization

Smoking Cessation

Smoking cessation programs are the cornerstone of helping patients slow the progression of COPD.

♦ Combining pharmacologic (e.g., nicotine replacement strategies and buproprion) and nonpharmacologic interventions (e.g., behavioral modification, psychological and social counseling) is more effective than either intervention used alone.
♦ See Table 21.3 for a common five-step strategy used to identify and assist patients with smoking cessation.
♦ A major pharmacologic intervention is nicotine replacement (substitution) therapy, using either nicotine gum, transdermal patches, nasal spray, or inhaler. All appear to be equally effective, but transdermal systems may be most convenient. See Table 21.4
  • Nicotine polacrilex chewing gum (Nicorette):
    —Gradual rise to serum nicotine levels of 8–12 ng/mL compared to high brain concentrations within 7–19 seconds and peak serum levels of 10–50 ng/mL in 5 minutes with cigarettes.
    —Avoid acidic beverages (impair buccal absorption): coffee, cola, wine, orange juice.
    —Side effects: nausea, stomach gas, belching, throat irritation, lightheadedness, hiccups.
  • Nicotine transdermal systems:
    —Gradual rise to serum levels of 6–17 ng/mL; more sustained level than with gum.
  • Nicotrol removed after 16 hours, all others after 24 hours. Less sleep disturbances?
  • Skin irritation: 35–45%.
  • Increased risk of cardiac effects if patient smokes while patch is in place.
    —Caution with both gum and patch in patients with angina or arrhythmias
♦ Bupropion (Zyban)
  • Inhibits neuronal uptake of norepinephrine and dopamine. Nicotine also activates epinephrine and dopamine release in CNS. Thus, buproprion may substitute for nicotine during withdrawal.
  • Equally effective or superior to nicotine replacement as monotherapy, possible additive effect in combination therapy.

- Start treatment 7 days before target quit date to allow gradual build up of blood levels.
- 150 mg sustained release tablet QD for 3 days, then 150 mg BID for 7–12 weeks.
- Side effects: agitation, anxiety, insomnia. Reduced by slow titration described above.
- Caution: seizure risk of 0.1% at 300 mg/day. Contraindicated if history of seizures.

Chronic Pharmacologic Management

See Chapter 20: Asthma for a description of the pharmacology, dosing, and side effects of respiratory drugs.

A general medication treatment algorithm for COPD patients is presented in Figure 21.1. The following differences between the pharmacotherapy in COPD and that for asthma should be noted.

♦ There is often no reversible (asthmatic) component, except during an acute exacerbation. Therefore, responses to bronchodilators are unpredictable. Changes in FEV_1 or peak flow rate after single-dose challenges with beta agonists or anticholinergics may not be predictive of clinical benefit. A 1- to 2-week trial of any drug should be tried. Both objective (pulmonary function) and subjective (symptomatic) responses should be considered when determining whether a drug is responsive in a given patient.

♦ Anticholinergic bronchodilators (e.g., ipratropium) should be added earlier in COPD than in asthma because of relatively greater responsiveness.

♦ For convenience, patients documented as having additive bronchodilation from albuterol and ipratropium may use the fixed-dose combination product: Combivent (18 μg ipratropium + 90 μg albuterol per puff.) For further titration, combined nebulized solutions of the two drugs may be used.

♦ Continuous use of short-acting beta-agonists (e.g., albuterol) has been associated with poor patient outcome and increased side effects in patients with asthma. It is not known whether this data can be extrapolated to COPD patients. There is increasing evidence that long-acting beta-agonists like salmeterol provide subjective relief to some COPD patients, even in the absence of improved pulmonary function.

♦ Theophylline may play a greater role in the treatment of COPD than asthma. Subjective benefit may be derived even in the absence of improved pulmonary function tests, possibly via a diaphragm stimulatory (inotropic) effect. See Chapter 20: Asthma for detailed descriptions of theophylline dosing and drug interactions. Factors to consider in COPD patients are age and heart failure (both slow metabolism), smoking status (induces metabolism), and interacting drugs.

♦ Although chronic bronchitis is an inflammatory disease, the underlying pathology is significantly different from asthma. Except during acute exacerbations, only 10–30% of COPD patients benefit from either inhaled or oral corticosteroids. As a result, inhaled steroids are added much later in the COPD algorithm than they are in asthma patients. Inhaled steroids may be most effective in patients with bronchodilator responsiveness (i.e., an "asthmatic" component.) A 2-week trial of oral or inhaled steroids is warranted if beta-agonists, anticholinergics, and theophylline fail to provide adequate relief. If responsive, begin chronic inhaled steroids.

♦ Oral steroids are used in "burst therapy," for COPD exacerbations as in asthma, but there is a high risk of dependence and side effects with chronic use.

♦ There is no role for cromolyn, nedocromil, or leukotriene modifiers in COPD management.

Acute COPD Exacerbations

Emergency department and hospital management of COPD patients is essentially the same as for acute asthma, but responses may be slower and less dramatic.

♦ Aggressive inhaled beta-agonist and anticholinergic bronchodilators plus systemic corticosteroids are all indicated.

♦ Add IV theophylline only if the above measures fail

♦ Discharge on a 1- to 4-week tapering course of oral steroids. Taper slower if on steroids prior to the exacerbation.

♦ Antibiotics

• Viral upper respiratory infections may trigger acute exacerbations.

• Bacterial infections may be superimposed.

• Evidence for empiric antibiotics for episodes of greater sputum production and sputum purulence (viscous and discolored) is controversial.

• A long-acting cephalosporin (e.g., ceftriaxone) plus a macrolide (erythromycin or azithromycin) will cover *Streptococcus pneumoniae* (including penicillin-resistant), *Hemophilus influenzae*, *Moraxella catarrhalis*, and *Mycoplasma pneumoniae*

• Other alternatives include amoxicillin/clavulanate, cefuroxime axetil, clarithromycin, and second-generation quinolones.

• Caution regarding increased resistance to amoxicillin, ampicillin, or trimethoprim-sulfamethoxazole.

• Caution re drug interactions between theophylline and clarithromycin, erythromycin, or ciprofloxacin.

Oxygen Therapy

♦ Indications for oxygen therapy include

• Hypoxemia: PaO_2 <55 mm Hg and/or O_2 saturation <88%.

• PaO_2 56–59 mm Hg and/or O_2 saturation 89%, combined with either polycythemia or cor pulmonale

♦ Goal of therapy: PaO_2 >60 mm Hg or O_2 saturation >90%

♦ Minimum of 18–24 hours per day of continuous O_2 administration via nasal cannula at flow rate of 2 to 3 L/min required to raise fraction of inspired air (FiO_2) to 27%, compared with 21% with room air.

Sleep Apnea

♦ **Definition.** Sleep apnea is a breathing disorder characterized by frequent or prolonged cessation of breathing during sleep.

• >15 seconds per episode; >30 apnea episodes per night

• Reduction in arterial O_2 saturation

♦ **Obstructive apnea** occurs when an occlusion in the upper airway (e.g., pharyngeal collapse) and/or obesity prevents airflow. Inspiratory effort is normal (chest wall moves), but expiration is blocked. Loud snoring, sleep fragmentation, obesity, daytime somnolence, morning headache, shortness of breath with exertion, and erratic behavior are common.

♦ **Central apnea** is mediated by decreased responsiveness of respiratory centers in the brain to hypercapnea and is characterized by a cessation of both inspiration (primary defect) and expiration. The patient begins breathing again when PaO_2 levels become too low.

◆ **Mixed apnea** is a combination of obstructive and central apnea

◆ Pulmonary vasoconstriction leads to pulmonary hypertension, right-sided heart failure, and left-sided heart failure.

◆ **Treatment** of sleep apnea is summarized in Table 21.5.

Notes:

Table 21.1 • Clinical Features of Obstructive Airways Disease

	Asthma[a]	Bronchitis[b]	Emphysema[c]
Primary symptom:	Minimal between attacks; marked during attacks	Cough and sputum production	Dyspnea
Degree of bronchospasm	A. Bronchospasm, wheezing B. Cough C. Dyspnea		
Reversible with β-agonists	Yes	No	No
Allergic component	Frequent, but not always	None	None
Inflammation	Yes	Yes	Alveoli only
Sputum production	During acute attack only	Copious, continuous	Scanty
Cough	Yes (nonproductive); morning cough may be a sign of nocturnal asthma	Yes (productive)	No
Age of onset	Often in childhood with allergies; older onset usually nonallergic	46–65 yr	55–75 yr
Chronicity	Episodic (e.g., pollen season) or continuous	Continuous	Continuous
Cigarette use	Uncommon	High incidence	High incidence
Body build	Varied	Obese	Thin, barrel chest
Hypoxia, CO_2 retention	During acute attack only	Yes (blue bloater)	No (pink puffer)
Other	Wheeze, cough, chest tightness, shortness of breath, mucous plugging, airway edema, difficulty exhaling. Often worse at night, or following exercise		

[a]Asthma is a chronic condition characterized by recurrent (intermittent) reversible bronchospasm. Reversibility may be spontaneous or after drugs. Airway inflammation and hyperresponsiveness to a variety of stimuli are important components of asthma.
[b]Chronic bronchitis is an inflammation of the bronchial tree. Chronic cough on most days for at least 3 months/yr for 2 yr. Thickened sputum and edematous bronchial walls obstruct airflow.
[c]Emphysema is a destruction of alveolar walls and capillaries by ↑ lung enzymatic activity.

Table 21.2 • Staging of COPD Based on Pulmonary Function Testing

Stage	FEV$_1$ (% of predicted)	FEV$_1$:FVC ratio	Clinical Features
Normal	>80%	>80%	No impairment of function
Stage I: mild obstruction	50–80% (ATS) 60–80% (BTS) 70–80% (ERS)	60–75%	"Smokers' cough"; little or no shortness of breath (breathlessness); minimal impact on quality of life; modest health care expenditures
Stage II: moderate obstruction	35–49% (ATS) 40–59% (BTS) 50–69% (ERS)	50–60%	Breathlessness (± wheezes) on moderate exertion; cough (± sputum); reduction in breath sounds and presence of wheezes on auscultation; significant impact on health-related quality of life; large health care expenditures
Stage III: severe obstruction	<35% (ATS) <40% (BTS) <50% (ERS)	<50%	Breathlessness on any exertion or at rest; prominent wheezing and cough; hyperinflated lungs, cyanosis, peripheral edema; profound impact on health-related quality of life; large health care expenditures

ATS, American Thoracic Society; BTS, British Thoracic Society; ERS, European Respiratory Society.

Table 21.3 • Five-Step Strategy to Assist in Smoking Cessation

1. **Ask:** Systemically screen all patients at every visit to identify all tobacco users

2. **Advise:** Strongly urge all smokers to quit. Explain the health risks of smoking and the health benefits of stopping smoking. Personalize to patients' current health problems, the impact of smoking on their family (especially children), and economic costs.

3. **Identify** smokers willing to attempt to quit. If they are not ready now, continue to advise them until they are ready to quit.[a]

4. **Assist** the patient in quitting by developing a personalized quit plan.[b]

5. **Arrange:** Schedule follow-up contact[c]

[a]Recognize the 5 stages of change or transition from smoking to nonsmoking: precontemplation, contemplation, preparation, action, and maintenance.
[b]Quitting "cold turkey" is more likely to be successful than gradual withdrawal. Helpful to set a "quit date" 1–2 weeks in the future as the first step in the actual intervention once the patient makes the personal decision to quit. This gives the patient time to prepare mentally and to inform family and friends, requesting their understanding and support.
[c]Follow-up face-to-face meetings or phone calls by a caregiver after the quit date, plus a strong social support system throughout the process, improves success.

Notes:

Table 21.4 • Nicotine-Replacement Dosing[a]

Brand Names and Strengths	FDA-approved Dosing Regimen	AHCPR-recommended Dosing Regimen[b]
Chewing Gum Nicorette (2 mg), Nicorette (4 mg) (nonprescription)	2 mg (4 mg for highly dependent patients,[c] patients with severe withdrawal symptoms, or patients who failed on 2 mg) chew and "park" the gum intermittently over 30 min whenever the patient feels the urge to smoke[d] or every 1–2 hr for 6 wk, then every 2 hr for 3 wk, then every 4–8 hr for 3 wk, not to exceed 24 pieces daily for 12 wk of therapy	2 mg (4 mg for highly dependent patients,[c] patients who request it, or patients who failed on 2 mg) chew and "park" between the cheek and gum intermittently over 30 min whenever the patient feels the urge to smoke or every 1–2 hr, not to exceed 30 2-mg pieces daily or 20 4-mg pieces daily, for 1–3 mo; dosing frequency then gradually reduced
Transdermal Systems (Patches)		
Habitrol (21, 14, or 7 mg/day over 24 hr)	*Otherwise healthy patients:* 21 mg/day for 4–8 wk, then 14 mg/day for 2–4 wk, then 7 mg/day for 2–4 wk *Other patients[f]:* 14 mg/day for 4–8 wk, then 7 mg/day for 2–4 wk	21 mg/day for 4 wk, then 14 mg/day for 2 wk, then 7 mg/day for 2 wk
Nicoderm (21, 14, or 7 mg/day over 24 hr)	*Healthy patients:* 21 mg/day for 6 wk, then 14 mg/day for 2 wk, then 7 mg/day for 2 wk *Other patients[f]:* 14 mg/day for 6 wk, then 7 mg/day for 2–4 wk	21 mg/day for 4 wk, then 14 mg/day for 2 wk, then 7 mg/day for 2 wk
Nicoderm (21, 14, or 7 mg/day over 24 hr) (nonprescription)	21 mg/day for 6 wk, then 14 mg/day for 2 wk, then 7 mg/day for 2 wk[g]	Not addressed
Nicotrol 15, 10, or 5 mg/day over 16 hr	15 mg/day for 4–12 wk, then 10 mg/day for 2–4 wk, then 5 mg/day for 2–4 wk	15 mg/day for 4 wk, then 10 mg/day for 2 wk, then 5 mg/day for 2 wk
Nicotrol (15 mg/day over 16 hr) (nonprescription)	15 mg/day for 6 wk[g,h]	Not addressed
Prostep (22 or 11 mg/day over 24 hr)	*Patients ≥100 lb:* 22 mg/day for 4–8 wk, then 11 mg/day for 2–4 wk *Patients <100 lb:* 11 mg/day for 4–8 wk	22 mg/day for 4 wk, then 11 mg/day for 4 wk

Nasal Spray

Nicotrol NS (10 mg/mL)

One or two 1-mg doses (each dose is two 0.5-mg sprays, one in each nostril) per hr initially; increased as needed, not to exceed 5 doses/hr or 40 doses/day, for up to 8 wk; then gradually decreased over 4–6 wk

Not addressed

[a]All therapies are by prescription except where indicated. Therapy should probably be stopped if the patient has not stopped smoking after 4 weeks of therapy, because such patients are unlikely to succeed in quitting on that attempt.
[b]Consider a small initial dosage for light smokers (i.e., people who smoke ≤10–15 cigarettes daily).
[c]Patients who smoke >25 cigarettes daily or score ≥7 on the Fagerstrom Tolerance Questionnaire (a series of questions about smoking behaviors).
[d]Clinical studies found greater efficacy in patients who chewed more than nine pieces per day.
[e]Patients with a history of severe withdrawal symptoms or who smoke >20 cigarettes daily or immediately upon wakening.
[f]Light smokers (i.e., people who smoke <10 cigarettes/day), patients who are small (e.g., weigh <100 lb), and patients who have cardiovascular disease.
[g]These doses are based on data presented to an FDA advisory board committee on April 19, 1996.
[h]Nonprescription transdermal systems do not require a tapered dosing regimen.
Originally published in the American Pharmaceutical Association Special Report, A review of the new smoking cessation strategies from the Agency for Health Care Policy and Research. Washington, DC: APhA, 1996.

Notes:

Table 21.5 • Treatment of Sleep Apnea

Obstructive Apnea
Weight loss

Avoid sedatives, hypnotics, alcohol, antihistamines

Continuous positive airway pressure (CPAP) while sleeping at 5-20 cm H_2O

Acetazolamide (Diamox) 250 mg QD-QID to produce metabolic acidosis and stimulate respiratory drive (normocapnic patients only)

Protriptyline (Vivactil) suppresses REM sleep. Start at 10 mg HS; titrate dose upward

Tracheostomy

Surgery of uvula, palate, or pharynx

Central Apnea
Low flow nocturnal O_2

Acetazolamide same as for obstructive apnea

Medroxyprogesterone (Provera) 20-40 mg BID-TID as respiratory stimulant. Patients with hypercapnia most responsive.

Notes:

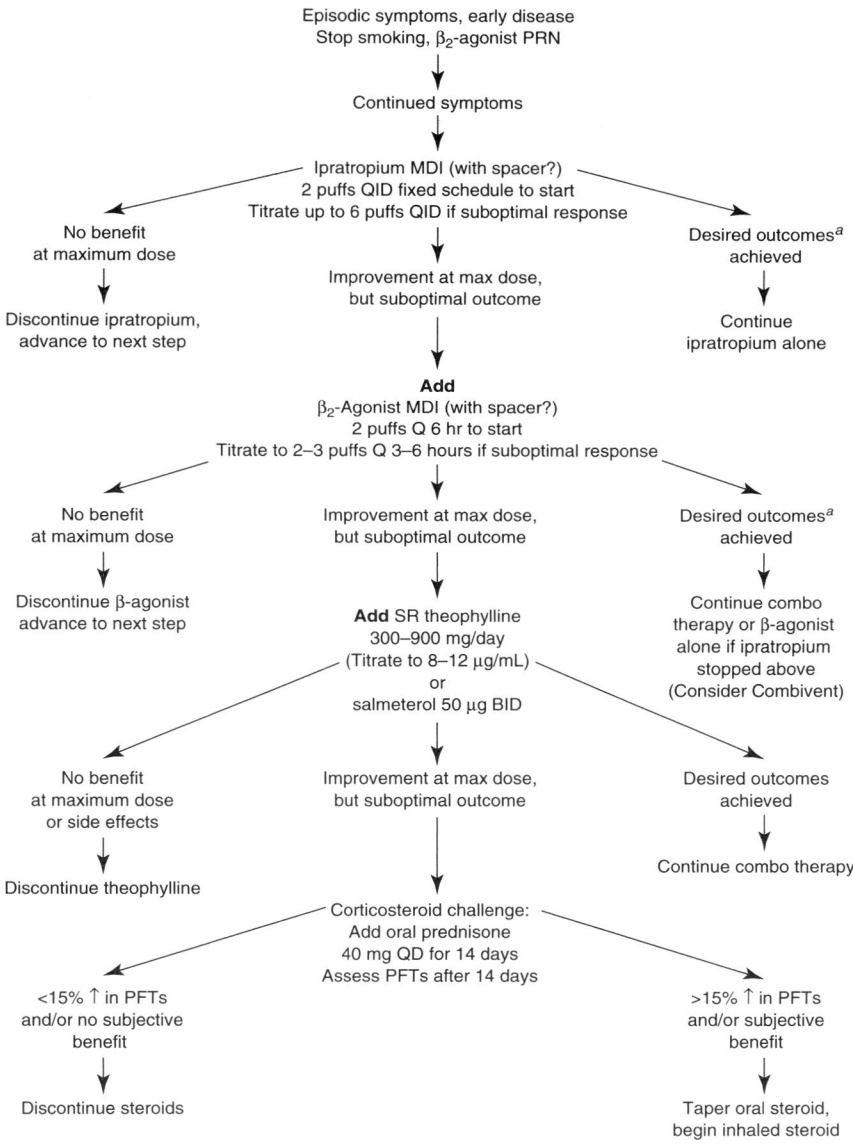

Episodic symptoms, early disease
Stop smoking, β_2-agonist PRN
↓
Continued symptoms
↓
Ipratropium MDI (with spacer?)
2 puffs QID fixed schedule to start
Titrate up to 6 puffs QID if suboptimal response

No benefit
at maximum dose
↓
Discontinue ipratropium,
advance to next step

Improvement at max dose,
but suboptimal outcome
↓

Desired outcomes[a]
achieved
↓
Continue
ipratropium alone

Add
β_2-Agonist MDI (with spacer?)
2 puffs Q 6 hr to start
Titrate to 2–3 puffs Q 3–6 hours if suboptimal response

No benefit
at maximum dose
↓
Discontinue β-agonist
advance to next step

Improvement at max dose,
but suboptimal outcome

Desired outcomes[a]
achieved
↓
Continue combo
therapy or β-agonist
alone if ipratropium
stopped above
(Consider Combivent)

Add SR theophylline
300–900 mg/day
(Titrate to 8–12 µg/mL)
or
salmeterol 50 µg BID

No benefit
at maximum dose
or side effects
↓
Discontinue theophylline

Improvement at max dose,
but suboptimal outcome

Desired outcomes
achieved
↓
Continue combo therapy

Corticosteroid challenge:
Add oral prednisone
40 mg QD for 14 days
Assess PFTs after 14 days

<15% ↑ in PFTs
and/or no subjective
benefit
↓
Discontinue steroids

>15% ↑ in PFTs
and/or subjective
benefit
↓
Taper oral steroid,
begin inhaled steroid

[a] Desired outcomes:
Subjective: Reduction or elimination of dyspnea, sputum production, nocturnal symptoms; increased exercise tolerance.
Objective: >15% improvement in peak flow or FEV_1. Consider single dose versus 2-week response. Also reduction in number of rescue β-agonist doses needed.

Fig. 21.1 COPD Treatment Algorithm.

The reader is referred to Chapter 22: Chronic Obstructive Pulmonary Disease, written by *Wayne Kradjan, Pharm. D.*, and *Dennis Williams, Pharm.D.*, in the seventh edition of **Applied Therapeutics: The Clinical Use of Drugs** for a more in-depth discussion. All notations to reference numbers are based on the reference list at the end of that chapter. The editors of this handbook express their thanks to Drs. Kradjan and Williams and acknowledge that this chapter is based upon their work.

Notes:

Chapter 22

Acute and Chronic Rhinitis

Definitions and Presenting Signs

♦ *Rhinitis* is an inflammation of the nasal mucus membranes characterized by nasal discharge, sneezing, and congestion. Vasodilation increases mucosal congestion and edema. Allergic forms of rhinitis also present with conjunctivitis and itching of the eyes, ears, nose, and palate. See Table 22.1 for classification of allergic and nonallergic rhinitis.

♦ Drugs capable of causing nasal disease are listed in Table 22.2.

Treatment Principles

♦ Nondrug therapies and environmental control provide symptomatic relief for all forms of rhinitis.

• Humidifiers, vaporizers, and drinking hot liquids can be used to hydrate airways.

• *Saline irrigation* can be used to soothe irritated tissues and moisture nasal mucosa.

• *Commercial nasal saline sprays* (e.g., Ayr, NāSal, Ocean, Saline X): 2 sprays 4–6 times daily. *For children <6 yr:* 2–6 drops in each nostril 4–6 times daily. *Self-prepared:* ½–1 tsp. salt to 6–8 oz water. Use as drops or spray or in WaterPik (1 tsp in 800 mL reservoir.)

• *Avoid precipitating factors* (especially in allergic rhinitis but also with vasomotor rhinitis) including allergens, molds, smoke, dust, cold air, and vasodilating drugs.

♦ *Antihistamines* are first line therapy of all forms of allergic rhinitis and NARES. (See Table 22.3 and Figure 22.1.)

• Control nasal discharge, sneezing, itching, and rhinitis with minimal decongestant effect.

• Most effective if taken before exposure and used continuously. (See Table 22.4.)

• First generation (sedating) antihistamines are least expensive. Slow dosage titration, nighttime dosing, and continuous (not intermittent) dosing may improve patient acceptance (See Table 22.4.)

• Switch to fexofenadine, loratadine, or cetirizine if intolerable sedation, interference with concentration, dry mouth, constipation, or urinary retention occur.

• Cetirizine is less sedating than first generation agents, but more sedating than fexofenadine and loratadine.

• Avoid first generation agents if patient has benign prostatic hyperplasia or narrow angle glaucoma.

• Antihistamines safe to use in asthma and in treated open-angle glaucoma.

• Use in viral infections (colds) and nonallergic rhinitis is debated. Primary benefit is drying due to anticholinergic-induced drying (also see ipratropium on page 22.3).

♦ **Intranasal antihistamines** are an alternative in patients with predominance of nasal itching, sneezing, and rhinorrhea.

- *Azelastine* (Astelin) intranasal solution, 125 μg/spray
- 2 sprays each nostril BID for adults or children > age 12
- Side effects: Bad taste (20%), somnolence (10–15%), headache (15–30%), nasal irritation, dry mouth, sore throat, epistaxis.

♦ **Topical ophthalmic antihistamines** are indicated for itchy eyes, burning, and tearing in patients with seasonal or perennial allergic rhinitis. See Table 22.5.

♦ **Decongestants** (alpha agonists) can be combined with antihistamines in patients with allergic rhinitis since antihistamines do not have a decongestant effect. Fixed-dose combinations are acceptable and cost effective. Use decongestants alone in nonallergic rhinitis, including vasomotor and viral. (See Table 22.6 for recommended dosages.)

- Use sprays and drops for short–term only (3–5 days) to avoid rebound.
- Use oral forms for chronic treatment. They are longer acting with no risk of rebound effects.
- *Caution:* May cause CNS stimulation (nervousness, tremor, dizziness, headache), tachycardia, or increased blood pressure.
- Urinary retention may add to that from first-generation antihistamines.
- *Ophthalmic decongestants* to reduce redness (vasoconstrictors) are available as combination products with an antihistamine (see Table 22.6). Use <3 days to avoid rebound conjunctivitis.

Anti-Inflammatory Therapy

♦ **Intranasal cromolyn** (Nasalcrom 4%) can be used for mild-to-moderate allergic rhinitis not adequately relieved by antihistamines and decongestants and when antihistamines or decongestants are contraindicated.

- Starting dose: 1–2 sprays in each nostril 4–6 times daily. Blow nose gently before each dose. Change dose no more often than Q 5–7 days.
- 2–4 week delay for full effect; congestion may be less responsive than other symptoms.
- Taper dose as symptoms improve; either seasonal or continuous therapy.
- Mild nasal burning or stinging in <10% of patients.
- See Table 22.5 for ophthalmic mast cell stabilizers. Indicated as an alternative to topical antihistamines.

♦ **Intranasal corticosteroids** are used for severe symptoms (see Table 22.7).

- Slightly faster onset (2–14 days) and more effective than cromolyn.
- Blow nose gently before each application.
- Taper dose as symptoms improve; either seasonal or continuous therapy.
- Side effects of burning, sneezing, itching, drying; nose bleeds may be less frequent with AQ formulations and fluticasone.
- To minimize burning and nose bleeds, direct stream of medication toward turbinates and away from the nasal septum. Point applicator nozzle straight and back, parallel to the septum.

♦ **Ophthalmic corticosteroids** are indicated if topical antihistamines and mast cell stabilizers are ineffective (see Table 22.5). Older formulations increase intraocular pressure or cause cataracts.

Other Pharmacologic Interventions

♦ **Oral corticosteroid** "bursts" (prednisone 40 QD or 1–2 mg/kg/day times 1 week) indicated for severe symptoms uncontrolled by maximal intranasal therapy. Do not exceed 3–4 courses/year.

♦ **Ipratropium** decreases nasal discharge by counteracting sympathetic over activity. Primarily a drying agent.

Atrovent 0.03% nasal spray. Two sprays BID-TID for symptomatic relief of allergic and nonallergic perennial rhinitis.

Atrovent 0.06% nasal spray. Two sprays TID-QID for symptomatic relief of rhinorrhea, associated with the common cold. Onset within 1 hr.

Side effects include nasal dryness, burning, nose bleeds, sore throat in 4%–8%. Dose- and duration-dependent.

♦ **Immunotherapy (desensitization)** is used for severe steroid-dependent allergic rhinitis. Dose: Give small concentrations (1 : 1,000,000–1 : 10,000,000) of the specific allergen subcutaneously; increase 1 or 2 times a week as tolerated.

Skin Testing

♦ Small quantities of specific allergens are applied by patch testing to confirm the diagnosis of allergic rhinitis. Because antihistamines may interfere with allergen responses, they should be discontinued before testing. Optimal timing is dependent on the half-life and duration of effect of the drug. (See Tables 22.8 and 22.9.)

Viral Upper Respiratory Infection

♦ **Antihistamines** may provide symptom relief via anticholinergic effects (dry secretions) but not from histamine blocking properties.

♦ **Topical (intranasal) and systemic decongestants** both provide symptom relief.

♦ **Ipratropium (Atrovent)** may provide symptom relief, but cost effectiveness is unknown. See section above for dosing information.

♦ **Antitussives** indicated for dry cough that keeps patient awake or disrupts activity. Do not suppress a productive cough.

• *Dextromethorphan* 60–120 mg/day in 3–4 doses (pediatric: 0.25–0.5 mg/kg per dose, not to exceed 30 mg/day if age 2–6 years, 60 mg/day if age 6–12 years). Caution with MAO inhibitors. Read labels carefully to find single-ingredient product (not combined with expectorant, analgesic, antihistamine, or decongestant).

• *Codeine* 10–20 mg q 4–6 hr not to exceed 120 mg/day (pediatric: 1–1.5 mg/kg/day divided into 3–4 doses, maximum 30 mg/day if age 2–6 years, 60 mg/day if age 6–12 years)

♦ **Expectorants** have limited if any value in reducing sputum volume or viscosity.

• *Guaifenesin* 300 mg 3–4 times per day

♦ **Analgesics and Antipyretics** may be unnecessary since myalgia and fever are not typical symptoms of the common cold. May give symptom relief of influenza illness

• *Acetaminophen* not to exceed 3 gm per day (see Chapter 6: Pain).

• *Aspirin* may increase viral shedding and spread in rhinovirus infection. Avoid in children due to association with Reyes syndrome.

• *Naproxen* reduced 5-day incidence of headache, malaise, myalgia, and cough in experimental colds without affecting duration of viral shedding.

♦ **Echinacea** may have immunostimulant properties to prevent and treat the common cold.

• Conflicting evidence of benefit for treatment. No value in long-term prophylaxis

• 300 mg 3–4 times daily at first sign of symptoms using preparation made from herbal leaf portion of the plant.

• Contraindicated in patients with autoimmune diseases or taking immunosuppressives

♦ **Zinc** salts may inhibit viral replication or bind intracellular adhesion molecule (ICAM)-1.

  • Conflicting evidence of benefit using zinc gluconate lozenges, 10 mg 5–6 times per day.

  • *Meta analysis* indicates a correlation between zinc ion absorption into oropharyngeal membranes and efficacy (shortened duration of cold symptoms). Additives and sweetening agents, such as citric acid, tartaric acid, mannitol, and sorbitol, may chelate or inactivate zinc.

  • *Side effects* include bad taste, nausea, mouth or throat discomfort, and diarrhea.

Table 22.1 • Possible Causes of Acute and Chronic Rhinitis

Acute	Chronic
Infectious	Allergic rhinitis[b]
Viral (common cold)	Seasonal ("hay fever")
Bacterial (rhinosinusitis)	Perennial (mold, dust mites, animal dander)
Foreign body	Nonallergic perennial rhinitis[c]
Drug-induced[a]—See Table 22.2	Idiopathic (vasomotor)
Hypothyroidism	NARES[d]
Pregnancy	Tumors
	Choanal atresia
	Nasal septal deviation
	Nasal polyps
	Enlarged adenoids and tonsils
	Chronic sinusitis
	CSF rhinorrhea[d]

[a]Includes "rebound" from overuse of decongestant nasal sprays ("rhinitis medicamentosa")
[b]Frequent coexistence of allergic rhinitis and allergic asthma. Both have acute and late phase reactions on exposure to allergens. Both responsive to anti-inflammatory medications.
[c]Nonallergic nasal mucosa may be hyperresponsive to various stimuli (e.g., cigarette smoke, perfumes, plants) that may mimic allergic responses.
[d]CSF = cerebrospinal fluid; NARES = nonallergic rhinitis with eosinophilia.

Notes:

Table 22.2 • Drugs Capable of Causing Nasal Congestion

Antihypertensives
  Enalapril
  Hydralazine
  Methyldopa
  Nadolol
  Prazosin
  Propranolol
  Reserpine

Psychotherapeutic Drugs
  Amitriptyline
  Perphenazine
  Thioridazine

Hormonal Products
  Estrogen
  Oral contraceptives

Rebound Vasodilation after Vasoconstriction
  Prolonged use of topical decongestants (*rhinitis medicamentosa*)

Direct Tissue Damage
  Cocaine

Miscellaneous
  Alprazolam
  Benzalkonium chloride
  Cromolyn sodium

From references 54 and 139.

Notes:

Table 22.3 • Oral Antihistamines: Classification and Dosage^a

Drugs/Preparations	Adult Dose^b (maximum daily dose)	Pediatric Dose^b (maximum daily dose)	Side Effects^c CNS^d	Anticholinergic	GI
Alkylamine					
Chlorpheniramine maleate (Chlor-Trimeton) 4-mg tab, 2-mg chewable tab, 8- and 12-mg SR tab, 2 mg/5 mL syrup, 8 and 12 mg + 75 mg phenylpropanolamine SR, 8 mg + 120 mg pseudoephedrine SR	2–4 mg Q 4–6 hr or 8–12 mg SR Q 12–24 hr^e	0.35 mg/kg/day^f (6–12 yr: 12 mg; >12 yr: 24 mg)	+	++	—
Brompheniramine maleate (Dimetane) 4-mg tab and liqui-gel, 4- and 6-mg SR tab, 2 mg/5 mL syrup, 16 mg + 240 mg pseudoephedrine 24-hr SR (Efidac 24)	4–8 mg Q 4–6 hr or 8–12 mg SR Q 12–24 hr^e	0.5 mg/kg/day^f (<6 yr: 6–8 mg; 6–12 yr: 12–16 mg; >12 yr: 24 mg)	+	++	—
Dexchlorpheniramine maleate (Polaramine) 2-mg tab, 2 mg/5 mL syrup	2 mg Q 4–6 hr or 4–6 mg SR HS^e	6–11 yr: 1 mg Q 4–6 hr; 2–5 yr: 0.5 mg Q 4–6 hr	+	++	—
Ethanolamine					
Diphenhydramine HCl (Benadryl) 25- and 50-mg tab/cap, 12.5-mg chewable tab, 6.25 and 12.5 mg/5 mL liquid, 12.5 mg/5 mL syrup/elixir/solution	25–50 mg Q 6–8 hr (300 mg)	6–11 yr: 12.5–25 mg Q 4–6 hr 2–5 yr: 6.25 mg Q 4–6 hr (6–11 yr: 150 mg; 2–5 yr: 37.5 mg)	+++	+++	+
Clemastine fumarate (Tavist) 1.34- and 2.68-mg tab, 0.67 mg/5 mL syrup, 1.34 mg + 75 phenylpropanolamine SR	1.34–2.68 mg Q 8–12 hr (8.04 mg)	6–12 yr: 0.67–1.34 mg Q 8–12 hr (4.02 mg)	++	+++	+
Ethylenediamine					
Tripelennamine HCl (PBZ) 25- and 50-mg tab, 100-mg SR tab	25–50 mg Q 4–6 hr or 100 mg SR Q 8–12 hr (600 mg)	5 mg/kg/day^f (300 mg)	++	±	+++
Phenothiazine					
Promethazine HCl (Phenergan) 12.5-, 25-, and 50-mg tab; 6.25 and 25 mg/5 mL syrup	25 mg HS or 12.5 mg Q 8 hr	0.5 mg/kg/dose HS or 0.1 mg/kg/dose Q 6–8 hr	+++	+++	—
Piperidine					
Cyproheptadine HCl (Periactin) 4-mg tab, 2 mg/5 mL syrup	4 mg Q 8 hr (0.5 mg/kg/day)	0.25 mg/kg/day^f (7–14 yr: 16 mg; 2–6 yr: 12 mg)	+	++	—

Azatadine maleate (Optimine) 1-mg tab	1–2 mg Q 12 hr	0.05 mg/kg/day^{f,g}	++	++	—
Phenindamine tartrate (Nolahist) 25-mg tab	25 mg Q 4–6 hr (150 mg)	6–12 yr: 12.5 mg Q 4–6 hr (75 mg)	±	++	—
Piperazine					
Hydroxyzine HCl (Atarax), pamoate (Vistaril) 10-, 25-, 50-, and 100-mg tab; 25-, 50-, and 100-mg (as pamoate) cap; 10 mg/5 mL syrup; 25 mg (as pamoate)/5 mL suspension	25 mg Q 6–8 hr	2 mg/kg/day^f	++	+	—
Cetirizine (Zyrtec)^a 5- and 10-mg tab, 5 mg/5 mL syrup	5–10 mg QD	6–12 yr: 5–10 mg QD 2–5 yr: 2.5–5 mg QD or 2.5 mg Q 12 hr	+	+	+
Second-Generation Piperidines^a					
Fexofenadine (Allegra) 30-, 60-, and 180-mg tab, 60 mg + 120 mg pseudoephedrine (Allegra-D)	60 mg Q 12 hr or 180 mg QD	6–11 yr: 30 mg Q 12 hr	±	±	—
Loratadine (Claritin) 10-mg tab, 1 mg/mL syrup, 10-mg rapidly disintegrating tab (Claritin Reditab), 5 mg + 120 mg pseudoephedrine 12-hr SR (Claritin-D), 10 mg + 240 mg pseudoephedrine 24-hr SR (Claritin-D 24)	10 mg QD	6–12 yr: 10 mg QD	±	±	+
Ebastine (investigational)	10–20 mg QD	<—^{g} >	±	±	—

^{a}All oral antihistamines are approximately equally effective. Because of higher cost, the following strategies should be considered before starting a nonsedating antihistamine: 1) titrate the dose of sedating antihistamines slowly [see Table 22.4], 2) use sedating antihistamines at night, and 3) encourage continuous (not intermittent) therapy. If these measures fail (continuing rhinitis symptoms or side effects), then start fexofenadine or loratadine [see Figure 22.1].

^{b}For patients <40 kg

^{c}Incidence: + + +, high; + +, moderate; +, low; ±, low to none; —, none.

^{d}Impaired psychomotor or cognitive ability may be present even in the absence of a subjective feeling of drowsiness. Tolerance to these effects may not always occur. Confusion or paradoxical agitation, especially in young children and elderly, is a manifestation of anticholinergic activity. Other anticholinergic effects are dry mouth, constipation, and urine retention (especially older males with prostate enlargement). Asthma is not a contraindication to antihistamine treatment; the risk of causing mucous plugging is minimal and they may have a small bronchodilating effect.

^{e}Sustained release (SR) formulations may be given as a single daily dose HS to reduce daytime sedation.

^{f}To be divided into 3–4 doses/day.

^{g}Not FDA-approved for children <12 years old.

CNS = central nervous system; GI = gastrointestinal; HS = bedtime; QD = every day.

Table 22.4 • H₁-Receptor Antagonist Titration Schedule

1. Start with a small dose (e.g., chlorpheniramine 4 mg or diphenhydramine 25 mg) HS only and continue with this dose for at least 3 days or until the patient feels no residual drowsiness in the morning.
2. Add a small dose in the morning. Do not increase the dose further for at least 3 days or until the patient is no longer drowsy on this dose.
3. Continue increasing the dose in this manner, adding to the bedtime dose alternately with the morning dose, until the desired therapeutic end point is achieved.
4. Do not discontinue the medication once symptoms improve. It is important to take the medication continuously to prevent symptoms and to avoid unwanted sedation caused by the medication.
5. A second-generation, H₁-receptor antagonist should be substituted for the traditional H₁-receptor antagonist when the patient cannot or will not adhere to therapy because of side effects (e.g., sedation) or inability to remember doses (inconsistent dosing requires starting the entire titration process over beginning with step 1.)

Table 22.5 • Topical Ophthalmic Drugs for Allergic Conjunctivitis

Drug/Concentration	Dose
Antihistamines	
Emedastine difumarate (Emadine) 0.05%	≥3 y/o: 1 drop QID
Levocabastine (Livostin) 0.05%	≥12 y/o: 1 drop QID for up to 2 wk
Antihistamine/Decongestant Combinations	
Antazoline phosphate 0.5% + Naphazoline HCl 0.05% (Vasocon-A)ᵃ	≥6 y/o: 1–2 drops up to QID
Pheniramine maleate 0.3% + Naphazoline HCl 0.025% (Naphcon-A)ᵃ	≥6 y/o: 1–2 drops up to QID
Mast Cell Stabilizers	
Cromolyn sodium (Crolom) 4%	≥4 y/o: 1–2 drops 4–6 times/day
Lodoxamide tromethamine (Alomide) 0.1%	≥2 y/o: 1–2 drops QID for up to 3 mo
Nedocromil (Alocril) 2%	Adults: 1–2 drops BID
Pemirolast (Alamast) 0.1%	Adults: 1–2 drops QID
Antihistamine/Mast Cell Stabilizers	
Ketotifen fumarate (Zaditor) 0.025%	≥3 y/o: 1 drop Q 8–12 hr
Olopatadine HCl (Patanol) 0.1%	≥3 y/o: 1–2 drops BID, Q 6–8 hr
Nonsteroidal Anti-inflammatory Drugsᵇ	
Ketorolac tromethamine (Acular) 0.5%	Adults: 1 drop QID
Corticosteroids	
Loteprednol etabonate (Alrex) 0.2%	Adults: 1 drop QID

ᵃNonprescription.
ᵇOther ophthalmic NSAIDs (diclofenac, flurbiprofen, suprofen) indicated for intraoperative miosis and/or postcataract surgery but not approved for allergic conjunctivitis.
BID, twice daily; QID, four times daily; y/o years old.

Notes:

Table 22.6 • Decongestants

Drug	Recommended Dosage[a,b]
Phenylamine Pseudoephedrine HCl (Sudafed)	*Adult:* 30–60 mg Q 4–6 hr 120 mg SR Q 12 hr *Pediatric:* 4 mg/kg/day divided Q 6 hr
Phenylpropanolamine HCl (Propagest)	*Adult:* 25 mg Q 4 hr to 50 mg Q 8 hr 75 mg SR Q 12 hr *Pediatric 6–12 yr:* 12.5 mg Q 4 hr *2–6 yr:* 6.25 mg Q 4 hr
Phenylephrine HCl (Neo-Synephrine)	*Adult (≥12 yr):* 2–3 actuations/nostril Q 3–4 hr *or* 2–3 drops 0.25–0.5% solution/nostril Q 3–4 hr *Pediatric 6–12 yr:* 2–3 actuations 0.25% spray/nostril Q 3–4 hr *or* 2–3 drops 0.25% solution/nostril Q 3–4 hr *6 mo–5 yr:* 1–2 drops 0.125% *or* 0.16% solution/ nostril Q 3 hr
Imidazoline Naphazoline HCl (Privine)	*Adult (≥12 yr):* 1–2 drops or sprays/nostril Q 6 hr
Oxymetazoline HCl (Afrin)	*Adult and Pediatric (≥6 yr):* 2–3 actuations/nostril Q 12 hr *or* 2–3 drops 0.05% solution/nostril Q 12 hr *Pediatric (2–5 yr):* 2–3 drops 0.025% solution/nostril Q 12 hr
Tetrahydrozoline HCl (Tyzine)	*Adult and Pediatric (≥6 yr):* 3–4 actuations/nostril Q 4 hr *or* 2–4 drops 0.1% solution/nostril Q 3–4 hr *Pediatric (2–6 yr):* 2–3 drops 0.05% solution/nostril Q 4–6 hr
Xylometazoline HCl (Otrivin)	*Adult (≥12 yr):* 2–3 actuations/nostril Q 8–10 hr *or* 2–3 drops 0.1% solution/nostril Q 8–10 hr *Pediatric (2–12 yr):* 2–3 drops 0.05% solution/nostril Q 8–10 hr

[a]Pediatric doses given for patients ≤40 kg; topical decongestants should not be used in any child <6 mo old.
[b]Therapy with any topical decongestant should not exceed 7–10 days.
[c]Phenylpropanolamine removed from the market following reports of increased incidence of strokes.
SR, sustained release.

Notes:

Table 22.7 • Intranasal Corticosteroid Preparations

Drug	Preparations	Dose/Actuation (µg)	Recommended Dosage[a]
Beclomethasone Dipropionate (Beconase, Vancenase)	Nasal inhaler with halogenated hydrocarbon propellants	42	*Adult:* 1 actuation/nostril BID–QID *Pediatric (6–12 yr):* 1 actuation/nostril TID
(Beconase AQ, Vancenase AQ) (Vancenase AQ 84 µg)	Aqueous nasal spray Aqueous nasal spray	42 84	*Adult and Pediatric (>6 yr):* 1–2 actuations/nostril QD
Budesonide (Rhinocort) (Rhinocort Aqua)	Nasal inhaler with halogenated hydrocarbon propellants Aqueous nasal spray	32 32	*Adult and Pediatric (>6 yr):* 2 actuations/nostril BID *or* 4 actuations/nostril Q AM
Dexamethasone (Decadron Phosphate Turbinaire)	Nasal inhaler with halogenated hydrocarbon propellants	84	*Adult:* 2 actuations/nostril BID–TID *Pediatric (6–12 yr):* 1–2 actuations/nostril BID
Flunisolide (Nasalide) (Nasarel)	Propylene glycol-based nasal spray Aqueous nasal spray	25 25	*Adult:* 2 actuations/nostril BID–TID *Pediatric (6–14 yr):* 1 actuation/nostril TID *or* 2 actuations/nostril BID
Fluticasone propionate (Flonase)	Aqueous nasal spray	50	*Adult:* 2 actuations/nostril QD *or* 1 actuation/nostril BID *Pediatric (4–11 yr):* 1–2 actuations/nostril QD
Mometasone furoate (Nasonex)	Aqueous nasal spray	50	*Adult:* 2 actuations/nostril QD *Pediatric (≥3 yr):* 1 actuation/nostril QD
Triamcinolone acetonide (Nasacort) (Nasacort AQ)	Nasal inhaler with halogenated hydrocarbon propellants Aqueous nasal spray	55 55	*Adult:* 2–4 actuations/nostril QD *Pediatric (6–12 yr):* 1–2 actuations/nostril QD

[a]Dosage should be reduced to the least effective dose once symptoms have been controlled.

Table 22.8 • Effects of H₁-Receptor Antagonists on Allergen Skin Tests

Drug	Extent of Suppression[a]	Half-Life[b]	Duration of Suppression (Days)
Astemizole	+ + +	13 days[c]	5–40
Brompheniramine	+	24.9	1–4
Cetirizine	+ + +	7.4–11 (7)	3–10
Chlorpheniramine	+	24.4 (11)	1–4
Clemastine	+ +	—	1–10
Cyproheptadine	±	16	1–4
Diphenhydramine	±	4–9	1–4
Ebastine	+/++	10–16[c] (10–14[c])	1–7
Fexofenadine	++	14 (18)	3–10
Hydroxyzine	+ +	20 (7.1)	1–10
Loratadine	+/++	11–24 (3.1)	3–10
Mizolastine	++	12–14	3–10
Promethazine	+	12	1–4
Tripelennamine	±	—	1–4

[a]+ + +, extensive; + +, moderate; +, mild; ±, minimal to none.
[b]Half-life in hours unless otherwise listed. Parenthetical numbers indicate half-life in children.
[c]Half-life of the active metabolite. Astemizole removed from the market.

Table 22.9 • Recommendations for Discontinuation of H₁-Antagonists before Allergen Skin Testing

1. Discontinue any short-acting antihistamine (i.e., those in Table 22.8 with a 1–4 day duration of suppression) 48–72 hours before skin testing. Remind the patient that, although allergic symptoms will return during the antihistamine-free period, reliable skin tests cannot be performed in a patient taking antihistamines.
2. Discontinue longer-acting H₁-antagonists at an interval appropriate to their duration of effect (e.g., for astemizole 2–4 weeks before skin testing; for hydroxyzine or clemastine 5–7 days before skin testing).
3. Before applying the full battery of skin tests, apply histamine (positive) control and glycerinated diluent (negative) control tests. A 1 mg/mL histamine base equivalent should yield wheal-and-flare diameters of 2–7 mm and 4.5–32.5 mm, respectively, to be considered a normal histamine reaction. A normal cutaneous reaction to histamine control suggests that accurate skin testing can be performed because hydroxyzine has been shown to equally suppress reactions to histamine and allergen.

Notes:

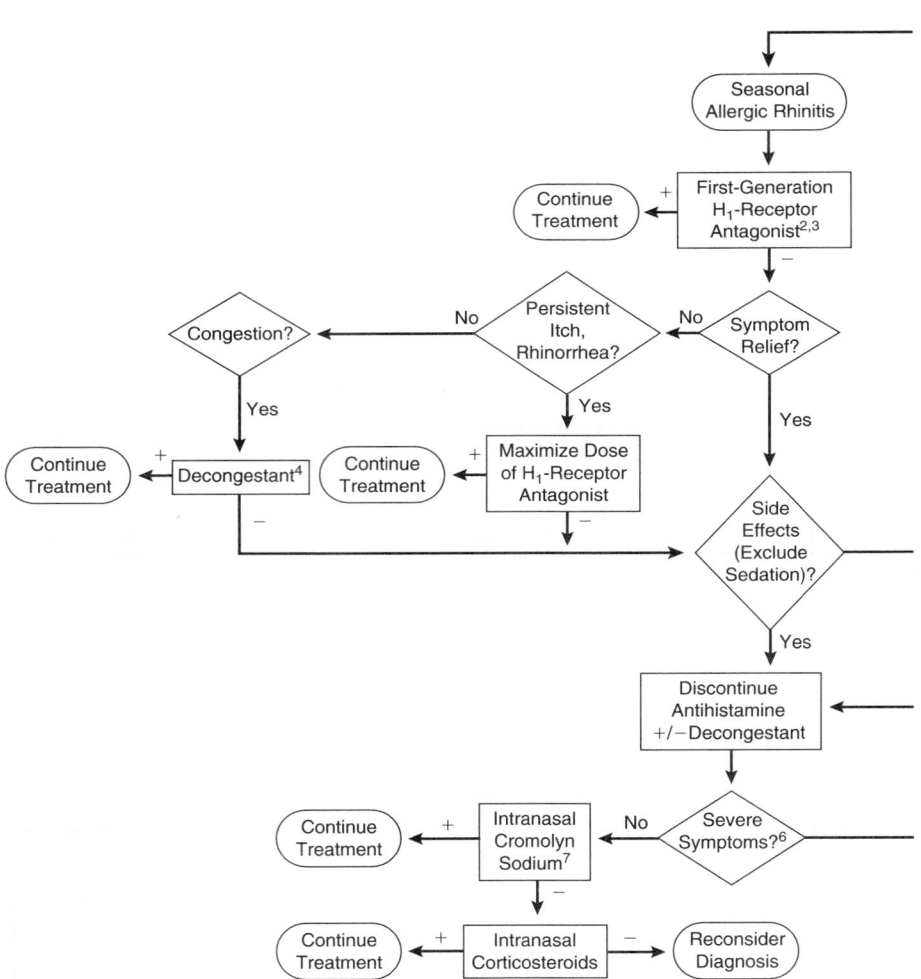

Fig. 22.1 Treatment Algorithm for Allergic Rhinitis: (1) Nonpharmacologic treatment includes avoidance, saline irrigation, and exercise. (2) Use of first-generation H_1-receptor antagonists is first-line therapy for seasonal allergic rhinitis if their use is not contraindicated (e.g., benign prostatic hyperplasia, narrow-angle glaucoma) and the patient agrees to therapy. (3) H_1-receptor antagonists must be started with a slow dosage titration *before* the season of sensitivity and discontinued at the end of the season. (4) Decongestants should be added to H_1-receptor antagonist therapy for patients with nasal congestion because antihistamines do not relieve this symptom. (5) Second-generation, nonsedating H_1-receptor antagonists are indicated if the patient experiences intolerable sedation while taking a first-generation H_1-receptor antagonist despite slow dosage titration and continuous dosing. (6) Severe symptoms are defined as those that interfere with daily activity such as work or sleep. (7) Intranasal cromolyn sodium is

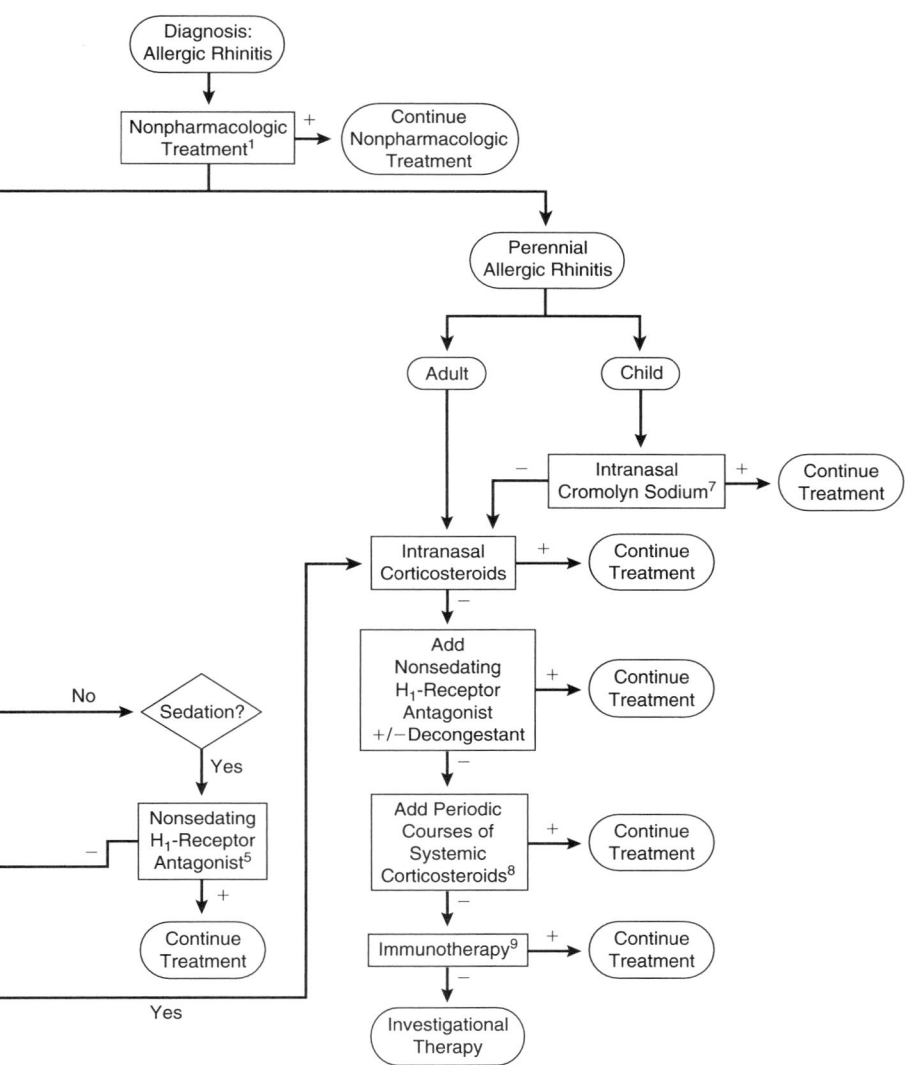

Fig. 22.1, cont'd effective for mild allergic rhinitis symptoms, but it must be administered very frequently, up to four times a day. Because of the low incidence of side effects, it is recommended as first-line treatment for children with perennial rhinitis. (8) Periodic or "burst" doses of oral corticosteroids are indicated for severe symptoms that are otherwise uncontrolled with maximal drug therapy. Corticosteroid bursts should be limited to fewer than four courses per year to limit systemic side effects. (9) Immunotherapy should permit dosage reduction for antiallergy medications and possibly elimination of some (but probably not all) medications. +, positive outcome of therapy defined as relief of symptoms, no interference with daily activities, and no adverse reactions to treatment; –, negative outcome of therapy defined as inadequate symptom relief, continued interference with daily activities, and/or adverse reactions to treatment.

The reader is referred to Chapter 23: Acute and Chronic Rhinitis, written by *Pamela A. Simon, Pharm. D.*, in the seventh edition of **Applied Therapeutics: The Clinical Use of Drugs** for a more in-depth discussion. All notations to reference numbers are based on the reference list at the end of that chapter. The editors of this handbook express their thanks to Dr. Simon and acknowledge that this chapter is based upon her work.

Notes:

Chapter 23

Drug-Induced
Pulmonary Disorders

Exposure to drugs and other chemicals can induce a variety of adverse effects on the lung including exacerbation of asthma, pulmonary edema, pulmonary fibrosis, pulmonary infiltrates with eosinophilia, and pulmonary hypertension. (See Table 23.1 for a partial list of drugs known to cause adverse effects on the lung, categorized by the type of reaction observed.) In particular, alkylating agents frequently are associated with pulmonary fibrosis. Drugs with only rare reports of pulmonary toxicity are not included but may be found in Chapter 24: Drug-Induced Pulmonary Disorders in the seventh edition of **Applied Therapeutics The Clinical Use of Drugs.**

Table 23.1 • Drug-Induced Pulmonary Disorders

Bronchospasm		
Acetaminophen	Rare	See aspirin for mechanism. Weak cyclo-oxygenase inhibitor; safer than aspirin.
ACE inhibitors	Common	Inhibit breakdown of bradykinin, prostaglandins, and/or substance P. Cough predominant symptom. Wheezing, ↓ pulmonary function tests rare
Acetylcysteine aerosolized (Mucomyst)	Uncommon	Nebulized solutions, metered-dose inhalers, and dry powder inhalers may produce cough or bronchospasm due to irritation from inhaled particles, propellants, and dispersants.
Albuterol (Proventil, Ventolin) and other bronchodilators given as MDI or nebulizer.	Rare	See Acetylcysteine
L-Asparaginase	Common	A manifestation of type I hypersensitivity reaction (anaphylaxis)
Aspirin[a]	Common	Inhibition of cyclooxygenase; diverts arachidonic acid metabolism through the lipo-oxygenase pathway leading to excess production of leukotrienes
β-adrenergic receptor blockers[b]	Common	Block sympathetic nervous system and cyclic AMP. Most evident in patients with asthma and COPD.
Beclomethasone (Beclovent, Vanceril) and other corticosteroids given as MDI.		See Acetylcysteine
Cephalosporins	Common	See L-Asparaginase.

(continued)

Table 23.1 • Drug-Induced Pulmonary Disorders (continued)

Bronchospasm (continued)

Cimetidine (Tagamet)	Rare	See L-Asparaginase.
NSAIDs[c]	Common	See aspirin for mechanism.
Penicillins	Common	See L-Asparaginase.
Pentamidine (aerosolized)	Uncommon	See Acetylcysteine
Sulfites[d]	Uncommon	H_2SO_4 produced on lung surface that stimulate afferent parasympathetic irritant receptors in the lung
Sulfonamides	Common	See L-Asparaginase.
Tartrazine[e] (FD & C yellow #5 dye)	Rare	Unknown
Tetracyclines	Uncommon	See L-Asparaginase.

Pseudolymphoma

Cyclosporine (Sandimmune)	Rare (3%–5%)	Inhibition of T-cell function with primary infection or reactivation of Epstein-Barr virus causing lympho-proliferation
Phenytoin (Dilantin)	Rare	Unknown

Pulmonary Edema

Contrast media	Rare	Cardiogenic osmotic effects
Epinephrine	Rare	Accidental overdose during anesthesia
Heroin[f]	Common	Due to outpouring of edema fluid into alveoli. Mechanism of ↑ capillary permeability unknown
Hydrochlorothiazide	Uncommon	Unknown mechanism. Not cardiogenic or immunologic
Interleukin 2 (IL-2; Aldesleukin)	Common	Dose-related ↑ in capillary permeability. 20% with respiratory distress; rare bronchospasm
Intravenous fluids	Common	Cardiovascular fluid overload
Methadone (Dolophine)	Common with overdose	Due to outpouring of edema fluid into alveoli. Mechanism of ↑ capillary permeability unknown
Muromonab CD_3 (OKT3)	Common	Release of mediators by damaged T-cells. Most common with first dose in volume overloaded patients
Propoxyphene (Darvon)	Uncommon (overdose)	Due to outpouring of edema fluid into alveoli. Mechanism of ↑ capillary permeability unknown. Also may be related to postictal pulmonary edema
Salicylates	Uncommon (overdose)	Noncardiogenic, ↑ vascular permeability to fluid and protein
Tocolytics [Ritodrine (Yutopar), terbutaline (Brethine)]	Uncommon	Peripheral vasodilation, cardiovascular fluid overload
Tricyclic antidepressants	Uncommon (overdose)	↑ capillary permeability with noncardiogenic pulmonary edema or adult respiratory distress syndrome

(continued)

Table 23.1 • Drug-Induced Pulmonary Disorders (continued)

Pulmonary Fibrosis (Cough, Dyspnea, Hypoxia)

Amiodarone (Cordarone)[g]	Common; 1–6% after 5–6 months	Amphiphillic compound (contains both hydrophilic and lipophilic portions) produces phospholipid storage disorder with inflammation and fibrosis resulting from breakdown of phospholipid-laden macrophages. Avoid chronic dose >400 mg/day.
BCNU (Carmustine)	Uncommon; usually after cumulative doses of 580–2100 mg/m^2 over 6 months–3 yr	Unknown; appears be dose related
Bleomycin (Blenoxane)[h]	Common; overall incidence estimated at 11%; 10% fatal	Direct cytotoxic injury to the lung epithelium probably due to free radical generation following binding of drug to DNA
Bromocriptine (Parlodel)	Rare	Vasoconstriction-induced ischemia resulting in pleural fibrosis (2%–3%) or pulmonary fibrosis
Busulfan (Myerlan)[i]	Common	Exact mechanism unknown; chemical alveolitis with proliferation of granular pneumocytes and fibrosis of alveolar walls
Chlorambucil (Leukeran)	Rare	Unknown; probably same as Busulfan
Cyclophosphamide (Cytoxan)	Rare	Unknown; probably same as Busulfan
Gold (Myochrysine)	Uncommon; usually after 300–400 mg total dose has been given	Unknown; does not appear to be immunologically mediated
Melphalan (Alkeran, uracil mustard)	Rare	Exact mechanism unknown; chemical alveolitis with proliferation of granular pneumocytes and fibrosis of alveolar walls
6-mercaptopurine (Purinethol)	Rare	Unknown
Methotrexate	Uncommon	Possibly an allergic reaction with fibrosis; noncaseating granuloma formation with lymphocytic infiltrates
Methysergide (Sansert)[j]	Common	Unknown
Mitomycin (Mutamycin)	Uncommon	Unknown. Similar reaction to bleomycin at cumulative doses as low as 400 mg/M^2.
Nitrofurantoin (Macrodantin)[k]	Rare	Both acute and chronic reactions[k]
Oxygen	Frequent; ↑ frequency as FiO_2 exceeds 50%	Formation of superoxide anions (O_2-) that are highly reactive and cytotoxic. These free radicals can oxidize sulfhydryl enzymes, inactivate DNA, and result in lipid peroxidation of cellular membranes
Paraquat (Chevron-Ortho Spot Weed and Grass Killer)[l]	Common; >120 deaths reported annually	O_2 toxicity by superoxide free radical production

(continued)

Table 23.1 • Drug-Induced Pulmonary Disorders *(continued)*

Pulmonary Fibrosis (Cough, Dyspnea, Hypoxia) *(continued)*

Penicillamine (Cuprimine)	Rare; 15 case reports	Unknown
Radiation—Cobalt irradiation in Hodgkin's and breast carcinoma	Common	An acute hypersensitivity reaction or a chronic dose-related toxicity when total dose >6000 rads
Tocainide (Tonocard)	Rare; 4 case reports	Unknown

Pulmonary Infiltrates with Eosinophilia

Carbamazepine (Tegretol)[m]	Rare	Unknown
Cromolyn sodium (Intal)	Rare	Allergic
Dantrolene (Dantrium)	Rare	Allergic reaction
Imipramine (Tofranil)	Rare	Allergy (?)
Minocycline (Minocin)	Uncommon	Allergic reaction
Nitrofurantoin[k]	Uncommon	Unknown
Para-aminosalicylic acid (PAS)	Common	Allergic reaction
Penicillin	Rare	Allergic reaction
Phenytoin (Dilantin)[m]	Rare	Unknown; most likely hyper-sensitivity
Procarbazine (Matulane)	Rare	Possibly allergic reaction
Sulfonamides	Rare	Allergic reaction

Pulmonary Hypertension

Dexfenfluramine (Redux)	Common	Pulmonary vasoconstriction via ↑ serotonin or potassium channel blockade
Magnesium trisilicate (talc)[o]	Common in drug abusers	Foreign body reaction

Respiratory Muscle Impairment (↓ Respiratory Rate or Drive)

Alcohol	Common (overdose)	Direct, dose-dependent respiratory drive inhibition
Aminocaproic acid	Rare	Drug-induced necrosis (necrotizing myopathy)
Aminoglycosides	Uncommon	Neuromuscular blockade like activity (additive to surgical neuromuscular blocking agents)
Amiodarone	Rare	Drug-induced neuropathy
Calcium channel blockers	Rare	Neuromuscular blockade
Captopril (Capoten)	Rare	Drug-induced neuropathy
Clofibrate	Rare	Drug-induced necrosis (necrotizing myopathy)
Corticosteroids	Rare	Myopathy with chronic use
Gold salts	Rare	Drug-induced neuropathy
Isoniazid	Rare	Drug-induced neuropathy (coupled with pyridoxine deficiency)
Neuromuscular blockers	Common	Direct pharmacologic effect
Opiates	Common (overdose)	Direct, dose-dependent respiratory drive inhibition
D-penicillamine	Rare	Neuromuscular blockade

(continued)

Table 23.1 • Drug-Induced Pulmonary Disorders *(continued)*

Respiratory Muscle Impairment (↓ Respiratory Rate or Drive) *(continued)*

Phenytoin	Rare	Drug-induced neuropathy
Sedative-hypnotics	Common (overdose)	Direct, dose-dependent respiratory drive inhibition
Vaccines (viral)	Rare	Drug-induced Guillain-Barré syndrome with respiratory muscle paralysis
Vincristine	Uncommon	Drug-induced neuropathy

[a]Classic description includes triad of severe asthma, nasal polyps, and aspirin intolerance. Bronchospasm typically occurs min to hr following ingestion; rhinorrhea, flushing of head and neck, and conjunctivitis.
[b]Only in patients with pre-existing bronchial hyperreactivity. May occur even with cardioselective agents. Also has occurred following topical administration of timolol ophthalmic solution.
[c]All NSAIDs that inhibit cyclo-oxygenase cross-react in aspirin-sensitive patients.
[d]Occurs in <10% of asthmatics. Sulfites and metabisulfites are common antioxidants used to preserve certain wines, foods, and drugs, including some bronchodilator aerosols.
[e]Appears to occur only in aspirin-intolerant patients with prevalence of 1%–5%.
[f]Mortality rate ≈ 10%. Usually after IV administration but also with nasal administration ("snorting"). Dyspnea, tachypnea, hypotension, cyanosis, tachycardia, and severe hypoxemia are common; marked respiratory distress and coma are common. Symptoms occur within 2 hr following administration; resolution is slow. Treatment consists of naloxone (Narcan), respiratory support, and oxygen therapy.
[g]1%–6% of patients; rarely occurs with doses <400 mg/day. Onset usually after 5–6 months; but as soon as 4 weeks and as late as 9 yr. May be an acute onset with rapid progression into respiratory failure, or symptoms may develop slowly over several months and improve when drug is discontinued or when dose is ↓ to 200–400 mg/day. Routine pulmonary function tests are not helpful for identifying patients of risk.
[h]Total cumulative dose of bleomycin should be restricted to <450 U.
[i]Symptoms begin after 3–4 yr of chronic use; dry hacking cough, tachypnea, cyanosis, dyspnea, and low grade fever. Clinical course is progression with no reversibility; corticosteroids are of little benefit.
[j]Fibrosis is pleuropulmonary rather than the more common interstitial fibrosis produced by other agents; may also produce chronic pleural effusion. Usually occurs after ≥6 months as a component of the retroperitoneal fibrosis.
[k]Chronic use for 6 months-6 yr has resulted in pulmonary fibrosis. This reaction is rare in comparison to acute reaction (i.e., pulmonary infiltrates with eosinophilia) described below. Clinical pattern consists of dry cough, exertional dyspnea, and fever.
[l]Oral ingestion of 15–20 cc can induce pulmonary fibrosis; mortality is 33%–50%. Pulmonary edema may appear several days after ingestion accompanied by progressive dyspnea. Inactivated by burning, toxicity should not occur from smoking marijuana sprayed with paraquat.
[m]Cough, fever, and dyspnea develop 3–6 weeks after initiation of therapy. Rash and lymphadenopathy usually present.
[n]Fever, chills, cyanosis, and dyspnea begin 2 hr–10 days following the initiation of therapy. May mimic pulmonary edema or acute asthma. Eosinophilia in ⅓ of patients. Symptoms regress within 24–48 hr after discontinuation.
[o]Talc is an inert ingredient in many oral dosage forms. When injected intravenously by drug abusers, arteritis and angiothrombosis of the pulmonary vasculature can develop. Cornstarch from dissolved tablets also implicated in granuloma formation and pulmonary hypertension.

The reader is referred to Chapter 24: Drug-Induced Pulmonary Disorders, written by *Phuong-anh (Baxi) Dang, Pharm.D., and Wendy Wilkinson, Pharm.D.,* in the seventh edition of **Applied Therapeutics: The Clinical Use of Drugs** for a more in-depth discussion. The editors of this handbook express their thanks to Drs. Dang and Wilkinson and acknowledge that this chapter is based upon their work.

Notes:

Notes:

Chapter 24

Upper Gastrointestinal Disorders

Dyspepsia

♦ General term describing upper abdominal pain or discomfort originating in the upper GI tract.

♦ May include symptoms of early satiety, postprandial bloating, nausea, and vomiting.

♦ Prevalence 25–55% of U.S. population

- 60% nonulcer dyspepsia
- 20% *peptic ulcer disease*
- 20% *gastroesophageal reflux disease*

Peptic Ulcer Disease (PUD)

♦ Peptic ulcer disease results from an imbalance between aggressive forces (primarily gastric acid and pepsin) and mucosal defensive factors that can be adversely affected by drugs (e.g., NSAIDs) and other variables (e.g., *cigarette smoking* and infection with *helicobacter pylori*). *Chronic PUD* is characterized by remission and recurrences. *Duodenal ulcers* and *gastric ulcers* are the most common types of chronic PUD. *Zollinger-Ellison syndrome* is a rare form of PUD caused by a gastrin-producing tumor.

♦ ***Clinical Presentation and Diagnosis.*** The most common and, in the majority of cases, the only symptom of an ulcer is *epigastric pain*. The pain associated with duodenal and gastric ulcers usually is not localized and usually is described as annoying, burning, gnawing, and aching.

- *Duodenal ulcer pain* commonly occurs when the stomach is empty and is relieved by food and antacids. This pain can be episodic with symptomatic periods lasting for weeks, followed by a period of no occurrence.
- *Gastric ulcer pain* occurs at any time during the day but often occurs immediately or within 1–3 hr after a meal.
- *Other symptoms* associated with both duodenal and gastric ulcers include nausea, vomiting, belching, bloating, anorexia, weight loss, melena (black, tarry stools), and hematemesis (coffee ground emesis).

  Clinical findings are relatively subjective, and an *endoscopy* to visualize directly the ulcer is needed for a definitive diagnosis.

♦ ***Helicobacter pylori (H. pylori) Infection***

- In the absence of NSAID exposure, 80–90% of duodenal ulcers and 60–80% of gastric ulcers are associated with *H. pylori* infection.
- 40–50% of general population tests positive for *H. pylori* infection, but only 15–30% of infected individuals develop PUD.

- *Carbon isotope urea breath tests*

  H. pylori produces ureases in the stomach that cause enzymatic hydrolysis of urea to produce ammonia and CO_2. The CO_2 is absorbed and partially excreted in the breath. Drink liquid containing ^{13}C (Meretek UBT) or ^{14}C-labeled urea, then measure for presence of $^{13}CO_2$ or $^{14}CO_2$ in the breath by mass spec (^{13}C) or scintillation counter (^{14}C).

  Positive only if organism present. Will revert to negative after infection eradicated.

- *Serologic testing: Enzyme-linked immunosorbent assay (ELISA)* detects antibody to *H. pylori* in serum.

  Simpler and less expensive than breath testing for screening but remains positive after infection eradicated.

- Direct biopsy and culture in patients undergoing endoscopy. Endoscopy indicated for new onset ulcer symptoms over age 45 or with alarm symptoms (weight loss, anemia, bleeding, dysphagia).

◆ Treatment Goals for Peptic Ulcer Disease

- Relieve symptoms
- Promote ulcer healing
- Prevent complications
- Eradicate *H. pylori* infection (Cure)
- Prevent recurrences

Treatment Guidelines

Symptom Relief

See Table 24.1 for indications and doses for *histamine$_2$ (H_2) antagonists, proton-pump inhibitors (PPIs),* and *gastromucosal protective agents (e.g., sucralfate)* used for symptomatic treatment and initial healing.

These agents are all ~70–95% effective in initial healing, but recurrence rates are high (up to 80%, especially in smokers). PPI have faster symptom relief and earlier healing than H_2 antagonists but higher cost.

Consider *H. pylori* testing and eradication in all patients to markedly reduce recurrence rate.

- ◆ Encourage all patients to stop smoking.
- ◆ **Duodenal Ulcer.** PRN antacids plus H_2 antagonists for 4–8 weeks **or** sucralfate for 4–8 weeks or PPI for 4 weeks
- ◆ **Gastric Ulcer.** PRN antacids plus H_2 antagonists for 8–12 weeks **or** PPI for 4 weeks.
- ◆ **Unhealed Ulcer.** Strongly consider endoscopy, *H. pylori* testing, and eradication. May continue therapy for 4 or more weeks at original doses.
- ◆ **Refractory Ulcer.** Strongly consider endoscopy, *H. pylori* testing and eradication. May use double doses of H_2 antagonists or PPI.
- ◆ **Zollinger-Ellison Syndrome.** High to very high dose PPI continued indefinitely (see Table 24.1). Titrate to end of drug dosing interval gastric acid secretion of <10 mEq/hr.

H. pylori Eradication

Effective eradication of *H. pylori* requires combination therapy. *The ideal regimen contains two antibiotics combined with either a PPI or bismuth.* See Table 24.2 for listing of representative *H. pylori* eradication regimens, dosing, and precautions.

Healed Ulcer Maintenance and Recurrence (Relapse)

- ◆ Maintenance treatment rarely necessary if *H. pylori* treated. Continued symptoms may be nonulcer dyspepsia or GERD. Use low dose, "on-demand" antacids or H_2 antagonists as indicated.

♦ If recurrence is suspected, retest for presence of *H. pylori*
  • Wait at least 30 days to retest. PPI may give false negative with breath test.
  • Serology may give continued-positive result after successful infection eradication.
  • If still *H. pylori*-positive, try a regimen with less potential for resistance (e.g., without metronidazole)
  • If *H. pylori* negative, repeat 4–8 week course of full-dose H_2 antagonist or PPI.

NSAID-induced Ulcer or Bleeding

♦ Discontinue NSAID and use acetaminophen (if possible). Use antacids or H_2 antagonist as indicated by symptoms. Reassess in two weeks.

♦ Treat *H. pylori* if present and/or give BID H_2 antagonists or PPI for 8 weeks. Possible better response in duodenal ulcer compared to gastric ulcer.

♦ Prevention (co-therapy in patients continuing to take NSAID):
  • Misoprostol 200 mcg QID (recent evidence that TID is effective with less side effects) in high-risk patients (age >70, hx of prior ulcer).
  • Proton pump inhibitors may be equal to or superior to misoprostol if NSAID must be continued.
  • H_2 antagonists more effective than placebo, but less effective than PPI.

♦ Probable lower risk with COX-2 inhibitors: celecoxib (Celebrex) or rofecoxib (Vioxx).

♦ Possibly lower risk with salsalate and nabumetone.

Acid Suppressants

Histamine$_2$ Antagonists (Cimetidine, Famotidine, Nizatidine, Ranitidine)

♦ **Mechanism.** Block gastric acid secretion by blocking the binding of histamine to H_2-receptors.

♦ **Indications and doses.** See Table 24.1

♦ **Adverse Effects and Drug Interactions.** Low incidence. Most common include GI (diarrhea, constipation); CNS alterations (mental confusion, headaches, dizziness, drowsiness); and rashes. Cimetidine has antiandrogen effects (gynecomastia, impotence) and is most likely to interact with other drugs (see Table 24.3). Famotidine has been associated with headaches and ranitidine with hepatotoxicity infrequently.

♦ **Pharmacokinetics.** The bioavailability, elimination, and other pharmacokinetic parameters are listed in Table 24.4.

Proton-Pump Inhibitors (Esomeprazole, Lansoprazole, Omeprazole, Pantoprazole, Rabeprazole)

♦ **Mechanism.** Irreversibly bind to H+-, K+-ATPase, and block acid secretion.

♦ **Indications and doses.** See Table 24.1

♦ **Adverse Effects and Drug Interactions.** Relatively negligible and comparable to H_2-antagonists. Most common include GI (nausea, diarrhea, abdominal pain), CNS alterations (dizziness, headache), and isolated reactions (skin rash, gynecomastia, increase in liver transaminases). See Table 24.5 for PPI drug interactions.

♦ **Pharmacokinetics.** See Table 24.6. All unstable in gastric acid requiring formulation in encapsulated enteric-coated granules or tablets. All are highly protein bound; metabolized in liver and excreted in bile and urine; and have short plasma half-lives, but long duration of action.

Sucralfate

♦ **Mechanism.** Binds to damaged and ulcerated tissue, forming a physical barrier to injury from aggressive forces.

+ **Indications and doses.** See Table 24.1
+ **Adverse Effects.** Relatively rare. Most common include constipation, dry mouth, nausea, and rashes.
+ **Pharmacokinetics.** Not absorbed systemically. Administer 30 min PC and HS and separated by a 2-hr interval from the administration of other drugs because sucralfate can interfere with absorption of drugs.
+ **Drug Interactions:** Reduced bioavailability or absorption of digoxin, phenytoin, ketoconazole, quinidine, quinolone antibiotics, and warfarin. Administer object drug 2 hours before or 6 hours after sucralfate.

Antacids

+ **Mechanism.** Neutralize acid and stimulate mucosal defenses. Administer PRN to relieve ulcer pain.
+ **Adverse Effects and Drug Interactions.** Diarrhea common in magnesium-containing products; constipation from calcium or aluminum. Avoid magnesium-containing antacids in renal failure. Space antacids 2–3 hr apart from ciprofloxacin, tetracycline, iron, and H_2-receptor antagonists.

Misoprostol

+ **Mechanism.** A synthetic prostaglandin E_1 analog with antisecretory and cytoprotective properties that can prevent ulcers in NSAID/aspirin users.
+ **Indications and Doses.** See Table 24.1.
+ **Adverse Effects.** Dose-dependent diarrhea, usually self-limiting with continued therapy. Contraindicated in pregnant patients.

Gastroesophageal Reflux Disorder (GERD)

+ **Pathogenesis.** GERD is a disorder in which the gastric contents are refluxed into the esophagus, causing irritation and injury to the esophageal mucosa. The disease is associated with a disruption of the balance between defense mechanisms and aggressive factors such as acid, pepsin, and bile salts. Three pathophysiological mechanisms predispose a patient to reflux:
  • A spontaneous transient relaxation of the lower esophageal sphincter (LES).
  • A low resting LES pressure.
  • An increase in abdominal pressure (e.g., bending over, hiatal hernia, pregnancy, obesity).
  • Often a chronic disease. May require treatment for years to lifetime.
+ **Clinical Presentation.** *Heartburn* (retrosternal burning that travels up the esophagus toward the pharynx), a bitter or acidy taste in the mouth (reflux), and possibly asthma symptoms.
  • 44% of adults at least monthly, 7% daily.
  • Drugs (e.g., progesterone, prostaglandins, calcium channel blockers, beta-adrenergic agonists, theophylline) and foods (e.g., chocolate, high-fat foods) can aggravate symptoms.
+ Esophagitis: Inflammation and tissue damage to esophagus detected on endoscopy
  • Graded from stage 1 (mild) to stage 4 (severe, *erosive* damage)
  • May or may not be associated with heartburn or other symptoms
  • Complications include strictures, hemorrhage, perforation, or Barrett's esophagus
+ Alarm Symptoms
  • Swallowing difficulty (pain, food sticking)

- Hoarseness, severe cough, asthma
- Weight loss, bleeding
♦ *Treatment Goals*
  - Raise gastric pH >4.0 throughout the day
  - Relieve pain or symptoms
  - Decrease frequency and duration of reflux
  - Promote healing if esophagitis is present
  - Avoid complications (Barrett's esophagus, cancer)
  - Prevent recurrence

TREATMENT

♦ *Classic ("Step-Up") Treatment Approach*
  - Step one (mild or episodic heartburn, no esophagitis)
    —Life-style changes: Eat small meals; avoid eating 3 hours before bedtime; weight loss; discontinue smoking; avoid food and drugs that lower LES pressure or pH (see list above); elevate the head of the bed by 6–8 inches.
    —PRN low dose antacids or H_2 antagonists, including nonprescription strengths (see Table 24.1 for doses). Antacids faster but shorter-acting than H_2 antagonists.
  - Step two (frequent or continued symptoms, stage 1–2 esophagitis)
    —Standard dose, prescription strength H_2 antagonists for 6–12 weeks plus PRN antacids for breakthrough symptoms. May require higher doses and longer duration (6–12 weeks) than for duodenal ulcer (see Table 24.1).
    —Cisapride (Propulsid) 10 mg QID equally effective to H_2 antagonists by increasing LES tone and improving esophageal peristalsis and gastric emptying (i.e., a "prokinetic agent"). Side effects (diarrhea, abdominal pain, nausea, constipation) are uncommon and appear to be free of extrapyramidal effects seen with metoclopramide (Reglan). However, *removed from market* due to risk of promoting torsade de pointe, especially if taken concurrently with CYP 3A4 inhibitors (erythromycin, clarithromycin, azole antifungals, quinidine) or if hypokalemic or hypomagnesemic.
  - Step three (continued symptoms or erosive esophagitis)
    —Double H_2 antagonist doses or use standard doses of a PPI (see Table 24.1 for doses). PPI faster symptom relief, longer duration acid suppression, and more complete acid suppression than high-dose H_2 antagonist. Combination of a H_2 antagonist plus a PPI is irrational. Combining a prokinetic agent with an acid suppressant is logical, but cisapride is no longer available.
  - Step four (refractory patients)
    —Double usual dose of PPI and/or esophageal sphincter surgery.
♦ *Alternative (Aggressive) Treatment Approach*
  - Step one. Start with life-style management and OTC acid suppressants
  - Step two. Failure of above, especially if erosive esophagitis suspected or documented. Start PPI before H_2 antagonist. Some even start with 5–10 days of very high dose PPI (e.g., omeprazole 40 mg BID or equivalent) as therapeutic challenge.
  - Step three. If respond to step two, try to "step down" or taper to lower dose of PPI or substitute an H_2 antagonist for longer-term suppression.
♦ *Maintenance.* Most patients with stage 3 or 4 esophagitis have high recurrence rates and require long-term maintenance H_2 antagonist or PPI. PPI more effective than H_2

antagonist in most severe cases. Standard dose PPI may be less expensive than high-dose H_2 antagonist.

Stress Ulcers

♦ Occur in specific clinical settings in critically ill patients and are distinctly different from chronic peptic ulcer disease in that they are not recurring and are unrelated to a previous history of ulcer disease.

♦ Can occur within hours of a major physiologic disturbance (e.g., severe burns, neurological injury, sepsis, hypotension, major surgery, multiple organ failure, thoracoabdominal or intra-abdominal injury) and progress over 24–48 hr.

♦ ***Prophylactic Therapy.*** Antacids, H_2-receptor antagonists, and sucralfate all can prevent stress ulcers.

  • *Antacids.* Aggressive dosing 30–60 mL every hour is effective but can be accompanied by diarrhea, metabolic disturbances, and cation accumulation in patients with renal dysfunction. The gastric pH should be measured before each dose and the dose doubled if the pH is <3.5 (a rather labor-intensive and inconvenient process).

  • *H_2-receptor antagonists* in doses to maintain gastric pH >4.
    —*Ranitidine.* 150–300 mg as a 24-hr continuous IV infusion. Some advocate a 50-mg ranitidine loading dose, followed by a 6–8 mg/hr continuous IV infusion.
    —*Cimetidine.* 300 mg as loading dose, followed by 37.5–50 mg/hr by continuous IV infusion.
    —*Famotidine.* 1.7 mg/hr as continuous IV infusion after a 20-mg loading dose.

  • *Sucralfate* 1 gm Q 6 hr is effective and, because it does not increase gastric pH, it may be less likely to allow the proliferation of GI bacteria. This may, in turn, reduce the likelihood of developing pulmonary infection.

Notes:

Table 24.1 • FDA Approved Indications and Doses for Antiulcer and GERD Medications[a]

Drug	Dosage Forms/Precautions	Approved Indications	Approved Dose
H$_2$ Antagonists			

Cimetidine (Tagamet, Tagamet HB,[b] generic)	100 mg tab (OTC)
	200, 300, 400, 800 mg tab
	300 mg/5 mL oral solution
	150 mg/mL IV injection soln.
	300 mg premix IV
	
	Reduce dose by 50% if Clcr <30 mL/min (e.g., 200 mg QD or 300 mg BID)
		Duodenal ulcer:
		  Active treatment
		  Maintenance
		Gastric ulcer: Active (benign)
		Hypersecretory (Zollinger-Ellison)
		
		GERD
		
		  Symptomatic[c]
		  Esophagitis (erosive[d])
		GI bleed prevention or treatment (critically ill)
			800 mg HS or 400 mg BID × 4–6 wks
			400 mg HS
			800 mg HS or 300 mg QID × 8 weeks
			300 mg QID to start, titrate to 2400 mg/day max
			
			200 mg up to BID (as 100-mg OTC tabs)
			800 mg BID or 400 mg QID × 12 weeks
			300 mg IV Q 6–8 hr or 50 mg/hr continuous IV up to 2400 mg/day

Famotidine (Pepcid, Pepcid AC[b])	10 mg tab and chewable (OTC)
	20 and 40 mg tab and disintegrating tab
	40 mg/5 mL oral suspension.
	10 mg/mL IV injection soln.
	
	Reduce dose by 50% if Clcr <10 mL/min (20 mg HS)
		Duodenal ulcer:
		  Active treatment
		  Maintenance
		Gastric ulcer: Active (benign)
		Hypersecretory (Zollinger Ellison)
		
		GERD
		
		  Symptomatic[c]
		  Esophagitis (erosive[d])
		  Maintenance
		GI bleed prevention or treatment (critically ill)
			40 mg HS or 20 mg BID × 4–6 weeks
			20 mg HS
			40 mg HS
			20 mg Q 6 hr to start, titrate to 160 mg Q 6 hr
			
			10–20 mg QD-BID (as 10 mg OTC tab)
			20 mg BID × 12 weeks
			20 mg QD
			20 mg IV Q 12 hr

Nizatidine (Axid, Axid AR[b])	75 mg cap (OTC)
	150 and 300 mg cap
	Reduce doses by 50% if Cl$_{cr}$ 20–50 mL/min (150 mg QD); if Cl$_{cr}$ <20 mL/min give 150 mg QOD
		Duodenal ulcer:
		  Active treatment
		  Maintenance
		Gastric ulcer: Active (benign)
		GERD
		
		  Symptomatic[c]
		  Esophagitis (erosive[d])
			300 mg HS or 150 mg BID × 4–6 wks
			150 mg HS
			300 mg HS or 150 mg BID × 8 weeks
			
			75 mg–150 mg QD-BID (as 75 mg OTC cap)
			150 mg BID × 12 weeks

(continued)

Table 24.1 • FDA Approved Indications and Doses for Antiulcer and GERD Medications[a] (continued)

Drug	Dosage Forms/Precautions	Approved Indications	Approved Dose
H₂ Antagonists *(continued)* Ranitidine (Zantac, Zantac 75[b], generic)	75 mg tab (OTC) 150 and 300 mg tab 150 mg gel cap, effervescent tab, or effervescent granules 15 mg/mL syrup 0.5 and 25 mg/mL IV injection solution Reduce dose by 50% if Cl$_{cr}$ <50 mL/min (150 mg Q 24 hr)	Duodenal ulcer: Active treatment Maintenance Gastric ulcer: Active (benign) Maintenance Hypersecretory (Zollinger-Ellison) GERD Symptomatic[c] Esophagitis (erosive[d]) Maintenance GI bleed prevention or treatment (critically ill)	300 mg HS or 150 mg BID × 4–6 wks 150 mg HS 150 mg BID × 8 weeks 150 mg HS 150 mg BID to start, titrate to 6 g/day max 75–150 mg up to BID (as 75 mg OTC tabs) 150 mg QID × 12 weeks 150 mg BID 50 mg IV Q 6–8 hr or 6.25 mg/hr continuous IV
Proton Pump Inhibitors Esomeprazole (Nexium)	20 and 40 mg ER capsules containing enteric-coated pellets Take 1 hour before AM meal. Swallow capsule whole; Do not open, crush, or chew. Contents of capsule may be placed in 1 tbsp. applesauce if difficulty swallowing. Do not chew.	Duodenal ulcer: H. pylori GERD Symptomatic[c] Esophagitis (erosive[d]) Maintenance	40 mg QD × 10 days (See Table 24.3) 20 mg QD × 4 weeks 20–40 mg QD × 4–8 wks. 20 mg QD
Lansoprazole (Prevacid)	15 and 30 mg DR capsules containing enteric pellets Take 1 hour before AM meal. Swallow capsule whole; do not open, crush, or chew. Contents of capsule may be placed in 1 tbsp. applesauce or other foods listed in package insert if difficulty swallowing. Do not chew. NG tube: Place intact granules in 40 mL apple juice. Flush tube to clear all drug.	Duodenal ulcer: Active treatment H. pylori Maintenance Gastric ulcer: Active (benign) Hypersecretory (Zollinger-Ellison) GERD Symptomatic Esophagitis (erosive[c]) Maintenance	15 mg QD × 4 wks 30 mg BID × 10–14 days (see Table 24.3) 15 mg QD 30 mg QD × 8 weeks 60 mg QD to start, titrate to 90 mg BID 15 mg QD 30 mg QD × 8 weeks; may give for additional 8 weeks. 15 mg QD

Drug	Dosage form/Instructions	Indication	Dosage
Omeprazole (Prilosec, generic)	10, 20, 40 mg DR capsules containing enteric pellets. Take 1 hour before AM meal. Swallow capsule whole; do not open, crush, or chew.	Duodenal ulcer:	
		Active treatment	20 mg QD × 4–8 wks
		H. pylori	20 mg BID × 10–14 days (See Table 24.3)
		Maintenance	10–20 mg QD
		Gastric ulcer:	
		Active (benign)	40 mg QD × 4–8 weeks
		Hypersecretory (Zollinger Ellison)	60 mg QD to start, titrate to 120 mg TID max
		GERD	
		Symptomatic[c]	20 mg QD × 4 weeks
		Esophagitis (erosive[d])	20–40 mg QD × 4–8 weeks
		Maintenance	20 mg QD
Pantoprazole (Protonix)	40 mg DR tablet. Can be taken with or without food. Do not crush, chew, or split tablets. 40 mg/vial IV injection solution	GERD	
		Esophagitis (erosive[d])	40 mg QD × 8 weeks, may give for additional 8 weeks
		GI bleed prevention or treatment (critically ill)	40 mg IV QD in 100 mL over 15 min
Rabeprazole (Aciphex)	20 mg DR enteric-coated tablet. Take 1 hour before AM meal. Do not crush, chew, or split tablets. Caution in patients with severe hepatic impairment	Duodenal ulcer:	
		Active treatment	20 mg QD × 4 wks
		Hypersecretory (Zollinger-Ellison)	Start at 60 mg QD, max dose not established
		GERD	
		Esophagitis (erosive[c])	20 mg QD × 4–8 weeks; may give for additional 8 weeks
		Maintenance	20 mg QD
Gastromucosal Protectant			
Sucralfate (Carafate)	1 g capsule. 1 g/10 mL oral suspension. Take 1 hour before meals (or antacids) and at bedtime.	Duodenal ulcer:	
		Active	1 g QID × 4–8 weeks
		Maintenance	1 gm BID

[a]BID = twice daily; Cap = capsule; Cl$_{cr}$ = creatinine clearance; DR = delayed release; ER = extended release; FDA = Food and Drug Administration; GERD = gastroesophageal reflux disease; HB = heartburn; hr = hour; HS = bedtime; IV = intravenous; OTC = over-the-counter (nonprescription); QD = once daily; QID = four times daily; QOD = every other day; Soln = solution; Tab = tablet; Tbsp = tablespoonful; TID = three times daily; wks = weeks.

[b]Nonprescription brand name.

[c]Symptomatic includes heartburn, acid indigestion, sour stomach, general dyspepsia without documented esophagitis.

[d]Esophagitis documented by endoscopy. Erosive esophagitis = stage 3–4.

Table 24.2 • Representative *H. pylori* Infection Eradication Regimens[a,b]

Amoxicillin + Clarithromycin + PPI (10–14 days)[c]
Amoxicillin 1 g BID with food
Clarithromycin 500 mg BID with food
PPI QD or BID on empty stomach (See footnote *d* for individual doses)[d]

Clarithromycin + Metronidazole + PPI (14 days)[e,f]
Clarithromycin 500 mg BID with food
Metronidazole 500 mg BID with food[e,f]
PPI BID on empty stomach[d]

Metronidazole + Tetracycline + Bismuth (14 days)[g]
Metronidazole 250 mg QID with food
Tetracycline 500 mg QID with food[h]
Bismuth subsalicylate 525 mg QID with meals and HS[i] (also add H_2 antagonist for 28 days)

Metronidazole + Tetracycline + Bismuth + PPI (14 days)
Metronidazole 250 mg QID or 500 TID with food
Tetracycline 500 mg QID with food[h]
Bismuth subsalicylate 525 mg QID with meals and HS[i]
Omeprazole 20 mg BID or lansoprazole 30 mg BID

Ranitidine-Bismuth Citrate + Clarithromycin (28 days)
Ranitidine-bismuth citrate[j] 400 mg BID for 28 days
Clarithromycin 500 mg TID with food for 14 days

[a]BID = twice daily; H_2 = Histamine 2; HS = At bedtime; PPI = Proton pump inhibitor; QD = Once daily; TID = Three times daily; QID = Four times daily.
[b]Only regimens containing two antibiotics plus either a PPI or bismuth are listed. Most with >90% eradication rates, if patient is compliant. Regimens of one antibiotic plus a PPI or two antibiotics without a PPI should not be used (eradication rates 75–90%).
[c]10-day regimens appear to be equally effective to 14-day regimens with better compliance, but further studies are required. 7-day regimens are less effective.
[d]Approved PPI doses in combination with amoxicillin and clarithromycin: esomeprazole 40 mg QD, lansoprazole 30 mg BID, omeprazole 20 mg BID. Omeprazole 40 mg QD, pantoprazole 80 mg QD, and rabeprazole 40 mg QD may also be effective. May continue up to 28 days if ulcer symptoms present at start of treatment.
[e]Alternative regimen for penicillin and amoxicillin allergic patients.
[f]The incidence of *H. pylori* resistance is higher for metronidazole than for clarithromycin, amoxicillin, or tetracycline. Resistance may be higher in women previously treated for vaginitis or urethritis with metronidazole. Concurrent use of metronidazole may cause flushing, nausea, vomiting (disulfiram like reaction.)
[g]Bismuth, metronidazole, tetracycline regimen known as "BMT." Compliance may be limited by QID dosing and large number of tablets taken daily. Helidac is a prepackaged blister pack to ease compliance but higher cost than using generic of each component.
[h]Food-drug interaction with tetracycline not a contraindication for this treatment. Conflicting data as to effectiveness of doxycycline as alternative to tetracycline.
[i]Bismuth subsalicylate as "Pepto Bismol" 264 mg chewable tablets or generic. Caution: may cause dark stools and possible salicylate sensitivity.
[j]Ranitidine-bismuth citrate available as Tritec, a complex of ranitidine 150 mg + bismuth citrate 240 mg. Not recommended since only one antibiotic, expensive and complex regimen. May be more effective by adding a PPI but very costly.

Notes:

Table 24.3 • Cimetidine Drug Interactions[a-c]

Major Significance: Well-Documented and Have the Potential to Be Harmful to the Patient[d]

Warfarin: R-warfarin metabolized by CYP 1A2, 2C19, and 3A4. S-warfarin metabolized by CYP 2C9. Cimetidine gradually ↑ the hypoprothrombinemia over 1–2 weeks; about 1 week is needed for the prothrombin time to return to precimetidine levels when cimetidine is discontinued. Drug interaction dose related.

Theophylline: A substrate for CYP 1A2 and 3A4. Cimetidine reduces theophylline elimination as soon as therapeutic serum levels of cimetidine achieved; a new steady-state serum theophylline level usually attained by the 2nd day. This dose-related interaction has resulted in theophylline toxicity and associated with fatalities.

Moderate Significance: More Documentation Needed and/or of Less Potential Harm to the Patient[d]

Alcohol: Cimetidine may produce small ↑ in blood alcohol levels and a slight ↑ in the degree of intoxication. May inhibit hepatic metabolism of alcohol (a CYP 2E1 substrate) and ↑ alcohol absorption by inhibiting gastric alcohol dehydrogenase (ADH).

Antidepressants (Tricyclic): Many metabolized by CYP 2C19 and 2D6. Imipramine also a substrate for CYP 1A2. Cimetidine inhibits the elimination of doxepin, imipramine, desipramine, and nortriptyline. Little clinical data available on amitriptyline, amoxapine, protriptyline, trimipramine, maprotiline, or trazodone, but theoretically, elimination of these should be ↓ as well.

Benzodiazepines: Diazepam metabolized by CYP 2C19 and 3A4. Others primarily by 3A4. Cimetidine appears to inhibit the hepatic metabolism of diazepam, chlordiazepoxide, desmethyldiazepam, and probably alprazolam and triazolam. Benzodiazepines that undergo glucuronidation (e.g., lorazepam, oxazepam, temazepam, triazolam) not affected. Ranitidine, famotidine, and nizatidine do not appear to interact clinically.

Beta Blockers: Propranolol metabolized by CYP 2D6. Cimetidine may ↑ plasma concentrations of beta blockers that undergo significant hepatic metabolism (e.g., alprenolol, oxprenolol, propranolol)

Calcium Channel Blockers: The metabolism of verapamil, nifedipine, and diltiazem is reduced by cimetidine. Mechanism is unclear since they are CYP 3A4 substrates, which is unaffected by cimetidine. ↑ in gastrointestinal pH can ↑ absorption and serum concentrations of nifedipine by 60–90%.

Carbamazepine: Cimetidine may transiently ↑ plasma carbamazepine concentrations, but effect appears to dissipate after about 1 week of cimetidine therapy. Mechanism is unclear since carbamazepine is a 3A4 substrate, which is unaffected by cimetidine.

Carmustine: Cimetidine ↑ the myelotoxicity of carmustine perhaps by inhibition of metabolism or additive effect on bone marrow.

Ketoconazole: Cimetidine ↓ GI absorption of ketoconazole by ↑ pH of GI tract.

Lidocaine: A CYP 1A2 substrate. Cimetidine modestly ↑ lidocaine serum concentrations, but not known how often this would cause lidocaine toxicity.

Meperidine: Cimetidine may ↑ the respiratory depression and sedation of narcotic analgesics. Morphine may be less likely to interact with cimetidine than other narcotics.

Phenytoin: A CYP 1A2, 2C9 substrate. Cimetidine ↑ serum phenytoin concentrations by inhibiting the hepatic metabolism of phenytoin. Phenytoin intoxication has occurred in some patients.

Procainamide: Cimetidine ↓ the renal tubular secretion of procainamide and its major metabolite (n-acetylprocainamide). Although cimetidine may significantly ↑ serum procainamide concentrations, incidence of procainamide toxicity from this interaction unknown.

Quinidine: Cimetidine inhibits the hepatic metabolism, may ↓ the renal clearance, and ↑ the plasma concentrations of quinidine. Mechanism is unclear since quinidine is a 3A4 substrate, which is unaffected by cimetidine.

[a]CYP = cytochrome P450.
[b]Cimetidine is a potent inhibitor of cytochrome P450 (CYP) isoenzymes 1A2, 2C9, and 2C6. This is a concentration-related, reversible effect. Ranitidine (Zantac) can inhibit cytochrome P450 in larger-than-normal doses; binds 4–10 times less avidly. Famotidine and nizatidine do not bind appreciably.
[c]Both cimetidine and ranitidine can inhibit renal excretion of drugs. Cimetidine ↑ serum creatinine by this mechanism. This does not represent nephrotoxicity.
[d]Although the pharmacokinetic characteristics of many of these drugs are significantly altered by cimetidine (primarily clearance), many of the interactions have been incompletely studied (e.g., single-dose studies in normal subjects). Therefore, even though a pharmacodynamic change may be undocumented, the clinician must watch for enhanced pharmacological and toxic effects of the affected drug.

Table 24.4 • Pharmacokinetic Comparison of H$_2$-Receptor Antagonists[a,b]

Variable	Cimetidine	Ranitidine	Nizatidine	Famotidine
Relative Potency	1	4–10	4–10	20–50
Absorption				
Bioavailability (%)[c]	30–80 (60)	30–88 (50)	75–100 (98)	37–45 (43)
Time to peak serum concentration (hr)	1–2	1–3	1–3	1–3.5
Volume of distribution (L/kg of body weight)	0.8–1.2	1.2–1.9	1.2–1.6	1.1–1.4
Elimination				
Total systemic clearance (mL/min)	450–650	568–709	667–850	417–483
Half-life in serum (hr)	1.5–2.3	1.6–2.4	1.1–1.6	2.5–4
Hepatic clearance (%)				
Oral	60	73	22	50–80
IV	25–40	30	25	25–30
Renal clearance (%)				
Oral	40	27	57–65	25–30
IV	50–80	50	75	65–80

[a]IV = Intravenous.
[b]Adapted with permission from Feldman M, Burton, ME. Histamine-receptor antagonists standard therapy for acid-peptic disease. N Engl J Med 1990; 323(24):1672.
[b]Average values are in parenthesis.

Notes:

Table 24.5 • Proton Pump Inhibitor Drug Interactions[a]

Object Drug[b]	Esomeprazole	Lansoprazole	Omeprazole	Pantoprazole	Rabeprazole
Caffeine (1A2)	Unknown	Unknown	Induce	No interaction	Unknown
Carbamazepine (3A4, 2C9?)	Unknown	Unknown	Inhibit, AUC ↑ 75%	No interaction	Unknown
Cyclosporine (3A4)	Unknown	No interaction	Unknown	No interaction	Unknown
Diazepam (2C19, 3A4)	Inhibit, ↓ clearance	No interaction	Inhibit, $t_{1/2}$ ↑ 130%	No interaction	No interaction
Digoxin	Reduced absorption	Unknown	AUC ↑ 10%	No interaction	AUC, Cmax, $t_{1/2}$ ↑
Lidocaine (3A4)	Unknown	Unknown	None	Unknown	Unknown
Ketoconazole	Reduced absorption	Reduced absorption	Reduced absorption	Reduced absorption	Reduced absorption
Metoprolol (2D6)	Unknown	Unknown	None	No interaction	Unknown
Phenytoin (1A2, 2C9, 2C19)	No interaction	No interaction	Inhibit, $t_{1/2}$ ↑ 27%	No interaction	No interaction
Prednisone (3A4)	Unknown	No interaction	No interaction	Unknown	Unknown
Propranolol (2D6)	Unknown	No interaction	No interaction	Unknown	Unknown
Theophylline (1A2, 2E1, 3A4)	Unknown	Inhibit, AUC ↑ 10%	No interaction	No interaction	No interaction
R-Warfarin (1A2, 2C19, 3A4)	No interaction	No interaction	Inhibit, ↓ clearance, 10% ↑ PT	No interaction	No interaction
S-Warfarin (2C9)	No interaction	No interaction	No interaction	No interaction	No interaction

[a]AUC = Area under the curve; C$_{max}$ = Maximum concentration; PT = Prothrombin time; $t_{1/2}$ = Half-life.
[b]Object Drug = potential interacting drug. Usual metabolizing P450 isoenzyme of object drug in parentheses.

Table 24.6 • Pharmacokinetic Comparison of Proton Pump Inhibitors

Drug	Bioavailability	$t_{1/2}$	Excretion	Metabolized by
Esomeprazole	64% (single dose, fasting)[a] 90% (repeated doses)	1.5 hr	Hepatic	2C19[c] (primary) 3A4 (secondary)
Lansoprazole	85%	0.5–2.5 hr	Hepatic, biliary	3A4 (primary) 2C19[c] (secondary)
Omeprazole	35–45% (single dose)[b] 60% (repeated doses)	0.5–1 hr	Hepatic	2C19[c] (primary) 3A4 (secondary)
Pantoprazole	77%[b]	0.9–1.9 hr	Hepatic	2C19[c] (primary) 3A4 (secondary)
Rabeprazole	52%[b]	0.9–1.7 hr	Hepatic	2C19[c] (primary) 3A4 (secondary) Sulfotransferase

[a] Esomeprazole absorption decreased 33–55% if taken with food.
[b] Food does not affect extent of absorption of omeprazole, pantoprazole, or rabeprazole, but rate of absorption slowed.
[c] 2C19 subject to genetic polymorphism. 5% of Caucasians and higher % of Asians are slower metabolizers.

The reader is referred to Chapter 25: Upper Gastrointestinal Disorders, written by *Candace Smith-Scott, Pharm.D.*, in the seventh edition of **Applied Therapeutics: The Clinical Use of Drugs** for a more in-depth discussion. All notations to reference numbers are based on the reference list at the end of that chapter. The editors of this handbook express their thanks to Dr. Smith-Scott and acknowledge that this chapter is based upon her work.

Notes:

Chapter 25

Inflammatory Bowel Disease

Inflammatory bowel disease is a generic classification for a group of nonspecific idiopathic inflammatory disorders of the gastrointestinal (GI) tract. Ulcerative colitis and Crohn's disease (granulomatous enteritis) are two major inflammatory bowel diseases that have similar clinical features but differ significantly in pathophysiology, anatomic distribution, and clinical course (see Table 25.1).

♦ **Ulcerative colitis** (UC) is an inflammation of the mucosal layer of the colon and rectum. The classic triad of symptoms is chronic diarrhea (watery and bloody), rectal bleeding, and abdominal pain. The volume of stool per day is reflective of the disease's severity.

Most patients with UC experience a chronic intermittent course with periods of normal function between exacerbations.

Complications include electrolyte depletion, dehydration, anemia, hypoalbuminemia, and the extraintestinal complications listed in Table 25.2.

♦ **Crohn's disease** (CD) is a patchy granulomatous inflammatory process that can involve any portion of the digestive tract. Inflammation is transmural with deep ulcerations, adhesions, and fistulas. See Table 25.1.

Symptoms. The classical triad of symptoms includes abdominal pain, diarrhea [partly formed, moderate (4–6 stools/day), and not grossly bloody], and weight loss (malabsorption).

The course of CD has no predictable pattern, ranging from a single episode to years of frequent relapses followed by complete remission to unremitting disease requiring surgery.

♦ Smokers are at a decreased risk of developing UC, but are at an increased risk for CD.

Goals of Therapy

♦ Relief of symptoms (induction of remission)
♦ Improve quality of life
♦ Maintain adequate nutritional status
♦ Reduce recurrent flairs (remission maintenance)
♦ Prevent complications (dehydration, perforation, anemia)

Pharmacotherapy Options

Aminosalicylates

♦ Most effective in patients with UC or colonic involvement from CD. Patients with ileal CD involvement may derive benefit from products that release active drug earlier (e.g., Asacol and Pentasa).

♦ **Sulfasalazine (Azulfidine).** Made up of sulfapyridine linked to 5-aminosalicylic acid (5-ASA) via an azo bond. The active moiety is 5-ASA (known generically as mesalamine), which has topical anti-inflammatory effects on the inflamed bowel. Sulfapyridine acts as a carrier to move 5-ASA past its primary absorption point in the upper intestine. The azo bond is cleaved by lower intestinal bacteria to release the active 5-ASA. Eighty percent of ASA remains in bowel; 90% of sulfapyridine absorbed systemically.

- *Side effects:* Systemic absorption of sulfapyridine is the major source of sulfasalazine side effects, especially at doses >4 g per day or in slow acetylators (serum concentrations >50 mg/mL.) Gastric distress, nausea, vomiting, diarrhea, headache, fever, arthralgias are common. Skin rashes in sulfa-allergic patients. Rare: leukopenia, agranulocytosis, hemolytic anemia, hepatotoxicity.

- ♦ *5-ASA (Mesalamine) Derivatives.* ASA is 90% absorbed in the upper intestine. Newer products delay release of 5-ASA in the upper intestine and deliver the active drug to the lower intestine without binding to sulfapyridine. All equal in efficacy to sulfasalazine but fewer side effects (abdominal cramps, belching, nausea, diarrhea, headache) and safe in patients allergic to sulfonamides. Rare: pancreatitis, hepatitis, renal dysfunction.

  - Delayed release tablets *(Asacol).* pH-sensitive, resin-coated tablet that releases mesalamine in distal ileum and colon (pH 7). Twenty-eight percent absorbed; 80% delivered to colon.

  - Controlled release capsules *(Pentasa).* Ethylcellulose-coated, acid-resistant microgranules of mesalamine that release 5-ASA in the duodenum, jejunum, ileum, and colon. Because Pentasa releases 5-ASA slightly earlier than Asacol, patients with upper intestinal CD may respond better to Pentasa, but adverse effects may be more frequent due to greater absorption.

  - Rowasa. Available as enema and suppositories that release 5-ASA into rectum and distal colon. Effectiveness limited to proctosigmoiditis.

- ♦ Balsalazide (Colazal). Prodrug delivered intact to colon, then cleaved to release 5-ASA.

- ♦ Osalazine (Dipentum). A delayed-release preparation created by linking two 5-ASA molecules by a unique azo bond. Cleave of the bond and release of 5-ASA occurs in the distal ileum and colon (2% absorbed, 98% reaches colon). Efficacy similar to Asacol and Pentasa but causes more diarrhea (5–30%), cramps, and nausea. Rare: pancreatitis and myocarditis.

Infliximab (Remicade)

A recombinant chimeric monoclonal antibody that binds to human tumor necrosis factor (TNFα) and neutralizes its activity by preventing its binding to cell membranes and in the blood. Based on the assumption that there is an overstimulation of the immune system by TNFα in inflammatory diseases. Also effective for rheumatoid arthritis, similar to etanercept (Enbrel).

- ♦ Approved for moderate-to-severe Crohn's disease, especially with fistula involvement. Eighty-two percent response rate at 4 weeks after single 5 mg/kg IV infusion over 2 hours. Sixty percent with decreased fistulae drainage. May repeat infusions at 2 and 6 weeks.

- ♦ Side effects: Infusion-related fever, chills, myalgia (16% over 2 hours). Headache (23%), nausea (17%), abdominal pain (12%), fatigue and fever (10%). Hypersensitivity reactions: hives, dyspnea, hypotension. Possible increased risk of infection and lymphoma, formation of autoimmune antibodies (ANA), and lupus-like syndrome

Ulcerative Colitis Treatment
Remission Induction (Exacerbations)
- ♦ *Severe Acute Exacerbations.* (i.e., >6 bloody stools/day), heart rate >90/minute, fever >99.5°F, anemia, increased erythrocyte sedimentation rate, and abdominal pain.
  - Monitor and replace fluids, electrolytes, vitamins, and minerals.

- Initiate total parenteral nutrition if needed.
- *Systemic Corticosteroids:* IV hydrocortisone 100 mg Q 6–8 hr or IV methylprednisolone 16 mg Q 6–8 hr (40–60 mg/day) or IV prednisolone 30 mg Q 12 hr. May increase dose if inadequate response. Once improvement has occurred, switch to PO prednisone 60–80 mg/day, then taper by 5–10 mg/week until the dose is 15–20 mg/day, then taper by 2.5–5 mg/week until discontinued.
- *Corticosteroid enemas.* Consider as an addition to parenteral steroids if distal colon or rectal involvement. See Table 25.3.
- *Sulfasalazine or 5-ASA derivatives.* May start during acute exacerbation or as soon as a response has been achieved. See Remission Maintenance section below for doses.
- Azathioprine (2–2.5 mg/kg/day PO), 6-mercaptopurine (1–1.5 mg/kg/day PO), or cyclosporine (4 mg/kg/day IV or PO) to be considered when corticosteroids fail to induce remission.
- Surgery may be indicated if no response in 72 hours.

♦ *Mild-to-Moderate Acute Exacerbations*
- Treat generally the same as for severe exacerbations, except one may use oral prednisone 40–80 mg/day divided in 3–4 doses instead of IV corticosteroids. Taper as described above. Begin sulfasalazine or other 5-ASA derivatives soon after starting corticosteroids.

♦ *Mild acute exacerbations,* limited to distal colon and rectum, can be treated topically.
- *Mesalamine* enema (4 gm/60 mL) HS or rectal suppositories (Rowasa 50 mg) for several weeks during and after the acute episode are as effective as rectal corticosteroids with fewer side effects. (Administration of enema: Instill total volume as a bolus with the patient in the supine position. Alternate position Q 20 minutes for 4 positions: supine to left decubitus to right decubitus to prone. Retain the contents for as long as possible. If the patient cannot retain the initial volume, it may be slowly dripped in over 20–30 minutes.) Up to 15% of the 5-ASA is absorbed systematically when given rectally.
- *Rectal corticosteroid* (see Table 25.3). Suppositories may be used for proctitis; enemas and foams for distal colitis or proctosigmoiditis. Up to 90% is absorbed. *Side effects* include adrenal suppression, growth retardation, osteoporosis, metabolic complications, increased risk of bowel weakening and perforation, cutaneous atrophy, and poor wound healing. Symptoms of abdominal or pelvic abscess may be masked.
- Antidiarrheals (e.g., loperamide) or analgesics may be given cautiously. Avoid opiates in severe attacks to decrease risk of toxic megacolon.

Toxic megacolon: All colonic activity ceases, leading to fluid retention and swelling of colon to several times its normal diameter with severe pain, fever, and risk of perforation.

Remission Maintenance

(Patients responding to acute treatment, with minimal or no continuing symptoms)
- ♦ Low-residue diet (avoid seeds, nuts, corn, raw fruits, and vegetables). Avoid milk if lactase insufficiency (Lactaid or Lactrase may be added to milk to increase tolerance).
- ♦ PRN antidiarrheals for short courses only during flairs.
- ♦ 5-ASA (Mesalamine derivatives). All of the following equally effective.
   - Sulfasalazine (Azulfidine or generic 500 mg tablets). Start at 500 mg QID. Adjust dose to 2–4 g per day during acute exacerbations, then taper to 1–2 g per day maintenance. Combinations with corticosteroids desired during acute exacerbation, but try to discontinue prednisone by 1–2 months.

- Asacol (400 mg tablets). Usual dose = 800 mg TID (2.4 g/day) × 6 weeks. Up to 4.8 g/day in acute exacerbations.
- Pentasa (250-mg capsules). Usual dose = 500 mg QID up to 8 weeks. Up to 3 g/day in acute exacerbation; 1 g/day for maintenance.
- Balsalazide (Colazal 750 mg capsules). Usual dose = 2.25 g TID (yielding 2.4 g/day of 5-ASA).
- Osalazine (Dipentum 250 mg tablets). Usual dose = 250 mg QID or 500 mg BID. Up to 500 mg QID in acute exacerbations.

Continued Symptoms After Exacerbation

◆ Continue treatments listed under remission maintenance as tolerated.

◆ Azathioprine 2–2.5 mg/kg/day or 6-mercaptopurine 1–1.5 mg/kg/day in patients unable to wean from corticosteroids. Monitor for nausea, fever, rash, and hepatitis. Bone marrow suppression is dose related. Pancreatitis may occur in 3–15% of patients.

◆ Cyclosporine 6–8 mg/kg QD PO for 6 months if required IV cyclosporine during exacerbation.

Crohn's Disease

Remission Induction (Acute Exacerbations).   Management of Crohn's disease is similar to acute ulcerative colitis but must be individualized to disease severity and anatomical lesions of the disease.

◆ **Corticosteroids** in the same doses as for UC exacerbations are effective for the treatment of active symptomatic Crohn's. They are most effective when the ileum alone or ileum and colon are involved (less effective when disease is confined to colon). When *disease is confined to small bowel,* use prednisone in a dose that has been adjusted according to disease severity and taper dose after remission. Chronic low doses (5–15 mg/day) may be required for remission induction (ineffective for remission maintenance of Crohn's). *Budesonide* (Entocort EC) 9 mg cap QD approved for mild to moderate Crohn's of ileum or ascending colon.

◆ **Sulfasalazine** 1 gm TID or QID (up to 6 g day) should be used for mild to moderately symptomatic Crohn's when *disease is confined to the colon.* Begin with 500 mg QD and increase gradually to minimize side effects. Improvement occurs in 4–6 weeks. Switch to oral prednisone if unresponsive. *Previously untreated patients with disease of the ileum and colon* should receive sulfasalazine. If no response in 1–2 months, switch to prednisone.

◆ **Asacol** (up to 8 g per day) or *Pentasa* (up to 4 g per day) may be more effective than sulfasalazine in patients with disease of lower ileum. None of the 5-ASA derivatives are reliable above the ileum

◆ Infliximab (Remicade) 5 mg/kg IV infusion over 2 hrs for patients failing corticosteroids, especially if fistulae drainage present. May repeat at 2 and 6 weeks. See page 25.2 for mechanism and side effects.

◆ Metronidazole (Flagyl) 400 mg BID or 250 mg QID if perianal involvement or fistulas. Expect response in 4–8 weeks.

◆ Azathioprine, 6-mercaptopurine, or cyclosporine may be tried, as for severe UC.

Remission Maintenance

(Patients responding to acute treatment, with minimal or no continuing symptoms)

No treatment is indicated. Sulfasalazine and corticosteroids are ineffective. Use may increase mortality and the need for surgical intervention.

Continued Symptoms After Exacerbation

♦ Diet and drug treatment similar to ulcerative colitis maintenance, except that sulfasalazine and 5-ASA derivatives are only effective for colonic or lower ileal involvements.

♦ Continued low-dose prednisone may be necessary, but attempt to taper and try other options below if possible.

♦ Continue metronidazole for 3–4 months if indicated (see Acute Exacerbations)

♦ Repeat infliximab at 2 and 6 weeks if indicated and response observed.

♦ Consider azathioprine 2–3 mg/kg/day, 6 mercaptopurine 1.5 mg/kg/day, cyclosporine 5–7.5 mg/kg/day, or methotrexate in refractory cases or if fistulas. Unclear as to superiority of one agent over the other, but there is more hepatotoxicity with methotrexate.

Table 25.1 • Pathophysiologic Differences Between Ulcerative Colitis and Crohn's Disease

Characteristic	Ulcerative Colitis	Crohn's Disease
Anatomical location	Colon and rectum (proctitis) only	Entire GI[a] tract (mouth to anus), especially ileum and colon
Distribution	Continuous, diffuse, mucosal	Segmental, focal, transmural
Bowel wall	Shortened, loss of haustral markings, generally not thickened	Rigid, thick, edematous, and fibrotic
Gross rectal bleeding, crypt abscesses	Common	Infrequent
Fissuring with sinus formation, noncaseating granulomas, strictures, abdominal mass	Absent	Common
Abdominal pain	Infrequent	Common
Toxic megacolon	Occasional	Rare
Risk of bowel carcinoma	Greatly ↑	Slightly ↑
Risk of recurrence after surgery	Low	High

[a]GI = Gastrointestinal.

Table 25.2 • Nonintestinal Complications of Ulcerative Colitis and Crohn's Disease

Manifestation	Ulcerative Colitis (%)	Crohn's Disease (%)
Arthritis/arthralgia	25	33
Erythema nodosum/pyoderma gangrenosum	4	5
Abnormal liver function tests	50	30
Iritis/uveitis	5	4
Ankylosing spondylitis	15	10
Growth retardation	18	13

Table 25.3 • Rectal Corticosteroids[a,b,c]

Product	Dose	Comments
Hydrocortisone hemisuccinate retention enema (Cortenema) 100 mg/60 mL	100 mg HS × 21 days (up to 2–3 months)	Relief in 3–5 days, but mucosal changes persist longer. Up to 50–90% absorbed, taper dose if prolonged therapy.
Hydrocortisone acetate rectal foam (Cortifoam) 90 mg/applicator	1 applicatorful 1–2 times/day for 2–3 weeks	Easier to retain than enemas, but absorption may be greater. Distribution not well studied
Proctofoam (1% hydrocortisone and 1% proxamine)	1 applicatorful 1–2 times/day for 2–3 weeks	Easier to use than enema. Proxamine is local anesthetic.

[a]Budesonide and beclomethasone enemas available outside of U.S. Possible less systemic absorption than hydrocortisone.
[b]Instill total volume as a bolus with the patient in the supine position. Alternate position every 20 minutes for 4 positions: Supine to left decubitus to right decubitus to prone. Retain the contents for as long as possible. If the patient cannot retain the initial volume, it may be slowly dripped in over 20–30 minutes.
[c]Side effects: May increase risk of bowel weakening and perforation. Cutaneous atrophy, decreased wound healing.

The reader is referred to Chapter 26: Inflammatory Bowel Disease, written by *Babette S. Duncan, Pharm.D.*, in the seventh edition of **Applied Therapeutics: The Clinical Use of Drugs** for a more in-depth discussion. All notations to reference numbers are based on the reference list at the end of that chapter. The editors of this handbook express their thanks to Dr. Duncan and acknowledge that this chapter is based upon her work.

Notes:

Chapter 26

Alcoholic Cirrhosis

Definitions

♦ *Cirrhosis* is a chronic liver condition characterized by widespread hepatocellular damage and nodular scarring within the liver. The liver nodules obstruct blood and biliary flow within the liver.

♦ *Portal hypertension* is an increased pressure in the portal vein (>12 mm Hg) subsequent to intrahepatic blood and biliary flow obstruction caused by liver nodule formation. The portal venous system collects blood from the abdominal portion of the digestive tract, pancreas, and spleen and transports the blood to the liver.

Clinical Presentation, Complications, and Treatment

♦ The symptoms of uncomplicated cirrhosis are nonspecific. Treatment is elimination of causative factors (especially alcohol) and nutritional support.

♦ More definitive therapies are directed at the major complications of cirrhosis and portal hypertension listed below. Treatment options for each of these complications are outlined in Table 26.1.

• Bleeding disorders.
• Esophageal varices.
• Ascites.
• Hepatic encephalopathy.
• Hepatorenal syndrome.

Notes:

Table 26.1 • Treatment of Complications of Cirrhosis

Complication/Drug Therapy	Dosing/Monitoring
Nonspecific Complaints Anorexia, nausea, abdominal discomfort, weight loss, weakness, fatigue	Abstinence from alcohol, adequate nutrition. Replace folic acid (1 mg/day), thiamine (100 mg/day). Normal protein intake of 35–50 gm/day unless encephalopathy present
Bleeding Disorders[a] Vitamin K (phytonadione)	10 mg QD SC or IV × 2–3 days. Monitor prothrombin time. If no response, extra doses probably of little value. IM may cause local bleeding. IV may cause fever, chills, sweating, and anaphylaxis. Infuse slowly at rate of 1–2 mg/min
Ascites[b] Na restriction/bedrest	10–20 mEq Na QD
Spironolactone (Aldactone)	*Dose:* Start at 50 mg QD, titrate dose to achieve 0.3–1 kg wt loss/day[c] or up to 400 mg QD. Slow onset (2–3 days). Wait 2–3 days before each dosage change *Monitor:* Abdominal girth, K (may cause hyperkalemia), BUN (↑ if overdiuresed), BP (avoid hypotension), precipitation of encephalopathy, urine electrolytes.[d] Gynecomastia with prolonged therapy. Can substitute triamterene or amiloride
Hydrochlorothiazide (HCTZ) *or* Furosemide	*Dose:* Start HCTZ at 25–50 mg, titrate to 0.3–1 kg wt loss/day. Start furosemide at 20–40 mg, titrate to 0.3–1 kg wt loss/day. Usually given when spironolactone fails; may start earlier while waiting for onset of spironolactone. Recent guidelines recommend furosemide as initial therapy, before or concurrent with spironolactone. Refractory cases may require large doses of furosemide combined with spironolactone *Monitor:* Same as spironolactone, except may cause hypokalemia. More likely to cause hypovolemia. No gynecomastia
Paracentesis *plus* albumin[e]	Remove 1–2 L ascitic fluid by paracentesis for relief of abdominal pain or respiratory distress. Large volume loss may cause cardiovascular collapse. 4–6 L/day paracentesis + 40–50 gm QD IV albumin better tolerated and clears ascites faster than diuretics
Surgery	Peritoneovenous (LeVeen or Denver) shunt to direct ascitic fluid back into vascular circulation. Complications include pulmonary edema, fever, wound infection, septicemia, and consumption coagulopathy. Investigational: Ascites filtration and reinfusion
Esophageal Varices[f] IV fluids/blood replacement	To maintain BP. Also balloon tamponade
Sclerotherapy (sodium tetradecyl sulfate)	*Dose:* 0.5–2 mL of 1%–1.5% solution injected into each varix 1–2 cm apart[g] *Monitor:* May cause chest pain, fever, local ulceration
Sclerotherapy (ethanolamine oleate) (Ethamolin)	*Dose:* 1.5–5 mL of 5% solution into varix *Monitor:* May cause chest pain. fever, local ulceration
Propranolol (Inderal)[h]	*Dose:* 20–80 mg QID PO for 6 months–1 yr. To ↓ portal pressure and hepatic blood flow *Monitor:* Reduce dose if pulse <60 beats/min or patient hypotensive
Nadolol	Nadolol used alone as alternative to propranolol for both primary[h] and secondary prevention[h]. *Dose:* 40 mg QD to start. Titrate to 20–25% decrease in HR or max of 160 mg QD
Isosorbide Mononitrate	May combine nadolol with isosorbide mononitrate. *Dose:* Start at 10 mg BID, then increase to 20 mg BID unless hypotension or severe headache. (Not for monotherapy)
Somatostatin[i]	50–250 µg bolus, then 250–500 µg/hr continous infusion
Octreotide (Sandostatin)[i]	50–100 µg bolus, then 25–50 µg/hr continous infusion

(continued)

Table 26.1 • Treatment of Complications of Cirrhosis (continued)

Complication/Drug Therapy	Dosing/Monitoring
Esophageal Varices[f] (continued)	
Endoscopic band ligation	Band placed around mucosa and submucosa of esophageal area containing the varix leads to strangulation, fibrosis, and obliteration of the vessel
Vasopressin (Pitressin) (if sclerotherapy, octreotide, and TIPS fails)	*Dose:* 20 U IV bolus, then 0.2–0.4 U/min IV infusion (*max:* 0.9 U/min). Intense vasoconstriction and antidiuretic hormone-like effect. Combination with IV (40–200 μg/min) or transdermal NTG (10 mg/day) have been tried to ↑ vasoconstriction and ↓ cardiac complications *Monitor:* May cause skin blanching, bradycardia, angina, myocardial or bowel infarct, GI cramping, dilutional hyponatrenia, or IV site phlebitis
Terlipressin (Glypressin)	Synthetic analog of vasopressin. Metabolized in vivo to lysine vasopressin. *Dose:* 2 mg IV bolus Q 6 hr *Monitor:* Same as vasopressin but fewer cardiac side effects
Transjugular intrahepatic portal systemic shunt (TIPS)	Expandable metal stent (tube) placed between a branch of the hepatic vein and the portal vein to decompress portal system within the liver
Surgery	Portacaval shunt. ↑ risk of encephalopathy
Hepatic Encephalopathy[j]	
Protein restriction	<30 g/day
Lactulose syrup[k] (10 g/15 mL) (Celphulac, Duphulac)	*Dose:* 10–30 g (15–45 mL) PO TID during acute episode. Also used chronically. Titrate to desired mental status or 2–3 soft stools/day. *Enema:* 300 mL of 50% lactulose in 700 mL tap water. Nonabsorbable disaccharide broken down by GI bacteria to lactic, acetic, and formic acids to ↓ bowel pH and prevent absorption of NH_3 *Side Effects:* Sweet taste, belching, flatulence, osmotic diarrhea
Neomycin[k]	*Dose:* 1–2 gm PO 4–6 × day or as 100 mL 1% enema. Sterilizes GI bacteria that produce NH_3 *Side Effect:* Diarrhea. 1%–3% absorbed; may cause ototoxicity or renal toxicity with prolonged use
Replacement of branched chain aminoacids (AAs)	*Hepatic-Acid:* 1–4 packs/day PO (Blend 1 pack with 250 mL H_2O to yield 15 gm protein, 98 gm carbohydrate, 12 gm fat, and 560 cal) *HepatAmine:* 8% AA TPN solution (high ratio of branched-chain AAs). High cost with lack of confirmed benefit; use only if above fails
Flumazenil (Mazicon)[l]	*Dose (Investigational Use):* Acute 0.2–0.4 mg IV Q 1–2 hr administered over 15–30 sec via a freely running IV infusion into a large vein. Chronic 25 mg BID *Side Effects:* Insufficient data for this use. Adverse reactions most frequently noted are dizziness, injection site pain, sweating, headache; the most serious is convulsions
Hepatorenal Syndrome[m]	Reduce diuretics. Dopamine 0.5–1 μg/kg/min IV infusion. Nearly 100% mortality

(continued)

Notes:

Table 26.1 • Treatment of Complications of Cirrhosis (continued)

Complication/Drug Therapy	Dosing/Monitoring
Disease Modification	
Colchicine (investigational use for anti-inflammatory and antifibrotic properties)	*Dose:* 0.6 mg BID *Side Effects:* Nausea, abdominal pain, diarrhea

[a]Increased risk of bleeding due to decreased production of the vitamin K-dependent clotting factors (II, VII, IX, and X) in the liver; prolonged prothrombin time. SC = Subcutaneous.

[b]Ascites is an accumulation of fluid in the abdominal (peritoneal) cavity. Contributing factors include: 1) renal sodium retention and volume expansion whereby excess fluid outflows into the peritoneal cavity from the congested portal system; 2) increased hydrostatic pressure in portal vein causing fluid to leak into the surrounding tissue; 3) decreased albumin production causing lowered plasma oncotic pressure; 4) exudation of fluid from the splanchnic capillary bed and liver surface directly into the abdominal cavity; and 5) leakage of albumin into the peritoneum. A relative decrease in vascular fluid volume stimulates the renin-angiotensin-aldosterone system leading to relative hyperaldosteronism, Na^+ rentention and urinary K^+ loss in some patients.

[c]Goals of therapy are to mobilize ascitic fluid; reduce abdominal girth; diminish abdominal discomfort and back pain; and prevent complications including bacterial peritonitis, respiratory distress, and hepatorenal syndrome. 0.3–1 kg/day wt loss based upon slow equilibration of ascitic fluid with serum. Larger weight loss (2 kg/day) may be acceptable if considerable peripheral edema also is present. Average dose of spironolactone: 200–400 mg QD. QD is acceptable due to long $t_{1/2}$ of active metabolite.

[d]Use of spironolactone assumes presence of hyperaldosteronism. Before treatment, urinary electolytes will show ↓ or absent Na^+ and ↑ K^+. Inhibition of aldosterone by spironolactone should restore normal urine electrolytes (i.e., more Na^+ than K^+). Addition of thiazide or furosemide ↑ urine Na^+, thereby invalidating urine electrolyte monitoring.

[e]Paracentesis = drainage of abdominal cavity via insertion of a needle or catheter.

[f]Portal hypertension causes distension and increased fragility of blood vessels in the esophagus that may rupture and bleed. These may be accompanied by gastric bleeding and hemorrhoids.

[g]Tetradecyl comes as a 3% solution. Dilute with equal parts of absolute alcohol and 50% dextrose in water for 1% solution.

[h]Primary prevention = Start propranolol when varices are visualized by endoscopy but before first episode of bleeding. Secondary prevention = Treatment after an acute bleed has been stopped by sclerotheropy, band ligation, or TIPS. Rebleeding incidence reduced but not mortality rate.

[i]Somatostatin reduces collateral blood flow by constricting splanchnic vessels. Octreotide is a long-acting synthetic analog of somatostatin. Both are investigational for this use.

[j]A metabolic disorder of the CNS with altered mental status (ranging from mild confusion to coma), asterixis (a flapping motion of the hands when wrist is hyperextended), and fetor hepaticus (a peculiar sweetish, musty odor of the breath). Encephalopathy is exacerbated by GI bleeding, metabolic and electrolyte abnormalities, volume depletion, and CNS depressant drugs. Three interrelated biochemical imbalances associated with hepatic encephalophathy are: 1) abnormal ammonia metabolism, 2) altered ratio of branched chain to aromatic amino acids and 3) possible increase in central nervous system GABAergic neurotransmission.

[k]Lactulose and neomycin equally effective. May be used in combination for additive effect. Theoretical interaction that sterilization of bacteria by neomycin may ↓ lactulose activation unproven.

[l]Benzodiazepine receptor antagonist.

[m]An episode of acute renal failure accompanying hepatic failure. Causes include unmetabolized toxins or volume depletion following overdiuresis.

The reader is referred to Chapter 27: Alcoholic Cirrhosis, written by *Ali Olyaei, Pharm.D.*, and *John Rabkin* in the seventh edition of **Applied Therapeutics: The Clinical Use of Drugs** for a more in-depth discussion. All notations to reference numbers are based on the reference list at the end of that chapter. The editors of this handbook express their thanks to Drs. Olyaei and Rabkin and acknowledge that this chapter is based upon their work.

Notes:

Chapter 27

Adverse Effects of Drugs on the Liver

Mechanisms of Hepatic Injury

The two major mechanisms by which drugs induce hepatic injury are *intrinsic hepatotoxicity* and *idiosyncrasy*. Intrinsic hepatotoxins predictably injure the liver. In contrast, idiosyncratic or unpredictable hepatotoxins cause hepatic damage in a small number of uniquely susceptible individuals. The major differences between these two types of drug-induced hepatic injury are listed in Table 27.1.

♦ *Acute Hepatic Injury*

Acute hepatic injury can be *hepatocellular* (also called cytotoxic injury; toxicity to liver parenchyma) or *cholestatic* (biliary obstruction, reduced bile flow) or a mixed presentation of both. Hepatocellular lesions can be due to necrosis (cellular destruction and death), steatosis (fat droplet deposition within hepatocytes), or a combination. See Table 27.2 for the clinical presentation and laboratory findings of acute liver injury.

♦ *Chronic Hepatic Injury*

The various forms of chronic drug-induced liver injury are listed in Table 27.3.

♦ *Risk Factors*

Several host factors affect the risk of drug-induced liver disease, including age, gender, dose, genetic factors, concurrent medications (including alcohol), and coexisting diseases. See Table 27.4.

♦ *Drug-induced Hepatotoxicity.* A listing of the more commonly described hepato-toxic drugs, the form of injury produced, and proposed mechanisms of the damage is presented in Table 27.5.

♦ *Herbals Associated with Liver Injury.* See Table 27.6.

Notes:

Table 27.1 • Characteristics of Intrinsic versus Idiosyncratic Hepatotoxins[a]

Intrinsic	Idiosyncratic (Hypersensitivity)
A distinctive histologic pattern observed for any given drug[a]	Variable histologic pattern of lesions[a]
Dose-dependent hepatotoxicity	Dose-independent hepatotoxicity
Elicited in all individuals	Only a small fraction of exposed individuals affected; requires "sensitization"
Reproducible in experimental animals	Cannot be reproduced in experimental animals
Predictable appearance of lesions and usually a brief latent period following exposure	Appearance of lesions bears no temporal relationship to the institution of drug therapy; delayed onset (1–5 weeks) on 1st exposure; rapid appearance on subsequent exposure
No extrahepatic manifestations of hypersensitivity	Lesions often accompanied by extrahepatic manifestations (e.g., fever, rash, eosinophilia). Allergic?

[a]Intrinsic reactions usually cytotoxic; idiosyncratic reactions may be cytotoxic, cholestatic, or mixed. See page 27.1 and Table 27.2 for definitions of cytotoxic and cholestatic.

Table 27.2 • Classification of Acute Hepatic Injury[a]

Type	Hepatocellular	Cholestatic
Morphology	Parenchymal destruction (cytotoxicity): necrosis and/or steatosis	Biliary obstruction[b]
Clinical manifestations	Hepatitis-like syndrome: jaundice, nausea, vomiting, right upper quadrant pain, fatigue. Lymphadenopathy with some drugs.	Jaundice, pruritus
Laboratory	Serum transferase $\uparrow$ 8–500 × normal	Serum transferase normal to 3× normal[b]
	Alkaline phosphatase normal to 3× normal	Alkaline phosphatase normal to 2–10× normal[b]

[a]Mixed injury (hepatocellular and cholestatic) can occur.
[b]Obstruction may be either of intrahepatic bile ducts (hepatocannicular) and/or within the extrahepatic biliary tree (cannicular). Cannicular lesions usually with transferase elevations less than 8× normal and alkaline phosphatase <3× normal. Higher elevations indicate hepatocannicular lesions and possible coexistent hepatocellular or portal tree inflammation.

Notes:

Table 27.3 • Forms of Drug Induced Chronic Hepatic Injury

Injury Type	Comments
Hepatocellular Injury	
Chronic hepatitis-like	Mimics viral or autoimmune hepatitis. Associated with highest transferase elevations.
Subacute hepatic necrosis	Toxic necrosis
Chronic hepatitis-like without inflammation	Antibodies against microsomal proteins (e.g., P450 enzymes)
Chronic steatosis	Usually macrovascular with fatty cirrhosis
Phospholipoidosis	
Fibrosis and cirrhosis	Mimics alcohol injury (pseudoalcoholic)
Cholestatic Lesions	
Chronic intrahepatic cholestasis	Resembles primary biliary cirrhosis but without anti-mitochondrial antibodies
Biliary sclerosis	
Vascular Lesions	
Hepatic vein thrombosis	Budd-Chiari Syndrome. Vascular injury to efferent portal blood flow.
Hepatic vein occlusion	Veno-occlusive disease; occlusion of terminal hepatic venules.
Peliosis hepatitis	Blood-filled cysts in the liver
Hepatoportal sclerosis	Pericellular or sinusoidal fibrosis causing portal hypertension without cirrhosis.
Granulomatous Hepatitis	
Hepatic Tumors	
Benign	
Adenoma	
Carcinoma	

Notes:

Table 27.4 • Risk Factors for Developing Drug-induced Liver Disease[9,10,28-39]

Factor	Examples of Drugs Affected	Comments
Age	Isoniazid, nitrofurantoin, halothane	Increased incidence/severity with age >60 yr
	Valproic acid, salicylates	Higher incidence in children
Sex	Halothane, methyldopa, nitrofurantoin	Higher incidence in females
	Flucoxacillin, azathioprine	Higher incidence in males
Dose	Acetaminophen, aspirin	Higher blood concentrations associated with risk of hepatotoxicity
	Methotrexate, vitamin A	Total dose, frequency, and duration associated with hepatotoxic risk
Genetic factors	Halothane, phenytoin, sulfonamides, isoniazid	Numerous familial cases; defective epoxide hydrolases increase susceptibility to phenytoin and halothane associated injury; acetylator phenotype may predispose to isoniazid hepatotoxicity
	Valproic acid	Familial cases, correlation with mitochondrial enzyme abnormalities
History of other drug reactions	Halothane, enflurane; erythromycins; diclofenac, ibuprofen	Rare incidence of cross-sensitivity reported between drug classes
Other drugs	Acetaminophen	Isoniazid, zidovudine may lower toxic dose threshold for hepatotoxicity
	Busulfan, azathioprine	Increased risk of hepatic veno-occlusive disease
	Valproic acid	Other antiepileptic drugs increase risk of hepatotoxicity
Excessive alcohol use	Acetaminophen	Lowered dosage threshold
	Isoniazid, methotrexate	Increased liver injury and enhanced fibrosis
Other diseases		
Obesity	Halothane hepatitis, methotrexate	Increased liver injury and enhanced fibrosis
Fasting	Acetaminophen	Increased risk of hepatotoxicity
Renal failure	Tetracycline, methotrexate	Increased liver injury and enhanced fibrosis
Pre-existing liver disease	Niacin (nicotinamide), methotrexate	Increased risk of liver injury
Organ transplantation	Azathioprine, busulfan	Increased risk of vascular toxicity
AIDS	Dapsone, trimethoprim-sulfamethoxazole, oxacillin	Increased risk of liver injury; hypersensitivity
Diabetes	Methotrexate	Increased risk of hepatic fibrosis

Table 27.5 • Drug-induced Hepatotoxicity[a]

Drug	Incidence	Morphology	Mechanism	Clinical Remarks
Acetohexamide (see chlorpropamide)				
ACE inhibitors (see Captopril)				
Acetaminophen	High with acute overdose >10 g. Chronic associated with prolonged high dosages (>4 g/day), concurrent alcoholism, fasting	Hepatocellular	Active metabolites, direct toxicity	Saturation of conjugation of pathways; shunting to P450 metabolism; accumulation of reactive metabolite
Alcohol	High with chronic exposure	Hepatocellular, cirrhosis	Direct toxicity	See Chapter 26: Alcoholic Cirrhosis
Allopurinol	Rare	Submassive or massive necrosis, cholestatic or granulomatous hepatitis	Hypersensitivity	*Onset:* 7 days–6 weeks. Generalized hypersensitivity symptoms have accompanied hepatitis
Amiodarone	Uncommon	Alcoholic hepatitis-like lesions	Phospholipidosis	↑ serum transferase in 40% of patients. Delayed onset. Also see peripheral neuropathy, corneal deposits, skin discoloration (bluish). May be related to polysorbate 80 added as surfactant to IV solution
Amitriptyline (see tricyclic antidepressants [TCAs])				
Amoxicillin-clavulanic acid	Uncommon	Cholestasis or mixed	Immunologic, idiosyncratic	*Onset:* 2–45 days. More in adults than children. Likely due to clavulanic acid or combination since rare with amoxicillin alone
Androgenic steroids	High incidence of hepatic dysfunction; low incidence of cholestatic jaundice	Cholestatic with minor or no portal inflammation; dilation of sinusoids; peliosis hepatitis; adenoma and carcinoma	Indirect intrinsic hepatotoxin	Only anabolic steroids with an alkyl group in the C-17 position have been incriminated. Testosterone, 19-nortestosterone, and their esters do not exhibit adverse effects on the liver

(continued)

Table 27.5 • Drug-induced Hepatotoxicity^a (continued)

Drug	Incidence	Morphology	Mechanism	Clinical Remarks
Aspirin and other salicylates	0.1–0.5% but high in certain subgroups	Focal hepatic necrosis; steatosis	Intrinsic hepatotoxicity	Up to 50% of patients with JRA, SLE, or rheumatic fever, and high salicylate levels (>25 mg/dL). May be a component of Reye's syndrome in children given aspirin during viral illnesses.
Azathioprine	Rare	Cholestasis: minor hepatocellular injury; veno-occlusive disorders (VOD)	Idiosyncrasy	Only a few isolated instances of cholestasis after 3 weeks to 6 months. ~20% of bone marrow and renal transplant patients develop VOD
Benoxaprofen (see nonsteroidal antiinflammatory drugs [NSAIDs])				
Captopril	Rare	Cholestasis or mixed	Hypersensitivity	*Onset:* 5 days–12 months. Also reported with enalapril and lisinopril
Bromfenac (see nonsteroidal antiinflammatory drugs [NSAIDs])				
Carbamazepine	<1%	Hepatocellular, cholestasis, or mixed	Hypersensitivity, possible toxic metabolite	Usually within first 8 weeks. Presents similar to phenytoin
Carmustine (BCNU)	Dose-related	Necrosis	Intrinsic hepatotoxin	Hepatic injury (presumably as an alkylating agent) in up to 25% of patients taking therapeutic doses
Chlorpromazine (CPZ) (also see prochlorperazine)	0.1%–0.2%	Cholestasis; scattered focal areas of necrosis	Hypersensitivity	In 80%, icterus develops between 1–4 weeks. Rare after 1st dose. Severe pruritus common. May occur with other phenothiazines as well.
Chlorpropamide (and other sulfonylurea hypoglycemics)	0.1%–0.5%	Mixed cholestatic-cytotoxic injury	Hypersensitivity, hepatotoxicity	*Onset:* Usually between 2–6 weeks. Much higher incidence with chlorpropamide than with other oral hypoglycemics

Drug		Mechanism	Comments
Chlortetracycline (see Tetracyclines)			
Ciprofloxacin (see Fluoroquinolones)			
Clarithromycin (see erythromycin)			
Cloxacillin (see oxacillin)			
Contraceptive steroids	*Four Types:* 1) Cholestasis	Dose-related	Indirect hepatotoxin; genetic predisposition?	Phenolic ring A and an alkyl group at C-17 of estrogen seem responsible. Progesterone has little or no adverse effect. Incidence of 1/10,000
	2) Adenoma, peliosis hepatitis			↑ in incidence of hepatic adenoma seems to have paralleled ↑ use of oral contraceptives
	3) Budd-Chiari syndrome			Rare: thrombosis and occlusion of hepatic vein
	4) Carcinoma?			Low incidence compared to widespread use
Cyclosporine	Cholestasis, venous occlusive disease	Uncommon, dose-related	Direct toxic effect on bile secretion	↑ Liver enzymes in 4%–7% of transplant patients with 1 month of treatment
Dantrolene	Chronic active hepatitis-like; submassive and massive necrosis	Hypertransferasemia without jaundice: 1.8%; overt hepatic jaundice: 0.6%	Idiosyncrasy; toxic metabolites	*Onset:* delayed ≥45 days in most cases. Doses ≤200 mg/day rarely lead to liver damage. Risk appears greater in females and patients >35 yr
Desipramine (see tricyclic antidepressants [TCAs])			
Didanoside (see zidovudine)			
Diltiazem	Granulomatous	Rare	Idiosyncrasy	Generally mild and reversible, occurring within 8 weeks. Also with nifedipine

(continued)

Table 27.5 • Drug-induced Hepatotoxicity[a] (continued)

Drug	Incidence	Morphology	Mechanism	Clinical Remarks
Erythromycin	2%	Cholestasis; mixed cholestatic-cytotoxic injury	Hypersensitivity; children less susceptible than adults.	Most often with estolate salt, but also with ethylsuccinate and propionate salts, clarithromycin, and roxithromycin. Onset 1–3 weeks with 1st exposure, faster on rechallenge.
Felbamate	<1%	Submassive necrosis	Idiosyncrasy	23 cases and 5 deaths. Now restricted use.
Fluconazole (see itraconazole and ketoconazole)				
Fluoroquinolones	Rare; high with trovafloxacin	Cholestasis; centrilobular necrosis	Idiosyncrasy	1.8%–2.5% of patients with mild elevations of LFTs. Reported with ciprofloxacin, enoxacin, ofloxacin, norfloxacin. 100 cases, 14 severe with trovafloxacin.
Fluoxetine	Very low	Cholestatic, hepatocellular	Hypersensitivity	3 reported cases
Fluphenazine	Rare	Cholestasis	Hypersensitivity	In 80%, icterus develops between 1–4 weeks. Rare after 1st dose. Severe pruritus common
Glibenclamide (see chlorpropamide)				
Glucocorticoids	Dose-related	Steatosis	Hepatotoxicity	Hepatic steatosis of little clinical consequence. Occasionally may lead to fat embolism in vascular bed of major organs (e.g., lung)
Haloperidol	0.2%–3%	Cholestasis	Hypersensitivity	
Halothane (also see methoxyflurane)	*Mild:* >25% *Severe:* Rare	*Mild:* Centrizonal necrosis, steatosis. *Severe:* Severe necrosis	Metabolic idiosyncrasy; hypersensitivity	Reactive metabolites cause mild self-limiting toxicity. Rare fulminate hepatitis may be autoimmune reaction to trifluoroacetyl acid metabolite. ↑ risk if prior exposure to halothane or isoflurane. Mortality: 14%–67% for severe forms

Drug	Incidence	Lesion	Mechanism	Comments
Ibuprofen (see NSAIDs)				
Imipramine (see tricyclic antidepressants [TCAs])				
Indinavir (see zidovudine)				
Isoflurane (see halothane)				
Isoniazid (INH)	1.2% (35–49 yr) 2.3% (>50 yr)	Similar to viral hepatitis	Direct hepatotoxicity of metabolite, monoacetyl hydrazine	10%–20% develop ↑ liver enzymes. Most common in 1st 3 months. Discontinue if AST >3–5× normal. *Risk factors*: age >35 yr, daily alcohol, pre-existing liver disease, other hepatotoxins
Itraconazole (also see ketoconazole)	Low	Mixed or cholestatic; rare fulminant hepatitis	Idiosyncratic, hepatocellular	24 cases of liver failure, 11 deaths
Ketoconazole (also see itraconazole)	0.03%–0.1%	Mixed or cholestatic hepatitis, rare fulminant hepatitis	Idiosyncratic, hepatocellular	↑ transferases in 8%–12% of patients without clinical symptoms. Lower incidence with fluconazole.
Lovastatin	Rare	Mild focal hepatitis	Hepatocellular	5%–7% with ↑ in transferases; usually clinically insignificant and reversible. Avoid in patients with liver disease or alcohol abuse. Also reported with pravastatin and simvastatin.
6-mercaptopurine (6-MP)	Dose-related (>2.5 mg/kg)	Cholestasis with fatty hepatic necrosis	Indirect intrinsic hepatotoxin	Reported in 6%–40% of leukemic patients; adults > children
Methimazole	Rare	Cholestasis	Hypersensitivity	1st 4 weeks–3 months. Can be accompanied by rash, fever, lymphadenopathy, or agranulocytosis
Methoxyflurane	Rare, but may be fatal.	Similar findings as in halothane hepatitis	Hypersensitivity; metabolic aberration?	Clinical syndrome and hepatic lesions from methoxyflurane very similar to those observed in halothane hepatitis. Halothane and methoxyflurane appear to crossreact in patients with history of halothane hepatitis

(continued)

Table 27.5 • Drug-induced Hepatotoxicity *(continued)*

Drug	Incidence	Morphology	Mechanism	Clinical Remarks
Methotrexate	Dose-related	Steatosis; necrosis; fibrosis; cirrhosis	Indirect intrinsic hepatotoxin	Fatty liver, fibrosis, or cirrhosis in >100 cases of patients with psoriasis
Methyldopa	Low	Cytotoxic injury: subacute or bridging necrosis; rare cholestasis; chronic active hepatitis	Hypersensitivity; toxic metabolite	↑ Liver enzymes in 1%–2%. In some, enzymes return to normal despite continued therapy. Cholestasis rare, severe cytotoxic injury <0.1%. CAH induced by methyldopa resembles "autoimmune" type CAH
Mithramycin (see Plicamycin)				
MAOIs (iproniazid, isocarboxazid, phenelzine)	Low	Hepatocellular damage	Metabolic idiosyncrasy	Encountered in patients given phenelzine for periods of 18 days–5 months. Findings indistinguishable from viral hepatitis. Incidence rare, but *mortality rate:* ≈15%. Tranylcypromine rarely causes jaundice
Naproxen (see NSAIDs)				
Nevirapine (see zidovudine)				
Niacin (nicotinic acid)	Occasional	Hepatocellular damage, cholestasis	Hypersensitivity	Possibly ↑ incidence with sustained release and >3 gm/day
Nifedipine (see diltiazem)				
Nitrofurantoin	Rare	Cholestasis; mixed cholestatic-cytotoxic injury; chronic active hepatitis	Hypersensitivity	*Onset:* usually abrupt with fever and eosinophilia. ⅔ have previous exposure to nitrofurantoin. *Latent period:* 2 days–5 months
NSAIDs	Low	Cholestasis, cytotoxic or mixed	Hypersensitivity; possible reactive metabolites	Most with benoxaprofen and bromfenac. Also diclofenac, ibuprofen, ketoprofen, naproxen, piroxicam, sulindac. Females >age 50 possibly higher risk.

Drug	Incidence	Mechanism	Lesions	Comments
Oral hypoglycemics (see Chlorpropamide)				
Oxacillin (also see penicillin)	Low	Hypersensitivity; idiosyncrasy	Anicteric hepatic dysfunction; rare cases of cholestatic jaundice reported	Also reported with cloxacillin and flucloxacillin. Risk factors: high dose, females, older age, >2 weeks exposure. Apparently no cross-hepatotoxicity between oxacillin and penicillin G or nafcillin.
Oxytetracycline (see tetracycline)				
Penicillin (also see oxacillin)	Very rare	Hypersensitivity	Necrosis; granuloma; "lupoid" hepatitis	Most cases associated with systemic hypersensitivity reactions (e.g., urticaria, rash, anaphylactic shock). Also carbenicillin, ampicillin
Phenelzine (see monoamine oxidase inhibitors [MAOIs])				
Phenylbutazone (also see NSAIDs)	0.25%	Hypersensitivity; intrinsic toxicity?	Local or diffuse parenchymal necrosis with or without cholestasis	*Onset:* within 4–6 months, occasionally after 12 months. *Fatality rate:* 12% with hepatic necrosis. Cholestasis and granulomatous lesions generally recover after 4 months
Phenytoin	Low; <1%	Hypersensitivity	Cytotoxic injury with varying degrees of cholestasis; necrosis	80% of cases involve adults age >20 yr. *Onset:* 1–5 weeks. Fever, rash, lymphadenopathy, and eosinophilia appear in most patients. *Fatality rate:* 40% due partly to exfoliative dermatitis
Piroxicam (see NSAIDs)				
Plicamycin (Mithramycin)	Dose-related	Intrinsic hepatotoxin	Necrosis	25%–100% of recipients on "full" doses; less with lower doses or alternate day. Rare in treatment of hypercalcemia
Pravastatin (see lovastatin)				

(continued)

Table 27.5 • Drug-induced Hepatotoxicity^a (continued)

Drug	Incidence	Morphology	Mechanism	Clinical Remarks
Prochlorperazine (also see chlorpromazine)	Rare	Cholestasis	Hypersensitivity	In 80%, icterus develops between 1–4 weeks. Rare after 1st dose. Severe pruritus common
Propylthiouracil (PTU)	Rare	Hepatocellular injury; chronic active hepatitis; cholestasis	Hypersensitivity	*Onset:* usually within 2–4 weeks
Quinidine	Rare	Mixed hepatocellular injury; granulomata	Hypersensitivity	*Onset:* mild hepatic injury within 6–12 days, usually heralded by fever
Pyrizinamide	Low	Hepatitis-like	Hypersensitivity	Usually in combination with rifampin and/or isoniazid
Rifampin	Low	Hepatitis-like	Direct hepatotoxicity or toxic metabolite	Often occurs in combination with isoniazid. Enzyme inhibition properties of rifampin may ↑ toxic isoniazid metabolites
Rosiglitazone (see troglitazone)				
Simvastatin (see lovastatin)				
Sulfonamides	0.5%–1%	Mainly cytotoxic injury; mixed hepatocellular injury; subacute hepatic necrosis with cirrhosis; chronic active hepatitis	Hypersensitivity; mild hepatotoxicity	*Onset:* often within 5–14 days, occasionally several months. ≈25% had prior exposure to sulfonamides. Includes cotrimoxazole
Tetracyclines	Low	Microvesicular fat droplets in hepatocytes; massive steatosis	Intrinsic hepatotoxicity	Chlortetracycline, oxytetracycline, and tetracycline have been reported to produce hepatic steatosis. 1.5 gm/day of tetracycline, especially when given IV to pregnant women or patients with renal disease

Drug	Frequency	Lesion	Mechanism	Comments
Tolbutamide (see chlorpropamide)				
TCAs (amitriptyline, imipramine, desipramine)	Rare to infrequent	Cholestasis; hepatic necrosis	Hypersensitivity + slight toxicity	Jaundice appears between 7th and 110th day
Trifluoperazine	Rare	Cholestasis	Hypersensitivity	In 80%, icterus develops between 1–4 weeks. Rare after 1st dose. Severe pruritus common
Terbinafine	Low	Mixed or cholestatic; rare fulminant hepatitis	Idiosyncratic, hepatocellular	16 cases of liver failure, 11 deaths
Troglitazone	Low	Hepatocellular, cholestasis	Idiosyncrasy	ALT >20× normal. *Onset:* mean 147 days; range 17–287 days. Removed from market after several patients required liver transplant. Two cases with rosiglitazone
Trovafloxacin (see fluoroquinolones)				
Valproic acid	0.05%–0.1%	Steatosis; focal or massive necrosis	Intrinsic hepatotoxicity; toxic metabolite (4 envalproate)	6%–44% of patients have elevated enzymes. Children age <2 yr at greatest risk for damage
Verapamil (see diltiazem)				
Vitamin A	Dose-related	Fatty liver: nonspecific hepatocellular degeneration; fibrosis; cirrhosis	Intrinsic hepatotoxin	Vitamin A intoxication results from large amounts (40,000 IU/day) for months to years
Zafirlukast (see zileuton)				
Zidovudine	Very low	Microvesicular steatosis	Idiosyncrasy	Usually after several months of therapy. Also reported with didanoside, nevirapine, and indinavir
Zileuton	Low	Unknown	Idiosyncrasy	~2%, usually in first 3 months. Discontinue if AST >3–5× normal.

aACE inhibitor = Angiotensin-converting enzyme inhibitor; CAH = Chronic active hepatitis; INH = Isoniazid; JRA = Juvenile rheumatoid arthritis; LFTs = Liver function tests; MAOIs = Monoamine oxidase inhibitors; NSAIDs = Nonsteroidal anti-inflammatory drugs; PTU = Propylthiouracil; SLE = Systemic lupus erythematosus; TCAs = Tricyclic antidepressants.

Table 27.6 • Selected Herbal Medications/Remedies Associated with Hepatic Injury

Herb	Proposed Use	Toxic Ingredient	Feature of Hepatic Injury
Comfrey Gordolobo yerba tea Mate tea	Health tonic	Pyrrolizidine alkaloids	Veno-occlusive disease
Chinese medicinal tea	Health tonic	T'u-san-chi'i (compositae)	Veno-occlusive disease
Jin Bu Huan	Sedative, analgesic	Lycopodium serratum	Hepatocellular injury: hepatitis, fibrosis, steatosis
Chinese herbs	Eczema, psoriasis	Many	Nonspecific hepatic injury
Germander (tea, capsules)	Weight reduction, health tonic	*Teucrium chamaedrys*	Hepatitis: necrosis, fibrosis
Chaparral leaf	Herbal remedy	*Larrea tridenta*	Hepatic necrosis
Mistletoe/skullcap/ valerian	Herbal tonic, cathartic	Senna, podophyllin, aloin	Elevated liver function tests
Margosa oil	Tonic	Melia azadirachta indica	Reye's syndrome
Pennyroyal oil (squawmint)	Abortifacient, herbal remedy	Labiatae plants (possibly diterpenes)	Elevated liver function tests
Oil of cloves	Dental pain	Unknown	Dose-dependent hepatotoxin

The reader is referred to Chapter 28: Adverse Effects of Drugs on the Liver, written by *Curtis Holt, Pharm.D.,* and *Lucia K. Jim, Pharm.D.,* in the seventh edition of **Applied Therapeutics: The Clinical Use of Drugs** for a more in-depth discussion. All notations to reference numbers are based on the reference list at the end of that chapter. The editors of this handbook express their thanks to Drs. Holt and Jim and acknowledge that this chapter is based upon their work.

Notes:

Chapter 28

Acute Renal Failure

Definitions

- ◆ *Acute renal failure* (ARF) is defined imprecisely to connote a rapid loss of renal function over days or weeks. Traditionally, ARF has been defined as an increase in serum creatinine (SrCr) of >0.5 mg/dL when baseline SrCr is <3.0 mg/dL, and an increase in SrCr of >1.0 mg/dL when the baseline SrCr is >3.0 mg/dL.
- ◆ *Subacute renal failure* occurs over weeks to months.
- ◆ *Chronic renal failure* occurs over months to years.
- ◆ Renal failure can also be described based upon site of renal lesions (e.g., tubular necrosis).

Clinical course of acute renal failure evolves through 3 phases.

- ◆ *1st Phase (Oliguric Phase).* Urine output decreased to 50–400 mL/day. Occurs within 1–2 days of renal insult and lasts a few days to a few weeks.
- ◆ *2nd phase (diuretic phase)* begins with recovery from 1st phase with increased urine volume. This phase may result, in part, from a return to normal GFR before tubular reabsorptive capacity has fully recovered. Lasts a few days, but patients remain markedly azotemic.
- ◆ *3rd phase (recovery phase)* begins with increased urine production and increased ability to concentrate urine. Recovery continues over weeks to months, depending upon severity of initial renal injury.

Pathogenesis

- ◆ The production and elimination of urine requires:
  1) delivery of blood flow to glomeruli;
  2) formation and processing of ultrafiltrate by the glomeruli and tubular cells; and
  3) urine excretion through the ureters, bladder, and urethra.
- ◆ Common causes of ARF are classified and linked to common clinical renal disorders in Table 28.1.
- ◆ *Prerenal azotemia* can develop when blood flow to the kidneys is reduced (e.g., hypotension, dehydration, hemorrhage, CHF)
- ◆ *Functional ARF* develops when medical conditions or drugs impair ultrafiltrate production or intraglomerular hydrostatic pressure (see Figures 28.1 and 28.2).
- ◆ *Intrinsic ARF* can occur in the microvasculature of the nephron (e.g., vasculitis); glomerulus (e.g., poststreptococcal glomerulonephritis); tubules (e.g., acute tubular necrosis from radiocontrast media, aminoglycosides); or interstitium (e.g., acute interstitial nephritis from methicillin).
- ◆ *Postrenal ARF* can develop when urine outflow is obstructed (e.g., calcium stones).

Assessments of Renal Function

♦ *Creatinine Clearance (Cl$_{Cr}$)*. Cockcroft-Gault formula:

$$Cl_{Cr} = \frac{(140 - Age)(LBW)}{(72)(SrCr)}$$

The LBW is an estimation of the patient's lean body weight in kilograms.

♦ Average serum creatinine method:

$$Cl_{Cr} = \frac{(U_V)(U_{Cr})}{0.5(SrCr_1 + SrCr_2)(Time)}$$

SrCr$_1$ and SrCr$_2$ are the serum creatinine concentrations at the start and end of a timed urine collection; and time is the urine collection interval in hours.

♦ *Urinalysis.* The types of urinary sediment and their diagnostic relevance are in Table 28.2. Urine indices to differentiate ARF into prerenal azotemia, acute tubular necrosis, or postrenal obstruction are in Table 28.3.

Prerenal and Functional ARF

♦ CHF is a major cause of functional ARF. Decreased cardiac output results in decreased effective circulating volume and decreased renal perfusion.

♦ NSAIDs cause ARF by inhibiting synthesis of prostaglandins (PGE$_2$ and PGI$_2$), which stimulate afferent arteriole vasodilation in response to decreased renal perfusion.

♦ Inhibition of the renin-angiotensin-aldosterone system in patients with compromised renal blood flow is common cause of functional ARF (e.g., ACE-inhibitors, angiotensin receptor blockers).

Intrinsic ARF-Poststreptococcal Glomerulonephritis

♦ Results from formation of antibodies against streptococcal antigens

♦ Onset usually 7–21 days after start of infection

♦ Diagnosis requires identification of a nephritogenic strain of Group A β-hemolytic streptococci, glomerular damage, and increased streptococcal antibody titers.

♦ Adequate treatment of underlying infection may not prevent poststreptococcal glomerulonephritis.

Tubulointerstitial Disease

♦ Radiocontrast media-induced ATN
  • Risk factors are listed in Table 28.4
  • Prevention strategies are listed in Figure 28.3
♦ Aminoglycoside-induced ATN
  • Risk factors are listed in Table 28.5
♦ Amphotericin-induced nephrotoxicity
  • Incidence as high as 80%
  • Sodium loading and lipid-based amphotericin B (Table 28.6) have minimized nephrotoxicity
♦ Drug-induced acute interstitial nephritis
  • Both humoral and cell-mediated
  • Humoral immune reactions occur within hours of exposure

- Cell-mediated injury can occur days to weeks after exposure
- Penicillins, cephalosporins, quinolones, and sulfonamides can cause.

Postrenal Acute Renal Failure

♦ Risk factors for nephrolithiasis are listed in Table 28.7
♦ Drugs associated with crystal-induced postrenal ARF are listed in Table 28.8

Table 28.1 • Causes of Acute Renal Failure	
Classification	Common Clinical Disorders
Prerenal azotemia	**Intravascular volume depletion** *Hemorrhage (surgery, trauma)* *Dehydration (gastrointestinal losses, aggressive diuretic administration)* *Severe burns* *Hypovolemic shock* *Sequestration (peritonitis, pancreatitis)* **Decreased effective circulating volume** *Cirrhosis with ascites* *Congestive heart failure* **Hypotension, shock syndromes** *Antihypertensive vasodilating medications* *Septic shock* *Cardiomyopathy* **Increased renal vascular occlusion or constriction** *Bilateral renal artery stenosis* *Unilateral renal stenosis in solitary kidney* *Renal artery or vein thrombosis (embolism, atherosclerosis)* *Vasopressor medications (phenylephrine, norepinephrine)*
Functional acute renal failure	**Afferent arteriole vasoconstrictors** *Cyclosporine* *Nonsteroidal anti-inflammatory drugs* **Efferent arteriole vasodilators** *Angiotensin-converting enzyme inhibitors* *Angiotensin II–receptor antagonists*
Intrinsic acute renal failure	**Glomerular disorders** *Glomerulonephritis* *Systemic lupus erythematosus* *Malignant hypertension* *Vasculitic disorders (Wegener's granulomatosus)* **Acute tubular necrosis** *Prolonged prerenal states* *Drug-induced (contrast media, aminoglycosides, amphotericin B)* **Acute interstitial nephritis** *Drug-induced (quinolones, penicillins, sulfa drugs)*
Postrenal acute renal failure	**Ureter obstruction (bilateral or unilateral in solitary kidney)** *Malignancy (prostate or cervical cancer)* *Prostate hypertrophy* *Renal calculi*

Notes:

Table 28.2 • Clinical Significance of Urinary Sediment in Acute Renal Failure

Cellular Debris	Clinical Significance
Red blood cells	Glomerulonephritis IgA nephropathy Lupus nephritis
White blood cells	Infection (pyelonephritis) Glomerulonephritis Acute tubular necrosis
Eosinophils	Drug-induced acute interstitial nephritis Pyelonephritis Renal transplant rejection
Hyaline casts	Glomerulonephritis Pyelonephritis Congestive heart failure
Red blood cell casts	Acute tubular necrosis Glomerulonephritis Interstitial nephritis
White blood cell casts	Pyelonephritis Interstitial nephritis
Granular casts	Dehydration Interstitial nephritis Glomerulonephritis Acute tubular necrosis
Tubular cell casts	Acute tubular necrosis
Fatty casts	Nephrotic syndrome
Myoglobin	Rhabdomyolysis
Crystals	Nonspecific

Table 28.3 • Urinary Indices in Acute Renal Failure

Component	Prerenal Azotemia	Acute Tubular Necrosis	Postrenal Obstruction
Urine Na^+ (mEq/L)	<20	>40	>40
FE_{Na+}	<1%	>2%	>1%
Urine/plasma creatinine	>40	<20	<20
Specific gravity	>1.010	<1.010	Variable
Urine osmolality (mOsm/kg)	Up to 1,200	<300	<300

Table 28.4 • Proven Risk Factors for Developing Radiocontrast Media–induced Acute Tubular Necrosis

Diabetic nephropathy
Chronic renal failure
Severe congestive heart failure
Volume depletion/hypotension
Dosage and frequency of contrast administration

Table 28.5 • Risk-factors for Developing Aminoglycoside Nephrotoxicity

Patient Factors
Elderly
Underlying renal disease
Dehydration
Hypotension/shock syndromes
Hepatorenal syndrome

Aminoglycoside Factors
Aminoglycoside choice: gentamicin > tobramycin > amikacin
Therapy >3 days
Multiple daily dosing
Serum trough >2 mg/L
Recent aminoglycoside therapy

Concomitant Drug Therapy
Furosemide
Amphotericin B
Vancomycin
Cisplatinum
Cyclosporine
Radiocontrast media
Foscarnet

Table 28.6 • FDA-approved Lipid-based Amphotericin B (AmB) Products and Indications

Product	FDA Indication
Abelcet	Invasive fungal infections in patients intolerant or refractory to standard AmB
AmBisome	Empiric therapy for presumed fungemia in immunocompromised patients; therapy in patients intolerant or refractory to standard AmB
Amphotec	Invasive aspergillosis in patients intolerant or refractory to standard AmB

Table 28.7 • Risk Factors for Nephrolithiasis

Low urine volume
Hypercalciuria
Hyperoxaluria
Hyperuricosuria
Hypercitruria
Chronically low or high urinary pH

Notes:

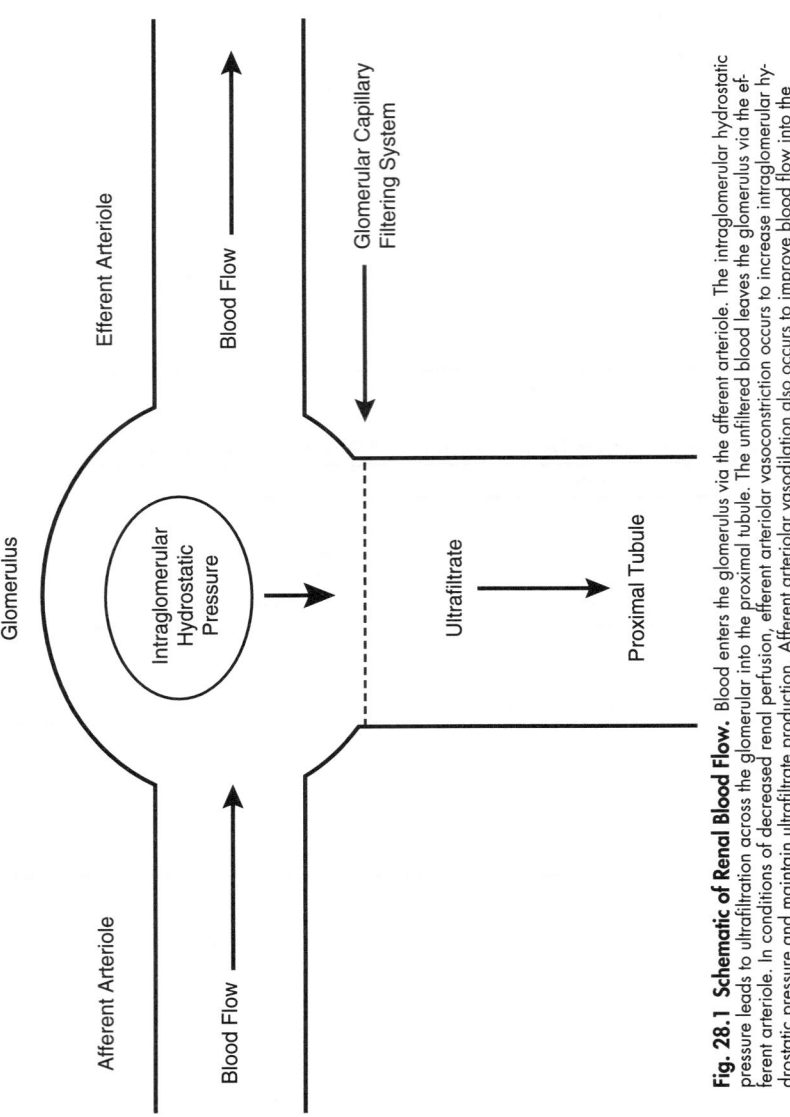

Fig. 28.1 Schematic of Renal Blood Flow. Blood enters the glomerulus via the afferent arteriole. The intraglomerular hydrostatic pressure leads to ultrafiltration across the glomerulus into the proximal tubule. The unfiltered blood leaves the glomerulus via the efferent arteriole. In conditions of decreased renal perfusion, efferent arteriolar vasoconstriction occurs to increase intraglomerular hydrostatic pressure and maintain ultrafiltrate production. Afferent arteriolar vasodilation also occurs to improve blood flow into the glomerulus.

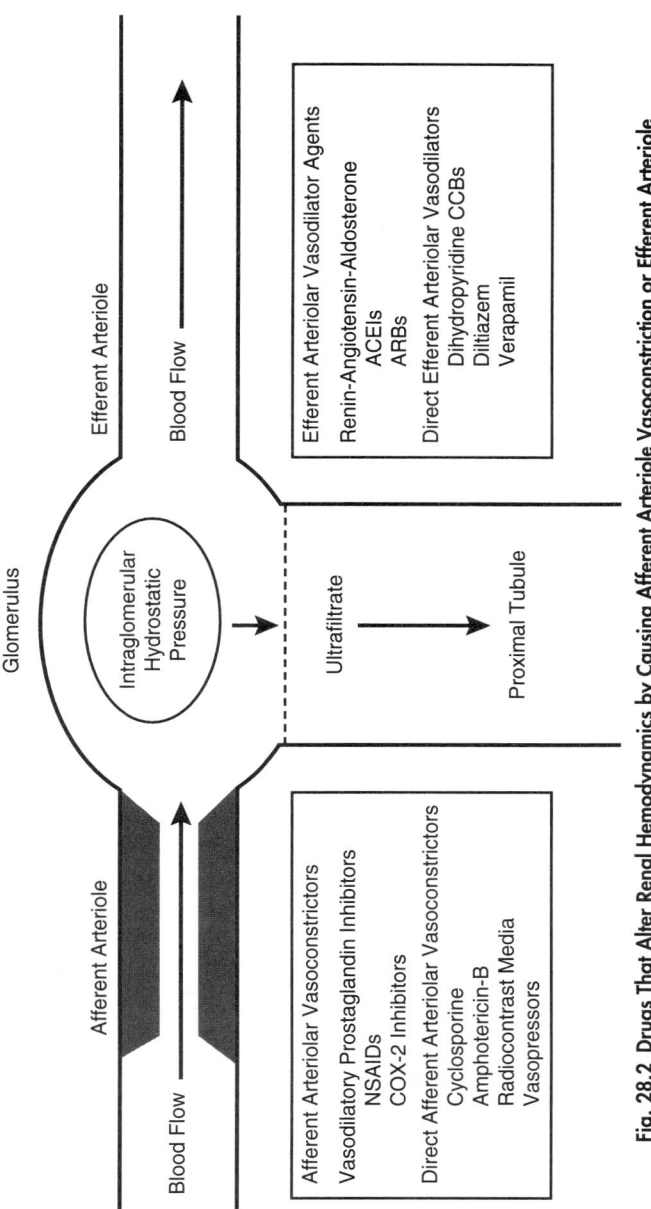

Fig. 28.2 Drugs That Alter Renal Hemodynamics by Causing Afferent Arteriole Vasoconstriction or Efferent Arteriole Vasodilation. ACEIs, angiotensin-converting enzyme inhibitors; ARBs, angiotensin II–receptor blockers; CCB, calcium channel blockers; NSAIDs, nonsteroidal anti-inflammatory drugs.

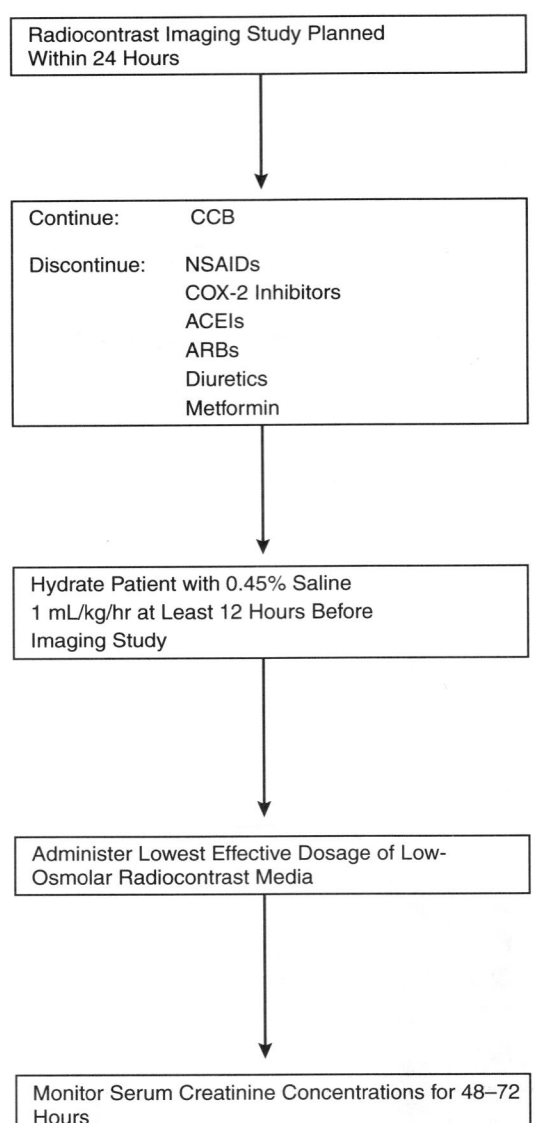

Fig. 28.3 Prevention of Radiocontrast-induced Acute Tubular Necrosis in High-Risk Populations. ACEIs, angiotensin-converting enzyme inhibitors; ARBs, angiotensin II–receptor blockers; CCB, calcium channel blockers; NSAIDs, nonsteroidal anti-inflammatory drugs.

The reader is referred to Chapter 29: Acute Renal Failure, written by *Donald R. Brophy, Pharm.D.,* in the seventh edition of **Applied Therapeutics: The Clinical Use of Drugs** for a more in-depth discussion. The editors of this handbook express their thanks to Dr. Brophy and acknowledge that this chapter is based upon his work.

Chapter 29

Chronic Renal Failure

Definitions

- ♦ **Chronic Renal Failure.** Progressive deterioration in renal function leading to irreversible damage to nephrons.
- ♦ **End-Stage Renal Disease (ESRD).** Chronic renal failure that necessitates dialysis to sustain life. Most common causes of ESRD are listed in Table 29.1
- ♦ **Renal Insufficiency.** A mild reduction in GFR in the absence of overt signs and symptoms.
- ♦ **Azotemia.** A laboratory diagnosis when nitrogenous wastes accumulate as GFR deteriorates.
- ♦ **Uremia.** Symptomatic renal failure.

Prevention

- ♦ ACE-inhibitors should be considered in patients with type 1 diabetes who are at high risk for nephropathy regardless of BP.
- ♦ Angiotensin II-receptor antagonists to prevent and slow progressive renal disease should prove to have benefits similar to ACE-inhibitors.
- ♦ Hyperlipidemia can contribute to progression of renal disease, and antihyperlipidemic drugs to prevent disease progression is advocated by many.

Clinical Features

- ♦ Most patients remain asymptomatic until GFR is <25% of normal.
- ♦ When GFR is <10%, symptoms of uremia appear.
- ♦ When GFR is <5%, dialysis or transplantation is required.
- ♦ Clinical manifestations and metabolic complications of uremia are listed in Table 29.2.

Diabetic Nephropathy (DN)

- ♦ Occurs in about 1/3 of all patients with diabetes and accounts for about 50% of ESRD in USA.
- ♦ Urine albumin excretion (UAE) correlates with rate of progression of renal disease and is useful in guiding therapy to prevent or delay progression of nephropathy.
- ♦ Functional stages of DN based primarily on GFR and UAE (Table 29.3).
- ♦ Poor glycemic control, systemic hypertension, and high-protein intake (>1.5 gm/kg body weight/day) are three primary risk factors for progression of renal disease.

♦ Intensive insulin therapy, ACE inhibitors, and limited protein diet are cornerstones of treatment.

Fluid and Electrolyte Management

♦ Most with ESRD require **sodium** and **fluid restriction** (about 100 mEq/day; 2000 mL/day) with modifications to special needs of patients. Loop diuretic in combination with another often is needed.

♦ Hyperkalemia is rare when GFR is >10 mL/min. Hyperkalemia can be treated with *calcium* (protects the myocardium but has no effect on K^+ concentration); *bicarbonate* (seldom effective and not advocated because of sodium load); *glucose plus insulin* (5–10 units IV insulin with 25–50 gm glucose); B_2 *agonists* (10–20 mg nebulized albuterol); *kayexalate* (15–30 gm PO) with sorbitol in a premixed formulation; or dialysis.

♦ Severe metabolic acidosis is rare because of compensatory hyperventilation. The stable ESRD patient typically has a mildly reduced serum bicarbonate, a reduced arterial P_{CO_2}, and slightly reduced arterial pH.

♦ **Renal osteodystrophy** is the term used to describe the skeletal complications of ESRD that primarily result from changes in calcium and phosphorus homeostasis in uremic patients. Treatment includes dietary phosphorus restriction (Table 29.5), phosphate-binding agents (Table 29.6), and vitamin (to prevent and treat secondary hyperparathyroidism).

♦ **Hypothyroidism** can occur because the kidney is involved in various aspects of thyroid hormone metabolism.

♦ **Glucose** and insulin clearance are altered in ESRD. Insulin doses should be adjusted.

♦ **GI abnormalities** are common (e.g., anorexia, nausea, vomiting, hiccups, abdominal pain, GI bleeding, diarrhea, constipation).

♦ **Uremic encephalopathy** (e.g., fatigability, daytime drowsiness, insomnia, slurred speech, impaired cognition, vomiting, emotional volatility), **peripheral neuropathies,** and abnormalities in **autonomic nervous system** are associated with CRF.

♦ **Dermatologic** abnormalities (e.g., hyperpigmentation, abnormal perspiration, dryness, persistent pruritus) also occur with CRF.

♦ **Leg muscle cramps** of unknown etiology frequently occur and can be treated with levocarnitine supplementation.

♦ **Immune suppression** enhance susceptibility to infections.

♦ Until Cl_{Cr} is <30 mL/min, magnesium is eliminated renally sufficient to maintain balance. Severe **hypermagnesemia** can depress cardiac conduction. Avoid magnesium containing antacids or laxatives.

Anemia Management

♦ Anemia characteristically is normocytic and normochromic in the absence of iron, folate, or B_{12} deficiency. Generally begins to develop when GFR <30 mL/min.

♦ Anemia is most commonly due to inadequate production of erythropoietin (EPO); increased presence of inhibitors of erythropoiesis; decreased RBC life-span; and blood loss (and secondary iron deficiency).

♦ Correct iron deficiency if present, then 200 mg/day of elemental iron (Table 29.4) during EPO therapy.

♦ Initial recommended doses for EPO are 120–180 μ/kg/week IV or 80–120 μ/kg/week SQ. Lower doses of EPO with SQ administration are needed to sustain targeted hematocrit.

Complications

- **Pericarditis** can develop and can be attributable to trauma, malnutrition, preceding infection, and severe uremia.
- **Hypertension** develops in an estimated 80% of hemodialyzed patients and 50% in those being peritoneally dialyzed.
- **Hyperlipidemia** is a common complication and may accelerate atherogenesis.

Table 29.1 • Main Causes of End-Stage Renal Disease, 1993–1997

Cause	% of New ESRD Cases
Diabetes	40.3
Hypertension	24.6
Glomerulonephritis	10.5
Interstitial nephritis	4.2
Cystic kidney disease	2.5
Others	17.9

Data from reference 1.
ESRD, end-stage renal disease.

Table 29.2 • Metabolic Effects of Uremia

Fluid, Electrolyte, and Acid-Base Effects
- Fluid retention
- Hyperkalemia
- Hypermagnesemia
- Hyperphosphatemia
- Hypocalcemia
- Metabolic acidosis

Hematologic
- Anemia
- Hemostatic abnormalities
- Immune suppression

Cardiovascular
- Hypertension
- Congestive heart failure
- Pericarditis
- Atherosclerosis
- Arrhythmias

Endocrine
- Calcium–phosphorous imbalances
- Hyperparathyroidism
- Metabolic bone disease
- Altered thyroid function
- Altered carbohydrate metabolism
- Hypophyseal-gonadal dysfunction
- Decreased insulin metabolism
- Erythropoietin deficiency

Musculoskeletal
- Renal bone disease
- Amyloidosis
- Extraskeletal calcifications

Gastrointestinal
- Anorexia
- Nausea, vomiting
- Delayed gastric emptying
- GI bleeding
- Ulcers

Neurologic
- Lethargy
- Depressed sensorium
- Tremor
- Asterixis
- Muscular irritability and cramps
- Seizures
- Motor weakness
- Peripheral neuropathy
- Coma

Dermatologic
- Altered pigmentation
- Pruritus

Psychologic
- Depression
- Anxiety
- Psychosis

Miscellaneous
- Reduced exercise tolerance

GI, gastrointestinal.

Table 29.3 • The Functional Stages of Diabetic Nephropathy

Stage	Onset from Diagnosis	Functional Abnormalities	Risk Factors for Progression
I: Clinically silent	Within 3 yr	↑ GFR	Hyperglycemia, intraglomerular hypertension, systemic hypertension, high protein intake
II: Incipient DN	7–15 yr	Microalbuminuria[a]; GFR starting to decline (may be normal or slightly ↑)	Hyperglycemia, systemic hypertension, high protein intake
III: Clinical DN	10–30 yr	Albuminuria[b]; GFR declining	Systemic hypertension, high protein intake
IV: ESRD	20–40 yr	GFR <10 mL/min	—

[a]Microalbuminuria = Urinary albumin excretion 30 to 300 mg/24 hr.
[b]Albuminuria = Urinary albumin excretion >300 mg/24 hr.
DN, diabetic nephropathy; ESRD, end-stage renal disease; GFR, glomerular filtration rate.

Notes:

Table 29.4 • Oral Iron Preparations

Preparation	Iron Form	Common Brand Names	Elemental Iron per Total Amount (mg/gm)	Commonly Prescribed Unit Size[a] (Amount Elemental Iron) (in mg)	Number of Units/Day to Yield 200 mg Elemental Iron
Ferrous sulfate	Ferrous	Feosol, Slow FE, Fer-In-Sol	200	325 (65)	3 tablets
Ferrous gluconate	Ferrous	Simron, Fergon	120	325 (38)	5 tablets
Ferrous fumarate	Ferrous	Femiron, Feostat	330	200 (66)	3 capsules
Iron polysaccharide	Ferric	Niferex, Nu-Iron	1,000	150 (150)	2 capsules

[a]Unit size reflects common tablet/capsule sizes prescribed and not necessarily that of the brand names listed.

Notes:

Table 29.5 • Phosphorus Content of Select High-Protein Foods

Food	Portion Size	Phosphorus Content (mg)
Black-eyed peas, cooked	1 cup	288
Cheese, American	4 ounces	1,200
Cheese, cheddar	4 ounces	545
Cheese, creamed cottage	4 ounces	150
Cheese, Swiss	4 ounces	800
Chicken, cooked	3½ ounces	190
Chocolate candy	2 ounces	130
Egg	1 large	100
Fish, cooked	4 ounces	400
Hamburger, ground sirloin	3½ ounces	186
Ice cream	8 ounces	163
Kidney beans, cooked	1 cup	278
Lamb	3½ ounces	200
Liver, chicken	3½ ounces	312
Milk, whole or skim	8 ounces (1 cup)	278
Peanut butter	2 tablespoons	118
Peanuts	3½ ounces	466
Pork tenderloin	3½ ounces	301
Salmon, canned	3½ ounces	344
Sardines, canned in oil	3½ ounces	434
Shrimp	3½ ounces	156
Soybeans	1 cup	322
Steak, sirloin	4 ounces	282
Tofu	3½ ounces	128
Tuna fish, canned	3½ ounces	250
Turkey	3½ ounces	200
Yogurt, plain	8 ounces	270

Data from reference 129.

Notes:

Table 29.6 • Phosphate-Binding Agents

Product	Select Available Agents[a]	Content of Elemental Mineral	Starting Dose
Calcium carbonate (40% calcium)	Tums	200, 300, 400 mg	0.8–2 g elemental Ca with meals
	Os-Cal-500	500 mg	
	Nephro-Calci	600 mg	
	Caltrate 600	600 mg	
	Calcarb HD (powder)	2,400 mg/packet	
	$CaCO_3$ (multiple preparations)	200–600 mg	
Calcium acetate (25% calcium)	Phos-Lo 667 mg	169 mg	2–3 tablets with meals
Calcium citrate (21% calcium)	Citracal (tablet and effervescent tablet)	200 mg 500 mg (effervescent tablet)	Not generally recommended
Aluminum hydroxide	AlternaGel (suspension)	600 mg/5 mL	300–600 mg with meals
	Amphojel (tablet and suspension)	300, 600 mg (tablet) 320 mg/5 mL (suspension)	
	Alu-Cap (capsule)	400 mg	
	Alu-Tab	500 mg	
	Basaljel (tablet, capsule, and suspension)	500 mg (tablet, capsule) 400 mg/mL (suspension)	
Magnesium carbonate	Mag-Carb (capsule)	70 mg	70 mg with meals
Magnesium hydroxide	Milk of Magnesia (tablet and suspension)	300, 600 mg (tablet) 400, 800 mg/5 mL (suspension)	300–400 mg with meals
Sevelamer hydrochloride (polymer-based)	Renagel (tablet, capsule)	403 mg (capsule) 400, 800 mg (tablet)	800–1,600 mg with meals

[a]Tablet unless noted otherwise.

The reader is referred to Chapter 30: Chronic Renal Failure, written by *Joanna Q. Hudson, Pharm.D.,* and *Curtis A. Johnson, Pharm.D.,* in the seventh edition of **Applied Therapeutics: The Clinical Use of Drugs** for a more in-depth discussion. All notations to reference numbers are based on the reference list at the end of that chapter. The editors of this handbook express their thanks to Drs. Hudson and Johnson and acknowledge that this chapter is based upon their work.

Notes:

Chapter 30

Renal Dialysis

Dialysis is a process to facilitate the removal of excess water and toxins from the body, which accumulate as a result of inadequate renal function.

Hemodialysis

♦ Process whereby a patient's anticoagulated blood and an electrolyte solution (dialysate) are perfused to opposite sides of a semipermeable membrane (artificial kidney).

♦ Metabolic waste products are removed from the blood by diffusing down a concentration gradient into the dialysate.

♦ Patients typically are dialyzed for 3–4 hr 3 times/week (e.g., Monday, Wednesday, Friday).

♦ Fluids ingested and produced through the metabolic process are retained in the patient between dialyses.

♦ Vascular access for dialysis requires an arteriovenous (AV) fistula or insertion of an artificial AV graft that connects the artery and vein.

♦ Patients without risk factors for heparin anticoagulation (e.g., bleeding disorder, recent surgery) are anticoagulated with heparin 2000 units IV 3–5 minutes before dialysis and with 1000 units/hr during dialysis. Monitor ACT hourly during dialysis.

♦ **Complications of Hemodialysis**

• *Hypotension* is primarily caused by excessive fluid removal at a rate exceeding mobilization of fluid stores, or occasionally, by excessive heating of the dialysate and subsequent vasodilation.

• *Hypersensitivity.* Anaphylaxis can develop secondary to dialyzer membrane or to ethylene oxide used to sterilize the dialyzer.

• *Dialysis Disequilibrium.* Rapid removal of urea lowers plasma osmolality, shifts free water into the brain, and induces cerebral edema.

• *Thrombosis* is the most common cause for loss of vascular access site.

• *Infection of the access site* is usually caused by *Staphylococcus aureus* or *Staphylococcus epidermidis.*

• *Aluminum toxicity* is caused by a high aluminum content in water or from excess aluminum used as binding agents for phosphate in the GI tract.

• *Amyloidosis* is caused by deposition of β_2-microglobulin in joints and soft tissues over prolonged periods. It occurs in about 50% after 12 years of dialysis.

• *Malnutrition.* Inadequate dietary intake, loss of amino acids by dialysis, a catabolic state induced by chronic renal failure, and multifactorial complications of end-stage renal disease contribute to malnutrition.

Peritoneal Dialysis

♦ Process whereby 2–3 L of sterile dialysate solution are instilled into the peritoneal cavity. Solution remains within the cavity for 3–8 hr before being drained and replaced with a fresh solution 3–4 times/day.

♦ Uremic toxins are removed by diffusion down a concentration gradient into the dialysate solution.

♦ Continuous ambulatory peritoneal dialysis and continuous cycling peritoneal dialysis are the dominant forms of chronic peritoneal dialysis. Less common forms are intermittent peritoneal dialysis and nocturnal intermittent peritoneal dialysis.

♦ Abdominal cavity access is through an indwelling catheter of silicone rubber or polyurethane.

♦ **Complications of Peritoneal Dialysis**

  • *Peritonitis* is the most significant complication. It is frequently caused by S. epidermidis (30%) or S. aureus (10%).

  • *Catheter exit-site infection* is most often caused by S. aureus and Pseudomonas species.

  • *Weight gain.* Dextrose in dialysate solutions serves as an osmotic agent for removal of fluid during each exchange and contributes about 500–1,000 calories absorbed from dextrose in peritoneal dialysis solutions.

Hemofiltration

♦ Process whereby blood is pumped under the influence of cardiac function through a hemofilter that serves as a site for fluid removal by ultrafiltration.

♦ It can be used for patients with acute renal failure in the acute care unit who have cardiovascular compromise such that hemodialysis is not a treatment option.

♦ Access to systemic circulation is through arteries (continuous arteriovenous hemofiltration) or veins (continuous venovenous hemofiltration).

♦ Lactated Ringer's usually is used to replace fluids to maintain adequate hydration and perfusion.

Dialysis of Drugs

♦ Drugs with high dialyzability are:

  • Low in molecular weight (MW <1 L/kg).

  • Hydrophilic.

  • Not highly protein-bound.

  • Have a small volume of distribution (a high Vd suggests extensive extravascular tissue binding and little drug available in the blood for dialysis clearance).

♦ The relative dialyzability of various drugs is listed in Table 30.1.

Notes:

Table 30.1 • Hemodialysis of Drugs

Dialyzable (50%–100%)

Acyclovir (Zovirax)	Ethanol	Methanol
Amikacin (Amikin)	Flucytosine (Ancobon)	Metronidazole (Flagyl)
Aspirin	Gentamicin (Garamycin)	Minoxidil (Loniten)
Ceftazidime (Fortaz)	Isoniazid	Neomycin
Chloral hydrate (Noctec)	Kanamycin (Kantrex)	Netilmicin (Netromycin)
Clavulanic acid	Lithium (Lithobid)	Tobramycin (Nebcin)

Moderately Dialyzable (20%–50%)

Acetaminophen (Tylenol)	Cefotaxime (Claforan)	Mezlocillin (Mezlin)
Acetazolamide (Diamox)	Cefoxitin (Mefoxin)	Nadolol (Corgard)
Amoxicillin (Amoxil)	Ceftizoxime (Cefizox)	Penicillin G
Ampicillin (Omnipen)	Cephalexin (Keflex)	Phenobarbital
Atenolol (Tenormin)	Cephalothin (Keflin)	Piperacillin (Pipracil)
Aztreonam (Azactam)	Cilastatin	Primidone (Mysoline)
Bretylium (Bretylol)	Cyclophosphamide (Cytoxan)	Procainamide (Pronestyl)
Captopril (Capoten)	Enalapril (Vasotec)	Sulfamethoxazole (Gantanol)
Carbenicillin (Geocillin)	Ethosuximide (Zarontin)	Ticarcillin (Ticar)
Cefaclor (Ceclor)	Fluconazole (Diflucan)	Tocainide (Tonocard)
Cefamandole (Mandol)	Imipenem (Primaxin)	Trimethoprim (Trimpex)
Cefazolin (Kefzol)	Meprobamate (Equanil)	

Slightly Dialyzable (5%–20%)

Amantadine (Symmetrel)	Cimetidine (Tagamet)	Pentobarbital (Nembutal)
Azathioprine (Imuran)	Erythromycin (E-mycin)	Quinidine
Cefonicid (Monocid)	Ethambutol (Myambutol)	Ranitidine (Zantac)
Cefoperazone (Cefobid)	Methaqualone (Quaalude)	Secobarbital (Seconal)
Cefotetan (Cefotan)	Methyldopa (Aldomet)	Tetracycline (Achromycin)
Chloramphenicol (Chloromycetin)	Methylprednisolone (Solu-Medrol)	

Not Dialyzable (0%–5%)

Ceftriaxone (Rocephin)	Flecainide (Tambocor)	Nafcillin (Unipen)
Chlordiazepoxide (Librium)	Flumazenil (Mazicon)	Oxacillin (Prostaphlin)
Clindamycin (Cleocin)	Flurazepam (Dalmane)	Oxazepam (Serax)
Clonidine (Catapres)	Ketoconazole (Nizoral)	Phenothiazines
Cloxacillin (Tegopen)	Lidocaine (Xylocaine)	Propoxyphene (Darvon)
Colchicine	Mebendazole (Vermox)	Propranolol (Inderal)
Diazepam (Valium)	Methicillin (Staphcillin)	Tolbutamide (Orinase)
Dicloxacillin (Dynapen)	Methotrexate (Mexate)	Valproate (Depakene)
Digitoxin (Crystodigin)	Metoclopramide (Reglan)	Vancomycin (Vancocin)
Digoxin (Lanoxin)	Miconazole (Monistat)	Verapamil (Isoptin)
Disopyramide (Norpace)	Midazolam (Versed)	Zidovudine (Retrovir)
Doxycycline (Vibramycin)	Minocycline (Minocin)	

The reader is referred to Chapter 31: Renal Dialysis, written by *Thomas J. Comstock, Pharm.D.,* in the seventh edition of **Applied Therapeutics: The Clinical Use of Drugs** for a more in-depth discussion. The editors of this handbook express their thanks to Dr. Comstock and acknowledge that this chapter is based upon his work.

Notes:

Notes:

Chapter 31

Dosing of Drugs in Renal Failure

Principles

♦ The elimination of drugs cleared by the kidney can be impaired significantly in patients with renal insufficieny (see Table 31.1).

♦ When a moderate (50%–75%) to large (75%) percentage of the drug is *excreted unchanged,* dosage adjustments usually will be required in patients with renal insufficiency. When less than 50% of a drug is eliminated in the urine as the parent compound, the need for dosage reduction is less clear.

♦ Some drugs are metabolized to active or toxic compounds that are then eliminated by the kidney (e.g., cyclophosphamide and meperidine). Normeperidine, the major metabolite of meperidine, accumulates in patients with renal insufficiency and has been associated with seizures.

Pharmacokinetics and Pharmacodynamics in Renal Failure

♦ Some drugs can be displaced from *tissue* binding sites in patients with renal failure and result in a decrease in the volume of distribution (Vd) and increases in serum concentrations of the drug. For example, digoxin Vd decreases from ≈500 L in normals to ≈225–250 L in patients with renal insufficiency.

♦ Some acidic, highly bound drugs (e.g., phenytoin) are displaced from serum proteins in renal insufficiency. This increases the percentage of free (unbound) drug and metabolic clearance. The net result of these two effects is that therapeutic serum levels (free plus bound) may be lower in patients with renal failure.

♦ Pharmacodynamics of drugs in renal failure require more study; patients can experience altered responses to some drugs (e.g., nifedipine, morphine).

Notes:

Table 31.1 • Pharmacokinetics and Dosing Guidelines for Drugs Commonly Used in Renal Failure [131]

Drug	Oral Availability (%)	Protein Binding (%)	Vd (L/kg)	Metabolism and Excretion	$t_{1/2}$ (hr)	Normal Dose Cl_{Cr} >50 mL/min	Dose Change with Renal Failure Cl_{Cr} (mL/min)	Effect of Dialysis
Acyclovir	15–30	15	0.7	76–82% excreted renally; 14% hepatic	Normal: 2.1–3.2 Anephric: 20	5 mg/kg Q 8 hr	10–50: 5 mg/kg Q 12–24 hr <10: 2.5 mg/kg Q 24 hr	Dialyzed; 80 mL/min
Allopurinol	90	0	0.6	Metabolized to active oxypurinol metabolite, which is excreted renally; 6–12% excreted unchanged renally	Normal: 1.1–1.6 Anephric: No change; 7 days oxypurinol	300 mg QD	10–50: 200 mg QD <10: 100 mg QD	Oxypurinol; moderately dialyzed
Amikacin	Parenteral	<5	0.2–0.3	94–99% excreted renally	Normal: 2–3 Anephric: 36–82	See section on aminoglycoside pharmacokinetics	See section on aminoglycoside pharmacokinetics	Dialyzed; 22–38 mL/min
Amphotericin B	Parenteral	90–95	4	95–97% hepatic metabolism or inactivation in body tissue; 3.5–5.5% excreted unchanged renally	Normal: Initial: 24–48; Terminal: 15 days Anephric: No change	0.3–1 mg/kg Q 24 hr	10–50: 100% Q 24 hr <10: 100% Q 24–48 hr (to minimize azotemia)	Not dialyzed: large Vd
Ampicillin	32–76	29	0.3	73–92% excreted renally; 12–24% hepatic metabolism or biliary elimination	Normal: 0.8–1.5 Anephric: 20	1–2 g Q 4–6 hr	10–50: 1–1.5 g Q 6 hr <10: 50% 1 g Q 8–12 hr	Moderately dialyzed
Atenolol	50	<5	1.2	75% excreted renally; 10% hepatic; 10% feces	Normal: 5–6 Anephric: 42–73	50–100 mg QD	10–50: ↓ 50% and titrate <10: ↓ 50% and titrate	Moderately dialyzed
Aztreonam	Parenteral	50–60	0.15–0.38	60–70% excreted renally; 12% hepatic	Normal: 1.3–2.2 Anephric: 6–9	1–2 g Q 6–8 hr	10–50: 1–2 g Q 8–12 hr <10: 1 g Q 12–24 hr	Moderately dialyzed

Drug	Route/Bioavailability	Protein binding (%)	Vd	Elimination	Half-life (hr)	Dose	Dosing adjustment	Dialysis
Captopril	65	30 (↓R)	0.7	36–42% excreted renally; 50% hepatic	*Normal:* 1.7–1.9 *Anephric:* 21–32	6.25–12.5 mg Q 8–12 hr	*10–50:* No change <*10:* ↓ 25% and titrate	Moderately dialyzed; 80–120 mL/min
Cefazolin	Parenteral	84–92	0.2	>95% excreted renally; 3–5% hepatic	*Normal:* 1.8–2.6 *Anephric:* 12–40	1–2 g Q 8 hr	*10–50:* 0.5–1.5 g Q 12 hr <*10:* 0.5–1 g Q 24 hr	Moderately dialyzed
Cefixime	50	69	0.1–1.0	20–40% excreted renally; 50% excreted by nonrenal mechanisms	*Normal:* 3.5 *Anephric:* ?	200–400 mg Q 12–24 hr	*10–50:* No change <*10:* 50% Q 12–24 hr	Not dialyzed
Cefoperazone	Parenteral	87–93	0.16	70–85% excreted unchanged in bile; 15–30% excreted renally	*Normal:* 1.6–2.6 *Anephric:* 2.5	1–2 g Q 8–12 hr	*10–50:* No change <*10:* ↓ with concurrent hepatic disease	Slightly dialyzed
Cefotaxime	Parenteral	38	0.22–0.36	40–60% hepatic (desacetyl active metabolite; 25% activity of parent compound); 40–65% excreted renally	*Normal:* 0.9–1.1 *Anephric:* 2.3–3.5, 12–20 (metabolite)	1–2 g Q 6–12 hr	*10–50:* 1–2 g Q 12 hr <*10:* 0.5–1 g Q 12 hr	Moderately dialyzed
Cefotetan	Parenteral	75–91	0.13	50–88% excreted renally; 12% excreted in bile	*Normal:* 3–4.2 *Anephric:* 13	1–2 g Q 12 hr	*10–50:* 1–2 g Q 24 hr <*10:* 0.5–1 g Q 24 hr	Slightly/moderately dialyzed
Cefoxitin	Parenteral	65–79	0.27	85% excreted renally; up to 15% biliary and/or hepatic	*Normal:* 0.7–0.8 *Anephric:* 12–24	1–2 g Q 6–8 hr	*10–50:* 1–2 g Q 12–24 hr <*10:* 0.5–1 g Q 24 hr	Moderately dialyzed

(continued)

Table 31.1 • Pharmacokinetics and Dosing Guidelines for Drugs Commonly Used in Renal Failure [31] (continued)

Drug	Oral Availability (%)	Protein Binding (%)	Vd (L/kg)	Metabolism and Excretion	t½ (hr)	Normal Dose ClCr >50 mL/min	Dose Change with Renal Failure ClCr (mL/min)	Effect of Dialysis
Ceftazidime	Parenteral	20–30	0.2–0.3	73–84% excreted renally	*Normal:* 1.6–2 *Anephric:* 13–25	1–2 g Q 8 hr	*10–50:* 1–2 g Q 12–24 hr *<10:* 0.5 g Q 24 hr	Dialyzed
Ceftizoxime	Parenteral	17–25	0.2–0.4	78–92% excreted renally	*Normal:* 1.4–1.7 *Anephric:* 19–30	1–2 g Q 8–12 hr	*10–50:* 1–2 g Q 12–24 hr *<10:* 0.5 g Q 24 hr	Moderately dialyzed
Ceftriaxone	Parenteral	83–96 (concentration-dependent)	0.1	40–67% excreted renally; 40% excreted in bile	*Normal:* 6.5–8.9 *Anephric:* 12	1–2 g Q 12–24 hr	*10–50:* 1–2 g Q 24 hr *<10:* 1–2 g Q 24 hr	Not dialyzed
Cefuroxime	40–50 (as axetil salt)	33	0.19	90–95% excreted renally	*Normal:* 1.1–1.7 *Anephric:* 15–17	0.75–1.5 g Q 6–8 hr	*10–50:* 50–75% Q 8–12 hr *<10:* 25–50% Q 24 hr	Moderately dialyzed
Cephradine	90–100	6–20	0.25–0.33	80–95% excreted renally; 5–20% hepatic metabolism or biliary/fecal elimination	*Normal:* 0.7–0.9 *Anephric:* 8–15	250–500 mg Q 6 hr	*10–50:* 250–500 mg Q 12 hr *<10:* 250–500 mg Q 24 hr	Moderately dialyzed
Cimetidine	62	20	0.9–1.1	40–80% excreted renally; some metabolism	*Normal:* 1.5 *Anephric:* 3.3–4.6	*PO:* 400 mg Q 12 hr *IV:* 300 mg Q 8 hr	*10–50:* ↓ 25% *<10:* ↓ 50%	Slightly dialyzed
Ciprofloxacin	50–85	22	2.2	62% excreted renally; the rest cleared hepatically, in the bile and via intestinal mucosa	*Normal:* 4 *Anephric:* 8.5	250–750 mg Q 12 hr (PO)	*10–50:* 250–500 mg Q 12 hr *<10:* 250–750 mg Q 24 hr	Slightly dialyzed

Drug					Normal/Anephric (hr)	Dose	10-50 / <10	Dialysis
Clindamycin	50	94	0.6	85% hepatic to active and inactive metabolites; 10% excreted renally; 5% feces	*Normal:* 2–4 *Anephric:* 1.6–3.4	600–900 mg Q 6–8 hr	*10–50:* No change *<10:* No change	Not dialyzed
Codeine	40–70	7	3–4	Hepatic with some active metabolites; little renal elimination (5–17%)	*Normal:* 2.9–4 *Anephric:* 19	No change	*10–50:* ↓ 25% and titrate *<10:* ↓ 50% and titrate	?
Cyclosporine	<5–89	>96	3.5	Extensively metabolized to active and inactive metabolites; <1% excreted renally	*Normal:* 6–13 *Anephric:* 16	No change	*10–50:* No change *<10:* No change	Not dialyzed
Digoxin	70	25 (↓R)	5–8 (↓R)	70% excreted renally	*Normal:* 36–44 *Anephric:* 80–120	No change	*10–50:* ↓ 50% *<10:* ↓ 75%	Not dialyzed
Enalapril[a]	36–44	<50	1	61% excreted renally; 33% excreted in feces	*Normal:* 5–11 *Anephric:* 36	No change	*10–50:* ↓ 50% and titrate *<10:* ↓ 50% and titrate	Slightly/moderately dialyzed
Erythromycin	30–65 (varies with salt)	84–90	0.9	85–95% hepatic to inactive metabolites; 5–15% excreted renally	*Normal:* 1.4–2 *Anephric:* 4	0.25–1 g Q 6 hr	*10–50:* No change *<10:* No change	Slightly dialyzed
Ethambutol	75–80	<5	1.6	65–80% excreted renally and 20% in feces; 8–15% hepatic	*Normal:* 3.1 *Anephric:* 18–20	15 mg/kg Q 24 hr	*10–50:* 7.5– 10 mg/kg Q 24 hr *<10:* 5 mg/kg Q 24 hr	Slightly dialyzed
Fluconazole	>85	11–12	0.8	70% excreted renally; some hepatic metabolism	*Normal:* 20–50 *Anephric:* 98	100–200 mg Q 24 hr	*10–50:* 50–200 mg Q 24 hr *<10:* 50–100 mg Q 24 hr	Moderately dialyzed

(continued)

Table 31.1 • Pharmacokinetics and Dosing Guidelines for Drugs Commonly Used in Renal Failure [13] (continued)

Drug	Oral Availability (%)	Protein Binding (%)	Vd (L/kg)	Metabolism and Excretion	t½ (hr)	Normal Dose Cl_Cr >50 mL/min	Dose Change with Renal Failure Cl_Cr (mL/min)	Effect of Dialysis
Foscarnet	Parenteral	14–17	0.4–0.7	>80% excreted renally	*Normal:* 2–3 *Anephric:* >100	*>80 mL/min:* 60 mg/kg Q 8 hr *50–80 mL/min:* 50 mg/kg Q 12 hr	*10–50 mL/min:* 60 mg/kg Q 24–48 hr *<10 mL/min:* 60 mg/kg Q 48 hr	Moderately dialyzed
Ganciclovir	Low	?	0.5	>90% excreted renally	*Normal:* 2.5–3.6 *Anephric:* 11.5–28	*>80 mL/min:* 5 mg/kg Q 12 hr *50–80 mL/min:* 2.5 mg/kg Q 12 hr	*10–50:* 1.25–2.5 mg/kg Q 24 hr *<10:* 1.25 mg/kg Q 24 hr	Dialyzed
Gentamicin	Parenteral	5–10	0.31	90–97% excreted renally	*Normal:* 1.5–3 *Anephric:* 20–54	See section on aminoglycoside pharmacokinetics	See section on aminoglycoside pharmacokinetics	Dialyzed; 24–50 mL/min
Ibuprofen	>80	99	0.15	Primarily metabolized; 45–60% excreted unchanged and as metabolites	*Normal:* 2 *Anephric:* No change	200–600 mg Q 4–6 hr	*10–50:* No change *<10:* No change	Not dialyzed
Imipenem	Parenteral	10–20	0.23–0.42	60–75% excreted renally; 22% hepatic to inactive metabolites	*Normal:* 0.8–1.3 *Anephric:* 2.9–3.7	5–10 mg/kg Q 6–8 hr	*10–50:* 5–10 mg/kg Q 8–12 hr *<10:* 5–10 mg/kg Q 12 hr	Moderately dialyzed
Indomethacin	98	90	0.26	Hepatic metabolism to inactive metabolites; <15% excreted unchanged	*Normal:* 2.6 *Anephric:* No change	25–50 mg Q 8–12 hr	*10–50:* No change *<10:* No change	?

Drug	Route/%	Protein binding	V_d	Metabolism/Excretion	Half-life	Dose	Dose adjustment	Dialysis
Ketoconazole	50–76	99	0.36	51% hepatic; 45% excreted unchanged in feces; 3% renally	*Normal*: 3–8 *Anephric*: No change	200–400 mg Q 24 hr (depends on severity of infection)	*10–50*: No change <*10*: No change	Not dialyzed
Labetalol	20–38	50	8–10	5% excreted renally; 95% hepatic	*Normal*: 5 *Anephric*: ? prolonged	No change	*10–50*: No change <*10*: No change	Not dialyzed
Lidocaine	Parenteral	50–70	1.7 (↑H)	Hepatic metabolism to inactive and active metabolites (glycylxylidide)	*Normal*: 1.5–1.8 *Anephric*: No change	Maintenance dose: 2–4 mg/min	*10–50*: No change <*10*: No change	Not dialyzed
Lithium	100	0	0.5–0.8	95% excreted renally	*Normal*: 22–29 *Anephric*: Prolonged	Variable (titrate with Cl_{Cr} to therapeutic levels of 0.4–0.8)	*10–50*: ↓ 25–50% <*10*: 50–75%	Moderately dialyzed/dialyzed
Meperidine	48–53	58	4.4	Hepatic hydrolysis and conjugation, active normeperidine metabolites; 10% excreted renally	*Normal*: 3–7 *Anephric*: ?	50–100 mg Q 3–4 hr (IV, IM)	*10–50*: 75–100% Q 6 hr <*10*: 50% Q 6–8 hr (Use cautiously)	?
Methotrexate	16–95 (dose-dependent)	50	0.4–0.8	>90% cleared renally; 10% metabolized to 7-OH-MTX	*Normal*: α 1.5–3.5; β 8–15 *Anephric*: Prolonged	No change	*10–50*: Adjust according to serum concentration <*10*: Avoid	Not/slightly dialyzed
Metoprolol	38	13	4	90% hepatic; 10% excreted renally	*Normal*: 3–4 *Anephric*: No change	50–200 mg QD	*10–50*: No change <*10*: No change	Metabolites dialyzed
Mezlocillin	Parenteral	26–42	0.2	45–65% excreted renally; 35–55% excreted hepatobiliary	*Normal*: 0.8–1.2 *Anephric*: 3–6	50 mg/kg Q 4–6 hr	*10–50*: 100% Q 6–8 hr <*10*: 50% Q 8 hr	Slightly/moderately dialyzed; 29 mL/min

(continued)

Table 31.1 • Pharmacokinetics and Dosing Guidelines for Drugs Commonly Used in Renal Failure[131] *(continued)*

Drug	Oral Availability (%)	Protein Binding (%)	Vd (L/kg)	Metabolism and Excretion	t½ (hr)	Normal Dose Cl$_{Cr}$ >50 mL/min	Dose Change with Renal Failure Cl$_{Cr}$ (mL/min)	Effect of Dialysis
Nadolol	34	20	2	75% excreted renally; 25% hepatic	*Normal:* 15–20 *Anephric:* 45	40–80 mg QD	*10–50:* ↓ 50% and titrate *<10:* ↓ 50% and titrate	Moderately dialyzed
Nafcillin	50	85–90	0.35	Up to 70% hepatic; 25–30% excreted renally	*Normal:* 1–1.5 *Anephric:* 1.9	1–2 g Q 4–6 hr	*10–50:* No change *<10:* No change	Not dialyzed
Nifedipine	45	98	0.8–1.1	100% hepatic	*Normal:* 2–4 *Anephric:* 3.8	No change	*10–50:* No change *<10:* No change (? ↑ response in renal failure patients)	?
Penicillin G	15–30	60	0.9–2.1	50% excreted renally; 19% hepatic	*Normal:* 0.4–0.9 *Anephric:* 4–10	2–3 MU Q 4 hr	*10–50:* Dose (MU/D) = 3.2 + Cl$_{Cr}$/7 *<10:* Dose (MU/D) = 3.2 + Cl$_{Cr}$/7	Moderately dialyzed; 46 mL/min
Pentamidine	Parenteral	?	12	<5% eliminated renally over 24 hr	*Normal:* 6 (5–9 days, urine data) *Anephric:* ?	4 mg/kg/day (IV)	*10–50:* No change *<10:* 100% QD–QOD	Probably not dialyzed
Phenobarbital	100	48–59	0.6	Hepatic metabolism; renal excretion: 10–40% unchanged and active metabolites	*Normal:* 100 *Anephric:* ?	No change	*10–50:* No change *<10:* Slight ↓	Moderately dialyzed/dialyzed

Drug			Route of excretion/metabolism	Half-life (hr)	Dose	Dosage adjustment for GFR	Dialysis
Phenytoin	>90	85–95 (↓R, H)	0.5–0.7 (↑R)	Hepatic metabolism; <5% excreted unchanged; 75% as inactive p-HPPH metabolites; concentration-dependent kinetics	*Normal:* 10–30 *Anephric:* 6–10	300–400 mg QD (titrate)	*10–50:* No change *<10:* No change (lower therapeutic level)	Not dialyzed
Piperacillin	Parenteral	16–22	0.2–0.47	50–60% excreted renally; up to 30–40% excreted in bile	*Normal:* 0.8–1.4 *Anephric:* 4–6	50 mg/kg Q 4–6 hr	*10–50:* 100% Q 6 hr *<10:* 50–75% Q 8 hr	Moderately dialyzed
Procainamide	75–95	15	1.7–2.3	Hepatic metabolism to active NAPA; 50–60% excreted renally	*Normal:* 2.5–4.7 (NAPA: 6) *Anephric:* 11–16 (NAPA: 42)	0.5–1.5 g Q 4–6 hr	*10–50:* 100% Q 6–12 hr *<10:* 100% Q 12–24 hr	Moderately dialyzed
Propranolol	36–40	88–94	2.9	Primarily hepatic; <1% excreted renally	*Normal:* 3–5 *Anephric:* No change	10–40 mg Q 6 hr (PO) and titrate	*10–50:* No change *<10:* No change	Not dialyzed
Ranitidine	52	15	0.8–1.1	70% excreted renally; some hepatic	*Normal:* 1.4–2.4 *Anephric:* 5–10	300 mg Q HS	*10–50:* ↓ 25% *<10:* ↓ 50%	Slightly dialyzed
Sulfamethoxazole	90–100	50–70 (↓R)	0.14–0.36 (↑R)	65–80% hepatic to inactive compounds; 20–30% excreted renally	*Normal:* 7–12 *Anephric:* 10–50	Q 6–12 hr	*10–50:* Q 12–24 hr *<10:* Q 24 hr	Slightly/moderately dialyzed
Tobramycin	Parenteral	<10	0.33	90–97% excreted renally	*Normal:* 2.5 *Anephric:* 33–70	See section on aminoglycoside pharmacokinetics	See section on aminoglycoside pharmacokinetics	Dialyzed: 50–60 mL/min

(continued)

Table 31.1 • Pharmacokinetics and Dosing Guidelines for Drugs Commonly Used in Renal Failure [131] (continued)

Drug	Oral Availability (%)	Protein Binding (%)	Vd (L/kg)	Metabolism and Excretion	t½ (hr)	Normal Dose ClCr >50 mL/min	Dose Change with Renal Failure ClCr (mL/min)	Effect of Dialysis
Trimethoprim	85–90	40–70	1–2	53–80% excreted renally; 20–35% hepatic	*Normal:* 8–16 *Anephric:* 24–62	Q 6–12 hr	*10–50:* Q 12–24 hr *<10:* Q 24 hr	Slightly/moderately dialyzed
Vancomycin	<10	10–55	0.5–0.7	80–90% excreted renally; 10–20% hepatic metabolism	*Normal:* 4–9 *Anephric:* 129–190	See section on vancomycin pharmacokinetics	See section on vancomycin pharmacokinetics	Conventional: not dialyzed; high flux: moderately dialyzed
Zidovudine	64	34–38	1.4	Primarily hepatic to inactive GAZT metabolite; 18% excreted renally	*Normal:* 0.8–2.9 *Anephric:* No change	100–200 mg Q 8 hr	*10–50:* No change *<10:* Possible ↓	Not dialyzed

[a]Pharmacokinetic values are for the active enalaprilat metabolite.

Notes:

The reader is referred to Chapter 32: Dosing of Drugs in Renal Failure, written by *Francesca T. Aweeka, Pharm.D.*, in the seventh edition of **Applied Therapeutics: The Clinical Use of Drugs** for a more in-depth discussion. All notations to reference numbers are based on the reference list at the end of that chapter. The editors of this handbook express their thanks to Dr. Aweeka and acknowledge that this chapter is based upon her work.

Notes:

Notes:

Chapter 32

Solid Organ Transplantation

Solid organ transplant has become the therapy of choice for patients with end-stage heart, liver, lung, and kidney disease. One-year patient survival for these major organs is approximately 80% to 90%, with some being >90%.

Organ Compatibility

♦ Histocompatibility antigens are located on the surface of cell membranes. These are encoded by the major histocompatibility complex (MHC) genes. The MHC in humans is called the human leukocyte antigen (HLA).

♦ Serologic, cytometric, genetic, and cellular assessments of donor and recipient serum and lymphocytes are needed before organ transplantation, because the genetic compatibility between donor and recipient affects graft survival.

♦ ABO blood typing is one of the most critical of all evaluations when determining the genetic compatibility for all solid organ transplants. Transplantation of an organ with ABO incompatibility would result in a hyperacute rejection and destruction of the graft.

Immunosuppressive Drugs

♦ Figure 32.1 summarizes the mechanisms of action of approved and investigational immunosuppressive agents.

♦ Approved immunosuppressives are listed in Table 32.1, which also identifies dosage forms, usual doses, and approximate costs.

♦ *Cyclosporine* has been the single most important drug in the current success of organ transplantation. Its use has increased patient and graft survival, has reduced morbidity associated with rejection and infection, and has extended the types and numbers of organ transplantations performed. Tables 32.2 and 32.3 list clinically significant pharmacokinetic and pharmacodynamic interactions with cyclosporine and tacrolimus.

♦ *Tacrolimus* (formerly FK506) is as effective as cyclosporine in liver, kidney, heart, and lung transplant patients as the primary immunosuppressant in combination with corticosteroids and/or mycophenolate or azathioprine.

♦ *Sirolimus* (formerly rapamycin) is the newest agent for prevention of acute rejection in kidney transplantation.

♦ *Antithymocyte Globulin* (Atgam, Thymoglobulin) can rapidly deplete circulating T cells, often within 24 hours of the initial dose.

♦ *Muromonab-CD3 (Orthoclone, OKT3),* a murine monoclonal antibody, suppresses T cell-mediated rejection. It is used for induction therapy (prophylaxis) or to treat acute graft rejection. Common OKT3 adverse effects are listed in Table 32.4.

♦ *Daclizumab (Zenapax) and basiliximab (Simulect)* are monoclonal antibodies used in combination with other immunosuppressives to prevent acute cellular rejection in kidney transplantation. They are not used to treat acute rejection.

Kidney Transplantation

 ♦ All patients with end-stage renal disease are potential candidates for kidney transplantation unless contraindicated. The relative or absolute contraindications are determined by the individual transplant centers.

 ♦ Less than 50% of patients who undergo kidney transplant experience an acute allograft rejection episode, and rates as low as 20% have been reported during the first year after transplantation.

 ♦ There is no consensus for the best immunosuppressive regimen.

 ♦ After kidney transplantation, the initial renal function can reflect excellent, moderate, or delayed graft function (DGF). DGF reduces kidney graft survival and complicates a patient's early management because of the need for dialysis, prolonged length of hospital stay, and increased costs of therapy. It also complicates the assessment of acute rejection because the patient already has impaired renal function.

 ♦ Rejection of a transplanted kidney can be categorized as hyperacute (within minutes to hours); accelerated (within 2-6 days); acute (within 7-10 days); or chronic (within 3 months to a year).

 ♦ High-dose corticosteroid therapy (e.g., methylprednisolone 250 to 1,000 mg/day IV for three doses) reverses the majority of acute rejection episodes and often is the first-line therapy of acute kidney rejection. Corticosteroid doses and regimens are as varied as the numbers of transplant programs. OKT3, Thymoglobulin, or ATG are other options for management of acute rejection episodes.

Heart Transplantation

 ♦ The criteria for the selection of patients for heart transplantation vary with the transplant center, but patients generally have NYHA functional class III or IV; intolerable symptoms in spite of maximal medical and surgical management; lack of reversible factors; and a 1-year life expectancy of <50%. An ejection fraction of <20% alone is not an indication for transplant.

 ♦ Most heart transplant recipients recover rapidly from the procedure, and most are extubated and off vasopressor/inotropic support within 24 to 48 hours.

 ♦ Inotropes and chronotropes usually are started in the operating room when the new heart is being reperfused and cardiopulmonary bypass is being discontinued. The choice of agent or combination of agents is based on hemodynamic parameters, which are monitored continuously. *Isoproterenol* and *epinephrine* are used to maintain the HR of 110–130 beats/min to maximize cardiac output. *Dobutamine* is used to increase CO, reduce LV dysfunction, and reduce SVR. *Dopamine,* at low doses, can improve renal blood flow. *NTG* or *nitroprusside* are used to reduce pulmonary arterial pressure and afterload, and if ineffective, *prostaglandin E_1* or a mechanical assist device can be used.

 ♦ Sinus node dysfunction, seen as nodal or sinus bradycardia and episodes of sinus arrest, is common in the early postoperative period. The donor sinus node serves as the heart's pacemaker, but because it is denervated, the transplanted heart cannot respond to cholinergic or vagal stimulation (e.g., atropine). Isoproterenol or a pacemaker may be needed.

 ♦ Immunosuppression with 3 or 4 drugs is administered aggressively during the early transplant period because the risk of organ rejection is greater during this time. Various regimens of drugs listed in Table 32.1 are used.

 ♦ Organ rejection can be classified as hyperacute, accelerated, acute, vascular, or chronic. Acute cardiac rejection can be further described as mild, moderate, or severe, with or without hemodynamic symptoms based on histologic findings. This classification serves as the basis for selection of pharmacological management. Drugs, doses, routes, and regimens vary from program to program. High-dose corticosteroids (e.g., IV methylprednisolone 1 gm/day × 3 days) commonly are used for moderate-to-severe rejection.

Lung Transplantation

♦ Primary indications for a single-lung transplant are emphysema, idiopathic pulmonary fibrosis, and alpha$_1$-antitrypsin deficiency. Cystic fibrosis, emphysema, and alpha$_1$-antitrypsin deficiency are primary indications for a double-lung transplant.

♦ The most common serious complications are airway complications, pulmonary edema, infection, and acute rejection.

♦ Pulmonary edema, which often is transient and mild, is thought to occur secondary to ischemia and reperfusion of the transplanted lung, impaired lymphatic drainage, and fluid resuscitation during the procedure. Treat with fluid restriction, diuretics, and low-dose dopamine if needed.

♦ Infection is the leading cause of death in the first 60 days after a lung transplant. At least 50% develop infection despite antibiotic prophylaxis based on the donor's previous bacterial cultures and sensitivities. The best prophylactic antibiotic regimen has not been established, but prophylaxis generally is directed against gram-negative organisms and staphylococci and based on the patient's previous antimicrobial experiences before transplant.

♦ Acute rejection occurs in >90% of patients within the first month despite aggressive immunosuppressive therapy and commonly is treated with IV methylprednisolone 500–1000 mg/day × 3 days. Chronic rejection (referred to as bronchiolitis obliterans) occurs after the first 3 months in at least 20% and is a major cause, along with infection, of late deaths.

Liver Transplantation

♦ The most common indication for liver transplant in adults is cirrhosis, but indications vary with each transplant center.

♦ Complications of liver transplantation include: primary graft nonfunction; coagulopathies and bleeding; hypocalcemia because of large amounts of citrate from blood transfusions; hypomagnesemia exacerbated by diuretics and cyclosporine; hypophosphatemia because of increased demand for phosphate for ATP; and CNS disturbances from high-dose corticosteroids.

♦ Acute liver rejection occurs within 1–6 weeks of transplant in about 50–70% of patients treated with either cyclosporine or tacrolimus and prednisone, and treatment generally is with 200–1000 mg/day of IV methylprednisolone. Chronic rejection manifests months to years after transplant in about 2–17% and is irreversible and unaffected by increased immunosuppressive therapy.

Post-Transplant Complications

♦ Organ rejection—acute or chronic.

♦ Post-transplant hypertension, hyperlipidemia, and osteoporosis. Management of these complications is described in Chapter 33 and throughout other chapters of *Applied Therapeutics: The Clinical Use of Drugs.*

♦ Secondary malignancies (e.g., post-transplant lymphoproliferative disorder) can be encountered.

♦ Common opportunistic infections are listed in Table 32.5.

♦ Ganciclovir, immune globulins, and foscarnet can be used for treatment of CMV. Ganciclovir, acyclovir, CMV hyperimmune globulin, and valacyclovir have been used in efforts to prevent the development of CMV.

Notes:

Table 32.1 • Immunosuppressive Agents

Drug	Dosage Form	Usual Dose[a]	Cost ($)
Azathioprine (Imuran)	50 mg tab 100 mg injectable	1–3 mg/kg/day	1.35/tab 81.60/100 mg vial
Azathioprine (generic)	50 mg tab		1.06/tab
Antithymocyte globulin (Atgam)	50 mg IgG/mL	10–20 mg/kg/day	284/5 mL
Basiliximab (Simulect)	20 mg/mL vial	20 mg × 2 doses	1067/20 mg dose
Cyclosporine (Sandimmune)	100 mg/mL oral solution 100 mg cap 25 mg cap 50 mg/mL IV solution	5–10 mg/kg/dose 5–10 mg/kg/dose 5–10 mg/kg/dose 1.5–2.5 mg/kg/dose	321/50 mL 6.40/cap 1.60/cap 283/5 mL
Cyclosporine (Neoral)	25 mg; 100 mg caps 100 mg solution 50 mL	4–5 mg/kg/day	1.30/cap; 4.90/cap 319/bottle
Daclizumab (Zenapax)	25 mg/5 mL vial	1 mg/kg × 5 doses	1047/70 mg dose
Gengraf (generic)	25 mg cap 100 mg cap		0.90/cap 3.56/cap
Methylprednisolone sodium succinate (various)	40, 125, 500 mg 1, 2 g injectable	10–1000 mg/dose	19.20/500 mg
Mycophenolate mofetil (Cellcept)	250 mg tab 500 mg cap 200 mg/mL susp IV 500 mg/vial	2–3.0 g/day	2.04/tab 4.10/cap 267/175 mL bottle 206/1 g dose
OKT3 (Orthoclone)	5 mg/5 mL injectable	2.5–5 mg/dose	720/5 mg
Prednisone (various)	1, 2.5, 5, 10, 20, 50 mg tab	5–20 mg/day	2.40/100 5 mg tab
Sirolimus (Rapamune)	1 mg/mL 1.0 or 150 mL	2–5 mg/day	328–822/bottle
Tacrolimus (Prograf)	0.5 mg cap 1 mg cap 5 mg cap	0.15–0.3 mg/kg/day	1.40/cap 2.39/cap 4.01/cap
Thymoglobulin	25 mg/vial	1.5 mg/kg/day	265/vial

[a]Usual dose is highly variable and depends on the transplanted organ and the transplant center.

Table 32.2 • Clinically Significant Pharmacokinetic Drug Interactions with Cyclosporine and Tacrolimus

Drug	Effect on Level
Diltiazem	↑
Verapamil	↑
Nicardipine	↑
Chloramphenicol	↑
Danazol	↑
Ketoconazole	↑
Miconazole	↑
Fluconazole	↑
Itraconazole	↑
Erythromycin	↑
Clarithromycin	↑
Tacrolimus	↑
Metoclopramide	↑
Grapefruit juice	↑
Octreotide	↓
Cholestyramine	↓
Antacids	↓
Rifampin	↓
Phenytoin	↓
Troglitazone	↓
Carbamazepine	↓
Phenobarbital	↓
Primidone	↓

Table 32.3 • Clinically Significant Pharmacodynamic Interactions with Cyclosporine and Tacrolimus

Drug	Effect
Aminoglycosides	Enhanced nephrotoxicity
Amphotericin B	Enhanced nephrotoxicity
NSAIDs	Enhanced nephrotoxicity
Cisplatin	Enhanced nephrotoxicity
Cyclosporine/tacrolimus	Enhanced nephrotoxicity
Minoxidil[a]	↑ hypertrichosis
Nifedipine[a]	↑ gingival hyperplasia
Lovastatin	Rhabdomyolysis

[a]Not applicable to tacrolimus.
NSAID, nonsteroidal anti-inflammatory drug.

Table 32.4 • Common OKT3-induced Side Effects

Symptom	Occurrence (%)
Fever	78
Tachycardia	68
Chills	60
Headache	40
Hypertension	31
Nausea	26
Vomiting	22
Tremor	21
Diarrhea	20
Chest pains	20
Dyspnea	20
Hypotension	15
Wheezing	12

Table 32.5 • Common Opportunistic Infections after Transplant

Organisms	Time of Onset after Transplant
CMV	1–4 mo
HSV	2 wk–2 mo
EBV	2–6 mo
VZV	2–6 mo
Fungal	1–6 mo
Mycobacterium	1–6 mo
PCP	1–6 mo
Listeria	1 mo–indefinitely
Aspergillus	1–4 mo
Nocardia	1–4 mo
Toxoplasma	1–4 mo
Cryptococcus	4 mo–indefinitely

CMV, cytomegalovirus; EBV, Epstein-Barr virus; HSV, herpes simplex virus; PCP, *Pneumocystis carinii* pneumonia; VZV, varicella-zoster virus.

Notes:

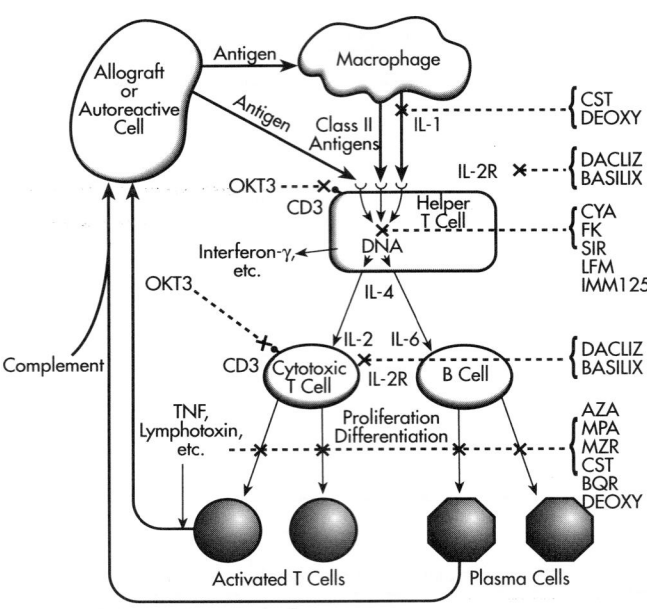

Fig. 32.1 Schematic Representation Summarizing the Mechanisms of Action of Approved and Investigational Immunosuppressive Agents. AZA, azathioprine; BASILIX, basiliximab; BQR, brequinar; CD, cluster of differentiation; CST, corticosteroids; CYA, cyclosporine; DACLIZ, daclizumab; DEOXY, deoxyspergualin; FK, tacrolimus; IL, interleukin; IMM125, Sandoz IMM125; LFM, leflunomide; MPA, mycophenolic acid; MZR, mizoribine; SIR, sirolimus; TNF, tumor necrosis factor. (Reprinted with permission from Miller L et al. Treatment of acute cardiac allograft rejection with rapamycin: A multicenter dose ranging study. J Heart Lung Transplant 1997; 16:44.)

The reader is referred to Chapter 33: Solid Organ Transplantation, written by *Robert E. Dupuis, Pharm.D.*, in the seventh edition of **Applied Therapeutics: The Clinical Use of Drugs** for a more in-depth understanding. The editors of this handbook express their thanks to Dr. Dupuis and acknowledge that this chapter is based upon his work.

Notes:

Chapter 33

Adult Enteral Nutrition

Enteral nutrition refers to the general delivery of nutrients into the GI tract but most commonly refers to tube feeding.

Indications

♦ Patients generally are considered at nutritional risk when patients' nutritional intake is inadequate to meet requirements for >7 days or when weight loss >10% preillness weight.

♦ More than 90% of institutions have a screening protocol to identify patients at nutritional risk.

♦ Tube feeding is the route of choice for malnourished patients who have a functional GI tract and no contraindications to its use.

Digestion

Table 33.1 lists the major steps in the preparation of ingested food for digestion.

Tube Placement

♦ Figure 33.1 illustrates the two basic types of tube placement—nasal versus ostomy— and the sites available for formula delivery (i.e., gastric, duodenal, jejunal).

♦ **Nasal** placement is preferred for short-term tube feeding when nasal, pharyngeal, or esophageal passages are not blocked. Mucosal bruising of the esophagus and hypopharynx are common with NG tube placement.

♦ **Tracheobronchial** placement can cause hemothorax, pneumothorax, or bronchopleural fistula if pleura is perforated by the procedure. Radiographic confirmation of tube placement is mandatory to rule out perforation or pulmonary intubation in unconscious patients.

♦ **Feeding ostomies** (e.g., gastrostomy, jejunostomy) usually are reserved for long-term tube feeding.

Site of Enteral Delivery

♦ The stomach is the preferred site for enteral formula delivery.

♦ Transpyloric delivery of nutrients into the duodenum or jejunum may be preferable in presence of gastric dysfunction, obstruction, or disease.

♦ Duodenal delivery preserves some degree of osmoregulation and causes less gastroesophageal reflux.

Formula Selection

♦ Enteral formula selection is based upon total nutrient requirements, fluid restrictions, and the extent to which normal digestion and absorption of nutrients are impaired.

♦ Table 33.2 categorizes enteral formulas into 4 "generic" groups to simplify formula selection. The relative cost of enteral formulas is shown in Table 33.3.

♦ **Polymeric formulas** require full digestive function and can be chosen based upon nutrient source, fiber content, caloric density, or protein content. Table 33.4 lists the fiber sources for selected enteral formulas.

♦ **Oligomeric formulas** require minimal digestive function, produce little residue in the colon, and can be chosen based upon protein source.

♦ **Specialized enteral formulas** are designed for specific disease states. These formulas have a good theoretical basis for use but lack conclusive clinical evidence of improved efficacy compared to standard formulas. Protein is the most frequently altered component of specialized enteral formulas. Table 31.3 lists high-protein enteral formulas with altered protein and/or fat sources.

♦ Table 33.5 lists enteral formulas with altered protein and/or fat sources.

Tube Feeding Regimens

♦ Route of feeding, selected formula, anticipated duration of feeding, location of patient (i.e., hospital, nursing home, home), and costs influence selection of feeding regimens.

♦ Scientific data to assist in the selection of the most appropriate enteral administration regimen are limited.

♦ **Continuous infusion** provides the daily volume of formula at a continuous rate over 24 hr/day. It is most commonly used in hospitalized patients.

♦ **Cyclic infusion** provides the daily volume of formula at a continuous rate for only several hours of the day. It is most commonly used for patients who are unable to consume a sufficient amount of nutrients.

♦ **Intermittent or bolus feedings** provide the daily volume of formula in a specified number of daily feedings. These feedings are more physiological than continuous feeding and more convenient for patients in nursing homes and for patients at home.

Monitoring Enteral Feedings

♦ **Adverse Effects.** The mechanical, GI, and metabolic complications of enteral feeding are described in Tale 33.6.

♦ **Efficacy.** Weight and fluid status reflect adequacy of caloric intake, especially with long-term treatment.

Medication Administration via Feeding Tube

♦ Generally better to administer medications separate from the enteral formula.

♦ Medications should be given by a route other than feeding tube to avoid drug interactions but also to avoid potential occlusion of the feeding tube.

Notes:

Table 33.1 • Functional Units of the GI Tract[a]

Functional Unit	Major Steps	Conditions/Diseases
Mouth and oropharynx	Chew and lubricate food; swallow	Amyotrophic lateral sclerosis, muscular dystrophy, severe RA, CVA, end-stage Parkinson's disease, paralysis, coma, anorexia due to other disease: cardiac or cancer cachexia, renal failure and uremia, liver failure, neurologic disease
Esophagus	Transport food to the stomach	Esophageal disease: ulcer, cancer, obstruction, fistula, esophagectomy, CVA
Stomach	Hold food for mixing and grinding; add acid and enzymes; release chyme to small bowel; osmoregulation	Severe gastritis or ulceration, gastroparesis, gastric outlet obstruction, gastric cancer, severe gastroesophageal reflux
Duodenum	Osmoregulation; neutralize stomach acid	Severe duodenal ulcer, duodenal fistula, cancer: gastric, pancreatic
Small bowel: jejunum and ilium	Digestion; absorption	Enterocutaneous fistula, severe enteric infection, malnutrition, malabsorption, Crohn's disease, celiac sprue, ileus and dysmotility syndrome
Pancreas	Secretion of digestive enzymes	Pancreatitis, pancreatic cancer, pancreatic injury, pancreatic fistula
Colon	Absorb fluid; ferment soluble fiber and unabsorbed carbohydrate; absorb water	Ulcerative colitis, Crohn's disease, colon cancer, colocutaneous fistula, colovaginal fistula, diverticulitis, colitis of any etiology, colon surgery

[a]CVA = Cerebrovascular accident; GI = Gastrointestinal; RA = Rheumatoid arthritis.

Table 33.2 • "Generic" Groups and Subgroups of Enteral Formulas[a]

Polymeric Formulas
  Nutrient Source
    Blenderized
    Milk based
    Lactose free
  Fiber Content
    Fiber free
    Low to moderate fiber (1–8 gm/L)
    Moderate to high fiber (>8 gm/L)
  Caloric Density
    Standard density (1–1.2 kcal/mL)
    Moderate density (≈1.5 kcal/mL)
    Calorically dense (2 kcal/mL)
  Protein or Nitrogen Content
    Low nitrogen (≈6% of kcal)
    Standard nitrogen (11%–15% of kcal)
    High nitrogen (16%–25% of kcal)
Oligomeric Formulas
  Elemental
  Peptide based

Specialized Formulas
  Renal Failure
    Essential amino acid enriched
    Low protein and electrolytes
  Hepatic Failure
    BCAAs
  Stress/Critically Ill
    Branched chain enriched
    High nitrogen plus conditionally essential nutrients
    Immune modulating
  Pulmonary Disease
  Glucose Control

Modular Components
  Carbohydrate
  Protein
  Fat

[a]BCAAs = Branched-chain amino acids.

Table 33.3 • Relative Cost of Enteral Formulas[a]

Type of Formula	Relative Cost
Polymeric Formulas	
Blenderized	2.5
Milk-based	0.8
Lactose-free, standard caloric density, standard nitrogen content plus	
Fiber-free[b]	1.0
Low-to-moderate fiber (1–8 g/L)	1.2
Moderate-to-high fiber (>8 g/L)	1.3
Lactose-free, standard nitrogen content, fiber free plus	
Standard caloric density (1–1.2 kcal/mL)[b]	1.0
Moderate density ($\approx$1.5 kcal/mL)	0.8
Calorically dense (2 kcal/mL)	0.8
Lactose-free, standard caloric density, fiber free plus	
Low nitrogen (6–10% of kcal as protein); low electrolyte	3.9
Standard nitrogen (11–15% of kcal as protein)[b]	1.0
High nitrogen (16–25% of kcal as protein)	1.3
Oligomeric Formulas	
Elemental (free amino acids)	13.7
Peptide-based	12.4
Specialized Formulas	
Renal failure	
Essential amino acid enriched	13
Low protein and electrolytes	3.9
Hepatic failure (branched-chain amino acids)	26.4
Stress/critically ill	
Branched-chain enriched	21
High nitrogen plus conditionally essential nutrients	9.9
Immune modulating	23.3
Pulmonary disease	2.5
Glucose control	2.6

[a]Based on average cost per 1,000 calories for equivalent formulas on contract from 1996–1999.
[b]Index product; given a relative value of 1.

Notes:

Table 33.4 • Fiber Sources for Selected Enteral Formulas

Formula Name	Total Dietary Fiber (g/L)	Soy Fiber; Soy Polysaccharide	Cellulose Gum, Gel, or Microcrystalline	Oat Fiber	Gum Arabic	Acacia	Partially Hydrolyzed Guar Gum	Pectin	Fructo-oligo-saccharides
			Primarily Insoluble Fiber				Primarily Soluble Fiber		
Advera	8.9	X							
AMTF Basic	14.2				X			X	
AMTF Diabetic	15				X			X	
Boost with fiber	10		X			X			
Choice dm	14.4	X	X			X			
Complete Modified	4.2 from fruits and vegetables								
DiabetiSource	4.4 from fruits and vegetables								
Ensure with fiber	14.4	X							
FiberSource	10		X				X		
FiberSource HN	10						X		
Glucerna	14.1	X							
Glucerna OS	8.5	X	X		X				
Glytrol	15	X			X			X	
Impact with fiber	10	X					X		
IsoSource VHN	10	X					X		
Jevity Plus	12	X	X	X	X				X
NuBasics with fiber	14	X							
Nutren 1.0 with fiber	14	X							
Nutriflavor	14.2				X				
ProBalance	10	X			X			X	
Promote with fiber	14.4	X		X					
Protain XL	8	X							
Replete with fiber	14	X							
ReSource Diabetic	12.7		X				X		
Ultracal	14.4	X		X					

Table 33.5 • High-Protein Enteral Formulas with Altered Protein and/or Fat Sources[a,b]

Formula (Manufacturer)	kcal/mL (mOsm/kg)	% Free Water	Protein g/L (% kcal)	NPC:N Ratio	Protein Sources	ARG g/L	GLN g/L
Protain XL (Mead Johnson/Sherwood)	1.0 (340)	83	57 (22)	85:1	Calcium and sodium caseinates	2	5.5
TraumaCal (Mead Johnson)	1.5 (560)	78	82 (22)	91:1	Sodium and calcium caseinates	3.3	7.2–10.6
Replete (Nestle)	1.0 (300–350)	84	62.5 (25)	75:1	Calcium-potassium caseinate	2.4	5.4–8
Replete with fiber (Nestle)	1.0 (300–350)	84	62.5 (25)	75:1	Calcium-potassium caseinate	2.4	5.4
Perative (Ross)	1.3 (385)	79	66.6 (20.5)	97:1	Partially hydrolyzed sodium caseinate; lactalbumin hydrolysate; L-arginine	14.7	5.4
AlitraQ (Ross)	1.0 (575)	85	52.5 (21)	119:1	Soy hydrolysate; whey; lactalbumin hydrolysate; free amino acids	3–4	14.2–15.5
Impact (Novartis)	1.0 (375)	85	56 (22)	71:1	Sodium and calcium caseinates; nucleic acid L-arginine	14	5.9
Impact with fiber (Novartis)	1.0 (375)	87	56 (22)	71:1	Sodium and calcium caseinates; nucleic acid L-arginine	14	5.9
Immun-Aid (McGaw)	1.0 (460)	82	80 (32)	53:1	Hydrolyzed lactalbumin; BCAAs; nucleic acid	15	12.5
Advera (Ross)	1.28 (NA)	80	60 (18.7)	108:1	Soy protein hydrolysate; sodium caseinate	4.1	5.4–6.4
Crucial (Nestle)	1.5 (490)	NA	94 (25)	67:1	Hydrolyzed casein L-arginine	15	7.2
AMTF High-Protein (Nyer Nutritional)	1.0 (330)	77	59 (25)	81:1	Concentrated whey protein	NA	10.4
AMTF Trauma (Nyer Nutritional)	1.5 (390)	71	78 (22)	95:1	Concentrated whey protein	NA	13.3
Fibersource HN (Novartis)	1.2 (490)	81	53 (18)	115:1	Soy protein isolate and concentrate	2.0	5.9
Isocal HN Plus (Mead Johnson)	1.2 (400)	81	54 (18)	114:1	Milk protein concentrate	NA	NA
IsoSource HN (Novartis)	1.2 (490)	82	53 (18)	115:1	Soy protein isolate and concentrate	2.3	5.8
IsoSource 1.5 (Novartis)	1.5 (650)	78	68 (18)	113:1	Sodium and calcium caseinates	NA	NA
IsoSource VHN (Novartis)	1.0 (300)	85	62 (25)	75:1	Sodium and calcium caseinates	NA	NA
Jevity (Ross)	1.06 (300)	84	44 (16.7)	125:1	Sodium and calcium caseinates	1.5	4–5.8
Lipisorb Liquid (Mead Johnson)	1.35 (630)	80	57 (17)	125:1	Sodium and calcium caseinates	2.3	7.3
Optimental (Ross)	1.0 (540)	84	51 (20.5)	97:1	Soy protein hydrolysate; partially hydrolyzed sodium caseinate; free amino acids	5	NA
Osmolite HN (Ross)	1.06 (300)	84	44 (17)	125:1	Sodium and calcium caseinates; soy protein isolates	1.7	4–5.6
Osmolite HN Plus (Ross)	1.2 (360)	82	55.5 (18.5)	110:1	Sodium and calcium caseinates	NA	NA
Oxepa (Ross)	1.5	74	59 (16.7)	125:1	Sodium and calcium caseinates	NA	NA
Peptamen VHP (Nestle)	1.0 (300)	84	40	75:1	Hydrolyzed whey	1.9	10.5
ProBalance (Nestle)	1.2 (350)	82	45 (18)	114:1	Calcium and potassium caseinates	2	4.6–6.9
SandoSource Peptide (Novartis)	1.0 (490)	84	50 (20)	100:1	Casein hydrolysate; sodium caseinates	5	4.7
Subdue (Mead Johnson)	1.0 (330)	78	50 (20)	100:1	Hydrolyzed whey	NA	NA
Ultracal HN Plus (Mead Johnson)	1.2 (370)	81	54 (18)	114:1	Milk protein concentrate	NA	NA

[a]ARG = Arginine (listed values reflect added L-arginine, not the amount present in protein); BCAAs = Branched-chain amino acids; DHA = Docosahexanoic acid; EPA = Eicosapentaenoic acid; GLN = glutamine (listed values reflect both free and protein-bound glutamine); MCT = Medium-chain triglycerides; NA = Not available; NPC:N = Nonprotein calorie to nitrogen; ω-3FA = Omega-3 fatty acids; ω-6FA = Omega-6 fatty acids.
[b]Changes periodically occur in nutrient sources and/or content; therefore, this table should be used as a general reference only and not for specific patient care issues.
[c]Omega-3 fatty acids from linolenic acid reflect linolenic content of nonfish oils.

Approximate % of Protein as BCAAs	Fat g/L (% kcal)	Fat Sources	% Fat kcal as MCT %/ ω-3FA	ω3FA Source[c] (ω-3FA:ω-6FA)	Fiber g/L	Carnitine mg/L	Taurine mg/L
21	30 (26)	Canola oil; high oleic sunflower oil; MCT oil; corn oil	20/NA	Linolenic acid (4.8:1)	9.1	150	150
23	68 (40)	Soy oil; MCT	30/6.5	Linolenic acid (6.3:1)	None	None	None
21	34 (30)	Canola oil; MCT; lecithin	25/6.6	Linolenic acid (2.5:1)	None	100	100
21	34 (30)	Canola oil; MCT; lecithin	25/6.6	Linolenic acid (2.5:1)	14	100	100
18	37.4 (25)	Canola oil; MCT; corn oil	40/4.5	Linolenic acid (4.7:1)	None	140	140
18.5	15.5 (13)	Safflower oil; MCT	53/10	Linolenic acid (4.2:1)	None	112	200
17	28 (25)	Structured lipids with palm kernel and sunflower oils; menhaden oil	27/6.5	Menhaden oil; linolenic acid (1.4:1)	None	None	None
17	28 (25)	Structured lipids with palm kernel and sunflower oils; menhaden oil	27/6.5	Menhaden oil; linolenic acid (1.4:1)	10	None	None
36	22 (20)	Canola oil; MCT	50/5.5	Linolenic acid (1.8:1)	None	200	100
15.5	22.8 (15.8)	Canola oil; MCT; sardine oil	20/5.4	Sardine oil; linolenic acid (2.9:1)	8.9	127	212
17.5	67.5 (39)	Soy oil; MCT; fish oil; lecithin	50/6	Fish oil, linolenic acid (2:1)	None	150	150
NA	27 (25)	High oleic safflower oil; canola oil; MCT oil	20	Linolenic acid	4	144	144
NA	65 (40)	Canola oil; MCT oil	NA	Linolenic acid	None	144	144
20.9	39 (29)	Canola oil; MCT oil	50 (4.4)	Linolenic acid (2.4:1)	10	None	None
NA	40 (29)	Canola oil; MCT oil, high oleic sunflower oil; corn oil	NA	Linolenic acid	None	150	150
20.6	39 (29)	Canola oil; MCT oil	50 (4.4)	Linolenic acid (2.4:1)	None	None	None
NA	65 (38)	Canola oil; MCT oil; soybean oil	NA	Linolenic acid	8	110	110
NA	29 (25)	Canola oil; MCT oil	50 (4.4)	Linolenic acid (≈2.4:1)	10	80	80
19	35 (29)	High oleic safflower oil; canola oil; MCT oil; lecithin	20 (3.3)	Linolenic acid (4.7:1)	14	115	115
23	57 (35)	Soy oil; MCT oil	85 (<1)	Linolenic acid (≥8:1)	None	194	194
NA	28 (25)	Structured lipid with EPA, DHA, MCT; canola oil; soy oil	NA	EPA; DHA; linolenic acid	None	110	110
19	35 (29)	High oleic safflower oil; canola oil; MCT oil; lecithin	20 (3.0)	Linolenic acid (4.9:1)	None	115	115
NA	39 (29)	High oleic safflower oil; canola oil; MCT oil; lecithin	19	Linolenic acid (5:1)	None	115	115
NA	89 (55)	Canola oil; MCT oil; sardine oil; borage oil	NA	Sardine oil; borage oil; linolenic acid	None	172	300
21	39 (33)	Sunflower oil; MCT oil	70 (1.4)	Linolenic acid (7.4:1)	None	100	100
21	34 (30)	Canola oil; MCT oil; corn oil; lecithin	20 (5.5)	Linolenic acid (4:1)	8.3	83	83
30	17 (15)	MCT oil; soybean oil; lecithin	NA	Linolenic acid	None	100	200
NA	34 (30)	MCT oil; canola oil	50	Linolenic acid	None	80	101
NA	40 (29)	Canola oil; MCT oil; high oleic sunflower oil; corn oil	NA	Linolenic acid	10	150	150

Table 33.6 • Complications of Tube Feeding[a]

Complication	Cause/Contributing Factor	Treatment/Prevention
Mechanical Complications		
Aspiration	Deflated tracheostomy cuff	Inflate trach cuff before feeding; keep inflated 1 hr after feeding; consider small-bore feeding tube placed past the ligament of Treitz (into the jejunum)
	Displaced feeding tube	Reinsert tube and check placement; consider hand restraints or feeding tube bridle
	Reduced gastric emptying	Check residuals Q 4–6 hr for gastric tube; raise head of bed at least 30°; change to a formula with lower fat content; try a medication to stimulate gastric emptying; place feeding tube into small bowel
	Lack of gag reflex; coma	Place feeding tube into small bowel beyond the pylorus and ligament of Treitz (into the jejunum)
Nasal or pharyngeal irritation or necrosis; esophageal erosion; otitis media	Large-bore, polyvinyl chloride tube for long periods of time	Reposition the tube daily and change tape; use smaller-bore feeding tube; position tube to avoid pressure on tissues; moisten mouth and nose several times daily
Tube obstruction	Poorly crushed medications	Crush medications thoroughly and dissolve in water; use liquid medications whenever possible; check compatibility of medication with tube and formula
	Inadequate flushing after medications or thick formula	Flush tube with 50–150 mL water after medications or thick formula and Q 8 hr with 20 mL minimum
	Poorly dissolved or mixed formula	Use a blender to mix formula (check manufacturer's guidelines for mixing); check for formula clumping as it is poured into the container for administration
	Formula mixed with low pH substance	Avoid checking gastric residuals through small-diameter feeding tubes; use the larger-diameter nasogastric tubes for checking residuals; avoid administering acidic pharmaceutic products through small-diameter feeding tubes; consider a nonacidic therapeutic alternative; flush the tube with a minimum of 30 mL water before and after administration if the acidic product must be given
Metabolic Complications		
Hyperglycemia, glycosuria (can lead to dehydration, coma, or death)	Stress response High carbohydrate formula (e.g., elemental) Drug therapy (steroids) Diabetes mellitus	Monitor fingerstick glucose Q 6 hr and have sliding scale insulin ordered Monitor in's and out's accurately
Excess CO_2 production (high RQ)	High % of carbohydrate calories or excess calories from any source	$\uparrow$ fat calories and/or $\downarrow$ total calories
Hyponatremia	Dilutional (fluid excess, SIADH); inadequate sodium intake; excess GI losses	Use full-strength formula or change to concentrated formula with 1.5–2.0 kcal/mL; add salt to the tube feeding (1 tsp = 2 g Na = 90 mEq); use diuretics if appropriate; replace GI losses
Hypernatremia	Inadequate free water intake Excess water losses (diabetes insipidus; osmotic diuresis from hyperglycemia; fever)	Use diluted formula or change to 1.0 kcal/mL formula; monitor in's and out's accurately; temperature and weight daily Correct hyperglycemia and the underlying cause of fever or diabetes insipidus

(continued)

Table 33.6 • Complications of Tube Feeding *(continued)*

Complication	Cause/Contributing Factor	Treatment/Prevention
Metabolic Complications *(continued)*		
Hypokalemia	Medications (diuretics, antipseudomonal penicillins, amphotericin B) Intracellular/extracellular shifts (insulin therapy, acidosis) Excess GI losses (NG suction, small bowel fistula, diarrhea)	Monitor serum potassium carefully; give PO or IV potassium replacement PRN Correct the underlying problem
Hyperkalemia	Potassium-sparing medications (triamterene, amiloride, spironolactone, ACE inhibitors); potassium-containing medications (penicillin G potassium)	Monitor serum potassium carefully; change to medications that do not have a potassium-sparing effect or that are not potassium salts
	Renal failure	Monitor renal function; change to a formula with lower potassium content
Hypercoagulability	Warfarin antagonism due to high vitamin K content of formula	Change to a formula with lower vitamin K content; monitor coagulation status
GI Complications		
Diarrhea	Atrophy of GI microvilli; malabsorption (pancreatitis, short gut syndrome, Crohn's disease); low serum albumin	Use a peptide-based or free amino acid formula until nutritional status improves; start with isotonic dilution and progress slowly while increasing the rate, then strength of formula; change to a formula with lower fat content if fat malabsorption appears to be occurring
	Hypertonic formula	Dilute formula or change to an isotonic formula
	Formula started and/or advanced too rapidly	Reduce rate and/or strength temporarily; advance slowly once diarrhea is controlled; change to continuous drip if using bolus feedings
	Lactose intolerance	Use lactose-free formula
	Contaminated formula	Hang fresh formula Q 4–6 hr; do not add new formula to remaining formula; change feeding container and tubing every day; use clean technique; discard open containers of formula after 24 hr; avoid unnecessary manipulation of the feeding system; mix formulas using aseptic technique and sterile water
	Medications Magnesium-containing antacids	Alternate with, or change to, $Al(OH)_3$ or calcium carbonate
	Antibiotics	Give Lactobacillus (Lactinex) to replenish GI flora; check for *C. difficile* and treat if present; give an antidiarrheal agent
	Quinidine, methyldopa	Give $Al(OH)_3$ antacid; give an antidiarrheal agent
	Metoclopramide, cisapride	Reduce dose; discontinue if no longer required
	High-osmolality liquid medications; irritating medications (potassium)	Dilute the medication with water before giving and/or give water through the tube before giving the medication; use the liquid form with a lower osmolality and/or less irritating formulation if there is a choice (water base versus syrup versus alcohol/propylene glycol/sorbitol)

(continued)

Table 33.6 • Complications of Tube Feeding^a (continued)

Complication	Cause/Contributing Factor	Treatment/Prevention
GI Complications (continued)		
	Colchicine	Reduce colchicine dose; give antidiarrheal agents
	Cholinergics (bethanechol)	If diarrhea is a major problem, consider alternative medication/therapy
Nausea, vomiting, distention, cramping, hyperactive bowel sound	Too rapid administration	Slow administration rate (give bolus over longer time; ↓ continuous infusion rate)
	Intolerance to osmolality and/or volume	Reduce osmolality by diluting formula with water or by changing to an isotonic formula; reduce volume of feeds by ↓ amount/bolus or reducing rate of continuous feeds
	Formula too cold	Bring formula to room temperature before administering
	Gastric retention; poor GI motility	Raise head of bed >30°; check gastric residuals; hold formula if large residual; place feeding tube past the pylorus into the small bowel; consider medication to increase motility; reduce dose or discontinue medications that ↓ GI motility if this will not adversely affect the patient (morphine, anticholinergics)
	Lactose intolerance	Use lactose-free formula
Dumping syndrome (weakness, diaphoresis, palpitations)	Hyperosmolar load infused rapidly or bolused into the small bowel	↓ rate and dilute temporarily; do not bolus into the small bowel unless the patient has a jejunostomy specially made for bolus feedings; use an isotonic formula
	Formula strength increased too fast; formula rate too high	↓ rate and/or strength temporarily, then advance the rate or strength slowly
Constipation	Inadequate fluid/free water intake	Dilute formula if feeding continuously; give free water between or with bolus feedings
	Inadequate bulk/fiber	Use a fiber-containing/high-residue formula; give bulk-forming laxative (Metamucil) or fruit juice
	Fecal impaction	Administer a stool softener; use daily
	Reduced gastric/GI motility	Encourage ambulation; consider medication to improve motility if more conservative measures fail
	Medications (narcotics, anticholinergics)	Use the lowest effective dose of the medication; discontinue the medication when possible to do so without adversely affecting patient care; change to an alternate drug if an effective one is available with less GI side effects

^{a}ACE = Angiotensin-converting enzyme; Al(OH)$_3$ = Aluminum hydroxide; CO$_2$ = Carbon dioxide; GI = Gastrointestinal; IV = Intravenous; Na = Sodium; NG = Nasogastric; PO = Per os (orally); PRN = As needed; RQ = Respiratory quotient; SIADH = Syndrome of inappropriate secretion of antidiuretic hormone.

Notes:

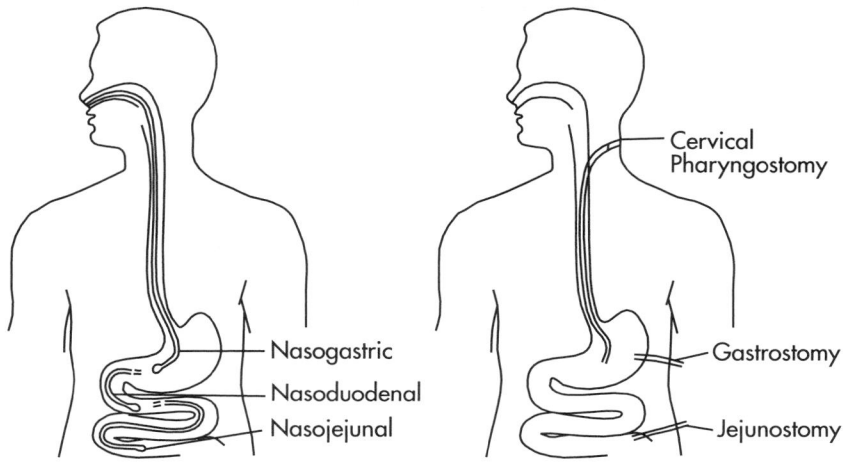

Fig. 33.1 Nasoenteric and Enterostomy Feeding Sites.

The reader is referred to Chapter 34: Adult Enteral Nutrition, written by *Carol J. Rollins, Pharm.D.,* in the seventh edition of **Applied Therapeutics: The Clinical Use of Drugs** for a more in-depth discussion. The editors of this handbook express their thanks to Dr. Rollins and acknowledge that this chapter is based upon her work.

Notes:

Notes:

Chapter 34

Adult Parenteral Nutrition

Malnutrition

- The *incidence* of malnutrition in hospitalized patients may be as high as 50%.
- Acute malnutrition occurs when nutrient intake is inadequate because of injury or stress (e.g., trauma, infection, major surgery). Acute stress or injury increases energy needs for the repair of tissues. When this energy is not provided exogenously, the body breaks down muscle to release amino acids for glucose production.
- Hospitalized patients with inadequate nutrient intake for >7 days or weight loss >10% should be considered for specialized nutrient support with parenteral or enteral nutrients.
- Whenever possible, nutrients should be provided enterally (see Chapter 33: Adult Enteral Nutrition) because enteral nutrients maintain gastrointestinal (GI) mucosal structure and function, is less costly and less invasive.

Patient Assessment

- **Nutritional History.** A nutritional history (Table 34.1) is needed to identify risks of malnutrition.
- **Weight Loss.** The pattern of weight loss must be evaluated (e.g., loss continuing, stabilizing, or reversing).
- **Physical examination** to include anthropometrics (measurements of subcutaneous fat and muscle).
- **Biochemical assessments** of visceral proteins (e.g., albumin, transferrin, transthyretin) are decreasd when intake of nutrients is inadequate or when nutritional substrates are shunted away during stress or injury to synthesize other proteins. Renal, hepatic, and cardiac dysfunction, hydration, and metabolic stress also decrease these serum proteins. The visceral proteins commonly used for nutritional assessments are summarized in Table 34.2
- **Immunocompetence** secondary to malnutrition may be assessed by determining the total lymphocyte count or by assessing delayed cutaneous hypersensitivity.
- Protein-calorie malnutrition can be classified as kwashiorkor, marasmus, or mixed.
- Estimations of basal energy expenditure and of total energy expenditure are shown in Table 34.3.
- Estimation of protein needs are summarized in Table 34.4.

Venous Access Sites

- **Peripheral.** When need for parenteral nutrition is for <10 days and patient has low energy and protein needs, parenteral nutrition can be delivered via peripheral veins. Venous access sites need to be rotated every 48–72 hr to minimize phlebitis. Low concentrations of dextrose (5%–10%) when mixed with amino acids (3%–5%) and lipids increase caloric density and minimize risk of phlebitis. *Midline venous access catheters* are longer, can be placed in a larger vein, can be left in place longer, can dilute the feeding formulation, and decrease phlebitis.

♦ **Central.** When a patient has limited peripheral venous access and a nonfunctional GI tract, nutrition can be delivered via a central venous catheter placed in the subclavian vein and threaded through to the superior vena cava, where rapid blood flow dilutes concentrated feeding formulations and phlebitis is minimized. Central venous access sites can remain in place for months without the need for rotation. Dextrose (20%–35%), amino acids (5%–10%), and lipids giving a caloric density of >1 kcal/mL and an osmolarity of >2000 mOsm/L can be administered.

Available Nutrients

♦ **Macronutrients.** The three required macronutrients (carbohydrate, fat, and protein) are available commercially. *Dextrose* is the most common carbohydrate for intravenous (IV) use and provides 3.4 kcal/gm. *Fat* for IV use is supplied as emulsions of either soybean oil or a mixture of soybean and safflower oils. Although fat has a caloric density of 9 kcal/gm, commercially available formulations, by the addition of glycerol and egg emulsifiers to adjust osmolarity, have a higher caloric density. Protein for parenteral administration is available as synthetic amino acids which have a caloric density of 4 kcal/gm. Table 34.5 summarizes available nutrients and their caloric density.

♦ **Micronutrients.** The micronutrients (electrolytes, vitamins, and trace minerals) are available as single products or may be administered as combination products. General guidelines for electrolyte requirements for parenteral feedings are included in Table 34.6. Most institutions use a multiple-vitamin product that contains 12 vitamins listed in Table 34.7. Recommended doses of trace elements are listed in Table 34.8.

Monitoring Metabolic Complications and Routine Monitoring Parameters

♦ **Hypokalemia** is a common metabolic abnormality because potassium moves intracellularly with dextrose and potassium is used in building lean body mass. Alkalosis also drives K+ into cells.

♦ **Hypophosphatemia** occurs quickly because phosphorus is used for synthesis of adenosine triphosphate which is an important energy carrier. Alkalosis also decreases phosphate stores by stimulating phosphorylation of carbohydrates.

♦ **Metabolic alkalosis** can arise secondary to nasogastric suctioning.

♦ **Hyperglycemia** is common because stress increases gluconeogenesis and because of the administration of hypertonic dextrose. Hyperglycemia can be minimized by gradually increasing the parenteral feeding formulation infusion, frequent monitoring of capillary blood glucose concentration, checking urine for glucosuria, and advancing therapy only when serum glucose is <200 mg/dL.

♦ **Elevations in liver function tests** may be noted as early as 1–2 weeks after initiation of therapy. They usually do not progress to significant liver dysfunction and resolve when therapy is discontinued.

♦ A suggested schedule for the routine monitoring of parenteral nutrition is provided in Table 34.9.

Amino Acid Composition in Available Formulations (See Table 34.10)

♦ Patients with cirrhosis and chronic hepatic failure have increased circulating concentrations of the aromatic amino acids (AAA; phenylalanine, tyrosine, and tryptophan) and decreased concentrations of branched-chain amino acids (BCAA; leucine, isoleucine, and valine). The AAA cross the blood-brain barrier and form false neurotransmitters which can impair neurotransmission and contribute to hepatic encephalopathy.

♦ Branched-chain amino acids have beneficial metabolic properties in patients in physiologic stress (multiple trauma, sepsis, major surgery). BCAA can increase protein synthesis in muscle and the liver, decrease excessive proteolysis in muscle, and normalize abnormal plasma amino acid profiles. Although BCAA have some advantages, clinical outcome may not be different.

Table 34.1 • Components of a Nutritional History

Medical history

Chronic illnesses

Surgical history

Psychosocial history

Socioeconomic status

History of gastrointestinal problems (nausea, vomiting, or diarrhea)

Diet history including weight-loss or weight-gain diets

Food preferences and intolerances

Medications

Weight history
  Increase or decrease
  Intentional or unintentional
  Time period for weight change

Functional capacity

Notes:

Table 34.2 • Visceral Proteins for Nutritional Assessment

Visceral Protein	Half-Life (Days)	Normal Serum Concentration
Albumin	18–21	3.5–5.0 g/dL
Transferrin	8–10	250–300 mg/dL
Transthyretin (prealbumin)	2–3	15–40 mg/dL
Retinol-binding protein	0.5	2.5–7.5 mg/dL

Table 34.3 • Estimation of Energy Expenditure

Basal Energy Expenditure (BEE)
Harris-Benedict Equations

BEE_{men} (kcal/day) = 66.47 + 13.75 W + 5.0 H − 6.76 A

BEE_{women} (kcal/day) = 655.10 + 9.56 W + 1.85 H − 4.68 A

or

    20–25 kcal/kg/day

Total Energy Expenditure (TEE)
TEE (kcal/day) = BEE × Stress factor × Activity factor

Stress or Injury Factors (% increase above BEE)

Major surgery	10–20
Infection	20
Fracture	20–40
Trauma	40–60
Sepsis	60
Burns	60–100

Activity Factors (% increase above BEE)

Confined to bed	20
Out of bed	30

or

No stress	28 kcal/kg/day
Mild stress	30 kcal/kg/day
Moderate stress	35 kcal/kg/day
Severe stress	40 kcal/kg/day

A, age in years; H, height in cm; W, weight in kg.

Table 34.4 • Estimation of Protein Requirements

U.S. RDA	0.8 g/kg/day
Hospitalized patient, minor stress	1.0–1.2 g/kg/day
Moderate stress	1.2–1.5 g/kg/day
Severe stress	1.5–2.0 g/kg/day

RDA, recommended dietary allowance.

Table 35.5 • Caloric Density of Intravenous Nutrients

Nutrient	kcal/g	kcal/mL
Amino acids	4.0	—
Amino acids 5%	—	0.2
Amino acids 10%	—	0.4
Dextrose	3.4	—
Dextrose 10%	—	0.34
Dextrose 50%	—	1.7
Dextrose 70%	—	2.38
Fat	10	—
Fat emulsion 10%	—	1.1
Fat emulsion 20%	—	2.0
Fat emulsion 30%	—	3.0
Glycerol	4.3	—
Glycerol 3%	—	0.129
Medium-chain triglycerides	8.3	—

Table 34.6 • Guidelines for Daily Electrolyte Requirements

Electrolyte	Amount
Sodium	80–100 mEq
Potassium	60–80 mEq
Chloride	50–100 mEq[a]
Acetate	50–100 mEq[a]
Magnesium	8–16 mEq
Calcium	5–10 mEq
Phosphorus (phosphate)	15–30 mmol

[a]As needed to maintain acid-base balance.

Notes:

Table 34.7 • Recommended Adult Daily Doses of Parenteral Vitamins

Vitamins	Dose
Fat-Soluble Vitamins	
A	3,300 IU (990 retinol equivalents)
D	200 IU (5 mg cholecalciferol)
E	10 IU (6.7 mg/dL-α-tocopherol)
K	—
Water-Soluble Vitamins	
Thiamine (B_1)	3.0 mg
Riboflavin (B_2)	3.6 mg
Pyridoxine (B_6)	4.0 mg
Cyanocobalamin (B_{12})	5.0 μg
Niacin	40.0 mg
Folic acid	0.4 mg
Pantothenic acid	15.0 mg
Biotin	60.0 μg
Ascorbic acid (C)	100.0 mg

34.8 • Recommended Daily Adult Doses of Parenteral Trace Elements

Trace Element	Dose
Zinc	2.5–4.0 mg
Copper	0.5–1.5 mg
Chromium	10–15 μg
Manganese	150–800 μg
Selenium	20–60 μg

Notes:

Table 34.9 • Routine Monitoring Parameters for Parenteral Nutrition

Before Initiating Therapy
Body weight
Serum electrolytes (Na, K, Cl, HCO_3^-, BUN, creatinine)
Glucose
Ca, Mg, P
Albumin, transthyretin
Triglycerides
Complete blood count
Liver-associated tests (AST, ALT, alkaline phosphatase, GGT, bilirubin)
Prothrombin time, INR

Daily
Body weight
Vital signs (pulse, respirations, temperature)
Fluid intake
Nutritional intake
Output (urine, other losses)
Serum electrolytes (Na, K, Cl, HCO_3^-, blood urea nitrogen, creatinine)
Glucose

2–3 Times a Week
CBC
Ca, Mg, P

Weekly
Albumin, transthyretin
Liver-associated tests (AST, ALT, alkaline phosphatase, GGT, bilirubin)
Prothrombin time, INR
Nitrogen balance

ALT, Alanine aminotransferase; AST, Aspartate aminotransferase; Ca, Calcium; Cl, Chloride; GGT, Gamma glutamyl transpeptidase; HCO_3^-, Bicarbonate; K, Potassium; Mg, Magnesium; Na, Sodium; P, Phosphorus.

Notes:

Table 34.10 • Amino Acid Product Comparison Table

Description	Product Name	Supplier	Available Concentrations (%)
Standard Formulations			
Contain essential[a] and nones-	Aminosyn, Aminosyn II	Abbott	3.5,[c] 5, 7,[c] 8.5,[c] 10,[c] 15
sential[b] amino acids, some	FreAmine III	B Braun	3, 8.5, 10
available with electrolytes[c]	Novamine	Baxter	15
	Prosol	Baxter	20
	Travasol	Baxter	3.5,[c] 5.5,[c] 8.5,[c] 10
Hepatic Failure Formulations			
Contain essential and nones-	HepatAmine	B Braun	8
sential amino acids with an	Hepatasol	Baxter	8
↑ proportion of branched-			
chain amino acids (leucine,			
isoleucine, valine)			
Renal Failure Formulations			
Contain primarily essential	Aminess	Baxter	5.2
amino acids; RenAmin also	Aminosyn-RF	Abbott	5.2
contains a complement of	Nephramine	B Braun	5.4
nonessential amino acids	RenAmin	Baxter	6.5
Stress Formulations			
Contain ↑ percentages of	Aminosyn HBC	Abbott	7
leucine, isoleucine, and	FreAmine HBC	B Braun	6.9
valine as well as all essential			
and nonessential amino acids			
Supplements			
Contain only branched-chain	BranchAmin	Baxter	4
amino acids (isoleucine,			
leucine, valine); must be			
used with a general			
formulation			

[a]Essential amino acids: isoleucine, leucine, lysine, methionine, phenylalanine, threonine, tryptophan, valine, histidine.
[b]Nonessential amino acids: cysteine, arginine, alanine, proline, glycine, glutamine, aspartate serine, tyrosine.
[c]These concentrations are available with or without electrolytes.

The reader is referred to Chapter 35: Adult Parenteral Nutrition, written by *Beverly J. Holcombe, Pharm.D.*, in the seventh edition of **Applied Therapeutics: The Clinical Use of Drugs** for a more in-depth discussion. The editors of this handbook express their thanks to Dr. Holcombe and acknowledge that this chapter is based upon her work.

Notes:

Chapter 35

Dermatotherapy

Dermatologic Drug Delivery Systems

♦ Drugs can be applied topically through various delivery systems (e.g., ointments, creams, lotions, aerosols) as listed in Table 35.1.

♦ The selection of the most appropriate delivery system is based upon the following:
  • If a lesion is wet, dry it.
  • If the lesion is dry, wet it.
  • Wet dressings are most useful in drying acute, inflamed lesions.
  • Ointment bases are most useful for chronic, fissured lesions.

♦ Examples of some *wet dressings* are listed in Table 35.2. Some of the more common commercially available *emulsions bases* are listed in Table 35.3. Average amounts of *cream* needed to cover various body parts are listed in Table 35.4.

♦ Drug absorption through the epidermis is enhanced by epidermal or stratum corneum injury, increased temperature, skin hydration, dermal circulation, and drug concentration.

Assessing the Dermatologic Patient

♦ **Determine onset and duration of lesion and potential exacerbating factors** (e.g., recent travel, stress, climate change).

♦ **Determine the type of dermatologic lesion** (i.e., scales, crusts, macules, purpura, petechiae, vesicles, bullae, nodule, cyst, atrophy, ulcer, pustule). If the patient presents with petechiae, cysts, atrophy, nodules, abscesses, or ulcers or if >1% of total body surface area (1% is about the size of the palm of your hand) is covered by purpura, pustules, bullae, or erosion, a physician should be contacted. Lesions extending into the dermis can lead to scarring. Figures 35.1–35.8 are pictures and drawings of various basic lesions. Table 35.5 details common diseases associated with specific lesion types.

♦ **Determine the Size of the Lesion.** Lesions with >25% of the patient's body affected should be referred to a physician. Less severe lesions (except for those mentioned above) are amenable to treatment with nonprescription medications.

♦ **Determine Part of Body Affected.** All lesions affecting the eyes and most lesions involving the mouth, face, genitalia, nails, and rectal areas should be evaluated by a physician.

♦ **Determine Age of the Patient.** Dermatological lesions in patients <2 yr or >65 yr of age may indicate systemic disease and should be evaluated by a physician.

♦ **Determine Presence of Systemic Symptoms.** Concurrent fever, orthostasis, ataxia, confusion, significant pain, difficulty breathing, or regional lymph node enlargement should be referred to a physician.

♦ **Determine the Presence of Allergies.** Most allergies can be traced to use of a new drug or product within the past 1 or 2 weeks.

♦ **Determine Past Dermatological and Medical History.** Patients with diabetes, renal disease, malnutrition, cancer, CHF, hepatitis, or alcoholism should have dermatological lesions referred to a physician, because these conditions might be adversely affected by inappropriate or inadequate OTC therapy.

♦ **Be reasonably sure of the diagnosis** before even considering OTC treatment.

♦ **Determine Efficacy of Previous Dermatological Treatments.** Previously ineffective medications are not likely to be effective.

♦ **Expectations for Improvement.** Generally most dermatological conditions amenable to OTC therapy should improve in a few days.

Topical Corticosteroids

♦ **Site of Application.** The penetration of topical corticosteroids varies with the site of application. Low-potency topical corticosteroids should be applied to areas of high blood flow (e.g., groin, axillae, face). High-potency steroids should be applied to areas of poor penetration (e.g., elbows, knees, palms, soles) to minimize systemic absorption.

♦ Table 35.6 lists common topical corticosteroids.

♦ Risk factors for systemic side effects from topical application of corticosteroids are presented in Table 35.7.

♦ General principles of topical corticosteroid therapy are listed in Table 35.8.

Topical Antibiotics

♦ Combination therapy with several antibiotics is effective in treating dermatologic infections that often are caused by more than one organism.

♦ Spectrum of activity of topical antibiotics is presented in Table 35.9.

Pruritus

♦ **Antihistamines.** *Topical* only provide a mild topical anesthetic effect and can cause allergic contact dermatitis. *Systemic* antihistamines also can relieve pruritus because of sedating effects. See Table 35.10 for minimizing sedation to hydroxyzine.

♦ **Atopic Eczema.** Recommendations for treatment of atopic eczema are shown in Table 35.11.

Dry Skin

General recommendations for the treatment of dry skin are presented in Table 35.12.

Drug Eruptions

♦ Medications commonly associated with drug eruptions are listed in Table 35.13.

Contact Dermatitis: Poison Ivy, Oak, and Sumac

♦ Urushiol oil is the common sensitizing agent in poison ivy, oak, and sumac.

♦ Erythematous and vesicular lesions appear 12–48 hours after exposure. They clear in 1–3 weeks.

◆ **Treatment.** Wash with soap within 15 minutes after exposure. Washing later with soap can prevent spread to other body parts. Clean under fingernails and wash clothing, shoes, or tools to avoid subsequent contamination.

Drug Therapy. Calamine lotion 2–4 times a day and topical hydrocortisone cream are helpful. Prednisone 50 mg/day is indicated if lesions are severe or if eyes, genitals, mouth, or respiratory tract are involved.

◆ A list of common contact sensitizers other than urushiol oil is found in Table 36.14.

Table 35.1 • Dermatological Drug Delivery Systems[a]

Delivery System	Function	Comment
Aerosols	Do not require direct mechanical contact with skin and useful when mechanical application would cause pain	Most expensive and inefficient method for application of dermatologicals. Shake well before application; avoid eyes and inhalation
Baths	Topical therapies can be applied to large areas of body through bathing. Useful in therapy of widespread eruptions	Bath oils (Lubath, Alpha-Keri) most useful for mild cases of dry skin. Colloidal (Aveeno,[b] Linit[b]) good for urticaria, pityriasis rosea, weeping eczemas
Creams	Most suited for nonacute, nonirritable dermatoses. Most are O/W and are intended to be rubbed in well until they vanish (vanishing cream)	Do not provide much occlusion. Most common mistake is failure to rub in fully or to use excessive amounts. Table 35.4 lists ≈ amounts needed
Emulsions	W/O emulsions most useful when dry skin conditions predominate; O/W emulsions similar to that for lotions	Water-soluble drugs should be dispersed in O/W emulsions and lipid-soluble drugs in W/O emulsions. See Table 35.3 for a list of emulsion bases
Gels	Nongreasy, nonstaining, nonocclusive, and quick drying. Useful for application to areas (face, hairy areas) where residue of a vehicle is cosmetically unacceptable	Thixotropic, becoming thinner with rubbing and usually contain propylene glycol and carboxypolymethylene
Lotions	Can lubricate, cool, or dry, depending upon formulation. Useful for superficial dermatoses and conditions with inflammation and tenderness	Suspensions of powder or liquid in an aqueous vehicle
Ointments	Provide occlusive covering. Most useful in relieving dryness, brittleness, and treating fissures. Spread more easily than creams but greasier	Consist of drugs or water droplets suspended in a continuous phase of oleaginous material. Should not be applied to intertriginous or hairy areas because occlusiveness traps heat and moisture
Powders	Absorb moisture by ↑ surface area for quicker evaporation. Useful in intertriginous areas to prevent friction	Useful in preventing bedsores; not to be applied to oozing lesions because of tendency to cake into granules that become difficult to remove
Wet dressings	Provide evaporative cooling, which causes vasoconstriction. Soothe and cool inflamed skin; dry oozing lesions, soften crusts, aid in cleaning and draining purulent wounds	Should be freshly prepared; store in closed containers[c] and do not reuse. Apply soaked cloth for 5–10 min, then resoak and reapply; continue for 30 min and repeat several times/day. See list of wet dressings in Table 35.2

[a]O/W = Oil-in-Water; W/O = Water-in-Oil.
[b]Aveeno = Colloidal Oatmeal; Linit = Hydrolyzed Starch.
[c]To avoid concentration of solution = secondary to evaporation.

Table 35.2 • Wet Dressings[4,7]

Agent[a]	Strength	Preparation (H$_2$O)	Germicidal Activity	Astringent Activity	Comments
Normal saline	0.9%	1 tsp NaCl to a pint	—	—	Inexpensive; easy to prepare
Aluminum acetate					
Burow's solution	5%	Dilute to 1:10–1:40 (0.5–0.125%).	Mild	+	—
Domeboro packets/tablets	—	One packet/tablet to a pint of water yields a 1:40 solution; two yields a 1:20 solution	Mild	+	—
Potassium permanganate	65- and 330-mg tablets	Dilute to 1:4,000–1:16,000; 65-mg tablet to 250–1,000 mL; 330-mg tablet to 1,500–5,000 mL	Moderate	—	Stains skin, clothing
Silver nitrate	0.1–0.5%	1 tsp of 50% stock solution to 1,000 mL will yield a 0.25% solution	Good	+	Stains; can cause pain
Acetic acid[b]	1%	Dilute 1:5 with standard 5% household vinegar	Good	+	Unpleasant odor; can be irritating

[a]Although many substances are added to wet dressings, the cleansing and drying effect of the water is the major benefit.
[b]Used primarily for *Pseudomonas aeruginosa* infections.

Table 35.3 • Commercially Available Emulsion Bases

Oil-in-Water	Water-in-Oil
Acid Mantle Cream	Aquaphor
Almay Emulsion Base	C-Solve
Aquaphilic	E-Solve
Cetaphil	Eucerin (Aquaphor and Water)
Dermabase	Hydrophilic Petrolatum USP
Dermovan	Hydrosorb
Hydrophilic Ointment USP	Hydrous Lanolin
Keri Lotion	Lubriderm
Lanaphilic	Nivea Cream
Multibase	Nutraderma
Neobase	Polysorb
Unibase	Qualatum
Vanibase	Vanicream
	Velvachol

Table 35.4 • Average Amounts of Cream Needed to Cover Various Parts of the Body[8]

Single Application (g)	Area (for Each Part Listed)	Amount Needed for 7 Days
2	Both hands, head, face, genital, anal	45 g (1.5 oz)
3	One arm, front or back of trunk	60 g (2 oz)
4	One leg	90 g (3 oz)
30–60	Whole body	1–2.5 kg (2.5–5 lb)

Notes:

Table 35.5 • Common Diseases Associated with Dermatologic Lesions

Macules and Papules

Psoriasis	Pityriasis rubra	Dermatophyte infections
Lichen planus	Pityriasis rosea	Secondary syphilis
Tinea versicolor	Diaper dermatitis	Eczema
Ichthyosis vulgaris	Erythroderma	Xerosis
Drug eruptions	Neurodermatitis	Actinic keratosis
Candidiasis	Lupus erythematosus	Sarcoidosis
Miliaria rubra	Seborrheic dermatitis	

Purpura and Petechiae Diseases

Senile purpura	Idiopathic thrombocytopenia	Purpura fulminans
Necrotizing vasculitis	Coumarin or heparin necrosis	Meningococcemia
Gonococcemia	Rocky Mountain spotted fever	Lupus erythematosus
Drug eruptions	Scurvy	Post-transfusion purpura
Disseminated intravascular coagulation	Leukemia	Lymphomas

Vesiculobullous (Blistering) Diseases

Pemphigus vulgaris	Staph-scalded skin syndrome	Toxic epidermal neurolysis
Varicella	Bullous pemphigoid	Herpes
Bullous impetigo	Contact dermatitis	Drug eruptions

Nodular and Cystic Diseases

Lymphoma	Sarcoidosis	Acne
Lipomas	Erythema nodosum	Vasculitis
Rheumatoid diseases	Polyarteritis nodosum	
Scabies	Xanthomas	

Ulcer (Skin) Diseases

Venous stasis	Arterial insufficiency	Anesthetic ulcer
Pyoderma gangrenosum	Decubitus ulcer	Syphilis
Chancroid	Lymphogranuloma venereum	Granuloma inguinale

Atrophy

Steroid use	Solar elastosis	Radiation dermatitis
Striae distensae	Lichen sclerosus	

Scales and Crusts
Very common with many chronic and acute dermatologic diseases

Pustules

Acne	Acne rosacea	Folliculitis
Candidiasis	Perioral dermatitis	Miliaria rubra
Impetigo	Psoriasis	

Notes:

Table 35.6 • Topical Corticosteroid Preparations

Corticosteroid	(Brand Name)	Vehicle
Low Potency		
Dexamethasone	(Decaspray) 0.04%	Aerosol
	(Decadron) 0.1%	Cream
	(Aeroseb–Dec) 0.01%	Aerosol
Hydrocortisone (generic)	(Cort-Dome) 0.5–2.5%	Towelettes, spray
	(Cortef) 0.5–2.5%	Aerosol
	(Penecort) 0.5–2.5%	Cream
	(Penecort) 0.5–2.5%	Gel, ointment
	(Synacort) 0.5–2.5%	Cream
	(Hytone) 0.5–2.5%	Lotion
Methylprednisolone acetate	(Medrol) 0.25%	Ointment
	(Medrol) 1.0%	Ointment
Alclometasone	(Aclovate) 0.05%	Cream, ointment
Betamethasone valerate	(Valisone, Decreased Strength) 0.01%	Cream
Clocortolone	(Cloderm) 0.1%	Cream
Desonide	(generic) 0.05%	Cream, ointment
	(DesOwen) 0.05%	Cream, lotion, ointment
	(Tridesilon) 0.05%	Cream, ointment
Fluocinolone acetonide	(generic) 0.01%	Cream
	(Synalar) 0.01%	Cream
	(FS Shampoo) 0.01%	Shampoo
Flurandrenolide	(Cordran, Cordran SP) 0.025%	Cream, ointment, solution
Triamcinolone acetonide	(generic) 0.025%	Cream, ointment
	(Aristocort) 0.025%	Cream, lotion, aerosol
	(Aristocort A) 0.025%	Cream
	(Kenalog) 0.025%	Cream, ointment, lotion
Medium Potency		
Betamethasone benzoate	(Uticort) 0.025%	Cream, gel, lotion
Betamethasone valerate	(generic) 0.1%	Cream, gel, lotion
	(Valisone) 0.1%	Cream, ointment
	(Psorion) 0.05%	Cream
Desoximetasone (generic) 0.05%	(Topicort) 0.05%	Cream, ointment, gel
Fluocinolone acetonide	(generic) 0.025%	Cream, ointment
	(Fluonid) 0.025%	Cream, ointment
Flurandrenolide	(Cordran, Cordran SP)	Tape, solution, cream, ointment
Fluticasone propionate	(Cutivate) 0.005% and 0.05%	Ointment, cream
Halcinonide	(Halog) 0.025%	Cream
Hydrocortisone valerate	(Westcort) 0.2%	Cream, ointment
Mometasone furoate	(Elocon) 0.1%	Cream, lotion, ointment
Triamcinolone acetonide	(generic) 0.1%	Cream, ointment, lotion
	(Aristocort) 0.1%	Cream, ointment
	(Aristocort A) 0.1%	Cream, ointment
	(Kenalog) 0.1%	Cream, ointment, lotion
High Potency		
Amcinonide	(Cyclocort) 0.1%	Cream, ointment, lotion
Betamethasone	(generic) 0.05%	Cream, ointment, lotion
dipropionate	(Alphatrex) 0.05%	Cream, ointment, lotion
	(Diprosone) 0.05%	Cream, ointment
	(Diprosone) 0.1%	Aerosol
Desoximetasone (generic) 0.25%	(Topicort) 0.25%	Cream, ointment,
Diflorasone diacetate	(Florone) 0.05%	Cream, ointment
	(Maxiflor) 0.05%	Cream, ointment
Fluocinolone	(Synalar HP) 0.2%	Cream
Fluocinonide	(generic) 0.05%	Cream, gel, ointment, solution
	(Lidex, Lidex-E) 0.05%	Cream, gel, ointment, solution

(continued)

Table 35.6 • Topical Corticosteroid Preparations (continued)

Corticosteroid	(Brand Name)	Vehicle
Halcinonide	(Halog, Halog-E) 0.1%	Cream, ointment, solution
Triamcinolone acetonide	(generic) 0.5%	Cream, ointment
	(Aristocort A) 0.5%	Cream
	(Aristocort) 0.5%	Cream, ointment
	(Kenalog) 0.5%	Cream, ointment
Very High Potency		
Betamethasone dipropionate	(Diprolene) 0.05%	Cream, ointment, gel, lotion
Clobetasol propionate	(generic) 0.05%	Cream, ointment
	(Temovate) 0.05%	Cream, ointment, gel
Diflorasone diacetate	(Psorcon) 0.05%	Cream
Halobetasol propionate	(Ultravate) 0.05%	Cream, ointment

Adapted from Drug Facts and Comparisons, 54th Ed. St. Louis: Facts and Comparisons, 2000.

Table 35.7 • Risk Factors for Systemic Side Effects from Topical Corticosteroids[69]

Duration of Application
- Limit to 3–4 wk

Potency of Corticosteroid
- Weak or moderately strong, 100 g/wk without occlusion
- Very potent, 45 g/wk without occlusion

Place of Application
- Thin stratum corneum results in easier penetration (eyelids, forehead, cheeks, armpits, groin, and genitals)

Age of Patient
- Very young children and elderly people have very thin epidermis

Manner of Application
- Occlusion

Presence of Penetration-enhancing Substances
- Propylene glycol
- Salicylic acid
- Urea

Condition of the Skin
- Normal or healthy

General Factors
- Liver status

Notes:

Table 35.8 • General Principles of Therapy

- Topical corticosteroids should be applied at least twice a day and up to four times a day. Increasing the frequency of application from once daily to three times daily clearly produces superior responses. Application six times daily is no more efficacious than three times daily.[7,10,11]
- An appropriate strength preparation should be used to bring the condition under control. It should be noted that 33 to 50% of all dermatologic conditions requiring topical corticosteroids can be managed with medium- or low-strength corticosteroid preparations.[7]
- After initial control, maintenance therapy should consist of the lowest strength formulation and the least number of application times per day to control the problem. It may be advisable to give the patient two different strengths of corticosteroid preparations; a mild one for routine use and a more potent one for flares or resistant lesions.[12]
- Occluded areas and certain areas of the body, such as the face and flexures, are more prone to the development of side effects. If corticosteroids must be used on the face or flexures, hydrocortisone should be used to reduce the probability of side effects.
- Children and patients with liver failure are at risk for systemic corticosteroid toxicities. In addition, patients who use the highest-potency preparations (Table 35.6) for >2 weeks are susceptible to systemic toxicity.[13]
- Preparations should be rubbed in thoroughly and, when possible, applied while the skin is moist (e.g., after bathing) to enhance the effect.[7]
- With chronic conditions such as atopic eczema, it is best to discontinue therapy gradually. This will reduce chances of rebound flares of topical lesions.[10,11]
- Generally, treatment should be initiated with a potent fluorinated corticosteroid with occlusion if tolerated. After the lesions are controlled, begin maintenance therapy with 1% hydrocortisone or a low-strength fluorinated corticosteroid such as triamcinolone acetonide 0.025%. Caution must be used when lesions are hot, acute, and/or inflamed, at which time one must cool the lesions down with wet-to-dry dressings before initiating steroid therapy.

Table 35.9 • Spectrum of Activity of Antibiotics Available for Topical Use

Bacitracin
Effective against all anaerobic cocci, most strains of streptococci, staphylococci, and pneumococci. Not effective against most Gram-negative organisms.

Gentamicin
Effective against most Gram-negative organisms (similar to neomycin), including *Pseudomonas* and many strains of *Staphylococcus aureus*.

Mupirocin
Very effective against *S. aureus* and does not interfere with wound healing. Currently, the only topical antibiotic that has been proven to be more effective than the vehicle based on FDA guidelines.

Gramicidin
Effective against most Gram-positive organisms. Not effective against most Gram-negative organisms.

Neomycin
Effective against most Gram-negative organisms (except *Pseudomonas*) and some Gram-positive organisms. Group A streptococci are resistant.

Polymixin B
Effective against most Gram-negative organisms (including *Pseudomonas*). Most strains of Proteus, Serratia, and Gram-positive organisms are resistant.

Notes:

Table 35.10 • Ways to Minimize Sedation from Hydroxyzine

1. Reduce the strength of hydroxyzine to 10-mg tablets.
2. Have the patient take the hydroxyzine on a scheduled basis, because some tolerance to the sedative properties probably will develop.
3. Switch to a less-sedating antihistamine. However, part of the benefit derived from antihistamines is related to their sedative action; this property helps the patient sleep and decreases the anxiety that is common with persistent pruritus.
4. If the previous three measures have been tried and sedation is still a problem, the patient must decide which is worse, the sedation or the pruritus, and make a decision whether or not to use the antihistamine.
5. A trial of one of the newer, nonsedating antihistamines (e.g., cetirizine) may be used if the previous measures fail.

Table 35.11 • Recommendations for Patients with Atopic Eczema or Other Irritant Dermatitis

1. Clothing should be soft and light. Cotton or corduroy is preferred. Wools and coarse, heavy synthetics should be avoided.
2. Heat should be avoided because it often makes the eczema worse. The environment should be well ventilated, cool, and low in humidity (30 to 50%). Rapid changes in ambient temperature should be avoided.
3. Bathing should be kept to a minimum (no longer than 5 minutes), and the patient should use a nonirritating soap (e.g., Basis soap). A colloid bath or the use of appropriate amounts of bath oil may be useful.
4. The skin should be kept moist with frequent applications of emollients (e.g., Keri, Lubriderm, Nivea, Aquaphor, Eucerin, or petrolatum).
5. Primary irritants such as paints, cleansers, solvents, and chemical sprays should be avoided.

Table 35.12 • General Recommendations for the Treatment of Dry Skin

1. Use room humidifiers.
2. Keep room temperature as low as comfortable to prevent sweating and water loss from the skin.
3. Keep bathing to a minimum (every 1 to 2 days) with warm, but not hot, water. After bathing, the patient should immediately apply an emollient (see Table 35.3). When the skin is soaked for 5 to 10 minutes, the stratum corneum can absorb as much as six times its weight in water. Application of an emollient immediately after bathing will trap the water in the skin and reduce dryness.
4. Eliminate exposure to solvents, drying chemicals, harsh soaps, and cleaners. These substances remove oils from the skin and reduce its barrier function. As the barrier function is lost, water loss from the skin is increased up to 75 times above normal. Exposure to cold, dry winds also will enhance water loss.
5. Apply emollients (see Table 35.3) three to six times a day. Many patients find the use of a urea-containing product to be effective and more cosmetically acceptable because it does not leave a greasy residue on the skin after application.
6. If scaling is a problem, keratolytic (Keralyt Gel) or a higher-strength, urea-containing preparation (20%) may be useful.
7. If inflammation is present, a mild to moderately potent topical corticosteroid may be very useful (see Table 35.6). An ointment vehicle is more effective than others.

Notes:

Table 35.13 • Medications Commonly Associated with Drug Eruptions[a]

Acneiform[b]
ACTH
Actinomycin D
Amoxicillin
Ampicillin
Androgens
Barbiturates
Carbamazepine
Cephalosporins
Chloral hydrate
Chloramphenicol
Contraceptives, oral[c]
Corticosteroids[c]
Ethambutol
Ethionamide
Iodides/bromides[c]
Isoniazid[c]
Lithium[c]
Naproxen
Phenytoin
Quinidine
Scopolamine
Streptomycin
Trimethadione

Alopecia[b]
Allopurinol
Anticoagulants[c]
Antimetabolites[c]
Bromocriptine
Captopril
Carbamazepine
Cimetidine
Clofibrate
Colchicine
Contraceptives, oral
Ethionamide
Gold
Indomethacin
Levodopa
Lithium
Propranolol
Quinacrine
Thallium
Trimethadione
Valproate sodium
Vitamin A (High Doses)

Bullous[b]
Aminosalicylic acid
Amiodarone
Ampicillin
Barbiturates[c]
Captopril
Cephalosporins
Chloral hydrate
Clonidine
Coumarins
Cytokines
Diclofenac

Gold
Iodides/bromides[c]
Lithium
Mesantoin
Nalidixic acid
NSAIDs[c]
Penicillins
Phenothiazines
Phenytoin
Promethazine
Sulfonamides
Tetracycline
Vancomycin

Eczematous[b]
Aminophylline
Antimetabolites
Chloral hydrate
Chlorpropamide
Chlorothiazide
Cephalosporins[c]
Codeine
Disulfiram
Gentamicin[c]
Gold
Iodides
Kanamycin
Meprobamate
Neomycin
Nitrofurantoin
Penicillins[c]
Procaine
Promethazine
Quinacrine
Streptomycin
Sulfonamides
Thiamine
Tolbutamide

Epidermal Necrolysis[b]
Ampicillin
Allopurinol[c]
Barbiturates
Carbamazepine[c]
Chlorpropamide
Hydantoin derivatives
Ibuprofen
Indomethacin
NSAIDs
Penicillins[c]
Pentamidine[c]
Phenylbutazone[c]
Phenytoin
Quinine
Sulfonamides[c]
Sulindac
Tolmetin

Erythema Multiforme[b]
Acetazolamide
Acetylsalicylic acid
Ampicillin
Barbiturates[c]

Bromides
Carbamazepine
Chloral hydrate
Chlorpropamide
Diflunisal
Griseofulvin[c]
Gold
Hydantoins[c]
Ibuprofen
Minoxidil
NSAIDs
Penicillins[c]
Phenolphthalein
Phenothiazines
Phenylbutazone
Procaine
Propranolol
Quinine
Rifampin
Salicylates
Sulfapyridine
Sulfonamides
Sulfonylureas
Sulindac
Thiazides
Tetracycline

Erythema Nodosum[b]
Aminosalicylic acid
Codeine[c]
Contraceptives, oral[c]
Iodides/bromides[c]
Penicillins[c]
Phenacetin
Salicylates
Sulfonamides

Exfoliative Dermatitis[b]
Actinomycin D
Allopurinol
Aminosalicylic acid
Barbiturates[c]
Bismuth
Captopril
Carbamazepine[c]
Chloroquine
Chlorpropamide
Cimetidine
Diltiazem
Gold
Griseofulvin
Hydantoins[b]
Iodides
Isoniazid
Lithium
Mesantoin
Nitrofurantoin
Penicillamine
Penicillins
Phenothiazines
Phenylbutazone
Phenytoin

Quinidine
Stilbestrol
Streptomycin
Sulfonamides
Sulfonylureas
Tetracycline
Thiouracil
Vitamin A

Fixed Drug[b]
Acetaminophen
Acetylsalicylic acid
Allopurinol
Amphetamines
Anticoagulants
Barbiturates[c]
Belladonna
Bismuth
Chloral hydrate
Chlordiazepoxide
Chloroquine
Clindamycin
Codeine
Contraceptives, oral[c]
Dapsone
Dextromethorphan
Digitalis
Diphenhydramine
Disulfiram
Epinephrine
Ergot
Ethchlorvynol
Griseofulvin
Gold
Hydralazine
Hydroxyurea
Ibuprofen
Indomethacin
Iodides/bromides
Ipecac
Meprobamate
Methenamine
Metronidazole
Morphine
Naproxen
Paclitaxel
Penicillins
Phenacetin
Phenophthalein[c]
Phenothiazines
Phenylbutazone
Quinidine
Reserpine
Saccharin
Salicylates
Stilbestrol
Streptomycin
Sulfonamides
Sulindac
Tetracyclines
Trimethoprim
Vermouth

(continued)

Table 35.13 • Medications Commonly Associated with Drug Eruptions[a] (continued)

Maculopapular
Aminosalicylic acid
Ampicillin[c]
Allopurinol[c]
Antimetabolites[c]
Atropine
Barbiturates[c]
Benzodiazepines
Busulfan
Carbamazepine
Cephalosporins[c]
Chloramphenicol
Chlordiazepoxide[c]
Chloroquine
Chlorothiazide
Chlorpromazine
Contraceptives, oral
Diazepam[c]
Erythromycin[c]
Ethionamide
Gentamicin[c]
Griseofulvin
Gold[c]
Hydantoin
    derivatives
Ibuprofen
Indomethacin[c]
Isoniazid[c]
Insulin
Lithium[c]
Meprobamate
Morphine
Naproxen
Nitrofurantoin[c]
NSAIDs[c]
Penicillamine[c]
Penicillins[c]
Phenothiazines
Phenylbutazone
Piroxicam
Promethazine
Quinacrine
Rifampin

Streptomycin
Sulfonamides
Sulfonylureas
Sulindac
Thiazides
Thiouracil
Tetracyclines
Tolmetin

Photosensitive
Amiodarone[b]
Ampicillin
Barbiturates
Carbamazepine
Chlordiazepoxide
Chlorothiazide
Chlorpropamide
Cimetidine
Ciprofloxacin
Coal tar
Contraceptives, oral
Dacarbazine
Diazepam
Enoxacin
Furosemide
Grepafloxacin
Griseofulvin[c]
Gold
Ketoprofen
Methoxsalen[c]
Methyldopa
Nalidixic acid[c]
Naproxen
Norfloxacin
Ofloxacin
Phenothiazines[c]
Phenylbutazone
Piroxicam
Promethazine
Proptriptyline[c]
Quinidine
Reserpine
Sparfloxacin

Sulfonamides
Sulfonylureas
Sulindac
Tetracyclines[c]
Thiazides[c]
Tolbutamide
Trovafloxacin
Vinblastine

Purpura
ACTH
Allopurinol
Barbiturates
Chlorothiazide
Corticosteroids
Coumarins[c]
Ephedrine
Gold[b]
Hydrochlorothiazide
Indomethacin
Iodides/bromides
Meprobamate
Penicillins
Quinidine
Sulfonamides

**Stevens-Johnson
Syndrome**
Ampicillin
Barbiturates[c]
Carbamazepine
Chloroquine
Chlorpropamide
Fansidar
Lithium
Meprobamate
Penicillins
Phenacetin
Phenothiazines
Phenytoin
Salicylates
Sulfonamides
Tetracycline
Trimethadione

Urticarial
ACTH
Ampicillin[c]
Allopurinol
Anticoagulants
Aspirin
Barbiturates
Cephalosporins
Chloral hydrate
Chlordiazepoxide
Chlorpromazine
Codeine[c]
Contraceptives, oral
Dextrans
Diazepam
Erythromycin
Fluorides
Griseofulvin
Gold
Hydralazine
Heparin
Ibuprofen
Indomethacin
Insulin
Iodides/bromides
Lithium
Morphine
Naproxen
Nitrofurantoin[c]
NSAIDs[c]
Penicillins[c]
Phenacetin
Phenylbutazone
Pilocarpine
Promethazine
Quinidine
Quinine
Reserpine
Saccharin
Sulfonamides
Sulindac
Thiouracil
Tolmetin

[a]ACTH, Adrenocorticotropic hormone; NSAIDs, Nonsteroidal anti-inflammatory drugs.
[b]Rash is more frequently reported.

Notes:

Table 35.14 •   Frequent Contact Sensitizers

Substance	Found In
Ammonia	Soaps, chemicals, hair dyes
Balsam of Peru	Cosmetics
Benzyl alcohol	Medications, cosmetics
Caine anesthetics	Medications
Carba	Rubber
Chromium	Jewelry
Epoxy resin	Glue
Ethylenediamine	Stabilizer in many topical products
Formaldehyde	Shoes, clothing, soaps, insulations
Mercaptobenzothiazol	Rubber
Naphthyl	Rubber
Neomycin	Topical medications
Nickel sulfate	Jewelry, fasteners
Paraben	Preservative in many topical products
Paraphenylenediamine	Hair dyes, leather
Potassium dichromate	Shoes, leather
Thiomersal	Preservatives, contact lens products
Thiram	Rubber products
Turpentine	Paint products
Wool alcohols	Lanolin-containing products, clothes

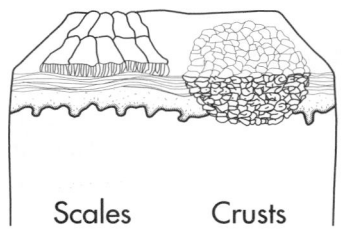

Scales   Crusts

Fig. 35.1 Scales and Crusts.

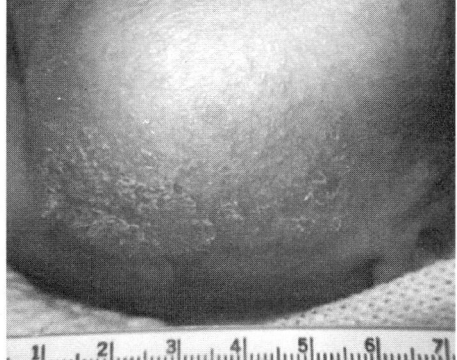

Notes:

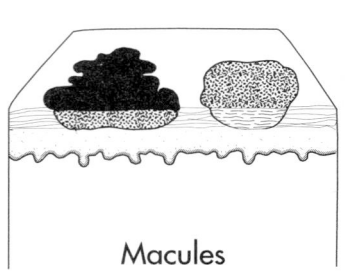

Macules

Fig. 35.2 Macules and Papules.

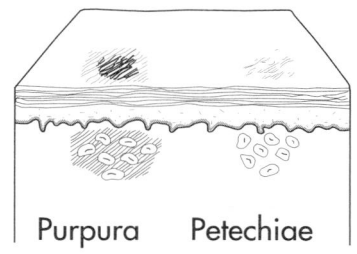

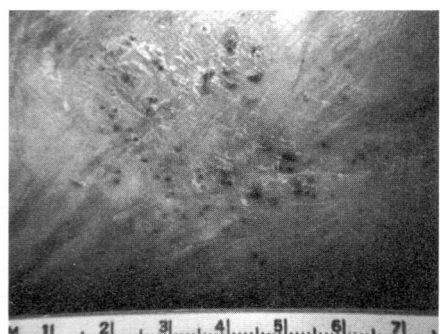

Purpura   Petechiae

Fig. 35.3 Purpura and Petechiae.

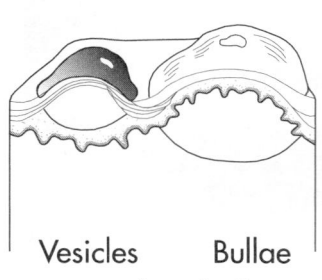

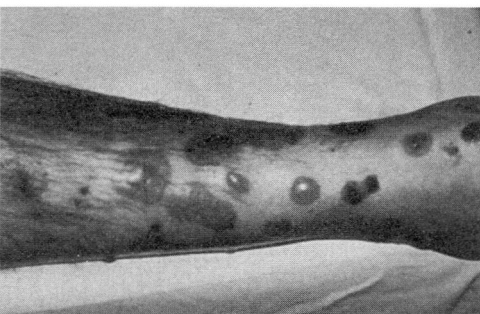

Vesicles   Bullae

Fig. 35.4 Vesicles and Bullae.

Notes:

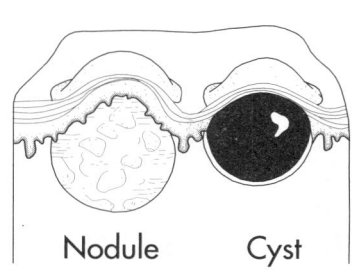
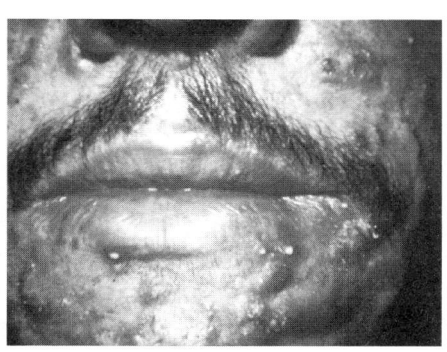

Fig. 35.5 Nodules and Cysts.

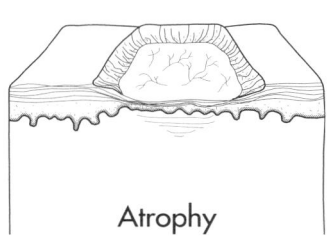
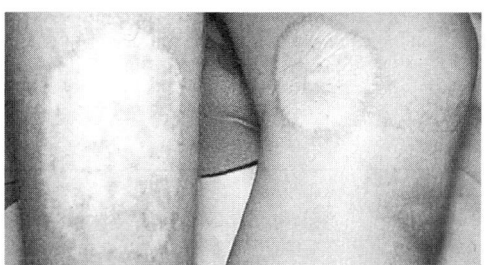

Fig. 35.6 Atrophy.

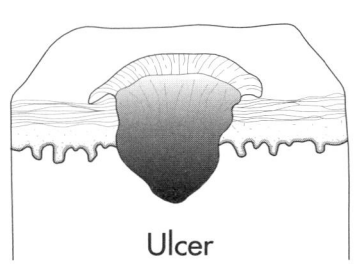
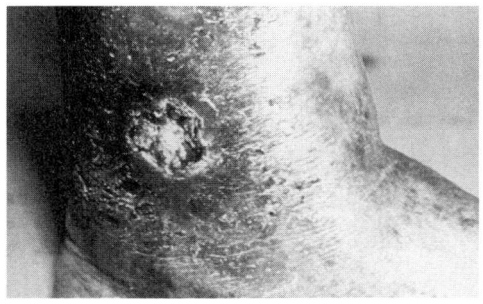

Fig. 35.7 Ulcer.

Notes:

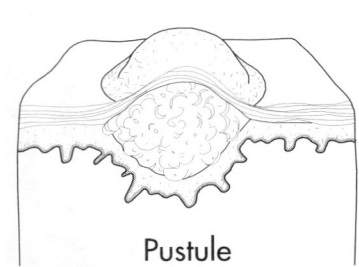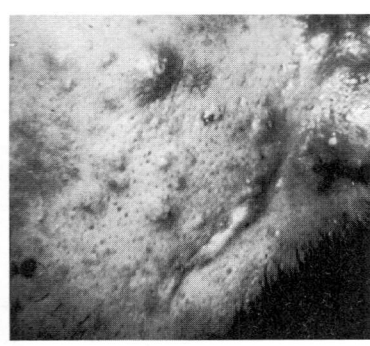

Fig. 35.8 Pustules.

The reader is referred to Chapter 36: Dermatotherapy, written by *T. A. Marek-Thompson, Pharm.D.*, and *C.A. Bond, Pharm.D.*, in the seventh edition of **Applied Therapeutics: The Clinical Use of Drugs** for a more in-depth discussion. All notations to reference numbers are based on the reference list at the end of that chapter. The editors of this handbook express their thanks to Drs. Marek-Thompson and Bond and acknowledge that this chapter is based upon their work.

Notes:

Chapter 36

Acne

Pathogenesis. Acne vulgaris is a self-limiting skin disorder involving the pilosebaceous follicles caused by increased sebum production, abnormal keratinization within the pilosebaceous canal, *Propionibacterium acnes* colonization, and an immune-mediated inflammatory reaction.

Lesions. The earliest lesions generally appear on the face, but the chest, back, or upper arms also may be affected. Noninflammatory lesions are closed comedones ("whiteheads") or open comedones ("blackheads"). Inflammatory lesions usually present as erythematous papules, pustules, cysts, or nodules. These lesions may be mild, or when severe, can cause scarring of tissue, disfigurement, and significant psychological distress.

Clinical Assessment. A detailed medical history (see Table 36.1) is critical to evaluation of acne and clinicians must take the time to assess the following:

- ◆ Distribution of lesions as to body sites such as the face, scalp, neck, shoulders, back, and arms.
- ◆ Provocative factors such as family history, work-related exposure, systemic or topical medications, or mechanical pressure on the skin.
- ◆ Hormonal factors such as absence of signs of virilization or atypical menstrual cycles.
- ◆ Whether the acne lesions are inflammatory or noninflammatory.

Treatment

- ◆ Treatment is primarily preventive; little can be done for existing lesions.
- ◆ At least BID washing with warm water and a mild soap (medicated soaps are not superior) removes excess sebum.
- ◆ Strongly discourage aggressive skin washing, abrasive cleansers, or squeezing and picking of lesions.
- ◆ Slow improvement over several weeks to months is the rule for *all* treatments.
- ◆ Treatment regimens should not be modified more often than every 2 months.
- ◆ Topical therapy generally is preferable for mild-to-moderate acne (Table 36.2).
- ◆ Drugs (see Table 36.3) generally are selected based upon increasing order of severity as follows: soap, benzoyl peroxide, topical antibiotics, systemic antibiotics, tretinoin, estrogens, and isotretinoin.
- ◆ Drug treatment of acne is based upon drug actions that:
  - • Normalize follicular keratinization (e.g., retinoids).
  - • Decrease sebum production (e.g., isotretinoin, hormones).
  - • Suppress bacterial *(P. acnes)* flora with antibiotics or benzoyl peroxide.
  - • Prevent inflammation (e.g., antibiotics, retinoids).
- ◆ Dermabrasion, cryotherapy, or ultraviolet light is used for severe cystic acne.

Notes:

Table 36.1 • Pertinent Historical Components to Be Obtained from a Patient with Acne

- Duration, including onset and peak severity
- Location and distribution
- Seasonal variation
- For *females*, relation to menstrual periods, pregnancy status, scalp hair thinning, contraceptive method if used
- Present and past treatments, topical and systemic, prescription and over-the-counter
- Family history, including severity
- Other skin disorders or medical problems
- Medications and drug allergies
- Occupational exposure to chemicals or oils
- Use of cosmetics, moisturizers, hairstyling products (pomades)
- Areas of skin friction or irritation

Table 36.2 • Choice of Topical Versus Oral Acne Therapy

Clinical Characteristics	Topical Therapy	Oral Therapy
Severity	Mild-to-moderate	Moderate-to-severe
Location	Face	Back, chest, arms
Treatment-resistant	In combination	Monotherapy or combined therapy
Likelihood of scarring	Not indicated	Indicated

Notes:

Table 36.3 • Drug Treatment of Acne

Drug	Efficacy and Indications	Mechanism	Adverse Effects	Comments
Benzoyl peroxide[a,b]	Improves 50%–75% of cases. Most effective and safest OTC[g] for mild to moderately severe acne. A topically applied 5% solution will ↓ FFAs[g] by 50%–60% and *P. acnes* by 98% after 2 weeks	Liberates free oxygen radicals that oxidize proteins and ↓ production of FFAs[g] in sebum caused by bacteria; loosens follicular plugs; comedolytic. Primary mechanism is its antibacterial activity	Dryness and irritation in most. In the fair skinned, wait until skin dries before applying; moist skin more sensitive to drying effect. Can discolor clothing. Avoid contact with hair. Keep away from eyes, mouth, nose, and mucous membranes. Allergic dermatitis 1%–3%. Pregnancy category C (not known if harmful to fetus when used during pregnancy)	Available in lotions, washes, creams, and gels. Formulations not equivalent in potency or irritant potential: alcohol base more potent than water base and causes more drying and stinging; gels most potent and require prescription (5% gel > potency than 10% cream or lotion)
Tetracycline[c]	Effective in moderate-to-severe acne. Inflammatory lesions ↓ and new lesions stop appearing 2–6 weeks after initiation of treatment	↓ FFAs[g] in skin, ↓ *P. acnes*, ↓ keratin production in sebaceous follicles	Minor with 250–500 mg/day dose. Antacids, iron, dairy products can ↓ absorption of drug	Oral antibiotic of choice because of low cost and low incidence of side effects. Erythromycin, clindamycin, cotrimoxazole, doxycycline, and minocycline also used. BID topical application of erythromycin or clindamycin should be tried for mild-to-moderate acne before systemic therapy
Tretinoin[d] (Retin-A)	Very effective prescription drug. Especially effective for "blackheads"	↑ follicle wall cell turnover; ↓ cohesiveness of cells; ↑ comedone extrusion; ↓ formation of new comedones	Erythema, irritation, and peeling common during 1st week. Especially irritating in the fair skinned. Initially may ↑ flare of acne before clearing	Creams < gels < solutions in potency or irritant potential. Use to ↓ age lines not FDA[g] approved and needs more study

(continued)

Table 36.3 • Drug Treatment of Acne (continued)

Drug	Efficacy and Indications	Mechanism	Adverse Effects	Comments
Isotretinoin[e,f] (Accutane)	Indicated for severe cystic acne unresponsive to conventional therapy. See guidelines in Table 36.4	↓ sebum production, ↓ sebaceous gland size, ↓ P. acnes, and normalized keratinization	Chelitis, skin desquamation, conjunctivitis, dry eyes, ↑ triglycerides, ↑ serum glucose, ↓ HDL,[g] teratogenic, hepatotoxic. See Table 36.5	Women must be tested for pregnancy before therapy, and effective contraception must be guaranteed because of very significant teratogenicity

[a] Cleansers: Wash QD or BID. Rinse thoroughly. Control amount of drying or peeling by altering frequency of application or application to moist skin (more sensitive to drying effect).

[b] Other dosage forms. Apply QD in small amount over affected area after cleansing skin, if dryness, redness, or peeling does not occur in 3 days, ↑ application to BID. Application causes mild stinging and warmth. Should result in mild dryness and erythema (NOT discomfort).

[c] Topical tetracycline (Topicycline), topical erythromycin (Eryderm, Staticin), and clindamycin (Cleocin-T) should be tried before use of systemic therapy. Topical tetracycline causes visible yellow tinting of skin, fluoresces in dark, and relatively less efficacy topically than clindamycin or erythromycin.

[d] Object of Therapy: Causes some erythema, peeling, and mild flushing; this is more important than set daily dosage (i.e., BID). Must be titrated; start with 0.05% for fair-skinned patients and 0.1% for others; no other topically applied therapy should be used initially, except for a mild soap; suggest applying at bedtime, 15–30 minutes after a shower/bath; avoid sun exposure; expect peeling in 1 week that should last 3–4 weeks; 3 months required for clearing (effectiveness cannot be judged for 6–8 weeks); water-based cosmetics are okay to use concomitantly.

[e] Initial Dose: 0.5–1 mg/kg/day in 2 daily divided doses for 15–20 weeks. After >2 months off therapy, a 2nd course can be initiated if warranted. Available in 10, 20, and 40 mg capsules.

[f] Table 34.3 provides guidelines for administration. Table 34.4 lists significant adverse effects.

[g] FDA = Food and Drug Administration; FFAs = Free fatty acids; HDL = High-density lipoproteins; OTC = Over-the-counter.

Notes:

Table 36.4 • Guidelines for Isotretinoin Use in Acne

Patient Selection
Severe cystic acne
Moderate acne but resistant to combination conventional therapies
Unusually severe acne variants (conglobata, fulminans)

Dosage
0.5–1 mg/kg/day
Use higher dosage in young patients, males, those with severe acne, patients with acne involving the trunk

Duration of Therapy
Cumulative dose of 120 mg/kg (usually 3–7 mo)

Relapse Rate
Repeat courses required in 15–20% of patients
Retreatment usually safe and effective
Very rarely, patients may require 3–5 courses

Table 36.5 • Adverse Effects of Systemic Retinoids[a]

Body System	Adverse Effect	Management
Common, Pharmacologic		
Skin	Dryness, peeling, pruritus. Photosensitivity	Moisturizers or emollients. Sunscreens, protective clothing
Hair, nails	Alopecia, nail fragility	None, discontinue drug if severe
Mucous membranes	Cheilitis Dry mouth, nose, eyes Blepharoconjunctivitis	Lip balms Sugarless gum/candy, saline nasal spray, artificial tears, or ophthalmic ointment ↓ dosage if severe or bothersome
Uncommon, Toxic		
Liver	↑ transaminases; hepatitis	Monitor if mild elevation. Avoid in patients with previous liver dysfunction. Discontinue drug if hepatitis occurs.
Bones	Pain	Monitor at each visit.
Muscle, ligaments	Pain, calcifications	Monitor; discontinue if severe.
Eyes	↓ night vision	Patients should use caution.
Metabolic	↑ triglycerides ↑ cholesterol ↑ VLDL, LDL	Reduce/eliminate alcohol; low-fat diet; consider dosage reduction or drug discontinuation.

[a]LDL = Low-density lipoprotein; VLDL = Very low-density lipoprotein.

The reader is referred to Chapter 37: Acne, written by *Terry L. Seaton, Pharm.D.*, in the seventh edition of **Applied Therapeutics: The Clinical Use of Drugs** for a more in-depth discussion. The editors of this handbook express their thanks to Dr. Seaton and acknowledge that this chapter is based upon his work.

Notes:

Notes:

Chapter 37

Psoriasis

Characteristics

♦ Psoriasis is a chronic proliferative skin disorder characterized by sharply defined erythematous patches covered with a distinctive silvery scale.

♦ Lesions of active psoriasis commonly develop on elbows, knees, scalp, gluteal cleft, fingernails, toenails, and at the site of epidermal trauma (e.g., scratches, sunburn, surgical wounds).

♦ Lesions usually are asymptomatic with about 20% experiencing pruritus.

♦ Most patients have chronic localized disease. but a small number have extensive disease *(erythrodermic psoriasis)*.

♦ Disease is lifelong with chronic recurrent exacerbations and remissions.

Treatment

♦ Many topical therapies (Table 37.1) are effective for localized psoriasis. The *severity* of psoriasis (extent or body involvement, *intensity* of scales and plaques): *type* of psoriasis (plaque, erythroderma, pustular); *location* of lesions (extensor surfaces, scalp, intertriginous areas); and *patient parameters* (age, size, personality, demographics) all affect the selection of the most appropriate therapy.

♦ Most patients begin treatment with high-potency steroid for limited psoriasis and add calcipotriene when response is inadequate. This is more effective and neater than tar or anthralin which usually requires concomitant UV light.

♦ Systemic therapies (methotrexate, etretinate) are reserved for severe (>20% involvement) psoriasis (Table 37.2).

♦ Drugs associated with exacerbation or precipitation of psoriasis are shown in Table 37.7.

Notes:

Table 37.1 • Topical Agents for the Treatment of Psoriasis (Mild to Moderate)[a]

Treatment Modality	Advantages	Disadvantages
Emollients	Basic adjunct of all treatments; safe; inexpensive; reduces scaling, itching, and related discomfort	Provides minimal relief alone
Keratolytics (salicylic acid, urea, α-hydroxy acids [i.e., glycolic and lactic acids])	Reduce hyperkeratosis; enable other topical modalities to better penetrate; inexpensive	Provide minimal relief individually; nonspecific; salicylism (tinnitus, nausea, vomiting) with salicylic acid if applied extensively
Topical corticosteroids	Rapid response; control inflammation and itching; best for intertriginous areas and face (lowest potency possible); convenient; not messy; most widely used topical treatment modality for psoriasis	Temporary relief; less effective with continued use (tachyphylaxis occurs); withdrawal can produce flares; atrophy, telangiectasia, and striae with continued use; expensive; adrenal suppression possible
Coal tar	Particularly effective for "flaky" scalp lesions; new preparations "pleasant"; efficacy enhanced in combination with UVB (i.e., Goeckerman regimen)	Effective only for mild psoriasis or scalp psoriasis; inconvenient—difficult to apply; stains clothing and bedding, not skin; strong smelling; folliculitis and contact allergy (bronchospasm in atopic patient with asthma after inhalation of vapor); carcinogenic in animals
Anthralin (dithranol in the United Kingdom)	Effective for widespread, refractory plaques; produces long remissions; short, concentrated programs preferred; enhanced efficacy in combination with UVB (i.e., Ingram regimen)	Purple-brown staining (skin, clothing, and bath fitments); irritating to normal skin and flexures; careful application required (inpatient?); can precipitate generalized psoriasis
Calcipotriene	As effective as topical corticosteroids, although slower, without long-term corticosteroid side effects; convenient; well tolerated	Slow onset; expensive; potential effects on bone metabolism (hypercalcemia); irritant dermatitis on face and intertriginous areas; contraindicated during pregnancy
Tazarotene	Extended response; convenient (QD, gel); maintenance therapy; effective on scalp and face; used in combination with topical corticosteroids	Slow onset; local irritation and pruritus; teratogenic (adequate birth control)
UVB	Effective as maintenance therapy; eliminates problems of topical steroids	Expensive (insurance reimburses); office-based therapy; sunburn (exacerbates psoriasis); photoaging; skin cancer

[a] <20% body involvement. UVB = ultraviolet B.

Table 37.2 • Agents for the Treatment of Severe Psoriasis[a]

Treatment Modality	Advantages	Disadvantages
UVA and psoralen (PUVA)	80% efficacy; "sun tan" cosmetically desirable	Time-consuming; expensive, office-based therapy (restrictive); sunburn (exacerbates psoriasis); photoaging; skin cancer; contraindicated during pregnancy and lactation. Table 37.3 lists measures to decrease toxicity of phototherapy.
Etretinate/acitretin	Not as effective as other systemic agents; efficacy enhanced if given with PUVA or UVB (i.e., RePUVA or ReUVB); less hepatotoxic than methotrexate; acitretin should replace etretinate[b]	Teratogenic (adequate birth control); contraindicated with liver or renal dysfunction, drug or alcohol abuse, hypertriglyceridemia, hypervitaminosis A. Monitoring recommendations are in Table 37.4.
Methotrexate	Gold standard for efficacy; effective for arthritis	Hepatotoxicity (periodic liver biopsy?); bone marrow toxicity; drug interactions; contraindicated during pregnancy and lactation, drug or alcohol abuse; caution during acute infections. Monitoring recommendations are listed in Table 37.5 and drug interactions in Table 37.6.
Hydroxyurea	Alternative to methotrexate (less hepatotoxicity)	Less effective than methotrexate; suppressive therapy (relapse occurs when discontinued); bone marrow suppression; caution during acute infections
Cyclosporine	Toxicity reputation and short-lived remissions have relegated use to extensive disease—not responsive to other agents; however, given changing pathophysiology and increasing experience at lower dosages, role in therapy changing; increasing role in rotational therapy to induce remissions	Renal impairment; suppressive therapy (relapse occurs when discontinued); increased risk of skin cancer, lymphomas and solid tumors; phototoxic; contraindicated during pregnancy and lactation, and with hypertension, hyperuricemia, hyperkalemia, acute infections

[a]>20% body involvement. UVA = Ultraviolet A; UVB = Ultraviolet B.
[b]Acitretin principle metabolite of etretinate; less lipophilic; shorter half-life; equal efficacy; less risk of toxicity.

Table 37.3 • Measures to Reduce the Toxicity of Photochemotherapy

Avoid long-term maintenance treatment and high cumulative dosages of radiation (approximately 200 treatments or a total UVA dose of 1,200 j/cm^2 is threshold for development of skin cancer).

Shield face and male genitalia during treatment.

Perform examinations to detect skin cancer at an early age.

Instruct patient to use sunscreen, protective clothing, and sunglasses.

Use rotational therapy (i.e., alternating monotherapies, allowing extended intervals off PUVA to allow skin recuperation before repeat exposure).

Use combination therapy (i.e., RePUVA) to reduce phototherapy dosage with superior efficacy.[37]

Notes:

Table 37.4 • Etretinate/Acitretin Therapy: Patient Monitoring

Type of Evaluation	Comments
Clinical evaluation (Psoriasis Area and Severity Index [PASI] score,[14] which includes the percent of body involvement and severity of lesions)	Performed twice in the first month, monthly for 6 mo, and Q 3 mo thereafter
Laboratory testing (CBC, UA, fasting glucose, renal function tests, calcium; *children:* calcium and phosphorus in blood and urine, vitamin D metabolism, osteocalcin, and parathyroid hormone)	Performed at each visit during first year and twice yearly thereafter; *children:* performed Q 6 mo
Liver function tests	Performed at each visit
Fasting lipids	Performed at each visit in first 4 mo and Q 2–3 mo thereafter; stop etretinate if serum triglycerides >800 mg/dL to reduce risk of pancreatitis
Pregnancy test	Performed before, monthly during, and for at least 1 yr after therapy
Radiographs	*Adults:* no routine radiograph monitoring if >40 years of age; *children:* yearly radiographic monitoring for long-term (>0.5 yr) treatment

Adapted from references 14 and 40–42. CBC = complete blood count; UA = urinalysis.

Notes:

Table 37.5 • Methotrexate Therapy: Patient Monitoring

Type of Evaluation	Comments
Clinical evaluation (Psoriasis Area and Severity Index [PASI] score,[14] which includes the percent of body involvement and severity of lesions)	Performed twice in the first month, monthly for 6 mo; then Q 3 mo thereafter
Laboratory testing	
CBC with differential and platelet count	Weekly for first 2 wk, biweekly for next month, then Q 1–2 mo
Renal function (serum creatinine, blood urea nitrogen, urinalysis)	Q 3–4 mo
Liver chemistry (AST, ALT, bilirubin, albumin)	Q 2 mo
Hepatitis A, B, C serologies	Baseline
Liver biopsy	Baseline (2–4 mo of therapy) only for high-risk patients; *first:* after 1–1.5 g cumulative dose; *repeat:* Q 1.5-g cumulative dose

ALT = Serum alanine aminotransferase; AST = Serum aspartate aminotransferase; CBC = Complete blood count.

Notes:

Table 37.6 • Methotrexate Drug Interactions

Mechanism	Drugs
Decreased renal elimination of methotrexate	Nephrotoxins (e.g., aminoglycosides, cyclosporine) Salicylates Sulfonamides Probenecid Cephalothin Penicillins Colchicine Nonsteroidal anti-inflammatory drugs
Additive or synergistic toxicity	Trimethoprim-sulfamethoxazole
Displacement of methotrexate from protein binding	Salicylates Probenecid Barbiturates Phenytoin Retinoids Sulfonamides Tetracycline
Intracellular accumulation of methotrexate	Dipyridamole
Hepatotoxicity	Retinoids Ethanol

Table 37.7 • Drugs Reported to Induce Psoriasis[a]

Anesthetics	Procaine
Antimicrobials	Amoxicillin, ampicillin, penicillin, sulfonamides, vancomycin, terbinafine, tetracycline
Anti-inflammatory drugs	Corticosteroids (following withdrawal), nonsteroidals (oxyphenbutazone, phenylbutazone, indomethacin, salicylates)
Antimalarials	Chloroquine, hydroxychloroquine[b]
β-Blockers	Propranolol
Cardiovascular drugs	Clonidine, digoxin, amiodarone, quinidine, calcium channel blockers (dihydropyridines, verapamil, diltiazem), acetazolamide, gemfibrozil, angiotensin-converting enzyme inhibitors
H_2 antagonists	Cimetidine, ranitidine
Hormones	Oxandrolone, progesterone
Narcotic analgesics	Morphine
Psychotropics	Lithium carbonate, stazepin, sodium valproate, fluoxetine
Miscellaneous	Potassium iodide, sulfapyridine gold, mercury, oxandrolone, progesterone, lithium

[a] Adapted from reference 56.
[b] Except for one case report, hydroxychloroquine (unlike chloroquine) does not adversely affect the course of psoriasis and usually induces a beneficial response in 75% of patients with psoriatic arthritis.

Notes:

The reader is referred to Chapter 38: Psoriasis, written by *Allan J. Ellsworth. Pharm.D.,* in the seventh edition of **Applied Therapeutics: The Clinical Use of Drugs** for a more in-depth discussion. All notations to reference numbers are based on the reference list at the end of that chapter. The editors of this handbook express their thanks to Dr. Ellsworth and acknowledge that this chapter is based upon his work.

Notes:

Chapter 38

Photosensitivity and Burns

UVR Radiation

♦ Photosensitivity reactions are closely linked to ultraviolet radiation (UVR) and include conditions such as sunburn, cataracts, photoaging, photodermatoses, phototoxicity, photoallergy, and photocarcinogenesis (e.g., squamous cell and basal cell carcinoma and malignant melanoma).

♦ **UV Index,** with a scale from 1 (minimal exposure) to 10 (very high exposure), forecasts the probable intensity of skin-damaging UVR expected to reach the surface at noon when the sun is highest in the sky. The amount of UVR exposure is affected by the elevation of the sun in the sky, amount of ozone in the stratosphere, and the amount of clouds.

♦ Excessive exposure of the skin to UVR results in an inflammatory erythematous reaction mediated by vasodilatory chemical mediators (e.g., histamine, prostaglandins, cytokines) that increase regional blood flow and cause erythema, increased sensation of warmth, tissue exudates, swelling, and the characteristic sunburn.

♦ The darker an individual's skin, the longer (or more UVR) is needed to cause erythema.

♦ Tanning, an adaptive mechanism of the skin to UVR, is the result of immediate pigment darkening and also of delayed tanning. Immediate pigment darkening results from oxidation of existing melanin in the skin and the skin type.

♦ Patients can be classified into six sun-reactive skin types based upon their response to initial sun exposure, skin color, tendency to sunburn, ability to tan, and personal history of sunburn (Table 38.1).

Photoprotection

♦ Sunscreens should be only one component of an overall program (acronym **C-H-E-S-S**) to reduce UV exposure and protect against long-term photodamage.

  • C = Clothing that is sun protective (i.e., tightly woven and in dark colors).

  • H = Hats with wide brims all around

  • E = Eyeglasses that block both UVA and UVB light

  • S = Sunscreen with a SPF of >15 applied appropriately

  • S = Shade, especially between 10 a.m. and 4 p.m.

♦ The effectiveness of a sunscreen formulation is based on its sun protection factor **(SPF)** and its **substantivity** (measure of a sunscreen's effectiveness including its ability to be adsorbed by, or adhere to, the skin while swimming or perspiring). A SPF of 8 signifies that an individual can be exposed eight times longer to UVB than without the sunscreen.

♦ Table 38.2 presents the common chemical classes of sunscreen agents and UV absorbance. Sunscreens should not be applied to children less than 6 months of age because of possible absorption and decreased ability to metabolize some chemicals.

♦ Prudent to avoid prolonged sun exposure, even with application of sunscreen. Sunscreen usage might promote melanoma by encouraging prolonged exposure to sunlight and to UVA rays insufficiently blocked by sunscreens.

♦ Sunscreens should be reapplied after profuse sweating or water activity.

♦ Table 38.3 lists sunscreens judged to be both safe and effective.

Treatment of Sunburn

♦ Sunburn is a self-limiting condition, and treatment is symptomatic (e.g., topical hydrocortisone cream or aloe vera gel, cooling compresses). NSAIDs (e.g., ibuprofen, naproxen) relieve pain and minimize prostaglandin-mediated inflammation. Topical anesthetics (e.g., benzocaine) provide transient relief (15 to 45 minutes) but can cause contact sensitization.

♦ Severe sunburn with symptoms (e.g., chills, nausea, vomiting, fever) should be seen by a physician. Prednisone 1 mg/kg/day × 3 days can be useful.

Photoaging

♦ Photoaging, or premature aging of the skin, results from a chronic inflammatory state induced by long-term exposure to sunlight and involves skin changes (wrinkled, yellowed, and sagging) that are different from those associated with normal chronologic aging.

♦ Tretinoin (transretinoic acid), available as a topical cream, gel, or liquid, can partially reverse some of the clinical and histological changes of photoaging. Generally is most effective for patients 50–70 years of age with moderate-to-severe photoaging.

♦ Adverse effects (e.g., erythema, peeling, burning, and stinging) and the clinical and histologic improvements appear to be dose dependent. Goal is to provide maximal benefit by using the highest-strength topical tretinoin while causing minimal skin irritation.

Phototoxicity and Photoallergy

♦ Phototoxicity, an immediate or delayed inflammatory reaction, occurs when a compound with photosensitizing ability absorbs a sufficient concentration of UV energy and transfers the energy to surrounding molecules, which then destroys surrounding tissue.

♦ Photoallergic reactions require prior or prolonged exposure to the photosensitizing compound and occur much less commonly than phototoxicity reactions. Photoallergy occurs by a similar mechanism as that of photosensitizing reactions, except that the immune system is involved and the rash generally is severe, intensely pruritic, and can spread to areas not exposed to sunlight.

♦ Photoallergies are not dose-related, and chemically related agents can also cause eruptions.

♦ Common drugs capable of inducing photosensitivity reactions are in Table 38.4.

Minor Burns

♦ Burn wounds are classified according to the depth of tissue damage, but it is often difficult to gauge the depth of the burn wound during the first 24–48 hours because of edema, tissue ischemia, or infection.

♦ First-degree burns result from injury to the superficial cells of the epidermis (e.g., mild sunburn). The burned skin does not form blisters and heals within 3–4 days without scarring.

♦ Second-degree burns often are erythematous, blistered, weeping, painful, and very sensitive to stimuli. Healing of deep second-degree burns occur slowly over about 35 days with eschar formation and possible severe scarring.

♦ Third-degree burns entail complete destruction of the full thickness of the skin. These are repaired most often by excision and grafting of the wound to prevent contractures of the skin.

♦ Fourth-degree burns are similar to third-degree burns, except that devitalized tissue extends into the subcutaneous tissue, fascia, and bone.

♦ American Burn Association treatment categories are listed in Table 38.5.

♦ Recommended criteria for transfer to burn centers are noted in Table 38.6.

Table 38.1 • Suggested SPF for Various Skin Types[a]

Complexion	Skin Type	Skin Characteristics	Suggested Product SPF
Very fair	I	Always burns easily; never tans	20–30
Fair	II	Always burns easily; tans minimally	15–20
Light	III	Burns moderately; tans gradually	10–15
Medium	IV	Burns minimally; always tans well	8–10
Dark	V	Rarely burns; tans profusely	8
Very dark	VI	Never burns; deeply pigmented	8

[a]SPF, Sun protection factor.

Notes:

Table 38.2 • Sunscreens and UVR Absorbance

Sunscreen	Absorbance
Anthranilates	
Menthyl anthranilate	260–380
Benzophenones	
Dioxybenzone	250–390
Oxybenzone	270–350
Sulisobenzone (Eusolex 4360)	260–375
Cinnamates	
Diethanolamine p-methoxycinnamate	280–310
Octocrylene	250–360
Octyl methoxycinnamate (Parsol MCX)	290–320
Dibenzoylmethanes	
Avobenzone (butyl methoxydibenzoylmethane, Parsol 1789)	320–400
Aminobenzoic Acid and Ester Derivatives	
Lisadimate (Glyceryl PABA)	264–315
Para-aminobenzoic acid (PABA)	260–313
Padimate O (octyl dimethyl PABA)	290–315
Roxadimate	280–330
Salicylates	
Homosalate	295–315
Octyl salicylate	280–320
Triethanolamine salicylate	260–320
Trolamine salicylate	260–320
Camphor Derivatives	
Benzoate-4 methylbenzylidene camphor	290–300
Mexoryl SX	290–400
Others	
Phenylbenzimidazole	290–340
Physical Sunscreens	
Red petrolatum	290–365
Titanium dioxide	290–700
Zinc oxide	290–700

Notes:

Table 38.3 • Examples of Commercially Available Sunscreen Products

Name (Active Ingredients)	Formulation	SPF
Aquaderm Sunscreen Moisturizer (octyl methoxycinnamate, oxybenzone)	Cream	15
Bain de Soleil All Day For Kids (octocrylene, octyl methoxycinnamate, oxybenzone, titanium dioxide)	Lotion	30
Bain de Soleil All Day Waterproof Sunblock (octocrylene, octyl methoxycinnamate, oxybenzone, titanium dioxide)	Lotion	15, 30
Bain de Soleil All Day Waterproof Sunfilter (octocrylene, octyl methoxycinnamate, titanium dioxide)	Lotion	4, 8
Bain de Soleil Mega Tan (octocrylene, octyl methoxycinnamate)	Lotion	4
Bain de Soleil Orange Gelée Sunfilter (octyl methoxycinnamate, octocrylene, oxybenzone, octyl salicylate)	Gel	4
Bain de Soleil Mademoiselle (octyl methoxycinnamate, octyl salicylate, titanium dioxide)	Lotion	30
Bain de Soleil SPF + Color (octocrylene, oxybenzone, octyl methoxycinnamate)	Lotion	8, 15, 30
Bain de Soleil Tropical Deluxe (octyl methoxycinnamate, octyl salicylate)	Lotion	4
Banana Boat Baby Block (octyl methoxycinnamate, octyl salicylate, oxybenzone, titanium dioxide)	Lotion	50
Banana Boat Cool Colorz Vanishing Sunblock (octyl methoxycinnamate, homosalate, octyl salicylate, oxybenzone)	Lotion	30
Banana Boat Faces Plus Sunblock (octyl methoxycinnamate, octyl salicylate, oxybenzone)	Lotion	23
Banana Boat Quik Blok Kids (octyl methoxycinnamate, homosalate, octyl salicylate, oxybenzone)	Lotion	25+
Banana Boat Sport Sunblock (octyl methoxycinnamate, octyl salicylate, oxybenzone)	Lotion	15, 30
Banana Boat Sport Sunblock (octyl methoxycinnamate, octyl salicylate, oxybenzone, octocrylene)	Lotion	50
BioSun Sunblock (octyl methoxycinnamate, oxybenzone, octyl salicylate, titanium dioxide)	Lotion	45
Blistex Regular (oxybenzone, padimate O)	Lip balm	10
Blistex Ultra Protection (homosalate, menthyl anthranilate, octyl methoxycinnamate, octyl salicylate, oxybenzone)	Lip balm	30
Bullfrog (octyl methoxycinnamate, oxybenzone)	Stick	18
Bullfrog Quik Stick (octyl methoxycinnamate, oxybenzone, octyl salicylate, octocrylene)	Stick	36
Bullfrog Body Lotion (octocrylene, octyl methoxycinnamate, oxybenzone, octyl salicylate)	Lotion	30
Bullfrog Body Lotion (octocrylene, octyl methoxycinnamate, oxybenzone)	Lotion	45
Bullfrog Body Gel (octocrylene, octyl methoxycinnamate, oxybenzone)	Gel	36
Bullfrog Extra Moisturizing (octocrylene, octyl methoxycinnamate, oxybenzone, octyl salicylate)	Gel	18
Bullfrog For Kids (octocrylene, octyl methoxycinnamate, oxybenzone)	Gel	18, 36
Bullfrog For Babies (octocrylene, octyl methoxycinnamate, oxybenzone, octyl salicylate, titanium dioxide, menthyl anthranilate)	Lotion	45
Bullfrog Magic Block—Disappearing Green (octyl methoxycinnamate, octyl salicylate, octocrylene, oxybenzone)	Lotion	30
Bullfrog Quik Gel (octyl methoxycinnamate, oxybenzone, octyl salicylate, octocrylene)	Gel	36
Bullfrog Sport (octocrylene, octyl methoxycinnamate, octyl salicylate, oxybenzone)	Lotion	18, 30

(continued)

Table 38.3 • Examples of Commercially Available Sunscreen Products (continued)

Name (Active Ingredients)	Formulation	SPF
Bullfrog Sunblock (octyl methoxycinnamate, oxybenzone, octyl salicylate)	Gel	18
Bullfrog Sunblock (octyl methoxycinnamate, oxybenzone, octyl salicylate, octocrylene)	Gel	36
Bullfrog Super Block (octocrylene, octyl methoxycinnamate, octyl salicylate, oxybenzone, titanium dioxide, menthyl anthranilate)	Lotion	45
Chap Stick (padimate O)	Lip balm	15
Chap Stick Ultra (octocrylene, octyl methoxycinnamate, oxybenzone, octyl salicylate)	Lip balm	30
Chap Stick Sunblock (oxybenzone, padimate O)	Lip balm	15
Chap Stick Sunblock 15 Petroleum Jelly Plus (oxybenzone, padimate O)	Ointment	15
Coppertone All Day Protection (homosalate, octyl methoxycinnamate, octyl salicylate, oxybenzone)	Lotion	45
Coppertone BUG & SUN for Adults (with insect repellent) (homosalate, octyl methoxycinnamate, octyl salicylate, oxybenzone)	Lotion	15
Coppertone BUG & SUN for Kids (with insect repellent) (octocrylene, octyl methoxycinnamate, oxybenzone)	Lotion	30
Coppertone KIDS 6 Hour Sunblock (homosalate, octyl methoxycinnamate, octyl salicylate, oxybenzone)	Lotion	15, 30, 40
Coppertone KIDS Sunblock (homosalate, octyl methoxycinnamate, octyl salicylate, oxybenzone)	Stick	30
Coppertone KIDS Colorblock Disappearing Colored Sunblock (Blue or Purple Formula) (octyl methoxycinnamate, octyl salicylate, oxybenzone, homosalate)	Lotion	30, 40
Coppertone KIDS Colorblock Disappearing Colored Sunblock (Blue Formula) (octyl methoxycinnamate, oxybenzone, octyl salicylate, homosalate)	Spray	30
Coppertone Lipkote (octyl methoxycinnamate, oxybenzone)	Lip balm	15
Coppertone Moisturizing Sunblock (octyl methoxycinnamate, octyl salicylate, octocrylene, oxybenzone)	Lotion	45
Coppertone Moisturizing Sunblock (octyl methoxycinnamate, octyl salicylate, homosalate, oxybenzone)	Lotion	25, 30
Coppertone Moisturizing Sunblock (octyl methoxycinnamate, oxybenzone)	Lotion	15
Coppertone Moisturizing Sunscreen (octyl methoxycinnamate, oxybenzone)	Lotion	6, 8
Coppertone OIL FREE Sunblock (homosalate, octyl methoxycinnamate, octyl salicylate, oxybenzone)	Lotion	8, 15, 30, 45
Coppertone Shade Oil-Free (homosalate, octyl methoxycinnamate, oxybenzone)	Gel	30
Coppertone Shade Sunblock (homosalate, octyl methoxycinnamate, octyl salicylate, oxybenzone)	Lotion	45
Coppertone Shade UVA Guard Sunblock (azobenzene, octyl methoxycinnamate, oxybenzone)	Lotion	30
Coppertone Sport (octyl methoxycinnamate, octyl salicylate, oxybenzone)	Lotion	4, 8, 15, 30
Coppertone Sport Ultra Sweatproof (octyl methoxycinnamate, oxybenzone, octyl salicylate)	Lotion	8, 15, 30, 48
Coppertone Water BABIES Sunblock (homosalate, octyl methoxycinnamate, octyl salicylate, oxybenzone)	Lotion	30, 45
DuraScreen (octyl methoxycinnamate, octyl salicylate, oxybenzone)	Lotion	15
DuraScreen (octyl methoxycinnamate, octyl salicylate, oxybenzone, phenylbenzimidazole, titanium dioxide)	Lotion	15, 30

(continued)

Table 39-3 • Examples of Commercially Available Sunscreen Products (continued)

Name (Active Ingredients)	Formulation	SPF
Eclipse Lip & Face Protectant (oxybenzone, padimate O)	Stick	15
Eclipse Original Suncreen (lisadimate, padimate O)	Lotion	10
Eucerin Dry Skin Therapy Facial Moisturizing (octyl methoxycinnamate, octyl salicylate, titanium dioxide, zinc oxide)	Lotion	25
Fisher-Price Waterproof Sunblock (titanium dioxide)	Cream	28
Hawaiian Tropic Baby Faces Sunblock (octocrylene, octyl methoxycinnamate, octyl salicylate, oxybenzone, titanium dioxide)	Lotion	35, 50
Hawaiian Tropic Just For Kids (homosalate, menthyl anthranilate, octyl methoxycinnamate, octyl salicylate, oxybenzone)	Lotion	30
Hawaiian Tropic Just For Kids (octocrylene, octyl methoxycinnamate, octyl salicylate, oxybenzone, titanium dioxide)	Lotion	45
Hawaiian Tropic Self-Tanning Sunblock (octyl methoxycinnamate, oxybenzone)	Cream	15
Hawaiian Tropic Sunblock (homosalate, menthyl anthranilate, octyl methoxycinnamate, octyl salicylate, oxybenzone)	Lotion	30^+
Hawaiian Tropic Sunblock (octocrylene, octyl methoxycinnamate, octyl salicylate, oxybenzone, titanium dioxide)	Lotion	45^+
Hawaiian Tropic Water Sport (octyl methoxycinnamate, octyl salicylate, titanium dioxide)	Lotion	15
Neutrogena Chemical-Free Sunblocker (titanium dioxide)	Lotion	17
Neutrogena Dry Oil (octyl methoxycinnamate, oxybenzone)	Spray	15
Neutrogena Healthy Skin Lotion (octyl methoxycinnamate, oxybenzone)	Lotion	15
Neutrogena Kids Sunblock (homosalate, octyl methoxycinnamate, oxybenzone, octyl salicylate)	Lotion	30
Neutrogena Sun Block (octyl methoxycinnamate, oxybenzone)	Lotion	15
Neutrogena Moisture Untinted (octyl methoxycinnamate, oxybenzone)	Lotion	15
Neutrogena Moisture with Sheer Tint (octyl methoxycinnamate, oxybenzone)	Lotion	15
Neutrogena Oil-Free Sunblock (homosalate, octyl methoxycinnamate, oxybenzone, octyl salicylate)	Lotion	30
Neutrogena Sensitive Skin Sunblock (titanium dioxide)	Lotion	17
Neutrogena Sunblock (menthyl anthranilate, octocrylene, octyl methoxycinnamate)	Cream	30
Neutrogena Sunblock (menthyl anthranilate, octyl methoxycinnamate, octyl salicylate, homosalate)	Spray	20
Neutrogena Sunblock Stick (octyl methoxycinnamate, octyl salicylate, oxybenzone)	Stick	25
Neutrogena UVA/UVB Sunblock (octyl methoxycinnamate, homosalate, octyl salicylate, oxybenzone, azobenzene)	Lotion	30, 45
Off! Skintastic with Sunscreen (octyl methoxycinnamate, octocrylene, oxybenzone, octyl salicylate)	Lotion	15, 30
PreSun Active Clear (octyl methoxycinnamate, octyl salicylate, oxybenzone)	Gel	30
PreSun Kids (octyl methoxycinnamate, octyl salicylate, oxybenzone)	Lotion	29
PreSun Lip Protector (oxybenzone, padimate O)	Lip Balm	15
PreSun Moisturizing (oxybenzone, padimate O)	Lotion	46
PreSun Moisturizing Sunscreen with Keri (octyl methoxycinnamate, octyl salicylate, oxybenzone)	Lotion	25
PreSun Sensitive Skin (octyl methoxycinnamate, octyl salicylate, oxybenzone)	Lotion	29

(continued)

Table 39-3 • Examples of Commercially Available Sunscreen Products (continued)

Name (Active Ingredients)	Formulation	SPF
PreSun Spray Mist (octyl methoxycinnamate, octyl salicylate, oxybenzone, padimate O)	Spray	23
PreSun Ultra (azobenzene)	Lotion	15, 30
PreSun Ultra (azobenzene)	Spray	27
Solbar PF (octyl methoxycinnamate, octocrylene, oxybenzone)	Cream	15, 50
Solbar PF (octyl methoxycinnamate, oxybenzone)	Liquid	15, 30
Solbar PF (octocrylene, octyl methoxycinnamate, oxybenzone)	Liquid	30
Solbar Plus (dioxybenzone, oxybenzone, padimate O)	Cream	15
Sundown Sport Sunblock (titanium dioxide, zinc oxide)	Lotion	15
Sundown Sunblock (octyl methoxycinnamate, octyl salicylate, oxybenzone, titanium dioxide)	Lotion	8, 15, 30
Sundown Sunscreen (octyl methoxycinnamate, octyl salicylate, oxybenzone, titanium dioxide)	Lotion	8
TI-Lite (octyl methoxycinnamate, titanium dioxide)	Cream	15
TI-Screen Baby Natural (titanium dioxide)	Lotion	16
TI-Screen Natural (titanium dioxide)	Lotion	16
TI-Screen (octocrylene, octyl methoxycinnamate, octyl salicylate, oxybenzone)	Lotion	30
TI-Screen (octyl methoxycinnamate, octyl salicylate, oxybenzone)	Gel	20+
TI-Screen (octyl methoxycinnamate, oxybenzone)	Lotion	8, 15+

Table 38.4 • Common Drugs Capable of Photosensitizing

Amiodarone	Furosemide	Naproxen	Piroxicam
Amitriptyline	Griseofulvin	Oral contraceptives	Sulfonamides
Dacarbazine	Isotretinoin	Oral hypoglycemics	Sulindac
Diphenhydramine	Ketoprofen	Phenothiazines	Tetracycline
Doxepin	Nalidixic acid	Phenylbutazone	Thiazides

Table 38.5 • Treatment Categories for Burn Injuries

- *Major burn injuries* are second-degree burns with >25% BSA involvement in adults (20% in children); all third-degree burns with ≥10% BSA involvement; all burns involving the hands, face, eyes, ears, feet, and perineum that may result in functional or cosmetic impairment; high-voltage electrical injury; and burns complicated by inhalation injury, major trauma, or poor-risk patients (elderly patients and those with debilitating disease).
- *Moderate, uncomplicated burns* are second-degree burns with 15 to 25% BSA involvement in adults (10 to 20% in children); third-degree burns with 2 to 10% BSA involvement; and burns not involving risk to areas of specialized function such as the eyes, ears, face, hands, feet, or perineum.
- *Major or moderate, uncomplicated burns* necessitate admission, and surgical referral is recommended for patients of all ages who have deep second- or third-degree burns covering ≥3% of the TBSA.
- *Minor burn injuries* include second-degree burns with <15% BSA involvement in adults (10% in children), third-degree burns with <2% BSA, and burns not involving functional or cosmetic risk to areas of specialized function. Patients with burns of this category may be treated on an outpatient basis if no other trauma is present; if circumferential burns of the neck, trunk, arms, or legs are not present; and if the patient is able to comply with therapy. After initial evaluation by a health care provider, patients may self-treat a second- or third-degree burn only if <1% BSA is involved.

Table 38.6 • Criteria for Transfer to Burn Centers

The American Burn Association and the American College of Surgeons recommend transfer to a burn center for all acutely burned patients who meet any of the following criteria[90]:

- Partial thickness burns ≥20% TBSA in patients aged 10 to 50 years old
- Partial thickness burns ≥10% TBSA in children aged 10 or adults aged 50 years old
- Full-thickness burns ≥5% TBSA in patients of any age
- Patients with partial- or full-thickness burns of the hands, feet, face, eyes, ears, perineum, and/or major joints
- Patients with high-voltage electrical injuries, including lightning injuries
- Patients with significant burns from caustic chemicals
- Patients with burns complicated by multiple trauma in which the burn injury poses the greatest risk of morbidity or mortality (in such cases, if the trauma poses the greater immediate risk, the patient may be treated initially in a trauma center until stable before being transferred to a burn center)
- Patients with burns who suffer an inhalation injury
- Patients with significant ongoing medical disorders that could complicate management, prolong recovery, or affect mortality
- Patients who were taken to hospitals without qualified personnel or equipment for the care of children
- Burn injury in those patients who will require special social/emotional and/or long-term rehabilitative support, including cases involving suspected child abuse, substance abuse, and so on

The reader is referred to Chapter 39: Photosensitivity and Burns, written by *Timothy J. Ives, Pharm.D.,* in the seventh edition of **Applied Therapeutics: The Clinical Use of Drugs** for a more in-depth discussion. The editors of this handbook express their thanks to Dr. Ives and acknowledge that this chapter is based upon his work.

Notes:

Notes:

Chapter 39

Gout and Hyperuricemia

GOUT

♦ Gout is a disorder of uric acid metabolism manifested by hyperuricemia or acute chronic recurrent arthritis, as well as deposits of monosodium urate. Gout should be considered a clinical diagnosis and hyperuricemia a biochemical one. These two terms are not synonymous and are not interchangeable.

♦ When 6 of the 11 criteria listed in Table 39.1 are present, an epidemiological diagnosis of gout has a specificity of 92.7% and a sensitivity of 84.8%. These criteria are useful when aspiration of a joint is not viable. The diagnosis of acute gout is confirmed only when large numbers of polymorphonuclear leukocytes and monosodium urate crystals are present in the synovial fluid aspirated from the affected joint.

Treatment

♦ ***Acute gouty arthritis*** can be treated effectively by any of the drugs listed in Table 39.2. The acute pain of an *initial* gout attack begins to recede about 4–8 hours after the initiation of treatment and the pain, redness, and swelling usually are resolved completely within 48–72 hours. There is considerable interpatient variation to this time frame for response, and subsequent gouty attacks may require a longer period of time to be resolved.

♦ ***Interval Treatment.*** After the initial attack of acute gout, the interval between subsequent attacks varies from a few days to several years. Antihyperuricemic drugs should be initiated only when gouty patients have frequent acute attacks, urate tophi, or evidence of renal damage. If these indications are absent, hypouricemic drug therapy should be withheld.

HYPERURICEMIA
Treatment

♦ ***Uricosuric drugs*** (e.g., probenecid, sulfinpyrazone) reduce the serum urate concentration by increasing the renal excretion of uric acid.

♦ ***Xanthine-oxidase inhibitors*** (e.g., allopurinol) decrease serum uric acid by inhibiting uric acid synthesis.

♦ Both allopurinol and probenecid are ineffective in the treatment of an acute gouty attack, and both can precipitate an acute gouty attack early in the course of therapy.

♦ Both are effective in the long-term management of hyperuricemia. (See Table 39.3.)

♦ ***Allopurinol Drug Interactions.*** See Table 39.4.

♦ ***Drug-induced hyperuricemia.*** See Table 39.5

Asymptomatic Hyperuricemia

- ◆ Individuals with high serum uric acid levels are more likely to develop acute gouty arthritis than normouricemic individuals, and the magnitude of the risk increases with increasing degrees of hyperuricemia.
- ◆ Hyperuricemia by itself has no deleterious effect on renal function.
- ◆ When financial costs, risk of adverse drug reactions, and patient compliance are considered, drug treatment of asymptomatic hyperuricemia is difficult to justify.

Table 39.1 • Criteria for Epidemiologic Diagnosis of Gout[10]

>1 acute attack of arthritis	Unilateral podagra
Exquisite pain involving joint	Tophi
Joint inflammation maximal within 1 day	Hyperuricemia
Oligoarthritis	Asymmetric swelling within a joint on a radiologic examination
Erythema over involved joints	
Podagra (first metatarsophalangeal joint)	Complete termination of acute attack

Notes:

Table 39.2 • Drugs Effective for Treatment of Acute Gout[a]

Drug	Dose	Comment
Colchicine	1 mg then 0.5 mg every other hour until relief of joint pain or onset of GI effects. Total dose/attack not to exceed 5 mg	↓ doses in elderly or patients with ↓ liver or ↓ renal function. GI toxicity (diarrhea, cramping) are predictable with therapeutic doses. Large overdoses are life-threatening, affecting multiple-organ systems (e.g., hepatic, hematopoietic, musculoskeletal, GI, neurological). IV doses of 2 mg diluted in 30 mL NS to be given over 5 min cause less GI distress but ↑ risk of phlebitis and serious extravasation. Least desirable benefit-to-risk ratio of all the drugs in this table.
Corticosteroids	Prednisone 20 mg BID, then 10 mg BID until attack quiescent. Taper dose over ensuing 10 days	Inconsistent results and rebound flares due to underdosage or premature discontinuation. Potential for relapse not greater than with other treatments when adequate doses used. Adverse effects not common with short courses of therapy, except for glucose and GI intolerance
Indomethacin	50 mg TID; gradually taper dose as attack subsides	Some consider to be drug of choice, but all drugs in this table are equally effective. GI distress, mental changes, headaches, and leukopenia more common with larger doses
NSAIDs	Fenoprofen (Nalfon) 800 mg TID-QID Flurbiprofen (Ansaid) 100 mg QID for 1 day, then 50 mg QID Ibuprofen (Motrin) 600 mg QID Ketoprofen (Orudis) 50 mg QID Meclofenamate (Meclomen) 100 mg TID-QID Naproxen (Naprosyn) 750 mg, followed by 250 mg Q 8 hr Piroxicam (Feldene) 40 mg QD Sulindac (Clinoril) 200 mg BID Tolmetin (Tolectin) 400 mg TID-QID	All are equally effective and commonly preferred over other drugs in this table. Adverse effects, except for GI effects, are uncommon with short-term treatment. Doses should be ↓ when attack subsides

[a] GI = Gastrointestinal; IV = Intravenous; NS = Normal saline; NSAIDs = Nonsteroidal anti-inflammatory drugs.

Table 39.3 • Treatment of Hyperuricemia

Drug	Initial Dose	Maintenance Dose	Adverse Effects
Allopurinol (Zyloprim)	100–150 mg/day for 2 weeks	300–400 mg/day[a]	Hypersensitivity (exfoliative dermatitis, toxic epidermal necrolysis, Stevens-Johnson Syndrome, hepatotoxicity, nephrotoxicity)
Probenecid (Benemid)	250 mg BID for 1–2 weeks	500 mg BID[a]	Hypersensitivity reactions; can precipitate urolithiasis. Aspirin (doses >600 mg QID) can completely negate 2 gm of probenecid

[a] ↑ or ↓ the dose as necessary to maintain serum uric acid concentration <6.5 mg/dL.

Table 39.4 • Allopurinol Drug Interactions[a]

Major Documentation

Azathioprine (Imuran). Metabolized to 6-mercaptopurine and then to inactive metabolites by xanthine oxidase. Allopurinol-inhibition of xanthine oxidase ↑ the serum concentration of 6-mercaptopurine and the risk of bone marrow depression. When a patient is stabilized on azathioprine (or 6-mercaptopurine), the azathioprine dose should be ↓ to ¼ of the recommended dose when allopurinol is added.[68]

Mercaptopurine (Purinethol). See as Azathioprine.

Moderate Documentation

ACE Inhibitors. May predispose patients to severe allopurinol-hypersensitivity reactions (e.g., Stevens-Johnson syndrome). Concurrent and subclinical renal impairment may be important variables.

Anticoagulants. Occasional patients on oral anticoagulants and allopurinol will develop enhanced anticoagulant effects; however, this interaction is unpredictable and primarily based on isolated case reports.

Cyclophosphamide. Allopurinol ↑ cyclophosphamide–bone marrow depression based on epidemiologic data and also possibly may inhibit cyclophosphamide clearance.

Anecdotal Documentation

Ampicillin. Dermatologic reactions occurred in 22.4% of 67 patients receiving concomitant allopurinol and ampicillin, as compared with 7.5% receiving only ampicillin and 2.1% receiving only allopurinol.[154] The observations from this epidemiologic report in 1972 have not been noted subsequently.

Antacids. Aluminum hydroxide inhibited the GI absorption of allopurinol in 3 patients on hemodialysis; however, the interaction can be avoided by administration of allopurinol ≥3 hr before aluminum hydroxide.

Chlorpropamide. Allopurinol or its metabolites might compete with chlorpropamide for renal tubular secretion and can result in an ↑ chlorpropamide effect in an occasional patient.

Cyclosporine. Cyclosporine toxicity was reported for one individual who had a cyclosporine blood level of 325 ng/mL (baseline, 110 ng/mL) 12 days following the addition of allopurinol 100 mg to a stable immunosuppressive regimen that included cyclosporine.[155]

Phenytoin. Allopurinol inhibits the hepatic metabolism of some drugs and seemed to inhibit the metabolism of phenytoin in 1 patient.

Probenecid. Allopurinol can inhibit the metabolism of probenecid, and probenecid can enhance the renal elimination of the active oxypurinol.

Theophylline. Allopurinol in high doses (300 mg Q 12 hr for 14 days) can ↑ mean theophylline AUC by approximately 27% and half-life by 25%; clearance can be ↓ approximately 21%. An active metabolite (1-ethylxanthine) also can accumulate.[156–158]

Vidarabine. An active metabolite of vidarabine is metabolized by xanthine oxidase and accumulation of this metabolite can ↑ neurotoxicity.

[a]ACE = Angiotensin-converting enzyme; AUC = Area under the concentration time curve; GI = Gastrointestinal. Adapted from reference 68.

Notes:

Table 39.5 • Drugs Commonly Associated with Hyperuricemia[a]

Drug	Mechanism	Comments
Acadesine[159-163]	?	Dose-dependent uric acid elevations and appearance of clinically relevant sequelae (crystalluria reported in 3 of 5 patients receiving doses of 0.2 to 0.38 mg/kg/minute).
Certain ACE-Inhibitors: (lisinopril, ramipril, trandolapril)[164-166]	Reduced urate renal clearance	Hyperuricemia and gout have occurred at therapeutic doses. Conversely, captopril and enalapril significantly reduce serum urate levels, as do angiotensin-II receptor blockers, except irbesartan.[167,168]
Cytotoxic Chemotherapy: aldesleukin, asparaginase, carboplatin, chlorambucil, cisplatin, cyclophosphamide, fludarabine, hydroxyurea, mechlorethamine, mercaptopurine, thioguanine, thiotepa, vinblastine, vincristine[169-182]	Rapid cell lysis	Occurs primarily with lymphomas and leukemias. Uric acid nephropathy, acute renal failure, and nephrolithiasis can result.
Cyclosporine[183,184]	Decreased urate renal clearance, either via a tubular mechanism or decrease in GFR	Cyclosporine-induced hyperuricemia may cause gout in patients with risk factors: renal dysfunction, concurrent diuretics, and male gender.
Diazoxide[185]	Decreased urate renal clearance	Not commonly encountered because drug generally used for short-term event.
Didanosine[186-188]	Catabolic effect	Uric acid blood increases of 0.5 to 5 mg/dL have occurred in patients receiving >9.6 mg/kg/day.
Diuretics: acetazolamide, bumetanide, chlorthalidone, ethacrynic acid, furosemide, indapamide, metolazone, spironolactone, thiazides, torsemide[189-194]	Secondary to volume contraction and increased uric acid reabsorption in the proximal tubules for all diuretics; thiazides may also competitively inhibit proximal tubular secretion	Dose- and duration-dependent elevations in uric acid.
Ethambutol[195]	Decreased urate renal clearance	Hyperuricemia has been demonstrated in a majority of patients receiving 20 mg/kg/day orally.
Ethanol[196]	Increased uric acid production	Purines in beer may also contribute to hyperuricemia.
Filgrastim[197]	Increased WBC production	Transient effect, seen more often with higher doses (30 to 60 μg/kg/day).
Fructose/Invert Sugar[198,199]	Diminished hepatic ATP synthesis and resultant acceleration of uric acid formation	Hyperuricemia seen with rapid infusion (500 mL/hr). Avoid in patients with gout and/or cirrhosis.
Glucocorticoids[200]	Tumor lysis	Seen when glucocorticoid is used as an antineoplastic agent.

(continued)

Table 39.5 • Drugs Commonly Associated with Hyperuricemia[a] (continued)

Drug	Mechanism	Comments
Levodopa[201]	Inhibition of urate excretion	Patients taking therapeutic doses have experienced hyperuricemia and gout. Secondarily, interference with colorimetric assay of uric acid may contribute a false-positive increment.
Methyldopa[202]	Interference with uric acid assay	False-positive elevation with phosphotungstate assay method. Questionable clinical significance, because studies have not demonstrated this effect in vivo at therapeutic doses.
Niacin[203]	?	Hyperuricemia and gout have occasionally occurred.
Pancreatic Enzymes: Pancreatin and Pancrelipase[204]	?	Hyperuricemia, hyperuricosuria, and uric acid crystalluria have occurred with high dosages.
Pyrazinamide[205]	Inhibition of renal tubular urate secretion	Hyperuricemia more common with daily than with intermittent administration. Gouty attacks have occurred in those with a history of gout. Asymptomatic hyperuricemia was the only manifestation seen in one trial of pediatric patients.
Salicylates (low dose)[206]	Inhibition of proximal tubular secretion of urate	Doses <2 g/day cause hyperuricemia.
Tacrolimus[207]	Reduced urate excretion	Hyperuricemia similar to that seen with cyclosporine.
Theophylline[208,209]	Interference with uric acid assay	False-positive elevation with automated Bittner adapted method. Interference does not appear to occur with phosphotungstate assay method.

[a]ACE = Angiotensin-converting enzyme; ATP = Adenosine triphosphate; GFR = Glomerular filtration rate; WBC = White blood cell.

Notes:

The reader is referred to Chapter 40: Gout and Hyperuricemia, written by *Lloyd Y. Young, Pharm.D.*, and *Keith D. Campagna, Pharm.D.*, in the seventh edition of **Applied Therapeutics: The Clinical Use of Drugs** for a more in-depth discussion. All notations to reference numbers are based on the reference list at the end of that chapter. The editors of this handbook express their thanks to Drs. Young and Campagna and acknowledge that this chapter is based upon their work.

Notes:

Notes:

Chapter 40

Rheumatic Disorders

RHEUMATOID ARTHRITIS (RA)

A chronic systemic inflammatory disorder characterized by potentially deforming polyarthritis and extra-articular manifestations (e.g., subcutaneous nodules, pleuritis, pneumonitis, pericarditis, myocarditis, vasculitis).

Diagnosis

- ♦ No specific test for diagnosis of RA; therefore, diagnosis primarily is based upon clinical criteria (see Table 40.1)
- ♦ Rheumatoid factor present in up to 75% of patients with RA but also present in healthy individuals and in some with diseases other than RA. Patients with RA typically have RF titers of at least 1:320.

Clinical Presentation

- ♦ Usually begins with nonspecific symptoms (fatigue, malaise, diffuse musculoskeletal pain, morning stiffness).
- ♦ Disease progression is highly variable.
  - Initial symptoms in about one-third are mild, intermittent, and resolve over several weeks to months. Patients may be symptom-free for several months and then experience symptoms more severe than those during initial onset.
  - Some experience sudden onset of symptoms followed by prolonged clinical remission of disease.
  - Others experience progressive uninterrupted disease and subsequent disabling joint deformities.
- ♦ RA-induced joint destruction begins with inflammation of the synovial lining. The pannus, a highly erosive enzyme-laden inflammatory exudate, invades articular cartilage, narrows joint spaces, erodes bone, and destroys ligaments and tendons resulting in joint deformities.
- ♦ Fig. 40.2 shows the frequency of involvement of different joint sites, and Fig. 40.3 show the characteristic finger deformities in RA.
- ♦ Table 40.2 lists the parameters used to assess disease activity, and Table 40.3 describes the criteria for clinical remission in RA.

Treatment

- ♦ Treatment involves combination of rest, exercise (physical therapy), emotional support, occupational therapy, and drugs. Goal of therapy is disease remission, but if not attainable, goals include control of disease activity, pain relief, maintenance of activities of daily living, and slowing of joint damage.

♦ The old standard for treatment of RA, known as the "pyramid approach" (shown in Fig. 40.1), was based on the assumption that RA is a slowly progressing, benign disease that is not life-threatening. RA, however, is not a benign condition for most patients, and the "pyramid approach" has not had a positive impact on improving function or in slowing of disease progression.

♦ The nonsteroidal anti-inflammatory drugs listed in Table 40.4 are commonly prescribed for RA but do not prevent or slow joint destruction.

♦ All patients with active RA not controlled by 3 months of NSAIDs or with poor prognosis RA (Table 40.5), are candidates for disease-modifying antirheumatic drugs (DMARDs).

♦ The DMARDS (hydroxychloroquine, sulfasalazine, methotrexate, leflunomide, gold, azathioprine, and d-penicillamine) have the potential to slow disease progression. Anticytokine therapies (e.g., Enbrel and Remicade) target the physiologic effects of TNF-α and presumably possess disease-modifying activity.

♦ The DMARD of choice is determined primarily by physician and patient preference, taking into consideration convenience of administration, monitoring requirements, medication and monitoring costs, time to therapeutic onset, and frequency and severity of adverse effects.

♦ Most patients with active RA receive at least one DMARD with an NSAID. Low-dose oral steroids often used "as needed" while awaiting the onset of DMARD action.

♦ Use of DMARDs in combination appears more effective than DMARD monotherapy.

♦ Drugs for management of RA are listed in Table 40.6.

JUVENILE RHEUMATOID ARTHRITIS (JRA)

Formerly all arthritis of childhood was referred to as JRA. New efforts are underway to delineate this disorder, and the term "chronic arthritis of childhood" is used increasingly to refer to many forms of childhood arthritis.

Clinical Presentation

♦ JRA begins before age 16. Onset is rare before 6 months of age, and peak age of onset is from 1–3 years.

♦ Children must be observed carefully for symptoms because of decreased ability to articulate complaints.

♦ Morning stiffness and joint pain can manifest as increased irritability, guarding of joints, or refusal to walk.

♦ Fatigue, low-grade fever, anorexia, weight loss, and failure to grow are other symptoms.

Treatment

♦ **Aspirin,** 60–80 mg/kg/day, in divided doses is treatment of choice for joint manifestations. Dose should be increased to achieve salicylate serum concentrations of 20–30 mg/dL.

• Monitor serum salicylate levels in similar manner as in adults.

• Salicylate-induced transaminitis (as opposed to hepatotoxicity) is dose and serum concentration dependent and can occur in >50% of children receiving large doses.

• Avoid salicylates during febrile illnesses that represent possible infection with either influenza or chicken pox because of possible induction of Reye's syndrome (hepatic injury and progressive encephalopathy).

+ **NSAIDs.** Up to two-thirds of JRA patients achieve good disease control with NSAIDs.
  - Tolmetin 15 mg/kg/day in divided doses (*max:* 30 mg/kg/day).
  - Naproxen 10–15 mg/kg/day in 2 daily divided doses.
  - Ibuprofen doses should not exceed 40–50 mg/kg/day.
  - Indomethacin 1–2 mg/kg/day (maximum of 200 mg/day).
  - Diclofenac 2–3 mg/kg/day in 2–4 daily divided doses.
+ **DMARDs** seldom are needed. Most DMARDs used for adult RA are not effective for JRA. MTX is clearly the DMARD of choice for JRA. Recommended MTX dose for JRA is 5–15 mg/m^2 each week.
+ Etanercept (Enbrel) 0.4 mg/kg (maximum 25 mg) SQ twice weekly is the only FDA-approved anticytokine for JRA. JRA patients should be current on immunizations before therapy is initiated.

Osteoarthritis (OA)

+ OA or degenerative joint disease is the single most common form of arthritis affecting >80% of people >60 yr of age.
+ Unlike RA, the symptoms of OA are limited to the involved joints and structures and reflect the "wearing out" of a joint.
+ **Etiology** and much of the pathophysiology remain unexplained.
+ **Treatment** is directed toward providing symptomatic relief with acetaminophen (up to 4 gm/day) initially followed by NSAIDs if joint symptoms persist.

Table 40.1 • Criteria for Diagnosis of RA^a

1. Morning stiffness in and around joints lasting at least 1 hr before maximal involvement[b]
2. Soft-tissue swelling (arthritis) of three or more joint areas observed by a physician[b]
3. Swelling (arthritis) of the proximal interphalangeal, metacarpophalangeal, or wrist joints[b]
4. Symmetric arthritis[b]
5. Subcutaneous nodules
6. Positive test for RF
7. Radiographic erosions or periarticular osteopenia in hand or wrist joints

[a]RA = Rheumatoid arthritis; RF = Rheumatoid factor.
[b]Criteria 1–4 must be present for at least 6 weeks; 4 or more criteria must be present.
Adapted from reference 3.

Table 40.2 • Parameters Used to Assess Disease Activity and Drug Response in RA^a

Duration and intensity of morning stiffness
Number of painful or tender joints
Number of swollen joints; severity of joint swelling
Range of joint motion
Time to onset of fatigue
ESR or CRP
Radiographic changes: osteopenia, joint space narrowing, bony erosions
Hgb/Hct
Subcutaneous nodules, pleuritis, pneumonitis, myocarditis, vasculitis
AIMS
HAQ

[a]AIMS = Arthritis impact measure scale; CRP = C-reactive protein; ESR = Erythrocyte sedimentation rate; HAQ = Health assessment questionnaire; Hct = Hematocrit; Hgb = Hemoglobin; RA = Rheumatoid arthritis.

Table 40.3 • Criteria for Complete Clinical Remission in RA[a]

A minimum of five of the following requirements must be fulfilled for at least 2 consecutive months in a patient with RA[b]:
1. Morning stiffness not >15 minutes
2. No fatigue
3. No joint pain
4. No joint tenderness or pain on motion
5. No soft-tissue swelling in joints or tendon sheaths
6. ESR (Westergren's) <30 mm/hr (females) or 20 mm/hr (males)

[a]ESR = Erythrocyte sedimentation rate; RA = Rheumatoid arthritis.
[b]Exclusions: Manifestations of active vasculitis, pericarditis, pleuritis, myositis, or unexplained recent weight loss or fever secondary to RA prohibit designation of complete clinical remission.
Adapted from reference 9.

Notes:

Table 40.4 • Nonsteroidal Anti-Inflammatory Drugs[a]

NSAID	Half-Life (hr)	Maximum Daily Dose (mg)	Cost Index[b]	Comments
Salicylate				
Aspirin	0.25–0.33	6,000[c]	1[d]	—
Choline salicylate (Anthropan)	3–20[e]	4,800[c]	2–3	Available as 870 mg/57 mL liquid formulation
Diflunisal (Dolobid)	8–12[e]	1,500	3[d]	—
Magnesium choline salicylate (Trilisate)	3–20[e]	4,800[c]	2[d]	Available as 650 mg/5 mL solution
Magnesium salicylate (Magan, Mobidin)	3–20[e]	4,800[c]	2–3	500 mg salicylate/tablet
Salsalate (Disalcid)	3–20[e]	4,800[c]	2[d]	Absorption/activation may be erratic
Sodium salicylate	3–20[e]	4,800[c]	1[d]	—
Propionic Acid				
Carprofen (Rimadyl)	—	—	—	Approved as second-line NSAID but not marketed
Fenoprofen (Nalfon)	2.5	3,200	2[d]	—
Flurbiprofen (Ansaid)	3–4	300	2[d]	—
Ibuprofen (Motrin, Rufen, Advil)	1–3	3,200	1[d]	100 mg/5 mL suspension approved for JRA
Ketoprofen (Orudis)	3–5	300	4[d]	—
Naproxen (Naprosyn)	13	1,500	4[d]	125 mg/15 mL suspension approved for JRA
Naproxen sodium (Anaprox)	13	1,375	4	—
Oxaprozin (Daypro)	56	1,800	3–4	—
Acetic Acid				
Diclofenac (Voltaren)	25–33	200	4[d]	Enteric-coated
Etodolac (Lodine)	7	1,200	4[d]	FDA-approved for OA only
Indomethacin (Indocin, Indocin SR)	2–5	200 SR: 1,500	1[d] 2	Also available as 25 mg/5 mL suspension

(continued)

Table 40.4 • Nonsteroidal Anti-inflammatory Drugs[a] (continued)

NSAID	Half-Life (hr)	Maximum Daily Dose (mg)	Cost Index[b]	Comments
Acetic Acid (continued)				
Ketorolac (Toradol)	6	40	6	Not FDA-approved for RA or OA
Nabumetone (Relafen)	24	200	3	Prodrug: Active metabolite 6-MNA
Sulindac (Clinoril)	18	400	2[d]	Prodrug: Active metabolite sulindac sulfide
Tolmetin (Tolectin)	1	2,000	4[d]	Approved for JRA. False-positive urinary protein by sulfosalicylic acid reagent assay
Anthranilic Acid				
Meclofenamate sodium (Meclomen)	2	400	2	Loose stools/diarrhea (dose-related)
Mefenamic acid (Ponstel)	2	1,000	4	Not indicated for chronic therapy
Oxicam				
Piroxicam (Feldene)	38–45	20	2[d]	—
Pyrazolone				
Oxyphenbutazone		400	1	Not indicated for chronic therapy
Phenylbutazone (Butazolidin, Azolid)		400	2–3	Oxyphenbutazone is also an active metabolite
Cyclooxygenase-2-Specific				
Celecoxib (Celebrex)	10	25–50	5	The COX$_2$-specific NSAIDs associated with relatively less GI adverse effects. Controversy developing as to possible cardiovascular effects
Rofecoxib (Vioxx)	17	400	5	—

[a] FDA = Food and Drug Administration; JRA = Juvenile rheumatoid arthritis; NSAIDs = Nonsteroidal anti-inflammatory drugs; OA = Osteoarthritis; RA = Rheumatoid arthritis.
[b] Source for cost data: Reents S, editor-in-chief. Clinical Pharmacology, Gold Standard Media, Inc., 1999. 1: <$10/mo, 2: $10–39/mo, 3: $40–59/mo, 4: $60–89/mo, 5: $90–199/mo, 6: >$200/mo.
[c] Highly variable; anti-inflammatory doses associated with serum concentrations of 15–30 mg/dL.
[d] Generic available.
[e] Half-life refers to metabolism to salicylic acid, which is dose-dependent.

Table 40.5 • Suggested Criteria for Disease-modifying Antirheumatic Drugs in RA*

1. Correct diagnosis along with one or more of the following:
   a. Persistently active disease despite NSAIDs reflected by:
      i. Elevated ESR or CRP
      ii. Falling Hgb
      iii. Thrombocytosis
      iv. Synovitis remains active or ↑ in intensity
   b. High titers of IgM RF
   c. Radiographic evidence of osteopenia, joint space narrowing, or new bony erosions
   d. Glucocorticoid dependency, 7.5 mg/day prednisone or equivalent
   e. Presence or development of extra-articular disease
      i. Subcutaneous nodules
      ii. Pleuritis/pneumonitis
      iii. Myocarditis
      iv. Uveitis
      v. Vasculitis
   f. Earlier age of onset (<50 years old)
   g. Swelling in >20 joints
2. No contraindications
3. Informed, cooperative patient

*CRP = C-reactive protein; ESR = Erythrocyte sedimentation rate; Hgb = Hemoglobin; RA = Rheumatoid arthritis; RF = Rheumatoid factor.
Adapted from reference 7.

Notes:

Table 40.6 • Drugs for Management of Rheumatoid Arthritis

Product	Formulation	Dosage	Comments
Aspirin	See Table 40.4	2.5–3 gm/day in divided daily doses. Adjust doses gradually to obtain serum levels of 15–30 mg/dL	Was formerly the traditional drug of 1st choice; 2 of 5 metabolic pathways are saturable at these serum concentrations and $t\frac{1}{2}$ ↑ to 18–24 hr. Adverse effects primarily are GI intolerance and ↓ platelet function. Enteric-coated products help ↓ GI intolerance. Should be avoided, if possible, during the last trimester of pregnancy.
Auranofin (Ridaura)	3 mg oral capsule	6 mg QD or 3 mg BID	Dermatological reaction in 15%–20% of patients; mild proteinuria and bone marrow suppression; urticaria; diarrhea. Objective benefits may not become apparent for up to 6 months or until the cumulative dose approaches 1 gm. Continue indefinitely to sustain remissions in patients who respond well. Low efficacy and rarely used.
Aurothioglucose (Solganal)	Oil suspension (50 mg/mL in 10 mL vials)	10 mg IM test dose; then 25 mg 1 week later; then 25–50 mg IM weekly until 1 gm; then 25–50 mg every other week; then Q 3–4 weeks	Shake thoroughly and use large-bore needle to withdraw suspension from vial. Lumps at injection site. *Adverse effects:* Dermatological reactions in 15%–20% of patients; mild proteinuria and bone marrow suppression; urticaria. *Objective benefits* may not become apparent for 3–6 months or until the cumulative dose approaches 1 gm. Gold sodium thiomalate and aurothioglucose are equally effective. Continue indefinitely to sustain remissions in patients who respond well. Screen for urine protein and get CBC before each injection.
Azathioprine (Imuran)	50 mg tab	1 mg/kg (50–100 mg) as single daily dose or twice daily divided dose. If no response, ↑ dose by 0.5 mg increments at 6- to 8-week intervals to maximum of 2.5 mg/kg/day. Can ↓ GI toxicity by giving after a meal	Benefits noted after 6–8 weeks of therapy. Discontinue if no benefit by 12 weeks. Reduce dose to $\frac{1}{3}$–$\frac{1}{4}$ if allopurinol administered concomitantly. Nausea and vomiting in ≈12%. Hematologic toxicities (leukopenia, thrombocytopenia) are dose related. Skin rashes, alopecia, and neoplasia also a potential. Baseline CBC, renal and liver function followed by CBC Q 1–2 weeks after dosage change and, then Q 1–3 months.
Etanercept (Enbrel)	25 mg inj	25 mg SQ twice weekly at least 3–4 days apart	Binds to both TNF-α and TNF-β. Rotate injection sites. Swirl diluent with powder for injection; do not shake. Clinical response in 1–2 weeks. Caution in patients at high risk for infections. The dissolved powder can be kept in refrigerator for no more than 6 hr before need to discard.
Glucocorticoids (various)	Various	Judicious use of low dose (<5 mg/day prednisone). Give as single daily dose in morning with food or milk	Do not alter course of disease. Long-term use of supraphysiological doses inevitably leads to adverse effects. Used for brief periods as "bridge therapy" while awaiting onset of effects of disease-modifying agents. Judicious use of low doses is important during flares of unremitting disease.

Gold sodium thiomalate (Myochrysine)	Aqueous solution 25 mg/mL in 1 mL ampules and 10-mL vials	10 mg IM test dose; then 25 mg 1 week later; then 25–50 mg IM weekly until 1 gm; then 25–50 mg every other week; then Q 3–4 weeks	*Adverse effects:* Dermatological reactions in 15%–20% of patients; mild proteinuria and bone marrow suppression; urticaria. Vasomotor reaction (nausea, weakness, flushing, tachycardia, syncope) in 5% of patients. Does not occur with other gold salts. Easier to administer than aurothioglucose. *Objective benefits may not become apparent for 3–6 months or until the cumulative dose approaches 1 gm.* Gold sodium thiomalate and aurothioglucose are equally effective. Continue indefinitely to sustain remissions in patients who respond well. Screen for urine protein and get CBC before each injection.
Hydroxychloroquine (Plaquenil)	200 mg tab (equivalent to 155 mg base)	200 mg BID-TID with food or milk. If positive benefit, ↓ dose by 50% to 200 mg QD-BID. Recommended doses are 2–6 mg/kg/day.	Usually takes 4–12 weeks before benefits apparent and sometimes as long as 6 months. Discontinuation rate high as 54% in 2 yrs due to inefficacy. *Irreversible retinopathy* (blind spots, photophobia, blurred distance vision, light flashes) is dose-related; occurs after years of therapy and unrelated to the less serious corneal deposits (benign, reversible, and occurs in about 10% of patients). Eye exams Q 6 months recommended. Avoid use in pregnancy and children.
Infliximab (Remicade)	100 mg inj.	Usual dose is 3 mg/kg IV at 0, 2, and 6 weeks, then Q 8 weeks thereafter.	Binds and neutralizes TNF-α. Must be given with MTX to prevent antibody formation to drug. May take 2–4 weeks before full benefit is seen. Serious adverse effects include serious injections. Fever, chills, and allergic reactions experienced should prompt contact of physician.
Leflunomide (Arava)	10 mg tab 20 mg tab 100 mg tab	100 mg/day × 3 days as loading dose followed by 20 mg QD. Can ↓ dose to 10 mg QD if not well tolerated.	Active metabolite responsible for almost all clinical effects, and serum half-life of MI metabolite in 2 weeks. Diarrhea (20%), rash (10%), alopecia (10–17%), but potential liver toxicity is greatest concern. Monitor ALT monthly after baseline for several months.
Methotrexate	2.5 mg tab	Optimal dosing regimen not yet established. Most common is 2.5 mg Q 12 hr × 3 doses administered once weekly. If no benefits by 6th week, gradually ↑ dose to 5 mg Q 12 hr × 3 doses once weekly. Do not exceed total weekly dose of 20 mg	MTX currently DMARD of choice especially for severe disease. Benefits begin in 3–6 weeks; continued improvement up to 12 weeks. ↓ dose to lowest possible effective dose. Emphasize to patient dose is *weekly*. Nausea, malaise and dizziness limited to days of dosing. Monitor hematology Q 4–8 weeks (leukopenia, thrombocytopenia, pancytopenia) and liver and renal function Q 4–8 weeks. Avoid in pregnancy (category X). Pulmonary toxicity begins with dry nonproductive cough, malaise, fever, then dyspnea. Patient should be advised to avoid alcohol.
NSAIDs	See Table 40.4	See Table 40.4	Larger doses than those listed for pain are sometimes needed for rheumatological disorders. Better tolerated than aspirin but more expensive. Up to 15% of RA patients stop NSAIDs due to dyspepsia. The COX-2 specific NSAIDs (Celebrex, Vioxx) associated with less GI adverse effects.

(continued)

Product	Formulation	Dosage	Comments
Penicillamine (Cuprimine, Depen)	125 mg cap 250 mg cap 250 mg tab	250 mg/day × 6 weeks, then ↑ to 500 mg/day by 125-250 mg/day at 4-8 week intervals until benefit noted or toxicity intervenes. Discontinue after 3-4 months at 1000 mg/day if no benefit noted. Take doses on empty stomach 1 hr before meal or 2 hr after meal	Up to 6 months of therapy needed before benefits are apparent. Reversible proteinuria (5%–26%) after 6–12 months of therapy; related to both duration of therapy and rate of dosage ↑. Rashes most common adverse effect; thrombocytopenia most common bone marrow effect. Loss of sensation, nausea, vomiting early in course of therapy. Potential for cross-reactivity in penicillin-allergic patients is possible but not likely. Adverse effects occur in 40%.
Sulfasalazine	500 mg tab	500 mg/day × 1 wk. ↑ by 500 mg/week to max of 1 gm BID or TID	Active moiety appears to be sulfapyridine. Onset of benefits delayed 1–2 months. Nausea, GI discomfort, skin rashes, and rare leukopenia (1-3%). CBC recommended Q 2-4 weeks for first 3 months, then Q 3 months thereafter.

Table 40.6 • Drugs for Management of Rheumatoid Arthritis (continued)

Notes:

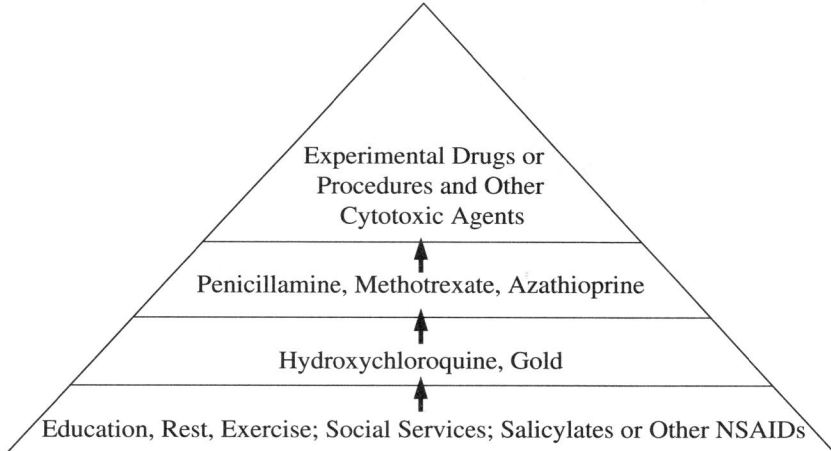

Fig. 40.1 Traditional Pyramid Approach for Treatment of Rheumatoid Arthritis. ↑ Indicates worsening disease.

Notes:

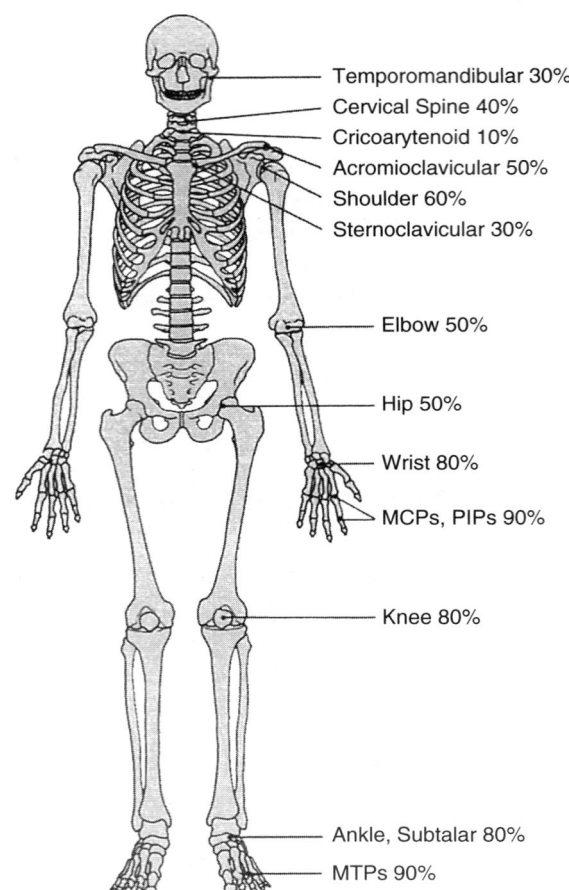

Temporomandibular 30%
Cervical Spine 40%
Cricoarytenoid 10%
Acromioclavicular 50%
Shoulder 60%
Sternoclavicular 30%

Elbow 50%

Hip 50%

Wrist 80%

MCPs, PIPs 90%

Knee 80%

Ankle, Subtalar 80%

MTPs 90%

Fig. 40.2 Frequency of Involvement of Different Joint Sites in Established RA.

Notes:

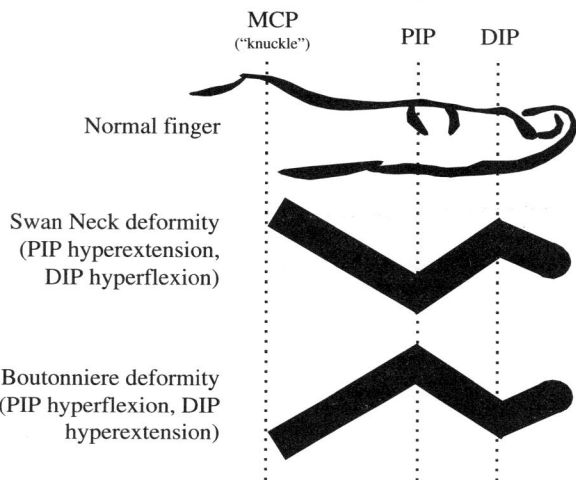

Fig. 40.3 Characteristic Finger Deformities in Rheumatoid Arthritis. DIP, distal interphalangeal joint; MCP, metacarpophalangeal joint; PIP, proximal interphalangeal joint.

The reader is referred to Chapter 41: Rheumatic Disorders, written by *Steven W. Chen, Pharm.D. and William C. Gong, Pharm.D.*, in the seventh edition of **Applied Therapeutics: The Clinical Use of Drugs** for a more in-depth discussion. All notations to reference numbers are based on the reference list at the end of that chapter. The editors of this handbook express their thanks to Drs. Chen and Gong and acknowledge that this chapter is based upon their work.

Notes:

Notes:

Chapter 41

Connective Tissue Disorders: The Clinical Use of Corticosteroids

Definitions

+ *Connective Tissue Disease* is a group of diseases of the tissues that support and connect other tissues and body parts. Connective tissue includes cartilage and bone, and diseases included in this category are cutaneous and systemic lupus erythematosus (SLE), scleroderma, polymyositis, dermatomyositis, and polyarteritis.

+ *Rheumatic or rheumatoid disorders* include arthritis (infectious, rheumatoid, and gouty); arthritis due to rheumatic fever or trauma; degenerative joint disease; neurogenic arthropathy; hydroarthrosis; myositis; bursitis; and fibromyositis.

+ *Rheumatism* is a general term for acute and chronic conditions characterized by inflammation, soreness, stiffness of muscles, and pain in joints and associated structures.

+ *Arthralgias* refers to pain in a joint.

+ *Arthritis* refers to the inflammation of a joint, usually accompanied by pain, swelling and, frequently, changes in structure.

+ *Arteritis* refers to the inflammation of an artery that can occur in association with rheumatoid arthritis or rheumatic fever.

Lupus Erythematosus

+ *Systemic lupus erythematosus* is an autoimmune disease in which various organs and cells are damaged by antibodies and immune complexes. *Discoid lupus* is characterized by chronic cutaneous lesions that occur in the absence of systemic manifestations.

• Criteria for classification of SLE are listed in Table 41.1.

• Clinical features of SLE vary with the organ system that is involved. Common features are listed in Table 41.2.

• At the onset, SLE may involve only one organ system. With time, multiple organ systems can be affected simultaneously. Most patients experience some form of arthralgias and myalgias and may develop intermittent arthritis.

• Course of disease can be mild and intermittent or persistent, severe, and fatal. Most experience exacerbations interspersed with periods of relative inactive disease.

• Treatment usually aimed at controlling acute symptoms because there is not a cure for SLE. NSAIDs are used to treat mild symptoms of arthralgias, myalgias, arthritis, and serositis. Corticosteroids and immunosuppressives are used for severe symptoms.

- Disease tends to wax and wane. Corticosteroid regimens for treatment of SLE are described in Tables 41.3 and 41.4.
- **Drug-induced lupus** presents similar to idiopathic SLE but with milder visceral involvement. Renal, lymph, GI, and CNS involvement are rare. Fever, rash, anemia, and cardiac problems occur slightly less frequently than with idiopathic lupus. Typically improves rapidly after discontinuation of the drug.

Scleroderma

- A chronic disease of unknown etiology that causes sclerosis of skin and organs (e.g., GI tract, lungs, heart, and kidneys).
- Dermatological changes (taut, firm, tough, leathery hyperpigmented skin firmly bound to subcutaneous tissue) usually precede the development of signs of visceral involvement.
- Prognosis is variable and unpredictable.
- No specific therapy. Because it is a multiorgan disease, therapy aimed at relieving affected organ systems with calcium channel blockers, ACE inhibitors, penicillamine, and steroids

Giant Cell Arteritis and Polymyalgia Rheumatica

- **Giant cell arteritis** is an inflammation of the medium- and large-sized arteries in the body.
  - The terms *"temporal arteritis"* or *"cranial arteritis"* are used when the temporal artery or other cranial arteries, respectively, are involved.
  - Local manifestations depend on the location of the involved artery and include: temporal headaches, blindness, scalp necrosis, tongue gangrene, and jaw claudication.
  - Corticosteroids must be instituted to alter the underlying histopathology and prevent blindness when the temporal artery is involved.
  - Prednisone, 40 to 60 mg/day for about 1 month, followed by gradual tapering of dose. Continue treatment for 1–2 years to minimize potential for relapse.
- **Polymyalgia rheumatica** is a syndrome characteristically associated with severe pain in the muscles of the neck, back, shoulders, upper arms, and thighs and with mild inflammation of large joints, such as the knees, hips, shoulders, and sternoclavicular joints.
  - Generally occurs in patients >50 years of age
  - Weakness is not prominent, but pain often makes it difficult to rise from a chair or get out of bed.
  - Absence of objective physical findings is dramatic. Indicators of inflammation include a high ESR (>40 mm/hr and sometimes as high as 100 mm/hr) and high serum concentrations of c-reactive protein and interleukin-b.
  - Clinical symptoms and laboratory findings are nonspecific, and diagnosis depends on differentiation from other similar disorders (e.g., polymyalgia associated with considerable muscle pain rather than the muscle weakness associated with polymyositis).
  - Polymyalgia sometimes is a manifestation of giant cell arteritis. Both can occur in the same patient, either concurrently or at different times.

Polymyositis and Dermatomyositis

◆ **Polymyositis** is an inflammatory disorder of skeletal muscles that is manifested by muscle weakness of the trunk, shoulders, hip girdles, upper arms, thighs, neck, and pharynx.

* The predominant symptom is muscle weakness in contrast to the pain of polymyalgia.

* Polymyositis can occur alone or in association with other collagen vascular diseases (e.g., SLE, scleroderma, and rheumatoid arthritis).

* It is associated with malignancy in about 10%.

* Treat with prednisone 1–2 mg/kg/day to bring symptoms under control.

* Treatment can take several months or years.

◆ **Dermatomyositis** is a term used when a dermatologic rash (often reddish purple, erythematous, scaly, and eczematous) accompanies the muscle involvement of polymyositis.

Clinical Use of Corticosteroids

◆ The corticosteroids (CS) are used primarily for their anti-inflammatory, immunosuppressive, or antiallergic activity. CS are used to treat, and more often, provide supportive therapy for treatment of many rheumatological disorders.

◆ The recommended dose of prednisone for most connective tissue diseases is 1 mg/kg/day in three to four divided doses.

◆ The equivalent potency, sodium-retaining potency, plasma half-life, and biologic half-life of several synthetic analogs of cortisol are listed in Table 41.5.

◆ The routes of administration of various corticosteroids are listed in Table 41.6.

◆ Doses of >5 mg/day of prednisone for an extended period of time is associated with adrenal insufficiency, and cortisol supplementation may be necessary during periods of stress (e.g., surgery).

◆ Common adverse effects of systemic corticosteroids are listed in Table 41.7.

Notes:

Table 41.1 • Revised Criteria for Classification of Systemic Lupus Erythematosus

Criteria	Explanation[a]
Malar rash	Classic red butterfly rash over bridge of nose and cheeks
Discoid rash	Disc-shaped, red, thick, scaly patches found anywhere on the body; occurs in approximately 15% of SLE patients; scarring may occur in older lesions
Photosensitivity	Skin rash resulting from an unusual reaction to sunlight as determined by patient history or observed by physician
Oral ulcers	Painless oral or nasopharyngeal ulcers observed by physician
Arthritis	Nonerosive arthritis involving two or more peripheral joints; characterized by tenderness, swelling, or effusion
Serositis	Evidence of inflammation of either the pleura or pericardium
Renal disorder	As manifested by persistent proteinuria (>0.5 g/day or $>3+$) or cellular casts
Neurologic disorder	Seizures or psychosis occurring without any other explanation
Hematologic disorder	Leukopenia ($<4,000/mm^3$), hemolytic anemia, lymphopenia ($<1,500/mm^3$), or thrombocytopenia ($<100,000/mm^3$)
Immunologic disorder	Positive LE cell test, presence of anti-(native) ds DNA antibody, anti-Sm antibody, or false-positive serologic test for syphilis (confirmed by FTA-Abs)
Antinuclear antibody	An abnormal ANA titer in the absence of drugs known to be associated with drug-induced lupus

[a]The diagnosis of systemic lupus erythematosus is made when a patient has 4 or more of the 11 criteria present, serially or simultaneously, during an interval of observation.
ANA, antinuclear antibody; anti-Sm, anti-Smith; ds, double-stranded; FTA-Abs, fluorescent treponemal antibody absorption; SLE, systemic lupus erythematosus.

Table 41.2 • Frequency of Lupus Manifestations During Course of Disease

Clinical Manifestations	Percent
Constitutional (general fatigue, malaise, fever, weight loss)	95
Musculoskeletal (arthralgias/myalgias/arthritis)	95
Hematologic abnormalities	85
Cutaneous (rashes, oral ulcers, alopecia, vasculitis)	80
Neurologic dysfunction and symptoms	60
Cardiopulmonary complications	60
Renal dysfunction	50
Gastrointestinal	45
Fetal loss	30
Thrombosis	15
Ocular	15

Notes:

Table 41.3 • The Multiple Uses of Corticosteroids in SLE

Indication	Corticosteroid Regimen
Cutaneous manifestations	Topical or intralesional corticosteroids
Minor disease activity	Prednisone (or equivalent) at a dosage of <0.5 mg/kg in a single or divided daily dose
Major disease activity	*Oral:* Prednisone (or equivalent) at a dosage of 1 mg/kg in a single or divided daily dose; duration should not exceed 4 wk without additional evaluation
	IV bolus: Methylprednisolone (1 g or 15 mg/kg) over 30 min; dose often repeated for 3 consecutive days

SLE, systemic lupus erythematosus.

Notes:

41.6   Arthritic Disorders

Table 41.4 • Corticosteroid Dosing Regimens[69]

Regimen	Indication	Rationale	Relative Efficacy[a]	Relative Side Effects[a]
Oral, QD low dose (≤10 mg prednisone)	Maintenance therapy	"Physiologic" dose, suppress symptoms	+	+
Alternate day moderate dose (>10 mg prednisone)	Nonsymptomatic manifestations of mild-to-moderate disease; maintenance therapy	Some adverse reactions less often; less adrenal suppression	++	+
QD moderate[b] to high dose	Control of active disease	Effective in many rheumatic diseases; less adverse reactions than split dose	++	++
Split daily dose	Rapid control of active disease	↑ efficacy over equivalent single dose	++	+++
"Minipulse"[c]	Rapid control of severe disease	More rapid control; possibly allows lower maintenance dose	+++	++
Parenteral IM deposteroids	Limited use as rescue (targeted injections preferred)	Temporary disease control	++	++
IV pulse	Severe/emergent life- or organ-threatening disease	Rapid control of severe disease; possibly ↓ maintenance dose	+++	+++

[a] Efficacy and side effects vary with the dose given.
[b] Given in morning to minimize adrenal suppression.
[c] For example, 100–200 mg/day prednisone for 2–5 days.
IM, intramuscular; IV, intravenous.

Table 41.5 • Comparison of Corticosteroid Preparations[34]

Compound	Equiv. Potency (mg)	Na-Retaining Potency (Mineralocorticoid Activity)	Plasma $t_{1/2}$ (min)	Biological $t_{1/2}$ (hr)
Short-Acting				
Cortisone	25	2+	30	8–12
Hydrocortisone (Cortisol)	20	2+	80–118	8–12
Prednisone	5	1+	60	18–36
Prednisolone	5	1+	115–212	18–36
Methylprednisolone	4	0	78–188	18–36
Triamcinolone	4	0	200	12–36
Long-Acting				
Dexamethasone	0.75	0	110–210	36–54
Betamethasone	0.6	0	300+	36–54

Table 41.6 • Routes of Administration of Various Corticosteroids

Corticosteroid	Route of Administration
Betamethasone	PO, IM, intra-articular, intrasynovial, intradermal, soft tissue injection
Cortisone	PO, IM
Dexamethasone	PO, IM, IV, intra-articular, intradermal, soft tissue injection
Hydrocortisone	IM, IV
Methylprednisolone	PO, IM, IV
Prednisolone	PO, IM, IV, intra-articular, intradermal, soft tissue injection
Prednisone	PO
Triamcinolone	PO, IM, intra-articular, intrasynovial, intradermal, soft tissue injection

IM, intramuscularly; IV, intravenously; PO, oral.

Table 41.7 • Adverse Effects of Systemic Corticosteroids[69]

	Short-Term, High-Dose	Long-Term Use
	Cerebral edema	Amenorrhea
	Diabetes mellitus	Aseptic necrosis of bone
	GI bleed	Cataracts
	Glaucoma	Centripetal obesity
	Hypertension	Growth failure
	Hypokalemic alkalosis	HPA suppression
	↑ BUN	Hyperlipidemia
	Mood disorders	Hypertension
	Pancreatitis	Immunosuppression
	Proximal myopathy	Mood disorders
	Sodium/water retention	Muscle weakness
		Osteoporosis
		Seizures

BUN, blood urea nitrogen; GI, gastrointestinal; HPA, hypothalamic-pituitary-adrenocortical axis.

The reader is referred to Chapter 42: Connective Tissue Disorders: The Clinical Use of Corticosteroids, written by *William C. Gong, Pharm.D.,* in the seventh edition of **Applied Therapeutics: The Clinical Use of Drugs** for a more in-depth discussion. All notations to reference numbers are based on the reference list at the end of that chapter. The editors of this handbook express their thanks to Drs. Chen and Gong and acknowledge that this chapter is based upon their work.

Notes:

Chapter 42

Contraception

Contraceptive Choices

- ♦ Social mores, religious beliefs, ease of use, availability, cost, convenience, effectiveness, mechanisms of action, and adverse effects influence the selection of a contraceptive method.
- ♦ Table 42.1 compares the first year failure rates of various birth control methods.
- ♦ Table 42.2 lists the available combination oral contraceptives (COCs)

Estrogens

- ♦ Inhibit ovulation by suppressing the hypothalamic release of follicle, stimulating hormone-releasing factor, luteinizing hormone-releasing factor, and the subsequent FSH and LH.
- ♦ Large postcoital doses of estrogens inhibit ovum implantation, accelerate ovum transport, decrease time available for fertilization, and break down the corpus luteum.
- ♦ The estrogen in all COCs is ethinyl estradiol.

Progestins

- ♦ Hamper transport of sperm by thickening cervical mucus; slow ovum transport and disturb the critical time sequence required for fertilization; inhibit activation of hydrolytic spermatic enzymes that are required for fertilization; inhibit implantation by altering FSH and LH peaks; and inhibit ovulation by disturbing hypothalamic-pituitary-ovarian function.
- ♦ All of the progestins (Table 42.3) have different progestational, estrogenic, antiestrogenic, and androgenic activities that vary from patient to patient. These pharmacological effects are described in Table 42.4.

Oral Contraceptives

- ♦ The initiation of COCs should be preceded by the gathering of patient information, which should include a routine physical examination and understanding of menstrual history and previous experiences with contraceptives (Table 42.5).
- ♦ Contraindications to COCs are listed in Table 42.6.
- ♦ Table 42.7 lists specific medical conditions of women who cannot safely use estrogens, but who may use progestin-only minipills, Depo-Provera, or Norplant.
- ♦ Choice of a COC begins with the selection of a product containing <35 μg ethinyl estradiol and a progestin containing either 1 mg norethindrone, 0.15 mg desogestrel, 0.15 mg levonorgestrel, or 0.25 mg norgestimate.

- Table 42.8 provides guidance on the selection of an initial COC and for alternative choices if adverse effects necessitate a change.
- Patients should be instructed on the early danger signs associated with COC use (Table 42.9).
- The remote risk that COCs might cause adverse effects in a nursing infant or might interfere with the quantity of breast milk can be obviated by use of progestin-only minipills (e.g., Micronor, Nor-Q.D.).
- The disadvantages of progestin-only minipills are listed in Table 42.10. Instructions to patients for use of the minipills are described in Table 42.11
- Drug interactions with oral contraceptives are listed in Table 42.12 and guidance for managing patients taking COCs and antibiotics are described in Table 42.13.
- Assessments of the risks associated with COCs (e.g., cervical dysplasia, cervical cancer, breast cancer, cardiovascular disease, thromboembolic events, hypertension, subarachnoid hemorrhage, diabetes, gallbladder disease, hepatic tumors, amenorrhea, galactorrhea, teratogenicity, headaches, and depression) require in-depth understandings and are beyond the scope of this Handbook.

Postcoital (Morning-After) Pills/Emergency Contraceptive Pills

- **Preven Emergency Contraceptive Kit** (4 blue tablets).—Patients are to read the instruction booklet, test for pregnancy, and if the pregnancy test is negative to take 2 tablets (containing levonorgestrel and ethinyl estradiol) within 72 hrs after unprotected intercourse and 2 more tablets exactly 12 hrs later.
- **Plan B** (2 white tablets)—The first progestin-only emergency contraceptive pill (0.75 mg levonorgestrel) is to be taken within 72 hrs of unprotected intercourse and the second exactly 12 hrs later. In the first 24 hrs after intercourse, Plan B can prevent 95% of expected pregnancies.
- Other postcoital estrogen and emergency contraceptive pill regimens are listed in Table 42.14.

Long-Acting Injections

- **Depo-Provera,** a long-acting progestin injectable, inhibits ovulation, thickens cervical mucus, and suppresses endometrial growth. Women likely to benefit from Depo-Provera contraception are described in Table 42.15. Instructions for the administration of Depo-Provera (DMPA) are outlined in Table 42.16.
- **Norplant** (six silastic capsules implanted under the skin of the upper arm) is formulated to release 20–30 µg/day of levorgestrel over 5 years and are to be replaced with new capsules in 5 years. The benefits of Norplant are most likely to occur in patients meeting the criteria for use as outlined in Table 42.17. Table 42.18 provides patient information on Norplant insertion. Table 42.19 describes Norplant removal to patients

Intrauterine Devices (IUDs)

- **Progestasert,** an IUD, contains 38 mg of progesterone and releases 65 mg/day for 1 year and must be replaced after 1 year.
- **ParaGard,** a polyethylene IUD wound with copper wire, may be left in place for 10 years. Precautions for the use of copper-bearing IUDs are described in Table 42.20.

♦ Patients must clearly understand the risks of IUDs, especially in light of the Dalkon Shield IUD, which was associated with tubal scarring and infertility. Patients using IUDs should be instructed to watch out for the early IUD danger signs as noted in Table 42.21.

Table 42.1 • Percentage of Women Experiencing an Unintended Pregnancy During the First Year of Typical Use and the First Year of Perfect Use of Contraception and the Percentage Continuing Use at the End of the First Year: United States

Method (1)	% of Women Experiencing an Unintended Pregnancy Within the First Year of Use		% of Women Continuing Use at One Year[c] (4)
	Typical Use[a] (2)	Perfect Use[b] (3)	
Chance[d]	85	85	
Spermicides[e]	26	6	40
Periodic Abstinence	25		63
Calendar		9	
Ovulation Method		3	
Symptothermal[f]		2	
Postovulation		1	
Cap[g]			
Parous Women	40	26	42
Nulliparous Women	20	9	56
Sponge			
Parous Women	40	20	42
Nulliparous Women	20	9	56
Diaphragm[g]	20	6	56
Withdrawal	19	4	
Condom[h]			
Female (Reality)	21	5	56
Male	14	3	61
Pill	5		71
Progestin only		0.5	
Combined		0.1	
IUD			
Progesterone T	2.0	1.5	81
Copper T 380A	0.8	0.6	78
LNg 20	0.1	0.1	81
Depo-Provera	0.3	0.3	70
Norplant and Norplant-2	0.05	0.05	88
Female Sterilization	0.5	0.5	100
Male Sterilization	0.15	0.10	100

(continued)

Notes:

Table 42.1 • Percentage of Women Experiencing an Unintended Pregnancy During the First Year of Typical Use and the First Year of Perfect Use of Contraception and the Percentage Continuing Use at the End of the First Year: United States (continued)

Method (1)	% of Women Experiencing an Unintended Pregnancy Within the First Year of Use		% of Women Continuing Use at One Year[c] (4)
	Typical Use[a] (2)	Perfect Use[b] (3)	

Emergency Contraceptive Pills

Treatment initiated within 72 hours after unprotected intercourse reduces the risk of pregnancy by at least 75%.[i]

Lactational Amenorrhea Method

LAM is a highly effective, *temporary* method of contraception.[j]

[a]Among *typical* couples who initiate use of a method (not necessarily for the first time), the percentage who experience an accidental pregnancy during the first year if they do not stop use for any other reason.
[b]Among couples who initiate use of a method (not necessarily for the first time) and who use it *perfectly* (both consistently and correctly), the percentage who experience an accidental pregnancy during the first year if they do not stop use for any other reason.
[c]Among couples attempting to avoid pregnancy, the percentage who continue to use a method for 1 year.
[d]The percentages becoming pregnant in columns (2) and (3) are based on data from populations where contraception is not used and from women who cease using contraception to become pregnant. Among such populations, about 89% become pregnant within 1 year. This estimate was lowered slightly (to 85%) to represent the percentages who would become pregnant within 1 year among women now relying on reversible methods of contraception if they abandoned contraception altogether.
[e]Foams, creams, gels, vaginal suppositories, and vaginal film.
[f]Cervical mucus (ovulation) method supplemented by calendar in the preovulatory and basal body temperature in the postovulatory phases.
[g]With spermicidal cream or jelly.
[h]Without spermicides.
[i]The treatment schedule is one dose within 72 hours after unprotected intercourse and a second dose 12 hours after the first dose. The Food and Drug Administration has declared the following brands of oral contraceptives to be safe and effective for emergency contraception: Ovral (1 dose is 2 white pills), Alesse (1 dose is 5 pink pills), Nordette or Levlen (1 dose is 4 light-orange pills), Lo/Ovral (1 dose is 4 white pills), Triphasil or Tri-Levlen (1 dose is 4 yellow pills).
[j]However, to maintain effective protection against pregnancy, another method of contraception must be used as soon as menstruation resumes, the frequency or duration of breast-feeds is reduced, bottle feeds are introduced, or the baby reaches 6 months of age.
Adapted with permission from Hatcher RA et al. Contraceptive Technology. 17th Ed. New York: Ardent Media, 1998: 216, Table 9.2.

Table 42.2 • Oral Contraceptives[a]

Product	Manufacturer	Progestin	Estrogen[b]
Low-Dose COCs			
Alesse *(pink, light green[c])*	Wyeth-Ayerst	0.10 mg LNG	20 μg
Apri *(light red, white[c])*	Duramed	0.15 mg DSG	30 μg
Brevicon *(blue, orange[c])*	Searle	0.5 mg NE	35 μg
Demulen *(white, pink[c])*	Searle	1.0 mg ED	50 μg
Demulen 1/35 *(white, blue[c])*	Searle	1.0 mg ED	35 μg
Desogen *(white, green[c])*	Organon	0.15 mg DSG	30 μg
Levlen *(light orange, pink[c])*	Berlex	0.15 mg LNG	30 μg
Levlite *(pink, light green)*	Berlex	0.10 mg LNG	20 μg
Levora *(white, peach[c])*	Watson	0.15 mg LNG	30 μg
Loestrin 1/20[c] *(white)*	Parke-Davis	1.0 mg NEAC	20 μg
Loestrin 1.5/30[c] *(green)*	Parke-Davis	1.5 mg NEAC	30 μg
Loestrin FE 1/20 *(white, brown[c])*	Parke-Davis	1.0 mg NEAC	20 μg
Loestrin FE 1.5/30 *(green, brown[c])*	Parke-Davis	1.5 mg NEAC	30 μg
Low-Ogestrel *(white, peach[c])*	Watson	0.3 mg DLNG	30 μg
Lo/Ovral *(white, pink[c])*	Wyeth-Ayerst	0.3 mg DLNG	30 μg
Modicon *(white, green[c])*	Ortho	0.5 mg NE	35 μg

(continued)

Table 42.2 • Oral Contraceptives^a *(continued)*

Product	Manufacturer	Progestin	Estrogen^b
Low-Dose COCs *(continued)*			
Necon 10/11 *(light yellow)*	Watson	0.5 mg NE (days 1–10)	35 μg
Necon 10/11 *(dark yellow, white^c)*	Watson	1.0 mg NE (days 11–21)	35 μg
Necon 1 + 35 *(yellow, white)*	Watson	1.0 mg NE	35 μg
Nordette *(light orange, pink^c)*	Wyeth-Ayerst	0.15 mg LNG	30 μg
Norinyl 1 + 35 *(orange, green^c)*	Watson	1.0 mg NE	35 μg
Norinyl 1 + 50 *(white, orange^c)*	Watson	1.0 mg NE	50 μg^e
Ortho-Cept *(orange, green^c)*	Ortho	0.15 mg DSG	30 μg
Ortho-Cyclen *(blue, green^c)*	Ortho	0.25 mg NGM	35 μg
Ortho-Novum 1/35 *(peach, green^c)*	Ortho	1.0 mg NE	35 μg
Ortho-Novum 1/50 *(yellow, green^c)*	Ortho	1.0 mg NE	50 μg^e
Ovcon-35 *(peach, green^c)*	Mead Johnson	0.4 mg NE	35 μg
Ovcon-50 *(yellow, green^c)*	Mead Johnson	1.0 mg NE	50 μg
Ovral *(white, pink^c)*	Wyeth-Ayerst	0.5 mg DLNG	50 μg
Biphasic COCs			
Jenest *(white)*	Organon	0.5 mg NE (days 1–7)	35 μg
Jenest *(peach, green^c)*	Organon	1.0 mg NE (days 8–21)	35 μg
Jenest 28 *(white, peach, green^c)*	Organon	0.5 mg NE (days 1–7)	35 μg
		1.0 MG NE (days 14–21)	(first 21 days)
Mircette *(white)*	Organon	0.15 mg DSG (days 1–21)	20 μg
Mircette *(green)*	Organon	Placebo (days 22–23)	—
Mircette *(yellow)*	Organon	— (days 24–28)	10 μg
Necon 0.5/35 *(light yellow, white^c)*	Watson	0.5 mg NE	35 μg
Ortho Novum 10/11 *(white)*	Ortho	0.5 mg NE (days 1–10)	35 μg
Ortho Novum 10/11 *(peach, green^c)*	Ortho	1.0 mg NE (days 11–21)	35 μg
Triphasic COCs			
Ortho Novum 7/7/7^f *(white)*	Ortho	0.5 mg NE (days 1–7)	35 μg
(light peach)		0.75 MG NE (days 8–14)	(first 21
(peach, green^c)		1.0 MG NE (days 15–21)	days)
Ortho Tri-Cyclen *(white)*	Ortho	0.18 mg NGM (days 1–7)	35 μg
(light blue)		0.215 MG NGM (days 8–14)	35 mg
(blue, green^c)		0.25 MG NGM (days 15–21)	35 mg
Tri-Levlen *(brown)*	Berlex	0.05 mg LNG (days 1–6)	30 μg
(white)		0.075 MG LNG (days 7–11)	40 mg
(light yellow, light green^c)		0.125 MG LNG (days 12–21)	30 mg
Tri-Norinyl^f *(blue)*	Watson	0.5 mg NE (days 1–7)	35 μg
(yellow-green)		1.0 MG NE (days 8–16)	(first 21
(blue, orange^c)		0.5 MG NE (days 17–21)	days)
Triphasil^f *(brown)*	Wyeth-Ayerst	0.05 mg LNG (days 1–6)	30 μg
(white)		0.075 MG LNG (days 7–11)	40 mg
(light yellow, light green^c)		0.125 MG LNG (days 12–21)	30 mg
Trivora *(blue)*	Watson	0.05 MG LNG (days 1–6)	30 mg
(white)		0.075 LNG (days 7–11)	40 mg
(pink)		0.125 LNG (days 12–21)	30 mg
Zovia 1 + 35E *(light pink, white^c)*	Watson	1.0 mg ED	35 μg
Zovia 1 + 50E *(pink, white^b)*	Watson	1.0 mg ED	50 μg
Constant Progestin Phasic Estrogen COC			
Estrostep Fe *(white, triangle-shaped)*	Parke-Davis	1.0 mg NEAC (days 1–5)	20 mg
(white, square-shaped)		1.0 mg NEAC (days 6–12)	30 mg
(white, round-shaped)		1.0 mg NEAC (days 13–21)	35 mg
(brown^c)		(days 22–28)	

(continued)

Notes:

Table 42.2 • Oral Contraceptives^a (continued)

Product	Manufacturer	Progestin	Estrogen^b
Minipill (Progestin-Only)			
Micronor *(lime)*	Ortho	0.35 mg NE	—
Nor-Q.D. *(yellow)*	Watson	0.35 mg NE	—
Ovrette *(yellow)*	Wyeth-Ayerst	0.075 mg DLNG	—

^{a}COC = Combination oral contraceptive; DLNG, d,l-norgestrel; DSG = Desogestrel; ED = Ethynodiol diacetate; LNG = Levonorgestrel; NE = Norethindrone; NEAC = Norethindrone acetate; NGM = Norgestimate.
^{b}Estrogen (ethinyl estradiol) in µg.
^{c}Placebo for 28-day cycles. (Parke-Davis products contain 75 mg of ferrous fumarate.)
^{d}Also available with 75 mg ferrous fumarate; pills are brown when they contain iron.
^{e}Estrogen (Mestranol) in mg.
^{f}These triphasics mimic the follicular, ovulatory, and luteal phases of the menstrual cycle. Hormonal side effects caused by insufficient progestin (e.g., late-cycle bleeding) are sometimes a problem. The estrogen dominance may be partly responsible for the minimal effects on lipids and the reduced prevalence of acne. Women with cardiovascular or metabolic abnormalities may benefit more from the triphasics because of reduced progestin content and the low estrogen content.

Notes:

Table 42.3 • Progestin Pharmacology and Contraceptive Pill Activity Listed According to Estrogen Content and Endometrial Potency^a

Drug	Endometrial Activity: % Spotting and Bleeding in Third Cycle of Use^b	Estrogenic Activity: μg Ethinyl Estradiol Equivalents/Day^c	Progestational Activity: mg Norethindrone Equivalents/Day	Androgenic Activity: Methyl Testosterone Equivalents (mg)/28 Days^e	Estrogenic Effect of Progestin^f	Antiestrogenic Effect of Progestin^g
50 μg Estrogen						
Ovral (DLNG)	4.5	42	1.3	0.80	0.00	18.5
Necon 1/50	10.6	32	1	0.34	1.00	2.5
Norinyl 1 + 50						
Ortho-Novum 1/50 (NE)						
Ovcon 50 (NE)	11.9	50^g	1	0.34	1.00	2.5
Zovia/Demulen 50 (ED)	13.9	26	1.4	0.21	3.44	1.0
<50 μg Estrogen Monophasic						
Alesse (LNG)/Levlite						
Apri/Desogen/Ortho-Cept (DSG)	13.1	30	1.5	0.17	—	Weak
Low-Ogestrel/Lo/Ovral (DLNG)	9.6	25	0.8	0.46	0.00	18.5
Ovcon 35 (NE)	11.0	40^g	0.4	0.15	1.00	2.5
Levlen/Levora/Nordette (LNG)	14.0	25	0.8	0.46	0.00	18.5
Ortho-Cyclen (NGM)	14.3	35	0.3	0.18	—	Weak
Brevicon/Modicon/Necon 0.5/35E (NE)	24.6	42	0.5	0.17	1.00	2.5
Necon 1 + 35						
Norinyl 1 + 35						
Ortho-Novum 1/35 (NE)	14.7	38	1.0	0.34	1.00	2.5
Mircette						
Loestrin 1.5/30 (NEAC)	25.2	14	1.7	0.8	1.52	25.0
Loestrin 1/20 (NEAC)	29.7	13	1.2	0.53	1.52	25.0
Zovia/Demulen 1/35 (ED)	37.4	19	1.4	0.21	3.44	1.0

(continued)

Table 42.3 • Progestin Pharmacology and Contraceptive Pill Activity Listed According to Estrogen Content and Endometrial Potency[a] (continued)

Drug	Endometrial Activity: % Spotting and Bleeding in Third Cycle of Use[b]	Estrogenic Activity: μg Ethinyl Estradiol Equivalents/Day[c]	Progestational Activity: Norethindrone Equivalents (mg)/Day[d]	Androgenic Activity: Methyl Testosterone Equivalents (mg)/28 Days[e]	Estrogenic Effect of Progestin[f]	Antiestrogenic Effect of Progestin[g]
<50 μg Estrogen Multiphasic						
Jenest 7/14 NE	14.1	39	0.8	0.28	1.00	2.5
Necon/Ortho-Novum 10/11 (NE)	19.6	40	0.8	0.25	1.00	2.5
Ortho-Novum 7/7/7 (NE)	14.5	48[g]	0.8	0.26	1.00	2.5
Ortho Tri-Cyclen (NGM)	17.7	35	0.3	0.15	—	Weak
Triphasil Tri-Levlen Trivora (LNG)	15.1	28[g]	0.5	0.29	0.00	18.5
Tri-Norinyl (NE)	25.5	40[g]	0.7	0.24	1.00	2.5
Estrostep (NEAC)						
Progestin Only						
Ovrette (DLNG)	34.9	0	0.08	0.12	0.00	18.5
Micronor/Nor Q.D.	42.3	1	0.12	0.12	1.00	2.5

[a]DLNG, dl-norgestrel; DSG = Desogestrel; ED = Ethynodiol diacetate; LNG = Levonorgestrel; NEAC = Norethindrone-acetate; NE = Norethindrone; NGM = Norgestimate.
[b]Information submitted to the U.S. FDA by the manufacturer. These rates are derived from separate studies conducted by different investigators in several population groups and, therefore, a precise comparison cannot be made.
[c]Estrogenic activity of entire tablet (mouse uterine assay).[14]
[d]Induction of glycogen vacuoles in human endometrium.[14]
[e]Rat ventral prostate assay.[14]
[f]Relative estrogen potencies of progestins on rat vaginal histology.[9,14]
[g]Relative antiestrogenic potencies of progestins.[9,14]
[h]Estimated.
Adapted with permission from Dickey RP. Managing Contraceptive Pill Patients. 8th Ed. Durant, OK: Essential Medical Information Systems, 1994:136, Table 5.

Table 42.4 • Estrogenic, Progestogenic, and Androgenic Effects of Oral Contraceptive Pills[a]

Estrogenic Effects	Progestogenic Effects	Androgenic Effects
• Nausea • Increased breast size (ductal and fatty tissue) • Cyclic weight gain due to fluid retention • Leukorrhea • Cervical eversion or ectopy • Hypertension • Rise in cholesterol concentration in gallbladder bile • Growth of leiomyomata • Telangiectasia • Hepatocellular adenomas or hepatocellular cancer (rare) • Cerebrovascular accidents (rare) • Thromboembolic complications including pulmonary emboli (rare) • Stimulation of breast neoplasia (exceedingly rare) **Nuisance Estrogenic Effects** • Corneal edema • Tear quality changes leading to visual refraction changes • Breast tenderness • Hypermenorrhea (Most pills with less than 50 μg of ethinyl estradiol do not produce troublesome estrogen-mediated side effects or complications.)	Both the estrogenic and the progestational components of oral contraceptives may contribute to the development of the following adverse effects: • Early or late cycle spotting or breakthrough bleeding • Breast tenderness • Chloasma • Headaches • Oligomenorrhea • Hypertension • Amenorrhea • Myocardial infarction (rare)	All low-dose combined pills suppress a woman's production of testosterone, which has a beneficial effect on acne, oily skin, and hirsutism. The progestin component may have androgenic as well as progestational effects: • Increased LDL cholesterol levels • Decreased HDL cholesterol levels • Decreased carbohydrate tolerance; increased insulin resistance • Pruritus **Nuisance Androgenic Effects** • Increased appetite and weight gain • Alopecia/hirsutism • Depression, fatigue, tiredness • Decreased libido and/or enjoyment of intercourse • Acne, oily skin • Increased breast tenderness or breast size

[a]HDL = High-density lipoprotein; LDL = Low-density lipoprotein.
Adapted with permission from Hatcher RA et al. Contraceptive Technology. 17th Ed. New York: Ardent Media, 1998:419, Table 19–4.

Table 42.5 • Patient Data to Be Considered Before Treatment with COCs[a]

Menstrual History
Age of menarche
Date of LMP
Duration of average menses
Regularity of menses or cycle length from month to month
Incidence of spotting (droplets of blood) and BTB in the time interval between periods
Incidence of premenstrual tension symptoms: breast tenderness and enlargement, nausea, fluid retention and bloating, weight gain, headaches, depression, anxiety, tension, irritability, or inability to concentrate

Contraceptive History
Use, response, side effects, and compliance

Routine Physical Examination Including
BP
Breast examination (teach patient to do self–breast examination)
Pelvic examination
Pap smear
Liver function evaluation
Family history
Social history

[a]BP = Blood pressure; BTB = Breakthrough bleeding; COCs = Combination oral contraceptives; LMP = Last menstrual period.

Notes:

Table 42.6 • Precautions in the Provision of COCs[a]

Precautions	Rationale/Discussion
Refrain from providing COCs for women with the following diagnoses (World Health Organization [WHO] category #4):	
DVT or PE, or a history thereof	Estrogens promote blood clotting. Thromboembolic events related to known trauma or an intravenous needle are not necessarily a reason to avoid use of pills.
Cerebrovascular accident (stroke), coronary artery or ischemic heart disease, or a history thereof	Estrogens promote blood clotting.
Structural heart disease, complicated by pulmonary hypertension, atrial fibrillation, or history of subacute bacterial endocarditis	Estrogens promote blood clotting.
Diabetes with nephropathy, retinopathy, neuropathy, or other vascular disease; diabetes of >20 years' duration	Estrogens promote blood clotting.
Breast cancer	Breast cancer is a hormonally sensitive tumor. In theory the hormones in COCs might cause some masses to grow.
Pregnancy	Current data do not show that hormonal contraceptives taken during pregnancy cause any significant risk of birth defects. However, hormonal contraceptives should not be given to pregnant women.
Lactation (<6 wk postpartum)	There is some theoretic concern that the neonate may be at risk because of exposure to steroid hormones during the first 6 wk postpartum. COCs can diminish the volume of breast milk.
Liver problems: benign hepatic adenoma or liver cancer or a history thereof; active viral hepatitis; severe cirrhosis	COCs are metabolized by the liver and their use may adversely affect prognosis of existing disease.
Headaches, including migraine, with focal neurologic symptoms	Focal neurologic symptoms, such as blurred vision, seeing flashing lights or zigzag lines, or trouble speaking or moving, may be an indication of an increased risk of stroke.
Major surgery with prolonged immobilization or any surgery on the legs	Increased risk for DVT and PE
>35 yr old and currently a heavy smoker (≥20 cigarettes a day)	Smoking increases the risk for cardiovascular disease.
Hypertension, 160+/100+ or with vascular disease	Hypertension is an important risk factor for cardiovascular disease.

(continued)

Table 42.6 • Precautions in the Provision of COCs^a (continued)

Precautions	Rationale/Discussion
Exercise caution if combined oral contraceptives are used or considered in the following situations and carefully monitor for adverse effects (WHO category #3):	
Postpartum <21 days	There is some theoretic concern regarding the association between COC use up to 3 wk postpartum and risk of thrombosis.
Lactation (6 wk to 6 mo)	In the first 6 mo postpartum, use of COCs during breast-feeding diminishes the quantity of breast milk and may adversely affect the health of the infant.
Undiagnosed abnormal vaginal/uterine bleeding	Although COCs are often used to manage heavy bleeding, clinicians should be sure that the cause of the bleeding is known before prescribing oral contraceptives.
>35 yr of age and light smoker (≤20 cigarettes/day)	Smoking increases the risk for cardiovascular disease. All smokers should be warned of this risk and should be encouraged and advised to stop smoking.
Past history of breast cancer but no evidence of recurrence for 5 yr	Breast cancer is a hormonally sensitive tumor.
Use of drugs that affect liver enzymes: rifampicin, rifabutin, and griseofulvin; anticonvulsants such as phenytoin, carbamazepine, barbiturates, topiramate, and primidone	COCs are metabolized by the liver. Drugs that affect liver enzymes could reduce the contraceptive effectiveness of COCs.
Gallbladder disease: medically treated and current biliary tract disease and history of COC-related cholestasis	Recent reports show that COCs may be weakly associated with gallbladder disease. There is also concern that COCs may worsen existing gallbladder disease.
Advantages generally outweigh theoretic or proven disadvantages and generally can be provided without restrictions in these conditions (WHO category #2):	
Severe headaches that definitely start *after* initiation of oral contraceptives; migraine headaches without focal neurologic symptoms	Migraine headaches with focal neurologic symptoms have been associated with an increased risk of stroke; any headaches clearly starting after initiation of pills may be related to pill use.
Diabetes mellitus: gestational diabetes or diabetes without vascular disease	Women with diabetes are at increased risk of heart disease and stroke, particularly if the woman smokes. Estrogens and progestins may slightly decrease glucose tolerance, but this is unlikely to happen with low-dose COCs.
Major surgery *without* prolonged immobilization	With the current low-dose pills, the problems associated with pill use and elective surgery have decreased.
Sickle cell disease or sickle C disease	Women with sickle cell disease are predisposed to occlusion of the microvasculature (because of abnormal, inflexible red blood cells). Studies of women with sickle cell disease have shown no significant differences between COC users and nonusers with regard to coagulation studies, blood viscosity measurements, or incidence or severity of painful sickle cell crises.
Moderate blood pressure: 140–159/100–109	Monitor blood pressure periodically. Hypertension is an important risk factor for cardiovascular disease.

Undiagnosed breast mass	Some clinicians and some clinical protocols suggest that women found to have a breast mass should not be provided COCs until cancer of the breast has been ruled out. Other clinicians are comfortable prescribing pills while the cause of the breast mass is being evaluated.
Cervical cancer awaiting treatment and cervical intraepithelial neoplasia	The risk of cervical cancer appears to be increased slightly in COC users. COC users may get Pap smears more regularly so that early dysplasia is more likely to be recognized. They also tend to have more sexual partners. Pill use may also alter susceptibility to infection with HPV, a known risk factor for cancer of the cervix.
Over 50 yr of age	Women >50 are at increased risk for heart and cerebrovascular disease.
Conditions likely to make it very difficult for a woman to take COCs consistently and correctly	Mental retardation, major psychiatric illness, alcoholism, other chemical abuse, and/or a history of repeatedly taking oral contraception or other medications incorrectly make compliance with taking COCs difficult.
Family history of hyperlipidemia	Some types of hyperlipidemia increase a woman's risk for heart disease. Routine screening is not recommended by WHO because of the rarity of the conditions and the high cost of screening.
Family history of death of a parent or sibling because of myocardial infarction before age 50	Myocardial infarction in a mother or sister is especially significant and suggests a need for lipid evaluation.

Do not restrict use of COCs for the following conditions (*WHO category #1*):

- Postpartum ≥21 days
- Postabortion after first or second trimester or immediately after postseptic abortion
- History of gestational diabetes
- Varicose veins
- Mild headaches
- Irregular vaginal bleeding patterns, *without* or *with* heavy or prolonged bleeding and no anemia
- Past history of PID
- Current or recent history (within last 3 mo) of PID
- Current or recent history (within last 3 mo) of STI
- Vaginitis without purulent cervicitis
- Increased risk of STI (e.g., multiple partners or partner who has multiple partners)
- HIV-positive, high risk of HIV, or AIDS
- Benign breast disease
- Family history of breast cancer

(continued)

Table 42.6 • Precautions in the Provision of COCs[a] (continued)

Precautions	Rationale/Discussion
Do not restrict use of COCs for the following conditions (WHO category #1): (continued)	
• Cervical ectropion	
• Endometrial or ovarian cancer	
• Viral hepatitis carrier	
• Uterine fibroids	
• Past ectopic pregnancy	
• Obesity	
• Thyroid conditions: simple goiter, hyperthyroidism, hypothyroidism	
• Benign or malignant gestational trophoblastic disease	
• Iron deficiency anemia	
• Epilepsy	
• Schistosomiasis (uncomplicated or with fibrosis of the liver)	
• Malaria	
• Current use of antibiotics	
• Nulliparity or parity	
• Severe dysmenorrhea	
• Tuberculosis, including pelvic	
• Endometriosis	
• Benign ovarian tumors	
• Prior pelvic surgery	

[a]COCs = Combined oral contraceptives; DVT = Deep venous thrombosis; HPV = Human papilloma virus; PE = Pulmonary embolism; PID = Pelvic inflammatory disease; STI = Sexually transmitted infection.
Adapted with permission from Hatcher RA et al. Contraceptive Technology. 17th Ed. New York: Ardent Media, 1998:420, Table 19.5.

Table 42.7 • Precautions in the Provision of Progestin-Only Contraceptives[a]

Precautions	Rationale/Discussion
Refrain from providing COCs for women with the following diagnoses (World Health Organization [WHO] category #4):	
Pregnancy	Although current data do not show an increased risk for birth defects caused by taking hormones during pregnancy, it is best to avoid any exposure of the fetus to hormones.
Unexplained abnormal vaginal bleeding suspicious for a serious underlying condition	Progestin-only contraceptives usually lead to irregular menses, increased days of light bleeding, or amenorrhea. These changes may mask an underlying problem such as pelvic inflammatory disease, cancer of the reproductive tract, or pregnancy. Until a diagnosis of the cause of unexplained vaginal bleeding is reached, do not inject Depo-Provera or insert Norplant. *(Exercise caution [WHO #3] in providing minipills.)*
Breast cancer	Some breast cancers are sensitive to progestins. Suspicious masses should be evaluated as soon as possible.
Exercise caution if COCs are used or considered in the following situations and carefully monitor for adverse effects (WHO category #3):	
Certain medications Antiseizure: phenytoin (Dilantin), carbamazepine, primidone, phenylbutazone Antibiotics: rifampin/rifampicin	Medications for epilepsy (except valproic acid) cause the liver to metabolize progestins more rapidly, decreasing already low blood levels of levonorgestrel, the hormone found in Norplant and minipills. *(Advantages generally outweigh theoretic or proven disadvantages [WHO #2] when providing Depo-Provera. See the next section.)*
Breast cancer with 5-year disease-free interval	Some breast cancers are sensitive to progestins. Evaluate suspicious masses as soon as possible.
Liver conditions such as severe decompensated cirrhosis, adenoma or cancer, active viral hepatitis	Progestin-only contraceptives are metabolized by the liver, and their use may adversely affect prognosis of existing disease. There is a concern that progestin-only contraceptives may increase the risk of hepatoma, as COCs do.
Cardiovascular conditions such as hypertension with or without vascular disease, current or history of ischemic heart disease, history of cerebrovascular accident (stroke)	HDL cholesterol levels fall in women using progestin-only contraceptives, especially Depo-Provera. There is also some concern regarding their hypoestrogenic effect. Although Norplant patient package inserts warn of cardiovascular complications, these concerns are based on past experience with high-dose COCs, not on data about Norplant. *(Advantages generally outweigh theoretic or proven disadvantages [WHO #2] when providing Norplant or minipills; see the next section.)*
Diabetes with nephropathy, retinopathy, and neuropathy	Exercise caution in providing Depo-Provera to women with diabetes complicated by other organic conditions. See the discussion on cardiovascular and liver conditions.

(continued)

Table 42.7 • Precautions in the Provision of Progestin-Only Contraceptives[a] (continued)

Precautions	Rationale/Discussion

Do not restrict use of progestin-only contraceptives because of the following conditions (WHO category #1) or
The advantages generally outweigh theoretic or proven disadvantages, and the method generally can be provided without restrictions in these conditions, although more use requires greater follow-up (WHO category #2):

	Depo-Provera	Norplant	Minipills
• Age: menarche to 16 years	2	2	2
• Age 16 or older	1	1	1
• Smokers, light or heavy, any age	1	1	1
• Over 16 years of age	1	1	1
• Obesity	1	1	1
Gynecologic or Obstetric Conditions			
• Breast-feeding: 6 wk postpartum and thereafter	1	1	1
• Immediately postpartum, not breast-feeding	1	1	1
• Postabortion: first or second trimester or septic	1	1	1
• History of pre-eclampsia or gestational diabetes	1	1	1
• Benign breast disease or family history of breast cancer	1	1	1
• Cervical ectropion	1	1	1
• Cholestasis of pregnancy	1	1	1
• Uterine fibroids or endometriosis	1	1	1
• Benign or malignant trophoblastic disease	1	1	1
• Nulliparous	1	1	1
• Benign ovarian tumors, including cysts	1	1	1
• Prior pelvic surgery	1	1	1
• Past ectopic pregnancy	2	1	1
• Irregular, heavy, or prolonged vaginal bleeding	2	2	2
• Undiagnosed breast mass	2	2	2
• CIN or cancer	2	2	2
Chronic Diseases or Other Conditions			
• Cholestasis while on combined pills	2	2	2
• History/current DVT or PE	1	1	1
• Major or minor surgery with or without immobilization	1	1	1

Condition		
• Superficial venous thrombosis (varicose veins or other)	1	1
• Valvular heart disease: uncomplicated or complicated	1	1
• Mild headaches	1	1
• Severe headaches including migraine *without* focal neurologic symptoms	2	2
• Gallbladder disease of any kind	1	1
• Thyroid: goiter, hypothyroid, hyperthyroid	1	1
• Iron deficiency anemia	1	1
• Epilepsy	1	1
• BP 140–179/90–109	2	2
• Hypertension by history that cannot be evaluated (except hypertension in pregnancy)	2	2
• BP 180+/110+	2	2
• Diabetes *without* vascular disease (noninsulin-dependent or insulin-dependent)	2	2
• Past elevated blood sugar levels during pregnancy	1	1
• Diabetes *with* nephropathy, retinopathy, and neuropathy	2	*
• Diabetes with other vascular disease or 20 years' duration	2	*
• Current or history of ischemic heart disease	2	*
• History of cerebrovascular accident (stroke)	2	*
• Severe headaches, including migraine *with* focal neurologic symptoms	2	2
• Mild (compensated) cirrhosis	2	2
• Rifampicin, griseofulvin, phenytoin, carbamezapine, barbiturates, primadone	2	*

Infections: STI and Other

Condition		
• PID, past or present	1	1
• Any STI, HIV-positive or AIDS	1	1
• Viral hepatitis carrier	1	1
• Schistosomiasis: uncomplicated or with fibrosis of liver (if severe, see cirrhosis); or malaria	1	1
• Antibiotics other than rifampicin and griseofulvin	1	1
• Tuberculosis (but also see antibiotics)	1	1

*See the previous section of this table.

CIN = Cervical intraepithelial neoplasia; DVT = Deep venous thrombosis; HDL = High-density lipoprotein; PE = Pulmonary embolism; PID = Pelvic inflammatory disease; STI = Sexually transmitted infection.

Adapted with permission from Hatcher RA et al. Contraceptive Technology. 17th Ed. New York: Ardent Media, 1998:479, Table 20.4.

Table 42.8 • Choosing a COC with <50 µg of Estrogen[a]

Start by Determining if the Woman Can Safely Use Estrogen

Step 1	Step 2

Is this person a good candidate for a pill with estrogen? → YES, she can use an estrogen.

In general, avoid prescribing a pill with estrogen to women with: → NO, it would be best if she did not use an estrogen. Therefore, you can consider:

- Current or a history of circulatory diseases caused by blood clots (including heart attack, stroke, or blood clots in deep veins) or cardiovascular disease caused by diabetes.
- Structural heart disease with complications such as atrial fibrillation or subacute bacterial endocarditis.
- Blood pressure of 160/100 or greater.
- Age of 35 or more who are smokers.
- Breast cancer or history thereof (exceptions may be made if no evidence of disease in past 5 yr).
- Active hepatic disease, including symptomatic viral hepatitis, severe or mild cirrhosis, or benign or malignant liver tumors.
- Past history of jaundice (cholestasis) related to oral contraceptives.
- Migraine headaches with neurologic impairment, such as blurred or lost vision, seeing flashing lights or zigzag lines, trouble speaking or moving.
- Diabetes and damaged vision (retinopathy), kidneys (nephropathy), or nervous system (neuropathy), or women who have had diabetes for 20 years or longer.
- Plan to undergo major surgery or any leg surgery requiring immobilization for several days or more. Estrogen-containing pills should be discontinued 4 wk before major surgery.

- Progestin-only pills, such as:
  - Micronor (0.35 mg norethindrone daily)
    NOR QD (0.35 mg norethindrone daily)
  - Ovrette (0.075 mg norgestrel daily)
- Norplant (5-year levonorgestrel implants)
- Depo-Provera (150 mg medroxyprogestrone acetate injection every 3 mo)
- Intrauterine device
  - Copper T 380-A
  - Levonorgestrel IUD
  - Progestasert System
- Condoms (male or female)
- Diaphragm, cervical cap, Reality female condom
- Foam, VCF Film, suppository
- Fertility awareness
- Male or female sterilization

Breast-feeding women, in general, should avoid estrogen until they start weaning the baby from breast-feeding.

Exceptions may be made in specific cases, and occasionally pills may be prescribed for women in the above categories, provided that the specialized (individualized) grounds are well documented in the record. For a fuller list of precautions see Table 42.6.

Most Women May Use Any of the Pills With <50 µg of Estrogen

Step 3

If there is no reason to avoid estrogen, you may choose between any of the following COCs based on:

- Number of micrograms of ethinyl estradiol
- Availability of pill
- Ease of understanding packaging of pills
- Price of pills to clinic**
- Price of pills to client**
- Prior experience of this individual woman or the clinician caring for this woman with a special pill

Pills are listed from the lowest to the highest number of micrograms of ethinyl estradiol:

Combined Pill	Estrogen (µg)	Availability/Cost in Your Clinic	Company
Loestrin 1/20	20	_____	Parke-Davis
Alesse	20	_____	Wyeth
Estrostep 21	20/30/35	_____	Parke-Davis
Loestrin 1.5/30	30	_____	Parke-Davis
*Apri	30	_____	Solvay
*Desogen	30	_____	Organon
Levora	30	_____	Watson
Low-Ogestrel	30	_____	Watson
Lo/Ovral	30	_____	Wyeth
Nordette	30	_____	Wyeth
Levlen	30	_____	Berlex
*Ortho-Cept	30	_____	Ortho
Tri-Levlen	30/40/30	_____	Berlex
Triphasil	30/40/30	_____	Wyeth
Ovcon 35	35	_____	Mead Johnson
Demulen 1/35	35	_____	Searle

Step 4

Other clinical considerations that might help in COC choice

A. To minimize the risk potential for *thrombosis* caused by estrogen in a woman 40–50 years of age or any woman at increased risk for thrombosis because of another cause (e.g., diabetic, very overweight woman, or a young woman who is a heavy smoker), prescribe:
   - Loestrin 1/20
   - Alesse

B. To minimize *nausea, breast tenderness, vascular headaches, and estrogen-mediated side effects*, prescribe:
   - Loestrin 1/20
   - Alesse/Levlite
   - Estrostep
   Or a 30 µg pill, such as:
   - Levlen/Levora
   - Loestrin 1.5–30
   - Lo/Ovral/Low-Ogestrel
   - Nordette

C. To minimize *spotting and/or breakthrough bleeding*, prescribe:
   - Lo/Ovral/Low-Ogestrel, Nordette, or Levlen
   - Estrostep
   - Ortho-Cyclen or Ortho Tri-Cyclen
   - Desogen, Ortho-Cept, or Apri

D. To minimize androgen effects such as *acne, hirsutism, oily skin, sebaceous cysts, pilonidal cysts, or weight gain*, prescribe:
   - Ortho-Cyclen or Ortho Tri-Cyclen
   - Desogen, Ortho-Cept, or Apri
   - Ovcon-35, Brevicon, Modicon, or Necon 0.5/35
   - Demulen 1/35 or Zovia 1/35

(continued)

Table 42.8 • Choosing a COC with <50 μg of Estrogen[a] (continued)

Most Women May Use Any of the Pills With <50 μg of Estrogen (continued)

Step 3

Combined Pill	Estrogen (μg)	Availability/Cost in Your Clinic	Company
Zovia 1/35	35	_____	Watson
Ortho-Cyclen	35	_____	Ortho
Ortho Tri-Cyclen	35	_____	Ortho
Ortho Novum 777	35	_____	Ortho
Ortho-Novum 1/35	35	_____	Ortho
Modicon	35	_____	Ortho
Necon 0.5/35	35	_____	Watson
Brevicon	35	_____	Watson
Necon 1/35	35	_____	Watson
Norinyl 1/35	35	_____	Watson
Tri-Norinyl	35	_____	Watson
**Nelova 1/35	35	_____	Warner-Chilcott
**Genora 0.5/35	35	_____	Phy Total Care
Genora 1/35	35	_____	Phy Total Care
Jenest	35	_____	Organon
Necon 10/11	35	_____	Watson

Step 4

E. To produce the most *favorable lipid profile*, prescribe:
- Ortho-Cyclen or Ortho Tri-Cyclen
- Desogen, Ortho-Cept, or Apri
- Ovcon-35, Brevicon, Modicon, or Necon 0.5/35

F. To use a combined pill as an emergency contraceptive:
- Ovral (2 within 72 hr, repeat in 12 hr)
- Lo/Ovral/Low-Ogestrel (4 within 72 hr, repeat in 12 hr)
- Levlen, Nordette Levora (4 within 72 hr, repeat in 12 hr)
- Triphasil, Tri-Levlen (4 yellow pills within 72 hr, repeat in 12 hr), Trivora (use pink tablets)

*Women using pills containing desogestrel may have an increased risk of venous thrombosis.

**The only pill costing pharmacists less than $10.00 per cycle:
Genora 0.5/35 ($8.59). Cost of most pills to pharmacists was $17.00 to $30.00 per cycle. In some clinics, pills may be purchased at prices as low as $0.50 to $1.00 per cycle.

[Source: Anonymous. 2000. Drug Topics Red Book. Average wholesale price listing.]

[a]© Robert A. Hatcher, MD, MPH April 1993. The following individuals assisted in the development of this flow chart: Marcia Angle, MD, MPH, Program for International Training and Health (INTRAH); James Bellinger, PAC, Emory University School of Medicine; Willard Cates, Jr., MD, MPH, Family Health International (FHI); John Guillebaud, MA, FRSCE, FRCOG, MFFP, Margaret Pyke Center, London; Robert A. Hatcher, MD, MPH, Emory University School of Medicine; Michael Policar, MD, MPH, Solano Partnership Health Plan; Sharon Schnare, CNM, MSN, FNP, DHHS/PHS-Region 10; Gary S. Stewart, MD, MPH, Planned Parenthood of Sacramento Valley; Susan Wysocki, RNC, BSN, NP, National Association of Nurse Practitioners in Reproductive Health. Adapted with permission from Hatcher RA, et al. Contraceptive Technology. 17th Ed. New York: Ardent Media, 1998:434, Table 19-3.

Table 42.9 • Pill Early Danger Signs (ACHES)

Signals	Possible Problem
Abdominal pain (severe)	Gallbladder disease, hepatic adenoma, blood clot, pancreatitis
Chest pain (severe), shortness of breath, or coughing up blood	Blood clot in lungs or myocardial infarction
Headaches (severe)	Stroke, hypertension, or migraine headache
Eye problems: blurred vision, flashing lights, or blindness	Stroke, hypertension, or temporary vascular problem
Severe leg pain (calf or thigh)	Blood clot in legs

Table 42.10 • Disadvantages of Minipill (Progestin Only)

Less effective than COCs
Dysmenorrhea
High incidence of irregular menses
Amenorrhea
Decreased menstrual flow and amount
Spotting and breakthrough bleeding
Concern about becoming pregnant

Table 42.11 • Minipill Patient Instructions

1. Begin the minipill on the first day of menstrual bleeding. Use a backup method of contraception for 48 hours if you start on any other day.
2. Take one pill every day at exactly the same time.
3. First-time users should use a backup method of contraception for the first cycle, because mistakes are more common then.
4. Use a secondary means of contraception if having regular periods on the minipill, because ovulation may be occurring.[9]
5. Take a pill as soon as you remember that you missed 1 and take the next pill at your regular time; use a secondary means of contraception for 48 hours. If you miss 2 pills, take 2 when you remember, 2 the next day, and use another method of contraception until your next period. If >2 pills are missed, discontinue, and restart on first day of menses or when pregnancy is ruled out.
6. Use a backup method of contraception for 2 days if you are >3 hours late taking a minipill.
7. Examine your breasts for lumps or other changes once each month when you start a new pill pack.
8. Be aware of early danger signs, ACHES,[9] and immediately notify your practitioner if any are noted (see Table 42.9).
9. Early resumption of ovulation may occur if Parlodel (bromocriptine mesylate) has been used for the prevention of lactation.
10. When switching from the minipill to a combined pill, begin on the first day of menses. No backup method is necessary.

Notes:

Table 42.12 • Oral Contraceptive Drug Interactions[a]

Interacting Drug	Net Effect
Drugs That May Reduce COC Enterohepatic Circulation	
Ampicillin[30–33,42,43,47,50]	Spotting, BTB, pregnancy
Cephalosporins[43,46]	Spotting, BTB, pregnancy
Chloramphenicol[37]	Spotting, BTB, pregnancy
Dapsone[43]	Spotting, BTB, pregnancy
Erythromycin[34,43]	Spotting, BTB, pregnancy
Isoniazid[34,37,38,52]	Spotting, BTB, pregnancy
Phenoxymethyl penicillin[34,43]	Spotting, BTB, pregnancy
Sulfonamides[43]	Spotting, BTB, pregnancy
Tetracyclines[36,43,46]	Spotting, BTB, pregnancy
TMP-SMX[31–35,43,46]	Spotting, BTB, pregnancy
Drugs That May Induce COC Liver Enzymatic Metabolism	
Butabarbital[43,48,49]	Spotting, BTB, pregnancy
Carbamazepine[43,48,49]	Spotting, BTB, pregnancy
Ethosuximide[43,48,49]	Spotting, BTB, pregnancy
Felbamate[50a]	Spotting, BTB
Griseofulvin[33,51]	Spotting, BTB, pregnancy
Mephobarbital[43,48,49]	Spotting, BTB, pregnancy
Nelfinavir[53]	Spotting, BTB, pregnancy
Phenobarbital or primidone[43,48,49]	Spotting, BTB, pregnancy
Phenytoin[43,48,49]	Spotting, BTB, pregnancy
Rifabutin[54]	Spotting, BTB, pregnancy
Rifampin[33–40,48,49,52]	Spotting, BTB, pregnancy
Secobarbital[55]	Spotting, BTB, pregnancy
St. John's Wort[55a]	Spotting, BTB
Miscellaneous Drug Interactions with COCs	
Anticoagulants[56,57]	↓ anticoagulation
Atorvastatin[58]	30% ↑ norethindrone; 20% ↑ ethinyl estradiol
Benzodiazepines[59,60]	Enhanced benzodiazepine effect
Cyclosporine[61]	Doubling of cyclosporine level
Insulin[62]	19% require ↑ insulin dosage
Phenytoin[48]	↑ serum phenytoin
Prednisolone[63]	50% reduction in prednisolone clearance
Ritonavir[64]	AUC of ethinyl estradiol ↓ 40%
Theophylline[65]	33% reduction in theophylline clearance
Tizanidine[66]	50% reduction in tizanidine clearance
Topiramate[67]	18–30% ↓ plasma ethinyl estradiol
Troglitazone[68]	30% ↓ in plasma ethinyl estradiol and norethindrone

[a]BTB = Breakthrough bleeding; COC = Combination oral contraceptives; TMP-SMX = Trimethoprim-sulfamethoxazole.

Table 42.13 • Managing Patients Taking COCs and Antibiotics[a,b]

Category A: Likely to Reduce COC Effectiveness
Rifampin, Rifabutin

Category B: Associated with COC Failure in 3 Case Reports
Ampicillin, amoxicillin, metronidazole, tetracycline

Category C: Associated with COC Failure in at Least One Case Report
Cephalexin, chloramphenicol, clindamycin, dapsone, erythromycin, griseofulvin, isoniazid, nitrofurantoin, phenoxymethylpenicillin, sulfonamides, sulfamethoxazole, trimethoprim

[a]COCs = Combination oral contraceptives.
[b]The author recommends a backup method of contraception until menses occurs after informing the patient of the limited evidence cited in this table and Table 42.12.

Table 42.14 • Postcoital Contraception

High-Dose Estrogens

Diethylstilbestrol	25 mg BID ×5 days
Ethinyl estradiol	2.5 mg BID ×5 days
Esterified estrogens	10 mg BID ×5 days
Conjugated estrogens	10 mg BID ×5 days
Estrone	5 mg ×5 days

FDA-approved Emergency Contraceptive Pills[a]

Alesse	5 pink tablets immediately followed by 5 tablets 12 hr later
Levlon/Nordette	4 light-orange tablets immediately followed by 4 tablets 12 hr later
Lo/Ovral	4 white tablets immediately followed by 4 tablets 12 hr later
Ovral[b]	2 white tablets immediately followed by 2 tablets 12 hr later
Trilevlen/Triphasil	4 yellow tablets immediately followed by 4 tablets 12 hr later[c]

Nonapproved Emergency Contraceptive Pill

Ovrette[222]	20 yellow tablets followed by 20 tablets 12 hr later

[a]Caution: Both Berlex and Wyeth-Ayerst have declined to submit new drug applications for their products to include emergency contraception and, therefore, the labeling does not cover it.
[b]Seems to be preferred because of low failure rate (0.16–1.7%) and low incidence of nausea and vomiting.
[c]Research on emergency contraception has only been reported for norgestrel products.

Table 42.15 • Depo-Provera Candidates

Candidates Are Patients in Whom:
Contraception of at least 1 year's duration is desired.
Estrogen should be avoided.
Compliance problems exist with other contraceptive methods.
Intrauterine devices should be avoided.
Barrier methods are undesirable.
Breast-feeding is desirable.
There is a history of seizure.
Amenorrhea is desirable.

Table 42.16 • DMPA Administration[a]

150 mg DMPA deep IM injection in the deltoid or gluteal site using a 1½-inch 21- to 23-gauge needle[b]

First injection during day 1–5 of cycle or after ruling out pregnancy

Reinjections given Q 12 wk ±14-day "grace period"

[a]DMPA, depo-medroxyprogesterone acetate; IM, intramuscular.
[b]Do not massage site after injection to avoid reduction of the depot.

Notes:

Table 42.17 • Norplant Candidates^a

Candidates Are Patients in Whom
Long-term ($\approx$5 years) contraception is desired.
Estrogen should be avoided.
Compliance with other contraceptive methods is problematic.
IUDs are not indicated.
Barrier methods are undesirable.
Seizures controlled by valproic acid or gabapentin are present.
Amenorrhea is undesirable.
Fertility on discontinuation needs to be prompt.

^aIUDs = Intrauterine devices.

Table 42.18 • Patient Information on Norplant Insertion

It is a minor surgical procedure performed under local anesthesia, lasting 5–10 min.

Minor discomfort is usually related to injection of local anesthesia. After adequate anesthesia, a pressure sensation is felt.

It is placed in the nondominant upper arm between days 1 and 7 of the cycle or after pregnancy is ruled out.

Bruising or tenderness at the site with touch or motion is common during the first 7–10 days after insertion. The use of an ice pack applied over the bandage for 20 min on the day of insertion and the application of warm moist heat decrease symptoms.

Complications are rare but include expulsion and infection.

Table 42.19 • Patient Information on Norplant Removal

Ease of removal depends on skill of clinician and proper insertion.^a

It is performed under local anesthesia, lasting 20–60 min.

Discomfort is minimal. Experienced sensations include burning with administration of local anesthetic and then pressure.

Complications include fracture of implant and, rarely, infections.

Levonorgestrel is metabolized rapidly after removal, so initiate another method of contraception on the day of removal.

^aDifficult removal is secondary to deep insertion or adhesions.

Notes:

Table 42.20 • Precautions to Use of Copper-Bearing Intrauterine Devices[a]

Refrain from providing an IUD for women with the following diagnoses (World Health Organization [WHO] category #4):

Precautions	Rationale/Discussion
Active, recent (within past 3 mo), or recurrent pelvic infection (acute or subacute): • Postpartum endometritis • Infection following an abortion • Active STI, including purulent cervicitis	IUD insertion increases the risk of upper genital tract infection and infertility. The IUD is unique among all models of contraceptives in its failure to prevent upper genital tract infection.
Known or suspected pregnancy	IUD insertion can lead to a spontaneous abortion with the possibility of septic abortion.
Severely distorted uterine cavity caused by anatomical abnormalities of the uterus including: • Leiomyomata • Endometrial polyps • Cervical stenosis • Bicornuate uterus • Small uterus	Severe distortions of the uterine cavity could cause difficulties in insertion and increase the chance of expulsion.

Exercise caution if an IUD is used or considered in the following situations and carefully monitor for adverse effects (WHO category #3):

Risk factors for PID: • Purulent cervicitis, until treated • Any history of gonorrhea or chlamydia (especially recent infections)	During IUD insertion, bacteria from a pre-existing STI can be introduced into the sterile uterine cavity, leading to PID. Most of the PID occurs in the initial 3 weeks following IUD insertion. A vaginal infection must be treated and resolved before an IUD is inserted. The woman and her partner(s) must be treated for STIs, if present, before considering IUD insertion.
Risk factors for an STI, including multiple sexual partners or a partner who has multiple sexual partners	IUDs fail to protect against STIs (in the vagina and cervix) that can ascend and cause an upper genital tract infection.
Impaired response to infection: • Steroid treatment • HIV infection and/or AIDS	Women with impaired immune response may be at greater risk for severe PID.
Risk factors for infection with HIV and AIDS	IUDs cause increased menstrual flow and a sterile inflammatory reaction in the uterus with increased numbers of white blood cells. If the woman is HIV positive, the IUD may increase the risk of HIV transmission to her sexual partner(s). Recommend condoms instead. The decreased immune response may increase the risk of PID.
Undiagnosed, irregular, heavy or abnormal vaginal bleeding; cervical or uterine malignancy (known or suspected), including unresolved Pap smear	Gynecologic problems should be diagnosed before an IUD is inserted. Because IUDs may cause uterine bleeding between periods and may increase menstrual flow, bleeding abnormalities could be attributed to the IUD in error, and the woman's true problem of cervical or uterine malignancy may be missed.
Previous problems with IUD: • Pregnancies • Expulsion • Perforation • Pain • Heavy bleeding	Monitor patient carefully.

(continued)

Table 42.20 • Precautions to Use of Copper-Bearing Intrauterine Devices[a] (continued)

Precautions	Rationale/Discussion
Past history of severe vasovagal reactivity or fainting	IUD use can occasionally cause a vasovagal reaction. This is most likely to occur in a nulliparous woman with a small uterus. Use of paracervical anesthesia (10 to 20 cc of 1% lidocaine) may decrease a woman's risk for severe pain or vasovagal reaction.
Difficulty obtaining emergency follow-up care and treatment for PID	PID with an IUD in place can be serious and, if untreated, can lead to hysterectomy or even death. Therefore, it is advisable to have a doctor nearby in case emergency care is needed.

Advantages generally outweigh theoretic or proven disadvantages and copper-bearing IUDs generally can be provided without restriction in these conditions (WHO category #2):

Valvular heart disease such as aortic stenosis *without* complications	Valvular lesions may make women more susceptible to SBE. Prophylactic antibiotics are recommended at time of IUD insertion. Mitral valve prolapse is generally not considered a reason to avoid IUD use.[a]

Advantages generally outweigh theoretic or proven disadvantages and copper-bearing IUDs generally can be provided without restriction in these conditions (WHO category #2): (continued)

Uterine fibroids, very narrow cervical canal, cervical lacerations, or other anatomic abnormality that does *not* distort the uterus	Severe distortions of the uterine cavity could cause difficulties in insertion and increased chance of expulsion of the IUD.
Heavy or prolonged menstrual bleeding *without* clinical signs of anemia	Increased menstrual blood loss from some IUDs can worsen anemia; however, the use of oral iron or nutritional counseling can reverse the effect.[c]
Woman who has never had a child	Other contraceptives (e.g., oral contraceptives, Depo-Provera, condoms) have a protective effect against PID and are better options for the woman who has never had a child and wants children in the future. Some studies demonstrate a slightly increased risk of infertility in women with a history of IUD use. Return of fertility, however, is excellent for most women following IUD use. Nulliparous women tend not to tolerate an IUD as well as women who have carried a pregnancy to term.[d]

(continued)

Notes:

Table 42.20 • Precautions to Use of Copper-Bearing Intrauterine Devices^a (continued)

Precautions	Rationale/Discussion

Do not restrict use of copper-bearing IUD because of these conditions (WHO category #1):

- Previous PID, has been pregnant since, and is not now at risk of STI
- Past ectopic pregnancy
- Irregular menstrual patterns *without* heavy bleeding
- IUD was removed because its period of effectiveness had ended
- IUD was expelled and client wants to try again
- Recent first-trimester abortion or miscarriage and no infection or risk of infection
- Breast-feeding
- Previous cesarean section
- Diabetes
- Current or past cardiovascular diseases or cardiovascular problems caused by diabetes; high blood pressure; stroke; deep or superficial venous thrombosis; pulmonary embolism; valvular heart disease without complications; ischemic heart disease; hyperlipidemia
- Headaches, including severe headaches and migraines
- Current or past breast cancer or benign breast disease
- Current or past liver or gallbladder disease
- Malaria; schistosomiasis; tuberculosis (other than pelvic tuberculosis); viral hepatitis
- Obesity
- Smoking
- Epilepsy
- Cervical intraepithelial neoplasia or cervical ectropion
- Thyroid conditions
- History of preeclampsia
- Benign ovarian tumors including cysts

^aIUD = Intrauterine device; PID = Pelvic inflammatory disease; SBE = Subacute bacterial endocarditis; STI = Sexually transmitted infection.
^bDajani AS et al. Prevention of bacterial endocarditis: recommendations by the American Heart Association. JAMA 1990;264:2919.
^cAndersson K, Rybo G. Levonorgestrel releasing intrauterine device in the treatment of menorrhagia. Br J Obstet Gynaecol 1990;97:690.
^dPeterson KR, Brooks L, Jacobsen B, Shonsky SO. Intrauterine devices in nulliparous women. Adv Contraception 1991;7:333.
Adapted with permission from Hatcher RA et al. Contraceptive Techology. 17th Ed. New York: Ardent Media, 1998: 517, Table 21.3.

Table 42.21 • IUD Early Danger Signs (PAINS)

Period late (pregnancy) or abnormal spotting or intermenstrual bleeding

Abdominal pain or pain with intercourse

Infection exposure (e.g., gonorrhea) or abnormal vaginal discharge

Not feeling well, fever, chills

String missing, shorter, or longer

The reader is referred to Chapter 43: Contraception, written by *Ronald J. Ruggiero, Pharm.D.*, in the seventh edition of **Applied Therapeutics: The Clinical Use of Drugs** for a more in-depth discussion. All notations to reference numbers are based on the reference list at the end of that chapter. The editors of this handbook express their thanks to Dr. Ruggiero and acknowledge that this chapter is based upon his work.

Notes:

Chapter 43

Obstetrics

Inside . . .

Definitions

   ♦ ***Gravida, Parity, and Pregnancy***

   Gravida refers to the number of pregnancies.

   Nulligravida is a woman who has never been pregnant.

   Primigravida is a woman who has been pregnant once.

   Multigravida is a woman who has been pregnant ≥2 times

   Parity refers to the number of deliveries after 20 weeks gestation, regardless of the outcome or the method of delivery.

   Nullipara describes a woman who has never delivered a fetus >20 weeks gestation.

   Primipara is a woman who has delivered a fetus or fetuses beyond 20 weeks gestation.

Multipara describes a woman who has had ≥2 deliveries beyond 20 weeks. For example, a woman who has had 2 spontaneous abortions and 3 normal deliveries would be described as "gravida 5, para 3."

♦ **Four-digit numerical designation** (e.g., 3–0–1–3) also can be used to describe a woman's obstetrical history.
- *First Digit.* Number of term infants delivered (>37 weeks).
- *Second Digit.* Number of preterm infants delivered (20–37 weeks).
- *Third Digit.* Number of abortions (<20 weeks).
- Fourth Digit. Number of live children delivered.

♦ **Pregnancy** is usually divided into 3 trimesters of 13 weeks each. It is more precise to use weeks gestation: number of weeks since last menstrual period (LMP). Pregnancy also can be divided into developmental periods.
- *Prenatal Period.* 40 weeks long. Refers to period of *in utero* development.
- *Embryonic Period.* 0–8 weeks gestation; organogenesis occurs; fetus is most susceptible to teratogenic effects of drugs.
- *Fetal Period.* 9–26 weeks gestation; organs become functional.
- *Perinatal Period.* 27 weeks gestation through delivery.

♦ **Delivery terms** refer to the time of delivery.
- *Abortion.* Delivery before 20 weeks gestation.
- *Term Infant.* Fetus delivered after completion of 37 weeks gestation and before 43 weeks.
- *Preterm.* Delivery occurs between 20–37 weeks gestation.
- *Postterm.* Delivery occurs after the beginning of 43 weeks gestation.

PREGNANCY

♦ **Diagnosis.** Based upon symptoms, physical changes and biochemical test results. (See Table 43.1.)

♦ **Danger Signs.** The danger signs of pregnancy are listed in Table 43.2.

♦ **Gestational Age.** Average duration of pregnancy from conception to term is 266 days; however, date of conception is rarely known. Measured from first day of the last normal menstrual period (LMP), duration is 279–282 days.

Delivery date also can be estimated by adding 7 days to the first day of the LMP, counting back 3 months and adding 1 yr. Less accurate than above.

Uterine size also can be used: above pubic symphysis at 12 weeks after LMP; at 16 weeks it is midway between the pubic symphysis and umbilicus; at 20 weeks it reaches the umbilicus, and by 26 weeks it reaches the xiphoid process.

Ultrasound is most accurate when performed in first half of pregnancy. Gestational age is determined by measuring fetal parameters.

Nutrition

♦ **Weight Gain.** Ideal weight gain is described in Table 44.3. Weight gain should be minimal during 1st trimester (2–4 lb), and thereafter, ≈1 lb/week. An additional 300 kcal/day will be needed during the last 2 trimesters and protein requirements increase from 0.9–1.3 gm/kg. Vitamin and mineral requirements are summarized in Table 43.4.

Morning Sickness

♦ 70% of pregnant women complain of nausea and vomiting by 4–8 weeks of gestation; in most cases, this disappears by 14–16 weeks gestation.

♦ 50% of women have mild complaints that can be treated with psychological support and diet (light snack before arising; small, frequent carbohydrate-rich meals; sipping fluids; and avoiding foods or smells that evoke nausea). The other half have moderate symptoms that must be treated (Table 43.5). Medications to treat nausea and vomiting that have been studied in pregnancy include the phenothiazines, antihistamines, and promotility drugs. Most antiemetics are in pregnancy category B or C (Table 43.6).

Diabetes Mellitus During Pregnancy
Pre-Existing Diabetes Mellitus

♦ **Risks of uncontrolled diabetes** include an increased incidence of perinatal mortality, congenital defects, prematurity, macrosomia (birth weight >10 lb), dystocia (difficult delivery), and maternal morbidity and mortality (ketoacidosis, hypertension, microvascular complications, UTIs, hydramnios).

♦ **Goals.** Attempt to achieve euglycemia (Hgb A_{1c}, 7%–8% and mean glucose concentration <110 mg/dL) *before* conception and throughout pregnancy.

♦ **Treatment.** Use multiple daily doses of insulin. See Chapter 47, Diabetes Mellitus for details. Watch for hypoglycemia and starvation ketosis, especially during 1st trimester when nausea and vomiting are most prevalent. Fluctuations in insulin doses occur during labor and delivery. During this period, use glucose and insulin infusions.

Gestational Diabetes Mellitus (GDM)

♦ **Definition.** GDM is carbohydrate intolerance which develops during pregnancy, usually 3rd trimester. It occurs in 2%–3% of pregnancies, but it is estimated that many cases go undetected. All women should be screened between weeks 24 and 28 of pregnancy. Approximately 35%–50% of women with GDM develop diabetes mellitus within 15 yr of delivery.

♦ **Treatment.** Most patients respond to diet; others will require insulin (fasting plasma glucose >105 mg/dL and 2-hr postprandial >120 mg/dL). Oral hypoglycemic agents are potentially teratogenic and should not be used.

Thyroid Dysfunction During Pregnancy
Hyperthyroidism

♦ Signs and symptoms, diagnosis, and treatment of hyperthyroidism during pregnancy are covered in Chapter 46: Thyroid Disorders. Important points to consider follow.

♦ Thyroid-binding globulin (TBG) is increased during pregnancy, and this alters thyroid function tests. Free T_4 (FT_4), free T_3 (FT_3), and the free thyroxine index (FTI) are best indicators of thyroid function.

♦ **Thioamides** are treatment of choice, although surgery during 2nd trimester is an alternative. Radioactive iodine (RAI) is contraindicated. *Propylthiouracil (PTU)* is less teratogenic than methimazole and is considered by some the drug of choice.

♦ In cases of thyrotoxicosis, use propranolol and iodides on a short-term basis only, since both are associated with adverse fetal effects.

Hypothyroidism

Signs and symptoms, diagnosis, and treatment of hypothyroidism are covered in Chapter 46: Thyroid Disorders. Elevated TSH is the most reliable test, although FT_4, FT_3, and FTI can be used. Treat with thyroxine.

EPILEPSY AND PREGNANCY

♦ Management of seizures is covered in Chapter 51: Seizure Disorders. Points of particular importance in the management of a pregnant patient follow.

♦ *Seizure frequency* may increase during pregnancy, but noncompliance must be considered as a cause. Maternal seizures increase the risk of fetal hypoxia.

♦ *Phenytoin* used alone or with other anticonvulsants is associated with a 2–3 times higher incidence of fetal malformations (fetal hydantoin syndrome) than the general population. (See Chapter 51: Seizure Disorders and Chapter 44: Teratogenicity and Drugs in Breast Milk.) *Carbamazepine* (Tegretol) may be drug of choice for tonic-clonic seizures because of lower teratogenic risk. Therapeutic serum concentrations for phenytoin may be lower during pregnancy due to protein-binding alterations (i.e., free concentrations remain the same).

♦ *Folic acid supplements* are recommended for pregnant women taking anticonvulsants because folic acid deficiency may be correlated with fetal malformations and there is little risk associated with supplementation.

♦ *Vitamin K (phytonadione),* 1 mg IM, is recommended after birth for all infants of mothers taking phenytoin or phenobarbital because these agents are associated with hemorrhagic disease of the newborn. Observe infant for bleeding for 24–48 hr.

HYPERTENSION DURING PREGNANCY

♦ One of the major causes of maternal and fetal morbidity and mortality. Occurs in up to 10% of all pregnancies. Many are primigravida >35 yr old and teenagers.

♦ Systolic and diastolic BP decline during first 2 trimesters. A nadir of 15–20 mm Hg in SBP below prepregnancy levels may occur in 2nd trimester. Therefore, upper limit of normal is 130/80 anytime during pregnancy.

♦ *Definitions and Diagnostic Criteria.* See Tables 43.7 and 43.8.

♦ *Treatment.* See Table 43.9.

ISOIMMUNIZATION

Hemolytic disease of the newborn (HDN) can occur if the mother (exposed during pregnancy to a fetal blood group antigen she does not possess) produces IgG antibody to that antigen. IgG crosses the placenta to affect the fetus. There are over 100 blood group antigens of which the ABO and Rh systems are only two.

ABO Incompatibility

♦ *Incidence.* Occurs in 20%–25% of all pregnancies, but HDN presents clinically in 10% of fetuses.

♦ Occurs when a Blood Type O mother carries a blood type A or B baby. Mothers who are Type A or B predominantly produce IgM.

♦ *Clinical Presentation.* ABO incompatibility in the newborn presents as jaundice, hyperbilirubinemia, and hemolytic anemia. About 10% of infants require photo-therapy.

Rh Incompatibility

♦ The HDN associated with Rh incompatibility (erythroblastosis fetalis) is much more severe and is dependent on amount of antibody fetus exposed to *in utero.* Hemolysis, anemia, hyperbilirubinemia, and erythropoietic hyperplasia occur. The extreme form (anemia, anasarca, hepatosplenomegaly, heart failure, and circulatory collapse) is called hydrops fetalis.

♦ Severity of Rh-associated HDN increases with each pregnancy.

♦ **Frequency.** The chance that an Rh-negative woman will deliver an Rh-positive infant is 10% (white), 5% (black), and 1% (Asian). The probability of isoimmunization is 16%.

♦ **Prevention.** Maternal isoimmunization can be prevented by administration of RhoD immune globulin (Rho GAM, Gamulin Rh, HypRho-D) before or shortly after exposure to fetal Rh-positive RBCs. (See Tables 43.10 and 43.11.) Monitor Rh-negative mother for ABO and Rh status (indirect Coombs') at beginning of each pregnancy, at 28 weeks, 35 weeks, and postpartum.

Preterm Labor

♦ **Definition.** Labor that begins before 37 weeks gestation. Occurs in 5%-15% of pregnancies.

♦ **Etiology.** See Table 43.12.

♦ **Symptoms.** Painful uterine contractions, cramps, low back pain, vaginal spotting, increased vaginal discharge and/or pelvic pressure before 37 weeks gestation.

♦ **Diagnosis.** Persistent contractions (e.g., Q 5–8 min of at least 30 sec duration) and a dilated cervix of >2 cm, a change of >1 cm, or a positive fibronectin test are necessary to diagnose preterm labor. Using regular uterine contractions alone to diagnose preterm labor can be misleading.

♦ **Treatment** of spontaneous preterm labor is aimed toward preventing or prolonging delivery to try and improve neonatal outcomes. Prolonging pregnancy for just one week can decrease neonatal morbidity and mortality by up to 15%. Evaluate gestational age and fetal lung maturation to determine if delaying delivery will benefit fetus. Based on results of evaluations, management will be either expectant (i.e., no intervention, wait for spontaneous delivery) or active intervention (corticosteroids for fetal lung maturation and tocolytic agents to stop or prolong labor). Tocolytic agents include: magnesium sulfate, betamimetics, calcium channel blockers, ethanol, indomethacin, and other prostaglandin synthetase inhibitors.

   • *Magnesium sulfate* is the most frequently used parenteral tocolytic agent. It relaxes uterine smooth muscle, decreases myometrial contractility, and is effective in stopping contractions for 48–72 hrs in about 60–80% of women without premature rupture of the membranes. $MgSO_4$ 6 gm IV loading dose for 30 minutes followed by 2 gm/hr continuous IV infusion through a controlled infusion pump is a common regimen. The hourly rate can be increased by 1 gm/hr until the patient has <1 contraction/10 min or a maximum of 4 gm/hr is achieved. Deep tendon reflexes and respiratory rate should be monitored hourly and urine output measured every 2–4 hrs.

   • *β-adrenergic agonists* (e.g., terbutaline PO, IV, SQ) inhibit uterine smooth muscle contractility and are considered second-line agents for tocolysis because of high incidence of adverse effects.

♦ *Adverse Effects of Betamimetic Therapy*

Cardiovascular. Dose-related fetal and maternal tachyarrhythmias (80), maternal hypotension, MI.

Hyperglycemia occurs in first 24–48 hr and then generally resolves. Increased insulin doses may be needed.

Hypokalemia may develop in a few hours and then return to normal 10–20 hr after beta agonist therapy is discontinued. Due to intracellular shift of Na^+.

Pulmonary edema has become widespread with >80 cases and 14 maternal deaths. May be due to infection, increased cardiac demands of pregnancy, pre-existing cardiac disease, fluid overload, increased pulmonary capillary pressure, or decreased osmotic pressure. Therapy includes O_2, fluid restriction, stopping betamimetics, diuretics.

Other. Tremor, nausea, vomiting, erythema, and headaches (10%–15%).

Fetal Effects. Hypoglycemia, tachycardia, hypocalcemia, hypotension.

LABOR INDUCTION
Indications

Indications for labor induction are summarized in Table 43.13. If induced before 32 weeks, benefit of early delivery must outweigh risks to mother and unborn child.

Prostaglandin E₂ (PGE₂)

♦ *Action.* Ripens (dilates) cervix and may induce labor. Effectiveness: 50% go into labor; 25% require no oxytocin.

♦ *Administration.* Apply 0.5 mg (0.25–1 mg) Prepidil gel intracervically 4–24 hr (average 12 hr) before oxytocin. Repeat Q 6 hr PRN. Cervidil vaginal inserts release 0.3 mg/hr over a 12-hr period. The insert is contained within a pouch attached to a long string which can remove the insert at the beginning of active labor. Maintain bedrest. Monitor uterine contractions, fetal heart rate, and cervical ripening.

♦ *Commercial Products.* Prepidil (Upjohn) (dinoprostone 0.5 mg/2.5 mL gel to be administered endocervically. Cervidil (dinoprostone 10 mg for vaginal insertion).

♦ *Adverse Effects.* Uterine hyperstimulation (0.6%–6%), vulvar edema, and rarely, nausea, vomiting, fever, pyrexia, shivering.

Oxytocin

♦ *Action.* Stimulates uterine contractions. Response increases throughout pregnancy but becomes significant after week 30.

♦ *Administration.* Add 10 units to 1 L solution (10 mU/mL). Administer 0.5–2 mU/min. Increase by 1–2 mU/min Q 15–30 min until desired contraction pattern is achieved (usually occurs 20–60 min after starting IV therapy with doses of 2–8 mU/min). Doses >20 mU/min are rarely required. Discontinue if adequate uterine contractions do not result in satisfactory progress. Regimens are listed in Table 43.14.

♦ *Adverse Effects.* Uterine hypercontractility resulting in hemorrhage, uterine rupture, vaginal/cervical lacerations, abruptio placentae, and fetal distress.

♦ *Contraindications.* Multiple gestations, major vaginal bleeding, disproportional pelvis, unfavorable fetal presentation, uterine infection, preeclampsia, eclampsia, fetal distress.

POSTPARTUM HEMORRHAGE

♦ *General Measures.* Uterine massage or compression, blood products, surgery.

♦ *Oxytocin.* Infuse 20–40 mU/min or give 10 units IM after delivery of infant and placenta to control hemorrhage. Drug of choice.

♦ *Ergonovine Maleate (Ergotrate Maleate) or Methylergonovine Maleate (Methergine).* IM is preferred route because IV is associated with vomiting, hypertension, headaches, and cramping. Give 0.2 mg IV or IM and repeat Q 2–4 hr as necessary. Ergonovine tablets PO or SL, 0.2–0.4 mg BID or QID or methylergonovine tablets 0.2 mg TID or QID can promote involution of an atonic uterus. Many prefer carboprost tromethamine (Hemabate) to ergots when patients are unresponsive to oxytocin because of CV effects from ergot alkaloids.

Lactation

Stimulation and suppression of lactation are most often managed without drugs. Suckling stimulates lactation. For suppression, avoid breast stimulation, use binders, and restrict fluids to decrease milk production. Occasionally drugs are required.

Stimulation

+ **Metoclopramide (Reglan) and chlorpromazine (Thorazine),** although not approved for lactation induction, stimulate prolactin and have been used. Metoclopramide 10 mg TID × 1–2 weeks is effective but is of concern because of potential for adverse CNS effects in infants.

Suppression

+ The only drug therapy recommended by the FDA are analgesics for relief of breast pain. Bromocriptine is no longer used because of cardiovascular complications. Ice packs provide some symptom relief.

Table 43.1 • Diagnosis of Pregnancy

Presumptive Evidence
Absence of an expected menstrual period
Breast changes (tenderness and enlargement)
Discoloration of vaginal mucosa (Chadwick's sign)
Nausea and/or vomiting ("morning sickness")
↑ in urinary frequency
Perception of fetal movement
Fatigue
Changes in skin pigmentation

Probable Evidence
Enlargement of abdomen
Changes in the size, shape, and consistency of the uterus (Hegar's sign)
Cervical changes
Braxton-Hicks contractions
Palpation of the fetus
Endocrine tests

Positive Evidence
Identification of fetal heart sounds
Perception of active fetal movements by examiner
Recognition of the embryo or fetus by sonography or roentgenography

From reference 9.

Notes:

Table 43.2 • Danger Signs of Pregnancy

Vaginal spotting or bleeding	Oliguria
Leakage of fluid from vagina	Persistent vomiting
Abdominal pain or cramping	Chills or fever
Severe or continuous headaches	Dysuria
Change in vision	Marked changes in the intensity or frequency of fetal movement
Swelling of the fingers or face	

From references 8 and 9.

Table 43.3 • Recommended Weight Gain During Pregnancy

Prepregnancy Weight for Height (BMI)	Total Weight Gain Recommendations (lbs)
Low: <19.8	28–40
Normal: 19.8–26	25–35
High: 26.1–29	15–25
Obese: >29	≥15

BMI, body mass index = weight/height^2 (kg/m^2).
From reference 19.

Table 43.4 • Mineral and Vitamin Requirements During Pregnancy

Nutrient	Dose	Comment
Iron	30 mg elemental Fe/day during 2nd and 3rd trimester or last half of pregnancy. ↑ to 60–100 mg/day if patient is anemic or has a history of multiple pregnancies.	Iron is needed for placenta and fetus and to accommodate 20%–30% ↑ in maternal RBC volume. Advise patient of black stools. Watch for GI upset and constipation.
Folic acid	0.5–1 mg/day during last half of pregnancy is dose most commonly prescribed even though a dose of 400 µg/day to supplement diet is probably sufficient. RDA during pregnancy is 400 µg/day.	Additional FA is needed to accommodate ↑ RBC volume. Supplements definitely required for women with hemolysis, a history of multiple pregnancies, those taking anticonvulsants, and those with an inadequate dietary intake of FA.
Calcium	RDA is 1200 mg/day (≈1 quart of milk). Provide supplements during 3rd trimester for women who don't consume dairy products.	Needed for fetal teeth and bone. Maternal calcium stores greatly exceed requirements during pregnancy. For most women, supplements are optional.

Notes:

Table 43.5 • Drugs Used to Treat Morning Sickness

Drug	Dose	Comment
Meclizine (Antivert)	25–50 mg/day PO	Considered drug of choice because of low teratogenic risk
Dimenhydrinate (Dramamine)	50–100 mg Q 4 hr PO *or* 50 mg Q 3–4 hr IM	Low teratogenic risk
Metoclopramide (Reglan)	5–10 mg TID PO *or* 5–20 mg TID IV or IM	Teratogenic risk appears low, but poorly studied
Pyridoxine	50 mg/day	Ineffective
Phenothiazines		
Promethazine (Phenergan)	12.5–25 mg TID PO or IM	Teratogenic potential is inconclusive
Thiethylperazine (Torecan)	10–20 mg QD–TID PO or IM	Reserved for women unresponsive to other agents
Prochlorperazine (Compazine)	5–10 mg TID–QID PO or IM	Reserved for women unresponsive to other agents

Table 43.6 • Pregnancy Categories for Gastrointestinal Medications

Drug	Pregnancy Category
Cimetidine	B
Dimenhydrinate	B
Famotidine	B
Granisetron	B
Lansoprazole	B
Meclizine	B
Metoclopramide	B
Misoprostol	X
Nizatidine	C
Omeprazole	C
Ondansetron	B
Prochlorperazine	C
Promethazine	C
Ranitidine	B
Sucralfate	B
Trimethobenzamide	C

Category A: Controlled studies in women fail to demonstrate risk to the fetus.
Category B: Either animal studies have not demonstrated a risk and there are no controlled studies in women, or animal studies have shown a risk that has not been confirmed in humans.
Category C: Either studies in animals have shown an adverse effect on the fetus and there are no controlled studies in women, or no studies in women or animals are available.
Category D: There is evidence of fetal harm, but the benefit of the medication may outweigh the risk.
Category X: There is evidence of fetal harm and no benefit of the medication outweighs the risk.
From reference 41.

Table 43.7 • Hypertension During Pregnancy: Definition and Diagnostic Criteria[a]

Note: Measure BP on at least 2 separate occasions, at least 6 hr apart

Hypertension	>130/80 mm Hg anytime during pregnancy, but particularly in the first 2 trimesters: >140/90 during the latter part of pregnancy
	An ↑ prepregnancy baseline of >30 mm Hg systolic or >15 mm Hg anytime during pregnancy
Chronic hypertension	HBP occurring before conception or before 20th week of pregnancy
Preeclampsia	HBP with proteinuria (1 + dipstick; >300 mg/24 hr collection), edema, or both that occur after week 20
Preeclampsia superimposed on chronic HTN	Chronic hypertension with symptoms of preeclampsia above
HELLP	A preeclampsia variant accompanied by hemolytic anemia, elevated liver enzymes, and thrombocytopenia
Eclampsia	Convulsions or seizures that occur in a patient with preeclampsia
Transient HTN	Development of HBP during pregnancy or in the first 24 hr postpartum without signs or symptoms of preeclampsia in women without preexisting hypertension

[a]BP = Blood pressure; HBP = High blood pressure; HELLP = Hemolysis, elevated liver enzymes, and low platelet (count); HTN = Hypertension.

Table 43.8 • Omnious Signs and Symptoms Associated with Preeclampsia[a]

BP ≥110 mm Hg diastolic or ≥160 mm Hg systolic

Proteinuria ≥2 gm in 24 hr (2+ or 3+ upon qualitative examination)

SrCr >1.2 mg/dL (unless previously elevated)

Elevated liver enzyme tests

Platelet count <100,000/mm³

Headache or other visual or cerebral disturbances

Epigastric pain

Retinal hemorrhage, exudate, or papilledema

Pulmonary edema

[a]BP = Blood pressure; SrCr = Serum creatinine.

Notes:

Table 43.9 • Treatment of Hypertension During Pregnancy

Mild Preeclampsia (e.g., BP 140/95 mm Hg with no symptoms)
Bedrest
Relaxation techniques, limitation of activity, and reassurance
Home BP monitoring and urine dipstick measurements for proteinuria
Recording of fetal activity
Report CNS problems or epigastric pain
Have prenatal visits at least 2 times a week
Platelet counts and LFTs 2 times a week
Normal diet
Na^+ restriction is not useful

Moderate Preeclampsia
(e.g., BP >160/100 mm Hg with no symptoms or mild symptoms [e.g., edema])
Bedrest, hospitalization, and normal diet *plus* antihypertensives

Methyldopa (Aldomet)
   Dose: 250 mg TID–QID up to 2–3 gm
   Comment: Most commonly used because it is safe and effective. Lethargy and drowsiness, the most
      common adverse effects, subside in 4–5 days

Labetalol (Normodyne, Trandate)
   Dose: 100 mg TID–QID up to 1200 mg
   Comment: Advantages include ↑ uteroplacental blood flow, ↑ fetal lung surfactant production, and
      ↓ platelet consumption during preeclampsia. Crosses placenta, but fetal malformations have not
      been reported; bradycardia and hypotension have occurred. Adverse effects include headache,
      dizziness, myalgia, lassitude, and tremors

Beta Blockers: Atenolol (Tenormin), metoprolol (Lopressor), pindolol (Visken), propranolol (Inderal)
   Dose: See Chapter 11: Essential Hypertension
   Comment: This class does not appear to be associated with fetal malformations, but adverse effects
      to both mother and fetus are most commonly associated with propranolol, particularly doses
      >160 mg/day. This may reflect its more extensive use

Clonidine
   Comment: Limited experience in pregnancy. Category C teratogen. See Chapter 44: Teratogenicity
      and Drugs in Breast Milk

Calcium Channel Blockers
   Comment: Seems to lower maternal BP and uterine artery perfusion pressure, but does not appear
      to reduce uteroplacental blood flow. No effects on fetal heart rate, and thrombocytopenia seems to
      resolve in mothers. However, neuromuscular blockade and significant falls in maternal BP have
      been noted in patients also on $MgSO_4$. Controlled trials are needed

ACE Inhibitors
   Comment: May result in fetal renal effects, pulmonary hypoplasia, and possible growth retardation.
      Not recommended for use in pregnancy

Diuretics
   Comment: Not recommended because intravascular volume may ↓. This could ↓ uteroplacental
      blood flow

Severe Preeclampsia
(>160/110 with symptoms while patient is at bedrest. See Table 43.8)
↓ BP gradually to maintain uteroplacental blood flow

$MgSO_4$: Used to prevent and treat seizures
   Dose: No symptoms of cerebral edema: 10 gm IM, then 5 gm Q 4 hr in alternating buttocks.
      Cerebral edema (headaches, visual disturbances, scotoma, altered consciousness): 4 gm IV fol-
      lowed by 5 gm IM Q 4 hr or infusion of 1–3 mg/hr
   Comment: Anticonvulsant range is 4–7 mEq/L. Before each dose, evaluate patient for Mg toxicity:
      ↓ patellar reflex, ↓ respiratory rate, hypocalcemic tetany. Make sure urine output is >100 mL/hr.
      Neonatal toxicity (respiratory depression, hyporeflexia) unusual if Mg concentrations are in thera-
      peutic range and if route of administration is IM. Calcium can be given for Mg overdose or for
      concentrations in the toxic range (>12 mEq/L). Use with antihypertensives

(continued)

Table 43.9 • Treatment of Hypertension During Pregnancy (continued)

Hydralazine (Apresoline)
> *Dose:* May be administered IV (onset 20–30 min) or IM (onset 30–40 min). Typical dose is 5 mg IV slowly, then 5–10 mg Q 20–30 min until diastolic is 90–100 min Hg. Administer additional doses for diastolic >110 mm Hg
>
> *Comment:* Most commonly used because of its long history of safety. Avoid hypotension, which can compromise uteroplacental blood flow. Common adverse effects include nausea, vomiting, tachycardia, flushing, headache, and tremors

Labetalol
> *Dose:* 0.25 mg/kg up to 20 mg IV, followed by 40–80 mg IV Q 10–20 min to a total of 300 mg or until the BP is controlled. IV infusion of 1–2 mg/min also has been recommended
>
> *Comment:* Considered an alternative agent but may be as effective as hydralazine with fewer adverse effects

---

Table 43.10 • Indications for Prophylactic Administration of Rh₀(D) Immune Globulin in the Rh D–Negative Pregnant Woman Who Is Not Rh D Alloimmunized[a]

Should Definitely Be Given[b,c]:
Antepartum at about 28 weeks' gestation
Postpartum within 72 hours of delivery if newborn Rh D positive, weak D positive, or unknown
After spontaneous or elective abortion
After invasive procedures: amniocentesis, chorionic villus sampling, fetal blood sampling

Should Be Considered[b,c]:
Threatened abortion
Second or third trimester bleeding
Abdominal trauma

[a] Prophylaxis unnecessary if father known to be Rh D negative.
[b] First trimester events and procedures: give Rh₀ (D) immune globulin 50 μg.
[c] Second and third trimester events and procedures: give Rh₀ (D) immune globulin 300 μg.
From reference 49.

Notes:

Table 43.11 • Recommendations for the Administration of Rh$_o$ Immune Globulin to an Rh-Negative Female

Antepartum
Maternal Antibody Screen Negative Weeks 1–28

Father is Rh-positive
or
Paternal status unknown
↓
Rh$_o$(D) immune globulin 300 µg should be administered at 28–32 weeks; ↓ incidence of isoimmunization from 1%–2% to 0.1%

Father is Rh-negative
↓
Rh$_o$(D) immune globulin not indicated

Maternal Antibody Status: Positive Anytime During Pregnancy
Manage as if Rh sensitized

Postpartum
Maternal and Cord Blood Antibody Screen Negative

Infant status known:

Infant Rh-positive or Du-positive
↓
Give mother 300 µg Rh$_o$(D) immune globulin within 72 hours of delivery; isoimmunization may be prevented if administered within 28 days after exposure

Father is Rh-negative or Du-negative
↓
No Rh$_o$(D) immune globulin

Infant's Rh status unknown within 72 hours postpartum and:

Father is Rh-positive, Du-positive, or status unknown
↓
Give mother 300 µgRh$_o$(D) immune globulin

Table 43.12 • Etiologies for Preterm Labor[a]

PROM	Fetal death
Infection of amniotic fluid	Cervical incompetency
Previous preterm delivery or late abortion	Uterine anomalies
Faulty placentation (e.g., abruptio placentae and placenta previa)	Maternal disease
	Retained IUD
Overdistended uterus (e.g., hydramnios)	Elective induction of labor too early in gestation
Multifetal gestation	Unknown causes

[a]IUD = Intrauterine device; PROM = Premature rupture of the membranes.

Table 43.13 • Indications for Labor Induction[a]

Maternal	Fetal
Pregnancy-associated hypertensive diseases	IUGR
Diabetes mellitus	Macrosomia
Renal disease	Rh immunization
PROM	Chorioamnionitis
COAD	Oligohydramnios
Logistical problems (i.e., distance from hospital, risk of rapid labor)	Fetal death

[a]COAD = Chronic obstructive airways disease; IUGR = Intrauterine growth retardation; PROM = Premature rupture of the membranes.

Table 43.14 • Oxytocin Regimens for Induction and Augmentation of Labor

Regimen	Starting Dose	Incremental Increase	Dosage Interval	Maximum Dose	Reference
Low-dose	1 mU/min	1 mU/min up to 8 U/min, then 2 mU/min	20 min	20 mU/min	156
High-dose	6 mU/min	6 mU/min[a]	20 or 40 min	42 mU/min	155
	4 mU/min	4 mU/min	15 min	Until adequate contractility reached	157

[a]Uterine hyperstimulation: Reduce incremental increase to 3 mU/min; recurrent hyperstimulation: Reduce to 1 mU/min.

The reader is referred to Chapter 44: Obstetrics, written by *Fotini K. Hatzopoulos, Pharm.D., Rosalie Sagraves, Pharm.D.,* and *Jennifer Mitchell, Pharm.D.,* in the seventh edition of **Applied Therapeutics: The Clinical Use of Drugs** for a more in-depth discussion. All notations to reference numbers are based on the reference list at the end of that chapter. The editors of this handbook express their thanks to Drs. Hatzopoulos, Sagraves, and Mitchell and acknowledge that this chapter is based upon their work.

Chapter 44

Teratogenicity and Drugs in Breast Milk

Teratogenicity

♦ The safe use of a drug in a single pregnancy or even in a large number of pregnancies does not assure that the drug is safe in all pregnancies. Most maternal chemical exposures (i.e., fetal exposures) do not result in noticeable birth defects, and the present state of knowledge does not allow prediction with any degree of certainty when a particular drug will prove teratogenic to a particular fetus. Only relative risks can be described for a specific population, not specific risks for specific patients. Animal studies, while beneficial in determining the relative toxicity of an agent, usually cannot be extrapolated directly to humans. Only in a few cases has a consensus been reached that a specific agent is teratogenic. Table 44.1 lists those agents generally considered to be proven human teratogens.

♦ Taken in total, environmental chemicals and drugs may cause up to 6% of all congenital malformations.

♦ **FDA Categories.** The FDA has prepared guidelines by which drugs can be categorized according to their teratogenic risk (see Table 44.2).

♦ **Contraindicated Drugs.** Although numerous drugs have been associated with congenital anomalies, only in a few cases has a consensus been reached that a specific drug is contraindicated during pregnancy (Table 44.3).

♦ Drugs that should be used with caution during pregnancy are listed in Table 44.4. This list is not all-inclusive.

Fetal Syndromes

♦ **Fetal Alcohol Syndrome.** See Table 44.5.

♦ **Fetal Hydantoin Syndrome.** The signs and symptoms of fetal hydantoin syndrome as well as other adverse fetal effects of phenytoin are listed in Table 44.6.

♦ **Fetal Warfarin Syndrome.** See Table 44.7.

♦ **Fetal Trimethadione Syndrome.** See Table 44.8.

Drug Excretion in Breast Milk

♦ **Factors Affecting Excretion.** The passage of drugs into breast milk is a major concern of clinicians. Numerous factors affect the excretion of a drug into breast milk (see Table 44.9).

♦ Suggestions for reducing the risk of infants to the effects of drugs in breast milk are contained in Table 44.10.

♦ **Selected drugs contraindicated during breast feeding** are listed in Table 44.11.

♦ **The effects of selected drugs on the nursing infant** are described in Table 44.12.

♦ Herbs that should be avoided or used with caution during lactation are listed in Table 44.13.

Glossary

Aneuploidy: Any deviation from an exact multiple of the haploid number of chromosomes, whether few or more; individuals exhibiting aneuploidy are usually abnormal physiologically and morphologically.

Angioma: A tumor whose cells tend to form in blood or lymph vessels.

Aplasia cutis: Localized failure of development of skin, most commonly of the scalp, less frequently of the trunk and limbs; the defects are usually covered by a thin translucent membrane or scar tissue, or may be raw, ulcerated, or covered by granulation tissue.

Arthrogryposis: Persistent flexure or contracture of a joint.

Bifid xiphoid: Cleft of the xiphoid process into two parts.

Blastula: The usually spherical structure produced by cleavage of a fertilized ovum, consisting of a single layer of cells (blastoderm) surrounding a fluid-filled cavity (blastocele).

Blepharophimosis: Abnormal narrowness of the palpebral fissure in the horizontal direction, caused by lateral displacement of the inner canthi.

Brachycephaly: The fact or quality of having a short head, with a cephalic index of 81.0 to 85.4.

Calvaria hypoplasia: Failure of the domelike superior portion of the cranium to form.

Choanal atresia: Congenital bony or membranous occlusion of one or both choanae caused by failure of the embryonic bucconasal membrane to rupture.

Coloboma: An apparent absence or defect of some ocular tissue, usually resulting from a failure of a part of the fetal fissure to close.

Chorioretinitis: Inflammation of the choroid and retina.

Coronal: Pertaining to the crown of the head.

Corpus callosum: An arched mass of white matter found in the depths of the longitudinal fissure, composed of transverse fibers connecting the cerebral hemispheres.

Cryptorchidism: A developmental defect characterized by failure of the testes to descend into the scrotum.

Cutis laxa: A congenital hereditary disorder in which the skin and subcutaneous tissues hypertrophy, the skin hanging in folds as a result.

Dandy-Walker malformation: Congenital hydrocephalus caused by obstruction of the foramina of Magendie and Luschka.

Dermatoglyphics: The study of the patterns of ridges of the skin of the fingers, palms, toes, and soles; may be a clinical and genetic indicator, particularly of chromosomal abnormalities.

Diastasis recti: Separation of the rectus muscles of the abdominal wall.

Diplegia: Paralysis affecting like parts on both sides of the body; bilateral paralysis.

Ebstein's anomaly: A malfunction of the tricuspid valve, the septal and posterior leaflets being attached to the wall of the right ventricle to a varying degree, and the anterior leaflet being normally attached to the annulus fibrosis.

Ectromelia: Gross hypoplasia or aplasia of one or more long bones of one or more limbs; the term includes amelia, hemimelia, and phocomelia.

Encephalocele: Hernia of the brain, manifested by protrusion of brain substance through a congenital or traumatic opening of the skull.

Epicanthal folds: See Epicanthus.

Epicanthus: A vertical fold of skin on either side of the nose, sometimes covering the inner canthus; it is present as a normal characteristic in persons of certain races and sometimes occurs as a congenital anomaly in others.

Epididymal cyst: A cyst of the elongated cordlike structure along the posterior border of the testis, in the ducts of which the spermatozoa are stored.

Epispadias: A congenital defect in which the urethra opens on the dorsum of the penis.

Exencephaly: A developmental anomaly characterized by an imperfect cranium, the brain lying outside of the skull.

Hamartoblastoma: A tumor developing from a hamartoma.

Hamartoma: A benign tumorlike nodule composed of an overgrowth of mature cells and tissues that normally occur in the affected part, but often with one element predominating.

Hemangioma: A benign tumor made up of newly formed blood vessels.

Hydrocele: A collection of fluid in the tunica vaginalis of the testicle or along the spermatic cord.

Hydrocephalus: A condition characterized by abnormal accumulation of fluid in the cranial vault, accompanied by enlargement of the head, prominence of the forehead, atrophy of the brain, mental deterioration, and convulsions.

Hydronephrosis: Distention of the pelvis and calices of the kidney with urine, as a result of obstruction of the ureter, with accompanying atrophy of the parenchyma of the organ.

Hydrops fetalis: The abnormal accumulation of serous fluid in the entire body of the newborn infant.

Hydroureter: Abnormal distention of the ureter with urine or with a watery fluid.

Hypertrichosis lanuginosa: Excessive growth of hair on the body of the fetus.

Hypognathia: Having a protruding lower jaw.

Hypospadias: A developmental anomaly in the male in which the urethra opens on the under side of the penis or on the perineum.

Imperforate anus: Abnormally closed anus.

IUGR: Intrauterine growth retardation.

Klippel-Feil anomaly: A condition characterized by shortness of the neck resulting from reduction in the number of cervical vertebrae or the fusion of multiple hemivertebrae into one osseous mass; the hairline is low and motion of the neck is limited.

Macrosomia: Greatly increased body size.

Meckel's diverticulum: An abnormal appendage of the ileum derived from an unobliterated yolk stalk.

Megacolon: Abnormally large or dilated colon.

Meningoencephalocele: Hernial protrusion of the meninges and brain substance through a defect in the skull.

Meningomyelocele: Hernial protrusion of a part of the meninges and substance of the spinal cord through a defect in the vertebral column.

Microcephaly: Abnormal smallness of the head, usually associated with mental retardation.

Micrognathia: Unusual or undue smallness of the jaws.

Microphallus: Abnormal smallness of the penis.

Microphthalmia: Abnormal smallness of the eyes.

Microtia: Gross hypoplasia or aplasia of the pinna of the ear, with a blind or absent external auditory meatus.

Müllerian duct: Ductus paramesonephricus; either of the paired embryonic ducts arising as a peritoneal pocket, extending caudally to join the urogenital sinus, and developing into uterine tubes and uterus.

Myelomeningocele: Hernial protrusion of the spinal cord and its meninges through a defect in the vertebral canal.

Myeloschisis: A developmental anomaly characterized by a cleft spinal cord, owing to failure of the neural plate to form a complete tube.

Myoclonia: Any disorder characterized by myoclonus.

Myoclonus: Shocklike contractions of a muscle.

Myotomes: The muscle plate or portion of a somite that develops into voluntary muscle.

Neuropore: The open anterior end or the posterior end of the neural tube of the early embryo; openings gradually close as the tube develops.

Nevus: A circumscribed stable malformation of the skin and occasionally of the oral mucosa, which is not due to external causes; excess (or deficient) tissue may involve epidermal, connective tissue, adnexal, nervous, or bascular elements.

Ocular hypertelorism: Abnormal increase in the interorbital distance.

Oligodactyly: A developmental anomaly characterized by a smaller-than-usual number of fingers or toes.

Oligohydramnios: Characterized by <300 mL of amniotic fluid at term.

Omphalocele: Protrusion, at birth, of part of the intestine through a large defect in the abdominal wall at the umbilicus, the protruding bowel being covered only by a thin transparent membrane composed of amnion and peritoneum.

Oxycephaly: A condition in which the top of the head is pointed.

Palpebral fissures: The longitudinal opening between the eyelids.

Pectus carinatum: Undue prominence of the sternum; also called chicken or pigeon breast.

Pectus excavatum: Undue depression of the sternum; also called funnel breast or chest.

Philtrum: The vertical groove in the median portion of the upper lip, a part of the prolabium.

Phimosis: Tightness of the foreskin, so that it cannot be drawn back from over the glans; also the analogous condition in the clitoris.

Phocomelia: A developmental anomaly characterized by absence of the proximal portion of a limb or limbs, the hands or feet being attached to the trunk of the body by a single small, irregularly shaped bone.

Pierre Robin syndrome: Micrognathia in association with cleft palate and glossoptosis, and with absent gag reflex.

Placode: A platelike structure, especially a thickened plate of ectoderm in the early embryo, from which a sense organ develops.

Polydactyly: A developmental anomaly characterized by supernumerary digits (fingers or toes) on the hands or feet.

Polyhydramnios: An excess of amniotic fluid, called also hydramnios.

Potter facies. A facial condition resembling that seen in Potter syndrome (oligohydramnios caused by renal agenesis) and caused by a lack of amniotic fluid and resulting fetal compression.

Prognathia: Having projecting jaws.

Rathke's pouch: A diverticulum from the embryonic buccal cavity, from which the anterior lobe of the pituitary gland is developed.

Retrognathia: Position of the jaws in back of the frontal plane of the forehead.

Rhizomelic dwarfing: A dwarfing pertaining to or involving the hip joint and shoulder joint.

Sacculus: The smaller of the two divisions of the membranous labyrinth of the vestibule, which communicates with the cochlear duct by way of the ductus reuniens.

Scoliosis: An appreciable lateral deviation in the normally straight vertical line of the spine.

Simian crease: A single transverse palmar crease formed by fusion of the proximal and distal palmar creases.

Somite: One of the paired, blocklike masses of mesoderm, arranged segmentally alongside the neural tube of the embryo, forming the vertebral column and segmented musculature.

Spina bifida: A developmental anomaly characterized by defective closure of the bony encasement of the spinal cord through which the cord and meninges may or may not protrude.

Syndactyly: The most common congenital anomaly of the hand, marked by persistence of the webbing between adjacent digits, so they are more or less completely attached.

Synostosis: A union between adjacent bones or parts of a single bone formed by osseous material, such as ossified connecting cartilage or fibrous tissue.

Talipes: A congenital deformity of the foot, which is twisted out of shape or position; also called clubfoot.

Talipes equinovarus: A deformity of the foot in which the heel is turned inward from the midline of the leg and the foot is plantar flexed.

Tetralogy of Fallot: A combination of congenital cardiac defects consisting of pulmonary stenosis, interventricular septal defect, dextroposition of the aorta so that it overrides the interventricular septum and receives venous and arterial blood, and right ventricular hypertrophy.

Utriculus: The larger of the two divisions of the membranous labyrinth, located in the posterosuperior region of the vestibule; the major organ of the vestibular system.

Varicocele: A varicose condition of the veins of the pampiniform plexus, forming a swelling that feels like a "bag of worms," appearing bluish through the skin of the scrotum, and accompanied by a constant pulling, dragging, or dull pain in the scrotum.

Vermilion border: The exposed red portion of the upper or lower lip.

Wolffian duct: Ductus mesonephricus; mesonephric duct, an embryonic duct initiated in association with rudiments of the pronephric kidney, taken over as excretory duct by the mesonephros, developed into various ducts of the reproductive system in the male and into vestigial structures in the female.

Table 44.1 • Drugs Considered Proven Human Teratogens[a]

Aminopterin/methotrexate	Coumarin derivatives	Phenytoin
ACE inhibitors	Diethylstilbestrol	Polychlorinated biphenyls
Antineoplastics	Ethanol (high dose)	Retinoids
Antithyroids	Iodides and radioactive iodine	Tetracycline
Barbiturates	Lithium	Thalidomide
Carbamazepine	Methyl mercury (organic)	Valproic acid
Cocaine	Misoprostol	Vitamin A (>18,000 IU/day)
	Paramethadione/trimethadione	

[a]ACE = Angiotensin-converting enzyme.
From references 17 and 23–25.

Table 44.2 • FDA Categories: Teratogenic Risks of Drugs

Category	Risk Factors
A	Controlled studies in women fail to demonstrate a risk to the fetus in the first trimester (and no evidence indicates a risk in later trimesters), and the possibility of fetal harm appears remote
B	Either animal reproduction studies have not demonstrated a fetal risk (but there are no controlled studies in pregnant women); or animal reproduction studies have shown an adverse effect (other than a decrease in fertility) that was not confirmed in controlled studies in women in the first trimester (and no evidence indicates a risk in later trimesters)
C	Either studies in animals have revealed adverse effects on the fetus (teratogenic, embryocidal, or other) and no controlled studies in women are available; or studies in women and animals are not available. Drugs should be given only if the potential benefit justifies the potential risk to the fetus
D	Evidence of human fetal risk is positive, but the benefits from use in pregnant women may be acceptable despite the risk (e.g., if the drug is needed in a life-threatening situation or for a serious disease for which safer drugs cannot be used or are ineffective)
X	Studies in animals or human beings have demonstrated fetal abnormalities or there is evidence of fetal risk based on human experience or both, and the risk of the drug in pregnant women clearly outweighs any possible benefit. The drug is contraindicated in women who are or may become pregnant

Adapted from reference 26.

Table 44.3 • Drugs Considered Contraindicated During Pregnancy [a,b]

Drug/Drug Class	Fetal/Neonatal Effects
Acitretin	Acitretin is the active metabolite of etretinate. Use of ethanol with acitretin results in conversion of acitretin back to etretinate.[28] See etretinate.
Aminopterin	Structurally similar to MTX. Human teratogen when used as unsuccessful abortifacient in first trimester: meningoencephalocele, cranial anomalies, cleft lip/palate, low-set ears, abnormal positioning of extremities, hypoplasia of thumb and fibula, short forearms, brachycephaly, hydrocephaly, anencephaly, talipes, incomplete skull ossification, hypognathia, and retrognathia.[23,27]
Chenodiol	Contraindicated because of potential for hepatotoxicity.[23]
Clomiphene	Used to induce ovulation. Neural tube defects and other anomalies have been reported, but most studies indicate no association with malformations. Inadvertent use in early pregnancy may have resulted in one infant with a ruptured lumbosacral meningomyelocele, and one infant with esophageal atresia with fistula, congenital heart defect, hypospadias, and absent left kidney.[23,27]
Cocaine	Maternal cocaine abuse associated with in utero cerebrovascular accidents, bowel atresias, and congenital defects of the GU tract, heart, limbs, and face. Other fetal and newborn consequences of maternal abuse are fetal growth retardation, and ↑ morbidity and mortality, including a possible association with SIDS. Maternal complications include shorter gestations, premature delivery, spontaneous abortions, abruptio placentae, and death.[23]
Danazol	Use after the eighth week of gestation (the onset of androgen receptor sensitivity) may result in masculinization of the female fetus (i.e., pseudohermaphroditism); male fetuses usually not affected but one male had multiple anomalies after first trimester exposure.[23,29]
Diethylstilbestrol (DES)	An estimated 6 million pregnant women were exposed to DES from 1940–1971 to treat obstetric problems. Exposure resulted in reproductive system defects in both female and male offspring[23]: *Female:* Lower Müllerian tract: vaginal adenosis; cervical/vaginal fornix defects; cockscomb, collar, pseudopolyp, and hypoplastic cervix; vaginal defects exclusive of fornix; incomplete transverse and/or longitudinal septum. Upper Müllerian tract: uterine structural defects; fallopian tube structural defects *Male:* Altered semen (↓ count, concentration, motility, morphology); epididymal cysts; hypotrophic testis; microphallus; varicocele; capsular induration DES exposure increases risk of developing vaginal and cervical clear cell adenocarcinoma[30]: DES exposure has not been related to defects other than those found in the reproductive system.
Estrogen and related compounds	Contraindicated in pregnancy. A study found an association between estrogen exposure and cardiovascular defects, eye and ear anomalies, and Down syndrome. Further analysis of these data failed to support the association with cardiac malformations. Other studies also have failed in finding association with congenital defects.[23,31,32]
Ethanol	Heavy consumption during pregnancy associated with IUGR and a pattern of anomalies known as the "fetal alcohol syndrome" (see Table 44.5). No known safe levels in pregnancy. Potent fetal brain toxin.[23]
Etretinate	Teratogenic effects reported include meningomyelocele, meningoencephalocele, multiple synostoses, facial dysmorphia, syndactylies, absence of terminal phalanges, malformation of hip, ankle and forearm, low-set ears, high palate, decreased cranial volume, and alterations of the skull and cervical vertebrae.[28] Teratogenic potential can persist for years because of a long half-life of 100 days after prolonged use.[33]

(continued)

Table 44.3 • Drugs Considered Contraindicated During Pregnancy[a,b] (continued)

Drug/Drug Class	Fetal/Neonatal Effects
HMG-CoA reductase inhibitors	One case of first trimester exposure to lovastatin with subsequent birth of an infant with constellation of malformations termed the VATER association (vertebral anomalies, anal atresia, tracheoesophageal fistula with esophageal atresia, and renal and radial dysplasias).[34] An interim evaluation of lovastatin and simvastatin exposure during pregnancy in postmarketing surveillance failed to demonstrate an increased risk of fetal anomalies.[35] A theoretic concern is that the interference of cholesterol biosynthesis by HMG-CoA reductase inhibitors may adversely impact sex steroid biosynthesis.[27]
Isotretinoin	Critical period of exposure is 4–7 wk. Multiple defects involve the CNS, cranium and face, cardiovascular system, thymus gland, and miscellaneous other structures.[23,36]
Leuprolide	Teratogenic in animals; no adverse fetal effects in over 100 cases of human exposure; spontaneous abortions and IUGR may occur because drug suppresses endometrial proliferation.[23]
Lysergic acid diethyl-amide (LSD)	Pure chemical does not cause chromosomal abnormalities, spontaneous abortions, or congenital anomalies. Reported adverse fetal effects in maternal abusers probably caused by multiple factors, including reporting bias.[23]
Menadione	Use near term or close to delivery has resulted in marked hyperbilirubinemia and kernicterus in newborn. If vitamin K needed during pregnancy, use phytonadione (K_1).[23]
Methyl mercury	Organic mercury poisoning has occurred primarily in Japan and Iraq. Known as Minamata disease in Japan. Nonspecific neurologic symptoms after third trimester exposure were observed in about 72 known cases.[3]
Mifepristone	RU 486; antiprogesterone agent used to induce abortion; also used for cervical ripening before abortion and for induction of labor at term; data are too limited to determine whether it is a human teratogen.[23]
Misoprostol	Has abortifacient properties; teratogenic potential has not been determined.[30]
Phencyclidine	Persistent irritability, jitteriness, hypertonicity, and poor feeding reported in newborns.[37]
Ribavirin	Teratogenic and/or embryotoxic in nearly all animal species tested.[30] Human fetal exposure reported in one case with no apparent anomalies at 1 year of age.[38] CDC considers the use of ribavirin during pregnancy contraindicated and recommends alternate job responsibilities for women who are pregnant, or who may become pregnant, if their functions place them in direct contact with patients receiving ribavirin via oxygen tent or mist mask.[39]
Sodium iodide (^{125}I) and (^{131}I)	Administration at 12 weeks' gestation or later will cause partial or complete destruction of fetal thyroid gland; effect is dose dependent with toxic doses 10 mCi.[37]
Thalidomide	Over 12,000 birth defects have been linked to thalidomide use during pregnancy. Critical periods of gestational exposure have been identified[2]: Days 22 to 36: limb defects Days 27 to 30: upper extremity defects Days 30 to 33: upper and lower extremity defects Malformations include amelia, phocomelia, bone hypoplasticity, absence of bones, anotia, micropinna, auditory canal defects, facial palsy, anophthalmos, microphthalmos, congenital heart defects, and GI tract and genital abnormalities.[28]

(continued)

Table 44.3 • Drugs Considered Contraindicated During Pregnancy[a,b] (continued)

Drug/Drug Class	Fetal/Neonatal Effects
Vaccines, live	Most live, attenuated virus vaccines potentially can cause fetal infection. Vaccination with smallpox in first and second trimesters has resulted in fetal death.[23]
Vitamin A (high dose)	Both deficiency and excess are thought to be teratogenic. Prolonged high dosages (>25,000 IU/day) associated with: microtia, craniofacial and CNS anomalies, facial palsy, microphthalmia/anophthalmia, facial clefts, cardiac defects, limb reductions, GI atresia, and urinary tract defects.[23,40,41]

[a]This list is not all-inclusive. Most drugs listed have been designated FDA risk factor X. All drugs of abuse are contraindicated in pregnancy.
[b]A glossary is provided at the beginning of this chapter.
CDC = Centers for Disease Control and Prevention; CNS = Central nervous system; GI = Gastrointestinal; GU = Genitourinary; HMG CoA = Hydroxymethylglutaryl-CoA; IUGR = Intrauterine growth retardation; MTX = Methotrexate; SIDS = Sudden infant death syndrome.

Table 44.4 • Selected Drugs That Should Be Used with Caution During Pregnancy[a,b]

Drug/Drug Class	Risk Factor[c]	Fetal/Neonatal Effects
ACE inhibitors	C/D[d]	Use in second and third trimesters has been associated with a pattern of anomalies called ACEI fetopathy with renal tubular dysplasia as the major malformation. Other reported defects include hypocalvaria, IUGR, patent ductus arteriosus, oligohydramnios, pulmonary hypoplasia, and anuria.[42–45]
Aminoglycosides	C/D[e]	Potential for VIII cranial nerve toxicity with high dosages. Prolonged therapy with kanamycin produced VIII cranial nerve damage; 9 of 391 (2.3%) infants had hearing loss.[4,23] Short-term therapy with streptomycin (1 g/day for 4.5 days) combined with ethacrynic acid resulted in complete hearing loss in both mother and infant.[23]
Amiodarone	D	Complications reported include fetal hypothyroidism, low birth weight, prematurity, bradycardia, and QT prolongation.[46] Because the drug contains 75 mg iodine per 200-mg dose, newborn thyroid status should be closely monitored.[47]
Amitriptyline	D	Limb reduction defects reported, but analysis of 86 first-trimester exposures did not confirm association. Other defects observed in three infants include micrognathia, anomalous right mandible, left talipes equinovarus (1 case), swelling of hands/feet (1 case), and hypospadias (1 case). Urinary retention occurred in one newborn after nortriptyline use.[23]
Angiotensin II–receptor antagonists	C/D[d]	Acts on the renin-angiotensin system; see ACE inhibitors.
Aspirin	C/D[g]	Commonly used in pregnancy either as single agent or in combination products. Most studies do not indicate association with congenital malformations, but prolonged use of high dosages may be teratogenic.[23] Use in early pregnancy in one study associated with twofold increase over nonexposed controls for congenital heart disease (defects in septation of truncus arteriosus).[48] It has been used alone or in combination with β-mimetics to treat premature labor. Low dosages (e.g., 40–150 mg/day) have been used to prevent pregnancy-induced hypertension, pre-eclampsia, and eclampsia. Use near term of full-dose aspirin may prolong gestation and labor; may adversely affect clotting ability of newborn by reducing collagen-induced platelet aggregation and may increase risk in premature or low-birth-weight infants for intracranial hemorrhage.[23]

(continued)

Table 44.4 • Selected Drugs That Should Be Used with Caution During Pregnancy[a,b] (continued)

Drug/Drug Class	Risk Factor[c]	Fetal/Neonatal Effects
Benzodiazepines	D/X[e]	Exposure has been associated with cleft lip/palate, abnormalities of the lung, heart, abdomen, GI tract, musculoskeletal system, and defects in the feet and toes. Other studies reported no association. Neonatal withdrawal from alprazolam and diazepam has been reported.[49–51]
β-Blockers	B/C/D[e]	Reduced birth weight may result from use of some β-blockers in second and third trimesters, but effect also may be due to severe maternal disease. Use of acebutolol, atenolol, or nadolol near term has caused β-blockade in newborns.[23]
Bismuth subsalicylate	C	Hydrolyzed in GI tract to bismuth salts and sodium salicylate, absorption of bismuth salts is negligible, but chronic exposure to salicylates may present fetal risk (see Aspirin). Restrict use to first half of pregnancy and do not exceed recommended doses.[23]
Brompheniramine	C	Ten malformations after 65 first-trimester exposures in one study.[31] Use of antihistamines during last 2 wk of pregnancy has been associated with an increased risk of retrolental fibroplasia in premature infants.[52]
Busulfan	D	Used in 38 pregnancies, 22 in first trimester resulting in six infants with defects: unspecified malformations (aborted at 20 wk); anomalous deviation left lobe liver, bilobular spleen, and pulmonary atelectasis; pyloric stenosis; cleft palate, microphthalmia, cytomegaly, hypoplasia of ovaries and thyroid gland, corneal opacity, and IUGR; myeloschisis, aborted at 6 wk; IUGR, left hydronephrosis and hydroureter, absent right kidney and ureter, and hepatic subcapsular calcifications.[23]
Carbamazepine	D	May produce malformations similar to those seen with phenytoin (see Table 44.6).[23] ↓ head circumference observed in some infants. In one stillborn infant, multiple defects (closely set eyes, flat nose with single nasopharynx, polydactyl, atrial septal defect, patent ductus arteriosus, absent gallbladder and thyroid gland, and collapsed fontanel) were observed.[53] A 1989 study concluded that carbamazepine exposure in the first trimester is associated with a pattern of malformations whose main features are minor craniofacial defects, fingernail hypoplasia, developmental delay, and ↑ risk for NTDs.[54–56]
Chloramphenicol	C	Use with caution at term. Unconfirmed report of cardiovascular collapse (gray syndrome) in newborns exposed in final stage of pregnancy.[23,57]
Codeine	C	Normally combined with nonnarcotic analgesics or other drugs. First trimester use in 563 cases associated with: respiratory malformations (8 cases), GU tract defects other than hypospadias (7 cases), Down syndrome (1 case), tumors (4 cases), umbilical hernia (3 cases), inguinal hernia (12 cases).[31] After 2,522 exposures to codeine anytime in pregnancy, the following were noted: hydrocephaly (7 cases), pyloric stenosis (8 cases), umbilical hernia (7 cases), inguinal hernia (51 cases).[31] In four retrospective studies, inguinal hernias, cardiac and circulatory system defects, cleft lip/palate, dislocated hip, musculoskeletal defects, and alimentary tract defects were associated with maternal consumption of codeine.[23,37]
Diphenhydramine	C	Based on 2,948 pregnancy exposures, possible associations with congenital malformations found in 40 infants: GU defects (5 cases), hypospadias (3 cases), eye/ear defects (3 cases), syndromes (other than Down) (3 cases), inguinal hernia (13 cases), clubfoot (5 cases), any ventricular septal defect (5 cases), and defects of diaphragm (3 cases).[31] A second study found possible association with cleft palate.[37] Neonatal withdrawal reported in one newborn.[23]

(continued)

Table 44.4 • Selected Drugs That Should Be Used with Caution During Pregnancy[a,b] (continued)

Drug/Drug Class	Risk Factor[c]	Fetal/Neonatal Effects
Diphenoxylate	C	Limited use in pregnancy has not resulted in fetal toxicity. Potential for fetal addiction from prolonged use of paregoric.[23]
Ephedrine	C	No evidence of teratogenicity based upon 873 exposures; ↑ in fetal heart rate and beat-to-beat variability have been observed[23,31] (also see Epinephrine).
Epinephrine	C	Statistically significant association found between 189 first-trimester exposures and major or minor anomalies in one study. Association also found between use anytime in pregnancy and inguinal hernia. Data may reflect serious maternal conditions requiring use of drug. After 9,719 exposures, adrenergics as a group were associated with minor anomalies, inguinal hernia, and clubfoot.[31] Adrenergics, including epinephrine, are teratogenic in some animal species.[23]
Ergotamine	X/D[f]	Small, infrequent doses may not be teratogenic; large doses or frequent use may cause teratogenicity because of disruption of fetal blood supply; oxytocic properties of drug may cause dysfunctional labor marked by prolonged contractions resulting in fetal hypoxia.[23] If possible, should be avoided in pregnancy.
Fluconazole	C	Four case reports described anomalies with structural defects of the CNS, extremities, and cleft palate; features resembled a known recessive genetic disorder; exposure period was throughout pregnancy in three cases.[58]
Fosphenytoin	D	This is a prodrug of phenytoin. After parenteral administration, fosphenytoin is converted to phenytoin.[28] See phenytoin.
Ibuprofen	B/D[g]	No evidence of teratogenicity with first trimester use, but experience limited. Use after 34–35 weeks' gestation may cause premature closure of ductus arteriosus resulting in PPHN. Naproxen use at 30 weeks' gestation associated with PPHN in three infants.[23]
Imipramine	D	Bilateral amelia observed in one infant, but analysis of 161 first trimester exposures did not confirm association with limb reduction defects. Other defects reported in 7 infants: defective abdominal muscles (1 case); diaphragmatic hernia (2 cases); exencephaly, cleft palate, adrenal hypoplasia (1 case); cleft palate (2 cases); and renal cystic degeneration (1 case). Neonatal withdrawal has been observed.[23]
Indomethacin	B/D[g]	Used to treat premature labor; Oliguric renal failure, hemorrhage, and intestinal perforation have been reported in some premature infants exposed just before delivery. Reduced fetal urine output may be therapeutic in cases of polyhydramnios. May cause constriction of the fetal ductus arteriosus, with or without tricuspid regurgitation.[23,59]
Lithium	D	Congenital defects have been reported in 22 infants, 17 (77%) involving cardiovascular system; 5/17 had rare Ebstein's anomaly (tricuspid valve malformation). Transient lithium toxicity in newborn has been reported frequently: cyanosis, hypotonia, bradycardia, thyroid suppression with goiter, atrial flutter, hepatomegaly, ECG anomalies (T-wave inversion), cardiomegaly, GI bleeding, diabetes insipidus, and shock.[23]
Marijuana	C	Maternal use may be associated with fetal growth retardation, but other factors such as multiple drug use, lifestyles, diseases, socioeconomic status, and nutrition may play significant role. One report has associated in utero exposure to marijuana to the development of acute nonlymphoblastic leukemia in childhood.[23,60] Contraindicated if used as drug of abuse.

(continued)

Table 44.4 • Selected Drugs That Should Be Used with Caution During Pregnancy[a,b] (continued)

Drug/Drug Class	Risk Factor[c]	Fetal/Neonatal Effects
Mercaptopurine	D	Thirty-four fetuses were exposed in first trimester and 45 in second or third trimesters. When abortions or stillbirths were excluded, defects or toxicity found in four cases: cleft palate, microphthalmia, hypoplasia of ovaries and thyroid, corneal opacity, cytomegaly, and intrauterine growth retardation (1 case); neonatal pancytopenia (fetus exposed to six antineoplastic agents in third trimester) (1 case); microangiopathic hemolytic anemia (1 case); and transient severe bone marrow hypoplasia (1 case).[23]
Methimazole	D	Nine cases of aplasia cutis in infants exposed in utero to carbimazole or methimazole. Transposition of great arteries, umbilical defects, imperforate anus, bilateral cataracts, partial adactyly of foot, and nonspecified malformations also have been reported. When used close to term, may rarely produce small, nonobstructing goiters in the newborn.[23,61]
Methotrexate	D	Data available for 26 pregnancy exposures involving 10 first-trimester cases. Three of the latter exposures had congenital defects: unspecified anomalies (1 case); absence of lambdoid and coronal sutures, oxycephaly, absence of frontal bone, low-set ears, ocular hypertelorism, dextroposition of heart, absence of digits on feet, growth retardation, wide posterior fontanel, hypoplastic mandible, and multiple anomalous ribs (1 case); oxycephaly caused by absent coronal sutures, large anterior fontanel, depressed/wide nasal bridge, low-set ears, long webbed fingers, and wide-set eyes (1 case).[23] Use before pregnancy with retention in maternal tissues may have resulted in desquamating fibrosing alveolitis in one newborn.[62]
Methyldopa	C	No known association with congenital defects. Frequently used for treatment of pregnancy-induced hypertension.[23] A decrease in intracranial volume after first-trimester use has been reported but no relationship between small head size and retarded mental development at 4 years of age.[63–65]
Methylene blue	D	Intra-amniotic injection has caused hemolytic anemia, hyperbilirubinemia, methemoglobinemia, and possibly small bowel obstructions.[23]
Metronidazole	B	No confirmed evidence of teratogenicity, but agent is mutagenic in bacteria and carcinogenic in rodents. No evidence of human cancer. FDA data indicate an estimated relative risk for birth defects after exposure to metronidazole to be 0.92. Two women exposed during fifth to seventh weeks of gestation delivered infants with midline facial defects (holotelencephaly and unilateral cleft lip/palate). Excessive fetotoxicity and teratogenicity noted in mice when combined with alcohol.[23,66–70]
Nicotine Nicotine polacrilex	C/D[e]	Smoking during pregnancy can cause fetal growth retardation, increased risk of spontaneous abortion, and perinatal mortality.[30] Use of nicotine replacement in the third trimester has been associated with decreased fetal breathing.[28] Spontaneous abortion has been reported.
Nifedipine	C	Limited use in second and third trimesters not associated with fetal toxicity, but severe maternal hypotension may occur. Has been used for treatment of premature labor.[23] May potentiate neuromuscular blocking action of magnesium resulting in pronounced maternal muscle weakness and hypotension; of three fetuses, one was stillborn.[71–75]
Nitrofurantoin	B	Apparently safe but use with caution at term because of theoretic potential for hemolytic anemia in newborn.[23]

(continued)

Table 44.4 • Selected Drugs That Should Be Used with Caution During Pregnancy[a,b] (continued)

Drug/Drug Class	Risk Factor[c]	Fetal/Neonatal Effects
Penicillamine	D	In <100 pregnancies, five infants with connective tissue anomalies were observed after use of drug: cutis laxa (1 case); cutis laxa, hypotonia, hyperflexion of hips and shoulders, pyloric stenosis, vein fragility, varicosities, impaired wound healing, and death (1 case); cutis laxa, IUGR, inguinal hernia, simian crease, perforated bowel, and death (1 case); cutis laxa, mild micrognathia, low-set ears, and inguinal hernia (1 case); cutis laxa, and inguinal hernia (1 case). Miscellaneous defects observed in four other infants may have not been caused by drug. Some clinicians suggest keeping daily dose <500 mg/day to lessen incidence of toxicity; others recommend avoiding drug during pregnancy.[23,76]
Phenobarbital	D	May produce malformations similar to those seen with phenytoin when used in epileptic patients (see Table 44.6). May cause early HDN. Also may cause fetal/newborn addiction.[23]
Phenylephrine	C	Use in treatment of maternal hypotension could result in fetal hypoxia because of constriction of normally maximally dilated α-adrenergic receptors in uterus. Severe persistent maternal hypertension with possible rupture of a cerebral vessel may occur if used with oxytocics or ergot derivatives. Based on 1,249 first-trimester exposures, a possible association was found with malformations including: eye/ear defects, syndactyly, preauricular skin tag, and clubfoot. After 4,194 exposures during anytime of pregnancy, possible associations were found with congenital dislocation of hip, other musculoskeletal defects, and umbilical hernia[23,31] (also see Epinephrine).
Phenylpropanol-amine	C	See phenylephrine for potential problem with fetal hypoxia. Based upon 726 first-trimester exposures, a possible association was found with malformations including: hypospadias, eye and ear defects, polydactyly, cataracts, and pectus excavatum. After 2,489 exposures during anytime of pregnancy, 12 infants had congenital dislocation of the hip[23,31] (also see Epinephrine).
Phenytoin	D	See Table 44.6[23]
Progesterone and related compounds	D/X[e]	In 1977 the FDA restricted use in pregnancy based on reports of cardiac malformations, CNS defects, masculinization of female fetuses, and limb defects. Re-evaluation of some of these data and new, well-designed studies have failed to show an association between these defects and progesterones. Progesterone is used frequently to prevent imminent abortion during the first trimester. Use of hydroxyprogesterone or medroxyprogesterone during early pregnancy may have been associated with esophageal atresia, but the absolute risk was low (about 6/10,000 exposed lived births).[23,77]
Propylthiouracil (PTU)	D	Drug of choice for treatment of hyperthyroidism during pregnancy; anomalies reported in seven infants after in utero exposure, but no association between PTU and defects suggested. May produce mild hypothyroidism in fetus when used close to term, evident as a goiter and elevated levels of neonatal TSH. Goiters in two infants sufficiently massive to cause death in one infant and respiratory distress in the other.[23]
Quinolones	C	Erosions of cartilage and arthropathy have been reported in immature animals, but effects in human are unknown. Avoid during pregnancy if safer alternatives are available.[28,30]
Rifampin	C	Although not a proven teratogen, one report observed 9 defects in 204 pregnancies: anencephaly (1 case), hydrocephalus (2 cases), limb malformations (4 cases), renal tract defect (1 case), and congenital hip dislocation (1 case).[78] HDN observed in 3 infants; prophylactic vitamin K recommended.[23]

(continued)

Table 44.4 • Selected Drugs That Should Be Used with Caution During Pregnancy[a,b] (continued)

Drug/Drug Class	Risk Factor[c]	Fetal/Neonatal Effects
SSRIs	C	Most data available are for fluoxetine. Use of fluoxetine does not appear to be associated with major birth defects, but some cases reported increased risk for minor anomalies.[49,79] Other SSRIs (sertraline, paroxetine, fluvoxamine) do not appear to increase risk of major anomalies.[80] Exposure near term may cause withdrawal symptoms, including jitteriness in newborn.[49,81] Safety requires further investigation.
Sulfonylureas, oral	C	Use near term may result in prolonged hypoglycemia. Not recommended in pregnancy because it will not provide better control than diet alone. Insulin is the treatment of choice during pregnancy.[23]
Tetracyclines	D	Use after fifth month of gestation will result in permanent yellow-brown staining of teeth. Inhibition of fibula growth may occur in premature infants.[23] Based on 1,944 pregnancy exposures, possible associations with congenital anomalies found in 61 infants: hypospadias (5 cases), inguinal hernia (47 cases), limb hypoplasia (6 cases), and clubfoot (3 cases).[31]
Thiazides and related diuretics	C/D[e]	Many experts consider diuretics contraindicated in pregnancy, except for patients with heart diseases, because they do not prevent or alter course of toxemia and may ↓ placental perfusion. No evidence of teratogenicity. Neonatal thrombocytopenia in 11 newborns (with 2 deaths) following use near term of chlorothiazide, hydrochlorothiazide, and methyclothiazide. Hemolytic anemia in two newborns after chlorothiazide and bendroflumethiazide. Fetal electrolyte disturbances observed in a few cases when used during third trimesters.[23]
Trimethadione	D	Phenotype exists for fetal trimethadione syndrome (see Table 44.8). Use in nine families (36 pregnancies) resulted in 25 infants with wide spectrum of defects. Not recommended in pregnancy.[23]
Valproic acid	D	Risk for NTDs is 1–2% (exposure must occur between the seventeenth and thirtieth day after fertilization).[82] A valproic acid syndrome has been suggested to consist of anomalies involving the following: NTDs, craniofacial, digits, and urogenital. Retarded psychomotor development and low birth weight also have been observed.[23,83–85]
Warfarin	X/D[f]	Teratogenic; see Table 44.7.[23]

[a]This list is not all-inclusive. Selected drugs are listed by drug class and not by individual names.
[b]A glossary is provided at the beginning of this chapter. ACEI = Angiotensin-converting enzyme inhibitor; CNS = Central nervous system; ECG = Electrocardiogram; FDA = Food and Drug Administration; GI = Gastrointestinal; GU = Genitourinary; HDN = Hemolytic disease of the newborn; IUGR = Intrauterine growth retardation; NTDs = Neural tube defects; PPHN = Persistent pulmonary hypertension of the newborn; SSRIs = Selective serotonin reuptake inhibitors; TSH = Thyroid-stimulating hormone.
[c]Risk factors listed for most drugs are according to the manufacturers' ratings based on FDA definitions. When this is not available, the risk factor indicated is from reference 23.
[d]Rated risk factor C in first trimester, D in second and third trimesters.
[e]Drugs within the same class may have different pregnancy category ratings.
[f]Rated risk factor X by manufacturer, rated D in reference 23.
[g]Rated risk factor D in third trimester or near delivery.

Notes:

Table 44.5 • Fetal Alcohol Syndrome

Craniofacial

Eyes	Short palpebral fissures, ptosis, strabismus, epicanthal folds, myopia, microphthalmia, blepharophimosis
Ears	Poorly formed conchae, posterior rotation
Nose	Short, upturned hypoplastic philtrum
Mouth	Prominent lateral palatine ridges, thinned upper vermilion border, retrognathia in infancy, micrognathia or relative prognathia in adolescence, cleft lip or palate, small teeth with faulty enamel
Maxilla	Hypoplastic

Central Nervous System
Mild to moderate retardation, microcephaly, poor coordination, hypotonia, irritability in infancy and hyperactivity in childhood (both mental and motor development are delayed)

Growth
Prenatal (affecting body length more than weight) and postnatal deficiency

Cardiac
Murmurs, atrial septal defect, ventricular septal defect, great vessel abnormalities, tetralogy of Fallot

Renogenital
Labial hypoplasia, hypospadias, renal defects

Cutaneous
Hemangiomas, hirsutism in infancy

Skeletal
Abnormal palmar creases, pectus excavatum, restriction of joint movement, nail hypoplasia, radioulnar synostosis, pectus carinatum, bifid xiphoid, Klippel-Feil anomaly, scoliosis

Muscular
Hernias of diaphragm, umbilicus or groin, diastasis recti

Other Problems Associated with Heavy Alcohol Consumption in Pregnancy
Intrauterine growth retardation (IUGR), increased risk of spontaneous abortions, neonatal withdrawal

Data from reference 23.

Table 44.6 • Fetal Effects of Hydantoins[a]

Fetal Hydantoin Syndrome

Craniofacial	Broad nasal bridge, wide fontanel, low-set hairline, ocular hypertelorism, cleft lip/palate, epicanthal folds, coloboma, broad alveolar ridge, metopic ridging, short neck, microcephaly, abnormal or low-set ears, ptosis of eyelids, coarse scalp hair
Limbs	Small or absent nails, altered palmar crease, dislocated hip, hypoplasia of distal phalanges, digital thumb
Other	Impaired growth (physical and mental), congenital heart defects

Other Birth Defects/Toxicities Associated with Phenytoin

Multiple malformations	Nearly all possible types have been reported
Tumors	Neuroblastoma, ganglioneuroblastoma, melanotic neuroectodermal, extrarenal Wilms' tumor, mesenchymoma, lymphangioma, ependymoblastoma
HDN	Involves various organ systems

[a]HDN = Hemorrhagic disease of the newborn.
Data from reference 23.

Table 44.7 • Fetal Warfarin Syndrome

Exposure Sixth to Twelfth Weeks
Common Features
Nasal hypoplasia
Depressed bridge of nose
Stippling in uncalcified epiphyseal regions (axial skeleton, proximal femurs, and calcanei)

Less Common Features
Birth weight <10th percentile for gestational age
Developmental retardation
Congenital heart disease
Deafness/hearing loss
Death
Laryngeal calcification
Scoliosis
Seizures
Eye anomalies (blindness, optic atrophy, and microphthalmia)
Hypoplasia of extremities ranging from severe rhizomelic dwarfing to dystrophic nails and shortened
    fingers

Exposure in Second and Third Trimesters
CNS Anomalies
Dorsal midline dysplasia characterized by agenesis of corpus callosum, Dandy-Walker malformation,
    and midline cerebellar atrophy; encephaloceles
Ventral midline dysplasia characterized by optic atrophy

Effects of CNS Anomalies
Blindness
Deafness
Death
Growth failure
Hydrocephalus
Mental retardation
Scoliosis
Seizures
Spasticity

Adapted from references 23, 27, 30, and 144.

Table 44.8 • Fetal Trimethadione Syndrome

Cardiac	Septal defects	Patent ductus arteriosus
Limb	Simian crease, hand defects	Clubfoot
Craniofacial	Low-set, cupped/abnormal ears; high arched or cleft lip and/or palate; microcephaly; irregular teeth	Epicanthic folds, broad nasal bridge, strabismus, low hairline, facial hemangiomata
Growth/Performance	Prenatal/postnatal deficiency, speech disorder	Mental retardation, myopia, impaired hearing
Genitourinary	Kidney/ureter defects, hypospadias, clitoral hypertrophy	Inguinal hernias, ambiguous genitalia, imperforate anus
Other	Tracheoesophageal fistula	Esophageal atresia

Data from reference 23.

Notes:

Table 44.9 • Factors Affecting the Fate of Drugs in Milk and the Nursing Infant

Maternal parameters	• Drug dosage and duration of therapy • Route and frequency of administration • Metabolism • Renal clearance • Blood flow to the breasts • Milk pH • Milk composition
Drug parameters	• Oral bioavailability (to mother and infant) • Molecular weight • pKa • Lipid solubility • Protein binding
Infant parameters	• Age of the infant • Feeding pattern • Amount of breast milk consumed • Drug absorption, distribution, metabolism, elimination

From references 89 and 93–95.

Table 44.10 • Reducing Risk of Infant Exposure to Drugs in Breast Milk[90,91,98]

A drug should be used only if medically necessary and treatment cannot be delayed until the infant is ready to be weaned

Drug Selection
Consider whether the drug can be safely given directly to the infant.
Select a drug that passes poorly into breast milk with the lowest predicted M/P ratio.
Avoid long-acting formulations (e.g., sustained-release).
Consider possible routes of administration that can reduce drug excretion into milk.
Determine length of therapy and, if possible, avoid long-term usage.

Feeding Pattern
Avoid nursing during times of peak drug concentration.
If possible, plan breast-feeding before administration of the next dose.

Other Considerations
Always observe the infant for unusual signs or symptoms (e.g., sedation, irritability, rash, decreased appetite, failure to thrive).
Discontinue breast-feeding during the course of therapy if the risks to the fetus outweigh the benefits of nursing.
Provide adequate patient education to increase understanding of risk factors.

Notes:

Table 44.11 • Drugs Considered Contraindicated During Lactation[a,b]

Drug/Drug Class	Effects on Nursing Infants
Amphetamine[c]	Accumulate in breast milk and may cause irritability and poor sleep patterns.[23,99,100]
Antineoplastics	Potential for immune suppression; cytotoxic effects of drugs on dividing cells in infants unknown.[99]
Bromocriptine	Suppresses lactation[23,99]
Cocaine[c]	Excreted in milk; contraindicated because of CNS stimulation and intoxication.[23,99,101,102]
Ergotamine	Potential for suppressing lactation; vomiting, diarrhea, and convulsions have been reported.[23,99]
Ethanol	Contraindication is controversial. Passes freely into milk; high maternal intake may cause, in nursing infants, sedation, diaphoresis, deep sleep, weakness, $\downarrow$ in linear growth, and abnormal weight gain. Chronic exposure also may be related to retarded psychomotor development. $\downarrow$ in milk ejection reflex may occur. Infants of alcoholic mothers may be at risk for potentiation of severe hypoprothrombic bleeding and pseudo-Cushing's syndrome. AAP classifies as compatible but should be considered contraindicated.[23,99,103] One review suggested waiting 1–2 hr per drink before breast-feeding.[90]
Heroin[c]	Possible addiction if sufficient amounts ingested.[23,99]
Immunosuppressants	Potential for immune suppression.[99]
Lithium	Milk and serum concentrations average 40% of maternal serum levels causing potential for toxic reactions; contraindicated.[23,99]
Lysergic acid diethylamide (LSD)[c]	Probably excreted in milk.[23]
Marijuana[c]	Excreted in milk.[23,99,104–107]
Misoprostol	Excretion in milk has not been studied but contraindicated because of potential for severe diarrhea in infant.[23]
Nicotine	Contraindication is controversial; absorption via passive smoking is higher than through breast milk; smoking in general is not recommended while nursing[98]; $\downarrow$ milk production[108]
Phencyclidine[c]	Potent hallucinogenic properties.[23,99,109]
Phenindione	Massive scrotal hematoma and wound oozing after herniotomy in one infant; contraindicated.[23,99]
Requiring Temporary Cessation of Breast-Feeding	
Metronidazole (after single-dose therapy)	Diarrhea and secondary lactose intolerance in one infant; mutagenic and carcinogenic in some species; AAP recommends halting breast-feeding for 12–24 hr to allow clearance of drug from the milk if single-dose therapy is administered.[99,110,111]
Radiopharmaceuticals	Halt breast-feeding temporarily to allow clearance of radioactivity from milk; suggested times for individual agents are[99]: Gallium-67 (^{67}Ga) 2 wk; Indium-111 (^{111}In) 20 hr; Iodine-125 (^{125}I) 12 days; Iodine-131 (^{131}I) 2–4 days; Radioactive Sodium 96 hr; Technetium-99m (^{99m}Tc) 15 hr– 3 days; (^{99m}TcO$_4$) (^{99m}Tc macroaggregates) 15 hr–3 days.

[a]AAP = American Academy of Pediatrics; CNS = Central nervous system.
[b]This list is not all-inconclusive. Selected drugs are listed by drug class and not by individual names.
[c]All drugs of abuse are contraindicated during lactation.

Notes:

Table 44.12 • Selected Commonly Used Drugs and Breast-Feeding[a,b]

Drug/Drug Class	Effects on Nursing Infants
Acetaminophen	Maculopapular rash on upper trunk and face of a nursing infant has been reported. Compatible.[99,112]
Acyclovir	Concentrated in milk; compatible.[99,113,114]
Alprazolam	Apparent drug withdrawal after 9-month exposure via milk in one infant. Use of other agents in class during breast-feeding considered cause for concern by AAP.[23,51,99]
Amiodarone	Excreted in milk; not recommended because of long elimination half-life and high proportion of iodine contained in each dose.[23,115,116]
Aminoglycosides	Potential for disrupting infant's intestinal flora.[90,98]
Amitriptyline	No adverse effects reported, but AAP considers use as cause for concern.[99]
Aspartame	Excreted in milk; use with caution if infant has phenylketonuria.[23,99]
Aspirin	One case severe salicylate intoxication (metabolic acidosis); potential for platelet dysfunction and rash; AAP recommends using with caution.[23,99,117]
β-blockers	Observe exposed infants for signs of β-blockade (e.g., hypotension, bradycardia). Acebutolol, atenolol, and nadolol are concentrated in milk; β-blockade evidenced by hypotension, bradycardia, cyanosis, hypothermia, or tachycardia observed in infants exposed to acebutolol or atenolol in breast milk.[23,99,118,119]
Bismuth subsalicylate	Significant amounts of bismuth in milk not expected because of poor oral absorption[23]; salicylate portion excreted in milk (see Aspirin) and because of this, some advise that the drug should not be used during nursing.[120]
Brompheniramine	Symptoms observed in one infant exposed to brompheniramine and d-isoephedrine: irritability, excessive crying, and disturbed sleeping patterns. Compatible.[23,99,121]
Bupropion	Accumulates in milk; use with caution during breast-feeding.[23,122]
Caffeine	Accumulation may occur when mother is moderate-to-heavy consumer; irritability and poor sleeping habits observed. Compatible in usual amounts.[23,99]
Carbamazepine	Compatible.[99]
Cephalosporins	Potential for disrupting infant's intestinal flora; usually considered compatible.[90,98,99]
Chloramphenicol	Excreted in milk. Potential bone marrow depression exists; AAP recommends using with caution.[23,99]
Chlorpromazine	Excreted into milk; drowsiness and lethargy observed in one infant; AAP considers use a cause for concern because of these effects and potential for galactorrhea.[23,99,123]
Cimetidine	May accumulate in milk. Theoretic potential for suppression of gastric acidity, inhibition of drug metabolism, and CNS stimulation. Compatible.[23,99,124]
Clemastine	Drowsiness, irritability, refusal to feed, neck stiffness, and high-pitched cry in one infant. AAP recommends using with caution.[23,99,125]
Clindamycin	Grossly bloody stools in infant whose mother received clindamycin and gentamicin. Considered compatible by AAP.[23,99]
Codeine	Compatible.[99]
Diazepam	Lethargy and weight loss reported with diazepam; watch for accumulation in infant; considered cause for concern by AAP.[23,99]
Digoxin	Excreted in milk. Compatible.[23,99]
Diphenhydramine	Excreted in milk; no effects reported.[23]

(continued)

Table 44.12 • Selected Commonly Used Drugs and Breast-Feeding[a,b] (continued)

Drug/Drug Class	Effects on Nursing Infants
Estrogen and related compounds	Estrogens are excreted in milk. Potential for ↓ milk volume and ↓ nitrogen and protein content; chlorotrianisene and estradiol used to suppress postpartum breast engorgement in nonbreast-feeding women. Withdrawal vaginal bleeding observed. Use of oral contraceptives associated with shortened duration of lactation, ↓ infant weight gain, ↓ milk production, and ↓ milk content of nitrogen and protein; report of breast tenderness and hypertrophy in one infant exposed to large doses of oral contraceptives. Compatible once breast-feeding has started.[23,99]
Famotidine	Accumulates in milk but to lesser degree than either cimetidine or ranitidine[126]; may be preferred over the latter two drugs during breast-feeding.[23,90] Compatible.[99]
Fluoxetine	One case of colic in infant reported; use with caution.[23]
Ibuprofen	Small amounts excreted in milk. Compatible.[23,99,127–129]
Metformin	Effects on infants unknown; monitor for possible lactic acidosis and gastrointestinal effects (e.g., anorexia, nausea, diarrhea).[130]
Methimazole	May cause thyroid dysfunction (goiter) in nursing infant; small doses (10–15 mg/day) may be safe in thyroid function of infant monitored. Use propylthiouracil if antithyroid agent required; AAP considers compatible.[23,99]
Metoclopramide	Stimulates milk production. Mild intestinal upset observed. AAP considers use as a cause for concern because of potential potent CNS effects.[23,99,130–133]
Morphine	Compatible.[99]
Naproxen	Small amounts excreted in milk; no effects reported.[23,134,135] Compatible.[99]
Nitrofurantoin	Excreted in milk; compatible. Hemolytic anemia in infants with G6PD deficiency possible.[23,99]
Nizatidine	Excreted in milk; probably compatible.[23]
Penicillins	Potential for allergic sensitization and disruption of infants' intestinal flora; considered compatible.[23,99]
Phenobarbital	Excreted in milk; no effects reported.[23,99]
Phenytoin	Methemoglobinemia, drowsiness, and ↓ sucking activity in one infant; considered compatible by AAP.[23,99]
Propoxyphene	Compatible.[99]
Propylthiouracil (PTU)	Excreted in milk. Compatible.[99,136,137]
Pseudoephedrine	Excreted in milk. Compatible.[99,138]
Quinolones	Use with caution because of potential for arthropathy in infants[23,139–141]; consider temporarily halting nursing to decrease infant exposure.[23]
Ranitidine	Concentrated in milk; no effects reported.[23,142]
Sulfonamides	Excreted in milk; use caution in infants with jaundice, G6PD deficiency, or if premature. One case of bloody diarrhea observed with sulfasalazine. AAP advises using sulfasalazine with caution.[23,99]
Sulfonylureas, oral	Effects on infants unknown; caution against hypoglycemia in infants.
Tetracyclines	Although excreted in milk, absorption by infant is negligible; considered compatible.[23,99]

(continued)

Notes:

Table 44.12 • Selected Commonly Used Drugs and Breast-Feeding[a,b] (continued)

Drug/Drug Class	Effects on Nursing Infants
Thiazide diuretics	May suppress lactation; considered compatible.[23,99]
Valproic acid	Compatible.[99]
Vancomycin	Excreted in milk; no effects reported: Systemic absorption by infant poor.[23,143]
Vitamins	All vitamins are excreted in milk and classified as compatible. Maternal ingestion of pharmacologic doses of vitamin D may cause hypercalcemia in the nursing infant; monitor infant's serum calcium levels.[23,99]
Warfarin	Compatible.[99]

[a]AAP = American Academy of Pediatrics; CNS = Central nervous system.
[b]This list is not all-inconclusive. Most drugs listed in this table are known to be excreted in breast milk, but effects of drug exposure to the nursing infant may not always be known. Some drugs designated as "compatible" may have case reports of adverse effects to infants, but these may be rare or limited only to certain types of patients. Always consult the latest guidelines before recommending use.

Table 44.13 • Selected Herbs That Should Be Avoided or Used with Caution During Lactation[a,b]

Common Name	Scientific Name(s)[c]
Aloe	Aloe barbadensis; A. capensis
Black cohosh	Cimicifuga racemosa
Bladderwrack	Fucus vesiculosis
Borage	Borago officinalis
Bugleweed	Lycopus americanus; L. europaeus; L. virginicus
Buckthorn bark	Rhamnus catharticus
Cascara sagrada	Rhamnus purshiana
Coltsfoot	Tussilago farfara
Comfrey	Symphytum officinale
Ephedra	Ephedra gerardiana; E. equisetina; E. sinica
Garlic	Allium sativum
Guarana	Paullinia cupana
Kava Kava	Piper methysticum
Rhubarb	Rheum palmatum; R. officinale; R. tanguticum
Senna	Senna alexandrina; S. obtusifolia
Uva Ursi	Arctostaphylos uva ursi
Wormwood	Artemisia absinthium

[a]This list is not all inconclusive
[b]If indicated, use of these herbs should only be under the supervision of a qualified health care provider with expertise in medicinal plants.
[c]Most common names refer to numerous species within one genus. Selected scientific names are included and may not be inconclusive of all species.
Data from references 192 and 195.

Notes:

The reader is referred to Chapter 45: Teratogenicity and Drugs in Breast Milk, written by *Veronica S.L. Young, Pharm.D.*, in the seventh edition of **Applied Therapeutics: The Clinical Use of Drugs** for a more in-depth discussion. All notations to reference numbers are based on the reference list at the end of that chapter. The editors of this handbook express their thanks to Dr. Young and Mr. Gerald Briggs and acknowledge that this chapter is based upon their work.

Notes:

Notes:

Chapter 45

Gynecological Disorders

Vaginal Infections

♦ The most common vaginal infections are *Candida* vulvovaginitis (20%–25%), bacterial vaginosis (30%–35%), *Trichomonas* vaginitis (10%), and mixed infections (15%–20%).

♦ **Candida vulvovaginitis (CV)** usually is caused by C. *albicans* in 80%–92%, with the remainder caused by C. *(Torulopsis) glabrata* and C. *tropicalis.*

   • Signs and symptoms associated with CV include vulvar and vaginal pruritus, vaginal soreness, vulvar burning, dyspareunia (painful intercourse), and a thick, white vaginal discharge that appears to be "curd-like."

   • Table 45.1 characterizes the vaginal secretions associated with CV, BV, and trichomoniasis. Differentiation of these vaginal infections can minimize the delay of treatment of noncandidal infections by women self-treating a presumed candidal infection with nonprescription medication.

   • Predisposing host factors for increased CV colonization include pregnancy; uncontrolled diabetes mellitus; use of high-estrogen-containing oral contraceptives, broad-spectrum antibiotics, cytotoxic agents, or corticosteroids; or being immunocompromised.

   • OTC & prescription drugs for treatment of CV are listed in Table 45.2.

♦ **Bacterial vaginosis (BV)** is usually polymicrobial primarily involving *Gardnerella vaginalis* in association with *Mycoplasma hominis,* and various species of *Mobiluncus, Prevotella, Bacteroides,* and *Peptostreptococcus.*

   • BV is classified as a vaginosis, rather than a vaginitis, because vaginal inflammation is absent (or minimal) and symptoms are mild. Diagnosis typically is based on criteria listed in Table 45.3.

   • CDC recommendations for treatment of BV in nonpregnant women include: 1) metronidazole (Flagyl) 500 mg orally BID × 7 days, or 2) clindamycin (Cleocin) cream 2%, one applicatorful (5 gm) intravaginally at bedtime for 7 days; or 3) metronidazole (MetroGel Vaginal) gel 0.75%, one applicatorful (5 gm) intravaginally BID for 5 days. Alternatives include metronidazole 2 gm orally as a single dose or clindamycin 300 mg orally BID × 7 days.

♦ **Trichomonas vaginalis** is described in Chapter 62 (Sexually Transmitted Diseases).

Toxic Shock Syndrome (TSS)

♦ TSS is an acute, life-threatening multisystem illness caused by a toxic shock-syndrome-toxin-1 (TSST-1), which is produced by *Staphylococcus aureus.*

♦ Tampon use is a risk factor for TSS because tampons create a more favorable environment for TSST-1 production.

♦ The CDC established a TSS case definition (Table 45.4) to aid in diagnosis.

♦ *Treatment* for TSS is primarily supportive (aggressive IV fluid and electrolyte therapy to maintain BP and organ perfusion) and should be individualized based on severity of illness. Most patients require up to 20 liters of crystalloid (normal saline or lactated Ringer's) during the first day. Colloids may be needed in severe cases. Antibiotics that have antistaphylococcal properties (e.g., nafcillin, vancomycin, cefazolin in combination with aminoglycosides) are appropriate; however, no study has shown that antibiotics improve the course of menstrual TSS.

Dysmenorrhea

♦ Primary dysmenorrhea is painful menstruation that occurs during ovulatory cycles and is caused by factors intrinsic to the uterus rather than underlying pelvic pathology.

♦ About 30–60% of women experience pain during menstruation, with 7–15% reporting severe pain that interferes with daily activity. The occurrence of primary dysmenorrhea is highest among women 17–24 years of age.

♦ Prostaglandins ($PGF_2\alpha$ and PGE_2) can produce pain and uterine contractions as well as nausea, vomiting, and diarrhea, which are common clinical findings in women with primary dysmenorrhea. Cold exposure and IUDs also may increase prostaglandin production.

♦ Patients often present with cramping pain in the suprapubic area that may radiate to the back or thighs. Dysmenorrhea pain typically begins within 12 hrs before menstrual flow, becomes most severe for next 2–24 hrs and continues for 24–72 hrs. Nausea and vomiting can occur in 89%, fatigue in 85%, diarrhea in 60%, backache in 60%, and headache in 45%.

♦ *Treatment* includes nondrug therapy (e.g., aerobic exercise, low-fat diets, relaxation techniques) and NSAIDs (Table 45.5). Combination oral contraceptives also can provide relief by reducing prostaglandin concentrations, either by decreasing the volume of menstrual fluid or suppressing ovulation.

Premenstrual Syndrome (PMS)

♦ PMS is an ill-defined problem with no standard definition. The term is applied broadly to several behavioral and somatic symptoms that occur cyclically about 7–14 days before menstruation and disappear shortly after the onset of menses.

♦ Over 150 nonspecific symptoms have been reported during the premenstrual phase and some of the more common ones are listed in Table 45.6.

♦ The term premenstrual dysphoric disorder (PMDD) describes a subset of women with PMS who experience primarily mood changes of comparable severity to those of a major depressive disorder. The diagnostic criteria for PMDD are shown in Table 45.7.

♦ *Treatment* of PMS is difficult because the cause is unknown. Most clinicians select drug therapy to relieve or diminish the most severe or troublesome symptoms. Table 45.8 lists drugs and dosing regimens that have been successful in the management of PMS.

Endometriosis

♦ Endometriosis is the presence of functioning, proliferating endometrial tissue outside of the uterine cavity. These can occur anywhere in the body, but most commonly are limited to the pelvic structures. The pathogenesis is unknown, but retrograde menstruation may lead to implantation of viable endometrial tissue.

♦ Typically occurs in nulliparous, menstruating women in their late 20s and early 30s; however, also occurs in about 30%–40% multiparous women.

♦ Progressive dysmenorrhea and dyspareunia are the most common presenting complaints of endometriosis. The pain may be an aching, a cramping, or a pressure sensation in the pelvic area and may occur premenstrually, menstrually, or throughout the menstrual cycle.

♦ Other symptoms associated with endometriosis depend on the organs affected. Table 45.9 lists the location of endometrial tissue and associated symptoms.

♦ Because symptoms and physical findings of endometriosis can be associated with other gynecologic conditions, a definitive diagnosis can be made only by laparoscopy or laparotomy, which allow direct visualization of the pelvic and abdominal structures.

♦ Goals of treatment are to relieve symptoms and, if desired, to preserve childbearing potential.

♦ *Treatment* modalities are: definitive and conservative surgery, hormonal therapy with estrogen-progestin combinations or progestins alone, danazol, or gonadotropin-releasing hormone agonists. *Definitive surgery* (total hysterectomy and bilateral salpingo-oophorectomy) eliminates the risk of disease recurrence. *Conservative surgery* (removal of endometriotic lesions and adhesions by laparoscopy or laparotomy) relieves symptoms, restores normal pelvic architecture, and preserves childbearing potential. Dosing regimens for *gonadotropin-releasing hormone agonists* are listed in Table 45.10. Danazol 400–800 mg/day for 6–9 months significantly improves dysmenorrhea in up to 95% of women with moderate-to-severe endometriosis; however, adverse effects (Table 45.11) are significant. Hormonal therapy to produce a pseudopregnancy or pseudomenopausal state is summarized in Table 45.12.

Climacteric & Postmenopause

♦ Climacteric (perimenopause) is the phase in the feminine aging process between the reproductive and nonreproductive years characterized by waning ovarian function and decreasing estrogen concentrations.

♦ Menopause (cessation of menstrual periods) may occur several years after the beginning of the climacteric.

♦ *Hot flushes,* episodic vasomotor symptoms (feelings of warmth in chest, neck, and face, often with visible red flushing), can be experienced by 50–85% of women in the climacteric years. Hot flushes respond to low doses of oral estrogen (e.g., 0.3–0.625 mg of conjugated estrogen). Women with an intact uterus should receive a progestin for at least 12 days/month along with estrogen to decrease the risk for endometrial hyperplasia. Before initiating estrogen, endometrial hyperplasia and adenocarcinoma should be ruled out. Discontinue estrogens (usually within 6–12 months) because hot flushes are self-limiting. Transdermal estradiol patch (with 0.05 mg/day) can be used alternatively for 3 weeks/month to relieve vasomotor symptoms. Clonidine 0.05 to 0.1 mg/day orally and transdermal (0.1 mg/day) is effective but less than estrogens. Megestrol acetate 20–40 mg/day and medroxyprogesterone acetate 10 mg/day can decrease hot flushes in women unable to take estrogens.

♦ *Genitourinary* atrophy, resulting from declining estrogen levels, often results in symptoms (e.g., vaginal dryness, dyspareunia, urinary incontinence, dysuria, frequency, urgency, nocturia) that respond to intravaginal estrogen creams (0.3–0.625 mg) and to transdermal and oral estrogens.

♦ Adverse effects and risks of estrogen replacement are listed in Table 45.13.

Postmenopausal Osteoporosis

♦ Osteoporosis is characterized by low bone mass and microarchitectural deterioration of bone tissue, leading to enhanced bone fragility and a consequent increase in fracture risk.

• Osteoporosis is classified as Type I, II, or III.
  • Postmenopausal (Type I) occurs primarily in women during first 3–6 yrs following menopause but can continue for 20 years after menopause.
  • Senile osteoporosis (Type II) occurs in both genders >75 years of age.
  • Secondary osteoporosis (Type III) occurs secondarily to use of medications or to disease states (Table 45.14).
• Adequate calcium and vitamin D intake with a weight-bearing exercise program can minimize the risk of osteoporosis. Table 45.15 lists the calcium content of some selected foods, and Table 45.16 lists the percentage of elemental calcium in selected calcium salts. Table 45.17 outlines strategies for prevention and treatment of postmenopausal osteoporosis.

Table 45.1 • Characteristics of Vaginal Discharge

Characteristics	Normal	Candidiasis	Trichomoniasis	Bacterial Vaginosis
Color	White or clear	White	Yellow-green	White to gray
Odor	Nonodorous	Nonodorous	Malodorous	Fishy smell
Consistency	Floccular	Floccular	Homogeneous	Homogeneous
Viscosity	High	High	Low	Low
pH	≤4.5	4–4.5	5–6.0	>4.5
Other characteristics	—	Thick, curd-like	Frothy	Thin

From references 16, 17, and 19.

Notes:

Table 45.2 • Products Available for the Treatment of Candida Vulvovaginitis[a]

Drug	Availability	Trade Names	Dosing Regimens
OTC Products			
Butoconazole	2% vaginal cream[b]	Femstat 3	*Nonpregnant women:* Administer 1 applicatorful intravaginally Q HS for 3 consecutive days; may extend to 6 days of therapy if necessary *Pregnant women during second and third trimesters:* Administer 1 applicatorful intravaginally Q HS for 6 consecutive days
Clotrimazole	1% vaginal cream	Gyne-Lotrimin 7; Mycelex-7; Sweet'n Fresh Clotrimazole 7; various generics	Administer 1 applicatorful intravaginally Q HS for 7 consecutive days
	100-mg vaginal tablets	Gyne-Lotrimin; Mycelex-7; Sweet'n Fresh Clotrimazole 7; various generics	Insert 1 tablet intravaginally Q HS for 7 consecutive days
	200-mg vaginal inserts	Gyne-Lotrimin 3	Insert 1 suppository intravaginally Q HS for 3 consecutive days
Miconazole	2% cream[b]	Monistat 7; Femizol-M; various generics	Administer 1 applicatorful intravaginally Q HS for 7 consecutive days
	100-mg vaginal suppositories[b]	Monistat 7	Insert 1 suppository intravaginally Q HS for 7 consecutive days
	100-mg vaginal suppositories[b] (with 2% topical cream)	Monistat 7 combination pack	Insert 1 suppository intravaginally Q HS for 7 consecutive days; apply topical cream to affected areas BID (morning and night) for 7 consecutive days
Tioconazole	6.5% vaginal cream[b]	Vagistat-1	Administer 1 applicatorful intravaginally at HS for 1 dose only
Prescription Products			
Clotrimazole	500-mg vaginal tablet	Mycelex-G	Insert 1 tablet intravaginally, preferably at HS for 1 dose only
	500-mg vaginal tablet (with 1% topical cream)	Mycelex Twin Pack	Insert 1 tablet intravaginally, preferably at HS, for 1 dose and apply topical cream to affected areas BID (morning and night) for 7 consecutive days
Fluconazole	150-mg oral tablet	Diflucan tablet	Take 1 tablet PO for 1 dose only
Miconazole	200-mg vaginal suppositories[b]	Monistat 3	Insert 1 suppository intravaginally Q HS for 3 consecutive days
	200-mg vaginal suppositories[b] (with 2% topical cream)	Monistat Dual-Pak; M-Zole 3 Combination Pack	Insert 1 suppository intravaginally Q HS for 3 consecutive days; apply topical cream to affected areas BID (morning and night) for 7 consecutive days

(continued)

Table 45.2 • Products Available for the Treatment of Candida Vulvovaginitis[a] (continued)

Drug	Availability	Trade Names	Dosing Regimens
Prescription Products (continued)			
Nystatin	100,000 U vaginal tablet	Mycostatin; Nystatin; various generics	Insert 1 tablet intravaginally Q HS for 14 consecutive days
Terconazole	0.4% vaginal cream	Terazol 7	Administer 1 applicatorful intravaginally Q HS for 7 consecutive days
	0.8% vaginal cream	Terazol 3	Administer 1 applicatorful intravaginally Q HS for 3 consecutive days
	80-mg vaginal suppositories[b]	Terazol 3	Insert 1 suppository intra-vaginally Q HS for 3 con-secutive days

[a] OTC = Over-the-counter.
[b] The Centers for Disease Control and Prevention states that the use of vaginally administered oil-based preparations may weaken latex products such as condoms and diaphragms.

Table 45.3 • Modified Amsel's Criteria for the Diagnosis of Bacterial Vaginosis[a]

At least three of the following signs must be present for diagnosis:
Homogeneous discharge

Fishy amine odor when 10% KOH is added (sniff test)

Clue cells (i.e., >20% on wet mount)

Vaginal pH >4.5

No lactobacilli on wet mount

[a] KOH = Potassium hydroxide.
From reference 20.

Table 45.4 • CDC Case Definition for TSS

Fever (>38.9°C)

Rash (diffuse macular erythroderma)

Desquamation of rash (1–2 wk after onset of illness, particularly palms and soles)

Hypotension (systolic BP <90 mm Hg for adults; <5th percentile by age for children; orthostatic syncope)

Plus involvement of at least three of the following organ systems:
   Mucous membranes (oropharyngeal, conjunctival, or vaginal)
   Muscular (severe myalgia or creatine phosphokinase level >2 times UNL)
   GI (vomiting or diarrhea)
   Renal (BUN or SrCr >2 times UNL or >5 WBC/HPF without UTI)
   Hepatic (total bilirubin, AST, or ALT >2 times UNL)
   Hematologic (platelets <100,000/mm^3)
   CNS (disorientation, altered mental status when temperature and BP are normal)
   Negative blood, throat, and cerebrospinal fluid cultures
   Negative serology for Rocky Mountain spotted fever, measles, and leptospirosis

ALT = Alanine aminotransferase; AST = Aspartate aminotransferase; BP = Blood pressure; BUN = Blood urea nitro-gen; CDC = Centers for Disease Control and Prevention; CNS = Central nervous system; GI = Gastrointestinal; HPF = High-powered field; SrCr = Serum creatinine; TSS = Toxic shock syndrome; UNL = Upper normal levels; UTI = Urinary tract infection; WBC = White blood cell.
From references 44 and 45.

Table 45.5 • NSAIDs and Dosing Regimens for Primary Dysmenorrhea[a]

Groups	Drugs	Dosages	Dosing Regimen/Maximum Daily Dose	Approved for Primary Dysmenorrhea
Salicylic acids	Aspirin Various[b]	325, 500, 650, 975 mg	500–600 mg PO Q 4–6 hr	No
Indole acetic acids	Diclofenac Cataflam[c]	50 mg (as potassium)	50 mg PO TID; some patients may need a first dose of 100 mg followed by 50 mg TID (max, 150 mg/day, may give 200 mg on first day)	Yes
Propionic acids	Ibuprofen Advil[b] Motrin IB[b] Nuprin[b] Motrin[c]	200 mg 200 mg 200 mg 200 mg 300, 400, 600, 800 mg	400 mg PO Q 4–6 hr[d] (max, 3.2 g/day)	Yes
	Ketoprofen Orudis KT,[b] Actron[b]	25, 50, 75 mg 12.5 mg	25–50 mg Q 6–8 hr[e] (max, 300 mg/day)	Yes
	Naproxen Naprosyn[c] and other Rx products	250, 375, 500 mg	500 mg PO first dose; 250 mg PO Q 6–8 hr (max, 1,250 mg/day)	Yes
	Naproxen sodium Aleve[b] Anaprox[c] and other Rx products	200 mg (220 mg naproxen sodium) 250 mg (275 mg naproxen sodium) 500 mg (550 mg naproxen sodium)	550 mg (naproxen sodium) PO first dose; 275 mg (naproxen sodium) PO Q 6–8 hr (max, 1,375 mg/day [naproxen sodium][e])[f]	Yes

(continued)

Table 45.5 • NSAIDs and Dosing Regimens for Primary Dysmenorrhea[a] (continued)

Groups	Drugs	Dosages	Dosing Regimen/Maximum Daily Dose	Approved for Primary Dysmenorrhea
Fenamates	Flufenamic acid	Only available in Europe	100–200 mg PO Q 8 hr	No
	Meclofenate sodium Meclomen[c]	50, 100 mg	100 mg TID for up to 6 days (max, 300 mg/day)	Yes
	Mefenamic acid Ponstel[c]	250 mg	500 mg PO first dose; 250 mg PO Q 6 hr for 2–3 days (max, 1 g/day; may give 1.25 g on first day)	Yes
Cox-2 Selective Agents	Rofecoxib, Vioxx[c]	12.5, 25 mg	50 mg Q 24 hr (max, 50 mg/day)	Yes

[a]NSAID = Nonsteroidal anti-inflammatory drug; OTC = Over-the-counter.
[b]OTC product, available without prescription.
[c]Rx product available by prescription.
[d]Dosing recommended for dysmenorrhea when using the prescription product is higher than the OTC dosing of 200 mg Q 4–6 hr; may wish to start with the OTC dosing when an OTC product is used.
[e]Dosing recommended for dysmenorrhea when using the prescription product is higher than the OTC dosing of 12.5 Q 6–8 hr; may wish to start with the OTC dosing when an OTC product is used.
[f]Dosing recommended for dysmenorrhea when using the prescription product is higher than the OTC dosing of 220 mg Q 8–12 hr; may wish to start with the OTC dosing when an OTC product is used.
From references 59, 67, and 68.

Table 45.6 • Common PMS Symptoms

Physical Complaints	Behavioral and Psychologic Complaints
Abdominal bloating	Anger
Acne	Anxiety
Ankle edema	Crying
Backache	↓ efficiency or work performance
Breast swelling and/or tenderness	↓ judgment
Constipation	↓ feeling of well-being
Diarrhea	Depression, sadness, or hopelessness
Fatigue, hypersomnia, insomnia	Difficulty concentrating
Headache	Irritability
Joint and muscle pain	Loneliness, social withdrawal
↑ cravings for sweet or salty foods	Restlessness, agitation
Nausea and vomiting	Tension
Weight gain	

PMS = Premenstrual syndrome.
From reference 94.

Table 45.7 • Diagnostic Criteria for Premenstrual Dysphoric Disorder

A. In most menstrual cycles during the past year, symptoms listed in B occurred during the last week of the luteal phase and remitted within a few days after onset of the follicular phase. In menstruating females, these phases correspond to the week before and a few days after the onset of menses. (In nonmenstruating females who have had a hysterectomy, the timing of the luteal and follicular phases may require measurement of circulating reproductive hormones.)

B. At least 5 of the following symptoms have been present for most of the time during each symptomatic late luteal phase, with at least 1 of the symptoms being either number 1, 2, 3, or 4:
   1. Marked affective lability (e.g., feeling suddenly sad, tearful, irritable, or angry)
   2. Persistent and marked anger or irritability
   3. Marked anxiety, tension, feelings of being "keyed up" or "on edge"
   4. Significantly depressed mood, feelings of hopelessness, or self-deprecating thoughts
   5. Decreased interest in usual activities (e.g., work, friends, hobbies)
   6. Easily fatigued or significant lack of energy
   7. Subjective sense of difficulty in concentration
   8. Marked change in appetite, overeating, or specific food cravings
   9. Hypersomnia or insomnia
   10. Other physical symptoms (e.g., breast tenderness or swelling, headaches, joint or muscle pain, a sensation of "bloating," weight gain)

C. The disturbance seriously interferes with work or with usual social activities or relationships with others.

D. The disturbance is not merely an exacerbation of the symptoms of another disorder, such as major depression, panic disorder, dysthymia, or a personality disorder (although it may be superimposed on any of these disorders).

E. Criteria A, B, C, and D are confirmed by prospective daily self-ratings during at least 2 symptomatic cycles (the diagnosis may be made provisionally before this confirmation).

Adapted from reference 96.

Notes:

Table 45.8 • Psychotropic Drugs for the Management of PMS[a]

Drug (Brand Name)	Daily Dosing Regimen (mg)	Intermittent Dosing Regimen (mg)[b]
SSRIs		
Citalopram (Celexa)	20	10–30
Fluoxetine (Prozac)	20	20
Fluvoxamine (Luvox)	100	NS
Paroxetine (Paxil)	5–30	NS
Sertraline (Zoloft)	50–150	100
Other Serotonergic Antidepressants		
Nefazodone (Serzone)	200–600	NS
Venlafaxine (Effexor)	50	NS
Tricyclic Antidepressants		
Clomipramine (Anafranil)	25–75	25–75
Nortriptyline (Aventyl, Pamelor)	50–125	NS
Anxiolytics		
Alprazolam (Xanax)	NS	1–2[c]
Buspirone (BuSpar)	NS	25–60

[a]NS = Not studied; SSRIs = Selective serotonin reuptake inhibitors.
[b]Day 14 until onset of menses.
[c]Dose to be tapered over 2 days after onset of menses to prevent withdrawal symptoms.

Table 45.9 • Location of Endometriosis and Associated Symptoms

Sites	Symptoms
Most Common	
Pelvic	
Cervix	Abnormal uterine bleeding
Ovaries	Dysmenorrhea
Peritoneum	Dyspareunia
Rectovaginal septum	Infertility
Uterosacral ligaments	Pelvic pain
Intestinal	
Abdominal scars	Intestinal obstruction
Sigmoid colon	Midabdominal pain
Small intestines	Nausea
	Painful defecation
	Rectal bleeding
Urinary Tract	
Bladder	Cyclic flank pain
Ureter	Hematuria
	Hydronephrosis
	Hydroureter
Least Common	
Miscellaneous	
Breasts	Hemoptysis
Diaphragm	Sciatica
Extremities	Subarachnoid bleeding
Gallbladder	
Pleura	
Sciatic notch	
Spleen	
Stomach	
Subarachnoid space	

From references 169 and 170.

Table 45.10 • GnRH Agonists

GnRH Agonist (Brand Name)	Strength	Dosage Form	Dosage Regimen
Nafarelin (Synarel)	2 mg/mL delivers 200 μg/spray	Intranasal	200–400 μg BID
Leuprolide (Lupron)	3.75, 7.5, 11.25 mg	IM depot	3.75 mg/month
Goserelin (Zoladex)	3.6 mg	SC implant	3.6 mg/month
Buserelin[b] (Suprefact)	300 μg/spray	Intranasal	300 μg BID to TID
Histrelin[b] (Supprelin)	120 μg/0.6 mL 300 μg/0.6 mL 600 μg/0.6 mL	SC injection	100 μg/day

[a]GnRH = Gonadotropin-releasing hormone; IM = Intramuscular; SC = Subcutaneous.
[b]Not available in the United States.
[c]Not FDA approved for treatment of endometriosis.

Table 45.11 • Incidence of Adverse Effects with Danazol

Androgenic Effects
Weight gain — 12–84%
Oily skin/hair — 11–45%
Acne — 15–39%
Hirsutism — 8–26%
Voice deepening — 3–12%

Antiestrogenic Effects
↓ breast size — 34–54%
Hot flushes — 5–50%
Vaginal dryness — 9%
Abnormal vaginal bleeding — 9%
Irritability — 3%

Miscellaneous Effects
Muscle cramps — 6–57%
Edema — 5–55%
Depression — 2–51%
↓ libido — 16%
Nausea — 13%
Skin rash — 2–9%
Headache — 3–6%
Diarrhea — 3%
Hair loss — 3%

From references 174, 183, and 204–206.

Notes:

Table 45.12 • Hormonal Therapy for Endometriosis[a]

Drug	Dose	Adverse Effects	Comments
Pseudopregnancy: Use for Women with Mild-to-Moderate Endometriosis Who Do Not Desire Pregnancy and Cannot be Treated Surgically			
Combination birth control pills	1 QD. ↑ Q 1–2 weeks by 1 tab/day until there is no breakthrough bleeding and amenorrhea established. Continue 6–9 months. *Range:* 1–5 tab QD	See Chapter 40: Contraception. Estrogenic side effects are associated with high-dose estrogen (50 μg/day) preparations	Use birth control pills containing strong progestogens plus ethinyl estradiol. Produces a state of hyperhormonal amenorrhea. Initially, symptoms may ↑, but these subside as endometrial tissue is absorbed. 2nd-line treatment. Young women with mild to moderate disease and severe dysmenorrhea are good candidates. Danazol therapy preferred because of adverse effects associated with high estrogens
Medroxyprogesterone (Provera)	10 mg TID PO × 3 months (up to 50 mg daily) 100 mg IM Q 2 weeks × 8 weeks, then 200 mg monthly	Breakthrough bleeding in 30%. Weight gain ≈1.5 kg (60%), edemal bloating (60%), anxiety and irritability (20%). Depo-Provera suppresses pituitary axis for 6–12 months after discontinuation. Use oral form in women who want to conceive	Pregnancy rates of 20%–40% are lower than those associated with conservative surgery or danocrine (Danazol). Reserve use for women who cannot tolerate Danazol or GnRH

Pseudomenopause

Drug	Dosage	Effects	Comments
Danazol (Danocrine) Synthetic derivative of 17-α-ethinyl testosterone. Suppresses LH and FSH from anterior pituitary. Many other effects	Start on day 1 of menstrual cycle with 200 mg BID. ↑ monthly by 200 mg/day until amenorrhea achieved or total daily dose is 800 mg/day. Continue for 6–9 months	Many androgenic effects.[b] Produces a hypoestrogenic, hypoprogestogenic state. 85%–94% experience side effects, but these are generally mild, transient, and well tolerated	Costly. 95% achieve symptomatic relief in 1–2 months. Pregnancy rates approximate conservative surgery. Use nonhormonal contraceptive concurrently. Use contraceptives for 3 months following therapy. Recurrence in ≈40% 6–9 months after therapy discontinued
GnRH agonists Prevent pulsed release of GnRH from hypothalamus resulting in ↓ FSH and LH		Most related to hypoestrogenic state. Antiestrogenic effects.[c] Can cause bone loss that is variably reversible within 6 months	Nafarelin and leuprolide only agents with approved FDA labeling for endometriosis. As effective as danazol for pain and implant shrinkage. Disease recurs after therapy is discontinued. Menses resumes 1–2 months after discontinuation
Leuprolide (Lupron) 3.75, 7.5 mg IM depot	3.75 mg IM/month × 6 months		
Nafarelin (Synarel) 2 mg/mL nasal spray	200–400 μg (1–2 sprays) Q 12 hr intranasally × 6 months		

[a]FDA = Food and Drug Administration; FSH = Follicle-stimulating hormone; GnRH = Gonadotropin-releasing hormone; LH = Luteinizing hormone.

[b]Androgenic Effects: 10–30 lb weight gain (12%–84%), oily skin/hair (11%–45%), acne (15%–39%), hirsutism (8%–26%), voice deepening (3%–12%), Antiestrogenic Effects: ↓ breast size (34%–54%), hot flushes (5%–50%), vaginal dryness (9%), abnormal vaginal bleeding (9%), Miscellaneous: Muscle cramps (6%–57%), edema (5%–55%), depression (2%–51%), ↓ libido (16%), nausea (13%), skin rash (2%–9%), headache (3%–6%), diarrhea (3%), hair loss (3%).

[c]Hot flushes (90%), sleep disturbances (72%), headache (19%), vaginal dryness (18%), emotional lability (15%), and ↓ libido (14%).

Table 45.13 • Adverse Effects and Risks of Estrogen Replacement Therapy (ERT)[a,b]

Adverse Effects
Nausea, vomiting, dizziness, weight gain, breast enlargement and tenderness. Occurs in 0.6%–10% of women taking ethinyl estradiol. Less frequent in women using synthetic estrogens

Dose-Related Bleeding. 2%–12% at 1.25 mg/day conjugated estrogens; 1%–4% at 0.625 mg. Progestins ↑ bleeding but normalize pattern and ↓ breakthrough bleeding

Established Risks
Endometrial Adenocarcinoma. Relative risk[c] in patients with intact uterus is 4–8 and is dose- and duration-related. Concurrent progestin ↓ risk by antagonizing proliferative effects of estrogens

Cholelithiasis. Relative risk is 2.5

Abnormal Glucose Tolerance. Rarely progresses to diabetes mellitus

Unestablished Risks
Cardiovascular Disease. ↓ risk for MI with relative risk of 0.4–0.9. May be related to ↓ LDL and ↑ HDL

Hypertension. No association established

Thromboembolic Disease. No association established

Breast Cancer. ERT probably does not ↑ risk. Caution in patients with other risk factors

Contraindications
Pregnancy

History of or current thrombophlebitis or thromboembolic disease

Known or suspected breast or endometrial cancer

Undiagnosed abnormal genital bleeding

Acute or active hepatic disease

Relative Contraindications
Hypertension

Diabetes mellitus

Severe varicose veins

Depression

Hepatic or renal disease

[a]HDL = High-density lipoprotein; LDL = Low-density lipoprotein; MI = Myocardial infarction.
[b]Risks associated with oral contraceptive use cannot be extrapolated to estrogen replacement in older, postmenopausal women.
[c]Relative risk is risk of developing the problem relative to a comparable population of women who are not taking estrogen replacement.

Table 45.14 • Risk Factors Associated with the Development of Osteoporosis

↑ age
Female gender
Caucasian or Asian
Family history
Small stature
Low weight
Early menopause or oophorectomy
Sedentary life-style
↓ mobility
Low calcium intake
Excessive alcohol problems
Cigarette smoking

Predisposing medical problems (e.g., chronic liver disease, chronic renal failure, hyperthyroidism, primary hyperparathyroidism, Cushing's syndrome, GI resection, or malabsorption)

Drugs (e.g., corticosteroids, long-term anticonvulsant therapy [e.g., phenytoin or phenobarbital], excessive use of aluminum-containing antacids, long-term high-dose heparin, furosemide, excessive levothyroxine therapy)

[a]GI = Gastrointestinal.

Table 45.15 • Calcium Content of Selected Foods

Food	Serving Size	Calcium (mg)
Dairy Products		
Milk, dry nonfat	1 cup	350–450
Yogurt, low fat	1 cup	345
Milk, skim	1 cup	300
Milk, whole	1 cup	250–350
Cheese, cheddar	1 oz	211
Cheese, cottage	1 cup	211
Cheese, American	1 oz	195
Cheese, Swiss	1 oz	270
Ice cream or ice milk	½ cup	50–150
Fish		
Sardines, in oil	8 med	354
Salmon, canned (pink)	3 oz	167
Vegetables		
Spinach, fresh cooked	½ cup	245
Broccoli, cooked	1 cup	100
Collards, turnip greens	½ cup	175
Soy beans, cooked	1 cup	131
Tofu	1 oz	75
Kale	½ cup	50–150

Table 45.16 • Percentage of Calcium in Various Salts

Salt	% Calcium
Calcium carbonate	40
Tricalcium phosphate (calcium phosphate, tribasic)	39
Calcium chloride	27
Dibasic calcium phosphate dihydrate	23
Calcium citrate	21
Calcium lactate	13
Calcium gluconate	9

Notes:

Table 45.17 • Prevention and Treatment of Osteoporosis[a]

Intervention	Comment
Primary Therapy	
Weight-bearing exercise	Prevents reduction of and helps restore cortical and trabecular bone loss (e.g., jogging, walking, running, bicycling, weight lifting)
Vitamin D	Improves calcium absorption. Maintain normal RDA of 200–400 IU/day. No evidence that high doses prevent osteoporosis. Do not exceed 600–800 IU without medical supervision
Calcium	Antiresorptive agent that $\downarrow$ bone demineralization. Maintain daily intake of 1200–1500 mg/day in adolescents and young adults up to age 24; 1000 mg in premenopausal women aged 25–50; and 1500 mg elemental Ca^+ in postmenopausal women and those >50 yr old. Calcium carbonate is inexpensive and has a high Ca^{++} content. Elderly may absorb calcium poorly due to $\downarrow$ gastric acid secretion and $\downarrow$ 1, 25 dihydroxy-vitamin D_3 concentration. Give them a soluble supplement such as Ca Citrate or $CaCO_3$ in divided doses with meals to $\uparrow$ absorption
Estrogen replacement	Most effective treatment for preventing and treating osteoporosis. Has antiresorptive activity and bone mass during initial phases. Initiate as soon as possible after menopause because of rapid bone loss postmenopausally. Conjugated estrogen (e.g., Premarin) 0.625–1.25 mg/day is effective.
Alternative Therapy	
Sodium fluoride	$\uparrow$ trabecular bone mass by directlv affecting osteoblasts: strengthens bone. 40–80 mg/day should be taken with calcium (1500 mg/day) to prevent mineralization abnormalities. Adverse effects: 30% experience GI irritation: others experience pain in lower extremities
Calcitonin (salmon: Calcimar, Miacalcin) (human: Cibacalcin)	Approved for type I $\downarrow$ bone resorption through direct effect on osteoclasts. Responses to 50–100 IU/day SC or IM have varied. 30% report flushing. Inconvenient and expensive
Calcitriol [1, 25 $(OH)_2$ D_3, Rocaltrol]	Not routinely used. Can normalize calcium absorption and $\downarrow$ vertebral fractures but can also cause hypercalcemia. *Dose:* 0.25–1 µg/day. Very expensive
Alendronate sodium (Fosamax)	A biphosphonate. Inhibits bone resorption. Dosed often at 5–10 mg/day. Other biphosphonates (e.g., Aredia, Actonel) also effective.
Etidronate (Didronel)	A biphosphate. Inhibits bone resorption mediated by osteoclasts. Repeated cyclic administration (400 mg/day × 2 weeks, 13 weeks drug-free) $\uparrow$ spinal bone density and $\downarrow$ rate of bone loss in postmenopausal osteoporosis
Raloxifene (Evista)	A selective estrogen receptor modulator. $\uparrow$s bone density by $\downarrow$ bone resorption and bone turnover. Usual dose is 60 mg QD. Can cause $\uparrow$ hot flushes and thromboembolic disease.

[a]GI = Gastrointestinal; RDA = Recommended daily allowance.

The reader is referred to Chapter 46: Gynecological Disorders, written by *Rosalie Sagraves, Pharm.D., Louise Parent-Stevens, Pharm.D.,* and *Jennifer Mitchell, Pharm.D.,* in the seventh edition of **Applied Therapeutics: The Clinical Use of Drugs** for a more in-depth discussion. All notations to reference numbers are based on the reference list at the end of that chapter. The editors of this handbook express their thanks to Drs. Sagraves, Parent-Stevens, and Mitchell and acknowledge that this chapter is based upon their work.

Chapter 46

Thyroid Disorders

Hormone Synthesis and Regulation

Triiodothyronine (T_3) and thyroxine (T_4) are the biologically active hormones produced by the thyroid gland. Low levels of thyroid hormone stimulate the release of thyrotropin-releasing hormone (TRH) from the hypothalamus which, in turn, stimulates the release of thyroid-stimulating hormone (TSH) from the pituitary.

♦ T_4 is the major circulating hormone secreted by the thyroid: 35%-40% is converted to T_3; 45% is converted to inactive reverse T_3 (rT_3). Some drugs and diseases can modify the conversion rate of T_4 to T_3. T_4 is very highly protein bound (99.97%): 70% to thyroxine-binding globulin (TBG); 15% to thyroxine-binding prealbumin (TBPA); and the rest to albumin. Binding accounts for the long half-life of 7 days.

♦ T_3 is 4 times more potent than T_4, but its concentration is lower. About 80% is derived from deiodination of T_4 peripherally. T_3 is less strongly bound to proteins (99.7%) accounting for its shorter half-life of 1.5 days.

Thyroid Function Tests

The principal tests recommended in the initial evaluation of thyroid disorders are the sensitive TSH and the free T_4 (FT_4). (See Table 46.1 for common tests and Table 46.2 for factors which can significantly alter thyroid function tests in euthyroid patients.)

Euthyroid Sick Syndrome

♦ Abnormal thyroid function tests occur in 37%-70% of chronically ill or hospitalized patients. Abnormal tests also are associated with starvation; acute infection; HIV disease; psychiatric disorders; and chronic cardiac, pulmonary, renal, hepatic, and neoplastic diseases. In general, the sicker the patient, the greater is the degree of abnormal thyroid function findings, even though the patient has no thyroid disease.

♦ TT_4 usually is low or normal; FT_4I is low or normal; TT_3 is low; rT_3 is high; and TSH and TRH are normal or near normal.

♦ T_4 and T_3 levels are not valuable in evaluating thyroid function in patients with significant nonthyroid illness. In these types of patients a normal, or near normal, TSH is necessary to establish euthyroidism.

Hypothyroidism

♦ Table 46.3 lists common symptoms, physical findings, and laboratory results. Hypothyroidism can present with minimal findings and atypically in the elderly.

♦ The common causes of hypothyroidism are described in Table 46.4.

Treatment

♦ *Goal.* The goal is to attain and maintain a euthyroid state with thyroid replacement therapy. Table 46.5 lists the common thyroid formulations and Table 46.6 outlines treatment regimens.

♦ Poor compliance or inadequate dose are the usual causes of lack of responsiveness to thyroid replacement therapy. Bioavailability and potency variability issues are becoming resolved with the FDA requirement that all manufacturers of T_4 must file for a NDA (new drug application).

Myxedema Coma

♦ Myxedema coma is the end stage of long-standing uncorrected hypothyroidism. It can be precipitated by cold weather, hypothermia, stress, illness, and medications.

♦ Signs and symptoms include hypothermia, delayed deep tendon reflexes, and altered sensorium (stupor to coma). Myxedema coma often occurs in the elderly and is difficult to distinguish from senility.

♦ Respiratory depressants (anesthetics, narcotics, phenothiazines, sedative-hypnotics) and diuretics can precipitate myxedema coma. Phenothiazines also can aggravate hypothermia. Hypothyroid patients are especially sensitive to the respiratory depressant effects of morphine (10 mg can induce coma or death in a patient who is already comatose).

♦ Treatment is based upon supportive therapy, correction of precipitating factors, and thyroid replacement. Give 400 μg of L-thyroxine initially to saturate TBG (200 μg in patients with cardiac problems). Regulate maintenance doses according to patient response. If the proper dose is given, consciousness, restoration of vital signs, and decreased TSH should occur within 24 hours. Administer 50–100 mg hydrocortisone Q 6 hr to treat possible secondary myxedema.

Hyperthyroidism

♦ Tables 46.8–46.10 list the clinical and laboratory findings, causes, and treatment, respectively, for hyperthyroidism.

♦ Surgery or thioamides are the treatments of choice for hyperthyroidism in pregnancy. Surgery is safe during 2nd trimester when preoperative preparation is adequate. Propylthiouracil generally preferred over methimazole during pregnancy.

Thyroid Storm

♦ Thyroid storm presents with an acute onset of high fever (sine qua non), tachycardia, tachypnea, and involvement of several organ systems: *Cardiovascular system:* tachycardia, pulmonary edema, hypertension, and shock; *CNS system:* tremor, emotional lability, confusion, psychosis, apathy, stupor, and coma; *GI system:* diarrhea, abdominal pain, nausea and vomiting, liver enlargement, jaundice, and nonspecific elevations of bilirubin and prothrombin time.

♦ Immediate treatment (Table 46.11) can minimize mortality. Direct toward 4 areas: decrease synthesis and release of hormones; reverse peripheral effects of hormones and catecholamines; maintain vital functions; and eliminate precipitating causes.

Ophthalmopathy of Graves' Disease

♦ *Signs and Symptoms.* Bilateral conjunctival edema; proptosis; incomplete lid closure; and decreased visual acuity, photophobia, tearing, and extreme irritation are some signs of ophthalmopathy.

♦ Fortunately, the severe form is rare (3%-5%). Ophthalmopathy can occur at any time and usually involves both eyes. Symptoms usually subside and remain stable once the patient is euthyroid but can progress.

♦ **Treatment** is symptomatic and empiric once euthyroidism is achieved. Gland ablation with RAI or surgical removal is the treatment of choice since the thioamides do not prevent progression. Concurrent radiation of the orbit and systemic steroids may be required: prednisone 35–80 mg/day PO (up to 100–140 mg/day) for days to weeks. The onset of action is 24 hours; taper initial large doses down as rapidly as possible. Subconjunctival or retrobulbar injections are not as effective.

Notes:

Table 46.1 • Common Thyroid Function Tests [a]

Tests	Measures	Normals [b]	Assay Interference	Comments
Measurement of Circulating Hormone Levels				
FT_4	Direct measurement of free thyroxine	*Dialysis method:* 9–24 pmol/L *Analog method:* 0.7–1.9 ng/dL (9–24 pmol/L)	No interference by alterations in TBG	Most accurate determination of FT_4 levels; might be higher than normal in patients on thyroxine replacement
FT_4I	Calculated free thyroxine index	T_4 *uptake method:* 6.5–12.5 $TT_4 \times RT_3U$ *method:* 1.3–3.9	Euthyroid sick syndrome (see Question 2)	Estimates direct FT_4 measurement; compensates for alterations in TBG
TT_4	Total free and bound T_4	5.0–12.0 mg/dL (64–154 mmol/L)	Alterations in TBG (see Table 46.2)	Specific and sensitive test if no alterations in TBG
TT_3	Total free and bound T_3	70–132 ng/dL (1.1–2.0 nmol/L)	Alterations in TBG levels; T_4 to T_3 (see Table 46.2). Euthyroid sick syndrome (see Question 2)	Useful in detecting early, relapsing, and T_3 toxicosis. Not useful in evaluation of hypothyroidism
RT_3U	Indirect measure of saturation of TBG binding sites; does not measure either T_3 or T_4 levels directly	26–35%	Alterations in TBG levels (see Table 46.2)	Can be used to calculate FT_3I and FT_4I
Tests of Thyroid Gland Function				
RAIU	Gland's use of iodine after trace dose of either ^{123}I or ^{131}I	5 hr = 5–15% 24 hr = 15–35%	False decrease with excess iodide intake; false elevation with iodide deficiency	Useful in hyperthyroidism to determine RAI dose in Graves'. Does not provide information regarding hormone synthesis
Scan	Gland size, shape, and tissue activity after ^{123}I or ^{99m}Tc	—	^{123}I scan blocked by antithyroid/ thyroid medications	Useful in nodular disease to detect "cold" or "hot" areas

Test of Hypothalamic-Pituitary-Thyroid Axis

Test	Description	Reference Range	Conditions	Comments
TSH	Pituitary TSH level	0.5– 4.7 mIU/L	Dopamine, glucocorticoids, metoclopramide, thyroid hormone, amiodarone (see Table 46.2)	Most sensitive index for hyper-thyroidism, hypothyroidism, and replacement therapy
Tests of Autoimmunity				
ATgA	Antibodies to thyroglobulin	<8%	Nonthyroidal autoimmune disorders	Present in autoimmune thyroid disease; undetectable during remission
TPO	Thyroperoxidase antibodies	<100 IU/mL	Nonthyroidal autoimmune disorders	More sensitive of the two anti-bodies. Titers detectable even after remission
TRab	Thyroid receptor IgG antibody	Titers negative	—	Confirms Graves' disease; detects risk of neonatal Graves[b]
Miscellaneous				
Thyroglobulin	Colloid protein of normal thyroid gland	5–25 ng/dL	Goiters; inflammatory thyroid disease	Marker for recurrent thyroid cancer or metastases in thyroidectomized patients

[a]ATgA = Antithyroglobulin; FT₄ = Free thyroxine; FTₐI = Free thyroxine index; IV = Intravenous; RAIU = Radioactive iodine uptake; RT₃U = Resin triiodothyronine uptake; T₃ = Triiodothyronine; T₄ = Thyroxine; TBG = Thyroxine-binding globulin; TPO = Thyroperoxidase; TRab = Thyroid-receptor antibodies; TSH = Thyroid-stimulating hormone; TT₃ = Total triiodothyronine; TT₄ = Total thyroxine.
[b]At University of California laboratories.

Table 46.2 • Factors That Can Significantly Alter Thyroid Function Tests in Euthyroid Patients[a]

	Drugs/Situations
↑ TBG Binding Capacity	
↑ TT_4	Estrogens,[3] tamoxifen[4]
↑ TT_3	Oral contraceptives[3]
↓ RT_3U	Heroin[5]
Normal TSH	Methadone maintenance[4]
Normal FT_4I, FT_4	Genetic ↑ in TBG
Normal FT_3I, FT_3	Clofibrate
	Active hepatitis[3]
↓ TBG Binding Capacity/Displacement T_4 from Binding Sites	
↓ TT_4	Androgens[3]
↓ TT_3	Salicylates,[3,6,7] disalcid,[7] salsalate[7]
↑ RT_3U	High-dose furosemide[3]
Normal TSH	↓ TBG synthesis-cirrhosis/hepatic failure[3]
Normal FT_4I, FT_4	Nephrotic syndrome[3]
Normal FT_3I, FT_3	Danazol[3]
	Glucocorticoids[3]
↓ Peripheral $T_4 \rightarrow T_3$ Conversion	
↓ TT_3	PTU
Normal TT_4	Propranolol[8]
Normal FT_4I, FT_4	Glucocorticoids[3]
Normal TSH	
↓ Pituitary and Peripheral $T_4 \rightarrow T_3$	
↓ TT_3	Ipodate, iopanoic acid[9–11]
↑ TT_4	Amiodarone[12,13]
↑ TSH (transient)	Euthyroid sick syndrome[3,14–18]
↑ FT_4I	
↑ T_4 Clearance by Enzyme Induction/↑ Fecal Loss	
↓ TT_4	Phenytoin[19–22]
↓ FT_4I	Phenobarbital[19]
Normal or ↓ FT_4	Carbamazepine[19]
Normal or ↓ TT_3	Cholestyramine, colestipol[23,24]
Normal or ↑ TSH	Rifampin[19]
↓ TSH Secretion	Dopamine[2]
	Levodopa[2]
	Glucocorticoids[2]
	Bromocriptine[3]
	Octreotide[3]
↑ TSH	Metoclopramide[2,3,25]
	Domperidone[26]

[a]FT_3 = Free triiodothyronine; FT_4 = Free thyroxine; FT_3I = Free triiodothyronine index; FT_4I = Free thyroxine index; PTU = Propylthiouracil; RT_3U = Resin triiodothyronine uptake; TBG = Thyroxine-binding globulin; T_3 = Triiodothyronine; T_4 = Thyroxine; TSH = Thyroid-stimulating hormone; TT_3 = Total triiodothyronine; TT_4 = Total thyroxine. From references 1 to 3.

Notes:

Table 46.3 • Clinical and Laboratory Findings of Primary Hypothyroidism[a]

Symptoms	Physical Findings	Laboratory
General: weakness, tiredness, lethargy, fatigue	Thin brittle nails	↓ TT_4
	Thinning of skin	↓ FT_4I
Cold intolerance	Pallor	↓ FT_4
Headache	Puffiness of face, eyelids	↓ TT_3
Loss of taste/smell	Yellowing of skin	↓ FT_3I
Deafness	Thinning of outer eyebrows	↑ TSH
Hoarseness	Thickening of tongue	Positive antibodies
No sweating	Peripheral edema	(in Hashimoto's)
Modest weight gain	Pleural/peritoneal/pericardial	RAIU <10%
Muscle cramps, aches, pains	effusions	↑ cholesterol
Dyspnea	↓ DTRs	↑ CPK
Slow speech	"Myxedema heart"	↓ Na
Constipation	Bradycardia (↓ HR)	↑ LDH
Menorrhagia	Hypertension	↑ AST
Galactorrhea	Goiter (primary hypothyroidism)	↓ Hct/Hgb

[a]AST = Aspartate aminotransferase; CPK = Creatinine phosphokinase; DTRs = Deep tendon reflexes; FT₃I = Free triiodothyronine index; FT₄I = Free thyroxine index; Hct = Hematocrit; Hgb = Hemoglobin; HR = Heart rate; LDH = Lactate dehydrogenase; Na = Sodium; RAIU = Radioactive iodine uptake; TT₃ = Total triiodothyronine; TT₄ = Total thyroxine.

Table 46.4 • Causes of Hypothyroidism

Nongoitrous (No Gland Enlargement)
Primary Hypothyroidism (Dysfunction of the Gland)
Idiopathic atrophy
Iatrogenic destruction of thyroid
    Surgery
    Radioactive iodine therapy
    X-ray therapy
Postinflammatory thyroiditis
Cretinism (congenital hypothyroidism)

Secondary Hypothyroidism
Deficiency of TSH due to pituitary dysfunction
Deficiency of TRH due to hypothalamic dysfunction

Goitrous Hypothyroidism (Enlargement of Thyroid Gland)
Dyshormonogenesis: defect in hormone synthesis, transport, or action
Hashimoto's thyroiditis[a]
Drug-induced: iodides, lithium,[b] thiocyanates, phenylbutazone, sulfonylureas,[c] amiodarone[d]
Congenital cretinism: maternally induced
Iodide deficiency
Natural goitrogens: rutabagas, turnips, cabbage

[a]Most common cause, an autoimmune disease; intra-thyroidal organo binding of iodine is blocked; can also present as hyperthyroidism
[b]Goiter with or without hypothyroidism can occur in a small percent of patients after 5 months–2 yr of therapy. Most affected individuals have personal or family history of thyroid disease. Inhibits release of thyroid hormone and also may affect the pituitary-thyroid axis. *Effect on thyroid tests:* low TT₄ and FT₄I; elevated TSH and RAIU. Goiter responds to discontinuation of lithium or suppression with thyroid. Discontinuation of lithium can unmask underlying hyperthyroidism.
[c]Large doses of tolbutamide or chlorpropamide (exceeding usual therapeutic range) can inhibit thyroid formation.
[d]Prevalence 6%–16%. Mechanism may be related to high iodine content (37.5 mg organic 1/100 mg) or altered metabolism of T₄ to reverse T₃. Rarely causes hyperthyroidism.

Notes:

Table 46.5 • Thyroid Preparations[a]

Drug/Dosage Forms	Composition	Dosage Equivalent	Comments
Thyroid USP (Armour) *Tab:* 0.25, 0.5, 1, 1.5, 2, 3, 4, and 5 gr	Desiccated hog, beef, or sheep thyroid gland. Standardized iodine content	1 gr[b]	Unpredictable T_4:T_3 ratio; supraphysiologic elevations in T_3 levels might produce toxic symptoms; Armour brand preferred
L-thyroxine (Levoxyl, Synthroid, Levothroid, various) *Tab:* 0.025, 0.050, 0.075, 0.088, 0.112, 0.125, 0.137, 0.15, 0.175, 0.2, and 0.3 mg *Inj:* 200 and 500 µg	Synthetic T_4	60 µg[b]	Stable, predictable potency; well absorbed; more potent than desiccated thyroid. When changing from >2 gr desiccated thyroid to L-T_4, a lower dosage of L-T_4 might be needed to avoid toxicity. Weight should be considered in dosing (1.6–1.7 µg/kg/day)
L-triiodothyronine (Cytomel) *Tab:* 5, 25, and 50 µg *Inj:* 10 µg/mL (Triostat)	Synthetic T_3	25–37.5 µg	Complete absorption; requires multiple daily dosing; toxicity similar to all T_3-containing products; see desiccated thyroid comments
Liotrix (Thyrolar) *Tab:* 0.25, 0.5, 1, 2, and 3 gr	60 µg T_4:15 µg T_3 50 µg T_4:12.5 µg T_3	Thyrolar-1	No need for liotrix because T_4 is converted to T_3 peripherally; expensive, stable, and predictable content

[a] gr = Grain; Inj = Injection; T_3 = Triiodothyronine; T_4 = Thyroxine; Tab = Tablet.
[b] 60 mg (1 gr) of desiccated thyroid = 60 µg of T_4.[36]

Notes:

Table 46.6 • Treatment of Hypothyroidism[a]

Patient Type/Complications	Dose (L-thyroxine)	Comment
Uncomplicated Adult	1.6-1.7 µg/kg/day; 100-125 µg/day average replacement dose; usual increment 25 µg Q 6-8 weeks	*Onset of action:* 2-3 weeks; *max effect:* 4-6 weeks. Reversal of skin and hair changes may take several months. An FT_4 or FT_4I and TSH should be checked 6-8 weeks after initiation of therapy because T_4 has a half-life of 7 days and 3-4 half-lives are needed to achieve steady state. Levels obtained before steady-state can be very misleading. Since 80% bioavailable, adjust IV doses downward. Small changes can be made by varying dose schedule (e.g., 150 µg QD except Sunday)
Elderly	1.6 µg/kg/day (50-100 µg/day)	Initiate T_4 cautiously. Elderly may require less than younger patients. Sensitive to small dose changes. A few patients >60 yr require ≤50 µg/day
Cardiovascular Disease (Angina, CAD)	Start with 12.5-25 µg/day. ↑ by 12.5-25 µg/day Q 2-6 weeks as tolerated	These patients very sensitive to cardiovascular effects of T_4. Even subtherapeutic doses can precipitate severe angina, MI, or death. Replace thyroid deficit slowly, cautiously, and sometimes even suboptimally.
Long-standing Hypothyroidism	Dose slowly. Start with 12.5-25 µg/day. ↑ by 12.5-25 µg/day Q 4-6 weeks as tolerated	Sensitive to cardiovascular effects of T_4. Steady state may be delayed because of ↓ clearance of T_4. Correct replacement dose is a compromise between prevention of myxedema and avoidance of cardiac toxicity.
Pregnant	Most will require 45% ↑ in dose to ensure euthyroidism	Evaluate TSH, TT_4, and FT_4I. *Goal:* normal TSH and TT_4/FT_4I in upper normal range to prevent fetal hypothyroidism
Pediatric 0-3 months	10 to 15 µg/kg/day	Hypothyroid infants can exhibit skin mottling, lethargy, hoarseness, poor feeding, delayed development, constipation, large tongue, neonatal jaundice, pig-like facies, choking, respiratory difficulties, and delayed skeletal maturation (epiphyseal dysgenesis). The serum T_4 should be increased rapidly to minimize impaired cognitive function. In the healthy term infant, 37.5 to 50 µg/day of T_4 is appropriate. Dose decreases with age (Table 46.7)

[a]CAD = Coronary artery disease; FT_4I = Free thyroxine index; TSH = Thyroid-stimulating hormone; T_4 = Thyroxine; TT_3 = Total triiodothyronine; TT_4 = Total thyroxine.
[b]In severely myxedematous patients, steady state may require ≥6 months. In patients who are clinically euthyroid but have ↑ TT_4 and FTI, use ↑ TT_3 and TSH as guide to dose adjustments.

Table 46.7 • T$_4$ Recommended Replacement Dose^a

Age	Daily µg/kg T$_4$
3–6 mo	10–15
6–12 mo	5–7
1–10 yr	3–6
>10 yr	2–4

^{a}T$_4$ = Thyroxine.

Table 46.8 • Clinical and Laboratory Findings of Hyperthyroidism^a

Symptoms
Heat tolerance
Weight loss common; or weight gain caused by ↑ appetite
Palpitations
Pedal edema
Diarrhea/frequent bowel movements
Amenorrhea/light menses
Tremor
Weakness, fatigue
Nervousness, irritability, insomnia

Physical Findings
Thinning of hair (fine)
Proptosis, lid lag, lid retraction, stare, chemosis, conjunctivitis, periorbital edema, loss of extraocular
   movements
Diffusely enlarged goiter, bruits, thrills
Wide pulse pressure
Pretibial myxedema
Plummer's nails^b
Flushed, moist skin
Palmar erythema
Brisk DTRs

Laboratory Findings
↑ TT$_4$
↑ TT$_3$
↑ FT$_4$I/FT$_4$
↑ FT$_3$I
Suppressed TSH
⊕ TRab
⊕ ATgA
⊕ TPO
RAIU >50%
↓ cholesterol
↑ alkaline phosphatase
↑ calcium
↑ AST

^{a}AST = Aspartate aminotransferase; ATgA = Antithyroglobulin antibody; DTRs = Deep tendon reflexes; FT$_4$ = Free
thyroxine; FT$_3$I = Free triiodothyronine index; FT$_4$I = Free thyroxine index; RAIU = Radioactive iodine uptake;
TPO = Thyroperoxidase antibody; TRab = Thyroid-receptor antibodies; TSH = Thyroid-stimulating hormone;
TT$_3$ = Total triiodothyronine; TT$_4$ = Total thyroxine.
^{b}The fingernail separates from its matrix, but only 1 or 2 nails generally are affected.

Notes:

Table 46.9 • Causes of Hyperthyroidism

Graves' disease (toxic diffuse goiter)

Toxic uninodular goiter (Plummer's disease)

Toxic multinodular goiter

Nodular goiter with hyperthyroidism caused by exogenous iodine (Jod-Basedow)

Exogenous thyroid excess through self-administration (factitious hyperthyroidism)

Tumors (thyroid adenoma, follicular carcinoma, thyrotropin-secreting tumor of the pituitary, and hydatidiform mole with secretion of a thyroid-stimulating substance)

Iatrogenic (iodides, amiodarone, interferon-α)

Notes:

Table 46.10 • Treatment for Hyperthyroidism[a]

Modality	Drug/Dosage	Mechanism of Action	Toxicity	Indication
Primary Treatment				
Thioamides				
PTU 50 mg tab; rectal formulation can be made[131]	100–200 mg PO Q 6–8 hr (*max*: 1,200 mg/day) for 6–8 weeks or until euthyroid; then maintenance of 50–150 mg QD PO	Blocks organification of hormone synthesis, blocks peripheral conversion of T_4 to T_3 (PTU only)	Skin rashes, GI symptoms, arthralgias, ↑ transaminases, hepatitis, agranulocytosis	DOC in pregnancy, thyroid storm, breast-feeding.
Methimazole (Tapazole) 5, 10 mg tab; rectal suppositories can be made[132]	Methimazole 30–40 mg PO QD or in 2 divided doses (*max*: 60 mg/day) for 6–8 wk or until euthyroid, then maintenance of 5–10 mg/day PO	Similar to PTU except does not block conversion of T_4 to T_3	Similar to PTU; cholestatic jaundice	Thioamide DOC because QD dosing and better compliance; alternative to PTU in pregnancy; not DOC in breast-feeding or thyroid storm
Surgery	Preoperative preparation with iodides, thioamides, ipodate, or propranolol before surgery; see specific operative agent	Subtotal or total thyroidectomy	Hypothyroidism, cosmetic scarring, hypoparathyroidism, risks of surgery, and anesthesia, vocal cord damage	Obstruction, choking, malignancy, pregnancy in second trimester, contraindication to RAI or thioamides
RAI	^{131}I radioactive isotope: 80–100 μCi/g thyroid tissue. Average dose, ≈10 mCi; pretreatment with corticosteroids indicated in patients with ophthalmopathy	Destruction of the gland	Hypothyroidism; worsening of ophthalmopathy; fear of radiation-induced leukemia; genetic damage; malignancy; rarely, radiation sickness	Adults, older patients who are poor surgical risks or have cardiac disease; patients with a history of prior thyroid surgery; contraindications to thioamide usage
Adjuncts to Primary Usage				
Iodinated contrast dye Ipodate (Oragrafin) Iopanoic acid (Telepaque)	0.5–1 g QD–QOD PO	Blocks T_4 to T_3 conversion; release of iodides to block hormone secretion from thyroid gland	Same as iodides	Alternative to thioamide for rapid control of hyperthyroidism, symptomatic relief of symptoms, adjuncts to surgery, thioamides, and possibly RAI; escape occurs with chronic usage

Drug	Dose	Action	Adverse Effects	Comments
Iodides Lugol's solution 8 mg/drop (5% iodine, 10% potassium iodide; Saturated [SSKI] 50 mg/drop)	5–10 drops TID PO for 10–14 days before surgery; minimum effective dose 6 mg/day	↓ vascularity of gland and ↑ firmness; blocks release of thyroid hormone	Hypersensitivity reactions, skin rashes, mucous membrane ulcers, anaphylaxis, metallic taste, rhinorrhea, parotid and submaxillary swelling; fetal goiters and death	Preoperative preparation before surgery; thyroid storm, provides symptomatic relief of symptoms. *Do not use before RAI or chronically during pregnancy.*
β-Blockers Propranolol or equivalent β-blocker. *Avoid* those with ISA	Propranolol 10–40 mg PO Q 6 hr or PRN to control HR <100 beats/min; IV 0.5–1 mg slowly	Blocks effects of thyroid hormone peripherally, no effect on underlying disease; blocks T_4 to T_3 conversion	Related to β-blockade; bradycardia, CHF, blocks hyperglycemic response to hypoglycemia, bronchospasm, CNS symptoms at high doses; fetal bradycardia	Symptomatic relief while awaiting onset of thioamides, RAI; preoperative preparation for surgery; thyroid storm
Calcium channel blockers	Diltiazem 120 mg TID–QID PO or verapamil 80–120 mg TID–QID PO PRN to control HR <100 beats/min	Blocks effects of thyroid hormone peripherally, no effect on underlying disease	Bradycardia, peripheral edema, CHF, headache, flushing, hypotension, dizziness	Alternative for symptomatic relief of hyperthyroid symptoms in patients who cannot tolerate β-blockers
Corticosteroids	Prednisone or equivalent corticosteroid 50–140 mg/day PO in divided doses; IV hydrocortisone 50–100 mg Q 6 hr or equivalent for thyroid storm	↓ TRab, suppression of inflammatory process; blocks T_4 to T_3 conversion	Complications of steroid therapy	Ophthalmopathy, thyroid storm (use IV steroid), pretibial myxedema, pretreatment before RAI therapy in patients with ophthalmopathy

^aCHF = Congestive heart failure; CNS = Central nervous system; DOC = Drug of choice; GI = Gastrointestinal; HR = Heart rate; ISA = Intrinsic sympathomimetic activity; IV = Intravenous; μCi = Microcurie; mCi = Millicurie; PTU = Propylthiouracil; RAI = Radioactive iodine; Tab = Tablet.

Table 46.11 • Treatment of Thyroid Storm^a

Drug	Dose	Comments
Thioamide	PTU 600–1200 mg/day Q 6 hr Methimazole 60–120 mg/day TID	No parenteral form available. Prepare rectal formulation of methimazole if NPO. PTU theoretical DOC since it has a more rapid onset
Iodides	Ipodate 1 gm/day *or* Lugol's solution, 30 drops/day PO	Blocks release of hormone. Administer at least 1 hr after thioamides to avoid blocking action
Propranolol	1 mg slow IV push Q 5 min until heart rate 90–110/min. *Maintenance infusion:* 5–10 mg/hr *or* 40 mg PO Q 6 hr. Double dose Q 12 hr until therapeutic response achieved	Used to ↓ symptoms of excess adrenergic stimulation (tachycardia, tremulousness, agitation). Preferred over reserpine and guanethidine
Hydrocortisone	100–200 mg IV Q 6 hr	Used to combat hypoadrenalism. Acutely depresses T_3 levels
Supportive therapy	Sedation, oxygen, glucose, hydration, antipyretics, antibiotics	—

^{a}DOC = Drug of choice; NPO = Nothing by mouth; FTU = Propylthiouracil.

The reader is referred to Chapter 47: Thyroid Disorders, written by *Betty J. Dong, Pharm.D.*, in the seventh edition of **Applied Therapeutics: The Clinical Use of Drugs** for a more in-depth discussion. All notations to reference numbers are based on the reference list at the end of that chapter. The editors of this handbook express their thanks to Dr. Dong and acknowledge that this chapter is based upon her work.

Notes:

Chapter 47

Diabetes Mellitus

Inside . . .

(continued)

Definition and Classification

Diabetes is a syndrome caused by an absolute or relative lack of insulin. Presenting symptoms, primarily are related to hyperglycemia and include the 3Ps (polyuria, polydipsia, polyphagia), weight loss, fatigue, and recurrent infections (e.g., vaginal candidiasis). Ketoacidosis signifies an absolute lack of insulin and, generally, type 1 diabetes due to autoimmune destruction of the pancreatic β cells. Type 2 diabetes is a heterogeneous disorder predominantly characterized by peripheral resistance to insulin action, increased hepatic glucose output, and progressive β cell failure. Long-term complications include retinopathy, nephropathy, painful peripheral neuropathy, autonomic neuropathy (impotence, gastroparesis, diarrhea), and macrovascular disease (hypertension, cardiovascular disease, strokes). See Table 47.1.

Diagnosis

For nonpregnant individuals of any age, a diagnosis of diabetes can be made when one of the following is present (see Table 47.3):

- ♦ Classical signs and symptoms of diabetes (polyuria, polydipsia, ketonuria, and rapid weight loss) combined with a random plasma glucose >200 mg/dL.
- ♦ An FPG ≥126 mg/dL.

♦ Following a standard oral glucose challenge (75 g glucose for an adult of 1.75 g/kg for a child), the venous plasma glucose concentration is ≥200 mg/dL at 2 hours and >200 mg/dL at least one other time during the test (0.5, 1, 1.5 hours); this is the oral glucose tolerance test (OGTT).

Treatment

The major components of treatment include diet, exercise, and drugs along with self-monitoring of blood glucose and self care made possible through intensive and continuous patient education. None of the key treatment elements should be modified in isolation of the others. See appropriate tables listed below.

Goals of Therapy

♦ Eliminate or diminish symptoms related to hyperglycemia (see above), hypoglycemia, and long-term complications.

♦ Slow and prevent long-term complications through euglycemia and elimination of cardiovascular risk factors (e.g., obesity, hypertension (<130/80 mm Hg), dyslipidemia, sedentary lifestyle, smoking).

♦ Maintain normal growth and development of children and adolescents; meet increased metabolic needs during pregnancy and lactation.

♦ Provide sufficient education and training to allow patient to be as self-sufficient in modifying behavior, diet, and medication to the extent possible.

Notes:

Table 47.1 • Type 1 and Type 2 Diabetes[a]

Characteristics	Type 1	Type 2
Other names	Previously, type I; insulin-dependent diabetes mellitus (IDDM); juvenile-onset diabetes mellitus	Previously, type II; noninsulin-dependent diabetes mellitus (NIDDM); adult onset diabetes mellitus
Percentage of diabetic population	5–10%	90%
Age at onset	Usually <30 yr; peaks at 12–14 yr; rare before 6 mo; some adults develop type 1 during the fifth decade	Usually >40 yr but increasing prevalence among obese children
Pancreatic function	Usually none, although some residual C-peptide can sometimes be detected at diagnosis, especially in adults	Insulin present in low, "normal," or high amounts
Pathogenesis	Associated with certain HLA types; presence of islet cell antibodies suggests autoimmune process	Defect in insulin secretion; tissue resistance to insulin; ↑ hepatic glucose output
Family history	Generally not strong	Strong
Obesity	Uncommon unless "overinsulinized" with exogenous insulin	Common (60–90%)
History of ketoacidosis	Often present	Rare, except in circumstances of unusual stress (e.g., infection)
Clinical presentation	Moderate-to-severe symptoms that generally progress relatively rapidly (days to weeks): polyuria, polydipsia, fatigue, weight loss, ketoacidosis	Mild polyuria, fatigue; often diagnosed on routine physical or dental examination
Treatment	Insulin Diet Exercise	Diet Exercise Oral antidiabetic agents (α-glucosidase inhibitors, biguanides, meglitinides, sulfonylureas, thiazolidinediones) Insulin

[a]HLA = Human leukocyte antigen.

Table 47.2 • Risk Factors for Gestational Diabetes Mellitus (GDM)[a]

- Maternal age >35 yr
- History of GDM
- History of polyhydramnios (excess amniotic fluid)
- Family history of diabetes (parents or siblings)
- Obesity: >20% IBW or BMI >27 kg/m^2
- Prior infant weight >9 lb at birth (macrosomia)
- Prior infant with congenital anomalies
- Previous unexplained fetal demise
- Ethnicity: Hispanic, Native American, Asian American, African American, or Pacific Islander

[a]GDM = BMI = Body mass index; IBW = Ideal body weight.

Table 47.3 • Normal and Diabetic Plasma[a] Glucose Levels in mg/dL for The Oral Glucose Tolerance Test (OGTT)

	Fasting	½, 1, 1½ hr	2 hr
Normal	<110 (6.1)	<200 (11)	<140 (7.8)
Impaired glucose tolerance (IGT)	<126 (7.0)	≥200 (11)	140–200 (7.8–11)
Impaired fasting glucose (IFG)	>110–125 (6.1–7.0)		
Diabetes (nonpregnant adult)	≥126 (7.0)	≥200 (11)	≥200 (11)

[a]Equivalent *venous whole blood* glucose concentrations are approximately 12 to 15% lower. *Arterial* samples are higher than venous samples postprandially because glucose has not yet been removed from peripheral tissues. *Capillary whole blood* samples contain a mixture of arterial and venous blood. Fasting levels will be equivalent to whole blood venous samples. One hour following a 100-g glucose load, capillary samples may be 30 to 40 mg/dL higher than venous samples.

Table 47.4 • Estimating Ideal Body Weight (IBW) and Body Mass Index (BMI)

Ideal Body Weight
1. Obtain height and weight.
2. Determine body frame (small, medium, or large).
3. Calculate ideal body weight:
   - Female: 100 lb (45 kg) for first 5 ft plus 5 lb (2.3 kg) for every inch over 5 ft
   - Male: 106 lb (48 kg) for first 5 ft plus 6 lb (2.7 kg) for each inch over 5 ft
   - Add 10% for large frame or subtract 10% for small frame

Body Mass Index
BMI = kg/m^2

$$BMI = \frac{Weight\ (in\ pounds) \div 2.2\ pounds/kg}{[Height\ (in\ inches) \times 2.5\ cm/inch \times 100]^2}$$

BMI (Healthy)	19–25 kg/m^2
BMI (Obese)	>27 kg/m^2
BMI (Morbid Obesity)	>30 kg/m^2

[a]The term *reasonable body weight* also is used. Reasonable body weight is defined as a weight that is achievable and maintainable for the patient, which may not be in the range considered desirable. Any weight loss, even 10 to 20 lb, may dramatically improve glycemic control. Weight goals should always be individualized. Adapted from reference 27.

Table 47.5 • Determining Caloric Needs

1. Determine basal energy expenditure (BEE) using the Harris-Benedict equation[27]:
   - Female: 655 + (9.6 × weight [kg]) + (1.9 × height [cm]) − (4.7 × age)
   - Male: 66 + (13.7 × weight [kg]) + (5 × height [cm]) − (6.8 × age)
2. Select appropriate activity factor:
   - Sedentary: Multiply by 1.3
   - Moderately active: Multiply by 1.45
   - Heavily active: Multiply by 1.6
3. Caloric needs = BEE × activity factor
4. For weight gain, add 500 calories to gain 1 lb/week. To lose weight, subtract 500 calories.

Notes:

Table 47.6 • Principles of Medical Nutritional Therapy

Calories
For young individuals, provide sufficient calories to maintain normal growth and development. For obese individuals, restrict caloric intake (500–1000 kcal below daily requirement) to improve tissue responsiveness to insulin. Avoid fad diets, extremely hypocaloric diets, fasts, and appetite suppressants

Content
Carbohydrates: 55%–60% of caloric intake. Emphasize complex carbohydrates. Modest amounts of simple sugars with meals may be allowed, depending on patient weight and metabolic control. Provide adequate carbohydrates at times that match the peak action of insulin

Fat: 30% of caloric intake with <10% from saturated fats and <10% from polyunsaturated fats. Restrict cholesterol intake to <300 mg/day to prevent cardiovascular disease and to <200 mg/day in people with elevated LDL

Protein: 10%–15% of caloric intake (0.8 gm/kg). May need to be restricted in patients with renal or hepatic failure or liberalized in children, elderly, and lactating women

Salt: 3000 mg/day. Restrict further in patients with hypertension, CHF, and certain renal diseases

Soluble Fiber: Emphasize foods high in fiber since these may slow carbohydrate absorption. Avoid in immobile or bedridden individuals

Alcohol: Modest amounts of unsweetened alcohol (e.g., 4 oz of dry white wine). No more than 2 drinks per day for men and one for women. Caloric content of alcohol must be considered

Distribution
Individuals treated with insulin must eat regularly scheduled meals and snacks to prevent hypoglycemic reactions

Patients with Type 2 diabetes treated with diet or sulfonylureas should attempt to space meals by 4–5 hr since normalization of postprandial glucose concentration is delayed. Do not skip meals if taking a long-acting sulfonylurea (e.g., glyburide)

Table 47.7 • Converting Plasma Glucose (mg/dL) to Whole Blood Glucose Values or to mmol/L

Converting to Equivalent Whole Blood Glucose Concentrations (mg/dL)
Whole blood glucose (mg/dL) = Plasma glucose (mg/dL) × 0.85

Conversion to mmol/L

$$\text{Plasma glucose (mmol/L)} = \frac{\text{Plasma glucose (mg/dL)}}{18}$$

Notes:

Table 47.8 • Factors Affecting HbA$_{1c}$[a]

Cause	Effect on HbA$_{1c}$
Alterations in RBC Survival	
• Hemoglobinopathies	Decreased
• Anemias	
Hemolytic	Decreased
Iron deficiency	Decreased[b]
• Blood loss	Decreased
Assay Interference	
• Uremia	Increased or no change[c,d]
• Hemodialysis	No change[c]
• Antioxidants	Decreased[e]

[a] HbA$_{1c}$ = Glycosylated hemoglobin; RBC = Red blood cell.
[b] For patients receiving iron replacement therapy. Normal levels would be expected in untreated patients.
[c] Interference seen in assays utilizing high-pressure liquid chromatography (HPLC) and electroendosmosis. Affinity chromatography appears unaffected.
[d] Carbamylated hemoglobin equaling 0.063% of total hemoglobin is formed for every 1 mmol/L of serum urea.
[e] Reported with vitamins C (1 g/day) and E (1,200 mg/day). Possible mechanism is competitive inhibition of hemoglobin glycosylation.

Table 47.9 • Insulin Pharmacokinetics[a]

Clearance

Total clearance	700–800 mL/min
Hepatic clearance	300–400 mL/min
Renal clearance	190–270 mL/min

IV Infusion
Elimination follows multicompartment model

Half-life for three compartments are as follows: 2.3–2.4 min, 14 min, 133 min

Insulin action most closely corresponds to last compartment. Therefore, it is unnecessary to adjust the dose more frequently than Q 2 hr

SC Administration of Regular Insulin[b]
Intermittent Boluses
Half-life (absorption, 70–120 min)

Half-life (elimination, 53 min)

SC Infusion
Steady state achieved in 6–8 hr

If infusion is discontinued, check for rise in glucose ketones after 2 or 3 hr. Because there is no SC pool, effects dissipate quickly

SC Administration of Intermediate-acting Insulins[b]
NPH half-life (absorption) 12–19 hr

[a] IV = Intravenous; NPH = Isophane insulin suspension; SC = Subcutaneous.
[b] Insulin absorption varies by 25% within the same individual and 50% among individuals. See Table 47.12 for factors that influence absorption.
Adapted from reference 46.

Notes:

Table 47.10 • Insulins Available in USA

Type/Duration of Action	Animal Source/ Manufacturing Process	Brand Name	Manufacturer
Rapid-acting			
Lispro	Recombinant DNA	Humalog	Lilly
Insulin aspart	Recombinant DNA	NovoLog	Novo Nordisk
Short-Acting			
Regular			
Purified	Pork	Regular Iletin II	Lilly
Human	Recombinant DNA	Humulin R	Lilly
		Novolin R[a]	Novo Nordisk
		Velosulin BR[b]	Novo Nordisk
Intermediate-acting			
NPH (Isophane Insulin Suspension)			
Purified	Pork	Pork NPH Iletin II	Lilly
Human	Recombinant DNA	Humulin N	Lilly
		Novolin N[a]	Novo Nordisk
Lente (Insulin Zinc Suspension)			
Purified	Pork	Lente Iletin II (Pork)	Lilly
Human	Recombinant DNA	Humulin L	Lilly
		Novolin L[a]	Novo Nordisk
NPH/Regular Mixture (70%/30%)			
Human	Recombinant DNA	Humulin 70/30	Lilly
		Novolin 70/30[b]	Novo Nordisk
NPH/Regular Mixture (50%/50%)			
Human	Recombinant DNA	Humulin 50/50	Lilly
NPL/Lispro Mixture (75%/25%)			
Human	Recombinant DNA	Humalog Mix75/25	Lilly
Long-acting			
Ultralente (Insulin Zn Suspension, Extended)			
Human	Recombinant DNA	Humulin U Ultralente	Lilly
Insulin glargine			
Human	Recombinant DNA	Lantus	Aventis

[a] These products also are available in 1.5-mL cartridges for use in "pen" delivery devices (Novolin Pen and as prefilled syringes).
[b] Phosphate-buffered product. Preferred for use in insulin pumps.

Table 47.11 • Insulin Pharmacodynamics[a]

Insulin	Onset (hr)	Peak (hr)	Duration (hr)	Appearance
Lispro	1/4	1/2–1 1/2	4–5	Clear
Insulin aspart	5–10 min	1–3	3–5	Clear
Regular	1/2–1	2–4	5–7	Clear
NPH	1–2	6–14	24+	Cloudy
Lente	1–3	6–14	24+	Cloudy
Ultralente[b]	6	18–24	36+	Cloudy
Insulin glargine	—	—	24	Clear[c]

[a] The onset, peak, and duration of insulin activity may vary considerably from times listed in this table. See text and Table 47.12.
[b] Human Ultralente may have a shorter duration of action. Some patients require twice-daily dosing.
[c] The only extended-duration insulin that is clear. It should not be mixed with other insulins or administered intravenously.

Table 47.12 • Factors Altering Onset and Duration of Insulin Action[a]

Factor	Comments
Route of Administration	Onset of action more rapid and duration of action shorter for IV>IM>SC[260–262] Intranasal insulin has more rapid onset and shorter duration than SC insulin, resembling IV pharmacokinetics[46,263,264]
Factors Altering Clearance Renal function	Renal failure ↓ insulin clearance. May prolong and intensify action of exogenous and endogenous insulin[36,37]
Insulin antibodies	IgG antibodies bind insulin as it is absorbed and release it slowly, thereby delaying and/or prolonging its effect[43]
Thyroid function	Hyperthyroidism ↑ clearance but also ↑ insulin action, making control difficult. Patients stabilize as they become euthyroid[265]
Factors Altering SC Absorption Site of injection	Factors that ↑ SC blood flow ↑ absorption rates of regular insulin. Effect on intermediate- and long-acting insulins minimal Rate of absorption fastest from the abdomen, intermediate from the arm, and slowest from the thigh[66] Less variation observed in type 2 patients. Less variation observed with lispro insulin *Site* *Half-Life Absorption (min)* Abdomen 87 ± 12 Arm 141 ± 23 Hip 153 ± 28 Thigh 164 ± 15
Exercise of injected area	Strenuous exercise of an injected area within 1 hr of injection can ↑ absorption rate. Rate of absorption of regular insulin ↑ but little effect on intermediate-acting insulin[46,266]
Ambient temperature	Heat (e.g., hot weather, hot bath, sauna) ↑ absorption rate. Cold has opposite effect[46,267]
Local massage	Massaging injected area for 30 min substantially ↑ absorption rate of regular insulin as well as longer-acting insulins[266]
Smoking	Controversial. Vasoconstriction may ↓ absorption rate[46]
Jet injectors	Insulin absorption more rapid, probably secondary to ↑ surface area for absorption[268]
Lipohypertrophy	Insulin absorption is delayed from lipohypertrophic sites[68]
Insulin preparation	More soluble forms of insulin are absorbed more rapidly and have shorter durations of action (see Table 47.11 and text). Human insulin may have shorter action than animal insulin
Insulin mixtures	The short-acting properties of regular insulin may be lost if mixed with Lente insulins (see Question 14)
Insulin concentration	More dilute solutions (e.g., U-40, U-10) are absorbed more rapidly than more concentrated forms (U-100, U-500)[40,44]
Insulin dose	Lower doses are absorbed more rapidly and have a shorter duration of action than larger doses

[a]IgG = Immunoglobulin G; IM = Intramuscular; IV = Intravenous; SC = Subcutaneous.

Notes:

Table 47.13 • Components of Intensive Insulin Therapy[a]

Multicomponent insulin regimen

Balance of carbohydrate intake, exercise, and insulin dosage

Daily, multiple self-monitoring of blood glucose levels

Patient self-adjustment of carbohydrate intake and insulin dosage with use of supplemental regular insulin according to a predetermined plan

Individualized target blood glucose and HbA_{1c} levels

Frequent contact between patient and diabetes team

Intensive patient education

Psychologic support

Regular objective assessment (as measured by HbA_{1c})

[a]HbA_{1c} = Glycosylated hemoglobin.
Modified from reference 54.

47.14 • Goals of Intensive Insulin Therapy[a,b]

Target Blood Glucose Values	Ideal[c] (mg/dL)	Acceptable[d] (mg/dL)	Pregnancy (mg/dL)
Fasting	70–120	70–140	60–90
Preprandial	70–105	70–130	60–105
1 hr postprandial	100–160	100–180	110–130
2 hr postprandial	80–120	80–150	90–120
2–4 AM	70–100	70–120	>60
HbA_{1c}[a]	<6%	≤7–8%	<6%
Urine ketones[e]	Absent	Rare	Rare

[a]HbA_{1c} = Glycosylated hemoglobin. Normal values vary; normalize to laboratory.
[b]Modified and extrapolated from references 17 and 59. Intensive insulin therapy is a complete therapeutic program of diabetes management and requires a team approach (see Table 47.13).
[c]Ideal values approximate those seen in nondiabetic individuals and are included for illustrative purposes only.
[d]Acceptable values should be individualized to levels that are attainable without creating undue risk for hypoglycemia. These results are similar to the results achieved in the DCCT trial. These values may be inappropriate for patients with hypoglycemic unawareness, counterregulatory insufficiency, angina pectoris, or other complicating features (see Table 47.17).
[e]Does not apply to type 2 diabetes patients.

Notes:

Table 47.15 • Examples of Flexible Insulin Regimens

AM	Noon	PM	Bedtime	Comments
Method 1				This regimen relies on the AM NPH or Lente to cover the noon meal and to provide basal insulin during the day. The evening NPH or Lente supplies basal insulin during the night. However, the evening NPH has peak activity at ≈ 2–4 AM when plasma glucose is at a physiologic nadir, predisposing the patient to nocturnal hypoglycemia. Empirically, some clinicians use a 1:2 ratio of Reg:NPH. If lispro or insulin glargine is used, we recommend basing the dose on an empiric insulin unit:grams carbohydrate ratio of 1:15 initially. See Table 47.16.
Reg/NPH	—	Reg/NPH	—	
Reg/Lente		Reg/Lente		
Lispro/NPH		Lispro/NPH		
Lispro/Lente		Lispro/Lente		
Aspart/NPH		Aspart/NPH		
Aspart/Lente		Aspart/Lente		
Method 2				See notes for Method 1. By shifting the NPH or Lente dose to bedtime, the peak action occurs in the early morning (5–7 AM), when the patient is awake and ready to eat. This also corresponds to the dawn phenomenon, a natural rise in the plasma glucose from growth hormone. See Method 1 comments for empirical doses.
Reg/NPH	—	Reg	NPH	
Reg/Lente		Reg	Lente	
Lispro/NPH		Lispro	NPH	
Lispro/Lente		Lispro	Lente	
Insulin aspart/NPH		Insulin aspart	NPH	
Insulin aspart/Lente		Insulin aspart	Lente	
Method 3				These methods provide premeal boluses of insulin. The evening dose of NPH, Lente, or insulin glargine provides basal levels at night to prevent lipolysis and suppress glycogenolysis and gluconeogenesis. Often, the intermediate- or long-acting insulins must be given twice daily to provide sufficient basal insulin throughout the day. When insulin glargine (Lantus) replaces two injections of NPH or Lente, the initial dose should be reduced by 20% from the previous day's total daily dose of intermediate-acting insulin. See regimens for Method 4.
Reg	Reg	Reg	NPH	
Reg	Reg	Reg	Lente	
Reg	Reg	Reg	Glargine	
Method 4				Lispro or insulin aspart is substituted for regular insulin in Method 3. Postprandial values are lower, but one may see preprandial hyperglycemia because the duration of action is too brief to supply sufficient levels of basal insulin during the day. To address this issue, some clinicians are combining lispro with regular insulin or very low doses of intermediate-acting insulin before meals (1 unit/hr). When lispro is used as the mealtime insulin, a minimum of two injections of intermediate-acting insulin is required. When insulin glargine (Lantus) replaces two injections of NPH or Lente, the initial dose should be reduced by 20% from the previous day's total daily dose of intermediate-acting insulin. See Method 6. Empirically, the lispro dose is based on the estimated CHO intake (1 unit/15 g). See Table 47.16.
Lispro/NPH	Lispro	Lispro	NPH	
Lispro/Lente	Lispro	Lispro	Lente	
Lispro	Lispro	Lispro	Glargine	
Aspart/NPH	Aspart	Aspart	NPH	
Aspart/Lente	Aspart	Aspart	Lente	
Aspart	Aspart	Aspart	Glargine	

(continued)

Table 47.15 • Examples of Flexible Insulin Regimens (continued)

AM	Noon	PM	Bedtime	Comments
Method 5				Because human Ultralente has a relatively short duration of action, it must be dosed twice daily to maintain smooth basal concentrations. However, because its onset is slow, a short-acting insulin must be given before the noon meal. Ultralente can be given at approximately 50% of the total daily dose with half of the dose given before breakfast and the other half given before dinner. Insulin glargine (Lantus), another long-acting insulin, cannot be mixed with other insulin because its pharmacodynamic profile could be altered. It may be given once daily.
Reg/Ultralente	Reg	Reg/Ultralente	—	
Lispro/Ultralente	Lispro	Lispro/Ultralente		
Aspart/Ultralente	Aspart	Aspart/Ultralente		
Method 6				Some patients achieve better control of fasting hyperglycemia by using NPH at bedtime to target early-morning insulin resistance while continuing to take Ultralente each morning.
Reg/Ultralente	Reg	Reg	NPH	
Lispro/Ultralente	Lispro	Lispro	NPH	
Aspart/Ultralente	Aspart	Aspart	NPH	

Reg, regular insulin.

Notes:

Table 47.16 • Empiric Insulin Doses[a,58]

Estimating Total Daily Insulin Requirements
These are initial doses only; they must be refined using SMBG results. Patients may be particularly resistant to insulin if their blood glucose concentrations are high (glucose toxicity); once glucose concentrations begin to drop, insulin requirements often decrease precipitously. The weight used is actual body weight. Insulin dose requirements can change dramatically over time, depending on circumstances (e.g., a growth spurt, modest weight gain or loss, illness).

Type 1 Diabetes
Initial dose	0.5–0.8 U/kg
Honeymoon phase	0.2–0.5 U/kg
With ketosis, during illness, during growth	1.0–1.5 U/kg

Type 2 Diabetes
With insulin resistance	0.7–1.5 U/kg

Estimating Basal Insulin Requirements
These are empiric doses only and should be adjusted using appropriate SMBG results (fasting or premeal). Basal requirements vary throughout the day, often increasing during the early morning hours. The requirement also is influenced by the presence of endogenous insulin, the degree of insulin resistance, and body weight. The range is 0.3 to 1.4 U/hr.
   Approximately 50% of total daily dose
   Approximately 0.7 U/hr for a 70-kg person (154 lb)

Estimating Premeal Insulin Requirements
Patients who are insulin resistant may require as much as 1 U for every 6 g of CHO ingested. Conversely, those who are exquisitely sensitive to insulin or have some endogenous insulin may require only 1 U for every 20+ g CHO. Use 1:10 for individuals >180 lb and 1:15 for individuals <140 lb.
   Approximately 1 U/10–15 g CHO

Estimating "Touch-Up" Doses of Lispro
Supplemental doses of rapid-acting insulin are administered to acutely lower glucose concentrations that exceed the target glucose concentration. These doses must be individualized for each patient and again are based on the degree of sensitivity to insulin action. For example, if the premeal or bedtime blood glucose target is 140 mg/dL and the patient's value is 190 mg/dL, an extra unit might be added to the premeal dose or an additional supplemental bedtime dose of lispro might be given. If the patient is resistant, doses as high as 1 U per 25 mg/dL may be required; ultrasensitive individuals may require 1 U per ≥60 mg/dL.
   1 U per approximately 50 mg/dL more than the plasma glucose goal is a conservative empiric dose

[a]CHO = Carbohydrate; SMBG = Self-monitored blood glucose

Notes:

Table 47.17 • Intensive Insulin Therapy: Indications and Precautions

Patient Selection Criteria
- Type 1, otherwise healthy patients (older than 13 yr of age) who are highly motivated and compliant individuals. Must be willing to test blood glucose concentrations four times daily and inject three to four doses of insulin daily
- Diabetic women who plan to conceive
- Pregnant diabetic patients
- Patients poorly controlled on conventional therapy (includes type 2 patients)
- Technical ability to test blood glucose concentrations
- Intellectual ability to interpret blood glucose concentrations and adjust insulin doses appropriately
- Access to trained and skilled medical staff to direct treatment program and provide close supervision

Avoid or Use Cautiously in Patients Who Are Predisposed to Severe Hypoglycemic Reactions or in Whom Such Reactions Could Be Fatal
- Patients with counterregulatory insufficiency
- Type 1 diabetes for ≥15 yr (not all patients)
- β-Adrenergic blocker therapy
- Autonomic insufficiency
- Adrenal or pituitary insufficiency
- Patients with coronary or cerebral vascular disease
  (*Note:* Counterregulatory hormones released in response to hypoglycemia may have adverse effects in these individuals)
- Unreliable, noncompliant individuals, including those who abuse alcohol or drugs and those with psychiatric disorders

Table 47.18 • Areas of Patient Education

Diabetes: Pathogenesis and the complications

Hyperglycemia: Signs and symptoms

Ketoacidosis: Signs and symptoms (see Table 47.28)

Hypoglycemia: Signs, symptoms, and treatment (see Table 47.27)

Exercise: Effect on blood glucose concentrations and insulin dose (see Table 47.25)

Diet: See Table 47.6

Insulins:
    Injection technique
    Types of insulin (animal source, NPH, regular)
    Onset and peak actions
    Storage
    Stability (look for crystallization and precipitation)

Therapeutic Goals: HbA_{1c}, blood glucose, cholesterol, triglycerides

Self-Monitored Blood Glucose Testing: See Table 47.19

Interpretation of self-monitored blood glucose testing results

Foot Care: Inspect feet daily; wear well-fitted shoes; avoid self-care of ingrown toenails, corns, or athlete's foot; see a podiatrist

Sick Day Management: See Table 47.26

Cardiovascular Risk Factors: Smoking, high blood pressure, obesity, elevated cholesterol

Importance of annual ophthalmologic examinations; tests for microalbuminuria

Notes:

Table 47.19 • Self-Monitored Blood Glucose Testing (SMBG): Patient Education

When and How Often to Test

Technique
- How and when to calibrate the machine
- Review all "buttons" and their purposes. Identify battery case. Review cleaning procedures

Preparation
1. Calibrate machine
2. Turn machine on
3. Prepare all materials: tissue, strip, lancet
4. Remember to close the lid of the strip container immediately. Strips exposed to air and moisture deteriorate rapidly
5. Wash hands with warm water. *Dry thoroughly.* A wet finger causes blood to spread rather than form a drop. Milk the finger from the base to ensure an adequate flow of blood. Some patients use a rubber band as a tourniquet
6. Lance the tip of the finger. Avoid the pads of the finger, where nerves are concentrated
7. Hold the finger *below* the heart with the lanced area pointing toward the floor
8. Once a sufficient amount of blood is available, *quickly* cover the *entire* pad or designated area with blood. Do not touch the pad with your fingers. Note: Many devices now require small quantities of blood.

Record Results in a Log Book and Bring to All Physician Visits. Include Relevant Information Regarding Unusual Alterations in Diet or Exercise

How to Use Results to Achieve Normoglycemia

Table 47.20 • Factors That Can Alter SMBG Results: Troubleshooting

- Machine improperly calibrated[a]
- Strips out of date or stored improperly[b]
- An inadequate amount of blood applied or smeared onto the strip[b]
- For strips that require blotting or wiping:
  Strip improperly blotted[a]
  Too much force applied to strip[b]
  Blood removed too early or contact time with reagent otherwise shortened[b]
  Blood removed beyond the specified time[c]
- Dirty meter[a]
- Low battery[a]
- Test performed outside of temperature and humidity operating conditions[a]
- Low[c] or high[b] hematocrit
- Dehydration[b]
- Hyperosmolar, nonketotic state[b]
- Lipemia[a]
- High levels of ascorbic acid or salicylates (rare)[b]

[a] Effect unpredictable.
[b] Values tend to be lower.
[c] Values tend to be higher.

Notes:

Table 47.21 • Interpreting Self-Monitored Blood Glucose Concentrations[a]

Test Time	Target Insulin Dose	Target Meal/Snack
Prebreakfast (Fasting)	Predinner/bedtime intermediate- or long-acting insulin	Bedtime snack
Prelunch	Prebreakfast regular insulin	Breakfast/midmorning snack
Predinner	Prebreakfast intermediate-acting insulin and/or prelunch regular insulin	Lunch/midafternoon snack
Bedtime	Predinner regular insulin	Dinner
2-hour postprandial	Premeal lispro insulin or insulin aspart	Preceding meal or snack
3 AM or later	Predinner intermediate-acting insulin	Dinner/bedtime snack

[a]Considerations: (1) Assumes a normal meal pattern. For patients who travel, have odd working or sleeping hours, or irregular meal patterns, these rules may not apply. (2) Assumes administration of regular insulin 30 to 60 minutes before meals or lispro insulin 15 minutes before meals and a normal pattern of insulin response (see Table 47.12 for factors that can alter insulin absorption and response). (3) If prebreakfast concentrations are high, rule out reactive hyperglycemia (Somogyi reaction or posthypoglycemic hyperglycemia). Consider contribution of dawn phenomenon as well. Whenever blood glucose concentrations are high, consider reactive hyperglycemia (excessive insulin doses). (4) Consider accuracy of reported test results: (a) Do they correlate with HbA$_{1c}$ and patient's signs and symptoms? (b) What is the patient's compliance? Could results be fabricated? (c) Is patient's technique appropriate? Check timing, adequate blood sample, machine, strips, calibration, and removal of blood (see Table 47.19). (d) Are insulin kinetics altered (see Table 47.19)? (e) Meals: consider content, quality, and regularity.

Table 47.22 • Factors That Can Alter Blood Glucose Control

Diet
Insufficient calories (e.g., alcoholism, eating disorders, anorexia, nausea, and vomiting)
Overeating (e.g., during the holidays)
Irregularly spaced or delayed meals
Dietary content (e.g., fiber, carbohydrate content)

Physical Activity
See Table 47.25

Stress
Infection
Surgery/trauma
Psychologic

Drugs
See Tables 47.38 and 47.39 for information about medications that affect blood glucose levels

Hormonal Changes
Menstruation: glucose concentrations may ↑ premenstrually and return to normal postmenses
Pregnancy
Puberty: hyperglycemia probably related to high growth hormone levels

Gastroparesis
Delays gastric emptying time. Peak insulin action and meal-related glucose excursions may become mismatched

Altered Insulin Pharmacokinetics
See Table 47.12

Insulin Injection Technique
Measuring
Timing
Technique

Inactive Insulin
Outdated insulin
Improperly stored insulin (heat or cold)
Crystallized insulin

Table 47.23 • Compatibility of Insulin Mixtures

Mixture	Proportion	Comments
Regular + NPH Regular + Lente	Any proportion <1 : 1	The pharmacodynamic profiles of regular and NPH insulin are unchanged when premixed and stored in vials or syringes for up to 3 months. In contrast, the rapid action of regular insulin is significantly blunted when mixed with Lente or Ultralente insulin. The excess zinc in Lente preparations binds the regular insulin, converting it into an intermediate-acting form. When the two insulins are mixed just before injection, the clinical importance of this effect appears to be minimal.
Lispro + NPH	Any proportion	The absorption rate and peak concentration of lispro is blunted when mixed with NPH; however, total bioavailability is unaltered. The manufacturer recommends mixing the two insulins just before injection.
Lispro + Ultralente	Any proportion	Ultralente does not alter the pharmacokinetics of lispro.
Regular + normal saline	Any proportion	Use within 2–3 hours of preparation.
Regular + insulin-diluting solution	Any proportion	Stable indefinitely.
Insulin glargine	Do not mix with other insulins	Pharmacodynamics could be modified.

Notes:

Table 47.24 • Guidelines for Dosing Insulin

Basic Insulin Dose
- First adjust the basic insulin dose (i.e., the dose that the patient will be instructed to take daily). This assumes that diet and physical activity are stable. Set a reasonable goal initially. This may mean the upper limits of the acceptable concentrations may be high initially (e.g., <200 mg/dL). Move toward a more ideal goal slowly.

- Only adjust insulin doses if a *pattern* of response is observed under stable diet and exercise circumstances. That is, the same response to insulin is observed for ≥3 days. It is important to verify the stability of diet and exercise. Consider adjusting these variables as well.

- Unless all levels are >200 mg/dL, try to adjust one component of insulin therapy at a time.

- Start with the insulin component affecting the fasting blood glucose concentration. This glucose level often is the most difficult to control and often affects all other glucose concentrations measured throughout the day.

- Adjust the basic insulin dose by 1–2 U at a time. The amount prescribed is based on the individual patient's response to insulin. This can be determined by looking at the patient's total daily dose on a U/kg basis (see the following and Table 47.16).

Supplementary Insulin Doses
- Once the basic dose of insulin has been established, supplemental doses of rapid- or short-acting insulin can be prescribed to correct excessive *preprandial* glucose concentrations. For example, if the goal is 140 mg/dL, and the glucose value is 190 mg/dL, administer an additional unit of lispro insulin. Supplemental doses also can be used when the patient is ill (see Table 47.26).

- Algorithms for supplemental doses are based on the patient's sensitivity to insulin. Generally, they are in the range of 1–2 U for every 50 mg/dL *above* the goal. If values ≥200 mg/dL, consider delaying the meal by another 20–30 min (i.e., 60 min after injection) (see Table 47.16).

- If premeal glucose concentrations are <60–70 mg/dL, the dose of lispro or regular insulin administered before the meal is ↓ 1–2 U; insulin administration is delayed until just before the meal; the meal should include an extra 15 g of glucose if the value is <50 mg/dL.

- If supplemental doses before a given meal are required for ≥3 days, the basic insulin dose should be adjusted appropriately. For example, if a patient taking lispro before meals requires an extra 2 U 2 hours after breakfast for ≥3 days, 2 U should be added to the prebreakfast dose.

Anticipatory Insulin Doses
- The basic insulin dose is increased or decreased based on the anticipated effects of diet or physical activity.

- Increase lispro or regular insulin by 1 U for each additional 15 g of carbohydrate ingested (e.g., holiday meal) or decrease the usual dose by 1–2 U if the meal is smaller than usual (see Table 47.16).

- See Table 47.25 for recommended insulin adjustments for exercise.

Table 47.25 • Exercise in Patients with Diabetes

1. Test blood glucose concentrations before, during, and after exercise.
2. For moderate exercise (e.g., bicycling or jogging for 30–45 min), ↓ the preceding dose of regular insulin by 30–50%. If glucose concentration is normal or low before exercise, supplement the diet with a snack containing 10–15 g of carbohydrate.
3. To avoid ↑ absorption of regular insulin by exercise, inject into the abdomen or exercise 30 min–1 hr following injection.
4. Individuals with low glycogen stores may be predisposed to the hypoglycemic effects of exercise. Examples include alcoholics, fasted individuals, or patients on extremely hypocaloric (<800 calories), low-carbohydrate (<10 g/day) diets.
5. Patients taking insulin are more susceptible to hypoglycemia than those taking sulfonylureas. Patients with type 2 diabetes mellitus treated with diet are unlikely to develop hypoglycemia.
6. Watch for postexercise hypoglycemia. Individuals who have been exercising during the day (e.g., skiing) should ↑ their carbohydrate intake and test their blood glucose concentration during the night to detect nocturnal hypoglycemia. Hypoglycemia can occur 8–15 hr following exercise.
7. If the glucose concentration is >240–300 mg/dL, the patient should not exercise. This indicates severe insulin deficiency. These patients are predisposed to hyperglycemia secondary to exercise.
8. Patients with severe proliferative retinopathy or retinal hemorrhage should avoid jarring exercise or exercise that involves moving the head below the waist.

Table 47.26 • Sick-Day Management

1. Continue taking your basic dose of insulin *even* if you are not eating well or have nausea or vomiting.
2. Test your blood glucose more frequently: every 3–4 hr.
3. If indicated, give yourself *supplemental* doses of lispro or regular insulin: for example, 1–2 U for every 30–50 mg/dL over an agreed-upon target glucose concentration (e.g., 150 mg/dL). Supplemental doses must be individualized based on the patient's sensitivity to insulin (see Table 47.16).
4. Begin testing your urine for ketones, especially when glucose readings exceed 300 mg/dL.
5. Try to drink plenty of fluid (½ cup/hr for adults) and maintain your caloric intake (50 g carbohydrate Q 4 hr). Foods such as Jell-O, noncarbonated soft drinks, crackers, soup, and soda may be used.
6. Call a physician if your blood glucose concentration remains >300 mg/dL or your urine ketones remain high after two or three supplemental doses of insulin.

Table 47.27 • Hypoglycemia[a]

Definition
- Blood glucose concentration <50 mg/dL; patient may or may not be symptomatic. Blood glucose <40 mg/dL; patient generally symptomatic. Blood glucose <20 mg/dL can be associated with seizures and coma.

Signs and Symptoms
- Blurred vision, sweaty palms, generalized sweating, tremulousness, hunger, confusion, anxiety, circumoral tingling and numbness. Patients vary with regard to their symptoms. Behavior can be confused with inebriation. Patients become combative and use poor judgment.

- *Nocturnal hypoglycemia:* nightmares, restless sleep, profuse sweating, morning headache, morning "hangover." In one study, 80% of patients with nocturnal hypoglycemia had no symptoms.

Clinical Considerations
- Irregular eating patterns
- ↑ physical exercise
- Gastroparesis: (delayed gastric emptying time)
- Defective counterregulatory responses
- Excessive oral sulfonylureas
- Drugs

Treatment
- 10–20 g rapidly absorbed carbohydrate. Repeat in 15–20 min if glucose concentration remains <60 mg/dL or if patient is symptomatic. Follow with complex carbohydrate/protein snack if meal time is not imminent.

- The following are examples of food sources that provide 10 g of carbohydrate:

Orange juice; regular, nondiet soda	½ cup
Apple juice	⅓ cup
Grape juice	¼ cup
Sugar	2 tsp or 2 cubes
Lifesavers	5–6 pieces
B/D glucose tablets	2 tablets

- If patient is unconscious the following measures should be initiated:
  Glucagon 1 mg SC, IM, or IV (Mean response time, 6.5 min)
  Glucose 25 g IV (Dextrose 50%, 50 mL)
  (Mean response time, 4 min)

[a]IM = Intramuscular; IV = Intravenous; SC = Subcutaneous.

Notes:

Table 47.28 • Diabetic Ketoacidosis (DKA): Patient Education

Definition: DKA occurs when the body has insufficient insulin.

Questions to Ask:
1. Has use been discontinued or a dose of insulin skipped for any reason?
2. If an insulin pump is being used, is the tubing clogged or twisted? Has the catheter become dislodged?
3. Has the insulin being used lost its activity? Is the bottle of regular insulin cloudy? Does the bottle of NPH appear frosty?
4. Have insulin requirements increased due to illness or other forms of stress (infection, pregnancy, pancreatitis, trauma, hyperthyroidism, or myocardial infarction)?

What to Look For:
1. Signs and symptoms of hyperglycemia: thirst, excess urination, fatigue, blurred vision, consistently elevated blood glucose concentrations (>300 mg/dL)
2. Signs of acidosis: fruity breath odor, deep and difficult breathing
3. Signs of dehydration: dry mouth; warm, dry skin; fatigue
4. Others: stomach pain, nausea, vomiting, loss of appetite

What to Do:
1. Review "Sick Day Management"
2. Test blood glucose four or more times daily
3. Test urine for ketones when blood glucose concentration is >300 mg/dL
4. Drink plenty of fluids (water, clear soups)
5. Continue taking insulin dose
6. Contact physician immediately

Table 47.29 • Common Laboratory Abnormalities in DKA[a]

Glucose	>700 mg/dL
Serum osmolarity	>340 in presence of coma
Sodium	Low, normal, or high[b]
Potassium	Normal or high
Ketones	Present in urine and blood
pH	<7.2
Bicarbonate	<15 mEq/L
WBC count	15,000–40,000 cells/mm, even without evidence of infection

[a] DKA = Diabetic ketoacidosis; WBC = White blood cell.
[b] Total body sodium is always low.

Notes:

Table 47.30 • Management of Diabetic Ketoacidosis (DKA)

Fluid Administration
- Use normal saline if patient is hypotensive or Na <140 mEq/L. If evidence of adequate perfusion (e.g., normal pulse and blood pressure, good skin turgor) and Na >150 mEq/L, use half normal saline.

- *Rate:* 1 L over 30 min–1 hr, followed by 1 L over second hr, then 500–1,000 mL/hr until corrected

Insulin
- Continuous IV infusion of regular insulin is preferred. Use IM route only if infusion is not available.

- *Loading Dose:* 0.1 U/kg IV (optional) *or* 20 U IM (advisable)

- *Maintenance Dose:* 0.1 U/kg/hr IV *or* 5–10 U/hr IM

- If no change in blood glucose level after 1 hr, double infusion rate.

- Once blood glucose <300 mg/dL, reduce infusion rate and change fluid to 5% dextrose (do not stop insulin infusion).

- When SC insulin can be initiated, administer dose 30 min before discontinuing IV infusion.

Potassium
- Add 20–40 mEq to IV fluids, except in patients with chronic renal failure, no urine output, or initial potassium level >6.0 mEq/L.

Phosphate
- Initiate if level <1 mg/dL. Use potassium phosphate salt, 40–60 mEq. Rarely needed.

Bicarbonate
- Replacement is controversial and may be dangerous.

Notes:

Table 47.31 • Oral Antidiabetic Pharmacokinetic Data^a

Drug (Brand Name) Available Tablet Strengths (mg)	Typical Dosing Regimen (mg)	Usual Minimum and Maximum Total Daily Dose/How Divided	Mean Half-Life	Approximate Duration of Activity	Bioavailability, Metabolism, and Excretion	Comments
α-Glucosidase Inhibitors						
Acarbose (Precose) 25, 50, 100 mg	25–100 mg with first bite of each meal. Begin with 25 mg; ↑ by 25 mg/meal every 4–8 weeks.	Minimum: 25 mg TID Maximum dose is 50 mg TID if <60 kg; 100 mg TID if >60 kg.	2.8 hr	Affects absorption of complex carbohydrates in a single meal	F = 0.5–1.7%; extensively metabolized by GI amylases to inactive products; 50% excreted unchanged in the feces	Titrate doses slowly to avoid GI effects
Miglitol (Glyset) 25, 50, 100 mg	25–100 mg with first bite of each meal. Begin with 25 mg; ↑ by 25 mg/meal every 4–8 weeks.	Minimum: 25 mg TID Maximum: 100 mg TID	2 hr	Affects absorption of complex carbohydrates in a single meal	Dose of 25 mg is completely absorbed; dose of 100 mg 50–70% absorbed; elimination by renal excretion as unchanged drug	
Biguanides						
Metformin (Glucophage) 500, 850 mg	Begin with 500 mg QD or BID; ↑ by 500 mg QD every 1–2 weeks.	0.5–2.5 g BID or TID	Plasma, 6.2 hr Whole blood, 17.6 hr	6–12 hr	F = 50–60%; excreted unchanged in urine	Avoid in patients with renal failure or those who could be predisposed to lactic acidosis (e.g. alcoholics, CHF, severe respiratory disorders, liver failure)
Metformin extended release (Glucophage XR) 500 mg	500–1,000 mg QD with evening meal; ↑ by 500 mg every 1–2 weeks.	1,500–2,000 mg QD	As for metformin, but active drug is released slowly	24 hr	As for metformin	As for metformin
Meglitinides						
Repaglinide (Prandin) 0.5, 1, 2 mg	If HbA$_{1c}$ is <8% or if this is first drug, begin with 0.5 mg with each meal. For others, begin with 1–2 mg/meal.	0.5–4 mg with each meal (16 mg/day) TID–QID	1 hr	C$_{max}$ is at 1 hr; duration is approximately 2–3 hr	F = 56%; 92% metabolized to inactive products by the liver; 8% excreted as metabolites unchanged in the urine	Take only with meals. Skip dose if meal is skipped.

Drug	Dose range	Dosing/titration	Half-life	Onset/Duration	Metabolism/Excretion	Comments
Nateglinide (Starlix) 60, 120 mg	60 or 120 mg TID	120 mg TID 1–30 min before meals; 60 mg TID for patients with near-normal HbA$_{1c}$ at initiation.	1.5 hr	Onset, 20 min; peak, 1 hr; duration, 2–4 hr	F = 73%; metabolized to inactive products (predominantly) that are excreted in the urine (83%) and feces (10%)	Skip dose if meal is skipped.
First-Generation Sulfonylureas						
Acetohexamide (Dymelor) 250, 500 mg	0.25–1.5 g QD or BID	250 or 500 mg QD; ↑ by 250 mg daily every 1–2 weeks.	5 hr (active metabolite)	12–18 hr	Activity of metabolite greater than parent drug. Metabolite excreted, in part, by kidney	Caution in elderly and patients with renal disease. Significant uricosuric effects
Chlorpropamide (Diabinese) 100, 250 mg	0.1–0.5 g QD	100 or 250 mg QD; ↑ by 100 or 250 mg every 1–2 weeks.	35+ hr	24–72 hr	Inactive and weakly active metabolites; 20% excreted unchanged; varies widely	Caution in elderly and patients with renal impairment. Highest frequency of side effects relative to other sulfonylureas
Tolazamide (Tolinase) 100, 250, 500 mg	0.2–1 g QD or BID	100–250 mg QD; ↑ by 100 or 250 mg every 1–2 weeks.	7 hr (4–25)	12–24 hr	Some metabolites with moderate activity excreted via kidney	Active metabolites may accumulate in renal failure
Tolbutamide (Orinase) 250, 500 mg	0.5–3 g BID or TID	250 mg BID before meals; ↑ by 250 mg daily every 1–2 weeks.	7 hr	6–12 hr	Metabolized to compounds with negligible activity	No special precautions. Shortest-acting sulfonylurea
Second-Generation Sulfonylureas						
Glimepiride (Amaryl) 1, 2, 4 mg	1–8 mg QD	1–2 mg QD initially; usual maintenance dose is 1–4 mg.	9 hr	24 hr	F = 100%; completely metabolized by liver. Principal metabolite is slightly active (30% of parent compound). Excreted by the urine (60%) and feces (40%)	Probably safe in patients with renal failure, but low initial doses are recommended for older patients and those with renal insufficiency. Incidence of hypoglycemia may be lower than other long-acting sulfonylureas
Glipizide (Glucotrol) 5, 10 mg	2.5–40 mg QD or BID[b]	2.5 mg QD in elderly, 5 mg QD in others; ↑ by 2.5 or 5 mg every 1–2 weeks.	2–4 hr	12–24 hr	Metabolized to inactive compounds	No special precautions. Daily dose >15 mg should be divided. Dose 30 min before meals

(continued)

Table 47.31 • Oral Antidiabetic Pharmacokinetics^a (continued)

Drug (Brand Name) Available Tablet Strengths (mg)	Typical Dosing Regimen (mg)	Usual Minimum and Maximum Total Daily Dose/How Divided	Mean Half-Life	Approximate Duration of Activity	Bioavailability, Metabolism, and Excretion	Comments
Second-Generation Sulfonylureas *(continued)*						
Glipizide extended-release (Glucotrol XL) 5 mg	5 mg QD; ↑ by 5 mg every 1–2 weeks.	5–20 mg QD	4–13 hr	24 hr	Same as glipizide	Use with caution in patients with pre-existing GI narrowing due to possible obstruction
Glyburide (Diabeta, Micronase) 1.25, 2.5, 5 mg	1.25 mg QD in elderly, 2.5 mg QD in others; ↑ by 1.25 or 2.5 mg every 1–2 weeks.	1.25–20 mg QD or BID^a	4–13 hr	12–24 hr	Metabolized to inactive/weakly inactive compounds; 50% excreted in urine and 50% in feces	Caution in elderly patients with renal failure and others predisposed to hypoglycemia. Daily doses >10 mg should be divided
Micronized Glyburide (Glynase PresTab) 1.5, 3 mg	1.5 mg QD; ↑ by 1.5 mg every 1–2 weeks.	1.0–12 mg QD	4 hr	24 hr	Metabolized to inactive/weakly inactive compounds; 50% excreted in urine and 50% in feces	Daily doses >6 mg should be divided. ↑ bioavailability relative to original formulation, resulted in reduced dose
Thiazolidinediones						
Rosiglitazone (Avandia) 2, 4, 8 mg	4 mg QD initially; ↑ to 8 mg QD (or 4 mg BID) in 12 weeks.	4–8 mg daily in single or divided doses	3–4 hr	Onset and duration poorly correlated with half-life because of mechanism of action. Onset at 3 weeks; max at 4+ weeks. Offset likely to be similar	F = 99%; extensively metabolized in liver into inactive metabolites; excreted ⅔ in urine and ⅓ in feces	Food has no effect on absorption. BID dosing may have greater HbA_{1c} lowering effect. No dose adjustments required in renal failure

Pioglitazone (Actos) 15, 30, 45 mg	15–30 mg QD; increase to 45 mg QD in 3–4 weeks. If used with insulin, ↓ insulin dose by 10–25% once FPG <120 mg/dL.	15–45 mg QD	3–7 hr (16–24 hr for all metabolites)	Same as previous	Extensively metabolized in liver. 15–30% excreted in urine, remainder eliminated in the feces	Food delays absorption but is not clinically significant. No dose adjustments required in renal disease

Combination Products

Glyburide/ Metformin (Glucovance)[c] 1.25/500, 2.5/500 mg 5.0/500 mg	2.5/500 mg QD or BID; ↑ by 2.5/500 mg every 1–2 weeks.	7.5/1,500–10/2,000 mg in two to three divided doses with meals	See metformin	See metformin	See metformin and glyburide	Effect should be similar to the two agents given in combination. Minimum dose of 1,500 mg metformin is needed for effect. No need to exceed 10 mg glyburide

[a]CHF = Congestive heart failure; C_{max} = Maximal clearance; F = Bioavailability; FPG = Fasting plasma glucose; GI = Gastrointestinal.
[b]These are maximum doses indicated by the manufacturers. Studies indicate that maximum insulin responses and glucose-lowering effects occur at doses of 10 mg/day.[132,133]
[c]FDA approval in August 2000.

Table 47.32 • Comparative Pharmacology of Antidiabetic Agents[a,b]

Agent Generic Name Brand Name Mechanism	FDA Indications	Efficacy	Adverse Effects	Comments
Insulin Replaces or augments endogenous insulin	Monotherapy; combined with any oral agent	$\downarrow$ HbA$_{1c}$ ∞ $\downarrow$ FPG ∞ $\downarrow$ PPG ∞ $\downarrow$ TG	Hypoglycemia, weight gain, lipodystrophy; local skin reactions.	Offers flexible dosing to match life-style and glucose concentrations. Rapid onset. Safe in pregnancy, renal failure, and liver dysfunction. Drug of choice when patients do not respond to oral agents.
Insulin-Augmenting Agents				
• *Meglitinides* Repaglinide (Prandin; NovoNorm) Nateglinide (Starlix) Stimulate insulin secretion.	Monotherapy; combined with metformin	$\downarrow$ HbA$_{1c}$ 1.7% $\downarrow$ FPG 61 mg/dL $\downarrow$ PPG 48 mg/dL	Hypoglycemia, weight gain.	Take only with meals. If a meal is skipped, skip a dose. Flexible dosing with life-style. Safe in renal and liver failure. Rapid onset.
• *Sulfonylureas* Various; see Table 47.33 Stimulate insulin secretion. May decrease hepatic glucose output and enhance peripheral glucose utilization.	Monotherapy; combined with metformin; combined with insulin (glimepiride)	$\downarrow$ HbA$_{1c}$ 1.5–1.7% $\downarrow$ FPG 50–70 mg/dL $\downarrow$ PPG 92 mg/dL	Hypoglycemia, especially long-acting agents; weight gain (4–22 lb). Rash, hepatotoxicity, alcohol intolerance, and hyponatremia are rare.	Very effective agents but cause hyperinsulinemia, which leads to hypoglycemia and weight gain. Some can be dosed once daily. Rapid onset of effect (1 week).
Insulin-Assisting Agents/Insulin Sensitizers				
• *α-Glucosidase Inhibitor* Acarbose (Precose) Miglitol (Glyset) Slow absorption of complex carbohydrates.	Monotherapy; combined with SFUs	$\downarrow$ HbA$_{1c}$ 0.5–1.0% $\downarrow$ FPG 20–30 mg/dL $\downarrow$ PPG 25–50 mg/dL	GI: flatulence, diarrhea. Elevations in LFTs seen in doses >50 mg TID of acarbose. Therefore, LFTs should be monitored every 3 months during the first year of therapy and periodically thereafter. Because miglitol is not metabolized, monitoring of LFTs is not required.	Titrate dose slowly to minimize GI effects. No hypoglycemia or weight gain. If used in combination with hypoglycemic agents, advise patients to treat hypoglycemia with glucose tablets, because absorption is not inhibited as with sucrose.

Insulin Sensitizers

• *Biguanides* Metformin (Glucophage) ↓ Hepatic glucose output; ↑ peripheral glucose uptake; ↓ or slowed CHO absorption.	Monotherapy; combined with SFUs	↓ HbA$_{1c}$ 1.5–1.7% ↓ FPG 50–70 mg/dL ↓ PPG 83 mg/dL ↓ TG 10–20% ↓ Total cholesterol 5–10% ↑ HDL (slight)	GI: cramping, diarrhea. Lactic acidosis (rare).	Titrate dose slowly to minimize GI effects. No hypoglycemia or weight gain; weight loss possible. Do not use in patients with ↓ renal or hepatic function or CHF requiring treatment.
• *Thiazolidinediones* Rosiglitazone (Avandia)	Monotherapy; or combined with metformin	↓ HbA$_{1c}$: Monotherapy: 0.8–1.5%[c] Combination: 0.7–1.2% ↓ FPG 25–60 mg/dL	Generally well tolerated. Mild anemia. 1.9% of patients on rosiglitazone, 2–3.5% of patients on pioglitazone. Mild-to-moderate edema with rosiglitazone and pioglitazone (4.8–9.1% of patients).	Pioglitazone/Rosiglitazone: LFTs must be measured at baseline, every 2 months during the first year, and periodically thereafter.
Pioglitazone (Actos)	Monotherapy; or combined with SFU, or metformin or insulin	↓ HbA$_{1c}$: Monotherapy: 0.6–1.9[c] Combination: 0.7–1.3% ↓ FPG 30–65 mg/dL *Effects on lipids (all):* ↓ TG 26% (variable with rosiglitazone) ↓ PPG 40–65 mg/dL ↑ HDL 8–14% ↑ LDL-C 5–19%[d] (variable with pioglitazone)	Weight gain: 1.2–3.5 kg with rosiglitazone, 2–8 kg with pioglitazone. Rare idiosyncratic cellular hepatotoxicity could be a problem as with troglitazone, which was removed from the market. Newer agents thought to be less hepatotoxic. Drug interactions reported with pioglitazone.	These agents can be used in renal failure. Slow onset (2–4 weeks).
"Insulin sensitizers"—enhance insulin action in the periphery. ↑ glucose utilization by muscle (primary) and ↓ hepatic glucose output.				

[a]CHF = Congestive heart failure; FDA = U.S. Food and Drug Administration; FPG = Fasting plasma glucose; GI = Gastrointestinal; HbA$_{1c}$ = Glycosylated hemoglobin; HDL = High-density lipoprotein; LFTs = Liver function tests; LDL = Low-density lipoprotein; LDL-C = Low-density lipoprotein cholesterol; PPG = Postprandial plasma glucose; SFU = Sulfonylurea; TG = Triglyceride.
[b]See text for expanded discussion and references.
[c]As monotherapy, no significant decrements in the HbA$_{1c}$ were observed. Significant therapeutic effects were observed for 600 mg only. Change in HbA$_{1c}$ and FPG values primarily reflect observations of troglitazone in combination with insulin or other oral agents.
[d]LDL/HDL ratio does not change. LDL particle may be "fluffier" type that is less subject to oxidation.

Table 47.33 • Pharmacokinetic Drug Interactions with Oral Antidiabetic Agents[a]

Drugs	Comments
Pharmacokinetic Drug Interactions with Sulfonylureas	
Drugs Increasing Sulfonylurea Effect	
• Antacids	Enhanced glyburide absorption due to increased gastric pH. Avoid concomitant administration.
• Chloramphenicol	↓ tolbutamide hepatic metabolism and ↑ $t_{1/2}$ 2- to 3-fold. Possible prolongation of chlorpropamide $t_{1/2}$.
• Cimetidime	↓ tolbutamide hepatic metabolism by 17% in one study. Ranitidine had no effect.
• Clofibrate	May displace sulfonylureas from proteins, ↓ insulin resistance, ↓ renal tubular secretion of chlorpropamide.
• Doxepin	Mechanism unknown. Monitor for hypoglycemia.
• Fluconazole	Increased plasma concentrations. Watch for hypoglycemia.
• Gemfibrozil	Possibly due to protein displacement. May need to reduce dose of sulfonylurea.
• Halofenate	Increases serum concentrations.
• Heparin	Heparin may have significantly prolonged glipizide hypoglycemia in one unconvincing case report. Confirmation needed.
• Methandrostenolone	Enhances hypoglycemic effect. Consider nandrolone and methenolone acetate.
• Methyldopa	↑ mean tolbutamide $t_{1/2}$ by 24% in one study.
• Nonsteroidal anti-inflammatory drugs	Sulfinpyrazone and phenylbutazone ↓ tolbutamide hepatic metabolism and ↑ $t_{1/2}$ 2- to 3-fold. Enhanced hypoglycemia secondary to acetohexamide (↓ renal excretion of active metabolite) and chlorpropamide also reported. Severe or fatal hypoglycemia can occur. Ibuprofen, naproxen, sulindac, and tolmetin do not affect sulfonylurea disposition.
• Salicylates	Limited and indirect documentation (primarily in vitro) that salicylates may ↑ sulfonylurea activity through protein-binding displacement or inhibition of active renal tubular secretion.
• Sulfonamide antimicrobials	Cotrimoxazole ↓ tolbutamide metabolism and ↑ $t_{1/2}$ by 30% in one study. Severe hypoglycemia with glyburide and chlorpropamide reported rarely. Sulfisoxazole also rarely associated with tolbutamide- and chlorpropamide-induced severe hypoglycemia.
• Warfarin	No evidence that warfarin affects sulfonylurea disposition; however, dicumarol ↑ tolbutamide (and possibly chlorpropamide) $t_{1/2}$ 3- to 4-fold, probably by ↓ hepatic metabolism. Sulfonylureas do not appear to alter patient response to the anticoagulants. Warfarin response should be monitored if glyburide is initiated, discontinued, or changed in dosage.
Drugs Decreasing Sulfonylurea Effect	
• Alcohol	Chronic ethanol use ↑ tolbutamide hepatic metabolism 2-fold. Conversely, short-term ethanol infusions ↓ tolbutamide clearance by 50%.
• Rifampin	↑ tolbutamide and glyburide metabolism, thereby ↓ $t_{1/2}$ and plasma drug concentrations.
Other Drugs	
• Cyclosporine	May compete with glipizide for cytochrome P450 hydroxylation. Necessitated a 20–30% dosage reduction of cyclosporine in two case reports.
• Phenytoin	Unknown effects on sulfonylureas; however, tolbutamide transiently ↑ free phenytoin concentrations through protein-binding displacement by approximately 45% in one study.

(continued)

Table 47.33 • Pharmacokinetic Drug Interactions with Oral Antidiabetic Agents^a (continued)

Drugs	Comments

Pharmacokinetic Drug Interactions with Metformin

- Alcohol — Potentiates the effects of metformin on lactate metabolism. Patients should avoid excessive alcohol intake.
- Cimetidine — Increase in peak metformin plasma concentrations. May necessitate a reduction in metformin dose.
- Erythromycin — Severe cholestatic hepatitis reported when used in combination with chlorpropamide. Monitor liver enzymes and bilirubin or use alternate antibiotic.
- Iodinated parenteral contrast dye — Can result in acute renal failure and metformin-induced lactic acidosis. Metformin should be withheld at least 48 hours before and 48 hours after the procedure. Reinstitute metformin only after renal function has been determined to be normal.

Pharmacokinetic Drug Interactions with α-Glucosidase Inhibitors

- Charcoal/digestive enzyme preparations — Intestinal adsorbents (e.g., charcoal) and digestive enzyme preparations (e.g., amylase, pancreatin) may reduce the effect of acarbose.
- Digoxin — Serum digoxin concentrations may be reduced, decreasing the therapeutic effects.
- Propranolol — Miglitol may significantly reduce the bioavailability of propranolol by 40%.
- Ranitidine — Miglitol may significantly reduce the bioavailability of ranitidine by 60%.

Pharmacokinetic Drug Interactions with Thiazolidinediones (excluding Rosiglitazone)

- Cholestyramine — Concomitant administration reduces troglitazone absorption by 70%.
- Ketoconazone — Ketoconazole appears to significantly inhibit the metabolism of pioglitazone. Glycemic control should be evaluated more frequently in patients taking these agents in combination.
- Oral contraceptives — Troglitazone and pioglitazone reduce plasma concentrations of oral contraceptives containing ethinyl estradiol and norethindrone. Result is a possible loss of contraception. Watch for symptoms of estrogen deficiency (e.g., hot flushes) in women taking estrogen hormone-replacement therapy.
- Terfenadine — Coadministration decreases plasma concentrations of terfenadine by 50–70%, possibly reducing terfenadine effectiveness. Proposed mechanism is induction of hepatic microsomal enzymes by troglitazone. Also may apply to concomitant use of troglitazone with cyclosporine, tacrolimus, and HMG-CoA reductase inhibitors.

^aHMG-CoA = 3-hydroxy-3-methyl-glutaryl coenzyme A; $t_{1/2}$ = Half-life.

Notes:

Table 47.34 • Assessment and Counseling Points: Type 2 Diabetes

For All Patients

- Educate about symptoms of *hyperglycemia,* including frequent urination, excessive thirst, unexplained weight loss, fatigue, and recurrent infections, which signal inadequate control.
- Educate about symptoms of *hypoglycemia,* including hunger, anxiety, rapid heart rate, sweatiness, morning headaches, and restless sleep. Skipped meals can predispose to hypoglycemia. May occur when antidiabetic agents are used in combination.
- Encourage patients to follow blood glucose concentrations according to *SMBG (self-monitoring of blood glucose).* Review physician's goals. Help patients interpret levels in context of diet, exercise, and drug therapy. *Periodically review patients' technique for appropriate meter use.*
- Reinforce principles of *diet, exercise,* and *smoking cessation.*
- Update *medication profile.* Include nonprescription medications, nutritional supplements, and alternative medicines. Review for drug–drug and drug–disease interactions.
- Review and reinforce *ADA Standards of Care,* including the following:
  - HbA$_{1c}$ quarterly for patients poorly controlled; semiannually for stabilized patients. Review target values.
  - Annual lipid panel
  - Annual evaluation for microalbuminuria
  - Annual retinal examination by an ophthalmologist
  - Annual foot examinations (*Note:* Patients with a history of previous lower extremity event should have monthly foot examinations.)
  - Blood pressure measurements *every visit.*

Sulfonylureas

- *First Generation:* Tolbutamide (Orinase), Chlorpropamide (Diabinese), Tolazamide (Tolinase), Acetohexamide (Dymelor)
- *Second Generation:* Glipizide (Glucotrol), Glyburide (Micronase, Glynase, DiaBeta), Glimepiride (Amaryl)
- This drug stimulates the release of insulin from the pancreas. The pancreas may not release insulin as rapidly as it should after one has eaten. The amount of insulin it releases may not be sufficient to lower blood glucose concentrations.
- Meals should *not* be skipped.
- Symptoms of hypoglycemia must be watched for.
- Weight gain is possible.

Repaglinide (Prandin), Netaglinide (Starlix)

- This drug stimulates the release of insulin from the pancreas. The pancreas may not release insulin as rapidly as it should after one has eaten. The amount of insulin it releases may not be sufficient to lower blood glucose concentrations.
- Dose should be taken up to 30 minutes before meals.

- Drug should *not* be taken if meal has been skipped.
- Symptoms of hypoglycemia must be watched for.
- Weight gain is possible.

Metformin (Glucophage)

- This drug decreases the production of glucose by the liver. The liver is probably producing more glucose than normal, and this is contributing to high blood glucose levels.
- Initially, gastrointestinal discomfort or diarrhea may be experienced. This usually *lessens* with time and can be minimized if taken with food and if doses are gradually increased.
- Any change in general health should be brought to the attention of the physician in charge of the patient's diabetes management. This applies particularly to problems affecting the heart, lungs, kidneys, or liver. *Unusual symptoms to be reported to the doctor include the following: severe fatigue, unexpected stomach discomfort, dizziness, shortness of breath, unexpected fluid retention, or sudden development of a slow or irregular heartbeat.*
- The drug may have to be discontinued temporarily if a special x-ray examination or radiologic procedure is needed. Under these circumstances, the radiologist or general physician must be reminded that metformin is being taken.

Thiazolidinediones (Rosiglitazone [Avandia], Pioglitazone [Actos])

- These drugs improve the ability of the muscle to respond to insulin. Insulin allows the muscle to take in glucose from meals and store it for future use.
- Drug should be taken once daily or twice daily with or without food.
- Rarely, rosiglitazone has been associated with liver problems. Blood tests should be checked for liver function every 1–2 months as directed by the physician. *Any unusual symptoms of fatigue, gastrointestinal distress, or increased abdominal girth should be reported to the physician.*
- Menstrual periods may resume, and pregnancy may occur. (For patients with polycystic ovarian syndrome only.)
- A birth control pill with higher amounts of estrogen may be required. A doctor should be consulted. (For patients taking low-dose oral contraceptives.)
- Any reappearance of menopausal symptoms, such as hot flushes, should be reported to the doctor. (For patients taking estrogen replacement therapy.)

α-Glucosidase Inhibitors (Acarbose [Precose], Miglitol [Glyset])

- These drugs slow the absorption of sugars and starches from the intestines. They do so by blocking the breakdown of these foods.
- *Each dose* should be taken with the first bite of each meal.

(continued)

Table 47.34 • Assessment and Counseling Points: Type 2 Diabetes (continued)

α-Glucosidase Inhibitors (Acarbose [Precose], Miglitol [Glyset]) (continued)

- When these drugs are begun, gas and soft stools or diarrhea may be experienced. This lessens with time and can be minimized by increasing the dose gradually as prescribed.
- Acarbose or miglitol by themselves do not cause hypoglycemia, but low blood glucose levels can occur if they are used in combination with other antidiabetic agents. Commercially available *glucose tablets* should be used to treat low blood sugar reactions because other carbohydrate sources, such as those containing sucrose or fructose, may not be absorbed quickly if acarbose or miglitol is being taken.

Insulin

- This drug is used to supplement the insulin secreted by the pancreas.
- Rapid- and short-acting insulins are designed to help cells utilize glucose from meals about to be eaten. Lispro insulin should be given 15 minutes before a meal. Eating should not be delayed. Regular insulin generally is given 30 minutes before the meal.
- NPH (or Lente) insulin can last for 12–24 hours, depending on the dose being used. This insulin is primarily used to maintain low

levels of insulin between meals. This insulin decreases glucose production by the liver.

- Ultralente insulin lasts 18–24 hours, and insulin glargine lasts 24 hours. Their functions are the same as those of NPH or Lente insulin.
- Normally, the body secretes just enough insulin to match sugar and starch (carbohydrate) intake from meals. When insulin is injected, sugar and starch intake must instead be matched to the dose and action of insulin. Therefore, it is very important to spread carbohydrate intake throughout the day and to eat regularly.
- The patient should be aware of when each insulin he or she uses will have its maximum effect. This is when he or she will be most vulnerable to low blood glucose or insulin reactions.
- The vial of insulin in use may be kept at room temperature. When a vial is opened, it should be dated. Some manufacturers recommend against use of the insulin 30 days after it has been opened.
- Inspect insulin vials for crystals or unusual particles. Regular lispro, aspart, and glargine insulins should appear as clear fluids. All other insulins are milky suspensions.
- Mixing, measuring, and injection techniques should be reviewed periodically.

Notes:

Table 47.35 • Treating Type 2 Diabetes Under Special Circumstances

Circumstance	Avoid	Consider
Patients with decreased renal function	Acarbose[a] Acetohexamide Chlorpropamide Glyburide Metformin	Glipizide Glimepiride Insulin Repaglinide Thiazolidinediones Tolazamide
Patients with impaired liver function	Acarbose[a] Acetohexamide Chlorpropamide Metformin Troglitazone ? Glyburide	Insulin Repaglinide[b] Miglitol
Patients who are obese or gaining excessive weight	Insulin[c] Sulfonylureas Repaglinide ? Thiazolidinediones[d]	Acarbose Miglitol Metformin
Patients experiencing hypoglycemia due to irregular eating patterns	Insulin Long-acting sulfonylureas	Acarbose Metformin Repaglinide Troglitazone

[a]This is a labeled recommendation. Although very little acarbose is absorbed into the systemic circulation, the small amount available relies on the kidneys for elimination. This accumulation and doses ≥300 mg daily rarely have been associated with elevated liver enzymes. Plasma concentrations of miglitol in renally impaired volunteers were proportionally increased relative to the degree of renal dysfunction.
[b]The manufacturer recommends more cautious dose titration in these cases.
[c]This recommendation presumes that the patient can be controlled on oral agents. Often by the time insulin is required in type 2 diabetes, pancreatic function may have deteriorated considerably.
[d]The effects of troglitazone on weight are negligible in some studies and considerable in others. When troglitazone is combined with sulfonylureas, a mean weight gain of 5.8 to 13.1 pounds was observed. Rosiglitazone is associated with mild weight gain (1.2 to 3.5 kg), and pioglitazone has been associated with mild-to-moderate weight gain (2 to 8 kg).

Table 47.36 • Presentation of Diabetes Mellitus in Elderly Patients Compared with Younger Patients

Metabolic Abnormality	Symptoms in Young Patients	Symptoms in Elderly Patients
↑ Serum osmolality	Polydipsia	Dehydration, confusion, delirium
Glycosuria	Polyuria	Incontinence
Catabolic state due to insulin deficiency	Polyphagia	Weight loss, anorexia

Notes:

Table 47.37 • Antihypertensive Agents: Important Adverse Effects in Patients with Diabetes

Drug	Blood Glucose[a]	Lipid Profile[a]	Impotence	Insulin Sensitivity	Proteinuria	Comments
Preferred Antihypertensive Agents[a]						
ACE inhibitors[b]	↑	Neutral	Rare	↑	→	May cause hyperkalemia in patients with impaired renal function
Calcium channel blockers	None	Neutral	Rare	No effect	Variable	Nifedipine potentially may worsen proteinuria
α-Adrenergic blockers	None or ↑	↓ LDL-C ↑ HDL-C ↓ TG	Rare	↑	Unknown	First-dose hypotension
Second-Line Antihypertensive Agents[c]						
Thiazide diuretics	↑	↑ Chol ↑ TG	+	→	→	Commonly used in low doses. Hypokalemia can ↓ insulin secretion, cause tissue resistance, and promote arrhythmias. Diabetogenic effects most prevalent in NIDDM. To minimize metabolic effects, do not exceed 25 mg/day HCTZ or use indapamide 2.5 mg/dL[a]
β-Adrenergic blockers	↓↑	↑ TG ↓ HDL	+	→	→	Can prolong and mask hypoglycemic symptoms (most important in patients on insulin and with long-term IDDM). Response to counterregulatory hormones may be exaggerated due to unopposed α effects (e.g., arrhythmias, hypertension). Cardioselective agents may be preferable. Hyperosmolar nonketotic coma may occur in patients with endogenous insulin. Unopposed α effects may ↓ peripheral circulation[a]
Central adrenergic inhibitors	None	None	++	No effect	No effect	Sedation, depression, dry mouth, sodium retention, orthostasis
Peripheral adrenergic inhibitors	None	None	+++	No effect	No effect	Orthostasis; sodium retention usually requires addition of thiazides
Vasodilators	None	None	Rare	No effect	No effect	Tachycardia and sodium retention require addition of thiazide and β-blocker

[a]ACE inhibitors = Angiotensin-converting enzyme inhibitors; Chol = Cholesterol; HDL-C = High-density lipoprotein cholesterol; LDL-C = Low-density lipoprotein cholesterol; NIDDM = Noninsulin-dependent diabetes mellitus; HCTZ = Hydrochlorothiazide; IDDM = Insulin-dependent diabetes mellitus; TG = Triglycerides. Agents are listed in general order of use; individualize selection to patient needs.
[b]These agents are preferred because they have minimal adverse metabolite effects.
[c]These agents are not contraindicated, but are not preferred because of adverse effects on glucose and lipid metabolism or sexual function.

Table 47.38 • Drugs That Can Increase Blood Glucose Levels[a,b]

Drug/Class Name	Clinical Significance[c]	Comments
Asparaginase	++	Generally resolves during or after asparaginase therapy is completed. Concomitant corticosteroids may increase the incidence and severity of glucose intolerance.
β_2-Agonists	++	Can induce maternal hyperglycemia when used as a tocolytic. For effect on infants, see Table 47.39.
β-Adrenergic blockers	++	Alternative antihypertensive therapy preferred, unless the benefits outweigh the risks (i.e., prevention of second myocardial infarction). Cardioselective β-blockers may cause fewer adverse effects than nonselective agents.
Calcitonin	+	Few case reports.
Calcium antagonists	+	Do not appear to cause clinically significant long-term adverse effects on carbohydrate metabolism.
Carbamazepine	+	One known case report.
Cimetidine	+	Few case reports.
Corticosteroids	+++	Glucose intolerance can occur within hours to days or after months of chronic therapy. The adverse effect generally is considered dose dependent and reversible upon discontinuation; the reversal may take several months.
Cyclosporine	++	May cause hyperglycemia and require insulin therapy during long-term therapy, whether or not concomitant corticosteroids are part of the immunosuppressant regimen.
Diazoxide	+++	Causes hyperglycemia predictably in most patients. Oral formulation used as therapeutic glucose-elevating agent.
Didanosine	+	Hyperglycemia without pancreatitis possible.
Diuretics	+++	All classes of diuretics, and in particular thiazides, have been reported to cause diabetes mellitus or worsen glucose control in people with diabetes; some may tolerate low doses (≤ 25 mg hydrochlorothiazide equivalent).
Encainide	+	Two known reports in the biomedical literature.
Imipramine	+	Few case reports.
Isoniazid	+	Few case reports.
Lithium	+	Conflicting data in the biomedical literature.
Marijuana	++	One case required 3-fold increase in insulin dose; another developed diabetic ketoacidosis after ingesting large amounts orally. Delta-9-tetrahydrocannabinol-impaired glucose tolerance in six subjects (6 mg IV).
Megestrol acetate	+	Few case reports.
Nicotinic acid	++	Alternative agents for hyperlipidemia preferred for people with diabetes.
Oral contraceptives	++	Appears to occur less frequently with an estrogen dose <50 μg.
Pentamidine	+++	Diabetes mellitus may occur days after initiation of therapy but more often is delayed by several weeks or even months. Initially, pentamidine may cause hypoglycemia (see Table 47.39).
Phenothiazines	+	Many case reports, most involving chlorpromazine. Controlled studies lacking.
Phenytoin	++	Predisposed individuals (family history, underlying insulin resistance, high doses) may develop hyperglycemia. Overall incidence very small.

(continued)

Table 47.38 • Drugs That Can Increase Blood Glucose Levels[a,b] (continued)

Drug/Class Name	Clinical Significance[c]	Comments
Pravastatin	+	One known case report.
Protease inhibitors	+++	Many cases of new-onset diabetes or worsening diabetes reported to the FDA. Some cases required hospitalization and were irreversible. Related to lipodystrophy and insulin resistance.
Rifampin	+	Few case reports.
Sympathomimetics	++	Clinically significant hyperglycemia infrequent, especially at usual doses.
Tacrolimus	++	May cause hyperglycemia and require insulin therapy during long-term therapy, whether or not concomitant corticosteroids are part of the immunosuppressant regimen.
Thyroid hormones	+	Adverse effect at excessive doses.

[a]The authors acknowledge Joanne M. Yasuda, Pharm.D., who updated this table using primary references. She is an assistant professor of Pharmacy Practice and Director of Drug Information at the College of Pharmacy, Western University of Health Sciences.
[b]This table does not include the many drugs that interact with the drugs used to treat diabetes (e.g., sulfonylureas).
[c]Clinical Significance:
+ Clinical significance possible. Limited or conflicting reports or studies.
++ Clinically significant. Primarily important under certain conditions.
+++ Clinically significant effect of substantial prevalence and/or magnitude.
Adapted from reference 254.

Notes:

Table 47.39 • Drugs That Can Decrease Blood Glucose Levels[a,b]

Drug/Class Name	Clinical Significance[c]	Comments
Anabolic steroids	+	Complex metabolic effects. Only certain steroids studied.
Angiotensin-converting enzyme (ACE) inhibitors	+	May increase peripheral sensitivity to insulin effects. Two case reports and one case-control study.
β-Adrenergic blockers	++	β-Blockers may prolong and mask the symptoms of hypoglycemia. Cardioselective β-blockers may cause less adverse effects than nonselective agents.
β2-Agonists	++	Can induce hypoglycemia in the infants of mothers who received these agents for tocolysis. For effect on mother, see Table 47.38.
Disopyramide	++	Elderly patients with liver and/or renal impairment appear to be the most susceptible to this serious adverse effect.
Ethanol	+++	Most often occurs in individuals chronically drinking large amounts of ethanol. The adverse effect can follow binge drinking and even moderate alcohol intake in fasting individuals. Symptoms of hypoglycemia may be mistaken for intoxication.
Fenfluramine (Pondimin)	+	Enhances peripheral utilization of glucose, thereby enhancing effect of antidiabetic agents on postprandial glucose concentrations. Hypoglycemia per se has not been reported.
Insulin	+++	Injectable solution or suspension used therapeutically to decrease glucose levels in people with diabetes.
Pentamidine	+++	Usually occurs several days to 2 weeks following initiation of therapy. It can be sudden, recurrent, and life-threatening. Pentamidine also may cause hyperglycemia (see Table 47.38).
Quinine/quinidine	++	Quinine 600–800 mg Q 8 hours for malaria may induce hypoglycemia in 10% of patients. Doses of 300 mg for leg cramps produce hypoglycemia infrequently.
Salicylates	++	Occurs with salicylate intoxication or anti-inflammatory doses (4–6 g/day in adults). Low doses unlikely to cause this adverse effect.
Sulfonamides	+	Rare reaction with renal failure and/or high doses.
Sulfonylureas	+++	Oral hypoglycemic agents used therapeutically to decrease glucose levels in people with type 2 diabetes.

[a]The authors acknowledge Joanne M. Yasuda, Pharm.D., who updated this table using primary references. She is an assistant professor of Pharmacy Practice and Director of Drug Information at the College of Pharmacy, Western University of Health Sciences.
[b]This table does not include the many drugs that interact with the drugs used to treat diabetes (e.g., sulfonylureas).
[c]Clinical Significance:
+ Clinical significance possible. Limited or conflicting reports or studies.
++ Clinically significant. Primarily important under certain conditions.
+++ Clinically significant effect of substantial prevalence and/or magnitude.
Adapted from reference 235.

Notes:

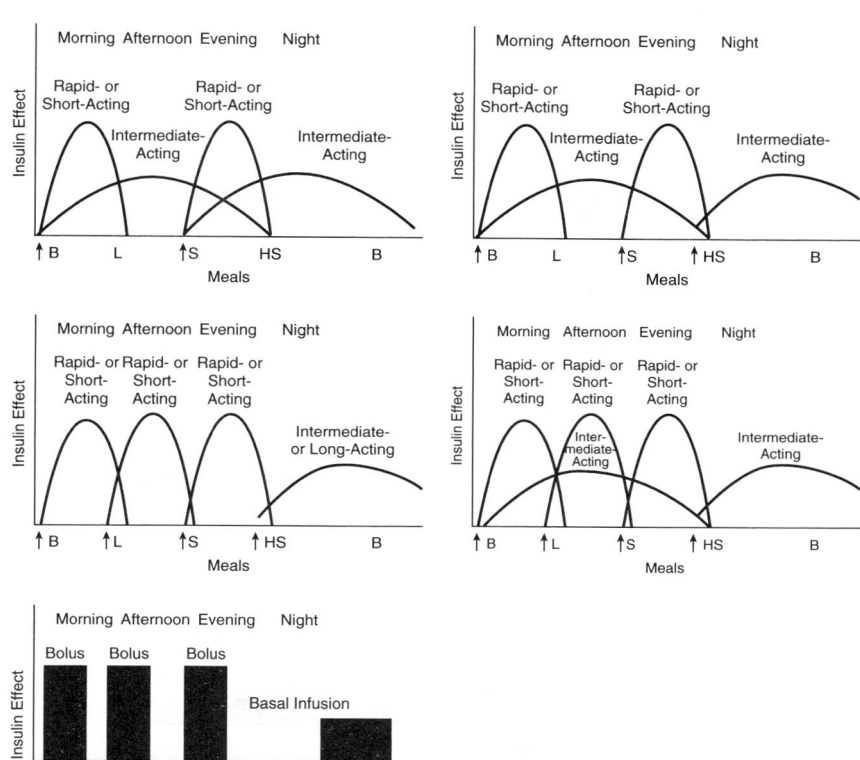

Fig. 47.1 Theoretical Insulin Effect Provided by Various Insulin Regimens. A. Two daily injections of short-acting (regular, lispro, insulin aspart) and intermediate-acting insulin (NPH or Lente). **B.** Morning injection of short-acting insulin and an intermediate-acting insulin, a presupper injection of short-acting insulin, and a bedtime injection of intermediate-acting insulin. Suggested for patients with early-morning hypoglycemia followed by rebound hyperglycemia or for patients with early-morning hyperglycemia (rebound phenomenon). **C.** Preprandial injections of short-acting insulin and intermediate-acting insulin at bedtime. A long-acting insulin (insulin glargine) may be used in place of intermediate-acting insulin. **D.** Preprandial injections of short-acting insulin and intermediate-acting insulin at breakfast and bedtime. **E.** Continuous subcutaneous insulin infusion. B, breakfast; HS, bedtime snack; L, lunch; S, supper. *Arrows,* time of insulin injection (30 minutes before meals). (Adapted from reference 270.)

Notes:

These drawings show areas of the body most suitable for insulin injections:

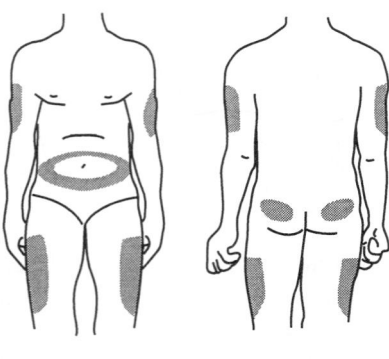

The actual point of injection should be varied each time within a chosen body area. Give injections at least one inch apart (Consult with your physician or diabetes educator about which area is most appropriate for you to use.)

Insulin is injected in the sub- cutaneous tissue (between the skin and the muscle layer). If the skin is pinched up and the needle is pushed all the way in, the needle will reach the proper space under the skin.

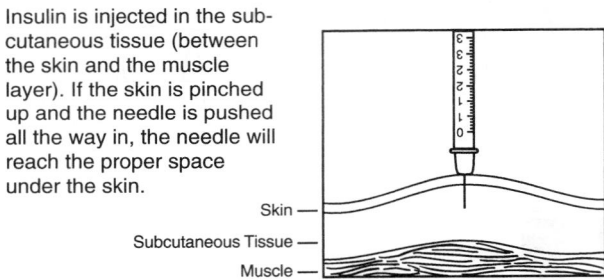

Skin ⎯
Subcutaneous Tissue ⎯
Muscle ⎯

Fig. 47.2 Selecting Insulin Injection Sites.

Notes:

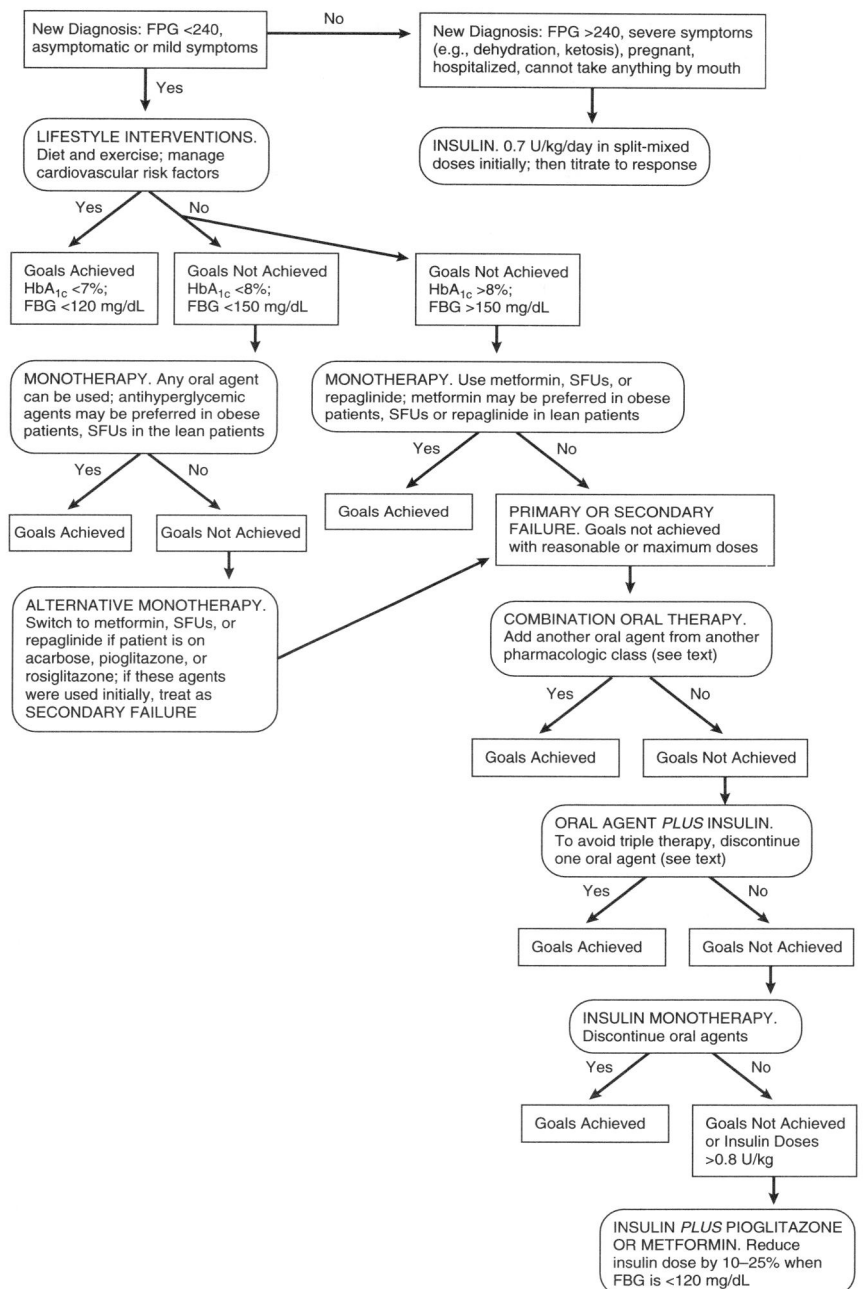

Fig. 47.3 Suggested Treatment Algorithm for Type 2 Diabetes. FBG, fasting blood glucose; FPG, fasting plasma glucose; SFUs, sulfonylureas.

The reader is referred to Chapter 48: Diabetes Mellitus, written by *Mary Anne Koda-Kimble, Pharm.D.,* and *Betsy A. Carlisle, Pharm.D.,* in the seventh edition of **Applied Therapeutics: The Clinical Use of Drugs** for a more in-depth discussion. All notations to reference numbers are based on the reference list at the end of that chapter. The editors of this handbook express their thanks to Drs. Koda-Kimble and Carlisle and acknowledge that this chapter is based upon their work.

Notes:

Chapter 48

Eye Disorders

Glaucoma

♦ **Definition and Classification.** Glaucoma, a medical condition characterized by increased intraocular pressure (IOP), primarily affects individuals >40 years of age, but can occur in other age groups including children. "Open-angle" glaucoma (elevated IOP due to decreased outflow or hypersecretion of aqueous humor) or "closed-angle" glaucoma (elevated IOP caused solely by closure of the anterior chamber angles) generally are associated with an IOP >22 mm Hg.

♦ **Pathophysiology.** Aqueous humor is produced by the ciliary processes of the eye. When aqueous humor production is excessive, or when its outflow through the trabecular meshwork of the eye is impaired, IOP is increased. The increase in pressure within the eye can result in loss of vision.

♦ **Primary Open-Angle Glaucoma (POAG)** is much more common than angle-closure glaucoma and accounts for ≈90% of cases. It is associated with a family history (i.e., genetic) and primarily affects those >40 yr. Loss of peripheral vision does not occur until late in the course of the disease.

Etiology. An increased IOP primarily results from decreased outflow of aqueous humor and is rarely due to increased aqueous humor production.

Onset usually is gradual and asymptomatic.

First-Line Treatment. POAG is treated primarily with topically applied **beta-blockers** (e.g., betaxolol), or alternatively with **α₂-adrenergic agonists** (e.g., brimonidine), **carbonic-anhydrase inhibitors** (e.g., dorzolamide), **miotics** (e.g., pilocarpine), or **mydriatics** (e.g., epinephrine). Systemic carbonic-anhydrase inhibitors are used adjunctively in some instances. Table 48.1 outlines topical agents commonly used to treat glaucoma. Figure 48.1 provides an algorithm for the medical management of glaucoma.

♦ **Angle-closure glaucoma** accounts for ≈5% of glaucoma cases and is a genuine medical emergency requiring immediate treatment. Acute attacks can end without treatment, but irreparable damage to the optic nerve occurs if the IOP remains elevated.

Etiology. The sole cause of increased IOP is closure of the anterior chamber angle, thus obstructing aqueous humor drainage.

Symptoms include a rapid increase in IOP which can result in sudden blurring or loss of vision, severe pain, and the appearance of halos around light.

Treatment. Permanent drug management is difficult and usually requires surgical correction. Drug therapy for acute angle-closure glaucoma includes:

• Pilocarpine 2%–4% 1 gtt Q 5 min for 6 doses if needed with punctal occlusion to avoid systemic side effects. (Timolol can be used concurrently.)

• *Plus* acetazolamide 500 mg IV.

• *Plus* mannitol IV 1–2 gm/kg *or* 50% glycerin PO 1–1.5 mg/kg.

◆ **Drug-Induced Glaucoma.** Drugs can precipitate glaucoma by increasing resistance to outflow of aqueous humor. Topical eye medications are more likely to cause this effect than systemic medications. (See Table 48.2: Ocular Effects of Medications.)

Ocular Effects of Medications

Table 48.2 lists the most common ocular side effects of many systemic medications.

Ocular Emergencies

◆ Pain, photophobia, blurred vision, loss of vision (sudden, complete, or transient), nystagmus, ocular hemorrhage, or a gritty, scratchy feeling complaint (i.e., suggestive of a foreign body) all require referral to an ophthalmologist.

◆ Chemical burns require immediate irrigation with the most accessible source of water (e.g., faucet, drinking fountain, shower) for at least 5 minutes before transport to the nearest emergency room.

Stye (Hordeolum)

◆ Infection of hair follicles or sebaceous glands of the eyelids most commonly caused by *Staphylococcus aureus*.

◆ Treat with hot, moist compresses and topical antibiotics (e.g., sulfacetamide). Over-the-counter (nonprescription) medications are not recommended.

Conjunctivitis

◆ Can be bacterial, fungal, parasitic, viral, or allergic in origin.

◆ Acute bacterial conjunctivitis ("pink-eye") often is treated empirically with topical ophthalmic antibiotic drugs or ointments (e.g., Neosporin). A culture should be obtained.

◆ Bacterial conjunctivitis often starts in one eye and is spread to the other.

◆ Allergic conjunctivitis can be treated with ophthalmic vasoconstrictors, antihistamines, or corticosteroids (see Table 48.3: Ophthalmic Corticosteroids).

Ocular Herpes Simplex

◆ Drugs available for treatment of ocular herpes simplex are listed in Table 48.4.

Notes:

Table 48.1 • Common Topical Agents Used in the Treatment of Open-Angle Glaucoma

Generic	Mechanism	Strength	Usual Dosage	Comments
Miotics				
Pilocarpine (Isopto-Carpine)	Parasympathomimetic	0.25–10% 4% (ointment) 20–40 µg/hr (Ocusert)	1–2 drops TID–QID ½ inch in cul-de-sac QD weekly	Long-term proven effectiveness. Little rationale for use of concentrations >4% or administration more frequently than Q 4 hr. Side effects of miosis with decreased vision and brow ache are frequent sources of patient complaints. Once-daily administration of ointment may ↑ compliance. Effectiveness over 24 hr should be assessed in patients receiving the ointment. Ointment may cause a visual haze and blurred vision.
Carbachol (Isopto-Carbachol)	Parasympathomimetic	0.75–3%	1–2 drops TID–QID	Used in patients allergic to or intolerant of other miotics. May be used as frequently as Q 4 hr. Corneal penetration is enhanced by benzalkonium chloride in commercial preparations. Side effects are similar to those of pilocarpine.
Echothiophate Iodide (Phospholine Iodide)	Anticholinesterase	0.03–0.25%	1 drop BID	Most used anticholinesterase agent. Long duration, although usually dosed BID, which enhances compliance. Solutions are relatively unstable. Side effects similar to those of pilocarpine, especially in concentrations >0.06%. ↑ cataract formation has been associated with its use.
Mydriatics				
Epinephrine (Glaucon, Eppy/N, Epitrate)	Sympathomimetic	0.25–2%	1 drop BID	Good response often seen with use of lower concentrations (0.5–1%). Bitartrate salt contains ½ labeled strength in epinephrine-free base equivalent. BID dosage enhances compliance. Cosmetic complaints associated with use include hyperemia and pigment deposits on the cornea and conjunctiva. Not recommended for use in aphakic patients because of 20–30% incidence of cystoid macular edema.
Dipivefrin (Propine)	Sympathomimetic	0.1%	1 drop BID	Prodrug of epinephrine associated with ↓ in systemic side effects if absorbed. BID dosage enhances compliance.
β-Blockers				
Betaxolol (Betoptic [solution], Betoptic S [suspension])	Sympatholytic	0.25% (suspension) 0.5% (solution)	1 drop BID	Effective with few associated ocular side effects. BID dosage enhances compliance. May be the ocular β-blocker of choice in patients with preexisting CHF or pulmonary disease, because of β₁ specificity. Patient response may be less than that seen with timolol.

(continued)

Table 48.1 • Common Topical Agents Used in the Treatment of Open-Angle Glaucoma (continued)

Generic	Mechanism	Strength	Usual Dosage	Comments
β-Blockers (continued)				
Carteolol (Ocupress)	Sympatholytic	1%	1 drop BID	Effective with few associated side effects. BID dosage enhances compliance. Use with caution in patients with pre-existing CHF or pulmonary disease.
Levobunolol (Betagan)	Sympatholytic	0.25–0.5%	1 drop QD–BID	Effective with few associated ocular side effects. QD–BID dosage enhances compliance. Use with caution in patients with pre-existing CHF or pulmonary disease.
Metipranolol (OptiPranolol)	Sympatholytic	0.3%	1 drop BID	Effective with few associated side effects. BID dosage enhances compliance. Use with caution in patients with pre-existing CHF or pulmonary disease.
Timolol (Timoptic)	Sympatholytic	0.25–0.5%	1 drop BID	Effective with few associated ocular side effects. BID dosage enhances compliance. Use with caution in patients with pre-existing CHF or pulmonary disease. Proven long-term effectiveness, with well-defined side effect profile.
Timoptic XE	Sympatholytic	0.25–0.5%	1 drop QD	New once-daily timolol formulation. The ophthalmic vehicle, gellan gum (Gelrite), prolongs precorneal residence time and ↑ ocular bioavailability, allowing QD administration.

α₂-Selective Adrenergic Agonists			
Apraclonidine (Iopidine)	Sympathomimetic	0.5–1%	1 drop preop and postop or 1 drop BID–TID	May be used preop and postop for the prevention of increased IOP after anterior-segment laser procedures. Use of NLO minimizes systemic side effects and allows for BID dosing. Does not penetrate the blood-brain barrier; therefore, negligible systemic hypotension. Local adverse effects fairly common. Tachyphylaxis may be observed.
Brimonidine (Alphagan)	Sympathomimetic	0.2%	1 BID–TID	Effective long-term monotherapy or adjunctive therapy. Use of NLO minimizes systemic side effects and allows for BID dosing. Penetrates the blood-brain barrier; therefore, may cause mild systemic hypotension and lethargy. Local adverse effects less common than with apraclonidine.
Topical Carbonic Anhydrase Inhibitor				
Brinzolamide (Azopt)	Decreased aqueous humor production	1%	1 drop TID	Effective long-term monotherapy or adjunctive therapy. Well tolerated with few systemic side effects. Less burning and stinging compared to dorzolamide.
Dorzolamide (Trusopt)	Decreased aqueous humor production	2%	1 drop TID	Effective long-term monotherapy or adjunctive therapy. Well tolerated with few systemic side effects.
Prostaglandin Analogs				
Latanoprost (Xalatan)	Prostaglandin F₂α agonist	0.005%	1 drop QHS	BID dosing may be less effective than QHS dosing. May cause increased pigmentation of the iris. Systemic side effects are rare but may cause muscle, joint, back pain, and skin rash. Effective monotherapy or adjunctive therapy.

Table 48.2 • Ocular Side Effects of Systemic Medications[a]

Drug Class	Effect(s)	Clinical Remarks
Analgesics Ibuprofen	Reduced vision	Rare; blurred vision has been reported in patients taking from four 200 mg tablets/wk to six tablets/day. Changes in color vision rarely have been reported.[158]
Narcotics, including pentazocine	Miosis	Miosis often with morphine in normal doses: slight with other agents. The effect is secondary to CNS action on the pupilloconstrictor center.[103,104]
	Tearing Irregular pupils Paresis of accommodation Diplopia	These effects are associated with narcotic withdrawal.[103,104]
Antiarrhythmics Amiodarone	Keratopathy	Dose- and duration-related; resembles chloroquine keratopathy. Corneal deposits are bilateral, reversible, and unassociated with visual symptoms. Patients taking 100–200 mg/day have only minimal deposits. Deposits will occur in almost 100% of patients receiving 400 mg/day.[103–106]
	Cataracts	Previously reported as insignificant, anterior subcapsular lens opacities have been associated with amiodarone therapy. Rarely, such opacities may progress, increasing in density and in the diffuse distribution of the deposits, ultimately covering an area somewhat larger than the undilated pupil's aperture. The mechanism for this effect is unclear, but like chlorpromazine, amiodarone is a photosensitizing agent. Given that the lens changes are limited largely to the pupillary aperture, light exposure may result in the lens changes.[159]
Anticholinergics Atropine Idicyclomine Glycopyrrolate Propantheline Scopolamine Trihexyphenidyl	Mydriasis Cycloplegia ↓ accommodation Photophobia	Systemic and transdermal anticholinergic agents may cause mydriasis and, less frequently, cycloplegia. Mydriasis may precipitate angle-closure glaucoma. Photophobia is related to the mydriasis. Accommodation ↓ for near objects.[103,104,160]
Anticonvulsants Carbamazepine	Diplopia Blurred vision	Ocular adverse reactions when dosage >1–2 g/day; disappear when dosage ↓.[103]
Phenytoin	Nystagmus Cataracts	Nystagmus in patients with high blood levels (>20 µg/mL); rarely occurs with other hydantoins. Cataracts may occur rarely with prolonged therapy.[103,104,161]
Trimethadione	Visual glare	A prolonged glare or dazzle occurs when eyes are exposed to light. The glare is reversible, occurs at the retinal level, and is more common in adolescents and adults; rarely in young children.[103,104]
Anesthetics Propofol	Inability to open eyes	6 of 50 patients undergoing ENT procedures using standardized anesthesia with propofol were unable to open their eyes either spontaneously or in response to verbal commands. This effect lasted between 3–20 min after the end of anesthetic administration. Two patients showed complete loss of ocular motility. This was a transient, myasthenic-like weakness.[162]

(continued)

Table 48.2 • Ocular Side Effects of Systemic Medications (continued)

Drug Class	Effect(s)	Clinical Remarks
Antidepressants		
Tricyclic antidepressants (TCAs)	Mydriasis Cycloplegia	Mydriasis is most common ocular side effect of TCAs. Cycloplegia is rare. Reports of precipitation of angle-closure glaucoma.[103,104]
Fluoxetine	Eye tics	Administration of fluoxetine 20–40 mg/day has been associated with paroxysmal contractions of the muscles around the lateral aspect of the eye. This effect occurred 3–4 wk after initiation of fluoxetine therapy and resolved within 2 wk of discontinuation.[163]
Antihistamines		
Chlorpheniramine	Blurred vision	Blurred vision occurs rarely (≈1% of patients taking 12–14 mg/day).[103,104]
	Mydriasis ↓ lacrimal secretions	Rare.[103,104]
Antihypertensives		
Clonidine	Miosis Dry itchy eyes	Miosis is seen in overdose.[104] Rare.[104]
Diazoxide	Lacrimation	About 20% experience lacrimation, which may continue after drug is discontinued.[103]
Guanethidine	Miosis Ptosis Conjunctivitis Blurred vision	Sporadically documented. One study reported a 17% incidence of blurred vision in patients taking guanethidine 70 mg/day.[103,104]
Reserpine	Miosis	Miosis is slight but can last up to 1 wk after a single dose.[103,104]
	Conjunctivitis	Common, secondary to dilation of conjunctival blood vessels.[103,104]
Anti-Infectives		
Amantadine	Corneal lesions	Diffuse, white punctate subepithelial corneal opacities have been reported, occasionally associated with superficial punctate keratitis. Onset has been 1–2 wk after initiation of therapy with dosages of 200–400 mg/day. Resolves with drug discontinuation.[164]
Chloramphenicol	Optic neuritis	Rare unless a total dose of 100 g and duration >6 wk are exceeded. Vision usually improves after the drug is discontinued.[103,104]
Chloroquine	Corneal deposits	Some patients using ordinary doses may develop corneal deposits in a few months. The deposits are visible with use of a biomicroscope, appear as white-yellow in color, but are of no consequence.[103,104]
	Retinopathy (macular degeneration)	Serious retinopathy when total dose >100 g. Usually develops after 1–3 yr; can occur in 6 mo. Visual loss may be peripheral, with progression to central vision loss and disturbance of color vision. Rarely effects such as blurred vision are seen earlier when larger doses (500–700 mg/day) are used. Macular changes may progress after drug is discontinued. These agents concentrate in pigmented tissue.[103,104]
Ethambutol	Retrobulbar neuritis	At dosages of 15 mg/kg/day, virtually void of ocular side effects. Such effects are rare at dosages of 25 mg/kg/day for a duration of a few months. Patients treated for prolonged periods should have routine visual examinations including visual fields. Most effects are reversible after the drug is discontinued.[103,104]
Gentamicin	Pseudotumor cerebri	Rare, but has been well documented with secondary papilledema and visual loss.[103,104]

(continued)

Table 48.2 • Ocular Side Effects of Systemic Medications (continued)

Drug Class	Effect(s)	Clinical Remarks
Anti-Infectives (continued)		
Isoniazid	Optic neuritis	Prevalence not well defined but appears to be significantly less than peripheral neuritis. Evaluation difficult because most patients malnourished, chronic alcoholics, or receiving multiple medications. Pre-existing eye disease does not appear to be a predisposing factor.[103,104]
Nalidixic acid	Visual sensations	Most common ocular side effect. Main feature a brightly colored appearance of objects; occurs soon after the drug is taken. Although quinolone antibiotics are nalidixic acid derivatives, they have rarely been associated with these ocular side effects.[103,104]
	Visual loss	Temporary effect (30 min–3 days).
	Papilledema	Primarily in infants and young children and secondary to ↑ intracranial pressure; reversible upon withdrawal of the drug.
Sulfonamides	Myopia	Acute and reversible; most common ocular side effect.[103,104]
	Conjunctivitis	Primarily with topical sulfathiazole, 4% incidence between the fifth and ninth days of therapy.[103,104]
	Optic neuritis	Even in low dosages. Usually reversible with complete recovery of vision.[103,104]
	Photosensitivity	Associated with use of sulfisoxazole lid margin therapy.[165,166]
Tetracyclines	Myopia	Appears to be acute, transient, and rare.[103,104]
	Papilledema	More common in children and infants than adults; rare.[103,104]
Anti-Inflammatory Agents (Also See Analgesics; Corticosteroids)		
Gold	Corneal Conjunctival deposits	Deposition in the conjunctiva and superficial cornea more common than in the lens or deep cornea. Incidence in cornea of 40–80% in total doses of 1.5 g; visual acuity is unaffected. One reported case after oral therapy.[103]
Indomethacin	↓ vision	Rare; also changes in color vision have been rarely reported.[103,104]
Phenylbutazone	↓ vision	Most common ocular side effect with this drug may be caused by ↑ lens hydration.[103,104]
	Conjunctivitis Retinal hemorrhage	Occurs less often than ↓ vision. The conjunctivitis may be associated with development of Stevens-Johnson syndrome or an allergic reaction.[103,104]
Antilipemic Agents		
Lovastatin	Cataracts	The crystalline lenses of hypercholesteremic patients were assessed before and after 48 wk of treatment with lovastatin 20–80 mg/day. Statistical analyses of the distribution of cortical, nuclear, and subcapsular opacities at 48 weeks showed no significant differences between placebo-treated and lovastatin-treated groups. Visual acuity assessments also were not significantly different among the groups.[167]

(continued)

Notes:

Table 48.2 • Ocular Side Effects of Systemic Medications (continued)

Drug Class	Effect(s)	Clinical Remarks
Antineoplastic Agents		
Busulfan	Cataracts	Reported with high dosages.[103,104]
Carmustine	Arterial narrowing Nerve fiber-layer infarcts Intraretinal hemorrhages	These ocular side effects are not well established. Evidence of delayed bilateral ocular toxicity developed in 2 of 50 patients treated with high-dose IV carmustine (800 mg/m²). Symptoms of ocular toxicity became evident 4 wk after IV treatment. Evidence of delayed ocular toxicity (mean onset 6 wk) ipsilateral to the site of infusion developed in 7 of 10 patients treated with intra-arterial carotid doses of carmustine to a cumulative minimum of 450 mg/m² in two treatments.[168]
Cytarabine	Keratoconjunctivitis Ocular burning Photophobia Blurred vision	Corneal toxicity and conjunctivitis have been reported with high-dose (3 g/m²) therapy.[169,170]
Doxorubicin	Conjunctivitis Excessive tearing	May last for several days after treatment.[103,104]
Fluorouracil	Ocular irritation Lacrimation	Reversible and seldom interfere with continued therapy.[103,104]
Tamoxifen	Corneal opacities ↓ vision Retinopathy	Generally occur in patients taking higher than normal doses for 12–18 mo.[193]
Vinca alkaloids (especially vincristine)	Extraocular muscle paresis (EMP) Ptosis	The onset of EMP or paralysis may be seen as early as 2 wk. Dose-related. Most recover fully when drug is discontinued.[103,104]
Barbiturates	Miosis Mydriasis Disturbances in ocular movement Ptosis	Most significant ocular side effects occur in chronic users or in toxic states. Pupillary responses are variable; miosis seen most frequently except in toxicity when mydriasis predominates. Nystagmus and weakness in extraocular muscles may be seen. Chronic abusers have a characteristic ptosis.[103,104]
Calcium channel blockers	Blurred vision Transient blindness	Primarily blurred vision; transient blindness at peak concentrations has been observed in several patients.[120]
Corticosteroids	Cataracts	Posterior subcapsular cataracts have been associated with systemic corticosteroids. ↑ in patients who have received >15 mg/day of prednisone or its equivalent daily for periods >1 yr.[103,104] Rare reports of bilateral posterior subcapsular cataracts associated with nasal aerosol or inhalation of beclomethasone dipropionate have been received. Most patients had received therapy for >5 yr, often in higher than the recommended dosage. About 40% of patients also were receiving systemic corticosteroids.[171] (Also see Question 14.)
	↑ intraocular pressure	More common with topical corticosteroids than with systemic therapy. Of little consequence in patients without pre-existing glaucoma. Glaucoma patients should be monitored routinely if receiving systemic corticosteroids.[103,104] (See Question 13.)
	Papilledema	Intracranial hypertension or pseudotumor cerebri from systemic corticosteroids has been well documented. The incidence appears to be greater in children than in adults; primarily associated with chronic therapy.
Digitalis	Altered color vision, visual acuity	Changes in color vision. A glare phenomenon and a snowy appearance in objects have been associated primarily with digitalis intoxication. In a small number of cases, reversible reduction in visual acuity has been noted. Also associated with changes in the visual fields.[103,104]
	↓ intraocular pressure	Digitalis derivatives can ↓ intraocular pressure, but clinical use for glaucoma is not practical because the therapeutic systemic dose for this effect is very near the toxic dose.[103,104]

(continued)

Table 48.2 • Ocular Side Effects of Systemic Medications *(continued)*

Drug Class	Effect(s)	Clinical Remarks
Diuretics Carbonic anhydrase inhibitors Thiazides	Myopia	Acute myopia that may last from 24–48 hr. Probably caused by an ↑ in the anteroposterior diameter of the lens, which may be reversible even if drug use is continued.[103,104]
Estrogens Clomiphene	Blurred vision Mydriasis Visual field changes Visual sensations	5–10% experience ocular side effects. Blurred vision is the most common effect, although visual sensations such as flashing lights, distortion of images, and various colored lights (primarily silver) may occur.[103,104]
Oral contraceptives (OCs)	Optic neuritis Pseudotumor cerebri Retrobulbar neuritis	Quite rare. In patients with retinal vascular abnormalities, use of OCs is questionable. Numerous other possible ocular side effects are associated with these agents, and further documentation is required.[103,104]
Hypouricemics Allopurinol	Cataracts	Conflicting reports have suggested allopurinol may be associated with anterior and posterior lens capsule changes and with anterior subcapsular vacuoles; 42 cases of cataracts have been reported; these have been observed primarily in age groups in whom normal lens aging changes would not be expected. No cause-and-effect relationship has been proven.[103,172–175]
Immune Modulators Interleukin-2	Visual deficits	Interleukin-2 visual complications have occurred during the first or second treatment cycle, usually within 5–6 days of initiation of therapy. Ocular symptoms included diplopia, binocular negative scotomata (isolated areas of varying size and shape in which vision is absent or depressed. These are not perceived ordinarily but would be apparent upon completion of a visual field examination), and palinopsia (abnormal recurring visual imagery). In most cases, treatment was continued for the entire planned duration of therapy. Symptoms resolved after discontinuation.[176]
Phenothiazines Chlorpromazine	Deposits on the lens	Rare when total dose <0.5 kg. Visible after a total dose of 1 kg in most cases; incidence may ↑ to 90% after ≥2.5 kg. Usually deposits do not affect vision appreciably. The cornea and conjunctiva may be affected after the lens shows pigment changes.[103,104]
	Retinal pigment deposits	The number of reported cases is small; further documentation is necessary.[103,104]
Thioridazine	Pigmentary retinopathy	Primarily associated with maximal daily dosages or average doses >1,000 mg. Daily dosages up to 600 mg are relatively safe; 600–800 mg is uncertain, but rarely suspect. If >800 mg/day is used, periodic ophthalmoscopic examinations may uncover problems before visual acuity is compromised.[103,104]
Therapy for Erectile Dysfunction Sildenafil (Viagra)	Disturbance of color vision. Increased brightness. Blurred vision.	Color vision alterations are mild to moderate. Blurred vision does not impair visual acuity. Visual alterations usually subside within 4 hr after the dose.[177]

*a*CNS = Central nervous system; ENT = Ear, nose, and throat.

Table 48.3 • Ophthalmic Corticosteroids

Low Potency	Intermediate Potency	High Potency
Dexamethasone 0.05% (Decadron Phosphate)	Clobetasone 0.1%[a]	Clobetasone 0.5%[a]
Dexamethasone 0.1% (Decadron Phosphate)	Dexamethasone alcohol 0.1% (Maxidex)	Fluorometholone acetate 0.1% (Flarex)
Medrysone 1% (HMS)	Fluorometholone 0.1% (FML)	Prednisolone acetate 1% (Pred Forte)
	Fluorometholone 0.25% (FML Forte)	Rimexolone 1% (Vexol)
	Loteprednol 0.2% (Lotemax)	
	Loteprednol 0.5% (Alrex)	
	Prednisolone acetate 0.12% (Pred Mild)	
	Prednisolone sodium phosphate 0.125% (Inflamase Mild)	
	Prednisolone sodium phosphate 1% (Inflamase Forte)	

[a]Not commercially available in the United States.

Notes:

Table 48.4 • Treatment of Ocular Herpes Simplex[a]

Drug	Formulation	Dose	Comment
Idoxuridine (Stoxil)	0.1% solution	1 gtt in each infected eye Q 1 hr during day and Q 2 hr throughout night until improvement confirmed by eye examination. Then, 1 gtt Q 2 hr during day and Q 4 hr throughout night for 3–5 days after healing complete	≈80%–85% of dendritic ulcers heal within 2 weeks. Does not penetrate cornea. No proven effectiveness in herpetic iritis or stromal keratitis. Incorporated into host DNA. Slows replication of noninfected cells. Emergence of resistant strains. *Side effects:* pain, irritation, inflammation, photophobia, contact dermatitis, keratopathy, follicular conjunctivitis, and thickening of lid margins
	0.5% ointment	Apply ½" 4–5 × day or as nighttime medication when drops used during day	
Vidarabine (Vira-A)	3% ointment	Apply into conjunctival sac ½" 5 × day (Q 3 hr) until healed, then BID × 7 days	Inhibits DNA. Effective for IDU-resistant strains or if allergic to IDU. Not effective for herpetic keratitis like IDU. Interferes less than IDU with growth of normal cells as corneal epithelium heals. *Side effects:* Pain, burning, inflammation, ↑ lacrimation
Trifluridine (Viroptic)	1% solution	1 gtt Q 2 hr while awake (*max:* 9 gtt/day). Then, 1 gtt Q 4 hr while awake (*max:* 5 gtt/day) for 7 days after healing completed. Do not use continuously for >21 days	*Drug of choice* for ocular herpes. ≈95% of herpetic corneal ulcers healed in 2 weeks. Penetrates cornea and potentially heals stromal keratitis and uveitis. Effective against IDU and vidarabine-resistant strains. Side effects might be less
Acyclovir		Investigational	High degree of viral specificity, lack of toxicity to normal host cells, and faster healing rate make it preferable to IDU or vidarabine. Trifluridine drug of choice since no ophthalmic preparation available

[a]IDU = Idoxuridine.

Notes:

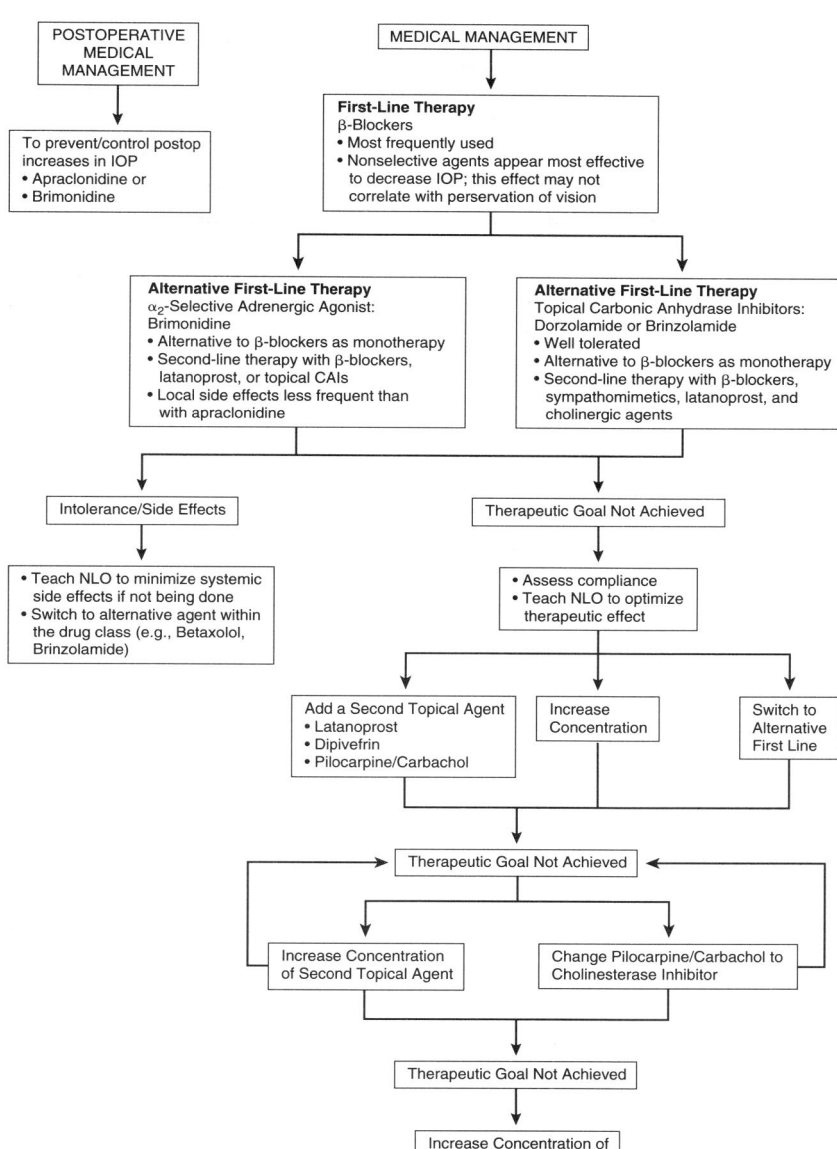

Fig. 48.1 Medical Management of Glaucoma.

Notes:

The reader is referred to Chapter 46: Eye Disorders, written by *Steven R. Abel, Pharm.D.*, and *Suellyn J. Sorensen, Pharm.D.*, in the seventh edition of **Applied Therapeutics: The Clinical Use of Drugs** for a more in-depth discussion. All notations to reference numbers are based on the reference list at the end of that chapter. The editors of this handbook express their thanks to Drs. Abel and Sorensen and acknowledge that this chapter is based upon their work.

Notes:

Chapter 49

Headache

For diagnostic and therapeutic purposes, headache can be categorized into one of two major types *(primary* and *secondary)* on the basis of the underlying etiology. *Primary headache disorders* are characterized by the lack of an identifiable and treatable underlying cause. Migraine, tension-type, and cluster headaches are examples of primary headache disorders. *Secondary headache disorders* are those associated with a variety of organic causes such as trauma, cerebrovascular malformations, and brain tumors. A comprehensive classification scheme of the different types of headaches, modified from the International Headache Society (HIS), is shown in Table 49.1.

Migraine

◆ Migraine is an idiopathic, recurring headache disorder manifesting in attacks lasting 4 to 72 hrs.

◆ ***Pathophysiology.*** Probably involves cerebrovascular changes as well as alterations in peripheral or central 5-HT activity. These effects may be mediated by a central mechanism involving brain stem noradrenergic and serotonergic neurotransmission. This forms the basis of drug action. For example, 5-HT, drugs that stimulate 5-HT_1 receptors (sumatriptan), drugs that antagonize 5-HT_2 receptors (methysergide), and drugs that inhibit 5-HT reuptake (amitriptyline) or 5-HT release (calcium channel blockers) relieve migraines.

◆ ***Epidemiology.*** Migraine is more common in females than males. Attacks can be precipitated by physiological and environmental factors as shown in Table 49.2

Signs and Symptoms

◆ Usually develop over minutes to hours progressing from a dull ache to a more intense pulsating pain that worsens with each pulse. If untreated can last from several hours to as long as 3 days.

◆ Attacks vary widely in intensity, frequency, and duration but are commonly unilateral and associated with nausea and vomiting.

◆ *Auras* or focal neurologic features precede (by 10–60 min) or accompany migraine in 10% of cases. Lightheadedness and photopsia (unformed flashes of light) are most common. Other visual disturbances include scotoma (an isolated area within the visual field where vision is absent); visual distortions; scintillating scotoma (scotomas surrounded by a shiny kaleidoscope-like pattern); and "fortification spectrum" (slowly enlarging scotoma surrounded by a bright zig-zag pattern resembling the top of a fort)

Treatment. Sleep and relaxation in a dark room accelerate pain relief. Minimize factors that precipitate migraine (see Table 49.2).

◆ *Abortive Therapy.* Table 49.3 lists drugs used to treat acute migraine headache.

• *Ergotamine tartrate* SL given at the first sign of a migraine attack is effective in 50%-70% of sufferers. Adjunctive therapy with *metoclopramide* can relieve nausea and vomiting and improve drug absorption.

- The "triptans" listed in Table 49.4 can be used for cases unresponsive to ergots and *NSAIDs*. These also relieve nausea, vomiting, and visual symptoms.
- *Dihydroergotamine* SQ, IM, or IV, "triptans" and potent narcotics are indicated for intractable migraine. *Chlorpromazine* and *corticosteroids* (prednisone 40–60 mg PO × 3–5 days or dexamethasone 4–19 mg IM) also may be tried.
- *Prophylactic therapy* in Table 49.5 is indicated when headaches are frequent (>2/month), resistant to treatment, and disabling. Therapy may reduce the frequency and severity of attacks and render headaches more susceptible to treatment.

Cluster Headache

♦ Cluster headache is a relatively infrequent vascular headache disorder with a characteristic periodic pattern of headache recurrence. Headaches tend to occur nightly over a relatively short period of time (i.e., several weeks or months). They occur most commonly in the spring and fall.

♦ Onset is abrupt, often waking the patient from sleep; reaches maximum intensity over 5–15 minutes and lasts 40–60 minutes.

♦ The pain is severe, throbbing, and affects the same side of the head, although it occasionally can affect the entire cranium.

♦ Associated symptoms include lacrimation, injected conjunctiva, rhinorrhea, and ptosis with miosis. Nausea, vomiting, and auras are not typical.

♦ **Precipitating factors** include alcohol, vasodilators, stress, warm weather, missed meals, and excessive sleep.

Treatment

♦ *Abortive therapy* includes oxygen and ergotamine as first-line agents. (See Table 49.6.)

♦ *Prophylactic therapy* aimed at prevention of cluster headaches during an active period should be considered if symptomatic therapy is ineffective, intolerable, or if headaches occur more frequently than twice daily. Table 49.7 lists drugs used for this purpose.

Tension Headaches

♦ Tension-type headache is the most common headache type with a lifetime prevalence of 88% in women and 69% in men.

♦ Dull aching sensation bilaterally which occurs in a hatband distribution around the head. Pain is usually mild to moderate in severity and is nonpulsating. Frequency varies widely, but some can have headache continuously for months or even years. Not associated with nausea and vomiting, aura, or photophobia.

Treatment

♦ *Analgesics* (aspirin, acetaminophen, NSAIDs) are the agents of choice for treatment of acute tension headache attacks.

♦ *Antihistamines, sedatives, anxiolytics, and skeletal muscle relaxants* can augment the effect of analgesics when analgesics afford insufficient relief alone.

♦ *Nondrug therapy* includes massage, hot baths, acupuncture, and a variety of relaxation techniques.

♦ *Amitriptyline* is considered the drug of choice for prophylaxis of tension-type and mixed-type headaches. The effective daily dose is 50–100 mg/day, although up to 300 mg/day may be required. Response does not require a history of depressive symptoms, and the benefit is noted in 2–10 days. Start with 25 mg at bedtime and increase gradually. Other drugs used prophylactically include doxepin, imipramine, maprotiline, protriptyline, fluoxetine, and desipramine.

Table 49.1 • Classification of Headache[7]

Migraine
Migraine without aura
Migraine with aura
Complicated migraine

Tension-Type Headache
Episodic tension-type headache
Chronic tension-type headache

Cluster Headache
Episodic cluster headache
Chronic cluster headache

Miscellaneous Headaches Unassociated with Structural Lesion (e.g., Cold Stimulus Headache, Benign Exertional Headache)

Headache Associated with Head Trauma
Acute posttraumatic headache
Chronic posttraumatic headache

Headache Associated with Vascular Disorders
Acute ischemic cerebrovascular disease (TIA or stroke)
Intracranial hematoma
Subarachnoid hemorrhage
Unruptured vascular malformation
Arteritis
Carotid or vertebral artery pain
Venous thrombosis
Arterial hypertension

Headache Associated with Nonvascular Intracranial Disorder (e.g., High or Low CSF Pressure, Intracranial Infection, or Neoplasm)

Headache Associated with Substances or their Withdrawal (e.g., Withdrawal from Alcohol, Caffeine, Ergotamine, Narcotics; Also see Table 49.2)

Headache Associated with Noncephalic Infection (e.g., Viral or Bacterial Infection)

Headache Associated with Metabolic Disorder (e.g., Hypoxia, Hypercapnia, Hypoglycemia, Dialysis)

Headache or Facial Pain Associated with Disorder of Cranium, Neck, Eyes, Ears, Nose, Sinuses, Teeth, Mouth, or Other Facial or Cranial Structures (e.g., Cervical Spine, Acute Glaucoma, Refractive Errors, Acute Sinus Headache)

Cranial Neuralgias, Nerve Trunk Pain, and Deafferentation Pain (e.g., Compression, Demyelination, Infarction, or Inflammation of Cranial Nerves)

Headache Not Classifiable

Notes:

Table 49.2 • Factors That May Precipitate Migraine Headache^a

Stress

Emotion

Glare

Hypoglycemia

Altered sleep pattern

Menses

Exercise

Alcohol

Carbon monoxide

Excess caffeine use or withdrawal

Foods containing:
  MSG (e.g., Chinese food, canned soups, seasonings [e.g., Johnny's Seasoning Salt])
  Tyramine (e.g., red wine, ripened cheeses)
  Nitrites (e.g., cured meat products)
  Phenylethylamine (e.g., chocolate, cheese)

Aspartame (e.g., artificial sweeteners, diet sodas)

Drugs
  Excess analgesic use or withdrawal
  Estrogens (e.g., oral contraceptives)
  Cocaine
  Nitroglycerin

^aMSG = Monosodium glutamate.

Notes:

Table 49.3 • Drug Treatment of Acute Migraine Headache[a]

Drug	Route	Dose	Contraindications	Adverse Effects	Comments
Ibuprofen (Motrin) or other NSAIDs	PO	400–800 mg	Aspirin or NSAID-related bronchospasm	N, V, bleeding, renal dysfunction	First-line therapy; acetaminophen may also be effective
Ergotamine tartrate (Cafergot, Ergostat)	PO, SL, PR	1–4 mg stat, then 1–2 mg Q 30 min to max of 6 mg/attack or 10 mg/wk	CV disease, sepsis, liver or kidney disease, arterial insufficiency, pregnancy, breast feeding, concomitant macrolide use	N, V, anorexia, limb paresthesias or pain	Use at HA onset for max effect; ↓ N and V by using smallest effective dose
Isometheptene/ dichloralphenazone/ acetaminophen (Midrin)	PO	2 cap stat, then 1 cap Q hr to max 5 cap/12 hr	See Ergotamine tartrate; avoid in patients taking MAOIs	N, V, dizziness, drowsiness	As effective as ergotamine tartrate
Sumatriptan (Imitrex)	PO, IN, SC	6 mg stat; may repeat in 1 hr	Ischemic heart disease, within 24 hr of ergot alkaloids	Heavy sensation in head or chest, tingling, pain at injection site	Effective and well tolerated; cost limits widespread use; reserve for intractable migraine or patients intolerant of other abortive agents
Chlorpromazine (Thorazine)	IM	1 mg/kg	CV disease, history of seizures	Extrapyramidal reactions, sedation, hypotension	For intractable migraine; also has antiemetic properties
Morphine (or meperidine)	IM	5–10 mg	↑ ICP or head trauma with funduscopic changes	Sedation, hypoventilation	For intractable migraine
Metoclopramide (Reglan)	PO, IM	10 mg stat	GI hemorrhage or obstruction; pheochromocytoma	Extrapyramidal reactions, sedation, restlessness	For adjunctive antiemetic therapy; prochlorperazine also effective

[a]See Table 49.4 for additional information on sumatriptan and other triptan agents. CV = Cardiovascular; GI = Gastrointestinal; HA = Headache; ICP = Intracranial pressure; IM = Intramuscular; IN = Intranasal; MAOIs = Monoamine oxidase inhibitors; N = Nausea; NSAID = Nonsteroidal anti-inflammatory drug; PO = Oral; PR = Rectal; SC = Subcutaneous; SL = Sublingual; V = Vomiting.

Table 49.4 • Clinical and Pharmacokinetic Features of the Triptans for Acute Migraine Headache[86,103,104,261–265a]

Drug	Route	Bioavailability (%)	T-max (hr)	Half-Life (hr)	Response Rate at 2 hr (%)	HA Recurrence Within 24–48 hr (%)	Dose/Attack (mg)
Sumatriptan (Imitrex)	PO	14	1.2–2.3	2	50–69	10–40	25–100
	IN	—	1–1.5	2	62–78	10–40	20–40
	SC	96	0.2	2	63–82	10–40	6–12
Zomitriptan (Zomig)	PO	40–46	1.5	2.5–3	62–67	32–37	2.5–10
Naratriptan (Amerge)	PO	60–70	3–5	6	43–49	27–39	1–5
Rizatriptan (Maxalt)	PO	40–45	1.3	1.8	60–77	30–47	5–20
Eletriptan (Relpax)	PO	50	1	4–5	54–68	16–30	20–80

[a]HA = Headache; IN = Intranasal; PO = Oral; SC = Subcutaneous.

Notes:

Table 49.5 • Drugs Commonly Used for Migraine Headache Prophylaxis[a]

Drug	Dose	Dosage Forms/Strengths	Effectiveness	Comments
Propranolol (Inderal)	20 mg BID–TID; gradually ↑ dose at weekly intervals to effect or max of 320 mg/day	Tab: 10, 20, 40, 60, 80, 90 mg ER Cap: 60, 80, 120, 160 mg	50–80% obtain complete or partial relief; comparable to methysergide	Drug of first choice for prophylaxis because of safety, efficacy, and tolerability; atenolol, metoprolol, nadolol, and timolol also effective
Amitriptyline (Elavil)	10–25 mg HS; ↑ by 10–25 mg/day at weekly intervals to max 150 mg/day; most should benefit from 50–75 mg/day	Tab: 10, 25, 50, 75, 100, 150 mg	Effectiveness comparable to propranolol and methysergide	Effective for prophylaxis of migraine and tension-type headache
Verapamil (Isoptin, Calan)	80 mg TID. If needed, ↑ dose gradually to max of 480 mg/day	Tabs: 40, 80, 120 mg ER Cap: 120, 240 mg ER Tab: 180, 240 mg	50% obtain complete or partial relief	Delay of 1–2 months for maximal effect; efficacy of nifedipine and diltiazem questionable
Valproate (Depakote)	250 mg BID; ↑ by 250 mg/day at weekly intervals to effect or adverse effects; most should benefit from 1,000–2,000 mg/day	Cap[b]: 250 mg DR Tab[c]: 125, 250, 500 mg SCaps: 125 mg	50% obtain complete or partial relief	Well tolerated; additional studies needed to confirm effectiveness
Methysergide (Sansert)	2–8 mg/day in 3–4 divided daily doses to be taken with food	Tab: 2 mg	60–70% obtain complete or partial relief	Use limited by propensity for frequent and sometimes severe adverse effects; drug holidays should be planned every 6 mo
Naproxen sodium	550 mg BID	Tab: 220, 275, 550 mg	30% obtain complete or partial relief	Modest efficacy; effective for menstrual migraine

[a]Cap = Capsules; DR = Delayed release; ER = Extended release; SCap = Sprinkle capsules containing coated particles; Tab = Tablets.
[b]Valproic acid capsules.
[c]Divalproex sodium delayed release tablets.

Table 49.6 • Drugs Commonly Used for Acute Treatment of Cluster Headache[a]

Drug	Route	Dose	Contraindications	Adverse Effects	Comments
Ergotamine tartrate (Ergostat, Cafergot)	SL, PR	1–2 mg at HA onset; may repeat in 5 min (SL only); do not exceed 6 mg/attack or 10 mg/wk	CV disease, sepsis, liver or kidney disease, arterial insufficiency, pregnancy, breast feeding, concomitant macrolide use	N, V, anorexia, limb paresthesias or pain	SL ergotamine may have faster onset of effect; ↓ N and V by using smallest effective dose. Effective in 70–80%
Oxygen	Inhalation	7 L/min for 15 min	—	—	Fast onset of effect; equally effective as ergotamine tartrate
DHE-45	SC, IM, IV	1 mg (SC, IM) or 0.75 mg (IV) stat; may repeat in 45 min	CV disease, sepsis, liver or kidney disease, arterial insufficiency, pregnancy, breast feeding	N, V, limb paresthesias or pain	More effective and faster onset than SL or PR ergotamine. Premedicate with antiemetic (e.g., metoclopramide or prochlorperazine)
Sumatriptan (Imitrex)	SC	6 mg at HA onset	Ischemic heart disease, within 24 hr of ergot alkaloids	Heavy sensation in head or chest, tingling, pain at injection site	Not an FDA-approved indication; costly but well tolerated

[a]CV = Cardiovascular; HA = Headache; IM = Intramuscular; IV = Intravenous; N = Nausea; PR = Rectal; SC = Subcutaneous; SL = Sublingual; V = Vomiting.

Table 49.7 • Drugs for Prophylaxis of Cluster Headache[a]

Drug	Dose/Day	Route	Comments
Ergotamine tartrate (Cafergot, Ergostat)[57]	0.25–0.5 mg BID–TID 5 days/wk 1–2 mg BID or HS for nocturnal HA; max 12 mg/wk	SC, PO, SL, PR	Effective when given 30 min before anticipated cluster HA
Indomethacin (Indocin)[57,258]	50 mg TID	PO	Effective for chronic cluster HA
Lithium carbonate[214,215,259]	600–1,500 mg	PO	Drug of choice for chronic cluster HA; effective in 80% of patients
Melatonin[213]	10 mg QD	PO	Efficacy demonstrated in 1 randomized controlled trial; patients with chronic cluster headache did not respond
Methylergonovine maleate[260]	0.2 mg TID-QID	PO	Effective in 75% of patients in one retrospective study
Methysergide (Sansert)[200,213]	2 mg TID–QID	PO	Effective in 65–70% of patients with episodic cluster HA; less effective for chronic cluster HA
Prednisone[57,200,212,213]	40 mg QID × 2 days, then taper by 5 mg/day to maintenance dose of 15–30 mg QID	PO	A first-line agent for episodic cluster HA; more effective and faster-acting than methysergide; benefits usually within 48 hr; best for short bouts of cluster HA because of long-term adverse effects
Triamcinolone (Aristocort)[57]	4–8 mg QID	PO	May be useful in patients unresponsive to prednisone
Valproate (Depakote)[220]	600–2000 mg/day divided TID–QID	PO	Effective in 73% of patients in 1 open trial
Verapamil (Isoptin, Calan)[145,216]	240–480 mg/day divided TID–QID	PO	Nifedipine and nimodipine also effective; further study needed to confirm efficacy

[a]HA = Headache; PO = Oral; PR = Rectal; SC = Subcutaneous; SL = Sublingual.

The reader is referred to Chapter 50: Headache, written by *Brian K. Alldredge, Pharm.D.*, in the seventh edition of **Applied Therapeutics: The Clinical Use of Drugs** for a more in-depth discussion. All notations to reference numbers are based on the reference list at the end of that chapter. The editors of this handbook express their thanks to Dr. Alldredge and acknowledge that this chapter is based upon his work.

Notes:

Notes:

Chapter 50

Parkinson's Disease

Definition and Etiology

♦ Parkinson's disease is a disorder of the extrapyramidal system of the brain involving, in particular, the basal ganglia. It is a chronic, progressive disorder of motor function primarily of middle to late life. It affects men and women equally. Death usually is not caused by the disease itself, but rather by immobility (e.g., aspiration pneumonia, cardiovascular disease).

♦ *Etiology* is unknown in most cases (idiopathic parkinsonism). In some cases, Parkinson's disease is associated with viral encephalitis, neurotoxins, neuroleptic drugs, and illicit drugs (e.g., MPTP).

Pathophysiology

♦ The pathologic hallmark of Parkinson's disease is Lewy bodies (i.e., intraneuronal inclusion bodies) within the dopaminergic cells of the substantia nigra.

♦ Clinical manifestations seem to be associated with a progressive decrease of dopamine, an inhibitory neurotransmitter, and the relative increase of acetylcholine, an excitatory neurotransmitter.

♦ Exposure to an environmental contaminant superimposed upon the normal loss of basal ganglia dopamine may result in the clinical manifestations of Parkinson's disease.

Clinical Presentation

♦ **The four classic features** of Parkinson's disease consist of tremor, muscle rigidity, slowness of movement, and postural disturbances.

Tremor. A "pin-rolling" type of tremor involving the thumb and index finger usually is the first noticeable symptom of Parkinson's. The tremor worsens when the patient is fatigued or under stress and disappears with purposeful movements.

Muscular Rigidity. A ratchet (catch-release) type of motion when extremities are moved passively, known as "cogwheeling," is attributable to action of opposing muscles.

Bradykinesia is a poverty of spontaneous movement which manifests as "masked facies" or a blank stare. The patient also experiences decreased eye blinking and decreased ability to initiate or terminate steps (festinating gait).

Postural disturbances such as a stooped posture and decreased postural reflexes also are present.

♦ **Associated Symptoms.** Symptoms associated with the clinical features of Parkinson's include handwriting abnormalities, drooling, seborrhea, speech disturbances (soft, monotone voice), dysphagia, and constipation. Other symptoms include sensory complaints (numbness and paresthesia) and psychiatric disturbances (anxiety, depression, dementia).

Staging of Disability

Staging helps to assess the degree of disability and to determine disease progression relative to treatment. (See Table 50.1.)

Treatment

♦ An overview of the management of patients with Parkinson's disease is presented in Figure 50.1. No cure is known for parkinsonism; therefore, treatment is only symptomatic.

♦ Development and implementation of a long-term individualized treatment plan usually is characterized by frequent dosage adjustments over time because of the chronic and progressive nature of this disease.

♦ Table 50.2 lists the dosing regimens and adverse effects of medications used for treatment of Parkinson's disease.

♦ Table 50.3 describes levodopa drug interactions.

♦ Table 50.4 compares the pharmacologic and pharmacokinetic properties of dopamine agonists.

♦ Table 50.5 compares the pharmacologic and pharmacokinetic properties of catechol-O-methyltransferase (tolcapone, entacapone).

Table 50.1 • Staging of Disability in Parkinson's Disease	
Stage I	Unilateral involvement only; minimal or no functional impairment
Stage II	Bilateral involvement, without impairment of balance
Stage III	Evidence of postural imbalance; some restriction in activities; capable of leading independent life; mild to moderate disability
Stage IV	Severely disabled, cannot walk and stand unassisted; significantly incapacitated
Stage V	Restricted to bed or wheelchair unless aided

From reference 2.

Notes:

Table 50.2 • Medications Used for the Treatment of Parkinson's Disease[a]

Generic (Trade) Name	Dosage Unit	Titration Schedule	Usual Daily Dose	Adverse Effects
Amantadine (Symmetrel)	100 mg capsule Liquid: 50 mg/5 mL	100 mg QD; increased by 100 mg 1–2 wk	100–300 mg	Orthostatic hypotension, insomnia, depression, hallucinations, livedo reticularis, xerostomia
Anticholinergic Agents				
Benztropine (Cogentin)	0.5, 1, and 2 mg tablets Injection: 2 mL (1 mg/mL)	0.5 mg/day increased by 0.5 mg Q 3–5 days	1–3 mg QD to BID	Constipation, xerostomia, dry skin, dysphagia, confusion, memory impairment
Procyclidine (Kemadrin)	5 mg tablet	0.75 mg TID increased by 2.5 mg Q 3–45 days up to 20 mg	2.5–5 mg TID to QID	Constipation, xerostomia, dry skin, dysphagia, confusion, memory impairment
Trihexyphenidyl (Artane)	2 and 5 mg tablets Liquid: 2 mg/5 mL	1–2 mg/day increased by 1–2 mg Q 3–5 days	6–15 mg divided TID to BID	Constipation, xerostomia, dry skin, dysphagia, confusion, memory impairment
Antihistamines				
Diphenhydramine (Benadryl)	25, 50 mg capsules Liquid: 12.5 mg/5 mL Injection: 50 mg/mL	As tolerated up to 50 mg QID	25–50 mg TID to QID	Slight to moderate drowsiness; thickening of bronchial secretions; changes in appetite; headache, xerostomia
Orphenadrine (Norflex)	100 mg tablet Injection: 30 mg/mL	As tolerated up to 100 mg BID	Oral: 100 mg BID Injection: 60 mg Q 12 hr	Drowsiness, blurred vision, rash, nausea, vomiting, decreased urination, facial flushing tachycardia
Dopamine Replacement				
Caribidopa-Levodopa (Regular) (Sinemet)	10/100, 25/100, and 25/200 tablets	25/100 BID, increased by 25/100 weekly to effect and as tolerated	30/300 to 150/1500 divided TID to QID	Nausea, orthostatic hypotension, confusion, dizziness, hallucinations, dyskinesias, blepharospasm
Carbidopa-Levodopa (CR) (Sinemet CR)	25/100 and 50/200 tablets	25/100 BID (spaced at least 6 hr apart), increased Q 3–7 days	50/200 to 500/2000 divided QID	Same as regular Sinemet

(continued)

Table 50.2 • Medications Used for the Treatment of Parkinson's Disease[a] (continued)

Generic (Trade) Name	Dosage Unit	Titration Schedule	Usual Daily Dose	Adverse Effects
Dopamine Agonists				
Bromocriptine (Parlodel)	2.5 mg tablet, 5 mg capsule	1.25 HS titrate slowly as tolerated over 4–6 weeks	10–40 mg divided TID	Orthostatic hypotension, confusion, dizziness, hallucinations, nausea, leg cramps
Pergolide (Permax)	0.05, 0.25, and 1 mg tablets	0.05 mg HS titrate slowly as tolerated over 4–6 wk	1–4 mg divided TID	Orthostatic hypotension, confusion, dizziness, hallucinations, nausea, leg cramps
Pramipexole (Mirapex)	0.125, 0.25, 0.50, 1, 1.5 mg tablets	0.375 divided TID; titrate weekly by 0.125–0.25 mg/dose	1.5–4.5 mg divided TID	Orthostatic hypotension, confusion, dizziness, hallucinations, nausea, somnolence
Ropinirole (Requip)	0.25, 0.5, 1, 2, 4, 5 mg tablet	Titrate weekly by 0.25 mg/dose	3–12 mg divided TID	Orthostatic hypotension, confusion, dizziness, hallucinations, nausea, somnolence
COMT Inhibitor				
Entacapone (Comtan)	200 mg tablet	One tablet with each administration of levodopa/carbidopa up to 8 tablets daily	3–8 tablets daily	Diarrhea, dyskinesias, abdominal pain, urine discoloration
Tolcapone (Tasmar)	100, 200 mg tablet	100–200 mg TID	300–600 mg divided TID	Diarrhea, dyskinesias, abdominal pain, urine discoloration, hepatotoxicity
MAO-B Inhibitor				
Selegiline (Eldepryl)	5 mg tablet, capsule	5 mg AM; may increase to 5 mg BID	5–10 mg (take 5 mg with breakfast and 5 mg with lunch)	Insomnia, dizziness, nausea, vomiting, xerostomia, dyskinesias, mood changes

[a]COMT = Catechol-O-methyltransferase.

Table 50.3 • Levodopa Drug Interactions[a]

Drug	Interaction	Mechanism	Comments
Anticholinergics[85]	↓ levodopa effect	↓ gastric emptying, thus ↑ degradation of levodopa in gut, and ↓ amount absorbed	Watch for ↓ levodopa effect when anticholinergics used in doses sufficient to ↓ GI motility. When anticholinergic therapy discontinued in a levodopa patient, watch for signs of levodopa toxicity. Anticholinergics can relieve symptoms of parkinsonism and might offset the reduction of levodopa bioavailability. Overall, interaction of minor significance.
Benzodiazepines[92]	↓ levodopa effect	Mechanism unknown	Use together with caution; discontinue if interaction observed.
Ferrous sulfate[93]	↓ levodopa oral absorption by 50%	Formation of chelation complex	Avoid concomitant administration.
Food	↓ levodopa effect	Large, neutral amino acids compete with levodopa for intestinal absorption	Although levodopa usually taken with meals to slow absorption and ↓ central emetic effect, high-protein diets should be avoided (see Question 15).
MAOIs[90,91,94] (e.g., phenelzine, tranylcypromine)	Hypertensive crisis	↑ peripheral dopamine and norepinephrine	Avoid using together; selegiline and levodopa used successfully together. Carbidopa might minimize hypertensive reaction to levodopa in patients receiving an MAOI.
Methyldopa[86,87]	↑ or ↓ levodopa effect	Acts as central and peripheral decarboxylase inhibitor	Observe for response, may need to switch to another antihypertensive.
Metoclopramide[95,96]	↓ levodopa effect	Central dopamine blockade	Avoid using together; domperidone, a peripheral dopamine-blocking antiemetic preferred.[b]
Moclobemide	↑ adverse effects (e.g., nausea, headache)	Not established	Although MAO-B is more important than MAO-A in the metabolism of dopamine, an MAO-A inhibitor such as moclobemide may have some effect on dopamine response.
Neuroleptics[88] (e.g., butyrophenones, phenothiazines)	↓ levodopa effect	Central blockade of dopamine neurotransmission	Important interaction, avoid using these drugs together.
Papaverine	↓ levodopa effect	Unknown; might block dopamine receptors	Should be avoided. Therapeutic response to levodopa returns 5–10 days after papaverine discontinued.

(continued)

Table 50.3 • Levodopa Drug Interactions^a (continued)

Drug	Interaction	Mechanism	Comments
Phenytoin[97]	↓ levodopa effect	Mechanism unknown	Avoid using together if possible.
Pyridoxine[84]	↓ levodopa effect	↑ peripheral decarboxylation of levodopa	Not observed when levodopa given with carbidopa.
Reserpine[86]	↓ levodopa effect	Central dopamine depletion	Clinical evidence lacking, best to avoid if possible.
Tacrine	↓ levodopa effect	↑ central cholinergic activity	Try to avoid combination. Doses of tacrine and/or antiparkinsonian drugs may need to be adjusted if used concomitantly.
TCAs[88,89]	↓ levodopa effect	↑ levodopa degradation in gut because of delayed emptying	TCAs and levodopa have been used successfully together; use with caution.

^aMAO-A = Monoamine oxidase A; MAO-B = Monoamine oxidase B; MAOI = Monoamine oxidase inhibitor; TCAs = Tricyclic antidepressants. For more information regarding these and other levodopa drug interactions, see Hansten PD, Horn JR. Drug Interactions & Updates Quarterly. Facts and Comparisons, St. Louis, 2001.
^bNot available in the United States.

Notes:

Table 50.4 • Pharmacologic and Pharmacokinetic Properties of Dopamine Agonists

	Bromocriptine	Pergolide	Pramipexole	Ropinirole
Type of compound	Ergot derivative	Ergot derivative	Nonergoline	Nonergoline
Receptor specificity	D_2, D_1,[a] α_1, α_2, 5-HT	D_2, D_1, α_1, α_2, 5-HT, β	D_2, D_3, D_4, α_2	D_2, D_3, D_4
Bioavailability	8%	20%	>90%	55% (first-pass metabolism)
Tmax (min)	70–100	60–120	60–180	90
Protein binding	90–96%	90%	15%	40%
Elimination route	Metabolic (hepatic)	Metabolic (hepatic)	Renal	Metabolic (hepatic)
Half-life (hr)	3–8	27	8–12	6

[a]Antagonist.

Notes:

Table 50.5 • Pharmacologic and Pharmacokinetic Properties of Catechol-O-Methyltransferase Inhibitors[a]

	Tolcapone	Entacapone
Bioavailability	65%	30–46%
Tmax (hr)	2.0	0.7–1.2
Protein binding	99.9%	98%
Metabolism	Glucuronidation; CYP 3A4, 2A6 Acetylation; methylated by COMT	Glucuronidation
Half-life (hr)	2–3	1.6–3.4
Time to reverse COMT inhibition (hr)	16–24	4–8
Maximum COMT inhibition at 200-mg dose	80–90%	60%
Increase in levodopa AUC	100%	30–45%
Increase in levodopa half-life	75%	60–75%
Dosing method	TID, spaced 6 hr apart	With every administration of levodopa

[a]COMT = Catechol-O-methyltransferase.

Notes:

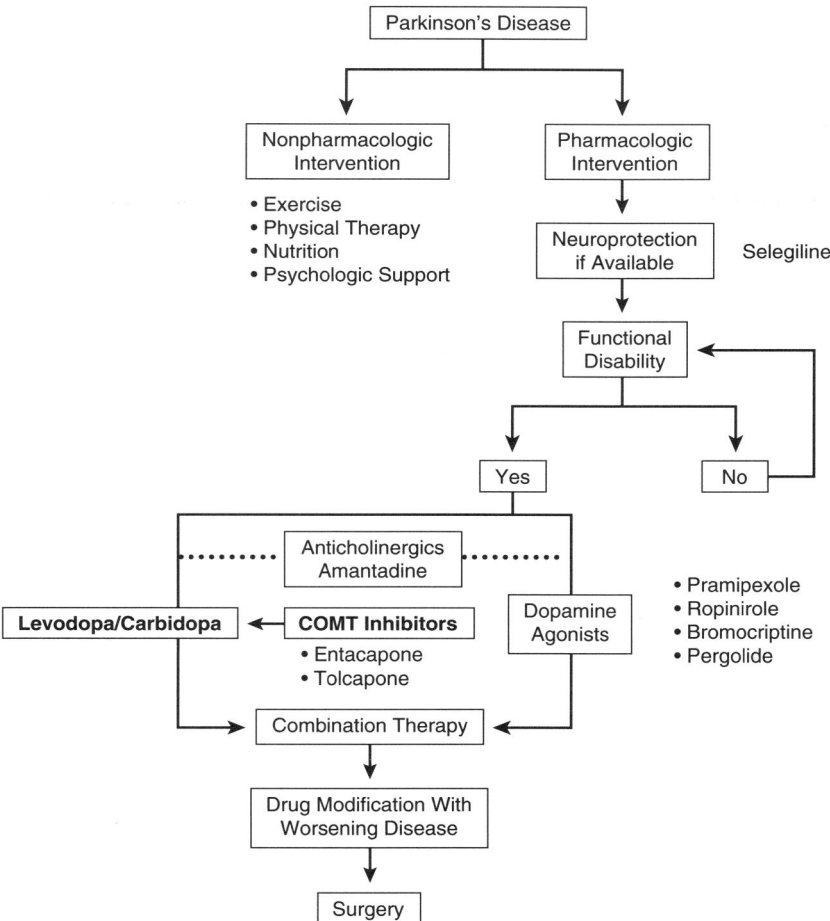

Fig. 50.1 Treatment Options in the Management of Parkinson's Disease. (Adapted with permission from Olanow CW et al. Neurology 1998;50[Suppl 3]:S1–7.)

The reader is referred to Chapter 51: Parkinson's Disease, written by *Mildred D. Gottwald, Pharm.D., John F. Flaherty, Pharm.D.* and *Barry E. Gidal, Pharm.D.,* in the seventh edition of **Applied Therapeutics: The Clinical Use of Drugs** for a more in-depth discussion. All notations to reference numbers are based on the reference list at the end of that chapter. The editors of this handbook express their thanks to Drs. Gottwald, Flaherty, and Gidal and acknowledge that this chapter is based upon their work.

Notes:

Notes:

Chapter 51

Seizure Disorders

Definition and Classification

+ ≈10% of the population will experience a seizure at some time.
+ ≈30% of seizures are caused by CNS disorders (e.g., meningitis, tumors, trauma, toxins). These seizures may recur, requiring long-term treatment.
+ Reversible insults to the CNS (e.g., alcohol withdrawal, fever, metabolic disturbances) can cause isolated seizures that do not require long-term therapy.
+ An epileptic seizure is the clinical manifestation of abnormal or excessive discharge of a set of neurons from the brain.
+ Epilepsy is a condition characterized by recurrent (>2) epileptic seizures unprovoked by any immediate cause.

Generalized Tonic Clonic (Grand Mal) Seizures

+ This is the most common seizure type.
+ Patient loses consciousness and falls at the onset. This may be accompanied by a cry. Tonic muscle spasms begin followed by a period of generalized, bilateral, repetitive clonic movements. Urinary incontinence is common.
+ Patient returns to consciousness but remains confused and lethargic (postictal state).

Absence (Petit Mal) Seizures

+ Absence seizures occur primarily in children and often disappear at puberty, although the patient may develop a second type of seizure.
+ Absence seizures consist of episodes of brief losses of consciousness, but patients do not generally fall, and consciousness returns immediately after the seizure.
+ Patients have no recall of events during the seizure and do not experience postictal confusion.
+ **Simple Absence Seizures.** Motor symptoms do not occur with simple absence seizures.
+ **Complex absence seizures** may be accompanied by muscle twitching, myoclonic jerking, or autonomic manifestations.

Simple Partial (Focal Motor or Sensory) Seizures

+ These are localized to a single cerebral hemisphere or a portion of a hemisphere. Brief; not associated with a loss of consciousness.
+ A variety of motor, sensory, or psychic manifestations may occur. A single limb may twitch, or there may be an abnormal sensory experience (e.g., an unusual smell).

Complex Partial (Psychomotor or Temporal Lobe) Seizures

♦ Complex partial seizures result from spread of abnormal focal discharges to the other cerebral hemisphere.

♦ Consciousness is impaired, and inappropriate behavior (e.g., lip smacking, tearing of clothing, or aimless wandering) may be exhibited.

♦ Brief postictal lethargy and confusion.

Epileptic Syndromes

♦ Seizures can be classified by type (Table 51.1), or they can be described as syndromes that include etiology, precipitating factors, age at onset, EEG patterns, severity, chronicity, family history, and prognosis.

♦ Identifying a syndrome can guide therapeutic decisions. Selected syndromes and their treatments can be found in Table 51.2.

Diagnosis

♦ Obtain history and description from family, teachers, and others: onset, duration, characteristics, behavior after seizure, deviation of eyes or head, localization of convulsive activity to one part of the body, impaired consciousness, and loss of continence.

♦ Neurological examination, medical history, CT scans, MRIs to locate brain lesions or anatomical defects, and EEG.

Treatment Principles

♦ Early control is important to normalize patient lives and decrease likelihood of seizure recurrence.

♦ **Nonpharmacologic treatment** includes surgery for some syndromes (e.g., Lennox-Gaustaut or Mesial Temporal Lobe Epilepsy), ketogenic diets, and avoidance of potential precipitants (e.g., stress, sleep deprivation. caffeine, alcohol).

♦ **Antiepileptic drug (AED) therapy** can completely control seizures in 60%–95% of patients.

♦ *Choice of AED.* Most AEDs have a narrow spectrum of efficacy; therefore, choice depends on accurate classification. Preferred drugs, typical dosing regimens, and adverse effects are listed in Tables 51.3, 51.4, 51.5, and 51.6.

♦ *Monotherapy Is Preferred Over Polytherapy.* Use of a single drug at optimum tolerated serum concentrations produces excellent results and minimal side effects in up to 80% of patients. Addition of a 2nd AED improves control in only 10%–20%. When substituting one AED for another, it is best to attain therapeutic concentrations of the new medication before attempting to discontinue the previous drug. Eliminating drugs in patients with long-standing seizure disorders lessens cognitive impairment and other side effects: seizure control may improve.

♦ *Therapeutic End Points.* Decreased seizure frequency and severity without producing significant dose-related side effects. Often, complete control is limited by intolerable side effects.

♦ *Duration of Therapy and Discontinuation.* AED therapy may be successfully withdrawn after a seizure-free period of 2–5 years. Seizures recur in only 12%–36%. Risk factors that may predict recurrence are listed in Table 51.6. Withdraw slowly over a period of at least 6 weeks and 1 drug at a time. Seizures occurring during withdrawal may be a symptom of withdrawal and do not necessarily necessitate reinstitution of therapy.

♦ There is poor correlation between "usual maintenance dose" and therapeutic concentrations due to interindividual variation in hepatic metabolism.

♦ Good correlation between concentration and therapeutic outcome and toxic symptoms. Therapeutic concentrations should only be considered guidelines since individuals differ dramatically in their response to specific concentrations. Seizure type also may influence concentrations required for control (e.g,. complex partial seizure requires higher levels of carbamazepine and phenytoin than do tonic-clonic seizures).

♦ Obtain serum drug concentrations in the following situations:

  • Uncontrolled seizures despite administration of higher-than-average doses.

  • Seizure recurrence in a previously controlled patient.

  • Documentation of intoxication.

  • Assessment of patient compliance.

  • Documentation of desired results from a dose change or therapeutic maneuver (e.g., loading dose).

  • Assessment of therapy in patient with infrequent seizures.

  • When precise dosage changes are required.

  • Frequent, routine determinations are costly and not warranted in stable patients.

♦ Factors that alter the relationship between AED serum concentrations and effect:

  • Laboratory variability.

  • Ranges not well established for some drugs (e.g., valproate and carbamazepine).

  • Inappropriate sample timing (wait 4–5 half-lives; measure A.M. trough level).

  • Interindividual variability in response to a given concentration.

  • Active metabolites are not measured.

  • Changes in serum protein binding.

AED Drug Interactions

♦ *Carbamazepine, phenobarbital, and phenytoin* are capable of inducing hepatic microsomal enzymes that are involved in the metabolism of various drugs (e.g., oral contraceptives). These anticonvulsants also interact with one another, as well as with valproic acid.

♦ *Valproic acid* interactions are especially complex because several pharmacokinetic parameters increase its likelihood for interacting with other drugs: extensive protein binding, ability to inhibit drug metabolism, and susceptibility to enzyme induction.

Phenobarbital. In the presence of valproic acid, serum phenobarbital levels rise considerably and necessitate reduction of the dose of phenobarbital.

Phenytoin. Total serum phenytoin levels tend to fall during the first several weeks of valproic acid administration, followed by a gradual return to prevalproic acid levels. Because free serum phenytoin levels are apparently not altered in most patients, alteration in phenytoin dosage is seldom required.

Carbamazepine. A potent enzyme inducer that makes it difficult to achieve adequate serum levels of valproate. Levels are often 50% of that normally expected. Conversely, valproate may inhibit epoxide hydrolase, causing accumulation of the active metabolite, carbamazepine epoxide. This can lead to carbamazepine intoxication. When carbamazepine is discontinued, taper by 10%–20% every 2 weeks.

Drugs That Reduce Serum Valproic Acid Levels. Serum valproic acid levels are reduced by phenytoin, carbamazepine, and possibly phenobarbital, and an increased dose of valproic acid may be required.

Clonazepam. Combined use of valproic acid and clonazepam may precipitate absence seizure.

♦ *AED-Oral Contraceptive Interaction.* AEDs can reduce the efficacy of oral contraceptives. This is manifested as breakthrough bleeding and pregnancy. Association with enzyme inducers such as phenobarbital, phenytoin, and carbamazepine. Not associated with valproate, lamotrigine, or gabapentin. Use of contraceptives with higher estrogen content may offset this interaction.

♦ *Carbamazepine-Erythromycin Interaction.* Inhibition of hepatic metabolism of carbamazepine by erythromycin may result in dramatic elevations in carbamazepine serum concentrations (up to 2 times) and precipitation of intoxication.

Febrile Seizures
Incidence and Classification

♦ Up to 5% of children have febrile seizures between 6 months and 6 yr of age.

♦ *Simple febrile seizures* occur with fever >38°C in normal children <5 yr of age. They last <15 minutes with no focal features.

♦ *Complex febrile seizures* show focal characteristics or are prolonged. Child may or may not have previous neurologic abnormalities.

♦ *Febrile status epilepticus* consists of continuous or serial tonic-clonic seizures lasting more than 30 minutes without return of consciousness. The fever does not originate in the CNS.

♦ *Seizures with fever* occur in association with febrile illnesses and may be of any type or duration. Neurologic status may or may not have been normal.

♦ Risk of recurrent afebrile seizures is 2–3 times greater than that for the general population. Risk factors include family history, complicated initial seizure, and pre-existing neurologic abnormalities.

Status Epilepticus
Definition and Characteristics

♦ Status epilepticus exists if there are more than 30 minutes of continuous seizure activity of 2 or more sequential seizures without full recovery of consciousness between seizures.

♦ In the absence of obvious precipitating factors (e.g., head trauma, CNS infection, hypoglycemia, or drug/alcohol abuse), the most common cause is noncompliance with maintenance AEDs.

♦ Uncontrolled seizures may cause severe metabolic and hemodynamic alterations, neurologic sequelae, and cardiovascular collapse. It is considered a medical emergency since mortality may be as high as 30%.

♦ Long-term consequences include cognitive impairment, memory loss, and worsening of seizure disorder.

Treatment

♦ *Immediate goal* is to ensure adequate ventilation and terminate current seizure activity. Place an airway (if airway placement is impossible, position patient on his side) and establish an IV line using normal saline. Obtain blood sample for electrolytes, glucose, AED concentrations, and toxicology screen.

♦ *Thiamine* 100 mg or B complex IV should be given before 25 gm *glucose* (50 mL of 50% dextrose solution) by IV push. Thiamine given first prevents Wernicke's encephalopathy.

♦ Treat seizure with IV diazepam or lorazepam [preferred because lower lipid solubility prevents rapid redistribution and accounts for longer effective duration of action (72 hr vs. 60 minutes)]. Side effects are short lived but include sedation, hypotension, and respiratory arrest.

♦ *Lorazepam* 0.1 mg/kg IV at 2 mg/minute mg, diluted with an equal volume of saline or water, IV push over 2 minutes. Repeat in 5–10 minutes if seizure activity has not stopped.

♦ *Diazepam* 0.2 mg/kg at 5 mg/minute IV to minimize cardiorespiratory toxicity related to propylene glycol solvent. Repeat in 5–10 minutes if necessary.

♦ *Phenytoin* (administered as either sodium phenytoin injection or as fosphenytoin) is a long-acting AED of choice for status epilepticus. A dose of phenytoin (20 mg/kg IV at 50 mg/minute) or fosphenytoin (20 mg/kg IV PE at 150 mg/minute is recommended).

Table 51.1 • International Classification of Epileptic Seizures

Partial Seizure (Local or Focal)
Simple Partial Seizures (Without Impairment of Consciousness)
Motor symptoms
Special sensory or somatosensory symptoms
Autonomic symptoms
Psychic symptoms

Complex[a] Partial Seizures (with Impairment of Consciousness)
Progressing to impairment of consciousness
    With no other features
    With features as in simple partial seizures
    With automatisms
With impaired consciousness at onset
    With no other features
    With features as in simple partial seizures
    With automatisms

Partial Seizures That Evolve to Generalized Seizures
Simple partial seizures evolving to generalized seizures
Complex partial seizures evolving to generalized seizures
Simple partial seizures evolving to complex partial seizures to generalized seizures

Generalized Seizures (Convulsive or Nonconvulsive)
Absence Seizures
Typical seizures (impaired consciousness only)
Atypical absence seizures

Myoclonic Seizures

Clonic Seizures

Tonic Seizures

Tonic-Clonic Seizures

Atonic (Astatic or Akinetic) Seizures

Unclassified Epileptic Seizures
All seizures that cannot be classified because of inadequate or incomplete data and some that cannot be classified in previously described categories

[a]Complex implies organized, high-level activity.
From references 1, 3, and 4.

Notes:

Table 51.2 • Selected Epileptic Syndromes[a]

Syndrome	Seizure Patterns and Characteristics	Preferred AED Therapy	Comments
Juvenile myoclonic epilepsy	Myoclonic seizures often precede generalized tonic-clonic seizures. Myoclonic and generalized tonic-clonic episodes upon awakening. Absence seizures also common. ↓ sleep, fatigue, and alcohol commonly precipitate seizures	Valproic acid. Phenytoin or carbamazepine as adjuncts to valproate in resistant cases. Carbamazepine reported to exacerbate seizures in some patients	5–10% of all epilepsies; 85–90% response to valproate. Lifelong therapy usually needed. High relapse rate with attempts to discontinue AED therapy
Lennox-Gastaut syndrome	Generalized seizures: atypical absence, atonic/akinetic, myoclonic, and tonic most common. Abnormal interictal EEG with slow spike-wave pattern. Cognitive dysfunction and mental retardation. Status epilepticus common	Valproic acid, benzodiazepines, lamotrigine. Topiramate may be effective. Felbamate also may be effective, but potential hematologic toxicity limits use. Poorly responsive to AEDs	Oversedation with aggressive AED trials may ↑ seizure frequency. Tolerance to benzodiazepines limits their usefulness
Childhood absence epilepsy (true petit mal)	Typical absences often in clusters of multiple seizures (pyknolepsy). Tonic-clonic seizures in ≈40%. Onset usually between ages 4 and 8. Significant genetic component. EEG shows classic 3-Hz spike-wave pattern	Ethosuximide or valproic acid	80–90% response rate to AED therapy. Good prognosis for remission. Tonic-clonic seizures may persist
Reflex epilepsy	Tonic-clonic seizures most common. Induced by flicker or patterns (photosensitivity) most commonly. Reading also may precipitate partial seizures affecting the jaw, which may generalize. Some cases involve precipitation of underlying seizures; some seem primary	AED specific to underlying seizures. Avoidance of precipitating stimuli when possible. Valproic acid usually effective for cases of spontaneous seizures precipitated by photosensitivity	Relatively rare. Seizures may be precipitated by television or video games
Temporal lobe epilepsy	Complex partial seizures with automatisms. Simple partial seizures (auras) common; secondary generalized seizures occur in 50%	Carbamazepine, phenytoin, valproic acid. Gabapentin, lamotrigine, topiramate, tiagabine	Often incompletely controlled with current AEDs. Emotional stress may precipitate seizures; psychiatric disorders seen with temporal lobe epilepsy; surgical resection often effective when AEDs fail

[a]AED = Antiepileptic drug; EEG = Electroencephalogram.
From references 9–14.

Table 51.3 • Antiepileptic Drugs Useful for Various Seizure Types[a]

Primary Generalized Tonic-Clonic	Secondarily Generalized Tonic-Clonic	Simple or Complex Partial	Absence	Myoclonic, Atonic/Akinetic
Most Effective with Least Toxicity				
Valproate	Carbamazepine	Carbamazepine	Ethosuximide	Valproate
Phenytoin	Oxcarbazepine	Oxcarbazepine	Valproate	Clonazepam
Carbamazepine	Phenytoin	Phenytoin		(Lamotrigene)[b]
Oxcarbazepine	Valproate	Valproate		(Topiramate)[b]
(Topiramate)[b]	(Gabapentin)[b]	(Gabapentin)[b]		
(Zonisamide)[b]	(Lamotrigine)[b]	(Lamotrigene)[b]		
	(Topiramate)[b]	(Levetiracetam)[b]		
	(Tiagabine)[b]	(Topiramate)[b]		
	(Zonisamide)[b]	(Tiagabine)[b]		
		(Zonisamide)[b]		
Effective, But Often Cause Unacceptable Toxicity				
Phenobarbital	Phenobarbital	Clorazepate	Clonazepam	(Felbamate)[c]
Primidone	Primidone	Phenobarbital	Trimethadione	
(Felbamate)[c]	(Felbamate)[c]	Primidone		
		(Felbamate)[c]		
Of Little Value				
Ethosuximide	Ethosuximide	Ethosuximide	Phenytoin	
Trimethadione	Trimethadione	Trimethadione	Carbamazepine	
			Phenobarbital	
			Primidone	

[a]Drugs are listed in general order of preference within each category. Recommendations by various authorities may differ, especially regarding the relative place of valproate and the role of phenytoin as a first-line AED. Many authorities now discourage the use of phenobarbital and primidone.
[b]The place of gabapentin, lamotrigine, levetiracetam, topiramate, tiagabine, and zonisamide is yet to be determined. They are placed on this table only to indicate the types of seizures for which they appear to be effective. Much more clinical experience is needed before their roles as possible primary AEDs are clarified.
[c]The place of felbamate is yet to be determined. It is placed on this table only to indicate the types of seizures for which it appears to be effective. Much more clinical experience is needed before felbamate's role as a possible primary AED is clarified. Felbamate has been associated with aplastic anemia and hepatic failure; until a possible causative role is clarified, felbamate cannot be recommended for treatment of epilepsy unless all other, potentially less toxic treatment options have been exhausted.
From references 26 and 28–30.

Notes:

Table 51.4 • Pharmacokinetic Properties of Antiepileptic Drugs[a]

Drug	Oral Absorption	Half-Life (hr)	Time to Steady State[b]	Dosage Schedule	Usual Therapeutic Serum Concentration	Plasma Protein Binding	Volume of Distribution (L/kg)
Carbamazepine	90–100%	*Chronic:* 5–25	2–4 days	BID to TID	5–12+ µg/mL	75% (50–90)	0.8–1.6
Ethosuximide	90–100%	*Pediatric:* 30 *Adult:* 60	5–10 days	QD (BID)	40–100 µg/mL	0%	0.7
Felbamate	>90%	12–20	3–4 days	BID to TID	Not determined	24%	0.7–0.8
Gabapentin	40–60%; ↓ with ↑ dose size	*Normal renal function:* 5–9; ↑ with ↓ renal function	*Normal renal function:* 1–1.5 days	TID to QID (Q 6–8 hr)	>2 µg/mL (proposed)	0%	≈0.8
Lamotrigine	90–100%	*Monotherapy:* 24–29 *Enzyme inducers:* 15 *Enzyme inhibitor (VPA*[b]*):* 59	4–9 days	QD	≤5 µg/mL (proposed)	55%	0.9–1.2
Levetiracetam	100%	*Normal renal function:* 6–8; ↑ with ↓ renal function	*Normal renal function:* 1–1.5 days	BID	Not determined	<10%	≈0.7

Drug							
Oxcarbazepine	100%	8–13	2–3 days	BID to TID	Not determined	40%	—
Phenobarbital	90–100%	2–4 days	8–16 days	QD	15–40 µg/mL	50%	0.5–0.6
Phenytoin	90–100%	Varies with dose	5–30+ days	QD (BID)	10–20 µg/mL	95%	0.5–0.7
Primidone	90–100%	3–12	12–48 hr	BID to TID	5–15 µg/mL (15–40 µg/mL for derived phenobarbital)	<50%	0.4–1.1
Tiagabine	90%	Monotherapy: 7–9 Enzyme Inducers: 4–7	1–2 days	TID to QID	Not determined	96%	1.1
Topiramate	≥80%	12–24	3–4 days	BID (QD)	Not determined	10–15%	0.7
Valproate	100%	10–16	2–3 days	BID to QID	50–150+ µg/mL	90+%	0.09–0.17
Vigabatrin	>60%	5–7	2–3 days	BID (QD)	Not helpful; irreversible inhibitor of GABA-transaminase	60–70%	—
Zonisamide	≈80%	Monotherapy: ≈60 Enzyme inducers: 27–36	2 wk	QD	Not determined	50–60%	1.3

a VPA = Valproic acid.
b Based on four half-lives. This lag time should allow determination of steady-state serum concentrations within limits of most assay sensitivities.

Table 51.5 • Drugs Used for the Treatment of Partial and Generalized Tonic-Clonic Seizures[a]

AED	Regimen	Adverse Effects	Comments
Carbamazepine (Tegretol)	Initial 200 mg BID (adults) or 100 mg BID (children) and ↑ weekly until therapeutic response or target serum concentrations. Usual maintenance doses 7–15 mg/kg/day in adults; 10–40 mg/kg/day in children.	GI upset, sedation, visual disturbance may limit dosage. Severe blood dyscrasias extremely rare (<1/50,000). Mild leukopenia more common. Laboratory monitoring of little value. Hepatotoxicity rare. May cause SIADH.	Usually little sedation and minimal interference with cognitive function or behavior. Preferred by most for partial or secondarily generalized seizures. Tegretol-XR or Carbatrol may allow less frequent dosing with fewer peak serum concentration–related side effects. These extended-release preparations may also facilitate compliance.
Phenytoin (Dilantin)	Initiate at maintenance dose of 4–5 mg/kg/day (300–400 mg/day). Titrate on basis of clinical response and target serum concentration. 3–4 weeks between dose ↑ recommended because of potentially slow accumulation.	Nystagmus, ataxia, sedation, mental changes usually predictable from serum concentrations. Gum hyperplasia, hirsutism common. Osteomalacia uncommon. Seizure frequency may ↑ with significantly ↑ serum concentrations. Peripheral neuropathy, pseudolymphoma, hypersensitivity with liver damage rare.	Clearance and $t_{1/2}$ change with dose. Small ↑ in dose (30 mg capsule dosage form) recommended as therapeutic range approached. Suspension and chewable tablets contain free-acid form of phenytoin; capsules contain sodium phenytoin (converts to 92% of free-acid form). Cautious use of suspension; dose measurement and potential mixing difficulties. IM administration not recommended. Potential precipitation in IV solutions. Dilute in small volume of normal saline and administer IV using 0.45–0.22 micron filter. Administer IV at <50 mg/min. Fosphenytoin (Cerebyx) recommended for IM and IV use. Can be diluted for IV infusion in saline or dextrose-containing fluids. Can be administered at up to 150 mg PE/minute IV. Lower rate of injection site complications.
Valproate (Depakene, Depakote)	See Table 51.6.		
Phenobarbital	Initial 1 mg/kg/day; titrate to therapeutic response or target serum concentration. 2–3 weeks between dose ↑.	Sedation (chronic), behavior disturbances common, especially in children. Possibly impairs learning and intellectual performance. Osteomalacia uncommon.	Considered outmoded for antiepileptic therapy in most patients. Questionable benefit for prophylaxis of febrile seizures; adverse effects outweigh benefits. IV use for refractory status epilepticus. 10–20 mg/kg IV at <100 mg/min; caution when used with diazepam for status epilepticus because of additive cardiovascular and respiratory depression.

Drug	Dosage	Side Effects	Comments
Primidone (Mysoline)	Initial 5–15 mg/kg/day; then titrate to therapeutic response or target serum concentration. 2–3 weeks between dose ↑.	Sedation, ataxia, GI toxicity common with initial therapy. Essentially similar profile to phenobarbital.	Considered outmoded for antiepileptic therapy in most patients. Most antiepileptic effects from phenobarbital as metabolite. Expensive with less favorable side effect profile.
Felbamate (Felbatol)	Initial 1,200 mg/day (15 mg/kg). ↑ Q 7 days by 1,200 mg/day (15 mg/kg/day). Current maximum recommended dose of 3,600 mg/day. Therapeutic serum concentrations not yet defined.	Nausea, anorexia, and headache common with initial add-on therapy; much less frequent with monotherapy. Insomnia may occur. Associated with cases of aplastic anemia and hepatotoxicity. Fatalities reported. Careful monitoring of patients necessary.	Significant inhibition of metabolism of other AEDs; doses of existing drugs should be ↓ 20–30% with addition of felbamate. May have positive effect on mental status and functioning.
Gabapentin (Neurontin)	Initial 300 mg/day with titration to 900–1,800 mg/day over 1–2 wk. Up to 2,400 mg/day or higher may be needed for some patients. Owing to short $t_{1/2}$ TID or QID dosing recommended.	Sedation, dizziness, and ataxia relatively common with initiation of therapy. Gabapentin therapy usually not associated with prominent side effects.	Primarily excreted unchanged by kidneys. No significant interactions with other AEDs or other drugs identified to date. Absorption dose dependent; fraction absorbed ↓ as size of individual dose ↑.
Lamotrigine (Lamictal)	*When added to enzyme inducers alone:* Initiate at 50 mg QD HS. May start at 50 mg BID. Daily dose can be ↑ by 50–100 mg Q 7–14 days. Usual maintenance doses of 400–500 mg/day. Doses up to 700 mg/day have been used. BID dosing may be necessary with enzyme inducer cotherapy. *When added to valproate alone:* Initiate at 25 mg QOD HS. Daily dose can be ↑ by 25 mg Q 14 days. Usual maintenance doses of 100–200 mg/day. *When added to valproate and enzyme inducers:* Initiate at 25 mg QOD HS. Daily dose can be ↑ by 25 mg Q 14 days. Usual daily doses of 100–200 mg/day.	Dizziness, diplopia, sedation, ataxia, and blurred vision. Common with initiation of therapy; limit speed of titration. Rash in ≈10% of treated patients; more common with coadministration with valproate and rapid dose escalation.	Significant ↑ in clearance of lamotrigine when coadministered with enzyme inducers such as carbamazepine. Significant ↓ in clearance when coadministered with valproate; valproate appears to inhibit metabolism of lamotrigine. ↑ CNS side effects when lamotrigine is used with carbamazepine. Slow, gradual titration of dose may reduce risk of skin rash.

(continued)

Table 51.5 • Drugs Used for the Treatment of Partial and Generalized Tonic-Clonic Seizures[a] (continued)

AED	Regimen	Adverse Effects	Comments
Tiagabine (Gabitril)	Initial 4 mg/day. ↑ by 4 mg/day at 7 days. Then ↑ daily dose by 4–8 mg Q wk. Maximum recommended dose of 32 mg/day in adolescents or 56 mg/day in adults. BID to QID dosing recommended.	Drowsiness, nervousness, difficulty with concentration or attention, tremor. Nonspecific dizziness described by some patients.	Increase clearance when given with enzyme inducers. TID or QID doses probably needed. Potential for protein-binding displacement interactions with other highly protein bound drugs (e.g., valproate). Significance of protein-binding displacement not known at present. Substrate for CYP 3A.
Topiramate (Topamax)	Initial 50 mg HS. ↑ daily dose by 50 mg Q 7 days. 200–400 mg/day recommended as target dosage range. Larger daily doses associated with increased CNS side effects without improved seizure control. BID dosing recommended.	Sedation, dizziness, difficulty concentrating, confusion. May be dose-related. Possible weight loss. Weak carbonic anhydrase (CA) inhibitor; may cause or predispose to kidney stones; CA inhibition also possibly related to paresthesias in up to 15%.	Approximately 70% renal elimination. Phenytoin and carbamazepine may reduce topiramate plasma concentrations and potentially increase dosage requirements. Topiramate may cause small ↑ in phenytoin plasma concentration and small ↓ in valproate concentrations. May ↓ effect of oral contraceptives.

[a]AEDs = Antiepileptic drugs; CNS = Central nervous system; GI = Gastrointestinal; PE = Phenytoin sodium equivalent; SIADH = Syndrome of inappropriate antidiuretic hormone secretion; $t_{1/2}$ = half-life.

Notes:

Table 51.6 • Common Drugs for the Treatment of Absence Seizures^a

AED	Regimen	Adverse Effects	Comments
Valproate (Depakene, Depakote)	Initial 5–10 mg/kg/day (sprinkle caps or syrup); then ↑ by 5–10 mg/kg/day weekly to therapeutic effect or target serum concentration. Manufacturer's recommended usual maximum dose of 60 mg/kg/day often must be exceeded clinically (especially for patients receiving enzyme-inducing AEDs) to achieve optimum clinical results	GI upset, appetite stimulation, and weight gain common. Serious hepatotoxicity extremely rare with monotherapy and in patients >2 yr	Enteric-coated tablets or capsules preferred oral dosage forms because of ↓ GI toxicity. Time to peak serum concentrations delayed for 3–8 hr with enteric coating; longer delay if given with food; serum concentrations must be interpreted carefully. Also effective against primarily generalized tonic-clonic seizures
Ethosuximide (Zarontin)	Initial 20 mg/kg/day or 250 mg QD or BID; then ↑ by 250 mg/day Q 2 wk to therapeutic effect or target serum concentration	GI upset and sedation common with large single dose, especially on initiation of therapy. Daily divided doses may be necessary despite long $t_{1/2}$. Leukopenia (mild, transient) in up to 7%; serious hematologic toxicity extremely rare	Parents/patient should be informed GI effects, and sedation may occur but tolerance usually develops. No good evidence that ethosuximide precipitates tonic-clonic seizures. Up to 50% of patients with absence may develop tonic-clonic seizures independent of ethosuximide

^aAED = Antiepileptic drug; GI = Gastrointestinal.

Notes:

The reader is referred to Chapter 52: Seizure Disorders, written by *Rex S. Lott, Pharm.D.*, and *James W. McAuley*, in the seventh edition of **Applied Therapeutics: The Clinical Use of Drugs** for a more in-depth discussion. All notations to reference numbers are based on the reference list at the end of that chapter. The editors of this handbook express their thanks to Dr. Lott and Mr. McAuley and acknowledge that this chapter is based upon their work.

Notes:

Chapter 52

Cerebrovascular Disorders

Definitions

♦ ***Cerebrovascular disease*** is a broad term encompassing a variety of disorders affecting the blood vessels of the CNS. These disorders result from either inadequate blood flow to the brain (i.e., cerebral ischemia) with subsequent infarction of the involved portion of the CNS or from hemorrhages into the parenchyma or subarachnoid space of the CNS and subsequent neurological dysfunction.

♦ ***Transient ischemic attack (TIA)*** is a temporary (<24 hr, usually 2–15 minutes) focal neurological deficit caused by cerebral ischemia, usually resulting from microemboli to the brain. The reversibility of symptoms is due to fibrinolytic dissolution of emboli and restoration of blood flow. See Table 52.1 for symptoms associated with TIAs.

♦ ***Reversible ischemic neurological deficit (RIND)*** is similar to TIA in that deficits are temporary: however, deficit improves over 72 hr and may not completely resolve. RIND is due to decreased blood flow to a portion of the brain, usually due to embolic or thrombotic clot. Clot slowly lyses or collateral blood flow results in resolution of symptoms.

♦ ***Cerebral infarction*** produces permanent neurological deficits caused by neuronal death in a focal area of the brain. Primary causes of persistent ischemia and infarction are atherosclerosis (which causes a *thrombus* or clot near the site of infarction) and *emboli,* which are clots that have migrated from a distant source (e.g., heart or carotid artery) to the cerebral arteries. A *stable (completed) infarction* is a permanent deficit that will neither improve nor deteriorate. An *improving infarction* is marked by a slow recovery of neurological function over days to weeks. A *progressive (evolving) infarction* describes continual deterioration of neurological function following the initial onset of symptoms.

♦ ***Cerebral hemorrhage*** involves escape of blood from a cerebral vessel to surrounding brain tissues: this decreases blood flow to focal areas of the brain; it accounts for 10% of strokes. Primary causes include subarachnoid hemorrhage, arteriovenous malformation, hypertensive hemorrhage, drug reactions, and trauma. Symptoms are similar to those of TIA and cerebral infarction.

♦ ***Stroke*** is a lay term to describe a sudden neurological change related to altered cerebral blood supply (e.g., cerebral ischemia, cerebral infarction, or cerebral hemorrhage). The presenting signs are slurred speech, difficulty swallowing, weakness, facial paralysis, or blindness. The exact symptoms are dependent upon the area of the brain that is affected.

Etiology of Cerebral Ischemia and Infarction

♦ Atherosclerotic diseases of the large arteries (60%);

♦ disease of penetrating arteries (20%);

♦ cardiac disease such as atrial fibrillation (15%);

♦ infection and inflammation (5%).

Treatment of TIAs

+ **Goals.** The immediate goal is to re-establish adequate blood flow. Longer range objectives are to prevent reocclusion, decrease risk of future TIAs, prevent cerebral infarction, and improve neurological function through rehabilitation.

+ **Prevention.** Control risk factors (see Table 52.2).

+ **Surgical interventions** are designed to remove the source of emboli or improve circulation to ischemic areas of the brain. *Carotid endarterectomy* (CEA) includes excision of atheromatous plaques: *balloon angioplasty* is used to expand a stenosed artery and improve blood flow. CEA is reserved for those with ulcerated lesions or stenotic clots that occlude >70% of blood flow. It is not indicated in those with permanent neurologic damage or 100% occlusion. Restenosis occurs in 25%; this is not prevented by aspirin and/or dipyridamole.

+ **Pharmacological management** requires precise diagnosis. An ischemic stroke should be differentiated from a hemorrhagic stroke because drugs can cause severe morbidity and mortality. Since platelets play a key role in the formation of atheromatous clots, various antiplatelet agents have been tried to prevent ischemic attacks. Anticoagulants are indicated in strokes related to atrial fibrillation (see Table 52.3).

  Aspirin reduces the risk of stroke and death in patients who have experienced a previous TIA or stroke. Effective doses range from 50–975 mg/day. Start with 50–75 mg/day and increase to BID-TID if there are recurrent TIAs. High doses of ASA can increase thrombotic tendencies.

  Dipyridamole has no apparent benefit in preventing TIA and stroke used alone. A precise role for the combination of dipyridamole and aspirin is yet to be determined.

  Sulfinpyrazone, used alone or in combination with ASA, does not reduce the incidence of TIAs and is no longer recommended for use in TIA.

  Ticlopidine is more effective than ASA in reducing the risk of TIAs and strokes in those with a prior cerebral thrombotic event by about 20%; even more so in nonwhites (48%). Less peptic ulcer and GI hemorrhage than ASA but causes diarrhea (20%), rash (12%–15%), and reversible neutropenia (1%–2%). The latter occurs in the first 3 months; a CBC is indicated Q 2 weeks over this period. Adverse effects and cost limit its use to those who have failed ASA. Dose is 250 mg BID.

  Clopidogrel (Plavix) inhibits platelet aggregation and may be more effective and safer than aspirin in preventing vascular occlusive events. More study is needed to determine effect on stroke. Aspirin remains the preferred drug for preventing ischemic stroke.

  Anticoagulants. Warfarin is indicated for those with TIAs or strokes arising from a clot of cardiac origin in patients with atrial fibrillation. There are no good studies comparing antiplatelets to anticoagulants in prevention of stroke in other situations. They may have a role in patients who continue to have TIAs or minor strokes despite adequate antiplatelet therapy and may be preferred when the affected region is the pons or medulla since further events could be devastating. Those with previous MI taking anticoagulants have fewer cerebrovascular events.

Cerebral Infarction and Ischemic Stroke

+ **Differential diagnosis** between hemorrhagic and ischemic stroke is vital, and therapy should not be initiated until an ischemic lesion has been confirmed (e.g., MRI, PET, CT).

+ **Supportive Therapy.** Maintenance of fluid and electrolyte balance is critical. Hyponatremia secondary to excessive hydration or inadequate sodium can increase damage and cause seizures. Serum glucose levels should be maintained <155 mg/dL with insulin if necessary, because hyperglycemia adversely affects outcomes. Finally, BP should be titrated to maintain optimal neurological function. Mild hypertension may be required for 1–2 days after stroke onset. Rapid drops in the BP can decrease cerebral blood flow and expand the region of ischemia and infarction.

♦ **Heparin.** Patients must be selected carefully for anticoagulant therapy based on the rate and extent of stroke progression, as well as etiology of the ischemia (i.e., embolic vs. thrombotic). Heparin is of questionable benefit for treatment of completed ischemic stroke and not advised for ischemic stroke due to embolism. Doses are similar to other indications: 50–70 units bolus followed by 10–25 units/kg/hr titrated to maintain the PTT 1.5–2 times baseline. Warfarin is given for 1–6 months at doses that increase INR to 2–3 times baseline.

♦ **Heparinoids** [low-molecular-weight heparin (LMWH)] are not indicated for acute ischemic stroke; however, LMWH may prevent further embolic events in some high-risk patients following ischemic stroke by reducing the incidence of deep venous thrombosis (DVT). Also see Chapter 13: Thrombosis.

♦ **Ancrod** leads to fibrinolysis and rarely is associated with significant bleeding complications. It shows promise for treatment of ischemic stroke, but further studies are needed to determine its role in treatment of ischemic stroke.

♦ **Thrombolytics.** Since the critical event in a thromboembolic stroke is development of an acute thrombus, thrombolytics (e.g., tPA or streptokinase) can improve neurological recovery by restoring blood flow. Thrombolytics, however, can cause life-threatening hemorrhage. Criteria for use of alteplase in the treatment of acute stroke are noted in Table 52.4.

Stroke Education. Patients should be instructed to get emergency medical treatment if experiencing paralysis, speech impairment, blurred or sudden loss of vision, or altered level of consciousness.

Subarachnoid Hemorrhage

♦ **Clinical Presentation.** Table 52.5 presents the Hunt and Hess Scale for rating the severity of subarachnoid hemorrhage. A CT scan demonstrates blood in the subarachnoid space. Three major complications are responsible for neurologic changes.

♦ **Treatment.** Therapy for managing the complications of subarachnoid hemorrhage are noted in Table 52.6.

Table 52.1 • Symptoms Associated with Transient Ischemic Attacks

Symptom	Right Carotid	Left Carotid	Vertebrobasilar
Aphasia	Possible	Yes	No
Ataxia	No	No	Yes
Blindness	Right	Left	Right or left side
Clumsiness	Yes	Yes	Yes
Diplopia	No	No	Yes
Dysarthria	Yes	Yes	No
Paralysis	Left side	Right side	Any limb
Paresthesia	Left side	Right side	Any limb
Vertigo	No	No	Yes

Table 52.2 • Definite Risk Factors for Stroke

Life-style Risk Factors	Pathophysiologic Risk Factors
Age (older)	Blood pressure differences between arms[a]
Alcohol abuse	Cardiac disease[b]
Cigarette smoking	Carotid bruit[c]
Drug abuse	Diabetes mellitus
Genetic factors	Hypertension
Males	↑ fibrinogen
	↑ hematocrit
	Migraine headaches[d]
	Sickle cell disease[e]
	Retinal emboli[f]
	Transient ischemic attacks (past history)

[a]This may indicate an aortic obstruction involving or before a carotid artery.
[b]Atrial fibrillation especially is associated with stroke due to the potential for embolism. However, the presence of cardiovascular disease is associated with peripheral and cerebrovascular disease.
[c]A carotid bruit indicates a blood flow defect in the carotid artery and usually is associated with a carotid artery thrombus. This increases the risk for small emboli to go to the brain.
[d]Migraine headaches are caused by strong vasoconstriction. In severe cases, the constriction of the cerebral arteries results in cerebral ischemia and stroke.
[e]Ischemic events are common in sickle cell disease due to clumping of red blood cells in arterioles and capillaries, restricting blood flow.
[f]Because the retinal artery is supplied from the carotid artery, an embolus to the retina usually is indicative of a carotid artery thrombus.

Table 52.3 • Drugs for Preventing Transient Ischemic Attacks and Ischemic Stroke[a]

Drug	Action	Dose	Adverse Effects
Aspirin	Antiplatelet	50–1,300 mg/day	Diarrhea, gastric ulcer, GI upset
Dipyridamole	Antiplatelet (use in combination with aspirin)	200 mg sustained release twice daily	GI upset
Ticlopidine	Antiplatelet	500 mg/day	Diarrhea, neutropenia, rash
Clopidogrel	Antiplatelet	75 mg/day	Thrombocytopenia, neutropenia
Warfarin	Anticoagulant	Titrate to INR 2–3	Bleeding, bruising, petechiae

[a]GI = Gastrointestinal; INR = International normalized ratio.

Notes:

Table 52.4 • Criteria for Alteplase Use in Treatment of Acute Stroke[a]

Inclusion Criteria	Exclusion Criteria
≥18 yr	Minor or rapidly improving symptoms
Clinical diagnosis of stroke with clinically meaningful neurologic deficit	CT signs of intracranial hemorrhage
Clearly defined onset within 180 min before treatment	History of intracranial hemorrhage
Baseline CT with no evidence of intracranial hemorrhage	Seizure at onset of stroke
	Stroke or serious head injury within 3 mo Major surgery or serious trauma within 2 wk GI or urinary tract hemorrhage within 3 wk Systolic BP >185 mm Hg, diastolic BP >110 mm Hg Aggressive treatment to lower BP Glucose <50 mg/dL or >400 mg/dL Symptoms of subarachnoid hemorrhage

[a]BP = Blood pressure; CT = Computed tomography; GI = Gastrointestinal.

Table 52.5 • Hunt and Hess Scale for Rating Severity of Subarachnoid Hemorrhage

Grade	Description
I	Minor headache, minor neck stiffness
II	Severe headache, severe neck stiffness, cranial nerve signs, photophobia
III	Drowsiness, confusion, mild paresis, mild dysphasia
IV	Stupor or sopor, moderate-to-severe hemiparesis, dysphasia
V	Coma, decerebrate rigidity, symptoms of acute midbrain syndrome

Table 52.6 • Therapy for Subarachnoid Hemorrhage Complications[a]

Rebleeding	Hydrocephalus	Delayed Ischemia
Surgical clip	Ventricular drain	Nimodipine 60 mg Q 4 hr for 21 days
Aminocaproic acid 5 g loading dose and 1 to 2 g/hr	Ventricular-peritoneal shunt	Hypervolemia PCWP 12–15 mm Hg
		Hypertension Systolic BP 170–220 mm Hg

[a]BP = Blood pressure; PCWP = Pulmonary capillary wedge pressure.

The reader is referred to Chapter 53: Cerebrovascular Disorders, written by *Timothy E. Welty, Pharm.D.*, in the seventh edition of **Applied Therapeutics: The Clinical Use of Drugs** for a more in-depth discussion. The editors of this handbook express their thanks to Dr. Welty and acknowledge that this chapter is based upon his work.

Notes:

Notes:

Chapter 53

Principles of Infectious Diseases

Inside . . .

The Approach to Treatment of Infections

♦ Evaluate evidence supporting an infection (e.g., fever, leukocytosis, erythema).

♦ Evaluate the potential of confabulating variables (e.g., drug fever, autoimmune disorders).

♦ Establish the severity of infection (e.g., hemodynamic, neurological, respiratory, and cellular changes).

♦ Determine the most likely site of infection by focusing on signs and symptoms.

♦ Determine pathogens commonly associated with specific sites of infection (see Table 53.1).

♦ Attempt to identify pathogens (e.g., cultures, Gram's stain).

♦ Determine isolate pathogenicity (e.g., colonization, contamination, infection).

♦ Determine susceptibility of pathogens to specific antimicrobials (see Tables 53.2, 53.3, and 53.4).

- ♦ Select an antimicrobial based on:
  - Clinical efficacy.
  - Adverse reaction profile.
  - Pharmacokinetic disposition.
  - Cost considerations.
- ♦ Determine dose by considering:
  - Usual dosing guidelines.
  - Age and body size.
  - Site of infection.
  - Anatomic or physiological barriers to antimicrobial access.
  - Route of elimination and organ function.
- ♦ Evaluate patient response to therapy by focusing on the evidence that indicates an infection.
- ♦ Evaluate the patient for adverse effects to selected antimicrobials.

Principles of Antimicrobial Therapy
Microbiology

- ♦ All organisms are classified according to morphology (e.g., cocci, bacilli), growth characteristics (e.g., aerobic versus anaerobic), and other qualities (e.g., Gram's stain positive or negative). The choice of antimicrobial therapy often is based on the morphology and growth patterns of these organisms. (See Table 53.1.)

Empiric Therapy

- ♦ Empirical therapy is often based on a working knowledge of the most likely pathogens expected to be found at the site of infection (see Table 53.2). Certain organisms are predictably associated with infection at certain sites and not in others. Certain host factors such as age, immunosuppression, prior antibiotic usage, and environment (e.g., hospital-versus community-acquired), help to predict the most likely organism.
- ♦ *Selection of an antimicrobial agent* for some infections can await the results of appropriate culture and sensitivity (C&S) testing. In many situations, however, treatment should be initiated immediately before C&S results are available. The selection of the most appropriate antimicrobial agent is, therefore, dependent upon knowledge of the pathogens most likely to cause infections in specific organs and tissues (see Table 53.2).
- ♦ *Classification of Antimicrobials.* See Table 53.3.

Treatment of Gram-Positive Infections (Table 53.4)
Staphylococci

- ♦ *Staphylococcus aureus* is generally susceptible to semisynthetic penicillins such as nafcillin, most first-generation cephalosporins, clindamycin, vancomycin, and TMP-SMX. Second- and third-generation cephalosporins generally have less predictable activity. However, cefuroxime and cefamandole appear to be as active as first-generation cephalosporins. Penicillin generally is ineffective against *S. aureus* due to production of beta-lactamase. Most methicillin-resistant (nafcillin-resistant) strains continue to be susceptible to vancomycin, cotrimoxazole, linezolid, and quinupristin-dalfopristin.

Streptococci

- ♦ With the exception of aztreonam and ciprofloxacin, streptococci generally are adequately covered by any of the agents listed in Table 53.4. Penicillin-resistant pneumococci are being encountered more frequently. The prevalence of intermediately susceptible strains in the U.S. is approximately 15–20%, and the prevalence of resistant isolates is 5–10%. If the isolate is a "susceptible" isolate, it generally is susceptible to a variety of agents, including most cephalosporins, macrolides, and doxycycline. If the organism is intermediately susceptible, high-dose penicillin is likely to be effective in pneumonia, however, not in meningitis. These intermediately susceptible isolates variably are inhibited by alternative agents, and laboratory susceptibilities should be documented. In cases of resistance vancomycin should be utilized; however, rifampin, imipenem, cefotaxime, and ceftriaxone may have some activity. Linezolid and Synercid are reliably active.

♦ **Enterococci,** primarily *Enterococcus faecalis* is usually susceptible to penicillin, ampicillin, piperacillin, and vancomycin. However, *Enterococcus faecium* often is resistant to ampicillin and vancomycin. Possible agents in the treatment of vancomycin-resistant enterococci (VRE) include quinupristin-dalfopristin (Synercid®) and linezolid, doxycycline, chloramphenicol, ± rifampin. Imipenem is active against some enterococci; however, resistance due to *E. faecium* is common.

Treatment of Gram-Negative Infections (Table 53.5)
Aerobic

♦ *First-generation and second-generation cephalosporins* have activity versus *E. coli, Proteus mirabilis,* and *Klebsiella pneumoniae* but have less predictable activity against more nosocomial organisms, such as *Citrobacter sp., Enterobacter sp.,* and *Pseudomonas aeruginosa.*

♦ *Aminoglycosides,* such as gentamicin, tobramycin, and amikacin, have excellent activity against cephalosporin-resistant organisms. Tobramycin usually is more active than gentamicin against *P. aeruginosa.* Gentamicin tends to have more activity than tobramycin against *Serratia marcescens.* Amikacin is likely to have activity against gentamicin and tobramycin-resistant Enterobacteriaceae.

♦ *Third-generation cephalosporins and aztreonam* have excellent activity against most Enterobacteriaceae, including aminoglycoside-resistant *E. coli* and *Klebsiella sp.* Aminoglycosides and TMP-SMX are superior agents to third-generation cephalosporins and/or aztreonam against *Enterobacter cloacae, Enterobacter aerogenes,* and *Citrobacter freundii.*

♦ *Ticarcillin, ureidopenicillins (piperacillin, mezlocillin), ceftazidime, and aztreonam* are effective antipseudomonal agents.

♦ Penems, cefepime, ciprofloxacin, and aminoglycosides are the most likely agents to be active versus third-generation cephalosporin-resistant isolates.

♦ *Haemophilus influenzae* is well covered by most of the listed agents, with the exception of ampicillin and first-generation cephalosporins. *H. influenzae* often produces beta-lactamase, averaging 30–40% in the U.S. In these cases, drugs such as ampicillin are inactive, and second- or third-generation cephalosporins, doxycycline, Augmentin, or Unasyn must be used.

Treatment of Anaerobic Infections (Table 53.6)
Anaerobic

♦ *Penicillin and ampicillin* have excellent activity against most anaerobes, including Peptococci, Peptostreptococci, and *Clostridia sp.* However, *Bacteroides fragilis* usually produces beta-lactamase and tends to be resistant to penicillin. Other Gram-negative anaerobes, including Prevotella, also can be beta-lactamase producers.

♦ *Cephalosporins,* while usually active against mouth anaerobes (e.g., peptococci and peptostreptococci) have only moderate activity for *Bacteroides* and *Prevotella* species.

♦ The most reliable antimicrobials against *B. fragilis,* the most important anaerobic intra-abdominal pathogen, include metronidazole, imipenem, and beta-lactamase inhibitor combinations (Timentin, Unasyn, Zosyn). Clindamycin, while generally effective, has a 75%–90% susceptibility, compared to nearly universal susceptibility for the above agents.

♦ *Aztreonam, ciprofloxacin, and the aminoglycosides* have little to no anaerobic activity. (See Table 53.4.)

Adverse Effects of Antimicrobials

♦ The adverse effects of commonly used antimicrobials are listed in Table 53.8.

♦ Table 53.7 summarizes the drugs of choice for various organisms. The selection of the drugs of choice takes into account the spectrum of activity, pharmacokinetic disposition, and clinical efficacy of the various agents.

Clinical Pharmacokinetics of Anti-Infectives

The bioavailability, distribution, and elimination of antimicrobial drugs are important considerations in the development of rational dosage regimens in the treatment of infection.

♦ *Bioavailability.* Oral treatment of serious aerobic Gram-negative infection generally is limited to trimethoprim-sulfamethoxazole (cotrimoxazole) and quinolones. Conditions such as inflammation (e.g., Crohn's disease, colitis), gastrectomy, and diarrhea may alter the oral bioavailability of some antimicrobials. Drugs that are normally minimally absorbed (e.g., oral vancomycin and aminoglycosides) may have increased bioavailability in certain disease states that are accompanied by inflammation.

♦ *Distribution.* Infections such as meningitis, endophthalmitis, and prostatitis are difficult to treat because of relatively impermeable barriers. Those antimicrobial agents that penetrate into these fluids generally should be used. Furthermore, increased doses of these agents are necessary for eradication of these infections.

♦ *Clearance.* Since most beta-lactam agents are eliminated by the kidney, clearance is often altered in renal failure (see Table 53.10). Exceptions to this rule include some semisynthetic penicillins (nafcillin, oxacillin, dicloxacillin, cloxacillin) and certain third-generation cephalosporins (ceftriaxone and cefoperazone), which also are eliminated via hepatic metabolism and/or biliary excretion. Aminoglycosides (gentamicin, tobramycin, amikacin), acyclovir, ganciclovir, flucytosine, and vancomycin also are extensively eliminated by the kidney. Drugs such as ciprofloxacin, cefotaxime, and piperacillin have mixed renal and metabolic clearance pathways, and thus accumulate to a lessee degree in patients with renal failure. Metronidazole, chloramphenicol, and clindamycin, among others, are eliminated almost exclusively by the liver.

♦ *Creatinine Clearance.* Renal function can be estimated using creatinine clearance. The following Cockcroft-Gault formula for estimation of renal function in males must be multiplied by 85% for females.

$$\text{Cl}_{\text{Cr}} \text{ (mL/min)} = \frac{(140 - \text{age})(\text{body weight in kg})}{(\text{SrCr mg/dL})(72 \text{ kg})}$$

Dosing reduction for hepatic failure is difficult to quantitate, given the lack of standardization in determining the degree of liver dysfunction. In certain cases, dosage reduction may be required independent of the route of elimination (e.g., amphotericin B-induced nephrotoxicity, erythromycin-associated cochlear toxicity in renal failure). Monitoring of serum levels is recommended for aminoglycosides (e.g., amikacin, gentamicin, and tobramycin), flucytosine, and vancomycin. In renal failure, metabolites of certain agents (e.g., metronidazole, cefotaxime, and nitrofurantoin) can accumulate.

♦ **Pharmacokinetic Antimicrobial Dosing Guidelines.** See Table 53.9.
♦ **Vancomycin Dosing in Patients with Renal Impairment.** Figure 53.1 is a reduced dosage nomogram for these patients.

Table 53.1 • Classification of Infectious Organisms

Bacteria
Aerobic
Gram-Positive
Cocci
  Streptococci: pneumococcus, *Streptococcus viridans,* group A streptococci
  Enterococcus
  Staphylococci: *Staphylococcus aureus, Staphylococcus epidermidis*
Rods (bacilli)
  Corynebacterium
  Listeria

Gram-Negative
Cocci
  Moraxella
  Neisseria (*Neisseria meningitidis, Neisseria gonorrhoeae*)
Rods (bacilli)
  Enterobacteriaceae (*Escherichia coli, Klebsiella, Enterobacter, Citrobacter, Proteus, Serratia, Salmonella, Shigella, Morganella, Providencia*)
  Campylobacter
  Pseudomonas
  Helicobacter
  Haemophilus (Coccobacilli morphology)
  Legionella

Anaerobic
Gram-Positive
Cocci
  Peptococcus
  Peptostreptococcus
Rods (bacilli)
  Clostridia (*Clostridium perfringens, Clostridium tetani, Clostridium difficile*)
  Propionibacterium acnes

Gram-Negative
Cocci
  None

Rods (bacilli)
  Bacteroides (*Bacteroides fragilis, Bacteroides melaninogenicus*)
  Fusobacterium
  Prevotella

Fungi
Aspergillus, Candida, Coccidioides, Cryptococcus, Histoplasma, Mucor, Tinea, Trichophyton

Viruses
Influenza, hepatitis A, B, C, D, E; human immunodeficiency virus; rubella; herpes; cytomegalovirus; respiratory syncytial virus; Epstein-Barr virus

Chlamydiae
Chlamydia trachomatis
Chlamydia psittaci
Chlamydia pneumoniae (TWAR)
LGV ([lymphogranuloma venereum] disease caused by *Chlamydia trachomatis* of immunotype L1-L3)

Rickettsiae
Rocky Mountain spotted fever, Q fever

Ureaplasma

Mycoplasmas
Mycoplasma pneumoniae, Mycoplasma hominis

Spirochetes
Treponema pallidum, Borrelia burgdorferi (Lyme disease)

Mycobacteria
Mycobacterium tuberculosis
Mycobacterium avium intracellulare

Notes:

Table 53.2 • Site of Infection: Suspected Organisms[a]

Site/Type of Infection	Suspected Organisms
Respiratory	
Pharyngitis	Group A streptococci
Bronchitis, otitis	*Haemophilus influenzae, Streptococcus pneumoniae, Moraxella catarrhalis*
Acute sinusitis	*Streptococcus pneumoniae, Haemophilus influenzae, Moraxella catarrhalis*
Chronic sinusitis	Anaerobes, *Staphylococcus aureus* (as well as suspected organisms associated with acute sinusitis)
Epiglottitis	*Haemophilus influenzae*
Pneumonia	
Community-Acquired	
Normal host	*Streptococcus pneumoniae*, viral, mycoplasma
Aspiration	Normal aerobic and anaerobic mouth flora
Pediatrics	*Streptococcus pneumoniae, Haemophilus influenzae*
COAD	*Streptococcus pneumoniae, Haemophilus influenzae*
Alcoholic	*Streptococcus pneumoniae, Klebsiella*
Hospital-Acquired	
Aspiration	Mouth anaerobes, Gram-negative aerobic rods, *Staphylococcus aureus*
Neutropenic	Fungi, Gram-negative aerobic rods, *Staphylococcus aureus*
AIDS	Fungi, Pneumocystis, *Legionella, Nocardia, Streptococcus pneumoniae*
Urinary Tract	
Community-Acquired	*Escherichia coli*, other Gram-negative rods, *Staphylococcus aureus, Staphylococcus epidermidis,* enterococci
Hospital-Acquired	Resistant Gram-negative rods, enterococci
Skin/Soft Tissue	
Cellulitis	Group A streptococci, *Staphylococcus aureus*
IV catheter site	*Staphylococcus aureus, Staphylococcus epidermidis*
Surgical wound	*Staphylococcus aureus*, Gram-negative rods
Diabetic ulcer	*Staphylococcus aureus*, Gram-negative aerobic rods, anaerobes
Furuncle	*Staphylococcus aureus*
Intra-Abdominal	*Bacteroides fragilis, Escherichia coli*, enterococci
Gastroenteritis	*Salmonella, Shigella, Helicobacter, Campylobacter, Clostridium difficile,* amoeba, Giardia, viral, enterotoxigenic-hemorrhagic *Escherichia coli*
Endocarditis	
Subacute	*Streptococcus viridans*
Acute	
IV drug abuser	*Staphylococcus aureus*, Gram-negative aerobic rods, enterococci, fungi
Prosthetic valve	*Staphylococcus epidermidis*
Osteomyelitis/ Septic Arthritis	*Staphylococcus aureus*, Gram-negative aerobic rods
Meningitis	
<2 months	*Escherichia coli*, group B streptococci, *Listeria*
2 months–12 years	*Streptococcus pneumoniae, Neisseria meningitidis, Haemophilus influenzae*
Adults	*Streptococcus pneumoniae, Neisseria meningitidis*
Hospital-acquired	*Streptococcus pneumoniae, Neisseria meningitidis*, Gram-negative aerobic rods
Postneurosurgery	*Staphylococcus aureus*, Gram-negative rods

[a]AIDS = Acquired immunodeficiency syndrome; COAD = Chronic obstructive airways disease; IV = Intravenous.

Notes:

Table 53.3 • Classification of Antibacterials

β-Lactam Antibiotics

Cephalosporins

First-Generation
Cefadroxil (Duricef)
Cefazolin (Ancef)
Cephalexin (Keflex)
Cephalothin (Keflin)
Cephapirin (Cefadyl)
Cephradine (Anspor)

Second-Generation
Cefaclor (Ceclor)
Cefamandole (Mandol)
Cefmetazole (Zefazone)
Cefonicid (Monocid)
Ceforanide (Precef)
Cefotetan (Cefotan)
Cefoxitin (Mefoxin)
Cefprozil (Cefzil)
Cefuroxime (Zinacef)
Cefuroxime axetil (Ceftin)

Third-Generation
Cefdinir (Omnicef)
Cefixime (Suprax)
Cefoperazone (Cefobid)
Cefotaxime (Claforan)
Cefpodoxime proxetil (Vantin)
Ceftibuten (Cedax)
Ceftizoxime (Cefizox)
Ceftriaxone (Rocephin)
Ceftazidime (Fortaz)

Fourth-Generation
Cefepime (Maxipime)

Carbacephems
Loracarbef (Lorabid)

Monobactams
Aztreonam (Azactam)

Penems
Carbapenems
Primaxin (imipenem plus cilastatin)
Meropenem

Penicillins
Natural Penicillins
Penicillin G
Penicillin V

Aminopenicillins
Ampicillin (Omnipen)
Amoxicillin (Amoxil)
Bacampicillin (Spectrobid)

Penicillinase-Resistant

Penicillins
Isoxazolyl penicillins (dicloxacillin, oxacillin, cloxacillin)
Nafcillin (Unipen)

β-Lactam Antibiotics

Penicillins (continued)

Carboxypenicillins
Carbenicillin (Geocillin)
Ticarcillin (Ticar)

Ureidopenicillins
Mezlocillin (Mezlin)
Piperacillin (Pipracil)

Combination with β-Lactamase Inhibitors
Augmentin (amoxicillin plus clavulanic acid)
Timentin (ticarcillin plus clavulanic acid)
Unasyn (ampicillin plus sulbactam)
Zosyn (piperacillin plus tazobactam)

Aminoglycosides
Amikacin (Amikin)
Gentamicin (Garamycin)
Neomycin (Mycifradin)
Netilmicin (Netromycin)
Streptomycin
Tobramycin (Nebcin)

Protein Synthesis Inhibitors
Azithromycin (Zithromax)
Clarithromycin (Biaxin)
Clindamycin (Cleocin)
Chloramphenicol (Chloromycetin)
Dalfopristin/Quinupristin (Synercid)
Dirithromycin (Dynabac)
Erythromycin (Erythrocin)
Linezolid (Zyvox)
Telithromycin (Ketec)
Tetracyclines (doxycycline, minocycline, tetracycline)

Folate Inhibitors
Sulfadiazine
Sulfadoxine (Fansidar)
Trimethoprim (Trimpex)
Trimethoprim-sulfamethoxazole (Bactrim, Septra)

Quinolones
Ciprofloxacin (Cipro)
Enoxacin (Penetrex)
Gatifloxacin (Tequin)
Gemifloxacin (Factive)
Levofloxacin (Levoquin)
Lomefloxacin (Maxaquin)
Moxifloxacin (Avelox)
Norfloxacin (Noroxin)
Ofloxacin (Floxin)
Trovafloxacin (Trovan)

Vancomycin (Vancocin)

Metronidazole (Flagyl)

Notes:

Table 53.4 • In Vitro Antimicrobial Susceptibility: Aerobic Gram-Positive Cocci

Drugs	Staphylococcus aureus	Staphylococcus aureus (MR)	Staphylococcus epidermidis	Staphylococcus epidermidis (MR)	Streptococci[a]	Enterococci[b]	Pneumococci
Ampicillin	+	–	+	–	++++	++	++++
Augmentin	+++	+	++++	–	+++	++	+++
Aztreonam	–	–	–	–	–	–	–
Cefazolin	++++	–	++++	–	++++	–	++
Cefepime	++	–	++	–	++++	–	++
Cefoxitin/Cefotetan	++	–	++	–	++++	–	+
Cefuroxime	++++	–	++++	–	++++	–	++
Ciprofloxacin[c]	+++	++	+++	++	+	+	++
Clindamycin	++++	+	+++	+	++	–	++
Cotrimoxazole	++++	+++	+++	+	++++	+	+
Erythromycin (azithromycin/clarithromycin)	++	–	+	–	+++	–	++
Imipenem	++++	+	++++	–	+++	++	+++
Levofloxacin (gatifloxacin, gemifloxacin, moxifloxacin)	++++	++	+++	++	+++	++	+++

Linezolid[f]	+++	+++	+++	+++	+++
Mezlocillin	+	—	+	+++	+
Nafcillin	+++	—	+++	+++	—
Penicillin	+	—	+	+++	+
Quinupristin/dalfopristin[d,f]	+++	+++	+++	+++	+++
Teicoplanin	+++	+++	+++	+++	+++
TGC[e]	++	—	++	+++	—
Ticarcillin	+	—	+	+++	+
Timentin	+++	—	+++	+++	+
Unasyn	+++	—	+++	+++	+
Vancomycin	+++	+++	+++	+++	+++
Zosyn	+++	—	+++	+++	+

[a]Nonpneumococcal streptococci.
[b]Usually requires combination therapy (e.g., ampicillin and an aminoglycoside) for serious infection.
[c]Levofloxacin (gatifloxacin, gemifloxacin, moxifloxacin) generally is more active than ciprofloxacin against staphylococci and streptococci.
[d]Active against E. faecium but unpredictable against E. faecalis.
[e]TGC = Cefotaxime, ceftizoxime, ceftriaxone, cefoperazone. Ceftazidime has comparatively inferior antistaphylococcal and antipneumococcal activity.
[f]Active versus vancomycin-resistant Enterococcus faecium.
MR, methicillin resistant

Table 53.5 • In Vitro Antimicrobial Susceptibility: Gram-Negative Aerobes[a]

Drugs	Escherichia coli	Klebsiella pneumoniae	Enterobacter cloacae	Proteus mirabilis	Serratia marcescens	Pseudomonas aeruginosa	Haemophilus influenzae	Haemophilus influenzae[b]
Ampicillin	++	−	−	+++	−	−	+++	−
Augmentin	+++	++	−	+++	−	−	+++	+++
Aztreonam	++++	++++	+	++++	++++	++++	++++	++++
Cefazolin	+++	+++	−	+++	−	−	+	−
Cefepime	+++	+++	+++	++++	++++	+++	++++	++++
Cefoperazone	+++	+++	+	++++	++++	++	++++	++++
Ceftazidime	+++	+++	+	++++	++++	+++	++++	++++
Cefuroxime	++	+++	+	+++	+	−	++++	++++
Cotrimoxazole	++	+++	+++	++++	+++	−	++	+++
Gentamicin	++++	++++	++++	++++	++++	+++	++	++
Imipenem/Meropenem	++++	++++	++++	+++	++++	++++	++++	++++
Mezlocillin	++	++	++	++	++	++	++	−
Piperacillin	++	+++	++	+++	+++	+++	+++	−
Quinolones[c]	++++	+++	++++	++++	++++	++	++++	++++
TGC	+++	+++	+	+++	+++	+	++++	++++
Ticarcillin	++	+	++	+++	++	++	++	−
Timentin	+++	++	++	+++	+++	++	+++	+++
Tobramycin	++++	++++	++++	++++	++	++++	+	++
Unasyn	++	++	−	++	++	−	+++	+++
Zosyn	++++	++++	++	+++	+++	+++	+++	+++

[a]TGC = Cefotaxime, ceftizoxime, ceftriaxone.
[b]β-Lactamase-producing strains.
[c]Ciprofloxacin has increased potency against P. aeruginosa compared with other quinolones.

Table 53.6 • Antimicrobial Susceptibility: Anaerobes

Drugs	Bacteroides fragilis	Peptococcus	Peptostreptococcus	Clostridia
Ampicillin	+	++++	++++	+++
Aztreonam	—	—	—	—
Cefazolin	—	++++	++++	—
Cefepime	+	++	++	+
Cefotaxime	++	+++	+++	+
Cefoxitin	+++	+++	++++	+
Ceftazidime	—	+	+	+
Ceftizoxime	+++	+++	+++	+
Ciprofloxacin	+	+	+	+
Clindamycin	+++	++++	++++	++
Gatifloxacin (moxifloxacin, trovafloxacin)	+++	++	++	+
Imipenem	++++	++++	++++	++
Metronidazole	++++	++++	++	+++
Penicillin	+	++++	++++	+++
Timentin	++++	+++	+++	+++
Unasyn	++++	++++	++++	+++
Vancomycin	—	+++	+++	+++
Zosyn	++++	++++	+++	+++

Notes:

Table 53.7 • Antimicrobials of Choice in the Treatment of Bacterial Infection

Organism	Drug of Choice	Alternatives	Comments
Aerobes			
Gram-Positive Cocci			
Streptococcus pyogenes (Group A streptococci)	Penicillin	Macrolide, cephalosporin	
Streptococcus pneumoniae	Penicillin	Macrolide, cephalosporin, trimethoprim-sulfamethoxazole, doxycycline	Although the incidence of penicillin nonsusceptible pneumococci continues to increase, high-dose penicillins remain active against most of these isolates. Penicillin-resistant pneumococci commonly demonstrate resistance to other agents, including erythromycin, tetracyclines, and cephalosporins.
Enterococcus faecalis	Ampicillin ± gentamicin	Vancomycin ± gentamicin; teicoplanin ± gentamicin	Most commonly isolated enterococcus (80–85%). Most reliable anti-enterococcal agents are ampicillin (penicillin, mezlocillin, piperacillin), vancomycin, and teicoplanin. Monotherapy generally inhibits but does not kill the enterococcus. Aminoglycosides must be added to ampicillin or vancomycin to provide bactericidal activity. Ampicillin resistance and, less frequently, vancomycin resistance are increasing. High-level aminoglycoside resistance takes place commonly.
Enterococcus faecium	Vancomycin ± gentamicin	Dalfopristin/Quinupristin (D/Q) Linezolid	Second most common enterococcal organism (10–20%) and is more likely than *E. faecalis* to be resistant to multiple antimicrobials. Most reliable agents are vancomycin D/Q and linezolid. Monotherapy generally inhibits but does not kill the enterococcus. Aminoglycosides must be added to cell wall active agents to provide bactericidal activity. Ampicillin and vancomycin resistance is common. High-level aminoglycoside is common. D/Q and linezolid are drugs of choice for vancomycin-resistant isolates.
Staphylococcus aureus	Nafcillin	Cefazolin, vancomycin, clindamycin, trimethoprim-sulfamethoxazole	≈10–15% of isolates inhibited by penicillin. Most isolates susceptible to nafcillin, cephalosporins, trimethoprim-sulfamethoxazole, and clindamycin. First-generation cephalosporins are equal to nafcillin. Most second- and third-generation cephalosporins adequate in the treatment of infection (exceptions include ceftazidime and cefonicid). Methicillin-resistant *S. aureus* must be treated with vancomycin or teicoplanin; however, trimethoprim-sulfamethoxazole, D/Q, linezolid, or minocycline can be used.
(Nafcillin-resistant)	Vancomycin	Teicoplanin, trimethoprim-sulfamethoxazole, minocycline	

Organism	First choice	Alternatives	Comments
Staphylococcus epidermidis	Nafcillin	Cefazolin, vancomycin, clindamycin	Most isolates are β-lactam-, clindamycin-, and trimethoprim-sulfamethoxazole-resistant. Most reliable agents are vancomycin, teicoplanin, D/Q, and linezolid. Rifampin active and can be used in conjunction with other agents; however, monotherapy with rifampin is associated with development of resistance.
(Nafcillin-resistant)	Vancomycin	Teicoplanin, quinolone	
Gram-Positive Bacilli			
Diphtheroids	Penicillin	Cephalosporin	
Corynebacterium jeikeium	Vancomycin	Erythromycin, quinolone	
Listeria monocytogenes	Ampicillin (± gentamicin)	Trimethoprim-sulfamethoxazole	
Gram-Negative Cocci			
Moraxella catarrhalis	Trimethoprim-sulfamethoxazole	Amoxicillin-clavulanic acid, erythromycin, doxycycline, second- or third-generation cephalosporin	
Neisseria gonorrhoeae	Quinolone, cefixime	Ceftriaxone	Second-generation cephalosporins also are active.
Neisseria meningitidis	Penicillin	Third-generation cephalosporin	
Gram-Negative Bacilli			
Campylobacter fetus	Imipenem	Gentamicin	
Campylobacter jejuni	Quinolone, erythromycin	Tetracycline	
Enterobacter	Trimethoprim-sulfamethoxazole	Quinolone, imipenem, gentamicin	Not predictably inhibited by most cephalosporins; imipenem, quinolones, trimethoprim-sulfamethoxazole, cefepime, and aminoglycosides are most active agents.
Escherichia coli	Third-generation cephalosporin	First- or second-generation cephalosporin, gentamicin	
Haemophilus influenzae	Third-generation cephalosporin	Second-generation cephalosporin, trimethoprim-sulfamethoxazole, β-lactamase inhibitor combinations	
Helicobacter pylori	Amoxicillin + clarithromycin + omeprazole	Tetracycline + metronidazole + bismuth subsalicylate	

(continued)

Table 53.7 • Antimicrobials of Choice in the Treatment of Bacterial Infection (continued)

Organism	Drug of Choice	Alternatives	Comments
Aerobes (continued)			
Gram-Negative Bacilli (continued)			
Klebsiella pneumoniae	Third-generation cephalosporin	First- or second-generation cephalosporin, gentamicin, trimethoprim-sulfamethoxazole	
Legionella	Erythromycin ± rifampin	Fluoroquinolone, doxycycline	
Proteus mirabilis	Ampicillin	First-generation cephalosporin, trimethoprim-sulfamethoxazole	
Other Proteus	Third-generation cephalosporin	β-Lactamase inhibitor combination, aminoglycoside, trimethoprim-sulfamethoxazole	
Pseudomonas aeruginosa	Antipseudomonal penicillin (or ceftazidime) ± aminoglycoside (or quinolone)	Quinolone or imipenem ± aminoglycoside	Most active agents include aminoglycosides, imipenem, ceftazidime, cefepime, aztreonam, quinolones, and the extended-spectrum penicillins.
Salmonella typhi	Quinolone	Ceftriaxone, trimethoprim-sulfamethoxazole	
Serratia marcescens	Third-generation cephalosporin	Trimethoprim-sulfamethoxazole, aminoglycoside	
Shigella	Quinolone	Trimethoprim-sulfamethoxazole, ampicillin	
Stenotrophomonas maltophilia	Trimethoprim-sulfamethoxazole	Ceftazidime, minocycline, quinolone, β-lactamase inhibitor combination	
Anaerobes			
Bacteroides fragilis	Metronidazole	Clindamycin, β-lactamase inhibitor combinations, imipenem	Most active agents (95–100%) include metronidazole, the β-lactamase inhibitor combinations (ampicillin-sulbactam, piperacillin-tazobactam, ticarcillin-clavulanic acid), and imipenem. Clindamycin, cefoxitin, cefotetan, cefmetazole, ceftizoxime, and the antipseudomonal penicillins (piperacillin, mezlocillin) have good activity but not to the degree of metronidazole. Aminoglycosides and aztreonam are inactive.

Organism	First choice	Alternative	Comments
Clostridia difficile	Metronidazole	Vancomycin	
Fusobacterium	Penicillin	Metronidazole, clindamycin	
Other Oropharyngeal			
Prevotella	Penicillin	Metronidazole, clindamycin	Most β-lactams active (exceptions include aztreonam, nafcillin, ceftazidime). If β-lactamase-producing, clindamycin should be added.
Peptostreptococcus	Penicillin	Clindamycin, cephalosporin	Most β-lactams active (exceptions include aztreonam, nafcillin, ceftazidime).
Other			
Actinomycetes			
Actinomyces israelii	Penicillin	Tetracycline	
Nocardia	Trimethoprim-sulfamethoxazole	Amikacin, minocycline, imipenem	
Chlamydiae			
Chlamydia trachomatis	Doxycycline	Erythromycin, azithromycin	
Chlamydia pneumoniae (TWAR strain)	Doxycycline	Erythromycin	
Mycoplasma			
Mycoplasma pneumoniae	Erythromycin, doxycycline	Azithromycin, clarithromycin	
Spirochetes			
Borrelia burgdorferi	Doxycycline	Ampicillin, second- or third-generation cephalosporin	
Treponema pallidum	Penicillin	Doxycycline	

Table 53.8 • Antibiotic Adverse Effects and Toxicities[a]

Antibiotic	Side Effects	Comments
β-Lactams, (penicillin, cephalosporins, monobactams, penems)	*Allergic*: anaphylaxis, urticaria, serum sickness, rash, fever	Many patients will have "ampicillin rash" with no cross-reactivity with any other penicillins. Most common in patients with mononucleosis or those receiving allopurinol. Likelihood of IgE-mediated cross-reactivity between penicillins and cephalosporins ≈3–7%. Extensive cross-reactivity between penicillins and imipenem. No IgE cross-reactivity between aztreonam and penicillins
	Diarrhea	Particularly common with ampicillin, Augmentin, ceftriaxone, and cefoperazone. Pseudomembranous colitis can occur with most antimicrobials
	Hematologic: anemia, thrombocytopenia, antiplatelet activity, hypothrombinemia	Hemolytic anemia more common with higher doses. Antiplatelet activity most common with the antipseudomonal penicillins and high serum levels of other β-lactams
		Hypothrombinemia more often associated with those cephalosporins with the methyltetrazolethiol side chain (cefamandole, cefotetan, cefoperazone, cefmetazole). Reaction preventable and reversible with vitamin K
	Hepatitis/Biliary	Most common with oxacillin. Biliary sludging and stones reported with ceftriaxone
	Phlebitis	
	Seizure activity	Associated with high levels of β-lactams, particularly penicillins and imipenem
	Potassium load	Penicillin G (K+)
	Sodium load	Ticarcillin, ticarcillin-clavulanic acid
	Nephritis	Most common with methicillin; however, reported for most other β-lactams
	Neutropenia	Nafcillin
	Disulfiram reaction	Associated with cephalosporins with methyltetrazolethiol side chain (cefamandole, cefotetan, cefoperazone, cefmetazole)
	Hypotension, nausea	Associated with fast infusion of imipenem
Aminoglycosides (gentamicin, tobramycin, amikacin, netilmicin)	Nephrotoxicity	Averages 10–15% incidence. Generally reversible, usually occurs after 5–7 days of therapy. *Risk factors*: dehydration, age, dose, duration, concurrent nephrotoxins, liver disease
	Ototoxicity	1–5% incidence, often irreversible. Both cochlear and/or vestibular toxicity occur.
	Neuromuscular paralysis	Rare, most common with large doses administered via intraperitoneal instillation or in patients with myasthenia gravis
Macrolides (erythromycin, azithromycin, clarithromycin)	Nausea, vomiting, "burning" stomach	Oral administration. Azithromycin and clarithromycin associated with less nausea than erythromycin
	Cholestatic jaundice	Reported for all erythromycin salts, most common with estolate
	Ototoxicity	Most common with high doses in patients with renal and/or hepatic failure
Clindamycin	Diarrhea	Most common adverse effect. High association with pseudomembranous colitis

Tetracyclines	Allergic	Rash, anaphylaxis, urticaria, fever
	Photosensitivity	
	Teeth/bone deposition and discoloration	Avoid in pediatrics
	Gastrointestinal	Nausea, diarrhea
	Hepatitis	Primarily in pregnancy or the elderly
	Renal (azotemia)	Tetracyclines have antianabolic effect and should be avoided in patients with $\downarrow$ renal function. Less with doxycycline
	Vestibular	Associated with minocycline
Vancomycin	Ototoxicity	Primarily with high serum levels (>50 μg/mL) while receiving concomitant ototoxins such as aminoglycosides
	Nephrotoxicity	Little to no nephrotoxicity observed with current preparations of vancomycin. May $\uparrow$ nephrotoxicity of aminoglycosides
	Hypotension, flushing	Associated with rapid infusion of vancomycin. Appears dose related (more common with 1-g dose compared with 500 mg)
	Phlebitis	Needs large volume dilution
Dalfopristin/ Quinupristin (D/Q)	Phlebitis	Generally requires central line administration
	Myalgia	Moderate to severe in many patients
	Increased Bilirubin	
Linezolid	MAO inhibition, tongue discoloration, thrombocytopenia, neutropenia, anemia	
Sulfonamides	Gastrointestinal	Nausea, diarrhea
	Hepatic	Cholestatic hepatitis, $\uparrow$ incidence in AIDS
	Rash	Exfoliative dermatitis, Stevens-Johnson syndrome. More common in AIDS
	Bone marrow	Neutropenia, thrombocytopenia. More common in AIDS
	Kernicterus	Caused by $\uparrow$ unbound drug in the neonate. Premature liver cannot conjugate bilirubin. Sulfonamide displaces bilirubin from protein, resulting in excessive free bilirubin and kernicterus
Chloramphenicol	Anemia	Idiosyncratic irreversible aplastic anemia (rare). Reversible dose-related anemia
	Gray syndrome	Caused by inability of neonates to conjugate chloramphenicol
Quinolones (ciprofloxacin, enoxacin, norfloxacin, ofloxacin)	GI	Nausea, vomiting, diarrhea
	Prolonged QT	Sparfloxacin, moxifloxacin; possibly all quinolones as a class
	Drug interactions	$\downarrow$ oral bioavailability with multivalent cations
	CNS	Altered mental status, confusion, seizures
	Cartilage toxicity	Toxic in animal model. Avoid in children; however, appears safe in cystic fibrosis
	Tendonitis/tendon rupture	Common in elderly, renal failure, concomitant glucocorticoids

(continued)

Table 53.8 • Antibiotic Adverse Effects and Toxicities *(continued)*

Antibiotic	Side Effects	Comments
Antifungals		
Amphotericin B	Nephrotoxicity	Common. May depend on patient Na load. ↓ dose or QOD dosing may result in improvement of renal function. Caution with concomitant nephrotoxins (e.g., aminoglycosides, cyclosporine)
	Hypokalemia	Predictable. Probably caused by renal tubular excretion of potassium. More common in patients receiving concomitant ticarcillin, mezlocillin, piperacillin
	Hypomagnesemia	Less commonly observed than hypokalemia
	Anemia	Long-term adverse effect. Similar to anemia of chronic disease. Treatable with transfusion
Flucytosine	Neutropenia, thrombocytopenia	Secondary to metabolism of flucytosine to fluorouracil. More commonly observed with flucytosine levels >100 μg/mL. More common in AIDS patients
	Hepatitis	Usually moderate ↑ in LFTs. Rarely clinical hepatitis
Ketoconazole (fluconazole, itraconazole)	Drug interactions	↓ oral bioavailability of ketoconazole and itraconazole with ↑ gastric pH
	Hepatitis	Ranges from mild ↑ in LFTs to occasional fatal hepatitis. May be less common with newer imidazoles/triazoles (e.g., fluconazole, itraconazole)
	Gynecomastia	More common with high dose (>400 mg/day). Less common with fluconazole and itraconazole. ↓ libido, azoospermia
Antivirals		
Abacavir	Hypersensitivity	Occurs in 3% of patients and includes fever, GI, malaise, rash. Repeated administration associated with severe reactions, including hypotension, respiratory distress
Acyclovir	Phlebitis	Caused by poor solubility of IV preparation. Reported in 1–20% of cases
	Renal failure	Low solubility of acyclovir associated with renal failure. Dehydrated patients, as well as rapid infusions, predispose to toxicity
	CNS	1% incidence in AIDS. ↑ incidence with dose in >10 mg/kg/day
Delavirdine (efavirenz, nevirapine)	Rash	
	Headache, insomnia, dizziness, nausea	Primarily with initiation of therapy with efavirenz

Drug	Adverse Effects	Comments
Didanosine (ddI)	Pancreatitis Peripheral neuropathy ↑uric acid	Fatalities reported Dose related
Foscarnet	Nephrotoxicity Mineral and electrolyte abnormalities Anemia Nausea, vomiting	Occurs in up to 60% of patients. May be prevented with normal saline bolus before dose. Frequent monitoring of renal function imperative ↑ and ↓ calcium/phosphate may be observed. Hypocalcemia, hypo- and hyperphosphatemia, hypomagnesemia, hypokalemia. ↑ risk of cardiomyopathy and seizures Anemia in 33%; usually manageable with transfusions and discontinuation of foscarnet
Ganciclovir	Neutropenia, thrombocytopenia Hepatitis	↑ incidence in AIDS. ↑ incidence with doses in excess of 10 mg/kg/day Usually mild to moderate ↑ in LFTs
Indinavir (amprenavir, lopinavir, nelfinavir, ritonavir, saquinavir)	Nausea, diarrhea, ↑ LFTs, hyperglycemia, fat wasting and redistribution, hyperlipidemia Paresthesia Nephrolithiasis	 Ritonavir Indinavir
Lamivudine (3TC)	Peripheral neuropathy	Adverse effects are uncommon
Stavudine (D4T)	Peripheral neuropathy	
Zalcitabine (ddC)	Peripheral neuropathy Mucocutaneous	Dose-related, delayed, often severe Early in the course of therapy
Zidovudine (AZT)	Anemia, neutropenia General	Anemia at 2–4 wk occasionally with ↑ MCV. Neutropenia appears later (6–8 wk) Severe headache, nausea, insomnia, myalgia, lethargy

^aAIDS = Acquired immunodeficiency syndrome; CNS = Central nervous system; GI = Gastrointestinal; IV = Intravenous; LFTs = Liver function tests; MCV = Mean corpuscular volume; Na = Sodium.

Table 53.9 • University of California San Francisco Adult Antimicrobial Dosing Guidelines[a]

Drug	Max Daily IV Dose[b]	Cl_Cr	Dialysis[c]	t_{1/2} (hr) Normal	t_{1/2} (hr) ESRD	Hepatic Failure Dosage
Acyclovir	30 mg/kg	>50 mL/min[d]: Herpes simplex infections: 5 mg/kg/dose Q 8 hr. HSV encephalitis/Herpes zoster: 10 mg/kg/dose Q 8 hr 10–50 mL/min: Herpes simplex infections: 5 mg/kg/dose Q 12–14 hr. HSV encephalitis/Herpes zoster: 10 mg/kg/dose Q 12–24 hr <10 mL/min[e]: Herpes simplex infections: 2.5 mg/kg Q 24 hr. HSV encephalitis/Herpes zoster: 5 mg/kg Q 24 hr	D[f]	2.3–3.2	20	No change
Amikacin[g]	1.5 mg/kg	>50 mL/min[d]: 0.3–1.0 mg/kg 10–50 mL/min: No change <10 mL/min[d]: No change	D[e]	2–3	36–82	No change
Amphotericin B			ND	15 days	Unchanged	No change
Ampicillin	12 g	>50 mL/min[d]: 1–2 g Q 6–8 hr 10–50 mL/min: 1–1.5 g Q 6 hr <10 mL/min[d]: 1 g Q 8–12 hr	MD[f]	1–1.3	20	No change
Aztreonam	8 g	>50 mL/min[d]: 1–2 g Q 6–8 hr 10–50 mL/min: 1–2 g Q 8–12 hr <10 mL/min[d]: 1 g Q 12–24 hr	MD[f]	1.3–2.2	6–9	No change
Cefazolin	8 g	>50 mL/min[d]: 1–2 g Q 8 hr 10–50 mL/min: 0.5–1.5 g Q 12 hr <10 mL/min[e]: 0.5–1.0 g Q 24 hr	MD[f]	1.8–2.6	12–40	No change
Cefotaxime	12 g	>50 mL/min[d]: 1–2 g Q 6–12 hr 10–50 mL/min: 1–2 g Q 8–12 hr <10 mL/min[e]: 0.5–1 g Q 12 hr	MD[f]	0.9–1.1	2.3–3.5	Limited data
Cefotetan	6 g	>50 mL/min[d]: 1–2 g Q 12 hr 10–50 mL/min: 1–2 g Q 24 hr <10 mL/min[e]: 0.5–1 g Q 24 hr	MD[f]	3–4.2	13	No change
Cefoxitin	12 g	>50 mL/min[d]: 1–2 g Q 6–8 hr 10–50 mL/min: 1–2 g Q 12–24 hr <10 mL/min[e]: 0.5–1 g Q 24 hr	MD[f]	0.7–0.8	12–24	No change

Ceftazidime	6 g	>50 mL/min[d]: 1–2 g Q 8 hr 10–50 mL/min: 1–2 g Q 12–24 hr <10 mL/min[e]: 0.5 g Q 24 hr	D[f]	1.6–2.0	13–25	No change
Ceftizoxime	12 g	>50 mL/min[d]: 1–2 g Q 8–12 hr 10–50 mL/min: 1–2 g Q 12–24 hr <10 mL/min[e]: 0.5 g Q 24 hr	MD[f]	1.4–1.7	19–35	No change
Ceftriaxone	4 g	>50 mL/min[d]: 1–2 g Q 12–24 hr 10–50 mL/min: 1–2 g Q 24 hr <10 mL/min[d]: 1–2 g Q 24 hr	ND	5–8	12–17[g]	Limited data
Cefuroxime	9 g	>50 mL/min[d]: 0.75–1.5 g Q 8 hr 10–50 mL/min: 0.75–1.5 g Q 12–24 hr <10 mL/min[e]: 0.75–1.5 g Q 24 hr	MD[f]	1.1–1.7	15–17	No change
Ciprofloxacin	800 mg	>50 mL/min[d]: 200–400 mg Q 12 hr 10–50 mL/min: 30–50 mL/min: No change. 10–30 mL/min: 100–300 mg Q 12 hr <10 mL/min[e]: 100–200 mg Q 12 hr	SD	4	8.5	No change
Clindamycin	4.8 g	>50 mL/min[d]: 600–900 mg Q 6–8 hr 10–50 mL/min: No change <10 mL/min[e]: No change	ND	2–4	1.6–3.4	600–900 mg Q 8–12 hr
Erythromycin	4 g	>50 mL/min[d]: 500–1,000 mg Q 6 hr 10–50 mL/min: No change <10 mL/min[e]: No change	SD	1.4–2.0	4	500–1,000 mg Q 8 hr
Ethambutol	25 mg/kg (PO)	>50 mL/min[d]: 15 mg/kg QD 10–50 mL/min: 7.5–10 mg/kg QD <10 mL/min[e]: 5 mg/kg QD	SD	3.1	98	No change
Fluconazole	400 mg	>50 mL/min[d]: 100–400 mg Q 24 hr 10–50 mL/min: 50–200 mg Q 24 hr <10 mL/min[e]: 50–100 mg Q 24 hr	MD[f]	30	98	No change
Flucytosine	150 mg/kg (PO)	>50 mL/min[d]: 12.5–37.5 mg/kg/dose Q 6 hr 10–50 mL/min: 25–50 mL/min: 12.5–37.5 mg/kg Q 12 hr 10–25 mL/min: 12.5–37.5 mg/kg Q 24 hr <10 mL/min[e]: 12.5–25 mg/kg Q 24 hr	D[f]	4–6	30–70	No change

(continued)

Table 53.9 • University of California San Francisco Adult Antimicrobial Dosing Guidelines[a] (continued)

Drug	Max Daily IV Dose[b]	Cl_Cr	Dialysis[c]	t½ (hr) Normal	t½ (hr) ESRD	Hepatic Failure Dosage
Ganciclovir	10 mg/kg	>50 mL/min[d]: >80 mL/min: 5 mg/kg/dose Q 12 hr; 50–79 mL/min: 2.5 mg/kg/dose Q 12 hr; 10–50 mL/min: 1.25–2.5 mg/kg/dose Q 12–24 hr; <10 mL/min[e]: 1.25 mg/kg Q 24 hr	D[f]	2.5–3.6	11.5–28	No change
Gentamicin[f]	(4 g)		D[f]	1.5–3.0	20–24	No change
Imipenem	50 mg/kg	>50 mL/min[d]: 5–10 mg/kg Q 6–8 hr; 10–50 mL/min: 5–10 mg/kg Q 8–12 hr; <10 mL/min[e]: 5–10 mg/kg Q 12 hr	MD[f]	0.8–1.3	2.9–3.7	No change
Isoniazid	300 mg	>50 mL/min[d]: 300 mg; 10–50 mL/min: No change; <10 mL/min[e]: No change	D[f]	0.5–4	8	200 mg QD
Ketoconazole	800 mg (PO)	>50 mL/min[d]: 200–400 mg QD; 10–50 mL/min: No change; <10 mL/min[e]: No change	ND	3.8	Unchanged	Limited data
Metronidazole	4 g	>50 mL/min[d]: 500 mg Q 8 hr; 10–50 mL/min: 500 mg Q 8 hr; <10 mL/min[e]: 500 mg Q 12 hr	D[f]	6–14	8–15	500 mg Q 12 hr
Nafcillin	12 g	>50 mL/min[d]: 1–2 g Q 4–6 hr; 10–50 mL/min: No change; <10 mL/min[e]: No change	ND	1–1.5	1.9	1–1.5 g Q 4–6 hr
Nitrofurantoin	400 mg (PO)	>50 mL/min[d]: 50–100 mg Q 6 hr; 10–50 mL/min: Avoid; <10 mL/min[d]: Avoid	N/A	N/A	N/A	N/A
Penicillin G	30 MU	>50 mL/min[d]: 2–3 MU Q 4 hr; 10–50 mL/min: 1–2 MU 4–6 hr; <10 mL/min[e]: 1 MU Q 6 hr	MD[f]	0.4–0.9	4–10	No change
Pentamidine	4 mg/kg	>50 mL/min[e]: 3–4 mg/kg Q 24 hr; 10–50 mL/min: No change; <10 mL/min[e]: No change	ND	5–9 days	No data	No change

Agent	Dose[b]	Dosage adjustment[d]	Dialyzability[c]	Half-life normal (hr)	Half-life ESRD (hr)	After dialysis
Piperacillin	24 g	>50 mL/min[d]: 3–4 g Q 4–6 hr; 10–50 mL/min: 3–4 g Q 6 hr; <10 mL/min[e]: 2–3 g Q 8 hr	MD[f]	0.8–1.4	3–6	Limited data
Pyrazinamide	35 mg/kg (PO)	>50 mL/min[d]: 20–25 mg/kg/day; 10–50 mL/min: No change; <10 mL/min[d]: No change	No data	9–10	Unchanged	ND
Rifampin	600 mg	>50 mL/min[d]: 600 mg QD; 10–50 mL/min: No change; <10 mL/min[e]: No change	ND	2.5–5	2–5	450 mg QD[i]
Tobramycin[g]	20 mg/kg TMP		D[f]	1.3–2.2	33–70	No change
Trimethoprim-sulfamethoxazole	20 mg/kg TMP	>50 mL/min[d]: Systemic GNR infection: 10 mg TMP/kg/day divided Q 6–12 hr. Pneumocystis carinii pneumonia: 12–20 mg TMP/kg/day divided Q 6–12 hr; 10–50 mL/min: Systemic GNR infection: 5–7.5 mg TMP/kg/day divided Q 12–24 hr. Pneumocystis carinii pneumonia: 10–15 mg TMP/kg/day divided Q 12–24 hr; <10 mL/min[e]: Systemic GNR infection: 2.5–5.0 mg TMP/kg/day Q 24 hr. Pneumocystis carinii pneumonia: 5–10 mg TMP/kg/day divided Q 24 hr	SD/MD	TMP: 8–12; SMX: 9–11	TMP: 24–62; SMX: 9–15; SMX-metabolite: 22–50	No change
Vancomycin	See Fig. 53.1		ND: conventional HD; MD: high flux[f]	9–11	129–190	No change

[a] Cl_Cr = Creatinine clearance; IV = Intravenous; N/A = Not available; PO = Oral; SMX = Sulfamethoxazole; TMP = Trimethoprim.

[b] Manufacturer's recommended maximum parenteral daily dose (unless other indicated).

[c] Dialyzability using conventional (Cuprophane) hemodialysis (ND, not dialyzed [>5%]; SD, slightly dialyzed [5–20%]; MD, moderately dialyzed [20–50%]; D, dialyzed [>50%]).

[d] Doses recommended for systemic infections commonly treated with this agent.

[e] For patients with minimal renal function or those with end-stage renal disease.

[f] Schedule dosing after hemodialysis. Some studies suggest dosing similar to conventional hemodialysis.

[g] The total daily dose of aminoglycosides can be administered as a single daily dose in patients with normal renal function (gentamicin or tobramycin: 5 mg/kg/day, amikacin 15 mg/kg/day). Patients with decreased renal function or abnormal body composition should have their doses adjusted according to serum levels.

[h] Changes in half-life in ESRD are caused by changes in protein binding, resulting in an increased volume of distribution without a change in the total clearance of the drug. Therefore, dosage adjustment in ESRD is not necessary. Limited data in a small number of patients with hepatic dysfunction do not support dosage reduction in hepatic disease. However, given that biliary elimination accounts for a significant amount of the total clearance of ceftriaxone, slight dosage reduction may be warranted with severe hepatic dysfunction.

[i] The half-life of rifampin in severe hepatic disease (cirrhosis, hepatitis) is increased from 2.8 to 5.4 hr; thus dosage reduction in severe hepatic disease is suggested.

Table 53.10 • Influence of Renal Disease on Antimicrobial Accumulation

None to Mild
Azithromycin, cefoperazone, ceftriaxone, chloramphenicol, clarithromycin, clindamycin, cloxacillin, dalfopristin/quinupristin, dicloxacillin, didanosine, doxycycline, erythromycin, ketoconazole, metronidazole, nafcillin, oxacillin, pentamidine, sulfamethoxazole, zalcitabine, zidovudine

Mild to Moderate
Cefotaxime, ciprofloxacin, clavulanic acid, imipenem, mezlocillin, norfloxacin, piperacillin, piperacillin-tazobactam

Significant
Acyclovir, amikacin, amoxicillin, ampicillin, ampicillin-sulbactam, aztreonam, cefadroxil, cefamandole, cefazolin, cefepime, cefixime, cefonicid, ceforanide, cefotetan, cefoxitin, ceftazidime, ceftizoxime, cefuroxime, cephalexin, cephalothin, flucytosine, foscarnet, ganciclovir, gentamicin, levofloxacin, methicillin, netilmicin, ofloxacin, penicillin G, teicoplanin, tetracycline, ticarcillin, tobramycin, trimethoprim, vancomycin

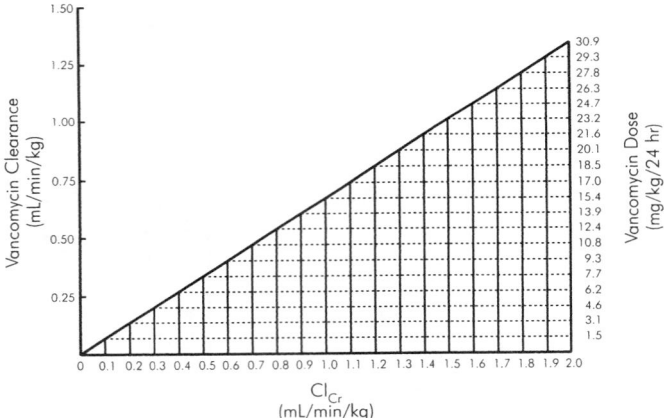

Fig. 53.1 Reduced Dosage Nomogram for Vancomycin in Patients with Impaired Renal Failure as derived by Moellering et al. Reprinted with permission from Ann Intern Med. 1981;94:343.

The reader is referred to Chapter 54: Principles of Infectious Diseases, written by *B. Joseph Guglielmo, Pharm.D.*, in the seventh edition of **Applied Therapeutics: The Clinical Use of Drugs** for a more in-depth discussion.

Notes:

Chapter 54

Antimicrobial Prophylaxis for Surgical Procedures

♦ Prophylactic antibiotics, when administered before some surgical procedures, can decrease the incidence of infection: this benefit must be balanced against potential adverse drug effects, superinfection, and risk of emergence of resistant strains.

♦ Antimicrobial prophylaxis is beneficial in high-risk gastroduodenal and biliary tract surgical procedures, colorectal surgery, appendectomy, vaginal hysterectomy, high-risk cesarean section, and most procedures involving implantation of prosthetic hardware (e.g., vascular graft, prosthetic hip).

♦ Prophylactic antibiotics reduce infections after cardiac surgery; however, the benefit is less conclusive than for the surgeries listed above.

♦ Clean surgical procedures with no placement of prosthetic material, low-risk gastro-duodenal and biliary surgery, and low-risk cesarean section do not appear to benefit from antibiotic prophylaxis.

♦ The risk of surgical infection for various procedures is summarized in Table 54.1.

♦ The choice of antibiotic prophylaxis should be directed against the most likely pathogens and need not eradicate every potential pathogen. Efficacy, safety, and cost also need to be considered. Antibiotic regimens are summarized in Table 54.2.

♦ In most cases, a single dose of parenteral antibiotic administered at the induction of anesthesia is sufficient. A second dose may be needed if a drug with a short half-life is used and surgery is prolonged, or if major blood loss occurs. Extending the duration of prophylaxis beyond the surgical period does not further reduce the rate of infectious complications.

Notes:

Table 54.1 • National Research Council Wound Classification[a]

Classification	Criteria	Infection Rate (%)
Clean	No acute inflammation or entry into GI, respiratory, GU, or biliary tracts; no break in aseptic technique occurs; wounds primarily closed	<5
Clean-contaminated	Elective, controlled opening of GI, respiratory, biliary, or GU tracts without significant spillage; clean wounds with major break in sterile technique	<10
Contaminated	Penetrating trauma (<4 hr old); major technique break or major spillage from GI tract; acute, nonpurulent inflammation	15–20
Dirty	Penetrating trauma (>4 hr old); purulence or abscess (active infectious process); preoperative perforation of viscera	30–40

[a]GI = Gastrointestinal; GU = Genitourinary.

Notes:

Table 54.2 • Suggested Prophylactic Antimicrobial Regimens for Surgical Procedures

Procedure	Predominant Organism(s)	Antibiotic Regimen (Alternative)	Adult Preoperative IV Dose
Clean			
Cardiac (all with sternotomy, cardiopulmonary bypass)	S. aureus, S. epidermidis	Cefazolin (Vancomycin)	1 g (1 g)
Vascular (aortic resection, groin incision, prosthesis)	S. aureus, S. epidermidis, Gram-negative enterics	Cefazolin (Vancomycin)	1 g (1 g)
Orthopedic (total joint replacement, internal fixation of fractures)	S. aureus, S. epidermidis	Cefazolin (Vancomycin)	1 g (1 g)
Neurosurgery	S. aureus, S. epidermidis	Cefazolin (Vancomycin)	1 g (1 g)
Clean-Contaminated			
Head and neck	S. aureus, oral anaerobes, streptococci	Cefazolin + metronidazole (clindamycin + gentamicin)	2 g cefazolin + 500 mg metronidazole (600 mg clindamycin + 1.5 mg/kg gentamicin)
Gastroduodenal (only for procedures entering stomach)	Gram-negative enterics, S. aureus, mouth flora	Cefazolin	1 g
Colorectal	Gram-negative enterics, anaerobes (B. fragilis)	Oral neomycin–erythromycin base (IV cefoxitin or cefotetan)	1 g each at 1 PM, 2 PM, and 11 PM day before surgery (1 g of either)
Appendectomy (uncomplicated)	Gram-negative enterics, anaerobes (B. fragilis)	Cefoxitin or cefotetan	1–2 g
Biliary tract (only for high-risk procedures)	Gram-negative enterics, Enterococcus faecalis, clostridia	Cefazolin	1 g
Cesarean section	Group B streptococci, enterococci, anaerobes, Gram-negative enterics	Cefazolin	2 g after umbilical cord clamped
Hysterectomy	Group B streptococci, enterococci, anaerobes, Gram-negative enterics	Cefazolin or cefotetan or cefoxitin	1 g

The reader is referred to Chapter 55: Antimicrobial Prophylaxis for Surgical Procedures, written by *Laurie L. Briceland, Pharm.D.* and *B. Joseph Guglielmo, Pharm.D.,* in the seventh edition of **Applied Therapeutics: The Clinical Use of Drugs** for a more in-depth discussion. All notations to reference numbers are based on the reference list at the end of that chapter. The editors of this handbook express their thanks to Drs. Briceland and Guglielmo and acknowledge that this chapter is based upon his work.

Notes:

Notes:

Chapter 55

Central Nervous System Infections

Anatomy and Physiology

- ♦ Brain and spinal cord are ensheathed by the meninges and suspended in cerebrospinal fluid
- ♦ Meninges consists of 3 layers: pia mater, arachnoid, dura mater
- ♦ Meningitis is inflammation of the subarachnoid space
- ♦ Abscess can be subdural (between arachnoid and dura) or epidural (outside dural space)
- ♦ Two barriers exist within the brain: the blood-CSF barrier and the blood-brain barrier (see Figure 55.1)
- ♦ Many antimicrobials pass the blood-CSF barrier; few pass the blood-brain barrier

Pathophysiology

- ♦ See Figure 55.2.

Meningitis

- ♦ Meningitis, an infection of the subarachnoid space, most commonly is caused by hematogenous spread of an organism to the meninges from a distal point.
- ♦ Age, seasonal variance, and underlying risk factors predispose individuals to specific microorganisms (see Table 55.1).
- ♦ Signs and symptoms of acute bacterial meningitis are listed in Table 55.2.
- ♦ Table 55.3 compares the typical findings when CSF is examined from patients with acute bacterial, fungal, or viral meningitis.
- ♦ Parenteral antimicrobial agents for the empirical treatment of meningitis are suggested in Table 55.4 and specific antimicrobials for specific pathogens are in Table 55.5. The dosing regimens for these antimicrobials are in Table 55.6.
- ♦ Antimicrobials that are lipophilic, have a small molecular weight, are in a unionized state, and have low protein binding are more likely to pass into the brain and CSF. Degree of meningeal inflammation also is an important determinant. The capability of various antimicrobials to penetrate into the CSF is described in Table 55.7.

Adjunct Therapy. Dexamethasone 0.15 mg/kg administered Q 6 hr reduces the incidence of hearing loss in children with *H. influenzae* meningitis.

Brain Abscess

♦ The most common pathogens associated with brain abscess include anaerobes, streptococci, staphylococci, and occasional gram-negative rods.

♦ Considering the more permeable barrier (blood-CSF barrier) associated with brain abscess, drug penetration is more likely than with meningitis.

♦ As with any abscess, surgical drainage often is the definitive therapeutic maneuver.

Table 55.1 • Microbiology of Bacterial Meningitis

Age Group or Predisposing Condition	Most Likely Organisms[a]
Neonates (<2 mo)	Group B streptococcus (*S. agalactiae*), *E. coli*, and other Gram-negative bacilli (*Klebsiella, Serratia* species), *L. monocytogenes*
Infants and children (2 mo–10 yr)	*H. influenzae*,[b] *S. pneumoniae*, *N. meningitidis*
Children and adults (>10–30 yr)	*N. meningitidis, S. pneumoniae*
Adults (30–60 yr)	*S. pneumoniae, N. meningitidis*
Elderly (>60 yr)	*S. pneumoniae, N. meningitidis, E. coli, Klebsiella* species, and other Gram-negative bacilli, *L. monocytogenes*
Postneurosurgical	*S. aureus*, Gram-negative bacilli (e.g., *E. coli, Klebsiella* species), *S. epidermidis*[c]
Closed head trauma	*S. pneumoniae, H. influenzae*
Open head trauma	*S. aureus*, Gram-negative bacilli (e.g., *E. coli, Klebsiella* species)

[a]Organisms listed in descending order of frequency.
[b]Need to consider this pathogen only in children not vaccinated with Hib.
[c]Most commonly seen in association with prosthetic devices (e.g., cerebrospinal fluid shunts).

Table 55.2 • Signs and Symptoms of Acute Bacterial Meningitis

Fever	Anorexia
Nuchal rigidity (stiff neck)	Headache
Altered mental status	Photophobia
Seizures	Nausea and vomiting
Brudzinski's sign	Focal neurologic deficits
Kernig's sign	Septic shock
Irritability[a]	

[a]Symptoms seen in infants with meningitis.

Notes:

Table 55.3 • CSF Findings in Various Types of Meningitis[a]

Microbial Etiology	WBC Count (cells/mm^3)	Predominant Cell Type	Protein	Glucose
Bacterial	>500	PMN	Elevated	↓
Fungal	10–500	MN	Elevated	Variable
Viral	10–200	PMN or MN	Variable	Normal

[a]CSF = Cerebrospinal fluid; MN = Mononuclear cells; PMN = Polymorphonuclear neutrophils; WBC = White blood cell.

Table 55.4 • Empiric Therapy for Bacterial Meningitis

Age Group or Predisposing Condition	Recommended Therapy	Alternative Therapy
Neonates (<2 mo)	Ampicillin and cefotaxime	Ampicillin and gentamicin
Infants and children (2 mo–10 yr)	Cefotaxime[a] + vancomycin	Cefotaxime[a] + rifampin
Older children and adults (10–60 yr)	Cefotaxime[a] + vancomycin	Cefotaxime + rifampin
Elderly (>60 yr)	Ampicillin, cefotaxime,[a] and vancomycin	Ampicillin, cefotaxime, and rifampin
Postneurosurgical	Nafcillin and cefotaxime[a] ± gentamicin	Vancomycin and cefotaxime[a] ± gentamicin
Open head trauma	Nafcillin and cefotaxime[a]	Vancomycin and cefotaxime[a]

[a]Ceftriaxone is an acceptable alternative.

Notes:

Table 55.5 • Definitive Therapy for Bacterial Meningitis[a]

Pathogen	Recommended Treatment	Alternative Agents
H. influenzae		
β-Lactamase–negative	Ampicillin	Cefotaxime[b]
β-Lactamase–positive	Cefotaxime[b]	Chloramphenicol
N. meningitidis	Penicillin G or ampicillin	Cefotaxime[c]
S. pneumoniae	*Penicillin-sensitive[c]:* Penicillin G or ampicillin	Cefotaxime[b]
	Intermediately penicillin-resistant[c]: Vancomycin + cefotaxime[b]	Cefotaxime[b] and rifampin
	Highly penicillin-resistant[c]: Vancomycin + cefotaxime[b] ± rifampin	
S. agalactiae	Penicillin G or ampicillin + gentamicin	Cefotaxime[b]
L. monocytogenes	Ampicillin ± gentamicin	TMP-SMX
Enterobacteriaceae		
E. coli, Klebsiella species	Cefotaxime[b]	Piperacillin + gentamicin[d]
Enterobacter, Serratia species	TMP-SMX	Piperacillin + gentamicin,[d] or ciprofloxacin,[e] or imipenem,[e] meropenem, cefepime[e]
P. aeruginosa	Ceftazidime + tobramycin[d]	Piperacillin + tobramycin, or ciprofloxacin,[e] or imipenem,[e] meropenem[b]
S. aureus		
Penicillinase-producing	Nafcillin or oxacillin	Vancomycin[d]
Methicillin-resistant (MRSA)	Vancomycin[e] ± rifampin	TMP-SMX[e] ± rifampin
S. epidermidis	Vancomycin[d] ± rifampin	TMP-SMX[e] ± rifampin

[a]MIC = Minimum inhibitory concentration; TMP-SMX = Trimethoprim-sulfamethoxazole.
[b]Ceftriaxone also may be used.
[c]Penicillin-sensitive strains defined as having MIC ≤0.1 μg/mL; intermediately resistant strains MIC >0.1–1.0 μg/mL; highly resistant strains MIC ≥2.0 μg/mL.
[d]Concomitant intrathecal therapy often required for optimal response.
[e]Limited experience or efficacy data for the agent against with this pathogen.

Table 55.6 • Suggested Antibiotic Dosing Regimens for Treatment of Central Nervous System Infections

| Antibiotic | Daily Dose[a] | | | Dosing Interval (hr) | |
	Neonates[b]	Children	Adults	Neonates	Children/Adults
Penicillins					
Ampicillin	100–200 mg/kg	200–300 mg/kg	12 g	8–12	4–6
Nafcillin	100–150 mg/kg	150–200 mg/kg	12 g	8–12	4–6
Penicillin G	0.1–0.2 million units/kg	0.15–0.2 million units/kg	20–24 million units	8–12	4–6
Piperacillin	150–300 mg/kg	250–300 mg/kg	16–20 g	8–12	4–6
Cephalosporins					
Cefotaxime	100–150 mg/kg	200–300 mg/kg	12 g	9–12	4–6
Ceftizoxime	100–150 mg/kg	200 mg/kg	12 g	8–12	6–8
Ceftriaxone	NR	100 mg/kg	4 g	—	12–24
Ceftazidime	100–150 mg/kg	150–200 mg/kg	8–12 g	8–12	6–8
Aminoglycosides[c]					
Gentamicin	5–7.5 mg/kg[d,e]	—	5–6 mg/kg[d,e]	12	8–12
Tobramycin	5–7.5 mg/kg[d,e]	—	5–6 mg/kg[d,e]	12	8–12
Amikacin	15–30 mg/kg[d,e]	—	15–25 mg/kg[d,e]	12	8–12
Chloramphenicol	NR	75–100 mg/kg	4–6 g	—	6
Metronidazole	—	30 mg/kg	1.5–2 g	—	6–8
TMP-SMX	—	12–15 mg/kg[f]	12–15 mg/kg[f]	—	8
Vancomycin	20–30 mg/kg	40–60 mg/kg[g]	2–3 g[g] or 20–30 mg/kg[g]	12	8–12

[a]Recommended daily dose when renal and hepatic function are normal.
[b]Infants <1 month old; lower end of dosage range applies to neonates ≤7 days old.
[c]Concurrent intrathecal doses of 5–10 mg (gentamicin, tobramycin), or 20 mg (amikacin) often required when treating Gram-negative bacillary meningitis.
[d]Dose should be individualized based upon serum level monitoring.
[e]Concurrent intrathecal therapy not recommended for neonatal meningitis.
[f]Dose is based upon the trimethoprim component.
[g]Concurrent intrathecal doses of 5–20 mg recommended if response to intravenous therapy is inadequate.

Table 55.7 • CSF Penetration Characteristics of Various Antimicrobials^a

Very Good^b
Chloramphenicol, metronidazole, rifampin, TMP-SMX

Good^c
Penicillins: Penicillin G, ampicillin, mezlocillin, nafcillin, piperacillin, ticarcillin
Other β-lactams: Aztreonam, clavulanic acid, imipenem, meropenem, sulbactam
Cephalosporins: Cefepime, cefotaxime, ceftazidime, ceftizoxime, ceftriaxone, cefuroxime
Fluoroquinolones: Ciprofloxacin, ofloxacin

Fair to Poor^d
Aminoglycosides: Amikacin, gentamicin, tobramycin
Other agents: Azithromycin, clarithromycin, clindamycin, erythromycin, vancomycin

^aCSF = Cerebrospinal fluid; TMP-SMX = Trimethoprim-sulfamethoxazole.
^bPenetrate CSF well, regardless of meningeal inflammation.
^cAdequate CSF penetration achieved when the meninges are inflamed.
^dPenetration often inadequate even when the meninges are inflamed.

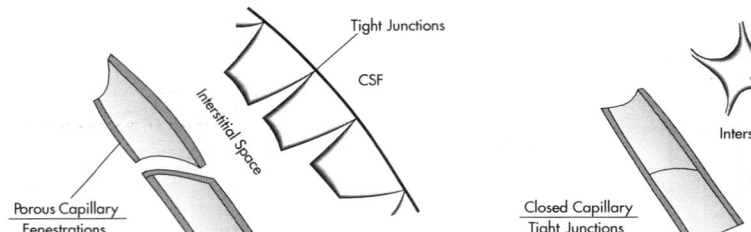

A. Capillary Surface Area = 1   B. Capillary Surface Area = 5,000

Fig. 55.1 The Two Membrane Barrier Systems in the Central Nervous System: The Blood-CSF Barrier (A) and the Blood-Brain Barrier (B). (Reproduced with permission from reference 15.)

Notes:

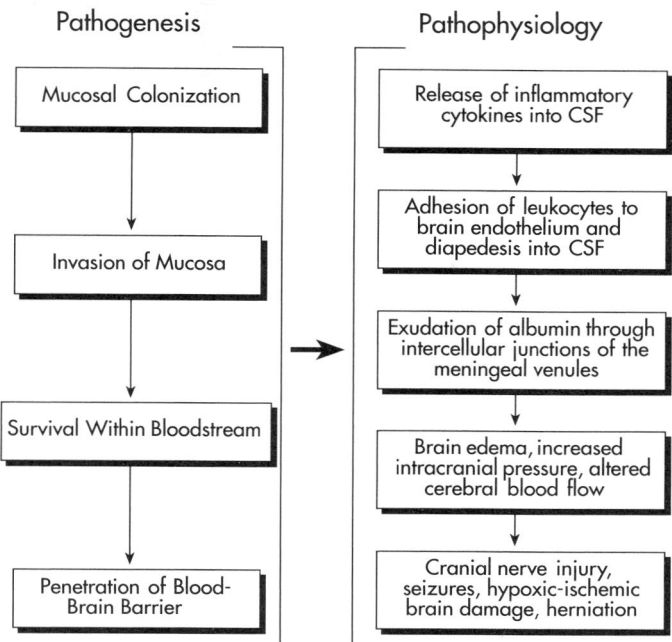

Fig. 55.2 Schematic Summary of the Pathogenesis and Pathophysiology of Bacterial Meningitis. (Adapted from references 2 and 4.)

The reader is referred to Chapter 56: Central Nervous System Infections, written by *Vicky J. Dadas, Pharm.D. and John F. Flaherty, Pharm.D.* in the seventh edition of **Applied Therapeutics: The Clinical Use of Drugs** for a more in-depth discussion. All notations to reference numbers are based on the reference list at the end of that chapter. The editors of this handbook express their thanks to Drs. Dadas and Flaherty and acknowledge that this chapter is based upon their work.

Notes:

Notes:

Chapter 56

Endocarditis

Pathogenesis

♦ In the past, endocarditis was classified as either "acute" or "subacute." However, there is significant overlap between acute and subacute relative to infecting organisms. Thus, the treatment regimens should be directed toward the likely pathogens (primarily *Streptococcus viridans, Staphylococcus aureus,* enterococci) rather than patient symptoms.

Epidemiology

♦ There are 10,000–15,000 new cases per year in the U.S.

♦ Mitral valve is the most commonly infected valve in infection due to *S. viridans;* the tricuspid valve is most likely to be infected with IV drug use.

♦ Primary risk factors include mitral valve prolapse, prosthetic valves, and IV drug abuse.

Clinical Presentation and Treatment

♦ ***Streptococcus viridans*** generally is associated with a more subacute clinical picture: symptoms often present for greater than 2–3 months. Signs and symptoms are nonspecific and subtle, but endocarditis should be suspected in any patient with a documented fever and heart murmur. Prior cardiac disease, peripheral embolic manifestations (e.g., petechiae, splinter hemorrhages), various laboratory abnormalities, and positive echocardiography strengthen the diagnosis, but microbiological documentation of bacteremia is most important. Susceptibility of all isolates to penicillin must be confirmed.

 Treatment regimens are in Table 56.1.

♦ ***Staphylococcus aureus*** is pathogenic in IV drug addicts and in patients with prosthetic cardiac valves. The organism is more virulent than *S. viridans* in that it less likely requires a cardiac defect for it to be infective. The course of the disease is of a more acute nature, requiring immediate initiation of antimicrobial therapy.

 Treatment (see Table 56.2) generally consists of 4–6 weeks of nafcillin or oxacillin. Three to 5 days of low-dose synergistic doses of an aminoglycoside may decrease the time to defervescence and time to resolution of bacteremia; however, the associated risks (ototoxicity, nephrotoxicity) of aminoglycoside therapy also must be considered. Two weeks of nafcillin plus low-dose aminoglycoside appears to be effective in the treatment of right-sided endocarditis in IV drug users. *S. aureus* infection of prosthetic valves should be treated with either nafcillin (or vancomycin if methicillin-resistant) plus rifampin (plus low-dose gentamicin for 2 weeks).

♦ ***Staphylococcus epidermidis,*** unlike *S. aureus,* is generally only infective in the presence of prosthetic material.

Treatment. The organism often is nafcillin (methicillin)-resistant; thus, vancomycin is the drug of choice with these isolates. The addition of rifampin and gentamicin for synergy also is recommended for treatment of infection by this organism. As with most infections of prosthetic hardware, removal of the infected cardiac valve often is necessary.

♦ ***Enterococcus faecalis* ond *Enterococcus faecium*** are inhibited but not killed by penicillin or vancomycin alone. Thus, a synergistic combination of these antibiotics with an aminoglycoside is necessary to produce the desired bactericidal effect (see Table 56.3). Cephalosporins and the penicillinase-resistant penicillins are *not* active versus enterococci, nor are they synergistic with the aminoglycoside and should not be used.

♦ ***HACEK Micro-Organisms.*** HACEK group accounts for 5%–10% of native valve endocarditis in patients who are not intravenous drug users. They are slow growing, fastidious gram-negative bacilli that often are difficult to culture. (See Table 56.4.)

Prophylaxis

Table 56.5 summarizes recommendations for prophylactic treatment of endocarditis.

Notes:

Table 56.1 • Suggested Regimens for Therapy of Native Valve Endocarditis Caused by *Streptococcus viridans* and *Streptococcus bovis*

Antibiotic	Dose[a] and Route[b]	Duration
Penicillin-susceptible (Minimum Inhibitory Concentration ≤0.1 μg/mL)		
Aqueous crystalline penicillin G[c]	*Adult:* 12–18 million U/24 hr IV, either continuously or in six equally divided doses *Pediatric:* 150,000–200,000 U/kg/24 hr IV (max: 20 million units/24 hr) either continuously or in 6 equally divided doses	4 wk
Ceftriaxone sodium[c]	*Adult:* 2 g once daily IV or IM	4 wk
Aqueous crystalline penicillin G	*Adult:* 12–18 million U/24 hr IV either continuously or in six equally divided doses *Pediatric:* 150,000–200,000 U/kg/24 hr IV (max: 20 million U/24 hr) either continuously or in 6 equally divided doses	2 wk
With gentamicin sulfate[d]	*Adult:* 1 mg/kg IM or IV (max: 80 mg) Q 8 hr *Pediatric:* 2–2.5 mg/kg IV (max: 80 mg) Q 8 hr	2 wk
Relatively Penicillin G Resistant (Minimum Inhibitory Concentration >0.1 μg/mL and <0.5 μg/mL)		
Aqueous crystalline penicillin G[e]	*Adult:* 18 million U/24 hr IV, either continuously or in six equally divided doses *Pediatric:* 200,000–300,000 U/kg/24 hr IV (max: 20 million U/24 hr) either continuously or in 6 equally divided doses	4 wk
With gentamicin sulfate[d]	*Adult:* 1 mg/kg IM or IV (max: 80 mg) Q 8 hr *Pediatric:* 2–2.5 mg/kg IV (max: 80 mg) Q 8 hr	2 wk
β-Lactam Allergic Patients		
Vancomycin hydrochloride[f]	*Adult:* 30 mg/kg/24 hr IV in two equally divided doses (max: 2 g/24 hr unless serum concentrations are monitored) *Pediatric:* 40 mg/kg/24 hr IV in 2 or 4 equally divided doses (max: 2 g/24 hr unless serum concentrations are monitored)	4 wk

[a]Pediatric dosages are adapted from reference 48.
[b]Antibiotic doses for patients with impaired renal function should be modified appropriately. Vancomycin dosage should be reduced in patients with renal dysfunction; cephalosporin dosage may need to be reduced in patients with moderate-to-severe renal dysfunction.
[c]Preferred in most patients >65 years of age and in those with impairment of the eighth nerve or renal function.
[d]Dosing of gentamicin on a mg/kg basis produces higher serum concentrations in obese patients than in lean patients. Therefore, in obese patients, dosing should be based on lean body weight. Other potentially nephrotoxic agents (e.g., nonsteroidal anti-inflammatory drugs) should be used cautiously in patients receiving gentamicin. A peak gentamicin serum concentration of 3 μg/mL and a trough concentration of <1 μg/mL are desirable.
[e]Cefazolin or other first-generation cephalosporins may be substituted for penicillin in patients whose penicillin hypersensitivity is not of the immediate type.
[f]Vancomycin dosage should be reduced in patients with impaired renal function. Vancomycin given on a mg/kg basis produces higher serum concentrations in obese patients than in lean patients. Therefore, in obese patients, dosing should be based on ideal body weight. Each dose of vancomycin should be infused over at least 1 hr to reduce the risk of the histamine-release "red-man" syndrome. Peak serum concentrations of vancomycin should be obtained 1 hr after completion of the infusion and should be in the range of 30–45 μg/mL. Trough concentrations should be obtained within half an hour of the next dose and be in the range of 5–15 μg/mL.
Adapted from Wilson WR et al. Antibiotic treatment of adults with infective endocarditis due to streptococci, enterococci, staphylococci, and HACEK microorganisms. JAMA 1995;274:1706–1713. Copyright 1995, American Medical Association.

Notes:

Table 56.2 • Treatment of Staphylococcal Endocarditis

Antibiotic	Dosage and Route[b]	Duration
Without Prosthetic Material[a]		
Methicillin-Susceptible Staphylococci		
Nonpenicillin-Allergic Patients		
Nafcillin	_Adult:_ 2 g IV Q 4 hr	4–6 wk
	Pediatric: 150–200 mg/kg/24 hr IV (_max:_ 12 g/24 hr) in 4–6 equally divided doses	
_or_		
Oxacillin	_Adult:_ 2 g IV Q 4 hr	4–6 wk
	Pediatric: 150–200 mg/kg/24 hr IV (_max:_ 12 g/24 hr) in 4–6 equally divided doses	
With optional addition of gentamicin[b,c]	_Adult:_ 1 mg/kg IM or IV (_max:_ 80 mg) Q 8 hr	3–5 days
	Pediatric: 2–2.5 mg/kg IV (_max:_ 80 mg) Q 8 hr	
Penicillin-Allergic Patients		
1. Cefazolin[d]	_Adult:_ 2 g IV Q 8 hr	4–6 wk
	Pediatric: 80–100 mg/kg/24 hr IV (_max:_ 6 g/24 hr) in equally divided doses Q 8 hr	
With optional addition of gentamicin[b]	_Adult:_ See Nonpenicillin-allergic patient	
	Pediatric: See Nonpenicillin-allergic patient	
2. Vancomycin[b,e,f]	_Adult:_ 30 mg/kg/24 hr IV in 2 or 4 equally divided doses (_max:_ 2 g/24 hr unless serum levels monitored)	4–6 wk
	Pediatric: 40 mg/kg/24 hr IV in 2 or 4 equally divided doses (_max:_ 2 g/24 hr unless serum levels monitored)	
Methicillin-resistant Staphylococci		
Vancomycin[b,e,f]	_Adult:_ 30 mg/kg/24 hr IV in 2 or 4 equally divided doses (_max:_ 2 g/24 hr unless serum levels monitored)	4–6 wk
	Pediatric: 40 mg/kg/24 hr IV in 2 or 4 equally divided doses (_max:_ 2 g/24 hr unless serum levels monitored)	
With Prosthetic Valve or Other Prosthetic Material[g]		
Methicillin-Resistant Staphylococci		
Vancomycin[b,e]	_Adult:_ 30 mg/kg/24 hr IV in 2 or 4 equally divided doses (_max:_ 2 g/24 hr unless serum levels monitored)	≥6 wk
	Pediatric: 40 mg/kg/24 hr IV in 2 or 4 equally divided doses (_max:_ 2 g/24 hr unless serum levels monitored)	
With rifampin[h]	_Adult:_ 300 mg PO Q 8 hr	≥6 wk
and	_Pediatric:_ 20 mg/kg/24 hr PO (_max:_ 900 mg/24 hr) in 2 equally divided doses	
With gentamicin[b,i,j]	_Adult:_ 1 mg/kg IM or IV (_max:_ 80 mg) Q 8 hr	2 wk
	Pediatric: 2–2.5 mg/kg/24 hr IV (_max:_ 80 mg) Q 8 hr	

Methicillin-Susceptible Staphylococci

Nafcillin or oxacillin[k]

Adult: 2 g IV Q 4 hr — ≥6 wk
Pediatric: 150–200 mg/kg/24 hr (*max:* 12 g/24 hr) in 4–6 equally divided doses

With rifampin[h]

Adult: 300 mg PO Q 8 hr — ≥6 wk
Pediatric: 20 mg/kg/24 hr PO (*max:* 900 mg/24 hr) in 2 equally divided doses

and

With gentamicin[b,i,j]

Adult: 1 mg/kg IM or IV (*max:* 80 mg) Q 8 hr — 2 wk
Pediatric: 2–2.5 mg/kg IV (*max:* 80 mg) Q 8 hr

[a]Antibiotic doses should be modified appropriately for patients with impaired renal function. For treatment of endocarditis caused by penicillin-susceptible staphylococci (MIC ≥0.1 mg/mL), aqueous crystalline penicillin G (Table 56.1, first regimen) should be used for 4–6 wk instead of nafcillin or oxacillin. Shorter antibiotic courses have been effective in some drug addicts with right-sided endocarditis caused by S. aureus. See text for comments on use of rifampin.

[b]Dosing of aminoglycosides and vancomycin on a mg/kg basis will give higher serum concentrations in obese than in lean patients.

[c]Benefit of additional aminoglycoside has not been established. Risk of toxic reactions because of these agents is increased in patients >65 years of age or those with renal or eighth nerve impairment.

[d]There is potential cross-allergenicity between penicillins and cephalosporins. Cephalosporins should be avoided in patients with immediate-type hypersensitivity to penicillin (see Chapter 4).

[e]Peak serum concentrations of vancomycin should be obtained 1 hour after infusion and be in the range of 30–45 μg/mL for BID dosing and 20–30 μg/mL for QID dosing. Trough serum concentrations should be obtained within half an hour of the next dose and be in the range of 5–15 μg/mL. Each vancomycin dose should be infused over 1 hour.

[f]See text for consideration of optional addition of gentamicin.

[g]Vancomycin and gentamicin doses must be modified appropriately in patients with renal failure.

[h]Rifampin is recommended for therapy of infections caused by coagulase-negative staphylococci. Its use in coagulase-positive staphylococcal infections is controversial. Rifampin increases the amount of warfarin sodium required for antithrombotic therapy.

[i]Serum concentration of gentamicin should be monitored, and dose should be adjusted to obtain a peak level of ≈3 μg/mL.

[j]Use during initial 2 wk. See text on alternative aminoglycoside therapy for organisms resistant to gentamicin.

[k]First-generation cephalosporins or vancomycin should be used in penicillin-allergic patients. Cephalosporins should be avoided in patients with immediate-type hypersensitivity to penicillin and those infected with methicillin-resistant staphylococci.

Adapted from reference 48 and Wilson WR et al. Antibiotic treatment of adults with infective endocarditis due to streptococci, enterococci, staphylococci, and HACEK microorganisms. JAMA 1995;274:1706–1713.

Table 56.3 • Therapy for Endocarditis Caused by Enterococci (or Streptococci viridans with an MIC ≥0.5 μg/mL)[a,b]

Antibiotic	Dose and Route	Duration
Nonpenicillin-Allergic Patient		
1. Aqueous crystalline penicillin G	*Adult:* 20–30 million U/24 hr IV given continuously or in 6 equally divided doses	4–6 wk
	Pediatric: 200,000–300,000 U/kg/24 hr IV (*max:* 30 million U/24 hr) given continuously or in 6 equally divided doses	
With gentamicin[c,d,e]	*Adult:* 1 mg/kg IM or IV (*max:* 80 mg) Q 8 hr	4–6 wk
	Pediatric: 2–2.5 mg/kg IM or IV (*max:* 80 mg) Q 8 hr	
or		
With streptomycin[c,e,f]	*Adult:* 7.5 mg/kg IM (*max:* 500 mg) Q 12 hr	4–6 wk
	Pediatric: 15 mg/kg IM (*max:* 500 mg) Q 12 hr	
2. Ampicillin	*Adult:* 12 g/24 hr IV given continuously or in 6 equally divided doses	4–6 wk
	Pediatric: 300 mg/kg/24 hr IV (*max:* 12 g/24 hr) in 4–6 equally divided doses	
With gentamicin[c,d,e]	*Adult:* 1 mg/kg IM or IV (*max:* 80 mg) Q 8 hr	4–6 wk
	Pediatric: 2–2.5 mg/kg IM or IV (*max:* 80 mg) Q 8 hr	
or		
With streptomycin[c,e,f]	*Adult:* 7.5 mg/kg IM (*max:* 500 mg) Q 12 hr	4–6 wk
	Pediatric: 15 mg/kg IM (*max:* 500 mg) Q 12 hr	
Penicillin-Allergic Patients[g]		
Vancomycin[h]	*Adult:* 30 mg/kg/24 hr IV in 2 or 4 equally divided doses (*max:* 2 g/24 hr unless serum levels monitored)	4–6 wk
	Pediatric: 40 mg/kg/24 hr IV in 2 or 4 equally divided doses (*max:* 2 g/24 hr unless serum levels monitored)	
With gentamicin[c,d,e]	*Adult:* 1 mg/kg IM or IV (*max:* 80 mg) Q 8 hr	4–6 wk
	Pediatric: 2–2.5 mg/kg IM or IV (*max:* 80 mg) Q 8 hr	
or		
With streptomycin[c,e,f]	*Adult:* 7.5 mg/kg IM or IV (*max:* 500 mg) Q 12 hr	4–6 wk
	Pediatric: 15 mg/kg IM or IV (*max:* 500 mg) Q 12 hr	

[a] Antibiotic doses should be modified appropriately in patients with impaired renal function.

[b] Choice of aminoglycoside depends on resistance level of infecting strain. Enterococci should be tested for high-level resistance (streptomycin: MIC ≥2,000 μg/mL; gentamicin: MIC ≥500 μg/mL).

[c] Serum concentration of gentamicin should be monitored and dosage adjusted to obtain a peak level of ≈3 μg/mL.

[d] Dosing of aminoglycosides and vancomycin on a mg/kg basis gives higher serum concentrations in obese than in lean patients.

[e] Serum concentrations of streptomycin should be monitored if possible and dose adjusted to obtain a peak level of ≈20 μg/mL.

[f] Desensitization should be considered; cephalosporins are not satisfactory alternatives.

[g] Peak serum concentrations of vancomycin should be obtained 1 hour after infusion and be in the range of 30–45 μg/mL for BID dosing and 20–30 μg/mL for QID dosing. Trough serum concentrations should be obtained within half an hour of the next dose and be in the range of 5–15 μg/mL. Each dose should be infused over 1 hour. Antibiotic treatment of adults with infective endocarditis due to streptococci, enterococci, staphylococci, and HACEK microorganisms. JAMA 1995;274:1706–1713.

Adapted from reference 48 and Wilson WR et al.

Table 56.4 • Therapy for Endocarditis due to HACEK Micro-organisms (*Haemophilus parainfluenza, Haemophilus aphrophilus, Actinobacillus actinomycetemcomitans, Cardiobacterium hominis, Eikenella corrodens,* and *Kingella kingae*)

Antibiotic	Dose and Route	Duration
1) Ceftriaxone[a]	2 gm Q 24 hr IM or IV	4 weeks
2) Ampicillin[b]	12 gm/24 hr IV, either continuously or in 6 equally divided doses	4 weeks
With gentamicin[c]	1 mg/kg IM or IV Q 8 hr	4 weeks

[a] Patient should be informed that IM injection of ceftriaxone is painful.
[b] Ampicillin should not be used if laboratory tests show beta lactamase production.
[c] For specific dosing adjustment and issues concerning gentamicin (obese patients, relative contraindications), see footnotes in Table 56.1.

Table 56.5 • Endocarditis Prophylaxis Regimen for Patients Who Are at Risk

Drug	Dosage
Dental, Oral, or Upper Respiratory Tract Procedures[a]	
Standard Regimen	
Amoxicillin	*Adult:* 2.0 g
	Pediatric: 50 mg/kg PO 1 hr before procedure
Allergic to Penicillin	
Clindamycin or	*Adult:* 600 mg
	Pediatric: 20 mg/kg PO 1 hr before procedure
Cephalexin or cefadroxil[b] or	*Adult:* 2.0 g
	Pediatric: 50 mg/kg PO 1 hr before procedure
Azithromycin or clarithromycin	*Adult:* 500 mg
	Pediatric: 15 mg/kg PO 1 hr before procedure
Unable to Take Oral Medications	
Ampicillin	*Adult:* 2.0 g IM/IV
(Allergic to penicillin)	*Pediatric:* 50 mg/kg IM/IV within 30 min before procedure
Clindamycin or	*Adult:* 600 mg
	Pediatric: 20 mg/kg IV within 30 min before procedure
Cefazolin[b]	*Adult:* 1.0 g
	Pediatric: 25 mg/kg IM/IV within 30 min before procedure
Genitourinary/Gastrointestinal (Excluding Esophageal) Procedures	
High-Risk Patients	
Ampicillin plus gentamicin	*Adult:* Ampicillin 2.0 g IM/IV plus gentamicin 1.5 mg/kg (*max:* 120 mg) within 30 min of starting the procedure; 6 hr later, ampicillin 1g IM/IV or amoxicillin 1 g PO
Moderate-Risk Patients	
Amoxicillin or ampicillin	*Adult:* Amoxicillin 2.0 g PO 1 hr before procedure or ampicillin 2.0 g IM/IV within 30 min of starting the procedure
Allergic to Ampicillin/Amoxicillin	
High-Risk	
Vancomycin plus gentamicin	*Adult:* Vancomycin 1.0 g IV over 1–2 hr plus gentamicin 1.5 mg/kg IV/IM (*max:* 120 mg); complete injection/infusion within 30 min of starting the procedure
	Pediatric: Vancomycin 20 mg/kg IV over 1–2 hr plus gentamicin 1.5 mg/kg IV/IM; complete injection/infusion within 30 min of starting the procedure
Moderate-Risk	
Vancomycin	*Adult:* Vancomycin 1.0 g IV
	Pediatric: 20 mg/kg IV over 1–2 hr; complete infusion within 30 min of starting the procedure

[a] Includes those with prosthetic heart valves and other high-risk patients.
[b] Cephalosporins should not be used in individuals with immediate-type hypersensitivity reaction (urticaria, angioedema, or anaphylaxis) to penicillins.
Reprinted from Dajani AS et al. Prevention of bacterial endocarditis. Recommendations by the American Heart Association. JAMA 1997;277:1794–1801. Copyright 1997, American Medical Association.

The reader is referred to Chapter 57: Endocarditis, written by *Annie Wong-Beringer, Pharm.D.*, in the seventh edition of **Applied Therapeutics: The Clinical Use of Drugs** for a more in-depth discussion. The editors of this handbook express their thanks to Dr. Wong-Beringer and acknowledge that this chapter is based upon her work.

Notes:

Chapter 57

Respiratory Tract Infections

Community-Acquired Respiratory Tract Infection

♦ Most community-acquired bacterial respiratory tract infections are caused by *Streptococcus pneumoniae* (pneumococci) (Table 57.2). The increased incidence of penicillin-resistant pneumococci has resulted in limited therapeutic options.

♦ "Susceptible" *S. pneumoniae* have an MIC of <0.1 µg/mL to penicillin. Isolates with MIC of 0.1–1 µg/mL are "intermediately susceptible," and those with MIC >1 µg/mL are "resistant."

♦ The prevalence of penicillin-susceptible isolates of pneumococci in the U.S. is 70%–85%. Intermediately susceptible isolates account for 10%–20% of organisms and 5%–10% are resistant.

♦ Penicillin-susceptible isolates of pneumococci can be treated with penicillin, cephalosporins, TMP-SMX, macrolides, and doxycycline. Intermediate strains are variably inhibited by these agents: high-dose penicillin or ampicillin probably is effective. Highly resistant isolates should be treated with IV vancomycin.

♦ Approximately 30%–40% of all isolates of *Haemophilus influenzae* and up to 100% of *Moraxella catarrhalis* are beta-lactamase producers, and these organisms respond best to 2nd- and 3rd-generation cephalosporins and beta-lactamase inhibitor combinations.

♦ Acute bronchitis should not be treated with antibacterials.

Croup Syndromes

♦ Features that distinguish viral croup from bacterial epiglottitis, bacterial tracheitis, and spasmodic croup are described in Table 57.3.

♦ Viral croup is caused by a parainfluenza virus and is not treatable with antimicrobial therapy.

♦ Epiglottitis is caused by bacteria *(H. influenzae, S. pyogenes, S. pneumoniae)* and should be treated with parenteral antibiotics. Epiglottitis can be a medical emergency requiring endotracheal intubation. Aggressive empiric treatment with intravenous agents active against beta-lactamase-producing *H. influenzae* (e.g., 2nd- or 3rd-generation cephalosporins) is warranted.

Community-Acquired Bacterial Pneumonias

♦ In the U.S., pneumonia is the sixth leading cause of death and the number one cause of death from infectious diseases. In the outpatient setting, the mortality rate from pneumonia is 1%–5% but approaches 25% in patients requiring hospitalization, especially if admitted to an ICU.

- Pneumonia is common among the elderly and those with coexisting illness (e.g., chronic obstructive lung disease, diabetes mellitus, renal insufficiency, CHF, chronic liver disease).
- Initial antimicrobial therapy usually is approached empirically because of limitations in diagnostic testing.
- Antimicrobial therapy for community-acquired pneumonias when the organism is known is described in Table 57.1.

Nosocomial Bacterial Pneumonia

- Associated with an increased colonization with aerobic gram negative pathogens, including *Pseudomonas aeruginosa, Enterobacter,* and others.
- Drugs that inhibit production of gastric acid increase colonization of the oropharynx.
- Nursing home residents should be considered at risk for nosocomial organisms.

Aspiration Pneumonia

- Depressed mental status, decreased gag reflex predispose
- Aspiration of oropharyngeal secretions predisposes to bacterial pneumonia
- In addition to usual pathogens associated with nosocomial or community pneumonia, mouth anaerobes are important pathogens.

Notes:

Table 57.1 • Comparison of Guidelines for Treatment of Community-Acquired Pneumonia in Hospitalized (Non-ICU) Patients

Infectious Diseases Society of America (2000)	Centers for Disease Control Working Group (1999)	American Thoracic Society (2001)
1. Extended Spectrum Cephalosporin *(Cefotaxime or Ceftriaxone)* **plus** **Macrolide** *(Azithromycin, Clarithromycin, Erythromycin)* **OR** **2. β-lactam/β-Lactamase Inhibitor** *(Ampicillin/Sulbactam, Piperacillin-Tozobactam)* **plus** **Macrolide** *(Azithromycin, Clarithromycin, Erythromycin)* **OR** **3. Fluoroquinolone Alone** *(Levofloxacin, Gatifloxacin, Moxifloxacin, Trovafloxacin)*	**1. IV β-Lactam** *(Cefuroxime, Cefotaxime, Ceftriaxone, or Ampicillin plus Sulbactam)* **plus** **Macrolide** *(Azithromycin, Clarithromycin, Erythromycin)* **OR** **2. Fluoroquinolone** *(e.g., Grepafloxacin, Levofloxacin, Sparfloxacin, or Trovafloxacin)* Criteria for use of fluoroquinolone: 1. Patients where above regime fails 2. Allergic to alternative agents 3. Documented infection with highly drug-resistant pneumococci	Depending upon underlying modifying risk factors: **1. IV β-Lactam** *(Cefotaxime, Ceftriaxone, Ampicillin/Sulbactam, high-dose Ampicillin)* **plus** **IV or oral Macrolide** *(Azithromycin, Clarithromycin)* or Doxycycline **OR** **2. IV New Fluoroquinolone Alone** If no modifying risk factors 1. IV Azithromycin alone (If macrolide allergy doxycycline plus β-Lactam)

Table 57.2 • Microbiology of Community-Acquired Pneumonia

Microbial Agent	Percentage
Bacteria	
S. pneumoniae	20–60
H. influenzae	3–10
S. aureus	3–5
Gram-negative bacilli	3–10
Atypical Agents	
Legionella species	2–8
M. pneumoniae	1–6
C. pneumoniae	4–6
Viral	2–15
No diagnosis	30–60

Notes:

Table 57.3 • Characteristics of the Different Classifications of Croup Syndrome^a

	Spasmodic Croup	Viral Croup	Bacterial Tracheitis	Supraglottitis
Synonyms	Subglottic allergic edema	Laryngotracheitis, laryngitis, LTB	Pseudomembranous croup, LTB	Epiglottitis
Frequency	Common	Most common	Less common	Rare
Age group	3 months–3 yr	3 months–3 yr	3 months–3 yr	2–8 yr
Common pathogens	None (parainfluenza), (influenza)	Parainfluenza, adenovirus, influenza	S. aureus, S. pyogenes, S. pneumoniae	H. influenzae, S. pyogenes, S. pneumoniae
Clinical Presentation				
Onset	Rapid, nocturnal	Gradual, preceding URI	Gradual, preceding URI	Rapid
Signs and symptoms	Afebrile, cough, stridor	Fever, cough, stridor	Fever, cough, stridor, "toxic" appearance	Fever, dysphagia, drooling, stridor, "toxic" appearance
Neck radiography	Normal	Subglottic narrowing (steeple sign)	Subglottic narrowing (steeple sign)	Swollen epiglottis (thumb sign)
Laboratory	Normal	↑ WBC count, no shift	↑ WBC count, left shift, ↑ CRP	↑ WBC count, left shift, ↑ CRP

^aCRP = C-reactive protein; LTB = Laryngotracheobronchitis; URI = Upper respiratory tract infection; WBC = White blood cell.

Table 57.4 • Microbiology of Nosocomial Pneumonia

Pathogen	Percentage of Cases (%)
Gram-Negative Bacilli	50–70
Pseudomonas aeruginosa	
Acinetobacter species	
Enterobacter species	
Staphylococcus aureus	15–30
Anaerobic bacteria	10–30
Haemophilus influenzae	10–20
Streptococcus pneumoniae	10–20
Legionella	4
Viral	10–20
Cytomegalovirus	
Influenza	
Respiratory syncytial virus	
Fungi	
Aspergillus	<1

Table 57.5 • Bacteriology of Aspiration Pneumonia

Community-Acquired Pneumonia

Streptococcus pneumoniae	*Fusobacterium* sp.
Peptococcus sp.	*Bacteroides melaninogenicus*
Peptostreptococcus sp.	*Bacteroides* sp.
Microaerophilic streptococci	*Streptococcus* sp.

Special Patients (Alcoholics, Diabetics [± Nursing Home Residents])

Staphylococcus aureus	*Escherichia coli*
Klebsiella pneumoniae	Anaerobes included above

Hospital-Acquired Pneumonia

Pseudomonas aeruginosa	*Escherichia coli*
S. aureus	*Enterobacter cloacae*
S. pneumoniae	*Serratia marcescens*
Anaerobes included above	Other Gram-negative bacilli

The reader is referred to Chapter 58: Respiratory Tract Infections, written by *Steven P. Gelone, Pharm.D. and George S. Jaresko, Pharm.D.,* and Chapter 94: Pediatric Infectious Diseases, written by *Nicholas Blanchard, Pharm.D.,* in the seventh edition of **Applied Therapeutics: The Clinical Use of Drugs** for a more in-depth discussion. The editors of this handbook express their thanks to Drs. Gelone, Jaresko, Blanchard, and Paap and acknowledge that this chapter is based upon their work.

Notes:

Chapter 58

Tuberculosis

♦ Tuberculosis is the leading global infectious killer with 2.9 million deaths annually.

♦ *M. tuberculosis* is an "acid-fast" bacillus (AFB) because of its resistance to decolorization by acid alcohol after staining with basic fuchsin. The organism thrives in environments with high oxygen tension (e.g., apices of the lung).

♦ **Transmission** of the bacillus is via aerosolized droplets from individuals infected with pulmonary tuberculosis. Thus, family contacts and those in close contact are at risk of infection.

♦ **Risk factors** for developing significant clinical disease after infection include immunosuppression (e.g., AIDS, malignancy, corticosteroid use), poor nutrition, diabetes, crowded living conditions, and various chronic diseases.

Preventive Therapy (Table 58.3)

♦ Patients with a recent conversion of PPD should be given isoniazid (INH) 300 mg/day (10 mg/kg/day in children) for 6–12 months (9 months for children) to prevent the development of clinical disease (see Figure 58.1 for preventive therapy guidelines). Patients who are immune suppressed (HIV, cancer) or with x-ray evidence of healed tuberculosis should receive therapy for 12 months.

♦ Considering the high incidence of hepatitis, isoniazid is not recommended for patients >35 yr of age who have a low risk of developing clinical disease.

Treatment of Active Tuberculosis

♦ The treatment of active TB requires multiple-drug therapy to prevent the development of resistance and to sterilize sputum and injected lesions quickly. Some experts recommend that all patients take drugs under direct observation.

♦ All isolates must be tested for antimicrobial susceptibility.

♦ Isoniazid, rifampin, pyrazinamide, and ethambutol are the primary drugs to treat tuberculosis. Regimen options for initial treatment of TB are listed in Table 58.1.

♦ Secondary antitubercular drugs (capreomycin, streptomycin, kanamycin, cycloserine, ethionamide, aminosalicylic acid) are reserved for treatment failures, drug-resistant organisms, extrapulmonary TB, or drug toxicity.

♦ **Possibly Resistant Organisms.** In those patients with risk factors for INH-resistant *M. tuberculosis,* an initial 4-drug combination of isoniazid, rifampin, pyrazinamide, and either ethambutol or streptomycin is recommended. Once full susceptibility is documented, the patient can be treated as described in Table 58.1. The dosing regimens for these drugs are listed in Table 58.2.

♦ **Documented Drug-Resistant Organisms.** Drug-resistant tuberculosis should be treated with ≥3 agents to which the organism is susceptible (see Table 58.4). Multidrug-resistant TB (isoniazid *and* rifampin resistant) should be treated for 12–24 months after cultures return negative.

♦ Rifamycins, particularly rifampin decrease serum levels of protease inhibitors. Protease inhibitors and delavirdine significantly inhibit the metabolism of rifabutin.

Table 58.1 • Regimen Options for the Initial Treatment of TB Among Children and Adults[a]

Without HIV Infection			TB With HIV Infection
Option 1	Option 2	Option 3	
Administer daily INH, RIF, and PZA for 8 wk followed by 16 wk of INH and RIF daily or 2–3 times/wk[b] in areas where the INH resistance rate is not documented to be <4%. EMB or SM should be added to the initial regimen until susceptibility to INH and RIF is demonstrated. Continue treatment for at least 6 months and 3 months beyond culture conversion. Consult a TB medical expert if the patient is symptomatic or smear or culture positive after 3 months	Administer daily INH, RIF, PZA, and SM or EMB for 2 wk followed by 2 times/wk[b] administration of the same drugs for 6 wk (by DOT), and subsequently, with 2 times/wk administration of INH and RIF for 16 wk (by DOT). Consult a TB medical expert if patient is symptomatic or smear or culture positive after 3 months	Treat by DOT, 3 times/wk[b] with INH, RIF, PZA, and EMB or SM for 6 months.[c] Consult a TB medical expert if patient is symptomatic or smear or culture positive after 3 months	Options 1, 2, or 3 can be used, but treatment regimens should continue for a total of 9 months and at least 6 months beyond culture conversion

[a]DOT = Directly observed therapy; EMB = Ethambutol; HIV = Human immunodeficiency virus; INH = Isoniazid; PZA = Pyrazinamide; RIF = Rifampin; SM = Streptomycin.
[b]All regimens administered 2 or 3 times/wk should be monitored by directly observed therapy for the duration of therapy.
[c]The strongest evidence from clinical trials is the effectiveness of all four drugs administered for the full 6 months. There is weaker evidence that SM can be discontinued after 4 months if the isolate is susceptible to all drugs. The evidence for stopping PZA before the end of 6 months is equivocal for the 3 times/wk regimen, and there is no evidence on the effectiveness of this regimen with EMB for less than the full 6 months.
From reference 26.

Notes:

Table 58.2 • Drugs Used in the Treatment of Tuberculosis[a]

Drug/Daily Dose	Twice Weekly Dose	Peak Serum Concentrations[41] (μg/mL)	Primary Side Effects	Dosage Adjustment in Renal Impairment	Comments
First-Line Drugs					
Isoniazid *Adult:* 5 mg/kg (*max:* 300 mg) *Child:* 10–20 mg/kg (*max:* 300 mg)	*Adult:* 15 mg/kg (*max:* 900 mg) *Child:* 20–40 mg/kg (*max:* 900 kg)	3–6	Peripheral neuropathy, hepatitis, skin rashes, fever, arthralgia, hypersensitivity reactions	No	Peripheral neuropathy preventable by pyridoxine 10–15 mg. ↑ serum levels of phenytoin. Hepatitis more common in older patients and alcoholics
Rifampin *Adult:* 600 mg *Child:* 10–20 mg/kg (*max:* 600 mg)	*Adult:* 600 mg *Child:* 10–20 mg/kg (*max:* 600 mg)	8–20	Hepatitis, thrombocytopenia, renal failure, "flu-like" syndrome, cutaneous reactions	No	Red discoloration of body secretions (perspiration, saliva, urine). Induces hepatic metabolism of warfarin, corticosteroids, diazepam, quinidine, oral contraceptives, methadone, ketoconazole, propranolol, sulfonylureas
Pyrazinamide *Adult:* 15–30 mg/kg (*max:* 2 g) *Child:* 15–30 mg/kg (*max:* 2 g)	50–70 mg/kg (*max:* 4 g)	20–60	Hepatitis, fever, skin rashes, arthralgia, GI disturbance, fever, hyperuricemia	Yes	AST monthly
Ethambutol *Adult:* 15–25 mg/kg (*max:* 2.5 g)	50 mg/kg	2–6	Optic neuritis, skin rashes, drug fever, hyperuricemia	Yes	Routine vision tests recommended; 50% excreted unchanged in urine
Second-Line Drugs					
Streptomycin *Adult:* 15 mg/kg IM (*max:* 1 g) ≥60 *years:* 0.5 g IM	25–30 mg/kg IM	35–45	Vestibular and/or auditory dysfunction or eighth nerve, renal dysfunction, skin rashes, neuromuscular blockade	Yes	Audiometric and neurologic examinations recommended; 60–80% excreted unchanged in urine. Monitor renal function

(continued)

Table 58.2 • Drugs Used in the Treatment of Tuberculosis[a] *(continued)*

Drug/Daily Dose	Twice Weekly Dose	Peak Serum Concentrations[41] (μg/mL)	Primary Side Effects	Dosage Adjustment in Renal Impairment	Comments
Second-Line Drugs *(continued)*					
Capreomycin *Adult:* 15–30 mg/kg IM (*max:* 1 g IM)		35–45	See streptomycin	Yes	See streptomycin
Kanamycin *Adult:* 15–30 mg/kg IM (*max:* 1 g)		35–45	Auditory dysfunction (see streptomycin)	Yes	See streptomycin
Cycloserine *Adult:* 15–20 mg/kg (*max:* 1 g)		20–35	CNS toxicity (psychosis and seizures), headache, tremor, fever, skin rashes	Yes	Contraindicated in epileptic patients. Some toxicity preventable by pyridoxine; 65% excreted unchanged in urine. Monitor serum concentrations
Ethionamide *Adult:* 15–20 mg/kg (*max:* 1 g)		1–5	GI irritation (50%), hepatitis (especially diabetics), gynecomastia, impotence, postural hypotension, difficulty in diabetic management	No	Must be given with meals and antacids. AST monthly
Para-aminosalicylic acid *Adult:* 4 g BID–TID *Child:* 75 mg/kg BID		40–70	GI upset (10%), anemia in G6PD-deficient patients, skin rashes, fever, hepatitis, hypothyroidism	Yes	Must be taken with acidic foods or beverage
Ciprofloxacin *Adult:* 750 mg BID		3–5	Nausea		
Ofloxacin *Adult:* 400–800 mg QD–BID		6–12	Nausea, mild CNS (insomnia)		
		6–12	Nausea, mild CNS (insomnia)		
Levofloxacin *Adult:* 500 mg–750 mg QD		6–12	Nausea, mild CNS		

[a]AST = Aspartate aminotransferase; CNS = Central nervous system; G6PD = Glucose-6 phosphate dehydrogenase; GI = Gastrointestinal; IM = Intramuscular.

Table 58.3 • High-Priority Candidates for Tuberculosis Preventive Therapy[a]

Preventive therapy should be recommended for the following persons with a positive tuberculin test, regardless of age:

1. Persons with known or suspected HIV infection[b]
2. Close contacts of persons with infectious TB[b]
3. Recent tuberculin skin test converters ($\geq$10 mm increase within a 2-yr period for those <35 yr of age; $\geq$15 mm increase for those $\geq$35 yr of age)
4. Persons with medical conditions that have been reported to increase the risk of TB (e.g., diabetes, prolonged corticosteroid therapy, immunosuppressive therapy, some IV hematologic and reticuloendothelial disease, IV drug use, end-stage renal disease, and clinical situations associated with rapid weight loss)

Preventive therapy should be recommended for the following persons in high-incidence groups with a positive tuberculin test who are <35 yr of age and do not have additional risk factors:

1. Foreign-born persons from high-prevalence countries (e.g., Latin America, Asia, and Africa)
2. Medically underserved low-income populations, including high-risk racial or ethnic minority populations, especially blacks, Hispanics, and American Indians/Alaska natives
3. Residents of facilities for long-term care (e.g., correctional institutions, nursing homes, and mental institutions)

Infected persons <35 yr of age with no additional risk factors for TB with a positive test (>15 mm) may also be considered for preventive therapy based on individual assessment of risk and benefits.

[a]HIV = Human immunodeficiency virus; IV = Intravenous; TB = Tuberculosis.
[b]Persons in these categories may be given preventive therapy in the absence of a positive tuberculin test in some circumstances.
Reprinted with permission from Snider DE. Recognition and elimination of tuberculosis. Adv Intern Med 1993; 38: 169.

Table 58.4 • Potential Regimens for Patients with Tuberculosis with Various Patterns of Drug Resistance

Resistance	Suggested Regimen	Duration of Therapy	Comments
Isoniazid, streptomycin, and pyrazinamide	Rifampin; pyrazinamide; ethambutol; amikacin[a]	6–9 months	Anticipate 100% response and <5% relapse rate[37]
Isoniazid and ethambutol ($\pm$ streptomycin)	Rifampin; pyrazinamide; ofloxacin or ciprofloxacin; amikacin[a]	6–12 months	Efficacy should be comparable to above regimen
Isoniazid and rifampin ($\pm$ streptomycin)	Pyrazinamide; ethambutol; ofloxacin or ciprofloxacin; amikacin[a]	18–24 months	Consider surgery
Isoniazid, rifampin, and ethambutol ($\pm$ streptomycin)	Pyrazinamide; ofloxacin or ciprofloxacin; amikacin;[a] plus 2[b]	20 months after conversion	Consider surgery
Isoniazid, rifampin, and pyrazinamide ($\pm$ streptomycin)	Ethambutol; ofloxacin or ciprofloxacin; amikacin[a]; plus 2[b]	24 months after conversion	Consider surgery
Isoniazid, rifampin, pyrazinamide, and ethambutol ($\pm$ streptomycin)	Ofloxacin or ciprofloxacin; amikacin[a]; plus 3[b]	24 months after conversion	Surgery, if possible

[a]If TB is resistant to amikacin, kanamycin, and streptomycin, capreomycin is a good alternative. Injectable agents usually are continued for 4–6 months if toxicity does not intervene. All of the injectable drugs are given daily (or twice or thrice weekly) and may be administered intravenously or intramuscularly.
[b]Potential agents from which to choose: ethionamide, cycloserine, or aminosalicylic acid. Others that are potentially useful but of unproved utility include clofazimine and amoxicillin-clavulanate. Clarithromycin, azithromycin, and rifabutin are unlikely to be active.
Reprinted with permission from Iseman MD. Drug Therapy: treatment of multidrug-resistant tuberculosis. N Engl J Med 1993;329:784–791. Copyright © 1993 Massachusetts Medical Society. All rights reserved.

Table 58.5 • Effects of Co-Administration of Rifamycins (Rifabutin, Rifampin) and HIV-1 Protease Inhibitors on the Systemic Exposure of Each Drug, Expressed as a Percentage Change in AUC of the Concomitant Treatment Relative to That of Treatment with the Drug Alone[a]

Protease Inhibitor (PI)	Rifabutin		Rifampin	
	Effect of Rifabutin on PI	Effect of PI on Rifabutin	Effect of Rifampin on PI	Effect of PI on Rifampin
Saquinavir[75]	45% decrease	NR	80% decrease	NR
Ritonavir[17,77]	NR	293% increase	35% decrease	Unchanged[a]
Indinavir[74]	34% decrease	173% increase	92% decrease	NR
Nelfinavir[19]	32% decrease	207% increase	82% decrease	NR
Amprenavir[76,78]	14% decrease	200% increase	81% decrease	NR

[a]AUC = Area under the serum concentration-time curve; NR = Not reported.
[b]Data from only two subjects.
These are average changes, but the effect of these interactions in individual patients may be substantially different. Rifampin is a potent inducer of CYP3A but is not itself a CYP3A substrate. For example, concomitant delavirdine, a potent CYP3A inhibitor, does not change serum concentrations of rifampin.[79] Therefore, although few data are currently available, it is likely that protease inhibitors will not substantially increase the serum concentrations of rifampin (the same is true of rifapentine).
No data exist regarding the magnitude of these bidirectional interactions when the rifamycin is administered twice or thrice weekly.
Reprinted with permission from Burman et al. Therapeutic Implications of Drug Interactions in the Treatment of Human Immunodeficiency Virus-Related Tuberculosis. Clin Infect Dis 1999;28:419–430. Copyright 1999 by the Infectious Diseases Society of America. All rights reserved.

Table 58.6 • Effects of Co-Administration of Rifamycins (Rifabutin, Rifampin) and Currently Approved Nonnucleoside Reverse Transcriptase Inhibitors on the Area Under the Serum Concentration-Time Curve of Each Drug[a]

NNRTI	Rifabutin		Rifampin	
	Effect of Rifabutin on NNRTI	Effect of NNRTI on Rifabutin (Predicted)[b]	Effect of Rifampin on NNRTI	Effect of NNRTI on Rifampin (Predicted)[b]
Nevirapine[98]	16% decrease	NR (decrease)	37% decrease	NR (unchanged)
Delavirdine[79,99,100]	80% decrease	342% increase	96% decrease	Unchanged
Efavirenz[101,102]	Unchanged	38% decrease	13% decrease	Unchanged

[a]AUC = Area under the serum concentration-time curve; NNRTI = Nonnucleoside reverse transcriptase inhibitor; NR = Not reported.
[b]Predicted using existing knowledge regarding metabolic pathways for the two drugs.[20]
Reprinted with permission from Burman et al. Therapeutic Implications of Drug Interactions in the Treatment of Human Immunodeficiency Virus-Related Tuberculosis. Clin Infect Dis 1999;28:419–430. Copyright 1999 by the Infectious Diseases Society of America. All rights reserved.

Notes:

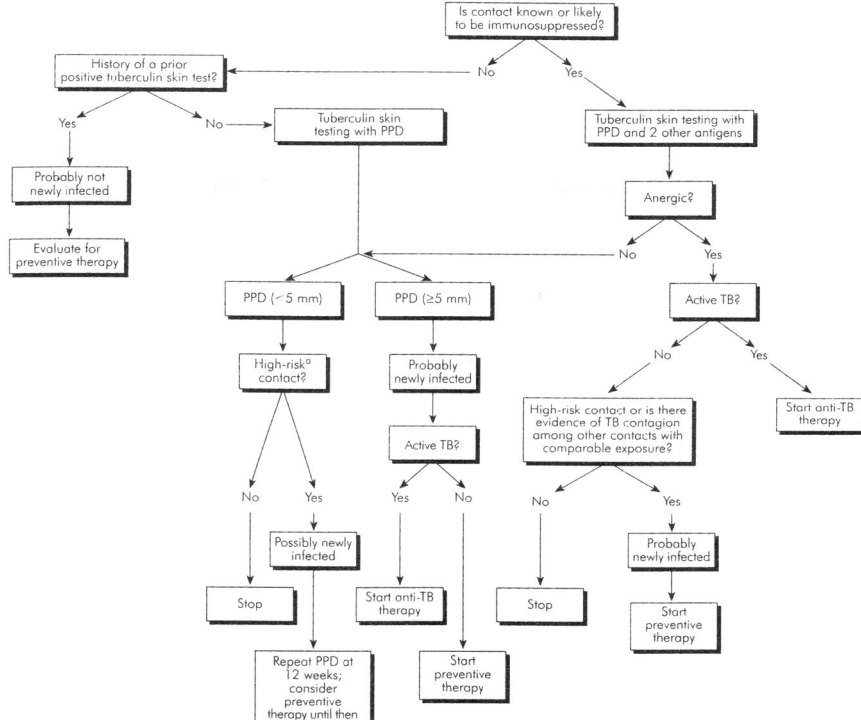

Fig. 58.1 Estimating the Likelihood of New Infection with *Mycobacterium tuberculosis* and Preventive Therapy Decision Making for Contacts of Infectious Tuberculosis Cases. PPD = Purified Protein Derivative. ᵃMembers of the immediate family, close social contacts, or others who shared the same indoor environment with an infectious TB patient for substantial periods.

The reader is referred to Chapter 59: Tuberculosis, written by *Shawn E. Berning, Pharm.D.,* in the seventh edition of **Applied Therapeutics: The Clinical Use of Drugs** for a more in-depth discussion. All notations to reference numbers are based on the reference list at the end of that chapter. The editors of this handbook express their thanks to Dr. Berning and acknowledge that this chapter is based upon his work.

Notes:

Notes:

Chapter 59

Infectious Diarrhea

♦ Diarrheal diseases are a leading cause of death, particularly in underdeveloped countries, and can be caused by bacterial, viral, or protozoal pathogens. Table 59.1 lists these common pathogens, symptoms, diagnostic evaluations, and therapy.

♦ Infection caused by toxin-producing bacteria (e.g., *Escherichia coli, Clostridium difficile*) can result in irritation, inflammation, and sloughing of bowel mucosa.

♦ Treatment of GI infections often requires antibacterial therapy; prevention and reversal of fluid and electrolyte losses are most critical. Antidiarrheal agents should be used only in mild cases and for no more than 3 days.

Traveler's Diarrhea

♦ Commonly is *defined by* the passage of >3 loose unformed stools/day plus at least one symptom of enteric infection (i.e., abdominal pain or cramps, nausea, vomiting, fever, dysentery, fecal urgency, tenesmus of >72 hr in duration).

♦ The *pathogenesis* of traveler's diarrhea is based upon the transmission of fecally contaminated sources that contain enterotoxins that are not inactivated by cooking or processing.

♦ The prophylaxis and therapy of traveler's diarrhea in adults are described in Table 59.2.

Pseudomembranous Colitis

♦ **Etiology.** Antibiotic-associated pseudomembranous colitis (AAPC) is a potentially serious infection caused by the enterotoxin-producing *C. difficile*. It is likely due to alteration of normal bowel flora as a result of antimicrobial use with subsequent overgrowth of *C. difficile*.

The most commonly implicated antibacterials in AAPC are ampicillin and clindamycin, but most agents have been implicated. Beta-lactams, as a class, most commonly predispose patients to AAPC.

♦ **Symptoms** include fever, elevated WBC count, abdominal cramping, and frequent loose stools.

If left untreated, sloughing of bowel mucosa can take place, resulting in secondary infection and dehydration.

♦ **Treatment.** Treat with oral metronidazole or vancomycin administered for 10 days.

Since the two agents appear to be equally effective, the less expensive metronidazole is recommended as the treatment of choice (see Table 59.3). Both, oral vancomycin and metronidazole may be associated with development of vancomycin-resistant enterococci.

If patients are unable to tolerate oral medications, parenteral agents or enemas can be considered; however, their efficacy is unknown.

Table 59.1 • Predisposing Factors, Symptoms, and Therapy of Gastrointestinal Infections[a]

Pathogen	Predisposing Factors	Symptoms	Diagnostic Evaluations	Drug of Choice[a]	Alternative[b]
Salmonella (nontyphoid)	Ingestion of contaminated poultry, raw milk, custards, and cream fillings; foreign travel	Nausea, vomiting, diarrhea, cramps, fever, tenesmus *Incubation*: 6–48 hr	Fecal leukocytes, stool culture	Fluoroquinolone, third-generation cephalosporins[c]	Ampicillin, amoxicillin, TMP-SMX, chloramphenicol, azithromycin
Salmonella (typhoid fever)				Fluoroquinolone, third-generation cephalosporins[c]	Chloramphenicol, TMP-SMX, ampicillin, amoxicillin[c]
Shigella	Ingestion of contaminated food, foreign travel Minimum infective dose: 10–100 organisms	Fever, dysentery, cramps, tenesmus *Incubation*: 12–24 hr	Fecal leukocytes	Fluoroquinolone[c]	Azithromycin, TMP-SMX, ampicillin, ceftriaxone[c]
Campylobacter	Day-care centers, contaminated eggs, raw milk, foreign travel	Mild-to-severe diarrhea; fever, systemic malaise *Incubation*: 24–72 hr	Fecal leukocytes, stool culture	Erythromycin, azithromycin, fluoroquinolone[c]	Tetracycline, aminoglycosides, third-generation cephalosporins, chloramphenicol
Clostridium difficile	Antibiotics, antineoplastics	Mild-to-severe diarrhea, cramps	*C. difficile* toxin, *C. difficile*, culture, colonoscopy	Metronidazole[c]	Vancomycin, exchange resins[c]

Disease	Epidemiology	Symptoms	Diagnosis	Treatment[b][c]	
Staphylococcal food poisoning	Contaminated meat, milk, exposed foods	Nausea, diarrhea; onset <4 hr, resolves in 24–48 hr; *Incubation:* 2–4 hr	Stool cultures	Supportive therapy only	
Travelers' diarrhea (*E. coli*)	Contaminated food (vegetables and cheese), water, foreign travel	Nausea, vomiting, mild-to-severe diarrhea, cramps; *Incubation:* 16–48 hr	Stool culture	See Table 59.2	
Enterohemorrhagic *Escherichia coli* (*E. coli* O157:H7)	Beef, raw milk, water	Diarrhea, headache, bloody stools; *Incubation:* 48–96 hr	Stool cultures on MacConkey's sorbitol	Supportive therapy only	
Cryptosporidiosis	Immunosuppression, day-care centers, contaminated water, animal handlers	Mild-to-severe diarrhea (chronic or self-limited); large fluid	Stool screening for oocytes, PCR, ELISA	Paromomycin	Spiramycin, HAART
Viral gastroenteritis	Community-wide outbreaks, contaminated food	Nausea, diarrhea (self-limited), cramps; *Incubation:* 16–48 hr	Special viral studies	Supportive therapy only	

[a]ELISA = Enzyme-linked immunosorbent assay; PCR = Polymerase chain reaction; TMP-SMX = Trimethoprim-sulfamethoxazole.
[b]See text for doses and duration of therapy.
[c]Not all cases require antibiotic therapy. See text for details.
From reference 14.

Table 59.2 • Prophylaxis and Therapy of Travelers' Diarrhea in Adults[a,b]

Drug	Prophylaxis[c]	Treatment
Bismuth subsalicylate	2 tablets chewed with meals and HS (8 tablets/day)	1 oz Q 30 min for a total dose of 8 oz/day
Loperamide	—	4-mg load, followed by 2 mg after each loose stool (max, 16 mg/day)
TMP-SMX	160–800 mg/day	320–1600 mg once, or 160–800 mg BID for 3 days
Doxycycline	100 mg/day	—
Trimethoprim	200 mg/day	—
Norfloxacin	400 mg/day	400 mg BID for 3 days
Ciprofloxacin	500 mg/day	500 mg BID for 3 days
Ofloxacin	300 mg/day	300 mg BID for 3 days
Levofloxacin	500 mg/day	500 mg QD for 3 days

[a] TMP-SMX = Trimethoprim-sulfamethoxazole.
[b] Many cases of travelers' diarrhea require neither prophylaxis nor therapy.
[c] While in endemic area, and continuing for 1 to 2 days after returning home, but not to exceed 3 weeks.
Adapted from references 7 and 140.

Table 59.3 • Costs of Drug Therapy for Antibiotic-Associated Pseudomembranous Colitis

Drug	Regimen	Cost[a]
Bacitracin solution	25,000 units QID × 10 days	$112/10 days
Metronidazole tablets (generic)	500 mg TID × 10 days	$9.95/10 days
Vancomycin capsules (Vancocin)	125 mg QID × 10 days	$215.12/10 days
Vancomycin solution[b] (generic)	125 mg QID × 10 days	$54.69/10 days

[a] AWP Red Book 1999.
[b] Prepared from intravenous formulation.

The reader is referred to Chapter 60: Infectious Diarrhea, written by *Larry H. Danziger, Pharm.D., Gail S. Itokazu, Pharm.D.,* and *David T. Bearden, Pharm.D.,* in the seventh edition of **Applied Therapeutics: The Clinical Use of Drugs** for a more in-depth discussion. All notations to reference numbers are based on the reference list at the end of that chapter. The editors of this handbook express their thanks to Drs. Danziger, Itokazu, and Bearden and acknowledge that this chapter is based upon their work.

Notes:

Chapter 60

Intra-Abdominal Infections

Intra-abdominal infections are contained within the peritoneum and present as localized infections (e.g., abscesses), diffuse inflammation throughout the peritoneum, or infections in visceral organs (e.g., liver, biliary tree, spleen). These infections usually occur as a result of external trauma, an inflammatory process, or spontaneously. The common pathogens in intra-abdominal infections are listed in Table 60.1.

Pathogenesis

♦ *Biliary tract infections* (cholangitis, cholecystitis). *Cholangitis* usually is an infectious inflammation of the biliary ductal system. *Cholecystitis* is an inflammation of the gallbladder. More severe disease requires surgical drainage of the biliary tree and antibiotic therapy. Antimicrobial concentrations in the biliary secretions vary with the antimicrobial; however, the importance of this pharmacokinetic property is not clear. Table 60.2 lists antimicrobial concentration in bile relative to serum.

♦ *Peritonitis* is an inflammation of the peritoneal lining in response to chemical irritation or bacterial invasion. *Primary* or "spontaneous" peritonitis develops independent of an apparent intra-abdominal event such as trauma (e.g., appendicitis) and occurs most commonly in patients with cirrhosis or postnecrotic liver disease, children with nephrotic syndrome, and some immunocompromised patients. *Secondary peritonitis* accounts for the majority of cases and often is secondary to contamination of the peritoneum by GI bacteria that have been released by inflammation, perforation, or trauma.

Treatment

♦ While antimicrobial therapy is critical in the treatment of intra-abdominal infections, surgical intervention often is the definitive therapy, particularly with abscess formation.

♦ Most antimicrobials do not penetrate readily into abscesses: thus, they often are ineffective without surgical drainage.

♦ The abscess normally is an anaerobic and acidic environment, which inactivates many antimicrobial agents.

♦ In most cases, therapy directed toward *B. fragilis* and *E. coli* (see Table 60.3) is sufficient to treat intra-abdominal infections, particularly secondary peritonitis and cholangitis.

♦ In selected patients who are seriously ill, additional antimicrobial therapy active against enterococcus should be considered.

♦ Monotherapy of secondary peritonitis is as effective (e.g., cephalosporins, beta-lactamase inhibitors) as multidrug therapy

Intraperitoneal Antibiotics

Peritonitis in patients undergoing chronic ambulatory peritoneal dialysis or intermittent peritoneal dialysis can be treated with intraperitoneal administration of antibiotics. Table 60.4 lists common loading and maintenance intraperitoneal antibiotic doses in the treatment of peritonitis.

Table 60.1 • Common Pathogens in Intra-Abdominal Infection

Disease	Pathogens	Comments
Primary peritonitis	E. coli, S. pneumoniae, Group A streptococci, occasional anaerobes	Predominately in spontaneous bacterial peritonitis in cirrhotics. Anaerobes less likely than aerobes
Secondary peritonitis	E. coli, B. fragilis, other aerobic gram-negative rods and anaerobes, enterococci	Generally polymicrobial with both aerobic and anaerobic pathogens. Enterococci are associated with chronic surgical infection, particularly in patients receiving broad-spectrum antimicrobials such as cephalosporins
Chronic ambulatory peritoneal dialysis	S. epidermidis, S. aureus, diphtheroids, gram-negative rods	
Cholecystitis, cholangitis	E. coli, anaerobes, other gram-negative rods	Necessity for antimicrobials that achieve high biliary concentrations is unknown

Table 60.2 • Concentration in Bile Relative to Serum[11]

Bile Less Than Serum	Bile Equal to Serum	Bile Greater Than Serum
Penicillin G	Ampicillin	Nafcillin
Phenoxypenicillins	Mezlocillin	Cefamandole
Amoxicillin	Cefazolin	Cefoxitin
Cefuroxime	Cefotaxime	Cephradine
Ceftazidime	Gentamicin	Cefoperazone
Ceftizoxime	Amikacin	Cefotetan
Vancomycin	Sulfamethoxazole	Ciprofloxacin
		Erythromycin
		Clindamycin
		Doxycycline
		Metronidazole
		Rifampin

Adapted from References 5 and 20.

Notes:

Table 60.3 • Treatment of Intra-Abdominal Infection

Regimen	Dosage
Combination Therapy[a]	
Metronidazole (or clindamycin)	500 (600) mg IV Q 8 hr
plus	
Aminoglycoside	5 mg/kg/day IV Q 24 hr
or	(normal renal function)
Metronidazole (or clindamycin)	500 (600) mg IV Q 8 hr
plus	
Aztreonam	1 gm Q 8 hr
or	
Metronidazole (or clindamycin)	500 (600) mg IV Q 8 hr
plus	
2nd- or 3rd-generation cephalosporin	(see below)
Monotherapy	
Cefotaxime (Claforan)[a,b,c]	1 gm Q 6 hr
Cefotetan (Cefotan)[a,b]	2 gm Q 12 hr
Cefoxitin (Mefoxin)[a,b]	2 gm Q 6 hr
Ceftizoxime (Cefizox)[a,b]	1 gm Q 8 hr
Ceftriaxone (Rocephin)[a,b,c]	1 gm Q 24 hr
Mezlocillin (Mezlin)[d]	4 gm Q 6 hr
Piperacillin (Pipracil)[d]	4 gm Q 6 hr
Imipenem-cilastatin (Primaxin)[a,e]	0.5 gm Q 6 hr
Meropenem (Merem)	1 gm Q 8 hr
Ticarcillin-clavulanic acid (Timentin)[a,f]	3.1 gm Q 6-8 hr
Ampicillin-sulbactam (Unasyn)[f]	3 gm Q 6 hr
Piperacillin-tazobactam (Zosyn)[f]	3.375 gm Q 8 hr

[a]Ampicillin or vancomycin may need to be added if enterococci are suspected. Use vancomycin in penicillin-allergic patients. This combination covers B. fragilis, E. coli, and enterococci.
[b]Cephalosporins have excellent activity against E. coli, moderate-to-good coverage of B. fragilis, and no activity against enterococci.
[c]Cefotaxime and ceftriaxone have limited anaerobic activity; thus, the addition of agents such as metronidazole may be necessary.
[d]The ureidopenicillins have moderate aerobic and anaerobic activity and excellent enterococcal activity. However, these agents should be reserved for suspected or documented pseudomonal infection.
[e]Imipenem has excellent activity versus B. fragilis; however, its activity against multidrug-resistant gram-negative bacilli such as Pseudomonas aeruginosa and Enterobacter cloacae, suggests that its use be restricted to the treatment of infection secondary to these organisms.
[f]Ampicillin-sulbactam, piperacillin-tazobactam, and ticarcillin-clavulanic acid have excellent activity versus B. fragilis, approaching that of metronidazole. Ticarcillin-clavulanic acid, however, has limited enterococcal activity whereas ampicillin-sulbactam has excellent activity against this organism but only moderate aerobic gram-negative activity. Piperacillin-tozobactam is active against both enterococcus and most gram-negative aerobes.

Table 60.4 • Antibiotics in CAPD Patients and Regimens for the Treatment of Peritonitis[46]

Drug	Intermittent Dosing (1 bag/day Unless Otherwise Specified)	Continuous Dosing (mg/L Unless Otherwise Specified)
Aminoglycosides		
Amikacin	2 mg/kg	LD 25, MD 12
Gentamicin	0.6 mg/kg	LD 25, MD 4
Netilmicin	0.6 mg/kg	LD 8, MD 4
Tobramycin	0.6 mg/kg	LD 8, MD 4
Cephalosporins		
Cefazolin	15 mg/kg	LD 500, MD 125
Cephalothin	15 mg/kg	LD 500, MD 125
Cephradine	15 mg/kg	LD 500, MD 125
Cephalexin	500 mg PO QID	NA
Cefamandole	1,000 mg	LD 500, MD 250

(continued)

Table 60.4 • Antibiotics in CAPD Patients and Regimens for the Treatment of Peritonitis[46,a] (continued)

Drug	Intermittent Dosing (1 bag/day Unless Otherwise Specified)	Continuous Dosing (mg/L Unless Otherwise Specified)
Cephalosporins (continued)		
Cefmenoxime	1,000 mg	LD 100, MD 50
Cefoxitin	ND	LD 200, MD 100
Cefuroxime	400 mg PO/IV QD	LD 200, MD 100–200
Cefixime	400 mg PO QD	NA
Cefoperazone	ND	LD 500, MD 250
Cefotaxime	2,000 mg	LD 500, MD 250
Cefsulodin	500 mg	LD 50, MD 25
Ceftazidime	1,000 mg	LD 250, MD 125
Cefizoxime	1,000 mg	LD 250, MD 125
Ceftriaxone	1,000 mg	LD 250, MD 125
Penicillins		
Azlocillin	ND	LD 500, MD 250
Mezlocillin	3,000 mg IV BID	LD 3 g IV, MD 250
Piperacillin	4,000 mg IV BID	LD 4 g IV, MD 250
Ticarcillin	2,000 mg IV VID	LD 1–2 g IV, MD 125
Ampicillin	ND	MD 125; or 250–500 mg PO BID; 250–500 mg PO QID
Dicloxacillin	ND	MD 125
Oxacillin	ND	MD 125
Nafcillin	ND	250–500 mg PO Q 12 hr
Amoxicillin	ND	
Quinolones		
Ciprofloxacin	500 mg PO BID	Not recommended
Fleroxacin	800 mg PO, then 400 mg PO QD	Not recommended
Ofloxacin	400 mg PO, then 200 mg PO QD	Not recommended
Others		
Vancomycin	15–30 mg/kg Q 5–7 days	LD 1,000, MD 25
Teicoplanin	400 mg IP BID	LD 400, MD 40[b]
Aztreonam	1,000 mg	LD 1,000, MD 250
Clindamycin	ND	LD 300, MD 150
Erythromycin	500 mg PO QID	LD ND, MD 150
Metronidazole	500 mg PO/IV TID	ND
Minocycline	100 mg PO BID	NA
Rifampin	450–600 mg PO QD or 150 mg IP TID–QID	NA
Antifungals		
Amphotericin	NA	1.5
Flucytosine	1 g QD PO or 100 mg/L IP each, exch for 3 days, then 50 mg/L/exch 200–800 mg PO QD	50 QD
Fluconazole	ND	ND
Ketoconazole		NA
Miconazole		LD 200, MD 100–200
Combinations		
Ampicillin/sulbactam	2 g Q 12 hr	LD 1,000, MD 100
Imipenem/cilistatin	1 g BID	LD 500, MD 200
Trimethoprim-sulfamethoxazole	320/1,600 Q 1–2 days PO	LD 320/1,600; MD 80/400

[a] BID = Twice a day; exch = Exchange; IP = Intraperitoneally; IV = Intravenous; LD = Loading dose; MD = Maintenance dose; NA = Not applicable; ND = No data; PO = Oral; QD = Once a day; QID = Four times a day; TID = Three times a day.

[b] This is in each bag for 7 days, then in two bags/day for 7 days, and then in 1 bag/day for 7 days.
The route of administration is intraperitoneal unless otherwise specified. The pharmacokinetic data and proposed dosage regimens presented here are based on published literature reviewed through January 1996. There is no evidence that mixing different antibiotics in dialysis fluid (except for aminoglycosides and penicillins) is deleterious for the drugs or patients.
Do not use the same syringe to mix antibiotics.
Note: CAPD patients with residual renal function may require increased doses or more frequent dosing, especially when using intermittent regimens.
Reprinted with permission from reference 46.

The reader is referred to Chapter 61: Intra-Abdominal Infections, written by *Jill S. Burkiewicz, Pharm.D.* and *Karen Kostiuk, Pharm.D.*, in the seventh edition of **Applied Therapeutics: The Clinical Use of Drugs** for a more in-depth discussion. All notations to reference numbers are based on the reference list at the end of that chapter. The editors of this handbook express their thanks to Drs. Burkiewicz and Kostiuk and acknowledge that this chapter is based upon their work.

Notes:

Notes:

Chapter 61

Urinary Tract Infections

Definitions

♦ **Urinary Tract Infection (UTI).** The presence of micro-organisms (viruses, fungi, but predominantly bacteria) in the urinary tract, including the bladder, prostate, kidneys, and collecting duct.

  • *Uncomplicated UTI:* Infections occurring in otherwise healthy persons, usually women, with no underlying risk factors.

  • *Complicated UTI:* Associated with conditions that increase risk for acquiring infections, increase the potential for serious outcomes, or increase the risk of failing therapy.

    • *Conditions:*
      —Men, children, pregnancy
      —Structural or neurologic abnormalities of urinary tract
      —Metabolic/hormonal abnormalities
      —Impaired host response

♦ **Pyuria.** White blood cells (WBCs) in the urine. A WBC count $\geq 8/mm^3$ of uncentrifuged urine or 2–5 per high-power field (hpf) in centrifuged urine sediment is consistent with a UTI.

♦ **Bacteriuria.** Bacteria cultured from urine when it is obtained by either suprapubic aspiration, catheterization, or from a freshly voided specimen. Asymptomatic bacteriuria exists if colony counts exceed $10^5/mL$ in a patient without UTI symptoms. Clinically significant bacteriuria probably exists if colony counts are $10^2/mL$ or more in patients with UTI symptoms.

♦ **Lower UTI.** An inflammation of the bladder and urethra, with dysuria, frequency, urgency, pyuria, and clinically significant bacteriuria.

♦ **Acute Pyelonephritis.** Inflammation of the kidney, with flank pain and tenderness, bacteriuria (often bacteremia), pyuria, and fever.

♦ **Chronic Pyelonephritis.** A chronic, inflammatory condition of the kidney with associated calyceal dilation and overlying cortical scarring. A nonspecific pathologic picture seen with many disease entities, only 1 of which is bacterial infection of the kidney.

♦ **Subclinical Pyelonephritis.** A kidney infection, but with lower UTI signs and symptoms only.

♦ **Urethritis.** Inflammation of the urethra, with dysuria. Etiologic organisms most commonly implicated are *Neisseria gonorrhoeae, Ureaplasma urealyticum, Chlamydia trachomatis,* and herpes simplex virus.

♦ **Prostatitis.** Inflammatory condition affecting the prostate. May be acute or chronic. Frequently, specific bacterial organisms cannot be detected.

◆ **Vaginitis.** Inflammation of the vagina, with dysuria and vaginal discharge. Common etiologic agents include *Candida albicans, Gardnerella vaginalis,* and Trichomonas.

Pathogenesis

◆ Most UTIs are caused by aerobic gram-negative bacilli originating from the intestinal tract, particularly, *Escherichia coli* (see Table 61.1).
◆ As with other infections, more resistant gram-negative organisms such as *Klebsiella sp.* and *Pseudomonas aeruginosa* are associated with hospital-acquired infection. (See Table 61.1.)

Clinical Presentation

◆ **Common symptoms of lower UTIs (cystitis)** include dysuria (burning), frequent urination, and suprapubic pain. However, signs and symptoms correlate poorly with the extent of infection.
◆ **Acute pyelonephritis symptoms** include loin pain, costovertebral angle (CVA) tenderness, fever, chills, nausea, vomiting, and hematuria. However, signs and symptoms correlate poorly with the extent of infection.

Diagnosis

◆ Diagnosis is confirmed by bacteria cultured from a midstream urine as determined by the dipstick method.
◆ The presence of >20 bacteria/hpf and >8 WBC/mm^3 of unspun urine or 2–5 WBC per hpf of centrifuged urine is common.
◆ WBC casts strongly suggest pyelonephritis.

Treatment

◆ **Drugs of choice** are listed in Tables 61.1 and 61.2.
◆ **Oral antimicrobials** are generally sufficient for the treatment of uncomplicated community or nosocomial cystitis. Complicated infections, such as pyelonephritis, are often treated initially with parenteral therapy; however, the majority of the course may be treated with oral antibiotics. (See Tables 61.1 and 61.2.)
◆ **Parenteral Agents.** In septic patients parenteral agents are mandatory. (See Table 61.3.)
◆ **Prophylaxis Against Recurrent UTI.** See Table 61.4.

Urine Concentrations of Antibiotics

◆ Most antibiotics concentrate in the urine, independent of the primary route of elimination. As a result, urinary tract infection caused by organisms classified as "resistant" relative to achievable plasma levels can still be treated in certain cases.

Antibiotic Penetration into the Prostate

◆ Most antibiotics do not readily cross the epithelium into the alkaline prostatic fluid.
◆ Trimethoprim, clindamycin, doxycycline, erythromycin, and the quinolones achieve high levels in prostatic secretions.

- **Acute Prostatitis.** As with other infections, acute prostatitis is associated with inflammation which increases antimicrobial penetration into prostatic secretions. Therefore, agents which do not normally cross the prostatic epithelium are effective in the acute, inflamed state.
- **Chronic Prostatitis.** In chronic prostatitis, inflammation is minimal, and most antibiotics do not readily cross the epithelium. Thus trimethoprim, quinolones, or like agents are necessary.

Table 61.1 • Urinary Tract Infections

Organisms Commonly Found	Antibacterial of Choice
Uncomplicated UTI	
Escherichia coli	TMP-SMX[c]
Proteus mirabilis	TMP-SMX[c]
Klebsiella pneumoniae	TMP-SMX[c]
Enterococcus faecalis	Amoxicillin
Staphylococcus saprophyticus	First-generation cephalosporin or TMP-SMX
Complicated UTI[a,b]	
Escherichia coli	First-, second-, or third-generation cephalosporin
Proteus mirabilis	First-, second-, or third-generation cephalosporin
Klebsiella pneumoniae	First-generation cephalosporin
Enterococcus faecalis	Ampicillin or vancomycin ± aminoglycoside
Pseudomonas aeruginosa	Antipseudomonal penicillin ± aminoglycoside; ceftazidime; cefepime; fluoroquinolone; carbapenem
Enterobacter	Fluoroquinolone; TMP-SMX; carbepenem
Indole-positive *Proteus*	Third-generation cephalosporin; fluoroquinolone
Serratia	Third-generation cephalosporin; fluoroquinolone
Acinetobacter	Carbepenem; TMP-SMX
Staphylococcus aureus	Penicillinase-resistant penicillin; vancomycin

[a]Oral therapy when appropriate.
[b]Drug selection based on culture and susceptibility testing when possible.
TMP-SMX = Trimethoprim-sulfamethoxazole; UTI = Urinary tract infection.
[c]Caution in communities with increased resistance (>10–20%). Fluoroquinolone, nitrofurantoin, cephalosporins should be used in areas with increased TMP-SMX resistance.

Notes:

Table 61.2 • Commonly Used Oral Antimicrobial Agents for Acute Urinary Tract Infections[1-3,5,35-37]

Drug	Usual Dose Adult	Usual Dose Pediatric
Amoxicillin	250 mg Q 8 hr	20–40 mg/kg/day in 3 doses
Amoxicillin + potassium clavulanate	500 + 125 mg Q 12 hr	20 mg/kg/day (amoxicillin content) in 3 doses
Ampicillin	250–500 mg Q 6 hr	50–100 mg/kg/day in 4 doses
Cefadroxil	0.5–1 g Q 12 hr	15–30 mg/kg/day in 4 doses
Cephalexin	250–500 mg Q 6 hr	15–30 mg/kg/day in 4 doses
Cephradine	250–500 mg Q 6 hr	15–30 mg/kg/day in 4 doses
Norfloxacin	400 mg Q 12 hr	Avoid
Ciprofloxacin	100–500 mg Q 12 hr	Avoid
Lomefloxacin	400 mg Q 24 hr	Avoid
Ofloxacin	200 mg Q 12 hr	Avoid
Levofloxacin	250 mg Q 24 hr	Avoid
Nitrofurantoin	50–100 mg Q 6 hr	5–7 mg/kg/day in 4 doses
Doxycycline	100 mg Q 12 hr	Avoid
Trimethoprim (TMP)	100 mg Q 12 hr	
TMP-SMX	160 + 800 mg Q 12 hr or 0.48 + 2.4 g single dose	10 mg/kg/day (TMP component) in 2 doses

Notes:

Table 61.3 • Parenteral Antimicrobial Agents Commonly Used in the Treatment of Urinary Tract Infections

Class	Drug	Average Adult Daily Dose UTI	Sepsis	Usual Dosage Interval[a]
Ampicillins	Ampicillin	2–4 g	8 g	Q 4–6 hr
	Ampicillin/sulbactam	6 g	12 g	Q 6 hr
Extended-spectrum penicillin	Ticarcillin	12 g	18 g	Q 4–6 hr
	Ticarcillin/ clavulanate	9–12 g	18 g	Q 4–6 hr
	Piperacillin	12 g	18 g	Q 4–6 hr
First-generation cephalosporins	Cefazolin	1.5–3 g	6 g	Q 8–12 hr
Second-generation cephalosporins	Cefoxitin	3–4 g	8 g	Q 4–8 hr
	Cefuroxime	2.25 g	4.5 g	Q 8 hr
	Cefotetan	1–4 g	6 g	Q 12 hr
Third-generation cephalosporins	Cefotaxime	3–4 g	8 g	Q 6–8 hr
	Ceftizoxime	2–3 g	8 g	Q 8–12 hr
	Ceftriaxone	1 g	2 g	Q 12–24 hr
	Ceftazidime	1.5–3 g	6 g	Q 8–12 hr
Fourth-generation cephalosporins	Cefepime	1–2 g	4 g	Q 12 hr
Carbapenems	Imipenem/cilastatin	1 g	2 g	Q 6 hr
	Meropenem	1.5–3 g	3 g	Q 8 hr
Monobactam	Aztreonam	1–2 g	6–8 g	Q 8–12 hr
Aminoglycosides	Gentamicin	3 mg/kg	5 mg/kg	Q 24 hr
	Tobramycin	3 mg/kg	5 mg/kg	Q 24 hr
	Amikacin	7.5 mg/kg	15 mg/kg	Q 24 hr
Quinolones	Ciprofloxacin	400–800 mg	800 mg	Q 12 hr
	Ofloxacin	400–800 mg	800 mg	Q 12 hr
	Levofloxacin	250–500 mg	500 mg	Q 24 hr

[a]Assuming normal renal function.

Table 61.4 • Antimicrobial Agents Commonly Used for Chronic Prophylaxis Against Recurrent UTIs[1–3,5,93]

Agent	Adult Dose
Nitrofurantoin	50–100 mg nightly
Trimethoprim	100 mg nightly
Trimethoprim 80 mg + Sulfamethoxazole 400 mg	0.5–1 tab nightly or 3 × per week
Norfloxacin	200 mg/day
Cephalexin	125–250 mg/day
Cefaclor	250 mg/day
Cephradine	250 mg/day
Sulfamethoxazole	500 mg/day

Notes:

The reader is referred to Chapter 62: Urinary Tract Infections, written by *Douglas N. Fish, Pharm.D.,* and *Jan V. Sahai, Pharm.D.,* in the seventh edition of **Applied Therapeutics: The Clinical Use of Drugs** for a more in-depth discussion. All notations to reference numbers are based on the reference list at the end of that chapter. The editors of this handbook express their thanks to Drs. Fish and Sahai and acknowledge that this chapter is based upon their work.

Notes:

Chapter 62

Sexually Transmitted Diseases

Gonorrhea, syphilis, and chlamydial infections are among the most commonly reported sexually transmitted diseases; however, viral infections (e.g., HIV, HBV, HPV, HSV), trichomoniasis, chancroid, and others also are commonly transmitted.

GONORRHEA
Clinical Presentation

♦ In *males,* a purulent discharge with dysuria is the first sign of infection occurring 1–7 days after contact with an infected source. Untreated gonococcal urethritis spontaneously resolves after several weeks: Most become asymptomatic carriers within 6 months.

♦ In *females,* the most common symptom is vaginal discharge due to mucopurulent cervicitis occurring within 10 days of exposure. Coexisting infection with *C. trachomatis* or *Trichomonas vaginalis* is very common.

Diagnosis

♦ Gram-negative diplococci *(Neisseria gonorrhoeae)* in exudate is diagnostic.
♦ Cultures for antimicrobial susceptibility are recommended.

Treatment

♦ CDC recommendations for treatment of uncomplicated gonorrhea are in Table 62.1.

CHLAMYDIA

♦ *Chlamydia trachomatis* is the most commonly sexually transmitted pathogen.
♦ Blinding trachoma is caused by serovars A, B, and C of *C. trachomatis.*
♦ Nongonococcal urethritis, cervicitis, endometritis, and salpingitis are caused by serovars D, E, F, G, H, I, J, and K.
♦ Lymphogranuloma venereum (LGV) is caused by serovars L_1, L_2, and L_3 of *C. trachomatis.*
♦ Genital *C. trachomatis* infections closely resemble those caused by *N. gonorrhoeae*. A high prevalence of *C. trachomatis* infection in patients with gonorrhea warrants empirical antichlamydial agents with gonococcal therapy.

Treatment

♦ **Urethritis/cervicitis/proctitis.** *Doxycycline* 100 mg PO BID for 7 days **or azithromycin** 1 gm PO for 1 dose are the therapies of choice. Erythromycin 500 mg PO QID for 7 days or ofloxacin 300 mg PO BID for 7 days are alternative therapies. Of the quinolones, only ofloxacin should be considered as an alternative.

♦ Sexual partners of patients with gonorrhea, syphilis, or chlamydia also should be treated.

♦ **LGV.** Doxycycline 100 mg PO BID for 21 days; alternatively, erythromycin 500 mg PO QID for 21 days.

SYPHILIS
Clinical Presentation

♦ Usual incubation period is 3 weeks (range: 10–90 days). *Treponema pallidum* can be found in blood at this time. A painless papule becomes ulcerated, indurated, and resolves spontaneously in 2–6 weeks.

♦ If untreated, a secondary stage with signs and symptoms develops about 6 weeks after the chancre first appears, followed by a latent stage and a subsequent tertiary stage with cardiovascular and neurological manifestations.

Treatment

♦ Most cases are treatable with IM benzathine penicillin G 2.4 MU once (see Table 62.3).

♦ HIV patients with early syphilis should have a repeat course of penicillin after 7 days.

GENITAL HERPES

♦ Herpes simplex virus consists of two antigenic serotypes, HSV_1 and HSV_2.

♦ HSV_1 is the primary cause of cold sores (herpes labialis), herpes keratitis, and herpes encephalitis.

♦ HSV_2 is the primary cause of genital herpes and neonatal herpes.

Clinical Presentation

♦ Tingling, itching, and genital burning beginning about 1 week after direct contact with active lesions, followed by appearance of numerous vesicles that eventually erupt, resulting in painful ulcerations.

♦ Lesions begin to heal in about 12 days, and symptoms abate in about 2–3 weeks after first appearance.

Treatment

♦ Most genital herpes infections are benign and heal spontaneously unless the patient is immunocompromised or lesions become infected.

♦ Although genital herpes is not curable, oral acyclovir analogues for 7–10 days decrease duration of pain, systemic symptoms, and time of viral shedding. Recurrence can be treated with these agents; however, they are less effective when compared to primary treatment.

♦ Suppressive therapy with acyclovir analogues reduces recurrent episodes. Toxicity and development of resistance of suppressive therapy of long duration, particularly in immunocompromised patients, must be considered.

♦ Acyclovir-resistant H. simplex has been associated with significant morbidity in the immunocompromised.

♦ Treatment guidelines for H. simplex are in Table 62.4.

Pelvic Inflammatory Disease (PID) (Table 62.2)

♦ PID occurs when vaginal or cervical microorganisms ascend to the fallopian tubes.

♦ *N. gonorrhoeae* and *C. trachomatis* are the major pathogens responsible for sexually transmitted PID. *Mycoplasma hominis, Ureaplasma urealyticum,* enteric gram-negative bacilli *(E. coli, Klebsiella sp.),* and a variety of anaerobic bacteria also have been implicated.

Treatment

Inpatient and outpatient regimens are listed in Table 62.5.

Vaginal Infections

♦ Trichomoniasis is a sexually transmitted disease caused by the protozoan, *Trichomonas vaginalis.*

♦ Bacterial vaginosis (formerly known as "nonspecific vaginitis") is associated with a malodorous increase in vaginal discharge. The role of sexual transmission is unclear for bacterial vaginosis or vaginal candidiasis.

Treatment

♦ Metronidazole is the only effective agent for the treatment of trichomoniasis. Recurrences or relapses can be treated with repeated courses, and higher doses may be needed.

♦ Treatment of vaginitis is found in Table 62.5.

Table 62.1 • Recommendations for Treatment of Uncomplicated Gonorrhea[a]

Drugs of Choice	Dosage	Alternatives
Cefixime	400 mg PO × 1	Spectinomycin 2 gm IM[c] × 1
or		
Ciprofloxacin[b]	500 mg PO × 1	
or		
Ofloxacin[b]	400 mg PO × 1	
or		
Ceftriaxone	125 mg IM × 1	

[a]Treatment of cervical, pharyngeal (not spectinomycin), rectal, and urethral disease.
[b]Contraindicated in pregnancy.
[c]Not effective in pharyngeal disease. Recommended only in pregnant penicillin-allergic patients.

Notes:

Table 62.2 • Antimicrobial Regimens Recommended by the CDC for Treatment of Acute Pelvic Inflammatory Disease

Inpatient

Cefoxitin (or cefotetan) plus doxycycline
Administer cefoxitin (2 gm IV Q 6 hr) or cefotetan (2 gm IV Q 12 hr) plus doxycycline (100 mg IV Q 12 hr) until improved. Continue doxycycline (100 mg PO BID) after discharge to complete 14 days of therapy

Clindamycin plus an aminoglycoside
Administer clindamycin (900 mg IV Q 8 hr) plus gentamicin (1.5–2 mg/kg IV Q 8 hr) until improved, followed by doxycycline 100 mg PO BID to complete 14 days

Outpatient

Cefoxitin or cefotetan plus probenecid (or ceftriaxone) and doxycycline
Administer cefoxitin (2 gm IM once) or cefotetan (2 gm IV once) plus probenecid (1 gm PO once) or ceftriaxone (250 mg IM once). Concomitantly administer doxycycline (100 mg PO Q 12 hr) for a total of 14 days

Ofloxacin plus metronidazole or clindamycin
Administer ofloxacin (400 mg PO BID) plus either metronidazole (500 mg PO BID) or clindamycin (450 mg PO QID) for a total of 10–14 days

---

Table 62.3 • Treatment Guidelines for Syphilis

Stage of Syphilis	Patients without Penicillin Allergy	Patients with Penicillin Allergy
Primary, secondary, or early latent	Benzathine penicillin G 2.4 MU single dose IM (1.2 MU in each hip)	Doxycycline 100 mg PO BID × 2 weeks
Late latent or latent of uncertain duration	Benzathine penicillin G 2.4 MU/week IM × 3 weeks	Doxycycline 100 mg PO BID × 4 weeks
Neurosyphilis (asymptomatic or symptomatic)	Aqueous penicillin G, 18–24 MU/day IV in 4–6 divided doses for 10–14 days. *or* Aqueous procaine penicillin G, 2.4 MU/day IM + probenecid 500 mg PO QID, both for 10–14 days.	No proven alternative to penicillin. Consider desensitization.
Congenital	Aqueous crystalline penicillin G 100,000–150,000 units/kg/day IV Q 8–12 hr for 10–14 days *or* Procaine penicillin G, 50,000 units/kg IM QD for 10–14 days	

Notes:

Table 62.4 • Antiviral Chemotherapy of Genital HSV-2 Infections

	Acyclovir	Valacyclovir[c]	Famciclovir	Duration	Comments
First clinical episode	400 mg PO TID or 200 mg PO 5 × per day	1 g PO BID	250 mg PO TID	7–10 days	May extend treatment duration if healing is incomplete
Episodic recurrent infection	400 mg PO TID or 200 mg PO 5 × per day or 800 mg PO BID	500 mg PO BID	125 mg PO BID	5 days	Most effective if initiated within the first 24 hr of the onset of lesions or during the prodrome
Daily suppressive therapy	400 mg PO BID[a]	500 mg PO QD[b] or 1 g PO QD	250 mg PO BID	Daily	Reduces the frequency of genital herpes recurrences by ≥75% among patients who have frequent recurrences (i.e., ≥6 recurrences per year); use should be re-evaluated at 1 yr
Severe disseminated	5–10 mg/kg/dose IV Q 8 hr	Not indicated	Not indicated	Variable	Hospitalize and treat until there is clinical resolution of symptoms

[a]Safety and efficacy up to 6 years has been documented with the use of acyclovir.
[b]Valacyclovir 500 mg QD appears less effective in patients with >10 episodes per year. Thus, 500 mg BID or 1 g QD should be used in these patients.
[c]Dosages up to 8 g/day have been used, but an association with a syndrome resembling either hemolytic uremic syndrome or thrombotic thrombocytopenic purpura was observed.

Table 62.5 • Treatment of Vaginitis^a

Trichomoniasis	*Drug of Choice:* Metronidazole 2 gm PO once *Alternative:* Metronidazole 500 mg tab or 375 mg cap PO BID × 7 days
Bacterial vaginosis	*Drug of Choice:* Metronidazole 500 mg PO BID × 7 days *Alternative:* Clindamycin 300 mg PO BID × 7 days *or* topical metronidazole *or* topical clindamycin
Candidiasis	*Drug of Choice:* Topical butoconazole, clotrimazole, miconazole, terconazole, or tioconazole *Alternative:* Fluconazole 150 mg PO once

^aAvoid oral metronidazole in 1st trimester in pregnancy.

The reader is referred to Chapter 63: Sexually Transmitted Diseases, written by *Jeffrey A. Goad, Pharm.D.*, in the seventh edition of **Applied Therapeutics: The Clinical Use of Drugs** for a more in-depth discussion. All notations to reference numbers are based on the reference list at the end of that chapter. The editors of this handbook express their thanks to Dr. Goad and acknowledge that this chapter is based upon his work.

Notes:

Chapter 63

Infections of Skin, Soft Tissue, and Bone

SKIN AND SOFT TISSUE INFECTIONS
Pathogenesis

+ Refers to infections involving skin, subcutaneous fat, fascia, or muscle.
+ Most skin infections (cellulitis, impetigo, furuncles) are due to streptococci and staphylococci (see Table 63.1). Necrotizing fascitis, diabetic ulcers, and bite wounds also commonly involve gram-negative bacilli and anaerobes.

Treatment

+ Oral penicillin is the drug of choice for streptococcal cellulitis and impetigo. In those instances in which mixed streptococcal/staphylococcal infection is being considered, oral dicloxacillin or cephalexin should be used (see Table 63.2).
+ More severe infection associated with mixed gram-positive, gram-negative, and/or anaerobic therapy should be treated with parenteral therapy.

BONE INFECTIONS
Pathogenesis

+ The most common organism associated with hematogenous osteomyelitis is *S. aureus;* however, gram-negative bacilli such as *E. coli* and *P. aeruginosa* occasionally are associated with disease.
+ Infection of orthopedic hardware most commonly is caused by *S. epidermidis.*
+ The bacteriology for septic arthritis is similar to that seen with hematogenous osteomyelitis, except for the increased prevalence of *N. gonorrhoeae.*

Clinical Features

+ Classic presentation includes fever with localized pain, tenderness, swelling, erythema, and decreased range of motion at the site of infection. Other features are listed in Table 63.3.
+ X-ray changes cannot be detected for 7–10 days after the onset of illness.

Treatment

+ Osteomyelitis must be treated with high-dose antibiotics to achieve adequate levels in infected bone. Early treatment enhances eradication of the infection. (See Table 63.4.)
+ Symptomatic response should be observed within 48–72 hr, but treatment should be extended for 6 weeks.

- While acute osteomyelitis is treatable with a 6-week course, chronic osteomyelitis may require prolonged therapy. Chronic osteomyelitis generally necessitates surgical intervention to remove infected or necrotic bone for cure.
- The importance of antibiotic penetration of bone and synovial fluid is unclear. All antimicrobials appear to penetrate bone to an acceptable level.
- Other factors, such as bone vascularity and presence of prosthetic hardware, have more important roles in the eradication of infection. Infection of hardware usually is not curable without removal of the prosthetic device.*
- Studies in the treatment of infectious arthritis indicate that almost all agents penetrate well into synovial fluid. Erythromycin and aminoglycosides penetrate to a lesser degree.

---

*The combination of ciprofloxacin with rifampin has been demonstrated to be effective in the treatment of infected arthroplasty without removal of hardware (methicillin-susceptible *S. aureus.*)

Notes:

Table 63.1 • Potential Organisms Causing Skin and Soft-Tissue Infections

	Gram-Positive		Gram-Negative			Anaerobes		
	Staphylococcal	Streptococcal	E. coli, Klebsiella, Proteus	Pasteurella multocida	Eikenella corrodens	Oral Anaerobes	Clostridium Species	Bacteroides fragilis
Cellulitis	X							
Diabetic soft tissue	X	X	X					X
Necrotizing infections	X	X	X			X	X	X
Erysipelas		X						
Animal bites	X	X	X	X		X		
Human bites	X	X	X		X	X		

Notes:

Table 63.2 • Spectrum of Activity for Antibiotics Useful in the Treatment of Skin and Soft-Tissue Infections

Antibiotics	Gram-Positive			Gram-Negative			Anaerobes		
	Streptococci Other Than Enterococcus	Enterococci	Staphylococci	E. coli, Klebsiella, Proteus	Pasteurella multocida	Eikenella corrodens	Oral Anaerobes	Clostridium Species	Bacteroides fragilis
Penicillin	++++	+++	+	—	+++	++++	++++	++++	—
Cloxacillin, nafcillin, flucloxacillin, dicloxacillin	++	—	++++	—	+	—	+++	+++	—
Amoxicillin-clavulanate, ampicillin-sulbactam	+++	+++	+++	++	+++	++	++++	+++	—
Piperacillin	++	+++	+	+++	++	++	+++	++++	+++
Piperacillin-tazobactam	+++	+++	++	++++	++	++	+++	++++	+++
Ticarcillin-clavulanate	+++	—	+++	++++	++	++	+++	++++	+++
Cephalexin, cefazolin	+++	—	++++	++	—	—	++++	+	—
cefoxitin, ceftrizoxime, cefotetan, cefmetazole	++	—	++	++	++	+	++	+	+++
Cefotaxime, ceftriaxone	++	—	+++	++++	++	++	+++	+	—
Clindamycin	++++	—	++++	—	—	—	++++	++	+++
Metronidazole	—	—	—	—	—	—	+++	+++	+++
Vancomycin	++++	+++	++++	—	—	—	+++	+++	—
Azithromycin	+++	—	++	—	++	++	++	++	—
Erythromycin	+++	—	++	—	+	+	++	++	—
Gentamicin	+	++	++	+++	—	—	—	—	—
Trimethoprim-sulfamethoxazole (co-trimoxazole)	+++	+	+++	++	++	+	—	—	—
Tetracycline, doxycycline	++	—	+++	+	++	++	++	+++	—
Ciprofloxacin	+	++	+++	+++	+++	+++	—	—	—
Levofloxacin	++	++	+++	++	+++	++	—	+	—

Table 63.3 • Features of Osteomyelitis

Feature	Hematogenous	Adjacent Site of Infection	Vascular Insufficiency
Usual age of onset (yr)	1–20; 50	50	50
Sites of infection	Long bones, vertebrae	Femur, tibia, skull, mandible	Feet
Risk factors	Bacteremia	Surgery, trauma, cellulitis; joint prosthesis	Diabetes, peripheral vascular disease
Common bacteria	*Staphylococcus aureus*, Gram-negative bacilli; usually one organism	*S. aureus*, Gram-negative bacilli; anaerobic organisms; often mixed infection	*S. aureus*, coagulase-negative staphylococci, Gram-negative and anaerobic organisms; usually mixed infection
Clinical findings			
Initial episode	Fever, chills, local tenderness, swelling; limitation of motion	Fever, warmth, swelling; unstable joint	Pain, swelling, drainage, ulcer formation
Recurrent episode	Drainage	Drainage, sinus tract	As above

Table 63.4 • Treatment Regimens in Acute Osteomyelitis[a]

Pathogen	Regimen	Dosage	Duration[b]
S. aureus (methicillin-susceptible)	Nafcillin	2 gm Q4–6H IV	6 wks
	or		
	Cefazolin	2 gm Q8H IV	6 wks
	or		
	Ceftriaxone	2 gm Q24H IV	6 wks
S. epidermidis (methicillin-susceptible)	Same as above		
Methicillin-resistant staphylococci[c]	Vancomycin	30 mg/kg/day IV	6 wks

[a]Septic arthritis involves same drugs for shorter duration.
[b]Chronic osteomyelitis requires longer treatment regimens

The reader is referred to Chapter 64: Osteomyelitis/Septic Arthritis, written by *Ralph H. Raasch, Pharm.D.*, and Chapter 65: Traumatic Skin and Soft Tissue Infections, written by *James P. McCormack, Pharm.D.* and *Glen Brown, Pharm.D.*, in the seventh edition of **Applied Therapeutics: The Clinical Use of Drugs** for a more in-depth discussion. The editors of this handbook express their thanks to Drs. Raasch, McCormack, and Brown and acknowledge that this chapter is based upon their work.

Notes:

Notes:

Chapter 64

Infections in
Neutropenic Patients

Patients may be immunocompromised as a result of a number of factors, including neutropenia, lymphocytic abnormalities (HIV, solid organ transplant), lack of humoral immunity, or damage to physical barriers.

Pathogenesis

♦ Table 64.1 lists the common bacterial, viral, fungal, and parasitic infections commonly encountered in immunocompromised patients.

♦ **Neutropenia** is associated with a significant risk of infection. This risk is both degree- and duration-related.

  • The lower the absolute neutrophil count (e.g., <500/mm³), the greater the likelihood of infection.

  • A duration of neutropenia >2 weeks also increases the risk of infection.

♦ Chemotherapeutic drugs that cause mucositis can facilitate systemic entry of bacteria or fungi from the GI tract.

♦ Indwelling intravenous catheters (e.g., Hickman) for long-term chemotherapy increase the risk of infection.

♦ With continued or new onset of fever, other pathogens must be considered. Among these pathogens include fungi, particularly *Candida* sp. and *Aspergillus* sp.

  • The most established choice for serious fungal infection is conventional amphotericin. Lipid-based products (ABLC, liposomal amphotericin) may be preferable in patients with renal insufficiency. Liposomal amphotericin has been shown to be associated with less breakthrough fungal infection than conventional amphotericin in febrile neutropenia.

  • Alternatives to amphotericin include azoles, such as fluconazole, itraconazole, voraconazole and others. Candins, such as caspofungin, also are useful in some patients with *Aspergillus* infection refractory or intolerant to amphotericin.

  • Treatment of systemic fungal infection is presented in Chapter 67: Fungal Infections.

Treatment

♦ An approach to the management of febrile neutropenic patients is shown in Figure 64.1; the antimicrobial therapy of these patients is in Table 64.2 and the modifications of therapy for these patients in Table 64.3. Monotherapy or combination therapy with a variety of agents has been used in the empirical treatment of febrile neutropenic patients (e.g., aminoglycosides) combined with either an antipseudomonal penicillin or third-generation cephalosporin or double beta-lactam therapy.

◆ Spectrum of activity, toxicity, development of resistance, and cost determine the regimen of choice.

◆ With documented blood cultures for *Staphylococcus epidermidis* and/or clinical evidence of an infected central line, vancomycin should be added to the antibacterial regimen.

◆ Suspected multidrug-resistant gram-negative infection requires the use of agents such as imipenem or ciprofloxacin.

◆ Anaerobic infection (e.g., perirectal abscess or mucositis) should be treated with metronidazole or clindamycin.

Notes:

Table 64.1 • Infections in Immunocompromised Patients

Immunologic Defect	Underlying Condition(s)	Bacteria	Fungi	Parasites	Viruses
Neutropenia	Chemotherapy; acute leukemia	*S. aureus*, coagulase-negative staphylococci, enterococci, *E. coli*, *K. pneumoniae*, *P. aeruginosa*	*Candida, Aspergillus, Fusarium*		Herpes simplex, varicella-zoster, cytomegalovirus
T-helper lymphocyte (cell-mediated immunity)	Immunosuppressive therapy; Hodgkin's disease; transplantation	*Listeria monocytogenes, Nocardia asteroides, Legionella, Salmonella,* mycobacteria	*C. neoformans, Aspergillus, Candida, H. capsulatum,* Mucoraceae	*P. carinii, T. gondii*	
Gamma-globulin (humoral immunity)	Splenectomy; chronic lymphocytic leukemia; hypogammaglobulinemia; bone marrow transplantation	*S. pneumoniae, H. influenzae, N. meningitidis*		*P. carinii, Babesia* sp.	
Damage to physical barriers	Surgical procedures	*S. aureus*; coagulase-negative staphylococci, *S. pyogenes*; Enterobacteriaceae; *P. aeruginosa, Bacteroides,*	*Candida*		
	Indwelling catheters; venipuncture	*S. aureus*, coagulase-negative staphylococci, *Corynebacterium*	*Candida*		
	Chemotherapy; endoscopy; radiation	*S. aureus*, coagulase-negative staphylococci, streptococci, Enterobacteriaceae, *P. aeruginosa, Bacteroides*	*Candida*		Herpes simplex
Microbial colonization	Chemotherapy; antibiotics; hospitalization	*S. aureus*, coagulase-negative staphylococci, Enterobacteriaceae, *P. aeruginosa, Legionella*	*Candida, Aspergillus*		
Transplantation	Bone marrow; solid organ	*S. aureus*, coagulase-negative staphylococci, Enterobacteriaceae, *P. aeruginosa, Legionella*	*Candida, Aspergillus*	*T. gondii, P. carinii*	Cytomegalovirus; hepatitis B and C; Epstein-Barr virus

Adapted from reference 6.

Table 64.2 • Antimicrobial Therapy in Neutropenic Patients[a]

Agent	Advantage/Disadvantages
Antibiotics	
Aminoglycosides	Broad-spectrum activity. Must be used in combination with β-lactams or fluoroquinolones. May cause nephrotoxicity.
Antipseudomonal penicillins	Broad-spectrum Gram-negative activity. Emergence of resistance if not combined with an aminoglycoside. Should not be used as monotherapy in neutropenic patients.
3rd-generation cephalosporins	Excellent Gram-negative,[a] suboptimal Gram-positive activity.[b] Superinfections and coagulopathies[c] may occur with some agents. Emergence of resistant *P. aeruginosa* if not combined with an aminoglycoside.
Carbapenems	Very broad-spectrum. Emergence of resistant *P. aeruginosa* if not combined with an aminoglycoside.
Monobactams	Alternative in β-lactam-allergic patients. Combine with vancomycin for empiric therapy. Add aminoglycoside to minimize development of resistance. Do not use as monotherapy.
Fluoroquinolones	Broad-spectrum Gram-negative activity. Alternative in β-lactam-allergic patients. Emergence of resistance can occur if used routinely for prophylaxis.
Glycopeptides[d]	Excellent Gram-positive activity. Empiric use common in centers with high incidence of methicillin-resistant staphylococci. Emergence of vancomycin-resistant enterococci is of increasing concern.
Antifungals	
Amphotericin B[e]	Agent of choice for empiric use and treatment of disseminated fungal infections. High incidence of adverse reactions, especially nephrotoxicity, fever/chills, and phlebitis.
Caspofungin	Active versus *Aspergillus* and *Candida*
Fluconazole	Effective for management of oropharyngeal and disseminated candidiasis. Prophylactic use in some centers has resulted in emergence of resistant Candida infections (e.g., *C. krusei*).
Itraconazole	Effective against *Aspergillus*. Disadvantages similar to those with ketoconazole.
Voriconazole	Drug of choice for Fusarium. Active versus *Aspergillus* and *Candida*.

[a]Ceftazidime, cefoperazone, and cefepime have the best antipseudomonal activity in this class.
[b]For example, ceftazidime.
[c]For example, cefoperazone.
[d]Includes vancomycin and teicoplanin (investigational).
[e]Lipid-based amphotericin is less nephrotoxic than conventional amphotericin. Liposomal amphotericin may be associated with less breakthrough fungal infection than the conventional product.
Adapted from reference 128.

Notes:

Table 64.3 • Therapeutic Modifications in Patients with Neutropenia and Fever[a]

Clinical Condition	Suspected Pathogen(s) and Type of Modification(s)
Fever (Persistent or Recurrent)	Undetected fungal infection: add empiric amphotericin B
Positive Blood Cultures	
Before antibiotic initiation	*Gm(+)*: Add vancomycin, pending further identification *Gm(–)*: If *P. aeruginosa* or *Enterobacter*, add aminoglycoside
Isolated while on empiric antibiotics	*Gm(+)*: Add vancomycin *Gm(–)*: If *P. aeruginosa* or *Enterobacter*, add aminoglycoside
Head, Eyes, Ears, Nose, Throat	
Necrotizing gingivitis	*Anaerobes*: Add clindamycin or metronidazole
Vesicular or ulcerative lesions	*Herpes Simplex* virus: Add antiviral (e.g., acyclovir)
Oral mucositis	*Candida*: Add oral clotrimazole, nystatin, or fluconazole
Sinus tenderness	*Aspergillus* or Mucormycosis: Add amphotericin B
Gastrointestinal Tract	
Esophagitis	*Candida* and/or *Herpes Simplex*: Add antifungal agent; if no response, add antiviral
Acute abdominal pain/perianal tenderness	*Anaerobes*: Add clindamycin or metronidazole to empiric regimen or switch to imipenem/cilastatin
Respiratory Tract	
Interstitial pneumonitis	*Pneumocystis carinii*: Institute trial of TMP-SMX or pentamidine *Legionella*: Add macrolide or quinolone *Cytomegalovirus*: Add ganciclovir
Focal lesion on chest radiograph	*Aspergillus*: Administer high-dose amphotericin B (1.0–1.5 mg/kg/day) or itraconazole or caspofungin
Central Venous Catheter Tunnel Infection	Remove catheter; treat appropriately, based on culture and susceptibility

[a]TMP-SMX = Trimethoprim-sulfamethoxazole.
Adapted from reference 141.

Notes:

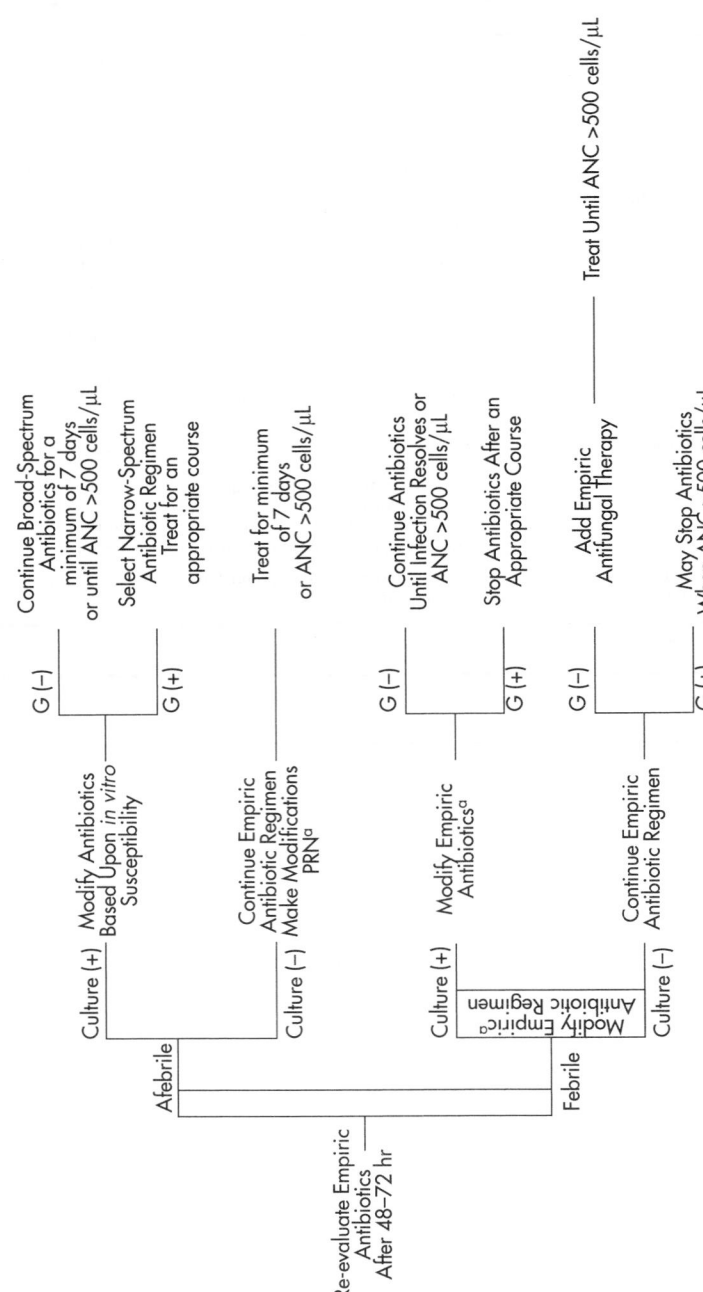

Fig. 64.1 Approach to Management of Febrile Neutropenic Patients. [a]See Table 64.2. G(+), ANC >500 µL; G(−), ANC <500 µL; SBT, serum bactericidal titer; F(+), temperature >38°C; F(−), afebrile; ANC, absolute neutrophil count.

The reader is referred to Chapter 66: Infections in Immunocompromised Hosts, written by *Hilary D. Mandler, Pharm.D.,* in the seventh edition of **Applied Therapeutics: The Clinical Use of Drugs** for a more in-depth discussion. All notations to reference numbers are based on the reference list at the end of that chapter. The editors of this handbook express their thanks to Dr. Mandler and acknowledge that this chapter is based upon her work.

Notes:

Notes:

Chapter 65

Pharmacotherapy of Human Immunodeficiency Virus Infection

Pathogenesis

♦ Transmission of HIV by direct exposure to contaminated body fluids
♦ HIV attaches to CD4 receptors on T-lymphocytes, releasing intracellular viral RNA
♦ Both dysfunction and depletion of lymphocytes results in the immunodeficiency state.

Epidemiology

♦ As of 2000, 36 million HIV-infected people worldwide with 5 million new infections per year and 3 million HIV-related deaths per year
♦ Sub-Saharan Africa has 25 million cases, with 4 million new infections per year and 2.5 million HIV-related deaths per year

Therapy

♦ Current recommendations for treatment (please see *www.hivatis.org* for the most up-to-date recommendations for the treatment of HIV).
♦ When to consider initiation of therapy (ATIS 2001)
  • Asymptomatic HIV-infected patient with CD4 <350
  • Asymptomatic HIV-infected patient with CD4 >350 but high levels of plasma HIV (more than 30,000 using branched DNA test or more than 55,000 using RT-PCR test.
  • All patients with acute HIV syndrome
  • All patients within 6 months of HIV seroconversion
  • All patients with symptoms ascribed to HIV infection (see surveillance case definition below)
♦ Recommended starting regimens (DHHS Guidelines)
  (One from Column A and from Column B in the "Preferred" category) (updated Aug/2001)

	Column A	Column B
Preferred	Efavirenz	d4T/3TC
	Indinavir	AZT/ddI
	Nelfinavir	AZT/3TC
	Ritonavir + Indinavir	d4T/ddI
	Ritonavir + Lopinavir (Kaletra)	ddI/3TC
	Ritonavir + Saquinavir (Fortovase)	

	Column A	**Column B**
Alternative	Abacavir	AZT/ddC
	Amprenavir	
	Delavirdine	
	Nevirapine	
	Ritonavir	
	Saquinavir (Fortovase)	
	Nelfinavir/Saquinavir (Fortovase)	
No recommendation	Hydroxyurea	
	Ritonavir + Nelfinavir	
Not recommended	All monotherapies	ddC/ddI
	Saquinavir (Invirase)	ddC/d4T
		ddC/3TC
		AZT/d4T

Characteristics of Antiretroviral Agents for the treatment of adult HIV infection. (See Table 65.2.)

♦ Monitoring of Therapy

- Adherence: Optimal results require 95% adherence. Barriers include toxicities, high pill burden, frequent dosing, food restrictions.
- Viral load: Check 4 weeks after starting therapy. Should decline 1.5–2.0 logs. Failure to achieve undetectable levels (<50 copies/ml) increases risk for breakthrough.
- CD4 lymphocytes: Response follows slower time course than viral load. Typically increases by 100–150 cells/mm^3 or more.
- Drug resistance testing
  —Genotypic (sequencing selected HIV genes for mutations producing drug resistance)
  —Phenotypic (testing for loss of viability or gene function)
  —Both methods are associated with improved clinical outcomes. Genotypic is less expensive and has faster turnaround time but is difficult to interpret.

Notes:

Table 65.1 • Conditions Included in the 1993 Surveillance Case Definition

Category A
Asymptomatic HIV infection
Persistent generalized lymphadenopathy
Acute HIV infection with accompanying illness or history of HIV infection

Category B
Bacillary angiomatosis
Candidiasis, oropharyngeal (thrush)
Candidiasis, vulvovaginal; persistent, frequent, or poorly responsive to treatment
Cervical dysplasia/carcinoma in situ
Constitutional symptoms, such as fever >38°C or diarrhea >1 mo
Hairy leukoplakia
Herpes zoster (shingles), involving at least two distinct episodes or more than one dermatome
Idiopathic thrombocytopenia purpura
Listeriosis
Pelvic inflammatory disease, particularly if complicated by tubo-ovarian abscess
Peripheral neuropathy

Category C
Candidiasis of bronchi, trachea, or lungs
Candidiasis, esophageal
Cervical cancer, invasive
Coccidioidomycosis, disseminated or extrapulmonary
Cryptococcosis, extrapulmonary
Cryptosporidiosis, chronic intestinal (>1 mo)
Cytomegalovirus disease (other than liver, spleen, or nodes)
Cytomegalovirus retinitis (with loss of vision)
Encephalopathy, HIV-related
Herpes simplex: chronic ulcer(s) (>1 mo); or bronchitis, pneumonitis, or esophagitis
Histoplasmosis, disseminated or extrapulmonary
Isosporiasis, chronic intestinal (duration >1 mo)
Kaposi sarcoma
Lymphoid interstitial pneumonia and/or pulmonary lymphoid hyperplasia[a]
Lymphoma, Burkitt's (or equivalent term)
Lymphoma, immunoblastic (or equivalent term)
Lymphoma, primary, of brain
Mycobacterium avium-intracellulare complex or *M. kansasii*, disseminated or extrapulmonary
Mycobacterium tuberculosis, any site (pulmonary[b] or extrapulmonary)
Mycobacterium, other species or unidentified species, disseminated or extrapulmonary
Pneumocystis carinii pneumonia
Pneumonia, recurrent[b]
Progressive multifocal leukoencephalopathy
Salmonella septicemia, recurrent
Toxoplasmosis of brain
Wasting syndrome resulting from HIV

[a]Children <13 yr old.
[b]Added in the 1993 expansions of the AIDS surveillance case definition for adolescents and adults.

Notes:

Table 65.2 • Characteristics of Antiretroviral Agents for the Treatment of Adult HIV Infection[5,9,299-301]

Drug	Dosage	Pharmacokinetic Parameters	Adverse Events	Administration Considerations
Nucleoside Reverse Transcriptase Inhibitors				
Zidovudine (AZT; ZDV) **Retrovir** *Preparations* Syrup: 10 mg/mL Capsule: 100 mg Tablet: 300 mg Injection: 10 mg/mL	300 mg BID or with 3TC as Combivir, 1 tablet BID or with 3TC and abacavir as Trizivir, 1 tablet BID	*Oral bioavailability:* 60% *Serum* $t_{1/2}$: 1.1 hr *Intracellular* $t_{1/2}$: 3 hr *Elimination:* hepatic glucuronidation; renal excretion of glucuronide metabolite	Bone marrow suppression (anemia and/or neutropenia); macrocytosis, myopathy (uncommon); hepatitis (uncommon); lactic acidosis with hepatic steatosis (rare)[a]; nail bed discoloration; subjective complaints with initiation of therapy (headache, nausea/vomiting, insomnia)	Can be administered without regard to meals (manufacturer recommends administration 30 min before or 1 hr after a meal)
Didanosine (ddI) **Videx** *Preparations* Pediatric powder for oral solution (when reconstituted as solution containing antacid): 10 mg/mL	>60 kg: 200 mg BID <60 kg: 250 mg QD; >60 kg: 400 mg QD	*Oral bioavailability:* 30–40% with tablet; 30% with powder *Serum* $t_{1/2}$: 1.6 hr *Intracellular* $t_{1/2}$: 25–40 hr *Elimination:* renal excretion ~50%	Pancreatitis, peripheral neuropathies (dose-related, reversible), nausea, diarrhea; lactic acidosis with hepatic steatosis (rare)[a]	Food decreases absorption (↓55%); administer ddI on an empty stomach (1 hr before or 2 hr after a meal)
Chewable tablets with buffers: 25, 50, 100, and 150 mg				When administering chewable tablets, at least 2 tablets per dose should be administered to ensure adequate buffering capacity
Buffered powder for oral solution: 100, 167, and 250 mg				Antacid buffer in tablets/powder may cause significant drug interactions with various medications; separate administration by at least 2 hr
Zalcitabine (ddC) **Hivid** *Preparations* Syrup: 0.1 mg/mL (investigational) Tablets: 0.375 and 0.75 mg	0.75 mg Q8H	*Oral bioavailability:* 85% *Serum* $t_{1/2}$: 1.2 hr *Intracellular* $t_{1/2}$: 3 hr *Elimination:* renal excretion ~70%	Peripheral neuropathy (dose-related, reversible), stomatitis, oral aphthous ulcers, pancreatitis (rare); lactic acidosis with hepatic steatosis (rare)[a]	Administer on empty stomach

Drug	Dose	Pharmacokinetics	Adverse effects	Administration
Stavudine (d4T) Zerit *Preparations* Solution: 1 mg/mL Capsules: 15, 20, 30, and 40 mg	>60 kg: 40 mg BID <60 kg: 20 mg BID	*Oral bioavailability:* 86% *Serum $t_{1/2}$:* 1 hr *Intracellular $t_{1/2}$:* 3.5 hr *Elimination:* renal excretion ~50%	Peripheral neuropathies, transaminase elevations; lactic acidosis with hepatic steatosis (rare)[a]	Can be administered without regard to meals
Lamivudine (3TC) Epivir *Preparations* Solution: 10 mg/mL Tablets: 150 mg	150 mg PO BID or with ZDV as Combivir, 1 tablet BID or with ZDV and abacavir, as Trizivir 1 tablet BID	*Oral bioavailability:* 86% *Serum $t_{1/2}$:* 3–6 hr *Intracellular $t_{1/2}$:* 12 hr *Elimination:* 70% unchanged in urine	Headache, nausea, fatigue, pancreatitis (rare; pediatric patients may be at increased risk)	Can be administered without regard to meals
Abacavir (1592) Ziagen *Preparations* Tablets: 300 mg Oral solution: 20 mg/mL	300 mg Q 12 hr or with ZDV and 3TC as Trizivir 1 tablet BID	*Oral bioavailability:* 83% *Serum $t_{1/2}$:* 1.5 hr *Intracellular $t_{1/2}$:* 3.3 hr *Elimination:* hepatic metabolism (noncytP450; alcohol dehydrogenase and glucuronyl transferase) with renal elimination of metabolites (82%)	Headache, nausea, vomiting, severe hypersensitivity reaction (~3–5%) characterized by nausea, malaise, abdominal pain and rash (can be fatal); patients with these symptoms should not be rechallenged with drug; lactic acidosis with hepatic steatosis (rare)[a]	Can be administered without regard to meals
Ribonucleotide Reductase Inhibitors				
Hydroxyurea Hydrea *Preparations* Capsules: 500 mg	500 mg BID	*Oral bioavailability:* 79% *Serum $t_{1/2}$:* 3.5–4.5 hr *Intracellular $t_{1/2}$:* unknown *Elimination:* hepatic metabolism with renal elimination	Bone marrow suppression, aphthous ulcers, hair loss, peripheral neuropathy	Administer on empty stomach; for those unable to swallow capsules, empty capsules into a glass of water and drink immediately
Nonnucleoside Reverse Transcriptase Inhibitors				
Nevirapine Viramune *Preparations* Suspension: 10 mg/mL (investigational) Tablets: 200 mg	200 mg PO QD ×7 days, then 200 mg PO BID (400 mg PO QD under investigation)	*Oral bioavailability:* >90% *Serum $t_{1/2}$:* 25–30 hr *Intracellular $t_{1/2}$:* unknown *Elimination:* metabolized by cytP450 (3A4 inducer) with 80% glucuronide metabolite being eliminated in urine	Rash (rare; can be severe, e.g., Stevens-Johnson syndrome),[a,b] hepatitis, elevated transaminases, nausea, vomiting, diarrhea	Can be administered without regard to meals

(continued)

Table 65.2 • Characteristics of Antiretroviral Agents for the Treatment of Adult HIV Infection[5,9,299-301] (continued)

Drug	Dosage	Pharmacokinetic Parameters	Adverse Events	Administration Considerations
Nonnucleoside Reverse Transcriptase Inhibitors (continued)				
Delavirdine **Rescriptor** *Preparations* Tablets: 100 mg	400 mg Q8H (four 100-mg tabs in 3 oz water to produce slurry) 600 mg BID (under investigation)	*Oral bioavailability:* 85% *Serum $t_{1/2}$:* 5.8 hr *Intracellular $t_{1/2}$:* unknown *Elimination:* metabolized by cytP450 (3A4 inhibitor) with 51% being eliminated in urine as metabolites	Rash (rare; can be severe, e.g., Stevens-Johnson syndrome),[a] nausea, headache, transaminase elevations	Can be administered without regard to meals
Efavirenz (DMP-266) **Sustiva** *Preparations* Capsules: 50, 100, and 200 mg	600 mg QHS	*Oral bioavailability:* 60–70% *Serum $t_{1/2}$:* 40–52 hr *Intracellular $t_{1/2}$:* unknown *Elimination:* hepatically metabolized (3A4 mixed inhibitor/inducer)	Rash (rare; can be severe, e.g., Stevens-Johnson syndrome),[a,b] dizziness, light-headedness, vivid dreams, headache, fatigue, nausea; false-positive cannabinoid test	Avoid taking with high-fat meals, levels ↑ 50% (increased risk for central nervous system toxicity)
Protease Inhibitors				
Indinavir **Crixivan** *Preparations* Capsule: 200 and 400 mg	800 mg Q 8 hr (BID dosing ineffective when sole protease inhibitor) 800 mg BID with 200 mg BID Ritonavir *or* 400 mg BID with 400 mg BID Ritonavir	*Oral bioavailability:* 65% *Serum $t_{1/2}$:* 1.5–2 hr *Intracellular $t_{1/2}$:* unknown *Elimination:* hepatically metabolized via cytP450 3A4 (inhibitor)	Nephrolithiasis, nausea, vomiting, asymptomatic hyperbilirubinemia, transaminases elevations, headache, taste disturbances, dry skin, thickening of nail beds, hyperglycemia,[a] lipodystrophies,[a] hypertriglyceridemia,[a] possible increased bleeding and factor VIII requirements in hemophiliacs[a]	Must be taken on an empty stomach (1 hr before or 2 hr after a meal); may take with skim milk or lowfat meal; adequate hydration necessary (at least 1.5 L of liquids per 24 hr) to minimize risk for nephrolithiasis
Lopinavir	133.3 mg with Ritonavir 33.3 mg as Kaletra 3 caps BID		Similar to Ritonvir (see below) but decreased frequency	Take with food

Drug/Preparations	Dosage	Pharmacokinetics	Adverse Effects	Administration
Ritonavir **Norvir** *Preparations* Oral solution: 80 mg/mL Capsules: 100 mg	600 mg Q 12 hr (days 1–2: 300 mg BID; days 3–5: 400 mg BID; days 6–13: 500 mg BID; day 14: 600 mg BID)	*Oral bioavailability:* unknown *Serum $t_{1/2}$:* 3–5 hr *Intracellular $t_{1/2}$:* unknown *Elimination:* extensive hepatic metabolism via cytP450 3A4 >2D6 (potent 3A4 inhibitor)	Nausea, vomiting, diarrhea (up to 50%); circumoral and extremities paresthesias; asthenia; hepatitis; taste perversions; transaminases elevations; elevated creatine phosphokinase levels; hyperglycemia[a], lipodystrophies[a]; hypertriglyceridemia[a]; possible increased bleeding and factor VIII requirements in hemophiliacs[a]	Take with food if possible to improve tolerability; dosage should be titrated upward to minimize gastrointestinal adverse events; refrigerate capsules
Nelfinavir **Viracept** *Preparations* Powder for oral suspension: 50 mg per one level scoop (200 mg per one level tsp) Tablet: 250 mg	750 mg TID or 1,250 mg BID	*Oral bioavailability:* 20–80% *Serum $t_{1/2}$:* 3.5–5 hr *Intracellular $t_{1/2}$:* unknown *Elimination:* hepatic metabolism via cytP450	Diarrhea (~20%), hyperglycemia,[a] lipodystrophies,[a] hypertriglyceridemia,[a] possible increased bleeding and factor VIII requirements in hemophiliacs[a]	Administer with meal or light snack (levels increased two to three times)
Saquinavir **Fortovase** (soft-gel capsules) **Invirase** (hard-gel capsules) *Preparations* Soft-gel capsules: 200 mg Hard-gel capsules: 200 mg	1,200 mg TID (soft-gel capsule) (1,600 mg BID of soft-gel capsule under investigation) Hard-gel cap should be used only in combination with ritonavir; 400 mg BID when used in combination with ritonavir (either formulation)	*Oral bioavailability:* 4% hard-gel capsule; soft-gel capsule not determined *Serum $t_{1/2}$:* 1–2 hr *Intracellular $t_{1/2}$:* unknown *Elimination:* hepatic metabolism via cytP450 3A4 (inhibitor)	Nausea, diarrhea, abdominal pain, dyspepsia, headache, transaminase elevations, hyperglycemia,[a] lipodystrophies,[a] hypertriglyceridemia,[a] possible increased bleeding and factor VIII requirements in hemophiliacs[a]	Take with full meal (levels increase sixfold); soft-gel capsules should be refrigerated or can be stored at room temperature for up to 3 mo
Amprenavir **Agenerase** *Preparations* Capsules: 50 and 150 mg Solution: 15 mg/mL	1,200 mg PO BID 450 mg BID in combination with 100 mg BID Ritonavir	*Oral bioavailability:* undetermined *Serum $t_{1/2}$:* 7.1–10.6 hr *Intracellular $t_{1/2}$:* unknown *Elimination:* hepatic metabolism via cytP450 3A4 (inhibitor)	Nausea, vomiting, diarrhea, rash (Stevens-Johnson syndrome has rarely been reported), circumoral paresthesias, hyperglycemia,[a] lipodystrophies,[a] hypertriglyceridemia,[a] possible increased bleeding and factor VIII requirements in hemophiliacs[a]	Can be taken without regard to meals; however, should not be taken with high-fat meals

[a]Although not conclusive, appears to be a class effect.
[b]In clinical trials, the nonnucleoside reverse transcriptase inhibitor (NNRTI) was discontinued because of rash in 7% of patients taking nevirapine, 4.3% of patients taking delavirdine, and 1.7% of patients taking efavirenz. Rare cases of Stevens-Johnson syndrome have been reported with all three NNRTIs.

Table 65.3 • Clinically Significant Drug–Drug Interactions with Antiretroviral Agents Used for Treatment of HIV[a,5,9,60,299,300,302]

Agent	Mechanism of Interaction	Interacting Drugs
Nucleoside Reverse Transcriptase Inhibitors		
Zidovudine (AZT; ZDV)	Decrease ZDV clearance: monitor for ZDV toxicity	Fluconazole, probenecid, nonsteroidal anti-inflammatory agents
	Additive toxicity: bone marrow suppression; monitor for toxicity	Dapsone, flucytosine, trimethoprim-sulfamethoxazole, chemotherapeutic agents, ganciclovir, interferon-alpha, acyclovir, hydroxyurea, primaquine, pyrimethamine, ribavirin, sulfadiazine, trimetrexate
Didanosine (ddI)	Decreased absorption of interacting drug because of antacid buffer of ddI (either chelation or increase in gastric pH); separate administration by at least 2 hr	Ketoconazole, itraconazole, tetracyclines, fluoroquinolones, delavirdine, indinavir, ritonavir, dapsone
	Decreased ddI serum levels: consider ddI dosage increase	Methadone
	Increased ddI absorption; potential for ddI toxicity: monitor carefully	H₂ blockers, antacids, omeprazole
	Additive toxicity; peripheral neuropathies: monitor carefully	d4T, vinca alkaloids, oral ganciclovir, isoniazid, metronidazole, hydroxyurea
	Decreased ddI clearance; increased risk for ddI toxicity (pancreatitis)	Ganciclovir (oral and IV)
Zalcitabine (ddC)	Additive toxicity; peripheral neuropathies: monitor carefully	d4T, vinca alkaloids, isoniazid, metronidazole, hydroxyurea
	Additive toxicity; pancreatitis: monitor carefully	Oral ganciclovir, d4T
	Potential for decreased renal clearance of ddC by interacting drug, increased risk for ddC toxicity: monitor carefully	Cimetidine, amphotericin, foscarnet, aminoglycosides
	Decreased absorption of ddC by interacting drug: separate administration	Antacids
Stavudine (d4T)	Additive toxicity; peripheral neuropathies: monitor carefully	ddI, ddC, vinca alkaloids, oral ganciclovir, isoniazid, metronidazole
Lamivudine (3TC)	None	None
Abacavir (1592)	Decreased metabolism of both abacavir and interacting drug: monitor for toxicity	Disulfiram, chlorzoxazone, chlorpromazine, isoniazid, chloral hydrate, ethanol
Nonnucleoside Reverse Transcriptase Inhibitors		
Nevirapine (NVP)	NVP-induced cytP450 enzyme metabolism; decreased plasma concentrations of interacting agent	Rifampin, rifabutin, oral contraceptives (use alternative or additional methods of birth control), triazolam, midazolam, protease inhibitors,[a] β-blockers, doxycycline, calcium channel blockers, methadone, quinidine, warfarin, digoxin

Drug	Mechanism	Interacting agents
Delavirdine (DLV)	DLV inhibition of cytP450 enzyme metabolism: increased plasma concentrations of interacting agent; monitor for toxicity	Protease inhibitors,[a] clarithromycin, quinidine, warfarin, dapsone
	cytP450 inhibition by interacting agent: increase in DLV plasma concentrations; monitor for DLV toxicity	Clarithromycin, ketoconazole, fluoxetine
	Decreased absorption of DLV: separate administration by at least 1 hr	ddI
	Decreased absorption of DLV by interacting drug	H_2 antagonists
Efavirenz (DMP)	DMP-induced cytP450 enzyme metabolism: decreased plasma concentration of interacting agent	Protease inhibitors,[a] clarithromycin (alternative recommended), rifabutin (increase rifabutin dosage to 450 mg QD)
	DMP inhibition of cytP450 enzyme metabolism: potential for interacting drug toxicity	Oral contraceptives (use alternative or additional methods of birth control)
Protease Inhibitors[b]		
Indinavir (IDV)	IDV inhibition of cytP450 enzyme metabolism: increased plasma concentrations of interacting agent; monitor for toxicity	Rifabutin (decrease dosage of rifabutin by 50%), protease inhibitors,[a] oral contraceptives, sildenafil, hemoglobin coacetyl-A reductase inhibitors, gemfibrozil, clarithromycin
	cytP450 induction by interacting agent: decreased plasma concentrations of IDV	Rifabutin (increase dosage of IDV to 1,000 mg TID), anticonvulsants, protease inhibitors[a]
	cytP450 inhibition by interacting agent: increased plasma concentrations of IDV	Ketoconazole/itraconazole (reduce dosage of IDV to 600 mg Q 8 hr), nonnucleoside reverse transcriptase inhibitors,[a] protease inhibitors[a]
	Decreased absorption of IDV: separate administration by at least 2 hr	ddI
Nelfinavir (NFV)	NFV induction of cytP450 enzyme metabolism: decreased plasma concentrations of interacting agent	Oral contraceptives (use alternative or additional contraceptive methods)
	NFV inhibition of cytP450 enzyme metabolism: increased plasma concentrations of interacting agent; monitor for toxicity	Protease inhibitors,[a] rifabutin (reduce dosage by 50%), sildenafil, hemoglobin coacetyl-A reductase inhibitors, gemfibrozil
	cytP450 induction by interacting agent: decreased plasma concentrations of NFV	Rifabutin (increase NFV to 1,000 mg TID), anticonvulsants, nonnucleoside reverse transcriptase inhibitors[a]
	cytP450 inhibition by interacting agent: increased plasma concentrations of NFV; monitor for toxicity	Ketoconazole/itraconazole, protease inhibitors[a]

(continued)

Table 65.3 • Clinically Significant Drug–Drug Interactions with Antiretroviral Agents Used for Treatment of HIV[a,5,9,60,299,300,302] (continued)

Agent	Mechanism of Interaction	Interacting Drugs
Protease Inhibitors[b] (continued)		
Ritonavir (RTV)	Substantial cytP450 enzyme inhibition by RTV: increased plasma concentration of interacting agent; monitor for toxicity	Protease inhibitors,[a] nonnucleoside reverse transcriptase inhibitors,[a] tricyclic antidepressants, serotonin receptor inhibitors (e.g., fluoxetine, sertraline), calcium channel blockers, β-blockers, lidocaine, ondansetron, quinine, prednisone, pravastatin, tamoxifen, tacrolimus, vinca alkaloids, haloperidol, hydrocodone, oxycodone, risperidone, thioridazine, tramadol, venlafaxine, nonsteroidal anti-inflammatory agents, glipizide, glyburide, warfarin, albendazole, cimetidine, desipramine (reduce dosage), cyclophosphamide, fluvastatin, gemfibrozil, ketoconazole/itraconazole/miconazole, methadone, pentoxifylline, phenobarbital, tocainide, prazosin, prochlorperazine, promethazine, rifabutin (decrease dosage to 150 mg QD) clarithromycin, sildenafil
	cytP450 enzyme induction by RTV: decreased serum concentrations of interacting agent	Oral contraceptives (use alternative or additional contraceptive methods), theophylline, methadone, sulfamethoxazole, zidovudine, divalproex, hydromorphone, lamotrigine, lorazepam, diphenoxylate
	Possible disulfiram-like reaction when coadministered with RTV (capsule and liquid contain alcohol)	Disulfiram, metronidazole
	Decreased absorption of RTV: separate administration by at least 2 hr	ddI
Saquinavir (SQV)	cytP450 induction by interacting agent: decreased plasma concentrations of SQV	Nonnucleoside reverse transcriptase inhibitors[a]; (Absolute Contraindications), dexamethasone, anticonvulsants
	cytP450 inhibition by interacting agent: increased plasma concentrations of SQV	Protease inhibitors,[a] nonnucleoside reverse transcriptase inhibitors,[a] ketoconazole/itraconazole, clarithromycin
	SQV inhibition of cytP450 metabolism: increased risk for toxicity of interacting drug; monitor carefully	Calcium channel blockers, clindamycin, clarithromycin, dapsone, quinidine, sildenafil, gemfibrozil
Amprenavir (AMP)	AMP inhibition of cytP450 metabolism: increased risk for toxicity of interacting drug; monitor carefully	Rifabutin (reduce rifabutin dosage by 50%), amiodarone, lidocaine, quinidine, warfarin, tricyclic antidepressants, hemoglobin coacetyl-A reductase inhibitors, sildenafil, dapsone, erythromycin, itraconazole/ketoconazole, alprazolam, clorazepate, diazepam, flurazepam, calcium channel blockers
	cytP450 enzyme induction by interacting drug: potential for decrease AmP concentrations	Anticonvulsants

[a]See Table 65.4 for Protease Inhibitor–Protease Inhibitor and Protease Inhibitor–Nonnucleoside Reverse Transcriptase Inhibitor Drug Interactions.
[b]Many potential drug–drug interactions with the protease inhibitors, nonnucleoside reverse transcriptase inhibitors have not been fully evaluated but have been identified based upon their potential for cytP450 isoenzyme interactions.

Table 65.4 • Drug Interactions Between Protease Inhibitors and Nonnucleoside Reverse Transcriptase Inhibitors[7,9,232,304,305,a]

	Indinavir (IDV)	Ritonavir (RTV)	Saquinavir (SQV)	Nelfinavir (NFV)	Nevirapine (NVP)	Delavirdine (DLV)	Efavirenz (DMP)
Indinavir (IDV)		IDV: ↑ 2–5× RTV: no effect Dosage: limited data for IDV 400 mg BID + RTV 400 mg BID; IDV 800 mg BID + RTV 200 mg BID; or IDV 800 mg BID + RTV 100 mg BID	SQV: ↑ 4–7× IDV: no effect Dosage: ND Antagonism in vitro	IDV ↑ 50% NFV: ↑ 80% Dosage: limited data for IDV 1,200 mg BID + NFV 1,250 mg BID	IDV ↓ 28% NVP: no effect Dosage: standard	IDV: ↑ 40% Dosage: IDV 600 mg Q 8 hr	IDV: ↓ 31% Dosage: IDV—1,000 mg Q 8 hr DMP—no change
Ritonavir (RTV)	IDV: ↑ 2–5× RTV: no effect Dosage: limited data for IDV 400 mg BID + RTV 400 mg BID; IDV 800 mg BID + RTV 200 mg BID; or IDV 800 mg BID + RTV 100 mg BID		RTV: no effect SQV: ↑ 20× Dosage: RTV—400 mg BID; SQV (hard-gel or soft-gel capsules)—400 mg BID	RTV: no effect NFV: ↑ 1.5× Dosage: limited data for 400 mg BID × NFV 500–750 mg BID	RTV: ↓ 11% NVP: no effect Dosage: standard	RTV: ↑ 70% Dosage: RTV—consider 400 mg BID	RTV: ↑ 18% DMP: ↑ 21% Dosage: RTV 600 mg BID (500 mg BID for intolerance)
Saquinavir (SQV)	SQV: ↑ 4–7× IDV: no effect Dosage: ND Antagonism in vitro	RTV: no effect SQV: ↑ 20× Dosage: RTV—400 mg BID; SQV (hard-gel or soft-gel capsules)—400 mg BID		SQV: ↑ 3–5× NFV: ↑ 20% Dosage: standard NFV, Fortovase 800 mg TID	SQV: ↓ 25% Dosage: ND	SQV: ↑ 5× DLV: ND Dosage: Fortovase 800 mg TID, DLV standard (monitor transaminase levels)	SQV: ↓ 62% DMP: ↓ 12% Coadministration not recommended

(continued)

Table 65.4 • Drug Interactions Between Protease Inhibitors and Nonnucleoside Reverse Transcriptase Inhibitors[7,9,232,304,305,a] (continued)

	Indinavir (IDV)	Ritonavir (RTV)	Saquinavir (SQV)	Nelfinavir (NFV)	Nevirapine (NVP)	Delavirdine (DLV)	Efavirenz (DMP)
Nelfinavir (NFV)	IDV: ↑ 50% NFV: ↑ 80% Dosage: limited data for IDV 1,200 mg BID + NFV 1,250 mg BID	RTV: no effect NFV: ↑ 1.5× Dosage: limited data for 400 mg BID + NFV 500–750 mg BID	SQV: ↑ 3–5× NFV: ↑ 20% Dosage: standard NFV, Fortovase 800 mg TID		NFV: ↑ 10% NVP: no effect Dosage: standard	NFV: ↑ 2× DLV: ↓ 50% Dosage: ND (monitor for neutropenic complications)	NFV: ↑ 20% DMP: no change Dosage: ND
Nevirapine (NVP)	IDV: ↓ 28% NVP: no effect Dosage: standard	RTV: ↓ 11% NVP: no effect Dosage: standard	SQV: ↓ 25% Dosage: ND	NFV: ↑ 10% NVP: no effect Dosage: standard		ND	ND
Delavirdine (DLV)	IDV: ↑ 40% Dosage: IDV 600 Q 8 hr	RTV: ↑ 70% Dosage: RTV—consider 400 mg BID	SQV: ↑ 5× DLV: ND Dosage: Fortovase 800 mg TID, DLV standard (monitor transaminase levels)	NFV: ↑ 2× DLV: ↓ 50% Dosage: ND (monitor for neutropenic complications)	ND		ND
Efavirenz (DMP)	IDV: ↓ 31% Dosage: IDV—1,000 mg Q 8 hr; DMP—no change	RIT: ↑ 18% DMP: ↑ 21% Dosage: RTV 600 mg BID (500 mg BID for intolerance)	SQV: ↓ 62% DMP: ↓ 12% Coadministration not recommended	NFV: ↑ 20% DMP: no change Dosage: ND	ND	ND	

aND = No data.

Table 65.5 • Antiretroviral Agents Used in the Treatment of Pediatric HIV Infection^{a,9}

Drug	Dosage	Special Instructions	Comments
Nucleoside Analog Reverse Transcriptase Inhibitors			
Zidovudine (AZT; ZDV)	*Premature infants:* 1.5 mg/kg Q 12 hr from birth until 2 wk of age, then increase to 2 mg/kg Q 8 hr (under investigation) *Neonatal dosage:* oral—2 mg/kg Q 6 hr; IV—1.5 mg/kg Q 6 hr *Pediatric usual dosage:* oral—160 mg/m^2 Q 8 hr; IV (intermittent infusion)—120 mg/m^2 Q 6 hr; IV (continuous infusion)—20 mg/m^2/hr *Pediatric dosage range:* 90–180 mg/m^2 Q 6–8 hr *Adolescent/adult dosage:* 200 mg TID or 300 mg BID	Can be administered with food (although manufacturer recommends administration 30 min before or 1 hr after meal) Infuse IV loading dose or intermittent infusion dose over 1 hr *For IV solutions:* dilute with 5% dextrose injection solution to concentration of 4 mg/mL; refrigerated diluted solution is stable for 24 hr	Decrease dosage in patients with severe renal impairment. Reduced dosage may be necessary in patients with substantial hepatic dysfunction. Some pediatric HIV experts would use a dosage of 180 mg/m^2 of body surface area Q 12 hr when using in drug combinations with other antiretrovirals compounds, but data on this dosing in children is limited.
Didanosine (ddI)	*Neonatal dosage (<90 days old):* 50 mg/m^2 Q 12 hr *Pediatric usual dosage:* 90 mg/m^2 Q 12 hr *Pediatric dosage range:* 90–150 mg/m^2 Q 12 hr *Adolescent/adult dosage:* >60 kg—200 mg BID; <60 kg—125 mg BID (dosages of 300–400 mg QD under evaluation)	Food decreases absorption: administer ddI on an empty stomach (1 hr before or 2 hr after a meal) *For oral solution:* Shake well and keep refrigerated; admixture is stable for 30 days When administering chewable tablets, at least 2 tablets should be administered to ensure adequate buffering capacity	Higher dosages may be necessary for central nervous system disease. ddI formulation contains buffering agent or antacids that may decrease the absorption of other drugs that require an acidic medium for absorption or chelate with the antacid buffer (see Drug Interaction Table 65.3); separate administration of agents by at least 2 hr.
Zalcitabine (ddC)	*Neonatal dosage:* unknown *Pediatric usual dosage:* 0.01 mg/kg Q 8 hr *Pediatric dosage range:* 0.005–0.01 mg/kg Q 8 hr *Adolescent/adult dosage:* 0.75 mg TID	Administer on empty stomach; antacids decrease absorption	Decrease dosage in patients with impaired renal function.
Stavudine (d4T)	*Neonatal dosage:* under evaluation *Pediatric usual dosage:* 1 mg/kg Q 12 hr (up to weight of 30 kg) *Adolescent/adult dosage:* >60 kg—40 mg BID; 30–60 kg: 30 mg BID	Can be administered with food *For oral solution:* Shake well and keep refrigerated; solution stable for 30 days	Decrease dosage in patients with renal impairment.
Lamivudine (3TC)	*Neonatal dosage (<30 days old):* 2 mg/kg BID *Pediatric usual dosage:* 4 mg/kg BID *Adolescent/adult dosage:* 150 mg BID	Can be administered with food *For oral solution:* Store at room temperature	Decrease dosage in patients with impaired renal function.

(continued)

Table 65.5 • Antiretroviral Agents Used in the Treatment of Pediatric HIV Infection[a,9] (continued)

Drug	Dosage	Special Instructions	Comments
Nonnucleoside Reverse Transcriptase Inhibitors			
Nevirapine	*Neonatal dosage (<90 days old; under investigation):* 5 mg/kg QD ×14 days, followed by 120 mg/m² Q 12 hr ×14 days, followed by 200 mg/m² Q 12 hr *Pediatric usual dosage:* 120–200 mg/m² Q 12 hr (initiate with 120 mg/m² QD ×14 days; increase to full dose Q 12 hr if there are no rash or other untoward events) *Adolescent/adult dosage:* 200 mg BID (initiate therapy at half dose ×14 days; increase to full dose if there are no rash or other untoward events)	Can be administered with food *For investigational suspension:* Must be shaken well; store at room temperature	To avoid potential for rash, titrate dosage over 2–4 wk. If rash occurs during the initial 14-day lead-in period, do not increase dosage until rash resolves. Nevirapine should be discontinued immediately in patients who develop severe rash accompanied by constitutional symptoms (e.g., fever, oral lesions, conjunctivitis, or blistering). Induces cytP450 3A enzyme system; potential for multiple drug interactions.[b]
Delavirdine	*Neonatal dosage:* unknown *Pediatric dosage:* unknown *Adolescent/adult dosage:* 400 mg TID	Can be administered with food; tablets can be dissolved in water and the resulting solution taken promptly	Inhibitor of cytP450 3A; potential for multiple drug interactions.[b]
Efavirenz (DMP-266)	*Neonatal dosage:* unknown *Pediatric dosage (age >3 yr; administer QD):* 10–<15 kg—200 mg; 15–<20 kg—250 mg; 20 –<25 kg—300 mg; 25–<32.5 kg—350 mg; 32.5–<40 kg—400 mg; >40 kg—600 mg *Adolescent/adult dosage:* 600 mg QD	Can be taken with and without food; however, efavirenz should not be taken with a high-fat meal (increased absorption resulting in potential for increased adverse events) Capsules may be opened and added to liquids or foods; grape jelly improves the palatability of efavirenz Administer dose at bedtime (particularly during the first 2–4 wk) to minimize central nervous system side effects	Efavirenz is a mixed inhibitor/inducer of cytP450 enzyme metabolism.[b]
Protease Inhibitors			
Indinavir	*Neonatal dosage:* unknown—due to side effect of hyperbilirubinemia, should not be given to neonates until further information available *Pediatric dosage:* 500 mg/m² Q 8 hr (under investigation) *Adolescent/adult dosage:* 800 mg Q 8 hr (1,000–1,200 mg BID under investigation)	Administer on an empty stomach 1 hr before or 2 hr after a meal (or can be taken with a light snack); adequate hydration is necessary to minimize risk for nephrolithiasis Capsules are sensitive to moisture and should be stored in original container with desiccant	Cytochrome P450 3A4 responsible for metabolism, potential for multiple drug interactions.[b] Decrease dosage in patients with hepatic insufficiency.

Drug	Dosage	Administration	Interactions
Nelfinavir	*Neonatal dosage:* 10 mg/kg TID (under investigation) *Pediatric dosage:* 20–30 mg/kg TID *Adolescent/adult dosage:* 750 mg TID (1,000–1,250 mg BID under investigation)	Administer with a meal or light snack *For oral solution:* Powder may be mixed with water, milk, pudding, ice cream, or formula (for up to 6 hr); do not mix with any acidic food or juice because of resulting poor taste Tablets readily dissolve in water and produce a dispersion that can be mixed with milk, chocolate milk; tablets can also be crushed and administered with pudding	Nelfinavir is an inhibitor of cytP450 3A4 metabolism; potential for multiple-drug interactions.[b]
Ritonavir	*Neonatal dosage:* unknown *Pediatric dosage:* 400 mg/m² Q 12 hr (to minimize nausea/vomiting, initiate therapy at 250 mg/m² Q 12 hr and increase dosage to full dose over 5 days) *Pediatric dosage range:* 350–400 mg/m² Q 12 hr *Adolescent/adult dosage:* 600 mg BID (400 mg BID when used in combination with saquinavir)	Administer with food Oral capsule must be kept in refrigerator *For oral solution:* Must be kept refrigerated and stored in original container, can be kept at room temperature if used within 30 days *To improve tolerance in children:* (1) Mix oral solution with milk, vanilla or chocolate pudding, or ice cream; (2) Have the child chew ice or eat frozen popsicles to dull the taste buds; (3) Have the child eat peanut butter before taking the dose; or (4) Have the child eat "strong-tasting" foods such as maple syrup or cheese before taking the dose	Ritonavir significantly interacts with a number of cytP450 isoenzymes, including 3A4; high potential for multiple drug interactions.[b]
Saquinavir	*Neonatal dosage:* unknown *Pediatric dosage:* unknown *Adolescent/adult dosage:* Soft-gel caps—1,200 mg TID; hard-gel caps—600 mg TID (400 mg BID [of either formulation] when used in combination with ritonavir)	Administer within 2 hr of a full meal to increase absorption; concurrent administration with grapefruit juice increases saquinavir concentrations; can cause photosensitivity reactions after sun exposure; sunscreen and/or protective clothing is recommended	Saquinavir interacts with cytP450 enzyme system; potential for multiple drug interactions (risk is substantially lower than that seen for ritonavir and nelfinavir).[b]

[a] See Table 65.2 for various dosage forms.
[b] See Tables 65.3, 65.4 for potential drug interactions.

Table 65.6 • HIV Internet Resources

Government Sites
Adult AIDS Clinical Trials Resources: http://www.actis.org/
American Foundation for AIDS Research: http://www.amfar.org
Centers for Disease Control: http://www.cdc.gov
Centers for Disease Control Prevention Information Network: http://www.cdcnac.org/
Community Provider AIDS Training Center: http://itsa.ucsf.edu/warmline/
Consensus Panel Guidelines On-line: http://www.hivatis.org/trtgdlns.html
CDC National AIDS Clearinghouse: http://www.cdcnac.org
Government HIV Mutation Charts: http://hiv-web.lanl.gov
Henry J. Kaiser Foundation: http://www.kff.org/archive/aidshiv.html
HIV/AIDS Treatment Information Network: http://www.hivatis.org
International AIDS Vaccine Initiative: http://www.iavi.org/
Morbidity and Mortality Weekly: http://www2.cdc.gov/mmwr/
MMWR AIDS resource: http://www.cdc.gov/nchstp/hiv_aids/pubs/mmwr.htm
National Institute of Allergy and Infectious Diseases: http://www.niaid.nih.gov
National Prevention Information Network: http://www.cdcnpin.org
Pediatric HIV Resource Page: http://www.pedhivaids.org
Post Exposure Prevention WebSite: http://epi-center.ucsf.edu/PEP/pepnet.html

United Nations AIDS WebSite: http://www.unaids.org/ University Sites
Harvard AIDS Institute: http://www.hsph.harvard.edu/hai.html
Johns Hopkins AIDS Service: http://www.hopkins-aids.edu
University of California, HIV/AIDS Program: http://hivinsite.ucsf.edu

Journal Sites
AIDS: http://www.aidsonline.com/
Annals of Internal Medicine: http://www.acponline.org
Antimicrobial Agents and Chemotherapy: http://aac.asm.org/
Journal of the American Medical Association: http://www.ama-assn.org
British Medical Journal: http://www.bmj.com
Clinical Infectious Diseases: http://www.journals.uchicago.edu/CID/
Journal of Antimicrobial Agents and Chemotherapy: http://www.oup.co.uk/jac/
Journal of Infectious Diseases: http://www.journals.uchicago.edu/JID/
The Lancet: http://www.thelancet.com
Nature: http://www.nature.com
Nature Medicine: http://medicine.nature.com/
New England Journal of Medicine: http://www.nejm.org
Science: http://sciencemag.org

AIDS Treatment/Advocacy Groups
AIDS Treatment Project United Kingdom: http://www.atp.org.uk/
Bulletin of Experimental Treatment for AIDS (BETA): http://www.sfaf.org/beta
Project Inform: http://www.projinf.org
San Francisco AIDS Foundation: http://www.sfaf.org/index.html
Treatment Action Group: http://www.aidsnyc.org/tag

Other Relevant Sites
The AIDS Map: http://www.aidsmap.com
AIDS Education Global Information System: http://www.aegis.com
Healthcare Communications Group: http://www.medscape.com
Immunenet: http://www.aids.org
Physician's Research Network: http://www.prn.org
The Body: http://www.thebody.com
Retroviral Conference: http://www.retroconference.org
Worlds AIDS Conference: http://www.aids98.ch/

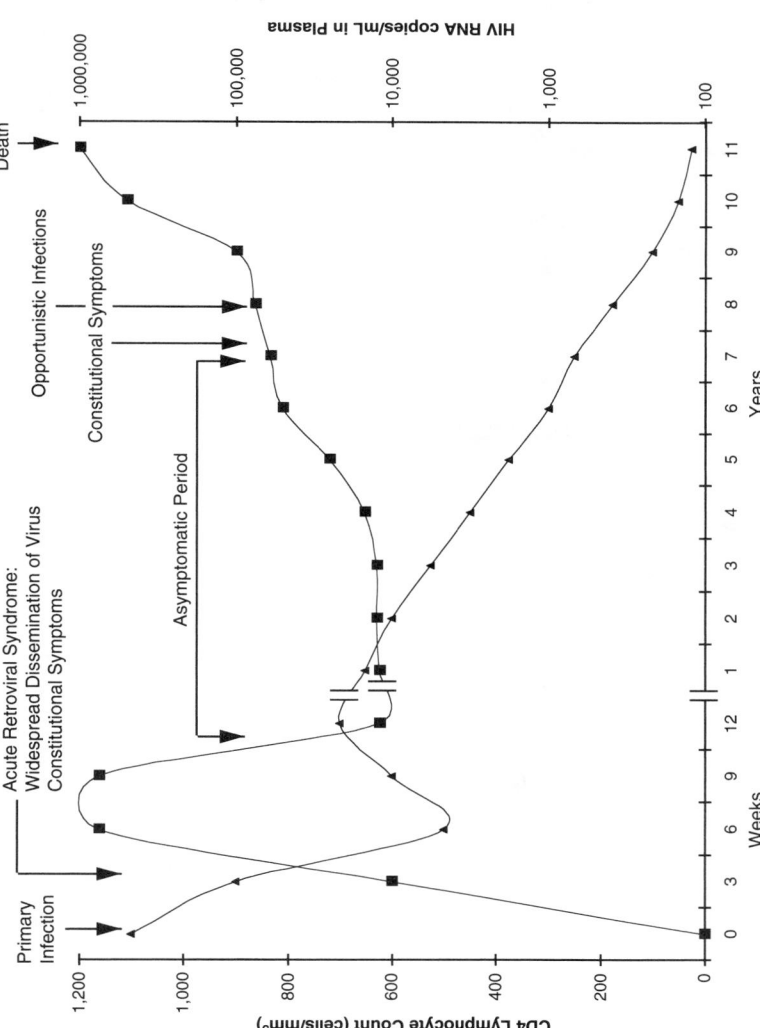

Fig. 65.1 Sample Disease Course for an Untreated HIV-Infected Individual Showing Relationship Among Immunologic, Virologic, and Clinical Outcomes Over Time; Constitutional Symptoms Include Fever, Night Sweats, and Weight Loss ■ **Viral Load Values;** ▲ **CD4 T Lymphocytes.** (Adapted from references 25 and 29.)

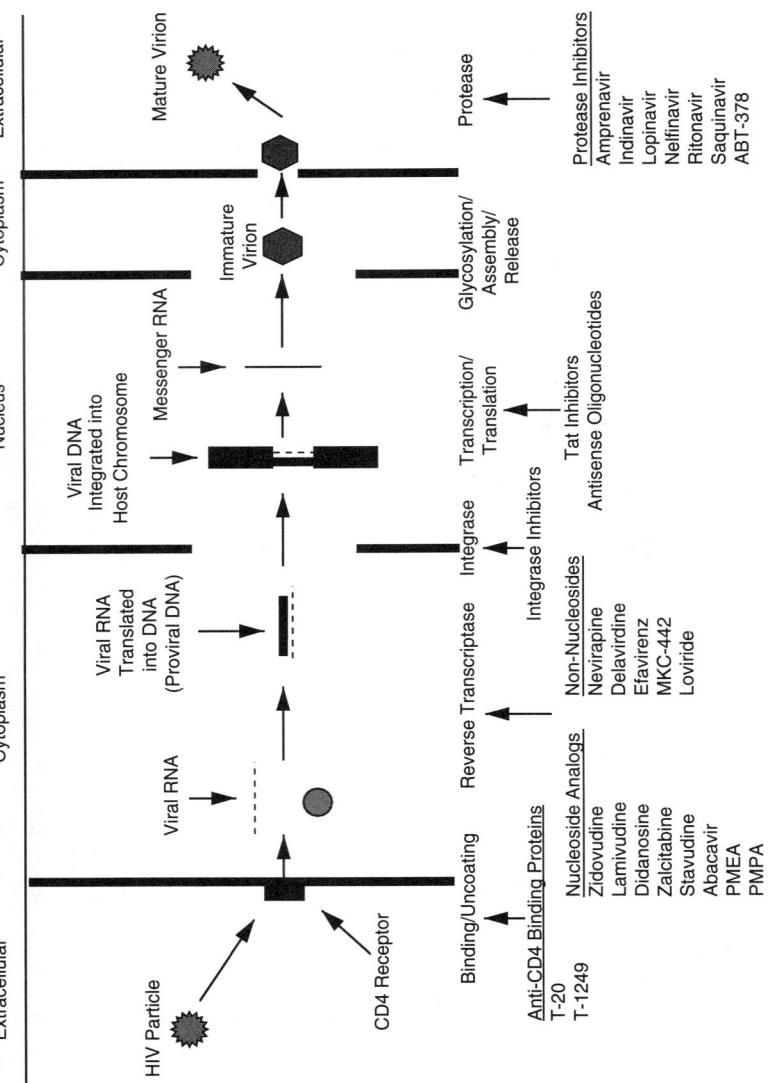

Fig. 65.2 Schematic Representation of HIV-1 Life Cycle Showing Sites of Activity for the Various Antiretroviral Agents. (Adapted and updated from reference 303.)

The reader is referred to Chapter 67: Pharmacotherapy of Human Immunodeficiency Virus, written by *Andrew D. Luber, Pharm.D.*, in the seventh edition of **Applied Therapeutics: The Clinical Use of Drugs** for a more in-depth discussion. All notations to reference numbers are based on the reference list at the end of that chapter. The editors of this handbook express their thanks to Dr. Luber and acknowledge that this chapter is based upon his work.

Notes:

Notes:

Chapter 66

Opportunistic Infections (OIs) in HIV Patients

♦ There is a close link between CD4 count and the likelihood of specific opportunistic infections in HIV+ patients (Fig. 66.1).

♦ HAART has decreased the incidence of several OIs. Discontinuation of prophylactic OI therapy can take place when CD4 lymphocytes rise above the threshold associated with risk for infection.

♦ Primary prophylaxis of OIs in HIV-infected patients (Table 66.1)

♦ Specific OIs: Treatment

• *Pneumocystis carinii* (Table 66.2)

• Cerebral toxoplasmosis

—Treatment of choice is pyrimethamine 100 mg; loading dose ×1, then 75–100 mg daily PO *plus* sulfadiazine 1–1.5 gm Q6H PO *plus* folinic acid 10–15 mg PO daily

—Primary toxicities include bone marrow suppression (pyrimethamine) and rash and crystalluria (sulfadiazine)

• Cytomegalovirus retinitis (Tables 66.3 and 66.4)

• Cryptococcal meningitis

—Treatment of choice is amphotericin 0.7 mg/kg/daily IV plus 100 mg/kg/daily PO divided in 4 doses.

—Once patient is stabilized, consolidation therapy with fluconazole 400 mg PO QD for 10 weeks is initiated.

—After consolidation therapy with fluconazole, daily suppression with fluconazole 200 mg PO QD is continued indefinitely.

• *Mycobacterium avium* complex (Table 66.5)

—Commonplace in endstage HIV

Notes:

Table 66.1 • Primary Prophylaxis of OIs in HIV-Infected Adults and Adolescents

Pathogen	Indication	Preventive Regimens		D/C Prophylaxis
		First Choice	Alternatives	
Strongly Recommended as Standard of Care				
Pneumocystis carinii	CD4+ count <200/μL or oropharyngeal candidiasis	Trimethoprim-sulfamethoxazole (TMP-SMX), 1 DS PO QD or TMP-SMX 1 SS PO QD	TMP/SMX 1 DS PO TIW; dapsone 50 mg BID or 100 mg/day; dapsone 50 mg QD plus pyrimethamine 50 mg QW plus leucovorin, 25 mg PO QW; dapsone, 200 mg PO plus pyrimethamine 75 mg PO plus leucovorin, 25 mg PO QW; aerosolized pentamidine, 300 mg QM via Respirgard II nebulizer, atovaquone, 1,500 mg PO QD	Patient on HAART with sustained ↑ in CD4 >200 cells for at least 3–6 months with sustained reduction in viral load for >3–6 months may discontinue PCP prophylaxis
Mycobacterium tuberculosis				
Isoniazid susceptible	Tuberculin skin test (TST) reaction ≥5 mm or prior positive result without treatment or contact with case of active tuberculosis	Isoniazid 300 mg PO plus pyridoxine 50 mg PO QD × 9 months or isoniazid 900 mg PO plus pyridoxine, 100 mg PO BIW × 9 months; rifampin 600 mg plus pyrazinamide 20 mg/kg PO QD × 2 months	Rifabutin 300 mg PO QD plus pyrazinamide, 20 mg/kg PO QD × 2 months; rifampin 600 mg PO QD × 4 months	
Isoniazid resistant	Same; high probability of exposure to multidrug resistance tuberculosis	Rifampin 600 mg PO plus pyrazinamide 20 mg/kg PO Q × 2 months	Rifabutin 300 mg plus pyrazinamide 20 mg/kg PO QD × 2 months; rifampin 600 mg PO QD × 4 months; rifabutin 300 mg PO QD × 4 months	
Multidrug resistant (INH and RIF)	Same; high probability of exposure to isoniazid-resistant tuberculosis	Choice of drugs requires consultation with public health authorities	None	

Toxoplasma gondii	IgG antibody to Toxoplasma and CD4+ count <100/µL	TMP-SMZ, 1 DS PO QD	TMP-SMZ, 1 SS PO QD: dapsone, 50 mg PO QD plus pyrimethamine, 50 mg PO QW plus leucovorin, 25 mg PO QW; atovaquone 1,500 mg PO QD with or without pyrimethamine 25 mg PO QD plus leucovorin, 10 mg PO QD	Insufficient patients evaluated to make a recommendation
Mycobacterium avium complex	CD4+ count <50/µL	Azithromycin 1,200 mg PO QW or clarithromycin 500 mg PO BID	Rifabutin 300 mg PO QD; azithromycin 1,200 mg PO QW plus rifabutin 300 mg PO QD	Patient on HAART with sustained ↑ in CD4 >100 cells for at least >3–6 months with sustained reduction in viral load for >3–6 months may discontinue MAC prophylaxis
Varicella-zoster virus (VZV)	Significant exposure to chickenpox or shingles for patients who have no history of either condition or, if available, negative antibody to VZV	Varicella zoster immune globulin (VZIG) 5 vials (1.25 mL each) IM administered ≤96 hr after exposure, ideally within 48 hr		
Generally Recommended				
Streptococcus pneumoniae	All patients	Pneumococcal vaccine 0.5 mL IM (CD4 ≥200/µL)	None	
Hepatitis B virus	All susceptible (Anti–HBc-negative) patients	Hepatitis B vaccine 3 doses	None	
Influenza virus	All patients (annually before influenza season)	Whole or split virus, 0.5 mL/IM/yr	Rimantadine 100 mg PO BID or amantadine 100 mg PO BID	
Hepatitis A virus	All susceptible (anti–HAV-negative) patients with chronic hepatitis C	Hepatitis A vaccine; two doses	None	

(continued)

Table 66.1 • Primary Prophylaxis of OIs in HIV-Infected Adults and Adolescents *(continued)*

Pathogen	Indication	Preventive Regimens		
		First Choice	Alternatives	D/C Prophylaxis
Not Recommended for Most Patients; Indicated for Use Only in Unusual Circumstances				
Bacteria	Neutropenia	Granulocyte colony-stimulating factor G-CSF) 5 μg/kg SC QD × 2–4 wk or granulocyte macrophage colony-stimulating factor (GM-CSF) 250 μg/m² IV over 2 hr QD × 2–4 w	None	
Cryptococcus neoformans	CD4+ count <50/μL	Fluconazole 100–200 mg PO QD	Itraconazole 200 mg PO QD	
Histoplasma capsulatum	CD4+ count <100/μL, endemic geographic areas	Itraconazole 200 mg PO QD	None	
Cytomegalovirus (CMV)	CD4+ count <50/μL and CMV antibody-positive	Oral ganciclovir 1 g PO TID	None	

Adapted from USPHS/IDSA Guidelines. MMWR Morbid Mortal Wkly Rep August 20, 1999;48(RR-10):1–66.

Table 66.2 • Treatment of *Pneumocystis carinii* Pneumonia[a]

Regimen	Dose	Route	Adverse Effects/Comments
Approved			
TMP-SMX	5 mg/kg TMP + 25 mg/kg SMX Q 6–8 hr × 21 days (2 DS tablets Q 8 hr)	IV, PO	Hypersensitivity, rash, fever, neutropenia ↑ LFTs, nephrotoxicity (15 mg/kg/day preferred to 20 mg/kg/day because of reduced toxicity)
Pentamidine isethionate	4 mg/kg IV daily over 60–90 min × 21 days	IV	Pancreatitis, hypotension, hypoglycemia, hyperglycemia, nephrotoxicity
Trimetrexate + leucovorin	45 mg/m^2 IV/day × 21 days 20 mg/m^2 PO or IV Q 6 hr × 24 days	IV PO/IV	Hematologic, GI, CNS, rash
Atovaquone[b]	750 mg BID with meals × 21 days (suspension)	PO	Headache, nausea, diarrhea, rash, fever, ↑ LFTs
Trimethoprim[b] + dapsone	15 mg/kg/day 100 mg/day × 21 days	PO PO	Pruritus, GI intolerance, bone marrow suppression Methemoglobinemia, hemolytic anemia (contraindicated in G6PD deficiency)
Clindamycin + primaquine	600 mg IV Q 8 hr or 300–450 mg PO Q 6 hr 15–30 mg (base) daily × 21 days	PO or IV PO	Rash, diarrhea Methemoglobinemia, hemolytic anemia (contraindicated in G6PD deficiency)
Prednisone	Within 72 hr of antipneumocystis therapy 40 mg Q 12 hr × 5 days, then 40 mg QD × 5 days, then 20 mg/day × 11 days	PO	Initiation in patients with moderately severe or severe disease Po$_2$ <70 mm Hg or A-a gradient >35 mm Hg
Investigational			
Difluoromethylornithine (DFMO, eflornithine)	400 mg/kg daily by continuous infusion or in four divided doses × 41–21 days, followed by 4–6 wk oral therapy	IV	Myelosuppression, GI toxicity

[a]CNS = Central nervous system; DS = Double strength; GI = Gastrointestinal; G6PD = Glucose-6 phosphate dehydrogenase; IV = Intravenous; PCP = *Pneumocystis carinii* pneumonia; PO = Oral; LFTs = Liver function tests; TMP-SMX = Trimethoprim-sulfamethoxazole.
[b]Used only in mild-to-moderate PCP.

Notes:

Table 66.3 • Treatment of CMV Retinitis[a]

	IV Ganciclovir	IV Foscarnet	Combination IV Ganciclovir and IV Foscarnet Sodium	IV Then Oral Ganciclovir	Intraocular Ganciclovir Implant	IV Cidofovir
Dosing regimens	Induction: 5 mg/kg Q 12 hr for 14–21 days Maintenance: 5 mg/kg QD Refractory disease: Induction: 7.5 mg/kg Q 12 hr for 14–21 days Maintenance: 10 mg/kg QD (Note: Dosage should be adjusted for creatinine clearance <70 mL/min; see Table 66.4.)	Induction: 90 mg/kg Q 12 hr for 14–21 days Maintenance: 90–120 mg/kg QD; 750–1,000 mL of 0.9% saline or D₅W solution with each dose	Prior ganciclovir: Induction: Both IV foscarnet 90 mg/kg Q 12 hr and IV ganciclovir 5 mg/kg QD for 14–21 days Maintenance: Both IV foscarnet 90–120 mg/kg and IV ganciclovir 5 mg/kg QD Prior foscarnet sodium: Induction: Both IV ganciclovir 5 mg/kg Q 12 hr and IV foscarnet 90–120 mg/kg QD Reinduction: IV ganciclovir 5 mg/kg and IV foscarnet 90 mg/kg Q 12 hr for 14–21 days	Induction: Same as IV ganciclovir Maintenance: 3,000–6,000 mg/day in 3 divided doses with food	Surgical: Intraocular implantation of ganciclovir (4.5 mg) implant releasing 1 μg/hr	Induction: 5 mg/kg every wk for 2 wk Maintenance: 5 mg/kg every 2 wk (Note: Dose reduction to 3 mg/kg for ↑ serum creatinine by 0.3–0.4 mg/dL above baseline; all doses given with probenecid and IV fluid)
Select adverse effects	Neutropenia; thrombocytopenia; catheter sepsis	Nephrotoxicity; electrolyte abnormalities; anemia; catheter sepsis; nausea/irritability; genital ulceration	Same as IV ganciclovir and IV foscarnet	Neutropenia; diarrhea/nausea	Surgical complications: transient blurred vision; infection; hemorrhage	Nephrotoxicity; neutropenia; probenecid adverse effects (rash, fever, nausea, fatigue); uveitis; alopecia; hypotonia

Important drug interactions	↑ Neutropenia; with zidovudine, cancer chemotherapy ↑ Didanosine levels	↑ Nephrotoxicity with other nephrotoxic drugs (e.g., amphotericin B, aminoglycosides, IV pentamidine)	Same as IV ganciclovir and IV foscarnet	Same as IV ganciclovir	Same as IV ganciclovir	↑ Nephrotoxicity with other nephrotoxic drugs (e.g., amphotericin B, aminoglycosides, IV pentamidine, NSAIDs) Probenecid: ↑ Level of most proximal tubular-excreted drugs
Adjunctive therapy	G-CSF/GM-CSF effective for neutropenia	IV or oral hydration essential; potassium, calcium/magnesium supplements, antiemetics may be required	Same as both IV ganciclovir and IV foscarnet	Same as IV ganciclovir	Systemic anti-CMV therapy recommended (oral ganciclovir 4,500 mg/day)	Probenecid and IV hydration essential; antiemetics, antihistamine, acetaminophen premedication commonly used for probenecid toxicity
Advantages	Systemic therapy; anti-HSV activity	Systemic therapy; anti-HSV (acyclovir-resistant) activity; anti-HIV activity	Increased efficacy compared with either IV ganciclovir or IV foscarnet alone; improved response for relapsed disease	Systemic therapy; oral administration; fewer catheter/sepsis complications	Longest time to retinitis progression in treated eye; no IV dosing or catheter required	Systemic therapy; no indwelling catheter required; infrequent dosing
Disadvantage	Hematologic toxicity; requires daily infusions; indwelling catheter	Nephrotoxicity; requires daily infusions/indwelling catheter; supplemental hydration required; prolonged infusion time; requires infusion pump or controlled rate infusion device	Same as IV ganciclovir and IV foscarnet; prolonged daily infusion time and impact on quality of life	Faster time to retinitis progression; high pill count; poor oral bioavailability (6%)	↑ Fellow eye and extraocular disease; requires surgery; postintraocular surgical complications	Requires probenecid and IV hydration; probenecid toxicity; nephrotoxicity (may be prolonged)

(continued)

Table 66.3 • Treatment of CMV Retinitis[a] (continued)

	IV Ganciclovir	IV Foscarnet	Combination IV Ganciclovir and IV Foscarnet Sodium	IV Then Oral Ganciclovir	Intraocular Ganciclovir Implant	IV Cidofovir
Monitoring requirement	Induction therapy: (a) CBC with WBC differential, platelet count weekly; (b) serum creatinine weekly. Maintenance therapy: (a) CBC with WBC differential, platelet count weekly; (b) serum creatinine every 2–4 wk	Induction therapy: (a) serum creatinine twice weekly; (b) serum Ca^{++}, albumin Mg^{--}, phosphates, and K^+ twice weekly; (c) hemoglobin and hematocrit weekly. Maintenance therapy: (a) serum creatinine weekly; (b) serum Ca^{++}, albumin Mg^{--}, phosphates, and K^+ weekly; (c) hemoglobin and hematocrit every 2–4 wk	Same as both IV ganciclovir and IV foscarnet	Induction therapy: IV ganciclovir. Maintenance therapy: oral ganciclovir (a) CBC with WBC differential, platelet count every 2 wk; (b) serum creatinine every 2–4 wk	No specific laboratory monitoring required for implant; if oral ganciclovir therapy is added, follow monitoring guidelines as outlined	Within 48 hr before each induction and maintenance: (a) serum creatinine quantitative proteinuria; (b) WBC with differential cell count; monitor intraocular pressure and slit-lamp examination at least monthly

Precautions and contraindications	Moderate-to-severe thrombocytopenia (platelet counts $<25 \times 10^9$/L)	Concomitant use with other nephrotoxic drugs (e.g., amphotericin B, aminoglycosides, or IV pentamidine) or in patients with pre-existing moderate-to-severe renal insufficiency (serum creatinine >168 µmol/L or creatinine clearance <50 mL/min)	Same as both IV ganciclovir and IV foscarnet	Use with caution in patients with immediately sight-threatening (zone 1) retinitis	External ocular or nasolacrimal infection; patients with ↑ risk of postoperative intraocular infection	Same as IV foscarnet, except parameters are baseline serum creatinine level (>1.5 mg/dL) or creatinine clearance (<55 mL/min), or 2+ proteinuria (after IV fluid) Discontinue therapy for 3+ proteinuria, if serum creatinine level increases by 0.5 mg/dL above baseline or intraocular pressure decreases by 50% of baseline value

[a]Fomivirsen intravitreal injection:
Induction therapy: 330 µg [0.05 mL] every other week for 2 doses (day 1 and day 15).
Maintenance dose: 330 µg [0.05 mL] once every 4 weeks (monthly).
Primary adverse effects: uveitis (ocular inflammation); increased intraocular pressure.
Adapted from Consensus Statement: International AIDS Society-USA: The treatment of cytomegalovirus diseases. *Arch Intern Med* 1998;158:957, and product information.

Table 66.4 • Dosage Adjustment for Cytomegalovirus Medications

Drug	Normal Dosage	CrCl (mL/min/1.73 m²)	Adjusted Dosage
Cidofovir	Induction dose: 5 mg/kg IV QW × 2 Maintenance dose: 5 mg/kg IV QOWK	Increase in serum creatinine of 0.3–0.4 above baseline Increase in serum creatinine of 0.5 above baseline or 3+ proteinuria Cidofovir is contraindicated in patients with pre-existing renal failure: 1. SrCr concentrations >1.5 mg/dL 2. Calculated CrCl of <55 mL/min 3. Urine protein ≥100 mg/dL (>2+ proteinuria)	3 mg/kg Discontinue cidofovir
Foscarnet	Induction dose: 60 mg/kg IV Q 8 hr to 90 mg/kg IV Q 12 hr Maintenance dose: 90–120 mg/kg IV QD	CrCl (mL/min/kg): >1.4 1.0–1.4 0.8–1.0 0.6–0.8 0.5–0.6 0.4–0.5 <0.4	*Induction Dose* Low Dose / High Dose 60 mg/kg Q 8 hr / 90 mg/kg Q 12 hr 45 mg/kg Q 8 hr / 70 mg/kg Q 12 hr 50 mg/kg Q 12 hr / 50 mg/kg Q 12 hr 40 mg/kg Q 12 hr / 80 mg/kg Q 24 hr 60 mg/kg Q 24 hr / 60 mg/kg Q 24 hr 50 mg/kg Q 24 hr / 50 mg/kg Q 24 hr Not recommended *Maintenance Dose* Low Dose / High Dose 90 mg/kg Q 24 hr / 120 mg/kg Q 24 hr 70 mg/kg Q 24 hr / 90 mg/kg Q 24 hr 50 mg/kg Q 24 hr / 65 mg/kg Q 24 hr 80 mg/kg Q 48 hr / 105 mg/kg Q 48 hr 60 mg/kg Q 48 hr / 80 mg/kg Q 48 hr 50 mg/kg Q 48 hr / 65 mg/kg Q 48 hr Not recommended
Ganciclovir	Oral (maintenance only): 1,000 mg PO TID IV: Induction dose: 5 mg/kg Q 12 hr Maintenance dose: 5 mg/kg QD or 6 mg/kg QD × 5 days/wk	CrCl (mL/min): ≥70 50–69 25–49 10–24 <10 CrCl (mL/min): >70 50–69 25–49 10–24 <10	Maintenance dose: 1,000 mg TID 1,500 mg QD or 500 mg TID 1,000 mg QD or 500 mg BID 500 mg QD 500 mg TIW after dialysis Induction dose: 5 mg/kg Q 12 hr 2.5 mg/kg Q 12 hr 2.5 mg/kg Q 24 hr 1.25 mg/kg Q 24 hr 1.25 mg/kg 3× Q wk following hemodialysis Maintenance dose: 5 mg/kg Q 24 hr 2.5 mg/kg Q 24 hr 1.25 mg/kg Q 24 hr 0.625 mg/kg Q 24 hr 0.625 mg/kg 3× Q wk following hemodialysis

Modified from reference 49 and product information.

Table 66.5 • Drugs Commonly Used in the Treatment of *Mycobacterium avium* Complex Infection[a]

Agents	Dose	Toxicities
Initial Therapy Agents		
Clarithromycin	500 mg PO BID[b]	Nausea, vomiting, diarrhea, abdominal pain, serum transferase elevations, bitter taste
Azithromycin	500 mg PO daily	Nausea, vomiting, diarrhea, abdominal pain, serum transferase elevations
Ethambutol	15–25 mg/kg/day PO	Optic neuritis,[c] nausea and vomiting
Rifabutin[d]	300 mg/day PO	Nausea, vomiting, diarrhea, serum transferase elevations, hepatitis, neutropenia, thrombocytopenia, rash, orange discoloration of body fluids, uveitis ↑ clearance of other drugs due to hepatic microsomal enzyme induction[e]
Secondary Agents		
Ciprofloxacin	500–750 mg PO BID	Nausea, vomiting, diarrhea, abdominal pain, headache, rare insomnia, hallucinations, seizures
Amikacin	10–15 mg/kg/day IV or IM	Nephrotoxicity, ototoxicity

[a]Macrolide + ethambutol +/− one or more of the drugs listed above.
[b]Clarithromycin dose >500 mg BID is associated with an increased mortality.
[c]Visual testing should be done monthly in patients receiving >15 mg/kg/day.
[d]Rifabutin dose 300–600 mg/day but should not exceed 300 mg/day if given with clarithromycin or fluconazole.
[e]Common drug interactions include protease inhibitors and clarithromycin.

Notes:

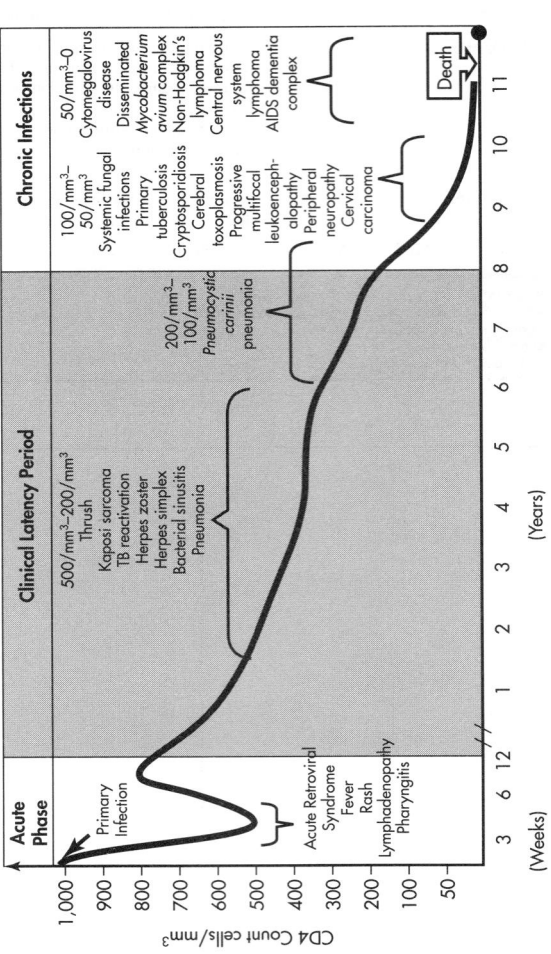

Fig. 66.1 Natural History of CD4+ Cell Count in the Average HIV Patient without Antiretroviral Therapy from Time of HIV Transmission to Death. (Illustrated by Mary Van, Pharm D.)

The reader is referred to Chapter 68: Opportunistic Infections (OIs) in HIV Patients, written by *Marjorie D. Robinson, Pharm.D.*, in the seventh edition of **Applied Therapeutics: The Clinical Use of Drugs** for a more in-depth discussion. All notations to reference numbers are based on the reference list at the end of that chapter. The editors of this handbook express their thanks to Dr. Robinson and acknowledge that this chapter is based upon her work.

Notes:

Notes:

Chapter 67

Fungal Infections

- ◆ Fungi exist in two forms: mold and yeast. Some (e.g., *Histoplasma capsulatum* and *Blastomyces dermatitidis*) grow as a mold in nature and convert to the yeast form in the infected host. *Aspergillus* sp. grow only as a mold form and *Cryptococcus neoformans* only as a yeast form.
- ◆ A morphological *classification* of fungi is presented in Table 67.1. A classification of fungal infections according to the area of body affected is listed in Table 67.2.
- ◆ Culture and histology remain the gold standard for *diagnosis*. Cultures take days to weeks to become positive. Radiographic diagnoses have limitations.
- ◆ Treatment decisions must include considerations for potential pathogenic fungi and the immunity of the host. Elderly patients with malnutrition can be mildly immunocompromised and susceptible to fungal infections as well as those with moderate or severe compromised immunity resulting from HIV, cancer chemotherapy, or organ transplantation.

Antifungal Drugs

- ◆ Table 67.3 lists the topical and systemic antifungal drugs approved for use in the U.S.
- ◆ Superficial and cutaneous mycoses and mucosal fungal infections (e.g., vaginal candidiasis) respond well to topical agents.
- ◆ More severe infection necessitates the use of systemic antifungal *treatment regimens* (Table 67.4). Adjunctive management issues, such as surgical drainage/excision and removal of central venous catheter, also need to be considered.
- ◆ Amphotericin, caspofungin, fluconazole, itraconazole, and voriconazole are the only effective parenteral treatments of disseminated fungal disease. Less severe disease can be treated with an oral azole.
- ◆ Amphotericin is active against most yeast, molds, and dimorphic fungi. The older azoles (ketoconazole, fluconazole) have a more limited *spectrum of activity*. Itraconazole and voriconazole differ from ketoconazole and fluconazole in that they are active against *Aspergillus* sp. The azoles are less active against certain nonalbicans *Candida* sp. including *C. glabrata* and *C. krusei*.
- ◆ The *pharmacokinetics* of systemically active antifungals are listed in Table 67.5.
- ◆ Formulations of amphotericin B are listed in Table 67.6.

Notes:

Table 67.1 • Organism Classification

Hyphae (Molds)
Hyalohyphomycoses
  Aspergillus species, *Pseudallescheria boydii*
  Dermatophytes: *Epidermophyton floccosum, Trichophyton* species, *Microsporum* species

Phaeohyphomycoses
  Alternaria species, *Anthopsis deltoidea, Bipolaris hawaiiensis, Cladosporium* species, *Curvularia geniculata, Exophiala* species, *Fonsecaea pedrosoi, Phialophora* species, *Fusarium* species

Zygomycetes
  Absidia corymbifera, Mucor indicus, Rhizomucor pusillus

Dimorphic Fungi
Blastomyces, Coccidioides, Paracoccidioides, Histoplasma, Sporothrix

Yeast
Candida species, *Cryptococcus neoformans*

Table 67.2 • Clinical Classification of Mycoses

Classification	Site Infected	Example
Superficial	Outermost skin and hair	Malasseziasis (Tinea versicolor)
Cutaneous	Deep epidermis and nails	Dermatophytosis
Subcutaneous	Dermis and subcutaneous tissue	Sporotrichosis
Systemic	Disease of ≥1 internal organs	
Opportunistic		Candidiasis, cryptococcosis, aspergillosis, mucormycosis
Nonopportunistic		Histoplasmosis, blastomycosis, coccidioidomycosis

Notes:

Table 67.3 • Antifungal Agents Approved for Use[a]

Agent (Brand Name)	Route of Administration
Systemic Agents	
Amphotericin B (generic, Abelcet, AmBisome, Amphotec)	IV
Caspofungin (Cancidin)	IV
Fluconazole (Diflucan)	IV, tablet
Fluorocytosine [Flucytosine] (Ancobon)	Capsule
Griseofulvin	Tablet
Itraconazole (Sporanox)	Capsule, oral solution, IV
Ketoconazole (Nizoral)	Tablet
Miconazole (Monistat)	IV, vaginal tablet, cream
Potassium iodide	Solution
Terbinafine (Lamisil)	Tablet
Voriconazole	IV, tablet
Primary Topicals, Class I	
Amphotericin B	Cream, lotion, ointment, oral suspension
Clioquinol (Vioform)	Cream, ointment
Clotrimazole	Cream, lotion, lozenge, pessary, solution, tablet
Miconazole	Aerosol, cream, lotion, pessary, spray, suppository, vaginal tablet
Naftifine (Naftin)	Cream, gel
Nystatin	Cream, lozenge, ointment, powder, suspension, tablet
Povidone iodine	Douche, gel, suppository
Tolnaftate	Cream, gel, powder, solution, spray
Undecylenic acid	Cream, foam, ointment, powder, soap
Topicals, Class I	
Butoconazole (Femstat)	Ointment
Ciclopirox (Loprox)	Cream, lotion
Econazole (Spectazole)	Cream
Haloprogin (Halotex)	Cream, solution
Ketoconazole (Nizoral)	Cream
Naftifine (Naftin)	Cream, gel
Oxiconazole (Oxistat)	Cream, lotion
Sulconazole (Exelderm)	Cream, solution
Terbinafine (Lamisil)	Cream
Terconazole (Terazol 7)	Cream, suppository
Tioconazole (Vagistat)	Ointment
Triacetin (Fungoid)	Cream, solution, spray

[a] IV = Intravenously.

Notes:

Table 67.4 • Recommended Treatment Regimens for Systemic Fungal Infection

Aspergillosis (disseminated)	Amphotericin B 1–1.5 mg/kg/day IV *Alternative:* Itraconazole 200 mg IV Q8H × 72 hrs, then 200 mg IV Q12H *or* Caspofungin 70 mg IV Q24H × 1 dose, then 50 mg IV Q24H
Blastomycosis	Itraconazole 200 mg PO BID
Candidiasis (deep-seated)	Fluconazole 400 mg PO/IV QD *or* Amphotericin B 0.5–0.7 mg/kg/day IV
Coccidioidomycosis	Fluconazole 400–800 mg PO/IV QD *or* Amphotericin B 0.5–1.0 mg/kg/day IV
Cryptococcosis (meningitis)	Amphotericin B 0.3–0.6 mg/kg/day IV with Flucytosine 100 mg/kg/day Q6H PO *Alternative:* Fluconazole 400 mg PO/IV QD
Histoplasmosis (acute immunocompromised)	Amphotericin 0.3–1.0 mg/kg/day IV *Alternative:* Itraconazole 200–400 mg QD PO

Other mycoses
  Mucor
  Fusarium
  Pseudoallescheria boydii
	Amphotericin B 1–1.5 mg/kg/day IV
	Voriconazole
	Itraconazole 200 mg IV Q12H

Notes:

Table 67.5 • Pharmacokinetic Properties of Systemically Active Antifungals[116,a]

Characteristic	Imidazoles		Triazoles		Terbinafine	Flucytosine
	Miconazole[b]	Ketoconazole[b]	Itraconazole[b]	Fluconazole[b]		
Absorption						
Relative bioavailability	<10	75[c]	99.8 (40)[c]	(85–92)[c]	70%	75–90[c]
C_{max} (µg/mL)	1.90	3.29	0.63	1.4	1.34–1.7	70–80
T_{max} (hr)	1.0	2.6	4.0	1.0–4.0	1.5	<2
AUC^d (µg/hr/mL)	ND	12.9 (13.6)	1.9 (0.7)	42	4.74–10.48	ND
Distribution						
Protein binding (%)	91–93	99	99.8	11	>99	2–4
CSF/serum concentration (%)	<10	<10	<10	60	<10	60
Excretion						
Beta $t_{1/2}$ (hr)	2.1	8.1[d]	17[d]	23–45	36	2.5–6.0
Active drug in urine (%)	1	2	<10	60–80	0	80

[a]AUC = Area under the concentration-time curve; C_{max} = Maximum concentration; CSF = Cerebrospinal fluid; ND = No data; T_{max} = Time of maximum concentration; $t_{1/2}$ = Half-life.
[b]Above parameters are estimated from the administration of currently recommended doses. Miconazole 7.4–14.2 mg/kg/day (500–1,000 mg) parenterally, ketoconazole 2.8 mg/kg/day orally (200 mg), itraconazole 1.4–2.8 mg/kg/day orally (100–200 mg), fluconazole 0.7–1.4 mg/kg/day orally, terbinafine 250 mg/day orally, and flucytosine 150 mg/kg/day parenterally.
[c]With meals (fasting), absorption altered by gastric acidity.
[d]Dose and/or infusion dependent.

Table 67.6 • Amphotericin B Formulations[a]

Category	Amphotericin B (Fungizone)	Amphotericin B Lipid Complex (ABLC, Abelcet)	Amphotericin B Colloidal Dispersion (Amphotec)	Liposomal Amphotericin B (AmBisome)
FDA-approved indication	Life-threatening fungal infections; Visceral leishmaniasis	Refractory/intolerant to AMB	Invasive aspergillosis in patients refractory/intolerant to AMB	Empirical therapy in neutropenic FUO; Refractory/intolerant to AMB; Visceral leishmaniasis
Formulation				
Sterol	None	None	Cholesterol sulfate	Cholesterol sulfate (5)[+]
Phospholipid	None	DMPC and DMPG (7:3)[+]	None	EPC and DSPG (10:4)[+]
Amphotericin B (Mole %)	34	33	50	10
Particle size (nm)	<10	1,600–11,000	122 (±48)	80–120
Stability	1 wk at 2–8°C or 24 hr at 27°C	15 hr at 2–8°C or 6 hr at 27°C	24 hr at 2–8°C	24 hr at 2–8°C
Dosage and rate	0.3–1.0 mg/kg/day over 1–6 hr	5.0 mg/kg/day at 2.5 mg/kg/hr	3.0–4.0 mg/kg/day over 2 hr	3.0–5.0 mg/kg/day over 2 hr
Lethal dose 50%	3.3 mg/kg	10–25 mg/kg	68 mg/kg	17 mg/kg
Pharmacokinetic parameters				
Dose	0.5 mg/kg	5.0 mg/kg × 7 days	5.0 mg/kg × 7 days	2.5 mg/kg × 7 days; 5 mg/kg × 7 days
Serum concentrations				
Peak	1.2 µg/mL	1.7 µg/mL	3.1 µg/mL	31.4 µg/mL; 83.0 µg/mL
Trough	0.5 µg/mL	0.7 µg/mL		4.0 µg/mL
Half-life	91.1 hr	173.4 hr	28.5 hr	6.3 hr; 6.8 hr
Volume of distribution	5.0 L/kg	131.0 L/kg	4.3 L/kg	0.16 L/kg; 0.10 L/kg
Clearance	38.0 mL/hr/kg	436.0 mL/hr/kg	0.117 mL/hr/kg	22.0 mL/hr/kg; 11.0 mL/hr/kg
Area under the curve	14 µg/mL · hr	17 µg/mL · hr	43.0 µg/mL · hr	197 µg/mL · hr; 555 µg/mL · hr

[a] + = Molar ratio of each component, respectively; AMB = Amphotericin B; DMPC = Dimyristoyl phosphatidylcholine; DMPG = Dimyristoyl phosphatidylglycerol; DSPG = Distearoylphosphatidylglycerol; EPC = Egg phosphatidylcholine; FUO = Fever of unknown origin; NA = Not applicable.

The reader is referred to Chapter 69: *Fungal Infections,* written by *John D. Cleary, Pharm.D., Stanley W. Chapman, M.D., Alice M. Clark, Ph.D.,* and *Helen, L. Lucia, M.D.,* in the seventh edition of **Applied Therapeutics: The Clinical Use of Drugs** for a more in-depth discussion. All notations to reference numbers are based on the reference list at the end of that chapter. The editors of this handbook express their thanks to Drs. Cleary, Chapman, Clark, and Lucia and acknowledge that this chapter is based upon their work.

Notes:

Notes:

Chapter 68

Viral Infections

TREATMENT OF VIRAL INFECTIONS
Antiviral Agents

Most antiviral agents must be administered parenterally in serious infections because their bioavailability is erratic (e.g., acyclovir 20%, oral ganciclovir 5%). Exceptions to this include amantadine, rimantadine, famciclovir, valacyclovir, and valganciclovir which are well absorbed.

- ◆ With the exception of rimantadine, oseltamavir, and zanamavir, the antivirals listed in Table 68.1 are eliminated primarily unchanged in the urine. Dosage adjustment is required in those patients with renal insufficiency.

- ◆ The normal half-life for acyclovir, famciclovir (penciclovir), and ganciclovir ranges from 2–3.5 hr, while for amantadine and rimantadine, it is 15–40 hr.

- ◆ Adverse effects of antiviral agents are described in Table 68.4.

Herpes Infections

- ◆ Herpes simplex and Herpes zoster commonly infect both the normal and immunocompromised patient. Genital herpes, a sexually transmitted disease, is treatable with oral acyclovir analogues. These agents do not eradicate the virus but reduce viral shedding, pain, and time to healing. Herpes simplex infection in immunocompromised patients can be disseminated, requiring parenteral therapy with 15 mg/kg/day of IV acyclovir.

- ◆ To ensure therapeutic brain tissue levels, H. simplex encephalitis should be treated with higher doses (30 mg/kg/day IV).

- ◆ H. zoster also requires achievement of higher acyclovir levels than H. simplex to inhibit growth of the organism; therefore, 30 mg/kg/day IV is recommended.

- ◆ Acyclovir has poor oral bioavailability, averaging 20%. As a result, the optimal oral dose in those patients who require suppressive or prophylactic therapy is not clear. However, doses of 200 mg BID have been used in the suppression of genital herpes and 400–800 mg 3–5 times a day in the prophylaxis of CMV infection in transplant patients. (See Table 68.3.)

- ◆ Famciclovir and valacyclovir are alternatives to acyclovir in the treatment of *H. zoster* in immunocompetent patients. Valacyclovir is effective in preventing infection in solid organ transplants.

Cytomegalovirus (CMV)

- ◆ CMV generally is treated with IV ganciclovir or foscarnet. Oral valganciclovir can be used in patients with normal absorption.

- ◆ ***Ganciclovir.*** Progression of CMV retinitis in AIDS patients is delayed with ganciclovir or foscarnet therapy. Bone marrow and solid organ transplant patients with asymptomatic pulmonary infection also benefit from the preemptive use of ganciclovir.

♦ **Foscarnet** is useful in the treatment of CMV retinitis. Unlike ganciclovir, foscarnet is not bone marrow toxic; renal toxicity is the dose-limiting toxicity of this agent.

Influenza

♦ **Oral amantadine** is effective in the prevention and treatment of uncomplicated infection due to Influenza A. The most commonly reported side effects with amantadine include nausea and CNS effects (e.g., psychosis, insomnia, irritability, confusion). The CNS side effects are dose-related and more common when doses exceed 300 mg/day.

♦ **Rimantadine** is active versus Influenza A and low toxicity, with protective efficacy rates similar to those with amantadine. Emergence of resistance is rapid with both amantadine and rimantadine.

The neuraminidase inhibitors, oseltamavir and zanamavir, are active against both influenza A and B. Development of resistance is rare, thus these agents are preferable in an outbreak situation. Both agents have been demonstrated to be effective in the prevention and treatment of influenza; however, they are substantially more expensive by acquisition cost.

Respiratory Syncytial Virus (RSV)

♦ Aerosolized ribavirin is the only agent approved for the treatment of RSV. The benefit of ribavirin is unclear at the present time. While early studies suggest some subjective and objective improvement with the use of the drug, the benefit of ribavirin in terms of morbidity and mortality is unclear.

♦ According to the manufacturer, ribavirin is teratogenic, embryolethal, carcinogenic, and mutagenic, depending upon the study model. The nature of these effects is unknown in humans.

♦ Considering the unknown toxicity and the widespread dissemination of the aerosolized drug, environmental precautions are recommended.

Notes:

Table 68.1 • Clinical Pharmacokinetics of Antiviral Drugs

Drug	Type of Patients	Total Clearance	Volume of Distribution	Elimination Half-Life (hr)	Comments
Acyclovir[a,15,18,20,30,178,179]	Adults	307 mL/min/1.73 m²	50 L/1.73 m²	2.5–3.0	Use 100% of recommended dose but extend dosage interval to 12 and 24 hr if Cl_{Cr} ranges from 25–50 and 10–25 mL/min/1.73 m², respectively; use 50% of recommended dose Q 24 hr if Cl_{Cr} ranges from 0–10 mL/min/1.73 m².
	Neonates	98–122 mL/min/1.73 m²	24–30 L/1.73 m²	3.2–4.1	
Amantadine[a,101,180]	Adults	2.5–10.5 L/hr	1.5–6.1 L/kg	22.6–37.7	Adjust doses in renal failure: 200 mg on day 1 and then 100 mg/day if Cl_{Cr} 30–50; 200 mg on day 1 and then 100 mg QOD if Cl_{Cr} 15–29; 200 mg Q 7 days if Cl_{Cr} <15 mL/min/1.73 m².
Famciclovir[162,163,181,182]	Adults	0.37–0.48 L/hr/kg	1.5 L/kg	2.2–3.0	Use 100% of recommended dose but extend dosage interval to 12 and 24 hr if Cl_{Cr} ranges from 40–59 and 20–39 mL/min, respectively; use 250 mg Q 48 hr if Cl_{Cr} <20 mL/min.
Ganciclovir	Adults	250–300 ml/min/1.73 m²	50 L/1.73 m²	2.5–3.0	
Oseltamivir[92,174]	Adults	18.8 L/hr (renal clearance)	NA	6.7–8.2	Use 75 mg/day in patients if Cl_{Cr} 10–30 mL/min. The effect of hepatic impairment has not been determined.
Rimantadine[170,173]	Adults	20–48 L/hr	25 L/kg	29–37	Because it undergoes extensive metabolism, dose may have to be adjusted in patients with severe liver disease. Dose adjustment may also be necessary in elderly and in those with severe renal failure (Cl_{Cr} ≤10 mL/min). Manufacturer recommends 50% reduction in dose in such cases.
Valacyclovir[165]	See acyclovir				Use 100% of recommended dose but extend dosage interval to 12 and 24 hr if Cl_{Cr} ranges from 30–49 and 10–29 mL/min, respectively; use 500 mg Q 24 hr if Cl_{Cr} <10 mL/min.
Zanamivir[91]	Adults	2.5–10.9 L/hr	15.9 L	2.5–5.1	4–17% of inhaled dose systemically absorbed. Although only limited studies with renal or hepatic impairment, dosing adjustment likely unnecessary.

[a]Bioavailability for oral acyclovir ranges from 0.15–0.30, for oral acyclovir ranges from 0.15–0.30, and for amantadine from 0.86–0.90.
NA = Data not available.

Table 68.2 • *In Vitro* Activity of Antiviral Agents

Drug	Herpes simplex	Herpes zoster	CMV	Influenza A	Influenza B
Acyclovir (Penciclovir)	++++	+++	+	—	—
Amantadine (Rimantadine)	—	—	—	++++	—
Foscarnet	++++	+++	+++	—	—
Ganciclovir	++++	+++	+++	—	—
Oseltamavir	—	—	—	++++	++++
Zanamavir	—	—	—	++++	++++

Notes:

Table 68.3 • Recommended Drugs for Various Viral Infections

Disease	Drug	Dosage (Age Group)	Route	Duration
Herpes encephalitis	Acyclovir (Zovirax)[a]	*Adults:* 10 mg/kg Q 8 hr *6 mo–12 yr:* 500 mg/m^2 Q 8 hr	IV	10 days
Neonatal herpes	Acyclovir (Zovirax)	10–20 mg/kg Q 8 hr	IV	14–21 days
Mucocutaneous herpes (immunocompromised patients)	Acyclovir (Zovirax)	*Adults:* 5 mg/kg Q 8 hr *<12 yr:* 250 mg/m^2 Q 8 hr	IV	7 days
Varicella-zoster (immunocompromised patients)	Acyclovir (Zovirax)[a]	*Adults:* 10 mg/kg Q 8 hr *Children:* 500 mg/m^2 Q 8 hr	IV IV	7 days
Herpes zoster (normal host)	Acyclovir (Zovirax) or Famciclovir (Famvir) or Valacyclovir (Valtrex)	800 mg 5 times/day 500 mg TID 1 g TID	PO PO PO	7–10 days 7 days 7 days
Varicella (chickenpox)	Acyclovir (Zovirax)[a]	*Adults and children >2 yr:* 20 mg/kg (≤800 mg) QID	PO	5 days
Herpes keratitis	Trifluridine 1% ophthalmic solution (Viroptic)	1 drop Q 2 hr; then 1 drop Q 4 hr	Topical	Until corneal ulcer reepithelialized; 7 days
Cytomegalovirus retinitis (immunocompromised patients)	Ganciclovir (Cytovene)	5 mg/kg Q 12 hr; then 5 mg/kg/day or 6 mg/kg, 5 days/wk	IV	14–21 days for induction; maintenance
Influenza A	Amantadine (Symmetrel)	*Adults and children >9 yr:* 100 mg BID *Children 1–9 yr:* 4.4–8.8 mg/kg/day but <150 mg/day	PO	10 days (treatment), 14–21 days (protection with vaccine), 90 days (protection without vaccine)
	Rimantadine (Flumadine)	*Adults and children ≥10 yr:* 100 mg BID *Children 1–10 yr:* 5 mg/kg/day (<150 mg/day)	PO	7 days (treatment), up to 6 wk for prophylaxis (not approved for treatment in children)
	Oseltamivir (Tamiflu)	*Adults:* 75 mg BID	PO	5 days treatment
	Zanamivir (Relenza)	*Adults and children >12 yr:* 10 mg (2 inhalations) BID	Inhalation	5 days treatment
Respiratory syncytial virus	Ribavirin (Virazole)	6 gm in 300 mL over 12–18 hr/day	Inhalation	3–7 days

[a]Foscarnet 40 mg/kg IV Q 8 hr is recommended for acyclovir-resistant herpes simplex virus or varicella-zoster virus.

Table 68.4 • Adverse Effects of Approved Antiviral Drugs

Drug	Adverse Effects
Acyclovir	Local irritation and phlebitis (9%); ↑ SrCr and BUN (5–10%); N/V (7%); itching and rash (2%); ↑ liver transaminases (1%–2%), CNS toxicity (1%)
Amantadine	Nausea, dizziness (light-headedness), and insomnia (5–10%); depression, anxiety, irritability, hallucination, confusion, dry mouth, constipation, ataxia, headache, peripheral edema, and orthostatic hypotension (1–5%)
Famciclovir	Headache (6–9%), nausea (4–5%), diarrhea (1–2%)
Oseltamivir	Nausea, vomiting (9–10%), vertigo (1%)
Ribavirin	Worsening of respiratory status, bacterial pneumonia, pneumothorax, apnea, ventilator dependence; cardiac arrest, hypotension; rash and conjunctivitis
Rimantadine	CNS (insomnia, dizziness, headache, nervousness, fatigue) and GI (N/V, anorexia, dry mouth, abdominal pain) (each 1–3%)
Trifluridine	Burning or stinging upon instillation (4.6%); palpebral edema (2.8%); keratopathy, hypersensitivity reaction, stromal edema, hyperemia, ↑ intraocular pressure
Valacyclovir	Headache (13–17%), nausea (10–16%), vomiting (1–7%), diarrhea (1–5%)
Vidarabine	Anorexia, N/V, diarrhea; ↓ in Hgb, Hct, WBC count, and platelet count; CNS toxicity; ↑ liver transaminases; rash, pruritus, and irritation at injection site
Zanamivir	Bronchospasm, decline in respiratory function, especially if underlying respiratory disease; nasal/throat irritation; headache (2%); cough (2%)

SrCr = Serum creatinine; BUN = Blood urea nitrogen; CNS = Central nervous system; GI = Gastrointestinal; Hgb = Hemoglobin; Hct = Hematocrit; N/V = Nausea and vomiting; WBC = White blood cell.

The reader is referred to Chapter 70: Viral Infections, written by *Milap C. Nahata, Pharm.D.* and *Neeta Bahal O'Mara, Pharm.D.*, in the seventh edition of **Applied Therapeutics: The Clinical Use of Drugs** for a more in-depth discussion. All notations to reference numbers are based on the reference list at the end of that chapter. The editors of this handbook express their thanks to Dr. Nahata and acknowledge that this chapter is based upon his work.

Notes:

Chapter 69

Viral Hepatitis

CAUSATIVE AGENTS AND CHARACTERISTICS (Table 69.1)

Definitions

Acute: Illness with discrete date of onset with jaundice or increased serum aminotransferase concentrations of >2.5 times the upper limit of normal.

Chronic: Inflammatory condition of the liver that involves ongoing hepatocellular necrosis for 6 months or more beyond the onset of acute illness.

♦ There are at least six etiologic forms of hepatitis virus: A, B, C, D, E, G (Table 69.2)

Hepatitis A Virus (HAV)

Treatment: Usually self-limiting with need only for supportive measures.

Prevention:

♦ Passive: immunoglobulin 0.06 mL/kg × 1

♦ Vaccine: (Table 69.3)

♦ Postexposure prophylaxis if within 2 weeks of exposure, immune globulin 0.02 mL/kg IM is protective.

Hepatitis B (HBV)

♦ *Serologic patterns* (Table 69.4)

♦ Within the first several weeks after exposure, HBsAg appears first in the blood and is present for weeks before symptoms or increased serum concentrations of aminotransferases. Antibody to HBsAg usually appears after a short window period during which time neither HBsAg nor anti-HBs are detectable.

♦ HBeAg is seen in the acute phase and persists in chronic infection. It is a marker of active viral replication and infectivity. The appearance of anti-HBe suggests resolution of HBV infection.

♦ Anti-HBc, the antibody directed against the core antigen, is the most sensitive diagnostic test for acute HBV infection.

Acute HBV

Treatment: Primarily supportive

Prevention:

♦ *Vaccination* (Table 69.5, 69.6)

♦ Who should be vaccinated?

 • All infants

 • High-risk groups: Health care workers with exposure to blood, staff of institutions for the developmentally disabled, hemodialysis patients, recipients of blood products, household and sexual contacts of HBV carriers, travelers to endemic areas, injecting drug users, sexually active homosexual men, inmates

- Postexposure prophylaxis: HBIG 0.06 mL/kg IM as soon as possible after exposure (Tables 69.7, 69.8)

Chronic HBV

Treatment: Symptom-free patients with moderate increased aminotransferases and liver biopsies demonstrating mild disease probably should not be treated.

♦ α interferon (5 million units daily or 10 million units three times a week × 16 wks) is moderately effective in treating chronic HBV, based upon clearance of viremia, normalization of aminotransferase values (Table 69.9)

  - Adverse effects are common (Table 69.10).

♦ Lamivudine 100 mg QD × 1 year for patients with compensated liver disease and evidence of active viral replication.

  - Well tolerated with most commonly reported adverse events including headache, fatigue, nausea.

Hepatitis D Virus (HDV)

- ♦ Present in some, but not all HBV patients
- ♦ Coinfection with HBV is correlated with higher risk of fulminant liver disease.
- ♦ HDV replication is dependent upon HBV replication; vaccination with HBV vaccine also prevents HDV infection.

Treatment:

- Primarily supportive with special attention to development of fulminant hepatic failure
- Antiviral therapy has not been found to be effective

Hepatitis C virus (HCV)

Acute HCV

Treatment: Limited data suggest patients with acute HCV receiving α interferon have a lower rate of chronic HCV.

Chronic HCV

- ♦ Symptomatic patients with compensated liver disease can be treated with α interferon or α interferon plus oral ribavirin or peg interferon.
- ♦ Combination of interferon 3 million units SC 3 × 1 wk + oral ribavirin (<75 kg 400 mg am and 600 mg pm; >75 kg 600 mg BID) is superior to interferon alone.

Notes:

Table 69.1 • Hepatitis Nomenclature[a]

Hepatitis Type	Antigen	Corresponding Antibody	Comments
A	Hepatitis A virus (HAV)	Hepatitis A antibody (anti-HAV)	RNA virus; present in stool and serum early in course of hepatitis A
B	Hepatitis B surface antigen (HBsAg)	Hepatitis B surface antibody (anti-HBs)	DNA virus; found in serum in >90% of patients with acute hepatitis B, anti-HBs appears following infection and confers immunity
	Hepatitis B core antigen (HBcAg)	Hepatitis B core antibody (anti-HBc)	Anti-HBc detected in serum during and after acute infection
	Hepatitis B envelope antigen (HBeAg)	HB envelope antibody (anti-HBe)	HBeAg correlates with infectivity; suggestive of active viral replication
C	Hepatitis C antigen (HCAg)	Hepatitis C antibody (anti-HCV)	RNA virus; previously known as post-transfusion NANB hepatitis
D	Hepatitis D antigen (HDAg)	Hepatitis D antibody (anti-HDV)	Defective RNA virus; requires presence of HBsAg
E	Hepatitis E antigen (HEAg)	Hepatitis E antibody (anti-HEV)	RNA virus present in stool; cause of enteric NANB hepatitis
G	Hepatitis G antigen (HGAg)	Not available	RNA-like virus; named GBV-A, GBV-B, and GBV-C; thought to be of tamarin origin

[a]NANB = Non-A, non-B hepatitis.

Table 69.2 • Comparison of the Etiologic Forms of Hepatitis A, B, C, D, E, and Gᵃ

Virus	HAV	HBV	HCV	HDV	HEV	HGV
Genome	RNA	DNA	RNA	RNA	RNA	RNA
Family	Picornavirus	Hepadnavirus	Flavivirus	Satellite	Calicivirus	Flavivirus
Size (nm)	27	42	30–60	40	32	Unknown
Incubation (days) [mean]	15–45 [30]	30–180 [80]	15–60 [50]	21–140 [35]	15–65 [42]	14–35 [na]
Transmission						
Oral	Yes	Rare	Rare	No	Yes, common	Unknown
Percutaneous	Rare	Common	Common	Common	Unknown	Yes
Sexual	No	Common	Common	No	No	Unknown
Perinatal	No	Common	Rare	Rare	Rare	Unknown
Onset	Sudden	Insidious	Insidious	Insidious	Sudden	Unknown
Clinical illness	70–80% adults 5% children	10–15%	5–10%	10%	70–80% adults	Unknown
Icteric presentation						
Children	<10%	30%	25%	Unknown	Unknown	Unknown
Adults	30%	5–20%	5–10%	25%	Common	Unknown
Peak ALT (U/L)	800–1,000	1,000–1,500	300–800	1,000–1,500	800–1,000	Unknown
Incidence of acute liver failure (%)	<1	<1	<1	2–7.5	<1; higher in pregnant women	Unknown

Serum diagnosis	HAV	HBV	HCV	HDV	HEV	HGV
Acute infection	Anti-HAV IgM	HBsAg Anti-HBc IgM	HCV-RNA (anti-HCV)	Anti-HDV IgM	Anti-HEV IgG (seroconversion)	HGV RNA
Chronic infection	NA	HBsAg Anti-HBc IgG	Anti-HCV (ELISA) RIBA	Anti-HDV IgG	NA	HGV RNA
Viral markers	HAV RNA	HBV-DNA DNA polymerase	HCV-RNA	HDV-RNA	Viruslike particles	HGV RNA
Immunity	Anti-HAV IgG	Anti-HBs	NA	NA	Anti-HEV IgG	Unknown
Virus	**HAV**	**HBV**	**HCV**	**HDV**	**HEV**	**HGV**
Case-fatality rate	0.1–2.7%	1–3%	1–2%	<1% coinfect	0.5–4% 1.5–21% pregnant women	Unknown
Complete recovery	>97%	85–97%	50%	90%	99%	Unknown
Incidence of chronic infection	0%	2–7% >90% neonates	50%	80% superinfect ≤5% coinfection	0%	Unknown
Carrier state	No	Yes	Yes	Yes	No	Unknown
Risk of hepatocellular carcinoma	No	Yes	Yes	Yes	No	No
Drug treatment	None	Interferon, lamivudine	Interferon, ribavirin + interferon	Interferon	None	Unknown

^{a}NA = Not applicable.

Table 69.3 • Recommended Doses of Hepatitis A Vaccines

Vaccinee's Age (yr)	Dose (Volume)[a]	Schedule (Months)[b]
Havrix		
Children 2–18 yr	720 EL.U. (0.5 mL)	0, 6–12
Adults >18 yr	1,440 EL.U. (1.0 mL)	0, 6–12
Vaqta		
Children 2–17 yr	25 U (0.5 mL)	0, 6–18
Adults >17 yr	50 U (1.0 mL)	0, 6

[a]Enzyme-linked immunosorbent assay (ELISA) units.
[b]Zero months represents timing of the initial dose; subsequent numbers represent months after the initial dose.
From reference 79.

Table 69.4 • Common Serologic Patterns of Hepatitis B Virus Infection

HbsAg	HbeAg	Anti-HBs	Anti-Hbe	Anti-HBc	Interpretation
+	+	–	–	±	Incubation period
+	+	–	–	+ (IgM)	Acute HBV infection (typical case); chronic HBV carrier with high infectivity
–	–	+	±	+ (IgG)	Recovery from HBV infection
+	±	–	±	+ (IgG)	Chronic HBV carrier; chronic hepatitis B
–	–	+	–	–	Successful immunization with HBV vaccine

Table 69.5 • Recommended Doses of Currently Licensed Hepatitis B Vaccines

Group[a]	Recombivax HB[b] Dose (µg) (m/L)	Engerix-B[a] Dose (µg) (m/L)
Birth to 10 yr	5 (0.5)	10 (0.5)
Children and adolescents 11–19 yr	5 (0.5)	10 (0.5) or 20 (1.0)
Adults ≥20 yr	10 (1.0)	20 (1.0)
Dialysis patients and other immunocompromised hosts	40 (1.0)[c]	40 (2.0)[d]

[a]HbsAg, hepatitis B surface antigen.
[b]Both vaccines are administered routinely in a 3-dose series at 0, 1, and 6 months. Engerix-B also has been licensed for a dose series administered at 0, 1, 2, and 12 months.
[c]Special formulation.
[d]Two 1.0-mL doses administered at 1 site, in a 4-dose schedule at 0, 1, 2, and 6 months.
Note: Effective 8/27/98, Merck Vaccine Division discontinued production of the 2.5-µg pediatric formulation of Recombivax HB. The 5-µg formulation is used instead to simplify and improve convenience of HBV vaccination.
From references 131–133.

Notes:

Table 69.6 • Recommended Schedules of Hepatitis B Vaccination for Infants Born to HBsAg (−) Mothers

Hepatitis B Vaccine	Age of Infant
Option 1	
Dose 1	Birth (before hospital discharge)
Dose 2	1–2 months[a]
Dose 3	6–18 months[a]
Option 2	
Dose 1	1–2 months[a]
Dose 2	4 months[a]
Dose 3	6–18 months[a]

[a]Hepatitis B vaccine can be administered simultaneously with diptheria-tetanus-pertussis, *Haemophilus influenza* type b conjugate, measles-mumps-rubella, and oral polio vaccines.
From reference 133.

Table 69.7 • Guide to Postexposure Immunoprophylaxis for Exposure to Hepatitis B Virus

Type of Exposure	Immunoprophylaxis
Perinatal	Vaccination + HBIG
Sexual	Vaccination + HBIG
Household contact	
Chronic carrier	Vaccination
Acute case	None unless known exposure
Acute case, known exposure	HBIG ± vaccination
Infant (<12 months) acute case in primary caregiver	HBIG + vaccination
Inadvertent (percutaneous/permucosal)	Vaccination ± HBIG

HBIG = Hepatitis B immunoglobulin.
From references 133 and 173.

Notes:

Table 69.8 • Recommendations for Hepatitis B Prophylaxis Following Percutaneous Exposure[133]

Exposed Person	Treatment When Source Is Found to Be		
	HBsAg-Positive	HBsAg-Negative	Unknown or Not Tested
Unvaccinated	Administer HBIG × 1[a] and initiate hepatitis vaccine	Initiate hepatitis B vaccine[b]	Initiate hepatitis B vaccine[b]
Previously vaccinated			
Known responder	Test exposed person for anti-HBs[c] 1. If inadequate, hepatitis B vaccine booster dose 2. If adequate, no treatment	No treatment	No treatment
Known responder	HBIG × 1[a] as soon as possible, repeat in 1 month *OR* HBIG × 1[a] plus 1 dose of hepatitis B vaccine	No treatment	If known high-risk-source, may treat as if source were HBsAg positive
Response unknown	Test exposed person for anti-HBs[c] 1. If inadequate, HBIG × 1[a] plus hepatitis B vaccine booster dose 2. If adequate, no treatment	No treatment	Test exposed person for anti-HBs[c] 1. If inadequate, hepatitis B vaccine booster dose 2. If adequate, no treatment

[a] HBIG dose 0.06 mL/kg IM.
[b] For dosing information see Table 69.5.
[c] Adequate anti-HBs is ≥10 mIU.

Table 69.9 • Factors Predictive of a Sustained Response to Interferon-Alpha in Patients with Chronic Hepatitis

Chronic hepatitis B
Short duration of disease
High serum aminotransferase concentrations[a]
Active liver disease with fibrosis[a]
Low HBV DNA concentrations
Wild-type (HBcAg positive) virus
Absence of immunosuppression

[a] One of the most commonly associated factors with a high degree of response to therapy.

Notes:

Table 69.10 • Serious Adverse Events Reported with Interferon-Alpha Therapy

Central Nervous System
Psychosis
Depression/suicide
Delirium/confusion
Extrapyramidal ataxia
Paresthesia
Seizures
Relapse in substance abuse

Hematologic
Granulocytopenia
Thrombocytopenia
Anemia

Dermatologic
Psoriasis
Erythema multiforme

Gastrointestinal
Autoimmune hepatitis
Primary biliary cirrhosis
Hepatic decompensation

Cardiovascular
Cardiac arrhythmias
Sudden death
Dilated cardiomyopathy
Hypotension

Other
Retinopathy
Hearing loss
Pulmonary interstitial fibrosis
Acute renal failure
Hyperthyroidism
Hypothyroidism
Systemic lupus erythematosus

From references 200, 214, and 215.

The reader is referred to Chapter 71: Viral Hepatitis, written by *Curtis D. Holt, Pharm.D.*, and *Robin L. Corelli, Pharm.D.*, in the seventh edition of **Applied Therapeutics: The Clinical Use of Drugs** for a more in-depth discussion. All notations to reference numbers are based on the reference list at the end of that chapter. The editors of this handbook express their thanks to Drs. Holt and Corelli and acknowledge that this chapter is based upon their work.

Notes:

Notes:

Chapter 70

Parasitic Infections

Infection secondary to parasites is observed throughout the world. Geographic location, immune status (AIDS, malignancy, immunosuppressive therapy), and other factors are associated with an increased likelihood of parasitic infection. Table 70.1 lists the drugs of choice for treatment of parasitic infection.

Notes:

Table 70.1 • Drug Therapy of Parasitic Infection[3,23,26,29,39–43,64,74,81,106,135,138,a]

Drug of Choice	Dosage	Adverse Effects
Amebiasis (Including Cyst Passers)		
Asymptomatic		
Iodoquinol	*Adult:* 650 mg PO TID × 20 days	Rash, acne, thyroid enlargement
	Pediatric: 30–40 mg/kg/day PO TID × 20 days	
or		
Diloxanide furoate	*Adult:* 500 mg PO TID × 10 days	Flatulence, abdominal pain
	Pediatric: 20 mg/kg/day PO TID × 10 days	
or		
Paromomycin	*Adult:* 500 mg PO TID × 7 days	Nausea, vomiting
	Pediatric: 25–30 mg/kg/day PO TID × 7 days	
Mild-to-Moderate Gastrointestinal Disease		
Metronidazole	*Adult:* 750 mg PO TID × 10 days	Nausea, headache, metallic taste, disulfiram reaction with alcohol, paresthesia
	Pediatric: 35–50 mg/kg/day PO TID × 10 days	
followed by		
Iodoquinol	*Adult:* 650 mg PO TID × 20 days	Rash, acne, thyroid enlargement
	Pediatric: 30–40 mg/kg/day PO TID × 20 days	
Severe Gastrointestinal Disease		
Metronidazole	*Adult:* 750 mg PO TID × 10 days	Nausea, headache, metallic taste, disulfiram reaction with alcohol, paresthesia
	Pediatric: 35–50 mg/kg/day PO TID × 10 days	
followed by		
Iodoquinol	*Adult:* 650 mg PO TID × 20 days	Rash, acne, thyroid enlargement
	Pediatric: 30–40 mg/kg/day PO TID × 20 days	
Alternatives		
Dehydroemetine	*Adult:* 1–1.5 mg/kg/day IM × 5 days (maximum, 90 mg/day)	Arrhythmias, hypotension, ECG: P-R, Q-T, QRS prolongation, and S-T depression
followed by	*Pediatric:* Same as adult	
Iodoquinol	*Adult:* 650 mg PO TID × 20 days	Rash, acne, thyroid enlargement
	Pediatric: 30–40 mg/kg/day PO TID × 20 days	
Amebic Liver Abscess		
Metronidazole	*Adult:* 750 mg TID × 10 days	Nausea, headache, metallic taste, disulfiram reaction with alcohol, paresthesia
	Pediatric: 35–50 mg/kg/day PO TID × 10 days	
followed by		
Iodoquinol	*Adult:* 650 mg PO TID × 20 days	Rash, acne, thyroid enlargement
	Pediatric: 30–40 mg/kg/day PO TID × 20 days	
Alternatives		
Dehydroemetine	*Adult:* 1–1.5 mg/kg/day IM × 5 days (maximum, 90 mg/day)	Arrhythmias, hypotension, ECG: P-R, Q-T, QRS prolongation and S-T depression
followed by	*Pediatric:* Same as adult	
Diloxanide furoate	*Adult:* 500 mg PO TID × 10 days	
	Pediatric: 20 mg/kg/day PO TID × 10 days	
or		
Paromomycin	*Adult:* 500 mg/kg/day PO TID × 7 days	Nausea, vomiting
	Pediatric: 25–30 mg/kg/day PO TID × 7 days	

Ascariasis (Roundworm)
Mebendazole — *Adult/Pediatric:* 100 mg BID PO × 3 days — Diarrhea, abdominal pain

Enterobiasis (Pinworm)
Albendazole — 400 mg PO × 1 and repeat in 2 weeks
or
Mebendazole — 100 mg PO × 1 and repeat in 2 weeks
or
Pyrantel pamoate — *Adult/Pediatric:* 11 mg/kg PO once (maximum, 1 g), repeat in 2 wk

Flukes (Trematodes)[b]
Praziquantel — *Adult/Pediatric:* 75 mg/kg/day in 3 doses × 1 day (*Exception: P. westermani* × 2 days) — Malaise, headache, dizziness, sedation, fever, eosinophilia

Giardiasis
Metronidazole[c] — *Adult:* 250 mg PO TID with meals × 5 days — Nausea, headache, metallic taste, disulfiram reaction with alcohol, paresthesia
Pediatric: 15 mg/kg/day PO TID × 5 days
or
Albendazole — 400 mg PO QD × 5 days — Diarrhea, abdominal pain, rarely hepatotoxicity, rare leukopenia

Hookworm
Mebendazole — *Adult/Pediatric:* 100 mg PO BID × 3 days — Diarrhea, abdominal pain
or
Albendazole — 400 mg PO × 1 — Diarrhea, abdominal pain

Lice
1% Permethrin (NIX) — Topical administration — Occasional allergic reaction, mild stinging, erythema

Malaria
All Plasmodia, except Chloroquine-Resistant
Parental Therapy
Quinidine gluconate — *Adult:* Loading dose 10 mg/kg of salt (6.2 mg base) diluted in 250 mL normal saline and infused IV over 2 hr, followed by a continuous IV infusion of 0.02 mg/kg/min (0.012 mg base) for 72 hr; should be switched to oral quinine 650 mg Q 8 hr as soon as possible — ECG findings: Q-T and QRS prolongation; hypotension, syncope, arrhythmias; cinchonism
Pediatric: Same as adult

(continued)

Table 70.1 • Drug Therapy of Parasitic Infection[3,23,26,29,39-43,64,74,81,106,135,138,a] (continued)

Drug of Choice	Dosage	Adverse Effects
Malaria (*continued*) Oral Therapy	*If chloroquine-susceptible: Chloroquine 1.0 gm (600 mg base) PO, 0.5 gm in 6 hrs, then 0.5 gm daily × 2 days *plus* Primaquine 26.3 mg (15 mg base) PO daily × 14 days	Primaquine needed only for *P. vivax* or *P. ovale* Check for G6PD
	*If chloroquine-resistant: 1) Quinine sulfate 650 mg PO Q 8 H × 3–7 days *plus* Doxycycline 100 mg PO BID × 7 days *or* 2) Mefloquine 750 mg PO × 1, then 500 mg 12 hours later	Central nervous system adverse effects
	*Prophylaxis (Adults) Mefloquine 250 mg PO weekly 1 week before, during, and 4 weeks after travel (If areas free of chloroquine resistance, give: chloroquine 500 mg PO per week, starting 1–2 weeks before travel, during, and 4 weeks after travel)	

Scabies

Drug	Dose/Administration	Adverse effects
5% Permethrin (Elimite cream)	Topical administration	Rash, edema, erythema
Alternatives		
Lindane (Kwell)	Apply topically once	Not recommended in pregnant women, infants, and in people with massive excoriated skin
Crotamiton 10% (Eurax)	Topically	Local skin irritation
Tapeworm[d]		
Praziquantel	*Adult/Pediatric:* 5–10 mg/kg PO × 1 dose	Malaise, headache, dizziness, sedation, eosinophilia, fever
Hydatid cysts[e]		
Albendazole	*Adult:* 400 mg BID × 8–30 days, repeat if necessary *Pediatric:* 15 mg/kg/day × 28 days, repeat if necessary (surgical resection may precede drug therapy)	Diarrhea, abdominal pain, rarely hepatotoxicity, leukopenia
Trichomoniasis		
Metronidazole	*Adult:* 2 g PO × 1 day or 250 mg PO TID × 7 days *Pediatric:* 15 mg/kg/day PO TID × 7 days	Nausea, headache, metallic taste, disulfiram reaction with alcohol, paresthesia

[a] ECG = Electrocardiograph; G6PD = Glucose-6-phosphate dehydrogenase.
[b] *Schistosoma haematobium, Schistosoma mansoni, Schistosoma japonicum, Clonorchis sinensis, Paragonimus westermani.*
[c] Quinacrine no longer is available in the United States or any other country at this time.
[d] *Diphyllobothrium latum* (fish), *Taenia saginata* (beef), *Taenia solium* (pork), and *Dipylidium caninum* (dog), except for *Hymenolepsis nana,* where dose is 25 mg/kg × 1 dose.
[e] *Echinococcus granulosus, Echinococcus multicularis.* For neurocysticercosis: 15 mg/kg/day in two divided doses × 8 days.

The reader is referred to Chapter 72: Parasitic Infections, written by *J.V. Anandan, Pharm.D.*, in the seventh edition of **Applied Therapeutics: The Clinical Use of Drugs** for a more in-depth discussion. The editors of this handbook express their thanks to Dr. Anandan.

Notes:

Chapter 71

Tick-Borne Diseases

Lyme Disease (Table 71.2)

Identification and pathology

- ◆ *Borrelia burgdorferi* is a spirochete that is transmitted to humans via tick bite.
- ◆ Lyme borreliosis is characterized as early localized, early disseminated, or chronic/persistent disease.
- ◆ Treatment is dependent upon stage of disease. (Table 71.3)

Endemic Relapsing Fever

- ◆ Caused by separate spirochetes, including *B. hispanica* and others
- ◆ Abrupt onset on high fever with occasional additional symptoms, including shaking chills, headache, tachycardia. Fever usually breaks in 3–6 days in untreated patients.
- ◆ After variable afebrile period of 3–36 days, cyclical periods of fever and symptoms appear.
- ◆ Treatment includes doxycycline 100 mg PO BID or erythromycin 500 mg PO QID, either continued for 5–10 days.

Tularemia

- ◆ Caused by a small gram-negative coccobacillus, *Francisella tularensis*
- ◆ 2 strains, A and B are recognized with type A fatal in 5–10% of cases
- ◆ 6 types of presentation, including ulceroglandular, glandular, typhoidal, oculoglandular, oropharyngeal, and pneumonic.
- ◆ Ulceroglandular accounts for 75–80% of cases, characterized by an ulcer at the site of the tick bite.
- ◆ After incubation of 3–6 days, patients have sudden onset of fever, chills, headache, and other symptoms; rare cases are associated with shock.
- ◆ Treatment is streptomycin 7.5–10 mg/kg IM or IV Q 12 H for 7–14 days.

Ehrlichiosis

- ◆ Ehrlichia chaffeensis is associated with human monocytic ehrlichiosis (HME); human granulocyte ehrlichiosis (HGE) is caused by an unknown ehrlichial species.
- ◆ Presents usually as a nonspecific, febrile, flu-like illness beginning 3–7 days after tick bite.
- ◆ Both HME and HGE are associated with fever 100% of the time.
- ◆ Malaise, myalgia, headache, rigors are common with HGE but less common for HME.
- ◆ Transaminitis, leukopenia, thrombocytopenia, anemia are often observed.

♦ Doxycycline 100 mg PO BID for 14 days is the drug of choice. If tetracyclines are contraindicated, rifampin 600 mg PO QD is the recommended alternative.

Rocky Mountain Spotted Fever (RMSF)

♦ The most prevalent, virulent rickettsial disease
♦ Observed only in Western Hemisphere but includes North, South, Central America.
♦ *Rickettsia rickettsii*
♦ After introduction into the body, associated with a generalized vasculitis, which in severe infection is associated with hypotension and intravascular coagulation.
♦ Dehydration is an early sign of RMSF; if the brain or lung is involved, fatalities have been reported.
♦ Arrhythmia occurs 10–15% of cases and confusion/lethargy in 25% of patients.
♦ Myalgia occurs in 75% of cases
♦ "Fulminant" RMSF is rapidly fatal.
♦ Treatment is doxycycline 100 mg PO/IV for 7 days or chloramphenicol 500 mg PO QID × 7 days.

Babesiosis

♦ Caused by a parasite, primarily *B. microti* in North America and *B. divergens* and *B. bovis* in Europe
♦ Diagnosis is confirmed by direct observation of the parasite inside the red blood cells.
♦ Most patients are asymptomatic with few sequelae from infection.
♦ Fevers, headache, sweats, myalgia, and hemolytic anemia are common in symptomatic patients.
♦ Treatment is (1) atovaquone 750 mg PO Q 12 H and azithromycin 500 mg × 1, then 250 mg/day × 7 days *or* (2) clindamycin 1.2 gm IV BID or 600 mg PO TID and quinine 650 mg PO TID × 7 days.

Colorado Tick Fever (CTF)

♦ Caused by a virus in the family Reoviridae
♦ Incubation period is 3–6 days after tick bite.
♦ Initial symptoms include headache, chills, myalgias. Rash is uncommon.
♦ Initial symptoms last about 2 days, followed by an afebrile period of 2 days, then recurrence of fever.
♦ CTF is usually self-limiting.

Notes:

Table 71.1 • Tick-Borne Diseases

Disease	Causative Agent	Tick Vector	Host	Region
Lyme	*Borrelia burgdorferi*	Ixodes	Wild rodents	Worldwide
Relapsing fever (endemic)	*Borrelia* species	Ornithodoros	Wild rodents	Worldwide
Tularemia	*Francisella tularensis*	Dermacentor Amblyomma	Rabbits	North America
Rocky Mountain spotted fever	*Rickettsia rickettsii*	Dermacentor	Wild rodents, ticks	Western hemisphere
Boutonneuse fever	*Rickettsia conorii*	Ixodes	Wild rodents, dogs	Africa, India, Mediterranean
North Asian tick typhus	*Rickettsia sibirica*	Ixodes	Wild rodents	Mongolia, Siberia
Queensland tick typhus	*Rickettsia australis*	Ixodes	Wild rodents, marsupials	Australia
Q fever	*Coxiella burnetii*	Dermacentor Amblyomma	Sheep, goats cattle, ticks, cats	Worldwide
Babesiosis	*Babesia* species	Ixodes	Mice, voles	Europe, North America
Ehrlichiosis				
HME	*Ehrlichia chaffeensis*	Amblyomma Dermacentor	Deer, mice, dogs	United States
HGE	*E. equi*–like bacteria	Ixodes Dermacentor	Deer, mice rodents	United States
Colorado tick fever	*Coltivirus* species	Dermacentor	Ticks	North America
Tick paralysis	Neurotoxin	Dermacentor	N/A	North America, Europe Australia, South Africa

Table 71.2 • Lyme Borreliosis Stages[4,19,20,31,32,90,a]

Early Localized Infection (Stage 1): Usually Days After Tick Bite
EM skin rash
Myalgia, arthralgia, headache, stiff neck, fatigue, lethargy
Viral-like syndrome, fever, chills

Early Disseminated Disease (Stage 2): Days to Months After Bite
Musculoskeletal: Fibromyalgia, Arthralgia
  Migratory arthritis
  Large or small joint swelling, especially the temporomandibular joint
  Painful, unilateral hand/finger swelling (Europe)
Heart (8% of Untreated Patients in the United States)
  Cardiomyopathy, CHF, myocarditis or pericarditis
  Conduction defects, varying degrees of AV, or bundle branch block, but permanent pacing is not
    indicated
  Arrhythmias
Nervous System (Neuroborreliosis)
  Cranial nerve (Bell's) palsy
  Meningitis, lymphocytic
  Radiculoneuritis, myelitis
  Sensory or motor peripheral neuropathy
  Ataxia
  Encephalomyelitis
Eye
  Iritis, conjunctivitis, choroiditis, uveitis, optic neuritis, retinal vasculitis, panophthalmitis, optic disk
    edema, keratitis
Lymph
  Generalized or localized lymphadenopathy
Skin
  Multiple secondary EM lesions in 50% with primary EM; lymphocytoma (lymphadenosis benigna
    cutis) rare in the United States but 1% in Europe
Liver
  Hepatitis, recurrent; Abnormal LFTs
Lung
  Acute respiratory distress syndrome
Kidney
  Microscopic hematuria or proteinuria
Testicle
  Orchitis

Chronic or Persistent Disease (Stage 3): Months to Years After Bite
Musculoskeletal (62% in the United States, less common in Europe)
  Chronic (10% of untreated in the United States) or intermittent arthritis of ≥1 large joints,
    especially the knee
Skin (10% in Europe, rare in the United States)
  Acrodermatitis chronica atrophicans (unique to Lyme borreliosis)
Fibromyalgia
Late Neurologic
  Peripheral neuropathy, subacute encephalopathy (memory impairment, sleep disturbance, dementia)
    and in Europe, progressive encephalomyelitis

[a]AV = Atrioventricular; CHF = Congestive heart failure; EM = Erythema migrans; LFTs = Liver function tests.

Notes:

Table 71.3 • Suggested Treatment Recommendation for Lyme Borreliosis[14,15,17,19,27-29,34,35,a]

Erythema Migrans, Early, Uncomplicated
Adult: Doxycycline (Vibramycin) 100 mg PO BID × 14–21 days (or 200 mg QD × 21 days)
or
Amoxicillin (Polymox) 500 mg PO TID × 14–21 days
or
Cefuroxime axetil (Ceftin) 500 mg PO BID × 14–21 days
Child (<8 yr): Amoxicillin 40 mg/kg/day PO in 3 divided doses × 14–21 days or cefuroxime 250 mg PO BID × 14–21 days

Erythema Migrans with Signs of Dissemination
Carditis
Adult: Ceftriaxone (Rocephin) 2 g IV QD × 14 days
or
Cefotaxime (Claforan) 2 g IV TID × 14 days
or
Penicillin G (Pfizerpen) 20 MU divided QID × 14 days
or
For mild cardiac involvement only: doxycycline or amoxicillin in doses as noted above × 21 days
Child: Ceftriaxone IV 100 mg/kg/day divided BID × 14 days
or
Cefotaxime IV 180 mg/kg/day divided TID × 14 days
or
Penicillin G IV 300,000 U/kg/day divided Q 6 hr × 14 days
Neurologic or Ocular Disease
Facial nerve paralysis as an isolated early finding: at dosages as noted above for early EM × 21–30 days
Meningitis, radiculitis, or encephalitis: IV drugs at dosages as noted above for carditis x × 0 days
or
Doxycycline 100 mg IV BID × 30 days

Chronic Disease
Lymphocytoma or Acrodermatitis
Oral regimens for 30 days
Arthritis
Adult: Doxycycline 200 mg/day PO × 30 days
or
Amoxicillin 500 mg PO QID × 30 days
or
Ceftriaxone or cefotaxime at dosages as noted above × 14–28 days
Child: Amoxicillin 50 mg/kg divided TID × 28 days
or
Ceftriaxone or cefotaxime (pediatric dosing) × 14–21 days

Pregnant/ Breast-Feeding
Amoxicillin 500 mg PO TID × 21 days; if evidence of dissemination: penicillin G IV 20 MU/day × 14–21 days (doxycycline contraindicated)
Ceftriaxone 2 g IV QD × 14 days

[a]EM = Erythema migrans.

Notes:

The reader is referred to Chapter 73: Tick-Borne Disease, written by *Tom B. Christian, RPh,* in the seventh edition of **Applied Therapeutics: The Clinical Use of Drugs** for a more in-depth discussion. All notations to reference numbers are based on the reference list at the end of that chapter. The editors of this handbook express their thanks to Dr. Christian and acknowledge that this chapter is based upon his work.

Notes:

Chapter 72

Anxiety Disorders

Definition. Unlike other mental disorders, anxiety can be both a normal emotion and a psychiatric illness. When anxiety is excessive for the situation or when the harmful effects of anxiety outweigh the beneficial, anxiety becomes a pathological disorder. It usually involves both *mental features* (e.g., worry, fear, difficulty concentrating) and *physical symptoms* (e.g., racing heart, shortness of breath, trembling, pacing).

Classification and Diagnosis. See Figure 72.1. Pathological anxiety is differentiated based on whether it occurs:

♦ As a primary anxiety disorder, which includes
  • Generalized anxiety disorder (GAD). See Table 72.1
  • Panic disorder. See Table 72.2
  • Phobic disorders. See Table 72.3
  • Obsessive-compulsive disorder (OCD). See Table 72.4
  • Posttraumatic stress disorder (PTSD). See Table 72.5
  • Acute stress disorder
  • Anxiety disorder not otherwise specified

♦ As a secondary anxiety disorder due to medical causes or substances. See Table 72.6

♦ In response to acute stress

♦ As a symptom in association with other psychiatric disorders

Comparative Drug Treatment of Anxiety Disorders. See Table 72.7. Psychological and behavioral strategies also are used.

GAD Treatment. See Table 72.8. Treatment is generally continued for 2–6 months.

♦ *Benzodiazepines (BZD)* are the most widely prescribed anxiolytics because they are efficacious and less toxic than older agents.
  • FDA approved indications and doses: See Table 72.9
  • Pharmacokinetics (PK). See Table 72.10
  • Physiologic variables affecting PK of BZDs. See Table 72.11
  • Drug interactions: See Table 72.12
  • Withdrawal symptoms: See Table 72.13. Onset 4–7 days for BZDs with long half-life. Symptoms generally mild if dose is tapered. Higher risk with high-potency agents such as alprazolam, lorazepam, and clonazepam.

♦ *Buspirone*
  • As effective as BZDs for GAD, but onset delayed 1–2 weeks. See Table 72.8.
  • Lacks CNS depressant, muscle relaxant, anticonvulsant and physical dependent effects associated with BZDs
  • Drug interactions. See Table 72.14

♦ *Venlafaxine XR and Other Antidepressants*
  • First antidepressant approved to treat GAD. As effective as BZDs. See Table 72.8
  • SSRIs effective in treating other anxiety disorders but not well studied in GAD

♦ *β Blockers* (e.g., propranolol) effectively reduce physical symptoms (tremor, flushing, tachycardia) associated with performance anxiety.

Panic Disorder Drug Treatment. See Table 72.15.

Phobic Disorders (Social Anxiety Disorder) Drug Treatment

♦ *Specific Serotonin Reuptake Inhibitors (SSRIs)* are primary treatment option.
   • Paroxetine is only medication approved by the FDA for treatment, but other SSRIs are likely to be effective.
   • Doses are similar to those used for depression
   • Response is gradual, and minimum trial is 8–10 weeks
♦ Other medications include MAOIs, BZDs, and β Blockers
♦ Cognitive and behavioral therapies are comparable to medications

PSTD and Acute Stress Disorder Treatment

♦ *SSRIs* are first-line treatment
   • Sertraline is only SSRI approved by FDA, but fluoxetine is also effective
   • Sertraline dose: 25 mg/day initially, gradually increased to 50–150 mg/day.
   • Onset 2 weeks, with continued improvement over 2–3 mos
   • Duration of therapy is 6–12 mos for acute cases and 12–24 mos for chronic cases (sxs present for >3 mos before treatment)
♦ Many other medications have been used. See Chapter 74 in **Applied Therapeutics: The Clinical Use of Drugs.**

OCD Drug Treatment

♦ *SSRIs* are first-line treatment
   • Efficacy documented for fluvoxamine (150 mg/day), fluoxetine (20 mg/day), paroxetine (40 mg/day), and sertraline (50 mg/day)
   • Use usual SSRI starting doses but allow 4 weeks before exceeding targeted minimally effective doses as noted above. See Chapter 75: Depression
♦ Many other medications (including clomipramine) and strategies have been used. See Chapter 74 in **Applied Therapeutics: The Clinical Use of Drugs.**

Table 72.1 • Diagnostic Criteria for GAD[a]

A. Unrealistic or excessive anxiety and worry about life circumstances for a period of at least 6 months, during which the person has been bothered more days than not by these concerns
B. The person has difficulty controlling the anxiety and worry
C. The anxiety and worry are associated with at least three of the following symptoms:
   1. Restlessness or feeling keyed up or on edge
   2. Being easily fatigued
   3. Difficulty concentrating or mind going blank
   4. Irritability
   5. Muscle tension
   6. Sleep disturbances
D. If another psychiatric disorder is present, the focus of the anxiety and worry is unrelated to it
E. The anxiety, worry, or physical symptoms cause significant distress or impairment in social, occupational, or some other important aspect of functioning
F. The disturbance is not due to the direct effects of a substance, medication, or general medical condition and does not occur only during the course of a mood disorder, a psychotic disorder, or a pervasive developmental disorder

Adapted from reference 1.
[a]GAD = Generalized anxiety disorder.

Table 72.2 • Diagnostic Criteria for Panic Disorder[a]

A. The presence of at least two unexpected panic attacks, characterized by at least four of the following symptoms, which develop abruptly and reach a peak within 10 min:
   1. Palpitations, pounding heart, or accelerated heart rate
   2. Sweating
   3. Trembling or shaking
   4. Sensations of shortness of breath or smothering
   5. Feeling of choking
   6. Chest pain or discomfort
   7. Nausea or abdominal distress
   8. Feeling dizzy, unsteady, lightheaded, or faint
   9. Derealization or depersonalization
   10. Fear of losing control or going crazy
   11. Fear of dying
   12. Numbness or tingling sensations
   13. Chills or hot flushes
B. At least one of the attacks has been followed by at least one of the following symptoms for a duration of at least 1 month:
   1. Persistent concern about having another attack
   2. Worry about the implications or consequences of the attack
   3. A significant change in behavior because of the attack
C. The symptoms are not due to the direct effects of a medication, substance, or general medical condition
D. The panic attacks are not better accounted for by another psychiatric or anxiety disorder (e.g., phobias, OCD)
E. May occur with or without agoraphobia (see text)

[a]OCD = Obsessive-compulsive disorder.
Adapted from reference 1.

Table 72.3 • Diagnostic Criteria for Phobic Disorders[a]

Social Anxiety Disorder
1. A marked and constant fear of one or more social situations where the person is exposed to unfamiliar people or possible scrutiny by others and the person fears humiliation or embarrassment
2. Exposure to the situation provokes an immediate anxiety response
3. The person realizes the fear is excessive or unreasonable (not required in children)
4. The situation is avoided or endured with intense anxiety or distress
5. The fear or avoidance significantly interferes with the person's normal routine or activities or causes marked distress
6. In individuals less than 18 years of age, the duration of the fear is at least 6 months
7. The anxiety or phobic avoidance are not better accounted for by another psychiatric disorder (e.g., fear of having a panic attack, obsessions that accompany OCD, or trauma related to PTSD)

Specific Phobia
1. A marked and persistent fear of a specific object or situation that is excessive or unreasonable
2. Other criteria (2–7) that are listed above for social anxiety disorder

[a]OCD = Obsessive-compulsive disorder; PTSD = Post-traumatic stress disorder.
Adapted from reference 1.

Notes:

Table 72.4 • Diagnostic Criteria for OCD[a]

A. The presence of either obsessions or compulsions:
   Obsessions:
   1. Recurrent and persistent ideas or thoughts that are experienced, at some time during the disturbance, as intrusive and senseless
   2. The thoughts, impulses, or images are not simply excessive worries about real-life problems
   3. The person attempts to ignore or neutralize the ideas or thoughts with some other thought or action
   4. The person realizes the obsessions are the product of his or her own mind
   Compulsions:
   1. Repetitive and intentional behaviors or mental acts performed in response to the obsession or according to rigid rules
   2. The behavior is designed to prevent or reduce distress or to prevent some dreaded event; however, the activity clearly is excessive and unrealistic to neutralize the situation
B. At some point during the disturbance, the person realizes that the obsessions and compulsions are excessive or unreasonable (not necessary in children)
C. The obsessions or compulsions cause marked distress, are time-consuming (>1 hr/day), or significantly interfere with some aspect of daily functioning
D. The content of the symptoms is not related to another psychiatric disorder, and the disturbance is not due to the direct effects of a substance, medication, or general medical illness

[a]OCD = Obsessive-compulsive disorder.
Adapted from reference 1.

Table 72.5 • Diagnostic Criteria for PTSD[a]

A. The person has experienced a traumatic event in which the individual witnessed, experienced, or was confronted with actual or threatened death, or serious injury to self or others and to which the person responded with intense fear, helplessness, or horror
B. The traumatic event is re-experienced persistently in some way (e.g., dreams, nightmares, flashbacks, recurrent thoughts or images), or intense distress is experienced on exposure to stimuli associated with the traumatic event
C. Persistent avoidance of stimuli associated with the event or numbing of general responsiveness (e.g., avoidance of thoughts, people, or places associated with the event, impaired recall of the event, anhedonia, feelings of detachment, restricted affect)
D. Persistent symptoms of increased arousal (not present before the event) that includes at least two of the following:
   1. Sleep disturbances
   2. Irritability or anger outbursts
   3. Difficulty concentrating
   4. Hypervigilance
   5. Exaggerated startle response
E. Duration of the disturbance (B, C, and D) of at least 1 month
F. The disturbance causes significant impairment in some aspect of daily functioning

[a]PTSD = Post-traumatic stress disorder.
Adapted from reference 2.

Notes:

Table 72.6 • Secondary Causes of Anxiety[a]

Medical Illnesses

Endocrine and metabolic disorders: hyperthyroidism, hypoglycemia, Addison's disease, Cushing's disease, pheochromocytoma, PMS, electrolyte abnormalities, acute intermittent porphyria, anemia

Neurologic: seizure disorders, multiple sclerosis, chronic pain syndromes, traumatic brain injury, CNS neoplasm, migraines, myasthenia gravis, Parkinson's disease, vertigo, essential tremor

Cardiovascular: mitral valve prolapse, CHF, arrhythmias, post-MI, hyperdynamic β-adrenergic state, hypertension, angina pectoris, postcerebral infarction

GI: PUD, Crohn's disease, ulcerative colitis, irritable bowel syndrome

Respiratory: COPD, asthma, pneumonia, pulmonary edema, respirator dependence, pulmonary embolus

Others: HIV infection, systemic lupus erythematosus

Psychiatric

Depression, mania, schizophrenia, adjustment disorder, personality disorders, delirium, dementia, eating disorders

Drugs

CNS stimulants: amphetamines, caffeine, cocaine, diethylpropion, ephedrine, MDMA (Ecstasy), methylphenidate, nicotine (and withdrawal), PCP, phenylephrine, phenylpropanolamine, pseudoephedrine

CNS depressant withdrawal: barbiturates, benzodiazepines, ethanol, opiates

Psychotropics: antipsychotics (akathisia), bupropion, buspirone, SSRIs, TCAs, venlafaxine

Cardiovascular: captopril, enalapril, digitalis, disopyramide, hydralazine, reserpine

Others: albuterol, aminophylline, baclofen, bromocriptine, cycloserine, dapsone, dronabinol, interferon alfa, isoniazid, isoproterenol, levodopa, lidocaine, mefloquine, metoclopramide, monosodium glutamate, nicotinic acid, NSAIDs, norfloxacin, pergolide, quinacrine, steroids, sumatriptan, theophylline, thyroid hormone, yohimbine

[a]CHF = Congestive heart failure; CNS = Central nervous system; COPD = Chronic obstructive pulmonary disease; GI = Gastrointestinal; MI = Myocardial infarction; NSAIDs = Nonsteroidal anti-inflammatory drugs; PCP = Phencyclidine; PMS = Premenstrual syndrome; PUD = Peptic ulcer disease; SSRIs = Selective serotonin reuptake inhibitors; TCAs = Tricyclic antidepressants.

Notes:

Table 72.7 • Summary of Comparative Medication Treatment Options for Anxiety Disorders

Disorder	First-Line Treatments[a]	Second-Line Treatments	Possible Alternatives
Generalized anxiety disorder	Venlafaxine XR Buspirone Benzodiazepines	Paroxetine Nefazodone	Tricyclic antidepressants[b] Fluoxetine Mirtazapine Hydroxyzine
Panic disorder	Paroxetine Sertraline Alprazolam Clonazepam	Fluvoxamine Citalopram Clomipramine Diazepam	Fluoxetine Venlafaxine Nefazodone Mirtazapine Imipramine Valproic acid
Social anxiety disorder	Paroxetine	Fluoxetine Fluvoxamine Sertraline Citalopram Clonazepam Alprazolam	Phenelzine[b] Venlafaxine Nefazodone Bupropion Buspirone[c] Ondansetron Gabapentin
Post-traumatic stress disorder	Sertraline	Fluoxetine Paroxetine Fluvoxamine Venlafaxine Nefazodone	Amitriptyline[b] Imipramine[b] Phenelzine[b] Mirtazapine Trazodone[c] Carbamazepine Valproic acid Lamotrigine Atypical antipsychotics[c]
Obsessive-compulsive disorder	Paroxetine Fluoxetine Sertraline Fluvoxamine	Clomipramine[b] Venlafaxine	Clonazepam[c] Antipsychotic agents[c] Buspirone[c] Phenelzine[b] Nefazodone Lithium[c]

[a]FDA-approved indications.
[b]Documented efficacy but not first-line because of undesirable clinical properties (side effects, potential toxicity, drug interactions).
[c]Adjunctive therapy.

Notes:

Table 72.8 • First-Line Treatment of Generalized Anxiety Disorders (GAD)

Drug (Brand Name) Dosage Forms	Usual Dose	Advantages	Disadvantages	Other
BZDs (various) See Table 72.9	See Table 72.9	• Effective • Rapid onset • Less dangerous relative to barbiturates • Superior to antidepressants in relieving somatic symptoms • Preferred for transient or intermittent anxiety (prn dosing)	• Sedation • Cognitive impairment • Psychomotor impairment • Abuse potential	• Most clinicians prefer shorter-acting agents (e.g. lorazepam or alprazolam) • High lipid solubility (e.g. diazepam) confers rapid onset but shorter duration despite long half-life. Can produce "drugged" effect.
Buspirone (BuSpar) 5, 10, 15 mg tabs Dividose Tabs: 15 mg can be bi- or trisected	• 20–30 mg daily in 2–3 divided doses. • Initial dose: 10–15 mg in 2-3 doses. Increase by 5 mg Q3–4 days.	• Effective • No CNS depressant effects. • Covers co-morbid psychiatric conditions (e.g. depression) • No sexual dysfunction • No dependence or abuse potential • Ideal for elderly, h/o drug abuse, mixed anxiety-depression, medically ill.	• Slow onset (1–2 wks; 2–4 wks for optimal effect) • Nausea, dizziness, headache, initial nervousness	• Caution in patients with kidney or liver dysfunction • Regular dosing required for efficacy • Use BZDs initially if rapid relief required • Antidepressant doses are higher (40–60 mg/day)
Venlafaxine XR (Effexor XR) 37.5, 75, 150 mg capsules	• 75–225 mg daily • Initial dose: 37.5–75 mg	• Superior to BZD in managing cognitive & psychiatric sxs • Covers co-morbid psychiatric conditions	• Slow onset (3–4 wks) • Nausea, dizziness, dry mouth, asthenia, sweating, sedation or insomnia initially. • Hypotension at higher doses.	• Anxious patients often require lower initial dose • Regular dosing required for efficacy • Use BZDs initially if rapid relief required

Table 72.9 • Clinical Comparison of Benzodiazepine Agents

Drug (Trade Name, Generic)	FDA-Approved Indications	Usual Dosage Range ≤65 Years of Age	Maximum Recommended Dosage ≥65 Years of Age	Approximate Dosage Equivalencies	Year Introduced
Chlordiazepoxide (Librium, Limbitrol,[a] Librax,[b] generic)	Anxiety, preoperative anxiety, acute alcohol withdrawal	15–100 mg/day	40 mg/day	50	1960
Diazepam (Valium, generic)	Anxiety, muscle relaxant, acute alcohol withdrawal, preoperative anxiety, anticonvulsant	4–40 mg/day	20 mg/day	10	1963
Oxazepam (Serax, generic)	Anxiety, alcohol withdrawal	30–120 mg/day	60 mg/day	30	1965
Flurazepam (Dalmane, generic)	Sedative-hypnotic	15–30 mg HS	15 mg HS	30	1970
Clorazepate (Tranxene, Tranxene-SD, generic)	Anxiety, alcohol withdrawal, anticonvulsant	15–60 mg/day	30 mg/day	15	1972
Clonazepam (Klonopin, generic)	Anticonvulsant, panic disorder	0.5–12.0 mg/day	3 mg/day	0.5	1975
Lorazepam (Ativan, generic)	Anxiety, anxiety associated with depression	2–6 mg/day	3 mg/day	1.5–2.0	1977
Alprazolam (Xanax, generic)	Anxiety, anxiety associated with depression, panic disorder	0.5–6.0 mg/day (up to 10 mg/day for panic disorder)	2 mg/day	1.0	1981
Halazepam (Paxipam)	Anxiety	60–160 mg/day	80 mg/day	60	1981
Temazepam (Restoril, generic)	Sedative-hypnotic	15–30 mg HS	15 mg HS	30	1981
Triazolam (Halcion)	Sedative-hypnotic	0.125–0.25 mg HS	0.125 mg HS	0.25	1983
Quazepam (Doral)	Sedative-hypnotic	7.5–15 mg HS	7.5 mg HS	15	1990
Estazolam (Prosom)	Sedative-hypnotic	1–2 mg HS	1 mg HS	2.0	1991

[a]Combination product containing amitriptyline.
[b]Combination product containing clidinium bromide.

Table 72.10 • Pharmacokinetic Comparison of Benzodiazepine Agents[a]

Drug	Elimination Half-Life (hr)[b]	Active Metabolites	Protein Binding	Pathway of Metabolism	Rate of Onset After Oral Administration
Chlordiazepoxide	>100	Desmethyldiazepam	96%	Oxidation	Intermediate
Diazepam	>100	Desmethyldiazepam	98%	Oxidation (CYP 3A4, CYP 2C19)	Very fast
Oxazepam	5–14	None	87%	Conjugation	Slow
Flurazepam	>100	Desalkylflurazepam, hydroxyethylflurazepam	97%	Oxidation	Fast
Clorazepate	>100	Desmethyldiazepam	98%	Oxidation	Fast
Lorazepam	10–20	None	85–90%	Conjugation	Intermediate
Alprazolam	12–15	Insignificant	80%	Oxidation (CYP 3A4)	Intermediate
Halazepam	>100	Desmethyldiazepam	97%	Oxidation	Slow
Temazepam	10–20	Insignificant	98%	Conjugation	Intermediate
Triazolam	1.5–5	Insignificant	90%	Oxidation (CYP 3A4)	Intermediate
Quazepam	47–100	2-oxoquazepam, desalkyloxoquazepam	>95%	Oxidation	Fast
Estazolam	24	Insignificant	93%	Oxidation	Intermediate
Clonazepam	20–50	Insignificant	85%	Oxidation, reduction (CYP 3A4)	Fast
Midazolam	1–4	None	97%	Oxidation (CYP 3A4)	NA

[a]NA = Not applicable.
[b]Parent drug + active metabolite.

Table 72.11 • Physiologic Factors Influencing Benzodiazepine Pharmacokinetics[a]

Factor	Physiologic and Pharmacokinetic Effects	Clinical Significance/Comments
Aging	Increased elimination half-life due to increased Vd of all benzodiazepines[65,235]	Lower benzodiazepine dosages, and possibly less frequent dosing intervals, recommended in the elderly
	Decreased clearance of benzodiazepines that undergo oxidative hepatic metabolism (see Table 72.9)[65,236]	Benzodiazepines that undergo conjugative metabolism (lorazepam, oxazepam) preferred in the elderly
	Decreased plasma proteins may lead to increased free fraction of highly protein-bound benzodiazepines (see Table 72.9)[65]	Possible increased clinical effects
	Decreased gastric acidity may lead to increased rate of benzodiazepine absorption[65]	Possible faster onset of clinical effects
Gender	Age-related decrease in hepatic oxidative metabolism of benzodiazepines more pronounced in males	Elderly males may require especially low benzodiazepine dosages
	Increased CYP 3A4 and CYP 2C19 activity in premenopausal women may result in higher clearance of drugs that undergo oxidative metabolism[15]	Possible decreased plasma benzodiazepine concentrations and shorter duration of clinical effects of oxidatively metabolized in premenopausal women
	Decreased glucuronidation in women may result in slower clearance of benzodiazepines metabolized by conjugation[15]	Women may have longer elimination half-lives of conjugated benzodiazepines and may require less frequent dosing
	Increased Vd in women due to lower lean body mass and higher adipose tissue[15]	Possible longer elimination half-lives in women, especially the elderly, and greater drug accumulation
	Lower plasma protein binding in women[15]	Clinical significance unknown
Obesity	Increased benzodiazepine elimination half-lives due to increased Vd[65]	Increased chance of drug accumulation in obese patients; dosage reductions may be indicated
Liver disease	Decreased clearance and increased elimination half-lives of long-acting benzodiazepines and alprazolam in cirrhosis and hepatitis; no changes with oxazepam or triazolam[103]	Avoid long-acting benzodiazepines, or use significantly lower doses to avoid drug accumulation
	Increased elimination half-life of lorazepam in cirrhosis but not acute hepatitis	Decreased lorazepam dose or increased dosing interval recommended in cirrhosis
Kidney disease	Decreased plasma protein binding may lead to increased free fraction of highly protein bound benzodiazepines (see Table 72.9)	Dosage reductions may be necessary
Ethnicity	Decreased oxidative metabolism (via CYP 2C19) of diazepam in Asians[106]	Asians may require lower doses of diazepam and possibly other benzodiazepines that are metabolized to desmethyldiazepam

[a]CYP = Cytochrome P450; Vd = Volume of distribution.

Notes:

Table 72.12 • Drug Interactions with Benzodiazepines[a]

Interacting Drug(s)	Effect on Object Drug	Clinical Significance/Comments
Hepatic enzyme inducers: carbamazepine, phenobarbital, phenytoin, and rifampin	Decreased Cps and clinical effects of benzodiazepines	Triazolam and midazolam may be ineffective in patients taking rifampin.[226] Carbamazepine greatly decreases the Cps and clinical effects of midazolam, alprazolam, and clonazepam, possibly rendering them ineffective.[227,228]
Hepatic CYP 3A4 inhibitors: ketoconazole, itraconazole, nefazodone, fluvoxamine, fluoxetine, erythromycin, isoniazid, clarithromycin, cimetidine, oral contraceptives, diltiazem, amprenavir, and nelfinavir	Significantly increased Cps of benzodiazepines that undergo oxidative metabolism (alprazolam, triazolam, diazepam, chlordiazepoxide, halazepam, clonazepam)	Benzodiazepine dosage reductions may be required because of increased clinical effects such as sedation and psychomotor impairment; effects are greatest on alprazolam, triazolam, and midazolam.[229] Ketoconazole and itraconazole should be avoided in patients taking alprazolam or triazolam.[230] Benzodiazepine dosage reductions are recommended when nefazodone, fluoxetine, or fluvoxamine are added to alprazolam, diazepam, or triazolam.[88,89]
Ritonavir	Initial inhibition of alprazolam and triazolam metabolism, followed by later induction of metabolism	Reduced benzodiazepine dosage is needed initially if ritonavir is added to therapy; a dosage increase may be required later.[231]
Grapefruit juice	Increased Cps of diazepam, alprazolam, and triazolam	Increased benzodiazepine clinical effects (sedation, psychomotor impairment) are possible.[229,232]
Omeprazole	Increased diazepam Cp	Increased benzodiazepine clinical effects (sedation, psychomotor impairment) are possible.[107]

(continued)

Table 72.12 • Drug Interactions with Benzodiazepines^a (continued)

Interacting Drug(s)	Effect on Object Drug	Clinical Significance/Comments
Antacids, ranitidine	Decreased rate of benzodiazepine absorption	Possible delayed onset of benzodiazepine clinical effects; separation of administration times is recommended.
Valproic acid, probenecid	Significantly decreased clearance of lorazepam	Lorazepam dosage reductions may be required.[233]
Estrogen-containing oral contraceptives	Decreased Cps of benzodiazepines that undergo conjugative metabolism (lorazepam, oxazepam, temazepam)	Decreased clinical effects of benzodiazepines are possible; a dosage increase may be required.[15]
Central nervous system depressants (alcohol, barbiturates, and opioids)	Increased central nervous system depressant effects of benzodiazepines (sedation, psychomotor impairment)	Avoid use of alcohol with benzodiazepines; exercise caution with use of other depressants.
Alprazolam	Increased digoxin Cp	Digoxin toxicity is possible; monitoring of digoxin level and possible digoxin dosage reduction are recommended.[234]
Benzodiazepines	Respiratory depression and adverse cardiovascular effects reported on addition of benzodiazepines in several patients taking clozapine	Avoid benzodiazepines in patients taking clozapine.[79]
Benzodiazepines	Possible decreased efficacy of levodopa in Parkinson's disease	Drug interaction is not well established; monitor for possible effect.
Benzodiazepines	Increased or decreased efficacy of neuromuscular blocking agents	Drug interaction is not well established; monitor for possible effect.

^aCp = Plasma concentration; CYP = Cytochrome P450.

Table 72.13 • Symptoms of Benzodiazepine Withdrawal

Common	Less Common	Rare
Anxiety	Nausea	Confusion
Insomnia	Depression	Delirium
Irritability	Ataxia	Psychosis
Muscle aches/weakness	Hyperreflexia	Seizures
Tremor	Blurred vision	Catatonia
Loss of appetite	Fatigue	

Table 72.14 • Buspirone Drug Interactions[108,a]

Interacting Drug(s)	Clinical Significance/Comments
CYP 3A4 inhibitors: nefazodone, fluoxetine, fluvoxamine, erythromycin, itraconazole, ketoconazole, diltiazem, verapamil, and grapefruit juice	Significant increases in buspirone Cp have been reported with these agents, but adverse clinical effects are not always apparent. Buspirone dosage reductions are recommended when coadministered with erythromycin, fluvoxamine, nefazodone, fluoxetine, or itraconazole.
Rifampin	Highly significant decreases in buspirone Cp; avoid concurrent use.
Haloperidol	Buspirone may increase haloperidol Cp, but one study found no interaction.
Monoamine oxidase inhibitors	Possible serotonin syndrome; avoid concurrent use.

^{a}Cp = Plasma concentration; CYP = Cytochrome P450.

Notes:

Table 72.15 • First-Line Therapy of Panic Disorders[a]

Drug (Brand Name) Dosage Forms	Usual Dose	Advantages	Disadvantages	Other
SSRIs (FDA approved) • *Paroxetine* (Paxil) 10, 20, 30, 40 mg tab • *Sertraline* (Zoloft) 25, 50, 100 mg tab	40 mg/day 10 mg initially 100–150 mg/day 25 mg initially Target dose: 125 mg	• Treatment of choice • Superior to TCAs • Slightly faster onset than TCAs • Preferred in patients with h/o depression, alcohol, or substance abuse	• Gradual onset (4–6 wks) • 10–12 wks needed to assess response • Initial anxiety, nausea, headache, insomnia or sedation. Subside after 1–3 wks	• Gradual dose increases needed to minimize side effects • Treatment duration is 12–24 mos
BZDs (FDA approved) • *Alprazolam* (generic, Xanax) 0.25, 0.5, 1, 2 mg tab • *Clonazepam* (generic, Klonopin) 1, 2 mg tab	4–6 mg (up to 10 mg) daily in 3–5 divided doses 1–3 mg daily in 2 divided doses	• Short onset	• Breakthrough attacks due to short duration of 3–5 hrs for alprazolam	• Higher doses needed than for other anxiety disorders
TCAs and MAOIs			• Anxiety, jitteriness, agitation	• Reserved for 2nd or 3rd line therapy • Clomipramine more effective than other TCAs

[a]BZDs = Benzodiazepines; MAOIs = Monoamine oxidase inhibitors; SSRIs = Specific serotonin reuptake inhibitors; TCAs = Tricyclic antidepressants.

Notes:

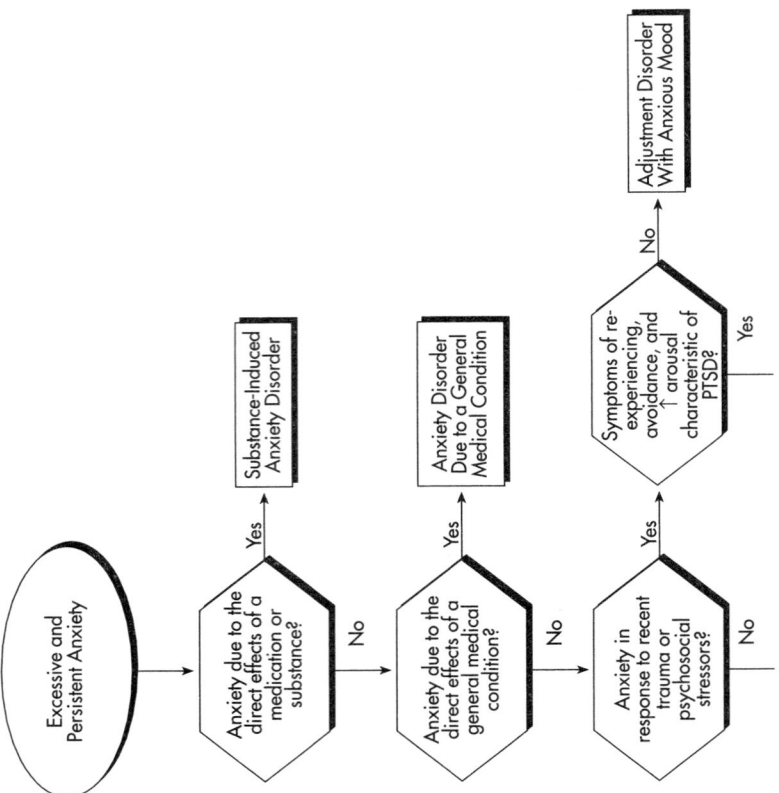

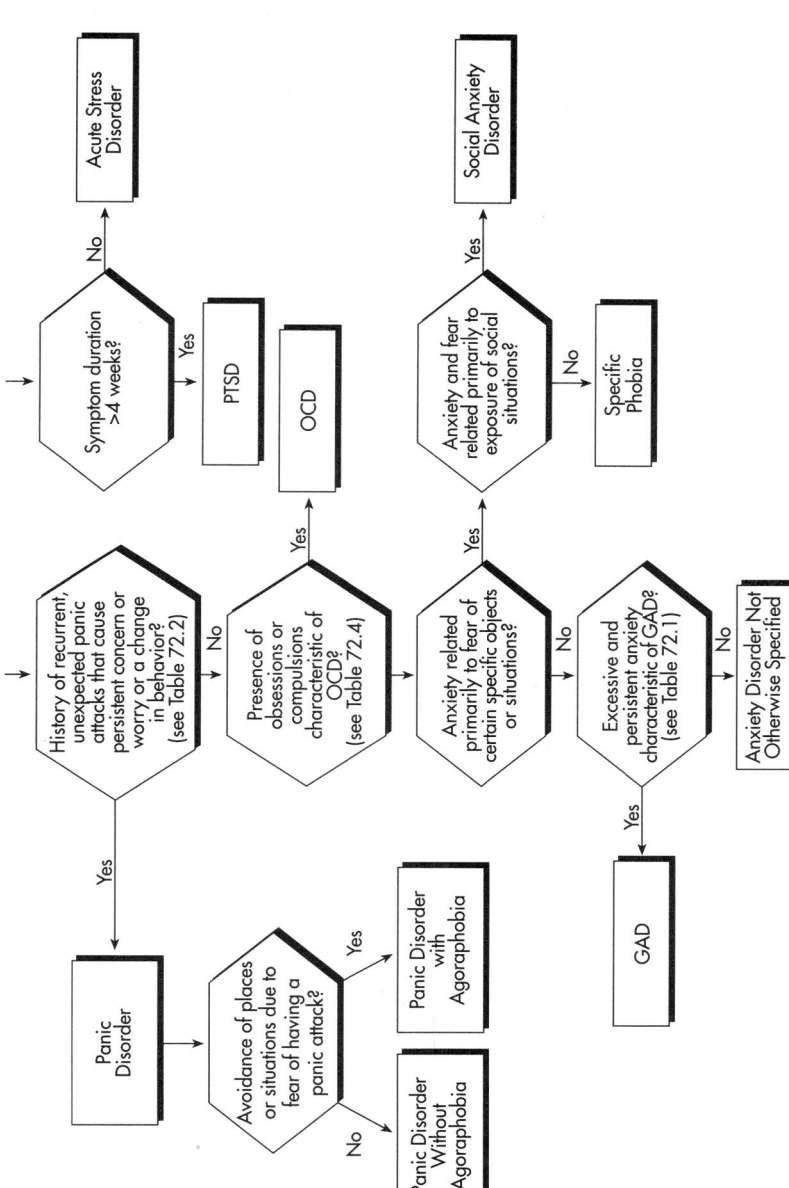

Fig. 72.1 Diagnostic Decision Tree for Anxiety Disorders. GAD, generalized anxiety disorder; OCD, obsessive-compulsive disorder; PTSD, post-traumatic stress disorder.

The reader is referred to Chapter 74: Anxiety Disorders, written by *Sara Grimsley Augustin, Pharm.D.*, in the seventh edition of **Applied Therapeutics: The Clinical Use of Drugs** for a more in-depth discussion. All notations to reference numbers are based on the reference list at the end of that chapter. The editors of this handbook express their thanks to Dr. Grimsley Augustin and acknowledge that this chapter is based upon her work.

Notes:

Chapter 73

Sleep Disorders

Prevalence

The prevalence of the major sleep disorders is listed in Table 73.1.

Classification

The DSM-IV classification of sleep disorders based upon pathophysiology and presumed etiology is listed in Table 73.2.

Causes

The potential causes of chronic sleep disorders are listed in Table 73.3.

Stages

The stages of sleep are commonly divided into the five stages shown in Table 73.4. Each stage serves a physiological function as individuals float into and out of these stages. Different age groups spend different amounts of time in each sleep stage.

Management of Insomnia

♦ Determine the nature of insomnia.
  • Difficulty falling asleep.
  • Difficulty maintaining sleep.
  • Early morning awakening.
  • Poor quality of sleep
  • Excessive daytime sleepiness (EDS)
  • Duration of insomnia (transient, short-term or <3 weeks, chronic)
♦ Consider possible medical, psychiatric, drug, social, and environmental etiologies (see Table 73.3).
♦ Initiate behavioral methods to improve sleep (see Table 73.5).
♦ Select a hypnotic as outlined in Table 73.6.
♦ The doses of commonly prescribed hypnotics are listed in Table 73.7, and the pharmacokinetic properties of hypnotics are presented in Table 73.8.

Notes:

Table 73.1 • Incidence of Major Sleep Disorders^a

Sleep Disorder	Incidence
Insomnia	30–35%
Transient	Few days
Short term	Up to 3 wk
Chronic	>3 wk
RLS	5–15%
PLMS (nocturnal myoclonus)	5–20%
Sleep apnea	2–4%
Narcolepsy	0.15%
Primary snoring	45%

^aPLMS = Periodic limb movements during sleep; RLS = Restless leg syndrome.

Table 73.2 • Classification of Sleep Disorders

Dyssomnias^a
Intrinsic: Idiopathic insomnia, narcolepsy, sleep apnea, periodic limb movements during sleep
Extrinsic: Inadequate sleep fitness, substance-induced sleep disorder
Circadian rhythm sleep disorders: Jet lag, shift work, delayed sleep phase syndrome

Parasomnias^b
Arousal: Confusional arousals, sleep walking, sleep terrors
Sleep/wake transition disorders: Sleep talking, nocturnal leg cramps
Associated with REM: Nightmares, sleep paralysis, impaired sleep-related penile erections
Other: Primary snoring, sudden infant death syndrome, sleep bruxism

Medical/Psychiatric/Substance-Induced Sleep Disorders
Associated with mental disorders: Mood disorders, anxiety disorders, psychotic disorders
Associated with neurologic disorders: Parkinson's disease, Huntington's disease, dementia
Associated with other medical disorders: Heart disease, renal insufficiency, pulmonary disease
Associated with a substance: Medication/substance abuse (e.g., phenylpropanolamine, cocaine)

Proposed Sleep Disorders
Menstrual-associated sleep disorder, pregnancy-associated sleep disorder, short or long sleeper

^aAny sleep pattern that is abnormal (e.g., insomnia or excessive sleepiness).
^bAny unusual behavior that emerges during sleep.
Adapted from references 31 and 32.

Notes:

Table 73.3 • Potential Causes of Chronic Sleep Disorders[68,71,a]

Psychiatric Disorders
Anxiety disorders
Bipolar disorder
Personality disorders
Organic mental disorders

Depressive disorders
Psychotic disorders
Somatoform disorders
Substance abuse

Medical/Neurologic Disorders
Angina pectoris
Bronchitis
Chronic fatigue
Cystic fibrosis
Huntington's disease
Parkinson's disease
Hypertension
Arthritis
Cardiac disease
Chronic pain
Cancer

Dementia
PUD
Hyperthyroidism and
hypothyroidism
Asthma
COAD
Epilepsy
Gastroesophageal reflux
Renal insufficiency
Connective tissue disease

Sleep Disorders
RLS
PLMS (nocturnal myoclonus)
Circadian rhythm sleep disorder (jet lag, shift
work, delayed sleep phase)

Sleep apnea (obstructive or central)
Primary snoring
Narcolepsy

Drugs Associated with Sleep Disturbance
Insomnia
Alcohol
Bupropion
Fluoxetine
Sertraline
MAOIs
TCAs
Thyroid supplements
Calcium channel blockers
Decongestants
Appetite suppressants
Theophylline
Corticosteroids
Dopamine agonists

Hypersomnia
Alcohol
Benzodiazepines
Antihypertensives
  Clonidine
  α-Adrenergic blockers
  ACE inhibitors
  β-Blockers
Anticonvulsants
Analgesics
Chloral hydrate
Antipsychotics
Antihistamines
Opioids

[a]ACE = Angiotensin-converting enzyme; COAD = Chronic obstructive airway disease; MAOIs = Monoamine oxidase inhibitors; PLMS = Periodic limb movements during sleep; PUD = Peptic ulcer disease; RLS = Restless leg syndrome; TCAs = Tricyclic antidepressants.

Notes:

Table 73.4 • Stages of Sleep

Stage I (NonREM)
- Transition between wakefulness and sleep
- Function is to initiate sleep
- Comprises about 2%–5% of sleep

Stage II (NonREM)
- Rapid wave (alpha) light sleep
- Thoughts are fragmented and short
- Provides rest for muscles and brain
- Comprises about 50% of sleep
- Arousal from sleep is highest during stages 1 and 2

Stages III and IV (NonREM)
- Short-wave (delta) deep restorative sleep
- Comprises about 15%–20% of sleep

Stage 5 (REM)
- Paradoxic sleep with aspects of both deep sleep and light sleep
- Dreaming is associated closely with REM sleep
- Physiological functions (breathing, temperature, heart rate, blood pressure, cerebral blood flow, metabolism, urine volume) are altered
- Purpose of REM sleep unknown, but REM sleep is essential
- REM deprivation causes profound psychological changes
- Many hypnotic drugs (except benzodiazepines in usual doses) ↓ REM
- Unknown if alteration of REM is better or worse than alteration of other stages

Table 73.5 • Sleep Fitness Guide[a]

- Keep the bedroom dark, comfortable, and quiet.
- Keep a regular sleep schedule; awaken at the same time daily.
- Avoid daytime naps even after a poor night of sleep.
- Do not live in bed: the bedroom should be reserved for sleep and sex.
- No eating, watching TV, or working in bed; it increases stress.
- Turn the face of the clock aside to minimize anxiety about falling asleep.
- If unable to sleep, get out of bed and do something to take your mind off sleeping.
- Establish a prebedtime ritual to condition your body for sleep.
- Relax before bedtime with soft music, mild stretching, yoga, or pleasurable reading.
- Exercise early in the day before dinner to alleviate stress; avoid exercising right before bedtime.
- Do not eat heavy meals before bedtime.
- Do not take any caffeine (e.g., coffee, tea, candy, soda) in the afternoon.
- Consult with a pharmacist, physician, or other primary care provider about your sleep problem because:
    A physical or mental condition can cause poor sleep.
    Prescribed medication and herbals can interfere with sleep.

[a]Also known as *sleep hygiene.*

Notes:

Table 73.6 • Stepwise Approach to Selecting a Hypnotic for Insomnia^a

Step 1. Determine type of insomnia: DFA, DMS, EMA; duration.
Step 2. Consider possible etiologies: medical, psychiatric, drug; treat causes.
Step 3. Sleep fitness ineffective or only partially effective; significant insomnia persists.
Step 4. Assess type of patient: age, size, diagnosis, organ function, drug interactions, abuse potential.

	Type of Insomnia		
Treatment Options	DFA	DMS	EMA
Antidepressants	*Duration of therapy:* Chronic use in depressive diagnosis *Onset and duration of effects:* Intermediate to long onset *Pharmacokinetic considerations:* See individual antidepressant *Clinical considerations:* Substance abuse; treatment-resistant insomnia		*Duration of therapy:* Chronic use in depressive diagnosis *Onset and duration of effects:* Intermediate to long onset *Pharmacokinetic considerations:* See individual antidepressant *Clinical considerations:* Substance abuse; treatment-resistant insomnia
Chloral hydrate	*Duration of therapy:* Short-term use, 2–7 days *Onset and duration of effects:* Rapid onset; intermediate duration *Pharmacokinetic considerations:* Major metabolite, trichloroethanol, is active *Clinical considerations:* GI side effects; rapid tolerance; no EEG effects; drug interactions		
Estazolam		*Duration of therapy:* Short-term and chronic *Onset and duration of effects:* Long onset; moderate duration *Clinical considerations:* Hepatic metabolism	

(continued)

Table 73.6 • Stepwise Approach to Selecting a Hypnotic for Insomnia^a (continued)

Treatment Options	Type of Insomnia		
	DFA	DMS	EMA
Flurazepam or quazepam	Duration of therapy: Short-term and chronic Onset and duration of effects: Rapid onset; long duration Pharmacokinetic considerations: Active metabolite Clinical considerations: Efficacy long term	Duration of therapy: Short-term and chronic Onset and duration of effects: Rapid onset; long duration Pharmacokinetic considerations: Active metabolite Clinical considerations: Efficacy long term	
Temazepam		Duration of therapy: Short-term and chronic Onset and duration of effects: Long onset; moderate duration Pharmacokinetic considerations: No hepatic metabolism	
Zolpidem, zaleplon, or Triazolam	Duration of therapy: Short-term use, 7–10 days Onset and duration of effects: Rapid onset; short duration Pharmacokinetic considerations: Short half-life Clinical considerations: Rebound insomnia; CNS side effects		

^{a}CNS = Central nervous system; DFA = Difficulty falling asleep; DMS = Difficulty maintaining sleep; EEG = Electroencephalogram; EMA = Early-morning awakening; GI = Gastrointestinal.

Table 73.7 • Hypnotic Dosing Comparison

Drug	Dose (mg)	Range (mg)
Midazolam (Versed)	15	10–30
Zaleplon (Sonata)	10	5–20
Zolpidem (Ambien)	10	5–20
Triazolam (Halcion)	0.25	0.125–0.25
Temazepam (Restoril)	15	7.5–30
Estazolam (ProSom)	1	1–2
Flurazepam (Dalmane)	15	15–30
Quazepam (Doral)	15	7.5–30

Notes:

Table 73.8 • Pharmacokinetic Properties of Hypnotics Acting at Benzodiazepine Receptors[a]

Active Substance	Lipid Solubility	T_{max} (hr)	Onset (min)	Half-Life (hr)	Duration (hr)[b]
Zaleplon	Moderate	1.1	30	1.1	1–2
Zolpidem	Low	1–2	30	2.5	2–4
Triazolam	Moderate	1	15–30	2–5	2–4
Temazepam	Moderate	1.5–2.0	60–120	10–20	8–12
Estazolam	Low	2	60–120	10–20	10–15
Flurazepam					
Hydroxyethyl-	Low	1	—	2–3	—
Aldehyde-	Low	1	—	1	—
N-desalkyl-	Moderate	10	30–60	50–100	10–30
Quazepam	High	2	30	20–40	10–30
2-oxo	High	2	30	20–40	—
N-desalkyl-flurazepam	Moderate	10	30–60	50–100	—

[a]T_{max} = Time of maximum concentration.
[b]Time the patient feels the effects after a single dose; usually approximates half-life with multiple doses; interindividual variability exists; and tolerance may develop with continued use, lessening the duration.

The reader is referred to Chapter 75: Sleep Disorders, written by *Julie A. Dopheide, Pharm.D.,* and *Glen L. Stimmel, Pharm.D.,* in the seventh edition of **Applied Therapeutics: The Clinical Use of Drugs** for a more in-depth discussion. Other topics covered in their chapter include management of insomnia in the medically ill psychiatric, pediatric, and elderly patients. Narcolepsy, sleep apnea, restless leg syndrome, despondence, rebound insomnia, and withdrawal also are addressed. All notations to reference numbers are based on the reference list at the end of that chapter. The editors of this handbook express their thanks to Drs. Dopheide and Stimmel and acknowledge that this chapter is based upon their work.

Notes:

Notes:

Chapter 74

Schizophrenia

Psychotic disorders are marked by deterioration in social functioning, loss of reality testing and perceptual deficits (including hallucinations and delusions), cognitive impairment, and affective or mood instability. Schizophrenia is the most common. For a glossary of commonly used terms, see Table 74.1.

Clinical Symptoms

♦ Most exhibit both positive and negative symptoms. See Table 74.2. Younger patients are more "positive" in presentation; older patients are more "negative" in presentation.

♦ Cognitive impairment is common and results in difficulty with community functioning, independent living, and learning new skills.

♦ Long-term outcome is poor, with a relapse and recurrence rate as high as 60% over 2 years after first hospitalization.

♦ High rate of functional deterioration, attempted suicide, and major affective disorder (usually depression).

Clinical Course

♦ Most alternate between acute psychotic episodes and stable episodes with some residual symptoms.

♦ Three phases, which tend to overlap
  • *Acute*—floridly psychotic and require hospitalization; positive symptoms most prominent
  • *Stabilization*—acute symptoms decrease in severity as the patient begins to stabilize. May last for 6 or more months.
  • *Stable*—a level of function considered optimal for the individual is attained. Complete symptom resolution is rarely attained. Negative and nonspecific symptoms (e.g., tension, mood instability) may persist.

♦ Predictors of good and poor prognoses. See Table 74.3.

Diagnosis

Criteria for schizophrenia. See Table 74.4.
Differential diagnosis. See Table 74.5.
Substance abuse is a common co-morbid disorder.

Treatment Principles

♦ A chronic disease for which there is no cure

♦ Treatment can decrease acute symptoms, decrease frequency and severity of psychotic episodes, and optimize functioning between episodes

♦ Target symptoms (see Table 74.2) are used to assess treatment response
♦ Nondrug therapy is additive to pharmacotherapy and improves long-term function

Antipsychotic Drug Therapy

♦ *Typical antipsychotic agents*
  • Subclassified into high- (e.g., haloperidol) or low-potency agents (e.g., chlorpromazine) based on their ability to block dopamine receptors; phenothiazines or nonphenothiazines; or by their potential for common adverse effects.
  • Equally effective; 40–75% improve after 6 weeks vs 20% placebo response.
  • More effective in improving positive than negative symptoms, which can be worsened by drug-induced akinesia
  • More favorable response may occur if baseline symptoms are severe and mainly positive in nature; significant improvement occurs in first few days of treatment; no dysphoria develops; plasma homovanillic acid levels decrease within first several weeks; CT scans show minimal brain atrophy
♦ *Atypical antipsychotic agents* (e.g., clozapine, risperidone)
  • Have less extrapyramidal effects, have no effect on serum prolactin
  • As effective as typical agents, may be more effective in reducing negative symptoms; clearly more efficacious for refractory schizophrenia
  • Initial treatment of choice (except clozapine) due to increased tolerability
♦ Relative incidence of adverse effects. See Table 74.6.
♦ Presentation and management of adverse effects. See Table 74.7.
♦ Relative potency. See Table 74.8.
♦ Acute and maintenance doses. See Table 74.8.
♦ Half-lives, cytochrome P450 pathway, plasma concentrations. See Table 74.9.
♦ Treatment is divided into three phases. See Table 74.10.

Notes:

Table 74.1 • Glossary of Commonly Used Terms in Schizophrenia

Affect: behavior (usually an expression of an emotion) that is observed by the interviewer. Common types of disturbances in affect include: *restricted*—mild decrease in range and intensity of the expression of emotion; *blunted*—significant decrease in intensity of the expression of emotion; *flat*—absence of expression of emotion; *inappropriate*—incongruency between patient's affect and mood or behavior; *labile*—abrupt shifts in expression of emotion.

Akathisia: syndrome consisting of subjective feelings of anxiety and restlessness, and objective signs of pacing, rocking, and an inability to sit or stand still for extended periods of time.

Akinesia: absence or decrease in voluntary movement; may be antipsychotic-induced (extrapyramidal side effects) or a manifestation of negative symptoms of schizophrenia.

Alogia: impoverished thinking usually manifested through speech and language deficits. Speech is brief and lacks spontaneity; replies to questions are very concrete (*poverty of speech*). *Poverty of content* refers to speech that is adequate in amount but is of little substance (overly abstract), repetitive, or stereotyped.

Anergy: lack of energy.

Anhedonia: loss of interest or pleasure.

Avolition: an inability to initiate and sustain goal-directed activities. The patient may sit for extended periods of time and show minimal interest in participating in social or work-related activities.

Circumstantiality: a form of disorganized speech characterized by "talking in circles" or taking an unusually long length of time in answering a question or expressing one's point of view.

Delusions: a false belief that is firmly held in spite of evidence to refute the belief. The belief does not qualify as a delusion if it is a cultural or religious belief accepted by a group of individuals. Types of delusions include grandiose, persecutory, and somatic type.

Executive function: the ability to design and carry out a solution to a plan when the solution is not obvious. Loss of executive function presents as failure to learn from past experience and failure to plan or organize life events.

Hallucination: a sensory perception (e.g., auditory, visual, somatic, tactile) experienced in the absence of external stimuli. Hallucinations may be recognized as false sensory perceptions in some, whereas others may believe that the experiences are reality based.

Loose associations: a form of disorganized, illogical speech characterized by unrelated words, phrases, and sentences used in a fashion that makes comprehension very difficult, if not impossible.

Mood: a pervasive and sustained emotion that is experienced by the patient. Examples include depressed, anxious, angry, or irritable mood.

Mood congruent delusions or hallucinations: delusions or hallucinations that are consistent with a mood or behavior (e.g., delusions/hallucinations of death, guilt, or punishment in the presence of a depressed mood).

Mood incongruent delusions or hallucinations: delusions or hallucinations that are not consistent with a mood or behavior (e.g., delusions/hallucinations of death, guilt, or punishment in the presence of mania).

Tangentiality: a form of disorganized speech in which answers are remotely or completely unrelated to questions and patients' thoughts frequently shift in an unconnected fashion.

Thought broadcasting: a delusion that one's thoughts are being broadcast to others (e.g., a patient feels that others can read his or her mind).

Thought disorder: a general term often used to describe any type of abnormal thought process (e.g., delusion, loose association, conceptual disorganization).

Thought insertion: a delusion that one's thoughts are being inserted into one's mind by others.

Table 74.2 • Positive and Negative Symptoms of Schizophrenia

Positive	Negative
Combativeness, agitation, and hostility	Psychomotor retardation
Tension	Affective flattening
Hyperactivity	Avolition
Hallucinations	Lack of socialization
Delusions	Alogia (poverty of speech)
Disorganized speech (loose associations, tangential, blocking)	Loss of emotional connectedness
Unusual behavior	Loss of executive functions

Table 74.3 • Prognosticators of Outcome for Schizophrenia Treated with Antipsychotics[a]

Feature	Good Prognosis	Poor Prognosis
Premorbid functioning	High	Low
Precipitating factors	Present	Absent
Age at onset	Older than average	Younger than average
Onset of symptoms	Sudden	Insidious
Family history	Positive for affective illness and negative for schizophrenia	Positive for schizophrenia
Interpersonal relationships	Married/stable home environment	Single
Affective symptoms	Present	Blunted affect
Behavioral features	Positive symptoms predominate	Negative symptoms predominate
CNS morphology by CT or MRI scan	Normal	Ventricular enlargement, cortical atrophy
Dopamine system	Hyperactive in limbic system	Hypoactive in frontal cortex
Response to typical neuroleptics	Good	Fair to poor

[a]CNS = Central nervous system; CT = Computed tomography; MRI = Magnetic resonance imaging.
Adapted from reference 25.

Notes:

Table 74.4 • DSM-IV-TR Criteria for Schizophrenia

A. Characteristic Symptoms
At least two of the following, each present for a significant portion of time during a 1-month period (or less if successfully treated):
1. Delusions
2. Hallucinations
3. Disorganized speech (e.g., frequent derailment or incoherence)
4. Grossly disorganized or catatonic behavior
5. Negative symptoms (i.e., affective flattening, alogia, or avolition)
Note: Only one "A symptom" is required if delusions are bizarre or hallucinations consist of a voice keeping up a running commentary on the person's behavior or thought, two or more conversations with each other.

B. Social/Occupation Dysfunction
For a significant portion of the time since the onset of the disturbance, one or more major areas of functioning such as work, interpersonal relationships, or self-care is markedly below the level achieved before the onset.

C. Duration
Continuous signs of the disturbance persist for at least 6 months. This 6-month period must include at least 1 month of symptoms (or less if successfully treated) that meet criterion A (i.e., active phase symptoms) and may include prodromal and/or residual periods when the "A criterion" is not fully met. During these periods, signs of the disturbance may be manifested by negative symptoms or by two or more symptoms listed in "criterion A" present in an attenuated form (e.g., blunted affect, unusual perceptual disturbances).

D. Schizoaffective Disorder and Mood Disorder Exclusion
Schizoaffective disorder and mood disorder with psychotic features have been ruled out because either (1) no major depressive, manic, or mixed manic episodes have occurred concurrently with the active phase symptoms or (2) if mood episodes have occurred during active phase symptoms, their total duration has been brief relative to the duration of the active and residual periods.

E. Substance/General Medical Condition Exclusion
The disturbance is not due to direct physiologic effects of a substance (drug of abuse or medication) or a general medical condition.

F. Relationship to a Pervasive Development Disorder
If there is a history of autistic disorder or another pervasive development disorder, the additional diagnosis of schizophrenia is made only if prominent delusions or hallucinations also are present for at least a month (or less if successfully treated).

Adapted with permission from American Psychiatric Association, Diagnostic and Statistical Manual of Mental Disorders—TR. 4th ed. (DSM-IV-TR). Washington, DC: American Psychiatric Press, 2000.

Table 74.5 • Differential Diagnosis for Schizophrenia (DSM-IV-TR)

Drug-induced Psychoses
Amphetamine
Cocaine
Cannabis (marijuana)
Phencyclidine (PCP)
Lysergic acid diethylamide (LSD)
Anticholinergics

Primary Psychiatric Disorders
Brief psychotic disorder
Schizophreniform disorder
Bipolar affective disorder, manic type
Mood disorder with psychotic features

Personality Disorders
Schizotypal
Schizoid
Paranoid

Table 74.6 • Relative Incidence of Antipsychotic Drug Adverse Effects

	Sedation	EPS	Anticholinergic	Orthostasis	Seizures	Prolactin Elevation	Cognitive Improvement	Weight Gain
Low Potency								
Chlorpromazine	+++	+++	+++	+++	++	++	[d]	++
Thioridazine	+++	++	+++	+++	++	++	[d]	+++
High Potency								
Trifluoperazine	++	++++	++	++	+++	+++	?	
Fluphenazine	++	++++	++	++	++	++++	?	
Thiothixene	+	++++	+	+	++	++++	?	++
Haloperidol	+	++++	++	+	++	++++	?	++
Loxapine	+++	++++	++	+++	++	++++	?	+
Molindone	+	+++	++	++	+		?	+
Atypicals								
Clozapine	+++	+	+++	+++	+++[c]	0	?/++	+++
Risperidone	+++	+[a]	++	++	++	0 to +++[c]	?/++	+++
Olanzapine	+++	+[b]	++	++	++	0	?	+++
Quetiapine	+++	+		++	++	0	[e]	++

[a] Very low at dosages <8 mg/day.
[b] With dosages <20 mg/day.
[c] Dose related.
[d] May worsen.
[e] Case report.
+, very low; ++, low; +++, moderate; ++++, high; +++++, very high; EPS, extrapyramidal side effects.
Adapted from references 23, 25, 49, 53, and 144.

Table 74.7 • Presentation and Management of Antipsychotic Adverse Events

Adverse Effect	Presentation	Causes and Risks	Management
Pseudoparkinsonism	Similar to idiopathic Parkinson's disease but reversible. Tremors and rigidity may be unilateral or bilateral. Onset is typically within 4 weeks of dose increase. Some develop tolerance, but 30% continue to have symptoms.	• Imbalance between dopaminergic and cholinergic systems in nigrostriatum. • Most common with high-potency typical antipsychotics. • Low risk with atypical agents • Elderly women most at risk	• Reduce dose if possible • Switch to atypical agent • Treat with antiparkinson drug: benztropine (Cogentin) 2 mg BID.
Acute Dystonia	Sudden onset of brief or sustained abnormal postures: tongue protrusion, oculogyric crisis, trismus, torticollis, etc	• Dysregulation of the dopamine system and imbalance between neurotransmitter systems caused by antipsychotics. • Young males taking high-potency antipsychotics at greatest risk	Benztropine 1–2 mg or diphenhydramine 25–50 mg IM; repeat in 15–20 minutes if unresponsive. Continue treatment with oral medications for 2 weeks.
Akathisia	Feelings of anxiety and restlessness, pacing, rocking, inability to sit or stand in one place. Can increase aggression; hard to distinguish from psychomotor agitation and worsening psychosis.	• Etiology poorly understood, but adrenergic system may be involved. • High-potency antipsychotics	• Propranolol 20 mg TID; increase by 20 mg every other day to max of 120 mg. • Benzodiazepines can be tried if no response after 1 week
Tardive Dyskinesia	Persistent, involuntary hyperkinetic abnormal movements (tics). Severity fluctuates and often remits during sleep. Prevalence 15–20%.	• Etiology not understood but probably involves dysfunction of several neurotransmitters. • Highest risk in first 5 years of treatment. • Elderly women at high risk (70%) • Large doses, long-term treatment, presence of EPS increases risk	• Slowly reduce dose of typical antipsychotic • Switch to atypical antipsychotic • Vitamin E 800 IU BID
Neuroleptic Malignant Syndrome	Rare (0.02–3.23%) but potentially lethal. Onset hours to months; symptoms develop over 24–72 hours. Muscular rigidity, hyperthermia (up to 41°C), autonomic dysfunction (e.g., tachycardia, labile BP, diaphoresis), altered consciousness.	• Associated with dopamine depletion. • Most commonly associated with typical agents	Dantrolene 50 mg QID plus a dopamine agonist: amantadine 100 to 200 mg two to three times daily or bromocriptine 2.5 to 15 mg TID. Supportive measures. Improvement should be noted in 24–72 hours. Switch to atypical agent.

(continued)

Table 74.7 • Presentation and Management of Antipsychotic Adverse Events (continued)

Adverse Effect	Presentation	Causes and Risks	Management
Hematologic Effects	• Mild, transient leukopenia occurs in 0.8% and recovers in about 2 weeks. • Agranulocytosis rare. Watch for fever and sore throat.	Associated with all agents. Risk of severe leukopenia higher with clozapine	• Continue medication if reduction is mild. • Discontinue if WBC count <300/mm^3 or ANC is <1500/mm^3.
Hyperprolactinemia	• Galactorrhea, amenorrhea, anovulation in women; azoospermia, impotence, gynecomastia in men • Bone loss.	Dopamine blocks release of prolactin. Thus, most common with typical agents	• Lower dose of typical agents • Treat with dopamine agonists such as amantadine or bromocriptine (see above). Symptoms usually improve in 15 days. • Switch to atypical agent
Hepatic Dysfunction	• Benign increase in AST or ALT <2 to 3 times normal. • Cholestatic jaundice usually develops within 1 month of therapy.	Jaundice most commonly associated with typical agents.	D/C phenothiazine. Jaundice resolves in 2 to 8 weeks. Elevated LFTs are benign.
Ocular Effects	• Corneal and lens changes visible by slit lamp but do not impair vision • Pigmentary retinopathy • Cataracts	• Associated with long-term use of phenothiazines and thiothixene • Associated with thioridazine >800 mg/day • Caused by quetiapine	Baseline slit lamp evaluation with repeat every 6 months recommended by FDA for patients taking quetiapine
Temperature Dysregulation	Poikilothermia—body temperature unable to respond to heat or cold leading to hyper- or hypothermia in hot and cold weather, respectively	Inhibition of hypothalamic temperature regulation exacerbated by anticholinergic effects of antipsychotics, including olanzapine and clozapine	Wear appropriate clothing, maintain hydration, stay in shade in hot weather and in warm areas when temperature is cold.

Dermatologic Effects	Photosensitivity, maculopapular rash, localized or generalized urticaria	Most common with phenothiazines (chlorpromazine) and thiothixenes	Wear protective clothing and sunscreens. Antihistamines usually provide relief when urticaria occurs, but drug may have to be discontinued.
Psychogenic Polydipsia	6 to 20% of mentally ill experience polydipsia and hyponatremia due to compulsive water drinking. Headaches, weakness, tremor cramps, seizures, coma, exacerbation of CHF	Altered antidiuretic hormone release secondary to stress, psychotropic drugs, nicotine, or mental illness. Anticholinergic drugs may exacerbate.	Restrict fluids, discontinue cigarettes and anticholinergic medications. Redouble efforts to control schizophrenia.
Sexual Dysfunction	Ejaculatory dysfunction most common; decreased libido, anorgasmia, impotence, and priapism	Multifactorial causes including α_2-adrenergic and calcium channel blockade, anticholinergic, endocrine, and sedative effects. Most common with thioridazine (60%) >300 mg, but also caused by atypical agents.	Change to high-potency antipsychotic agent or lower dose. May resolve with continued treatment. Reversible when drug is discontinued.
Seizures	Convulsions in patients who were seizure free	Lower seizure threshold. Risk increases with history of epilepsy or drug-induced seizures, perinatal problems, abnormal EEG, acute head trauma, rapid titration to high doses, and low-potency antipsychotics. Clozapine also causes seizures.	Use haloperidol in patients with risk factors. If clozapine is used, try to keep dose below 300 mg/day.
Weight Gain	3 to 15 pound weight gain, especially during first 12 weeks. Increases up to 25 pounds; common with clozapine.	Change in food preferences, increased food intake, carbohydrate craving, decreased activity, blockade of histamine and 5HT2C receptors.	Exercise, diet, and use of agents with lowest risks (e.g., haloperidol). Clozapine and olanzapine cause most weight gain; risperidone has intermediate risk.

Table 74.8 • Antipsychotic Relative Potency by Chemical Class and Adult Dosing

Drug and Chemical Class	Traditional Equivalence	Acute Phase Dosage (mg/day)	Maintenance/ Stable Phase Dosage (mg/day)
Phenothiazines			
Aliphatic Type			
Chlorpromazine (Thorazine)	100	300–1,500[a]	150–800
Piperidine Type			
Thioridazine (Mellaril)	100	300–800	150–600
Piperazine Type			
Perphenazine (Trilafon)	10	32–64[a]	8–48
Prochlorperazine (Compazine)	15	40–150[b]	
Trifluoperazine (Stelazine)	5	10–80	5–30
Fluphenazine (Prolixin)	2	5–80	2–20
Nonphenothiazines—Typical Agents			
Thioxanthene			
Thiothixene (Navane)	4	5–60[a]	5–30
Butyrophenone			
Haloperidol (Haldol)	2	5–100	2–20
Dibenzoxazepine			
Loxapine (Loxitane)	10	50–250[c]	25–100
Dihydroindolone			
Molindone (Moban)	10	25–225	25–100
Diphenylbutylpiperidone			
Pimozide (Orap)	1	10–30	2–6
Nonphenothiazines—Atypical Agents			
Benzisoxazole			
Risperidone (Risperdal)	1.5	2–16	2–8
Dibenzazepine			
Clozapine (Clozaril)	50	150–900	150–600
Thienobenzodiazepine			
Olanzapine (Zyprex)	4	10–20	c
Dibenzothiazepine			
Quetiapine (Seroquel)	N/A	300–750	b

[a]Dosages can be exceeded with caution, but high-dose therapy is rarely needed.
[b]Used as antinauseant and not routinely used as a maintenance drug.
[c]Insufficient data to determine.
N/A, not available.
Adapted from references 23, 25, 70, and 72.

Table 74.9 • Pharmacokinetic Comparisons of Antipsychotics

Antipsychotic Agent	Mean Half-Life (hr)	Major Cytochrome P450 Pathway	Plasma Concentration Range
Chlorpromazine	8–35	2D6	Not well defined
Thioridazine	9–30	2D6	Not well defined
Perphenazine	8–21	2D6	Not well defined
Fluphenazine	14–24	2D6	0.2–2.8 µg/mL
Fluphenazine decanoate	8 days	2D6	0.2–2.8 µg/mL
Thiothixene	34	2D6	2–15 µg/mL
Haloperidol	12–36	2D6	4–12 ng/mL
Haloperidol decanoate	21 days	2D6	4–12 ng/mL
Clozapine	16	1A2, 3A4	350–420 µg/mL suggested
Risperidone	22	2D6	Not well defined
Olanzapine	30	1A2	Not well defined
Quetiapine	7	3A4	Not well defined

Compiled from references 73, 103, 125, and 192.

Table 74.10 • Treatment Phases

Treatment Phase	Goal	Therapy	Onset and Duration
Acute	• Calm to prevent harm to selves or others	• High-potency antipsychotic (e.g. haloperidol or fluphenazine) • Benzodiazepine • Lorazepam (Ativan) 1–2 mg PO or IM Q 4–6 hrs as needed • Atypical agents not well studied	• Control may take 2–3 weeks and in some cases up to several months. • Therapeutic trial for a given dose is 3–8 weeks for people with little to no response and 5–12 weeks for partial responders.
Stabilization	• Reduce agitation • Control psychosis and thought disorder • Arrange psychosocial support	• Antipsychotic selected based on history of response (or that of a relative). • Atypical agents recommended as initial treatment and for breakthrough episodes.	
Stable	• Improve functioning and quality of life • Minimize long-term side effects • Reduce incidence of relapse	• Continuous antipsychotic therapy is essential • Use lowest effective dose but reduce by only 20% every 3–6 months to minimize risk for relapse. • Typical doses are risperidone 2–4 mg/day; fluphenazine 2.5 mg/day	• Treatment should be continued for at least 1 year. • Discontinuation can be considered if remission has been sustained for 1–2 years or 5 years in patients with a history of multiple episodes.
Inadequate Response or Treatment Resistance (30–33% of patients)	• Prevent hospitalizations and breakthroughs • Decrease persistent symptoms	• Change to different antipsychotic (except clozapine) • Clozapine only after failed trials with 3 other agents • Adjunctive treatment with anticonvulsants or lithium if clozapine fails or is not tolerated	• Lifelong therapy

The reader is referred to Chapter 76: Schizophrenia, written by *Patricia A. Marken, Pharm.D.*, and *Steven W. Stanislav, Pharm.D.*, in the seventh edition of **Applied Therapeutics: The Clinical Use of Drugs** for a more in-depth discussion of depot dosage forms, clozapine use (including hematological monitoring), use of plasma concentrations, and other details of drug therapy. All notations to reference numbers are based on the reference list at the end of that chapter. The editors of this handbook express their thanks to Drs. Marken and Stanislav and acknowledge that this chapter is based upon their work.

Notes:

Chapter 75

Mood Disorders I: Major Depressive Disorders

Classification. Depressive disorders and bipolar disorders (Chapter 76) are classified under "Mood Disorders" in the *Diagnostic and Statistical Manual of Mental Disorders,* Fourth Edition (DSM-IV). Depressive disorders include:

♦ *Major Depressive Disorder,* Single Episode (30–50% of cases)

♦ *Major Depressive Disorder, Recurrent* (average 6 episodes/lifetime). Other specifiers include:

  • With melancholic features (neurovegetative symptoms: early morning awakening, marked psychomoter agitation or retardation, anorexia or weight loss); lacks environmental triggers

  • With atypical features (e.g., weight gain, hypersomnia, leaden paralysis, or rejection sensitivity)

  • With psychotic features (e.g., hallucinations or delusions)

  • With catatonic features (stuporous) or with postpartum onset

♦ *Dysthymic Disorder.* Depression with fewer symptoms than major depression, but the course is more chronic with symptoms being present most of the time for at least two years.

♦ *Depressive Disorder Not Otherwise Specified*

Diagnosis, Assessment, and Clinical Presentation

  ♦ Rule out organic causes of depression induced or exacerbated by *medical conditions* (see Table 75.1) or *medications* (see Table 75.2)

  ♦ *Diagnostic criteria.* See Table 75.3

  ♦ *Elderly patients* may dwell on vague, chronic symptoms of physical illness with unclear etiology (e.g., headache, insomnia, joint pain, dizziness, or constipation), rather than sadness or melancholy.

  ♦ The structured *mental status examination* is a systematic way to assess a patient's mental health. See 75.4.

  ♦ *Target symptoms* of depression can be recalled by the pneumonic: D-SIG-E-CAPS. See Table 75.5.

Nondrug Management

  ♦ *Psychotherapy* is comparable to pharmacologic intervention for mild to moderate depression.

  ♦ *Electroconvulsive therapy* is recommended for treatment-resistant depression, severe vegetative depression, psychotic depression, and depression in pregnancy. Overall response is 70–90% in first week or two of treatments (2–3/week)

  ♦ *Other:* Phototherapy, sleep deprivation, exercise, herbs

Antidepressant Therapy

- ◆ All antidepressants are *equally effective* (60–70% respond).
  - • Selection is based on other factors. See Table 75.6.
  - • Specific serotonin reuptake inhibitors (SSRIs) usually the preferred drugs due to their favorable side effect profile
- ◆ *Onset of effect* for all antidepressants is about 4 to 6 weeks, although initial improvement can be seen in the first 2 weeks.
  - • Neurovegetative symptoms are first to subside (e.g., altered sleep or appetite, decreased energy, anxiety)
  - • Cognitive symptoms respond in 3 to 4 weeks (e.g., guilt, pessimism, poor concentration, hopelessness, sadness, decreased libido).
- ◆ *Pharmacology.* See Table 75.7.
- ◆ *Adverse Effects.* See Table 75.8.
- ◆ *Management of SSRI-Induced Sexual Dysfunction.* See Table 75.9.
- ◆ *Dose and Cost.* See Table 75.10.
- ◆ *Duration of Treatment.* See Table 75.11.
- ◆ *Discontinuation of Antidepressants and Withdrawal Symptoms.* See Table 75.12.
- ◆ *Antidepressant Drug Interactions.* See Table 75.13.
- ◆ *Foods Containing Tyramine.* See Table 75.14.
- ◆ *Treatment Augmentation for Partial Responders to SSRIs.* See Table 75.15.
- ◆ *Patient Education.* See Table 75.16.

Table 75.1 • Selected Medical Conditions That May Mimic Depression

Central Nervous System
Alzheimer's disease
Cerebrovascular accident (CVA)
HIV-associated dementia
Multiple sclerosis
Parkinson's disease

Cardiovascular
Cerebral arteriosclerosis
Congestive heart failure
Myocardial infarction

Endocrine
Addison's disease
Diabetes mellitus
Hypothyroidism

Women's Health
Perimenopause
Postpartum
Premenstrual dysphoric disorder

Other
Chronic fatigue syndrome
Chronic pain syndrome
Fibromyalgia
Irritable bowel syndrome
Malignancies (various)
Migraine headaches
Rheumatoid arthritis
Systemic lupus erythematosus

Notes:

Table 75.2 • Selected Medications That May Induce Depression

Cardiovascular Agents
β-Blockers
Clonidine
Methyldopa
Procainamide
Reserpine

Central Nervous System Agents
Barbiturates
Benzodiazepines (?)
Chloral hydrate
Ethanol
Phenytoin

Hormonal Agents
Anabolic steroids
Corticosteroids
Estrogen (?)
Progestins
Tamoxifen

Others
Indomethacin
Interferon
Narcotics

Table 75.3 • Diagnostic Criteria for Major Depressive Disorder

A. At least five of the following symptoms have been present during the same 2-week period and represent a change from previous functioning. One of the symptoms must be either depressed mood or loss of interest/pleasure.
   • Depressed mood most of the day, nearly every day
   • Loss of interest in pleasurable activities most of the day, nearly every day
   • Change in weight or appetite (increase or decrease) when not dieting
   • Insomnia or hypersomnia nearly every day
   • Fatigue or loss of energy nearly every day
   • Diminished ability to think or concentrate, or indecisiveness
   • Feelings of worthlessness or excessive or inappropriate guilt nearly every day
   • Psychomotor agitation or retardation nearly every day
   • Recurrent thoughts of death or suicidal ideation
B. Symptoms cause clinically significant distress or impairment in social, occupational, or other important areas of functioning.
C. Symptoms are not caused by an underlying medical condition or substance (e.g., medications or recreational drugs).

Table 75.4 • Mental Status Exam (AMSIT)

General Appearance, Behavior, Speech
• Apparent age; appear ill or in distress?
• Dress
• General reaction to examination, negativism
• Posture and gait
• Unusual movements
• Facial expression
• Signs of anxiety
• General level of activity
• Repetitious activities (stereotypy, mannerisms, compulsions)
• Disturbances of attention: distractibility
• Speech: mute, word salad, echolalia, klang, neologisms

Mood and Affect
• Quality of prevailing mood; intensity and depth
• Constancy of mood, patient-stated mood
• Affect: range, appropriateness, lability, flatness

Sensorium
• Orientation for time, place, person, situation
• Memory: recent and remote, immediate recall

Level of Intellectual Functioning
• An estimate of current intellectual functioning, not an estimate of original intellectual potential
• General fund of information: presidents, oceans, governor, large cities, current events. Why does the moon appear larger than the stars?
• Vocabulary
• Serial 7 substractions (also tests attention and sensorium)

Thought Processes
• Pattern of associations (tempo, rhythm, organization, distortions, excesses, deficiencies)
• False perceptions (hallucinations, illusions, delusions, distortions of body image, depersonalization)
• Thought content (what patient tells, main concerns, obsessive ideation)
• Abstracting ability (tests by similarities, proverbs)
• Judgment and insight

Table 75.5 • Depressive Disorder Target Symptom Mnemonic

D	SIG	E	CAPS
Depressed mood	Sleep (insomnia or hypersomnia) Interest (loss of, including libido) Guilt	Energy loss	Concentration (loss) Appetite (loss or gain) Psychomotor (agitation or retardation) Suicide (ideation)

From reference 246.

Table 75.6 • Factors to Consider in Selecting an Antidepressant

- History of prior response (personal or family member)
- Safety in overdose
- Adverse effect profiles
- Patient age
- Concurrent medical/psychiatric conditions
- Concurrent medications
- Convenience (e.g., minimal titration, once-daily dosing)
- Cost
- Patient preference

Notes:

Table 75.7 • Pharmacology of Antidepressant Medications

Medication	Serotonin	Norepinephrine	Dopamine	Bioavailability (Oral)	Protein Binding	Half-Life (Active Metabolite)
SSRI						
Fluoxetine (Prozac)	++++	0/+	0	80%	95%	24–72 (146)
Sertraline (Zoloft)	++++	0/+	+	>44%	95%	26 (66)
Paroxetine (Paxil)	++++	+	0	64%	99%	24
Citalopram (Celexa)	++++	0	0	80%	<80%	33
Tricyclics						
Desipramine (Norpramin)	+	++++	0/+	51%	90%	12–28
Nortriptyline (Pamelor)	++	+++	0	46–56%	92%	18–56
Amitriptyline (Elavil)	++++	+++	0	37–49%	95%	9–46 (18–56)
Imipramine (Tofranil)	+++	++	0/+	19–35%	95%	6–28 (12–28)
Doxepin (Sinequan)	+++	+	0	17–37%	68–85%	11–23
Others						
Bupropion (Wellbutrin)	0/+	+	+	>90%	85%	10–21
Venlafaxine (Effexor)	++++	+++	0	92%	25–29%	4 (10)
Nefazodone (Serzone)	+++	0	0	20%	99%	4–5 (4–18)
Mirtazapine (Remeron)	+++	++++	0	50%	85%	20–40

0, negligible; +, very low; ++, low; +++, moderate; ++++, high.

Table 75.8 • Adverse Effects of Antidepressant Medications

Medication	Sedation	Agitation/Insomnia	Anticholinergic Effects	Orthostasis	GI Effects (Nausea/Diarrhea)	Sexual Dysfunction	Weight Gain
SSRI							
Fluoxetine (Prozac)	+	+++	0/+	0/+	+++	+++	+
Sertraline (Zoloft)	+	+++	0/+	0	+++	+++	+
Paroxetine (Paxil)	++	++	+	0	+++	+++	++
Citalopram (Celexa)	++	++	0/+	0	+++	++	+
Tricyclics							
Desipramine (Norpramin)	++	+	++	+++	0/+	+	++
Nortriptyline (Pamelor)	++	+	++	++	0/+	+	++
Amitriptyline (Elavil)	+++	0/+	+++	++++	0/+	++	+++
Imipramine (Tofranil)	+++	0/+	+++	+++	0/+	++	++
Doxepin (Sinequan)	+++	0/+	+++	+++	0/+	++	++
Others							
Bupropion (Wellbutrin)	0	+++	+	0	+	0/+	0
Venlafaxine (Effexor)	++	++	+	0	+++	+++	+
Nefazodone (Serzone)	+++	+	+	++	++	0/+	0/+
Mirtazapine (Remeron)	+++	0	++	0/+	+	0/+	+++

0, negligible; +, very low; ++, low; +++, moderate; ++++, high.

Table 75.9 • Management of SSRI-Induced Sexual Dysfunction

- Patience (may improve after 2 to 4 wk)
- Reduced dosage (if possible)
- Drug holidays (sertraline, paroxetine only)
- Antidotes:
  - Bupropion 75–150 mg QD–BID
  - Nefazodone 50–200 mg HS
  - Mirtazapine 7.5–15 mg HS
  - Cyproheptadine 4–12 mg PRN (1 hr prior)
  - Methylphenidate 2.5–5.0 mg QD
  - Others: yohimbine, amantadine, buspirone, sildenafil, gingko
- Change of antidepressants (e.g., bupropion, nefazodone, mirtazapine)

Table 75.10 • Dosage Ranges and Costs of Antidepressant Medications

Medication	Brand Name	Starting Dose (mg/day)	Maximum Dosage (mg/day)	Usual Dosage (mg/day)	Relative Cost[a]
SSRI					
Fluoxetine	Prozac	10	80	10–20 mg QD	$$$$[c]
Sertraline	Zoloft	25	200	50 mg QD	$$$[b]
Paroxetine	Paxil	10	50	10–20 mg QD	$$$[b]
Citalopram	Celexa	10	60	20 mg QD	$$$[b]
TCA					
Desipramine	Norpramin	25	300	200 mg HS	$
Nortriptyline	Pamelor	10–25	150	100 mg HS	$
Others					
Nefazodone	Serzone	50	600	150 mg BID	$$$$
Bupropion	Wellbutrin	200	450	100 mg TID	$$$
Bupropion	Wellbutrin	150	400	150 mg BID	$$$
Mirtazapine	Remeron	15	45	15 mg HS	$$$$[b]
Venlafaxine	Effexor	25	375	50 mg BID	$$$$
Venlafaxine	Effexor XR	37.5	225	100 mg QD	$$$$

[a]Based on average wholesale prices for usual therapeutic doses (April 2000).
[b]AWP reduced by approximately 50% if half-tablets prescribed (e.g., ½ tab 100 mg Zoloft).
[c]Generic now available.
$, $0–25/month; $$, $25–50/month; $$$, $50–70/month; $$$$, >$70/month.

Notes:

Table 75.11 • Duration of Antidepressant Treatment

Acute Treatment Phase:	**3 mo**
Continuation Treatment Phase:	**4–9 mo**
Maintenance Treatment Phase:	**Variable**

- Acute *and* continuation treatment recommended for all patients with major depressive disorder (i.e., minimal duration of treatment = 7 mo)
- Decision to prescribe maintenance treatment is based on the following:
  - Number of previous episodes
  - Severity of previous episodes
  - Family history of depression
  - Patient age (worse prognosis if elderly)
  - Response to antidepressant
  - Persistence of environmental stressors
- Indefinite maintenance treatment is recommended if any one of the following criteria are met:
  1. Three or more previous episodes (regardless of age)
  2. Two or more previous episodes and age older than 50 yr
  3. One or more and age older than 60 yr

Table 75.12 • Discontinuation of Antidepressants

Withdrawal syndrome
- Worse with paroxetine, venlafaxine
- Symptoms: dizziness, nausea, paresthesias, anxiety/insomnia
- Onset: 36–72 hr
- Duration: 3–7 days

Taper schedule (for patients receiving long-term treatment)
- Fluoxetine: generally unnecessary
- Sertraline: decrease by 50 mg every 1–2 wk
- Paroxetine: decrease by 10 mg every 1–2 wk
- Citalopram: decrease by 10 mg every 1–2 wk
- Venlafaxine: decrease by 25–50 mg every 1–2 wk
- Nefazodone: decrease by 50–100 mg every 1–2 wk
- Bupropion: generally unnecessary
- Tricyclics: decrease by 10%–25% every 1–2 wk

Note: Risk of relapse greatest 1 to 6 months after discontinuation.

Notes:

Table 75.13 • Drug Interactions of the Cytochrome P450 System^a

	Relative Rank	CYP 1A2	CYP 2C	CYP 2D6	CYP 3A
Offending agent (i.e., inhibits enzyme)	**High**	Fluvoxamine	*Cyt 2C19* Fluvoxamine *Cyt 2C9* Fluoxetine Fluvoxamine	Paroxetine Fluoxetine	Fluvoxamine Nefazodone
	Moderate		*Cyt 2C19* Fluoxetine Sertraline	TCA Sertraline (high dose) Fluvoxamine	TCA (high dose)
	Low	Fluoxetine Paroxetine Sertraline (high dose) Venlafaxine Nefazodone Bupropion Mirtazapine Citalopram	*Cyt 2C19* Venlafaxine *Cyt 2C9* Sertraline	Venlafaxine Nefazodone Bupropion Citalopram (?)	Fluoxetine Sertraline Paroxetine Mirtazapine Citalopram
Other inhibitors		Quinolones (e.g., ciprofloxacin, enoxetine) Macrolides (erythromycin, clarithromicin)	Cimetidine (2C19) Omeprazole (2C19) Imidazoles (2C9, 2C19) (ketoconazole, fluconazole)	Fenfluramine Yohimbine Methadone Quinidine	Macrolides (erythromycin, clarithromicin) Cimetidine Calcium channel blockers (verapamil, diltiazem, nifed) Imidazoles (ketoconazole, fluconazole) Grapefruit
Other inducers		Cigarettes Caffeine St. John's Wort			Phenobarbital Phenytoin Carbamazepine Rifampin Prednisone St. John's Wort

(continued)

Table 75.13 • Drug Interactions of the Cytochrome P450 System[a] (continued)

Relative Rank	CYP 1A2	CYP 2C	CYP 2D6	CYP 3A
Affected agent (i.e., increased concentration)	TCA—tertiary amines (imipramine, amitriptyline) Phenothiazines (chlorpromazine) Thiothixene Haloperidol Clozapine Caffeine Theophylline Propranolol Tacrine	*Cyt 2C19* TCA—tertiary amines (imipramine, amitriptyline) Citalopram Barbiturates Propranolol Omeprazole *Cyt 2C9* Bupropion Phenytoin Tolbutamide Warfarin Nonsteroidal anti-inflammatory drugs	TCA—secondary amines (desipramine, nortriptyline) Fluoxetine Paroxetine Venlafaxine Nefazodone (mcpp metab) Amphetamines Risperidone Codeine Hydrocodone Dextromethorphan Chlorpheniramine β-Blockers (propranolol, metoprolol)	TCA—tertiary amines Fluoxetine Sertraline Venlafaxine Nefazodone Carbamazepine Quetiapine Buspirone Triazolobenzodiazepines Zolpidem Astemizole Cisapride Macrolides Calcium channel blockers Sex hormones (estrogen) Corticosteroids Lovastatin Protease inhibitors

[a]TCA = Tricyclic antidepressant.

Table 75.14 • Foods Containing Tyramine

High Amounts of Tyramine[a]
Smoked, aged, or pickled meat or fish
Sauerkraut
Aged cheeses such as Swiss and cheddar
Yeast extracts
Fava beans

Moderate Amounts of Tyramine[b]
Beer
Avocados
Meat extracts
Red wines such as Chianti

Low Amounts of Tyramine[c]
Caffeine-containing beverages
Distilled spirits
Chocolate
Soy sauce
Cottage and cream cheese
Yogurt and sour cream

[a]May not consume.
[b]May consume in moderation.
[c]May consume.
Adapted from Shulman KI et al. Dietary restriction, tyramine, and the use of monoamine oxidase inhibitors. J Clin Psychopharmacol 1989;9:397.

Table 75.15 • Partial Response to Antidepressant Treatment Augmentation Strategies (with SSRI)

Ensure completion of full therapeutic trial (4–6 wk).
Ensure optimal dose of antidepressant.
Consider combination therapies:
- Bupropion
- Nefazodone
- Lithium
- Thyroid supplements
- Pindolol (?)
- Buspirone
- Atypical antipsychotics
- Pramipexole

Notes:

Table 75.16 • Patient Education

Seven Things That Everyone Should Know About Depression
- **Depression is NOT a personality flaw or a weakness of character.**
  Depression has been associated with a chemical imbalance in the nervous system, which can be easily corrected with antidepressant medications and associated counseling.
- **All antidepressants are equally effective.**
  Approximately 65% of patients receiving a therapeutic trial of any antidepressant medication will have a beneficial response.
- **Most patients receiving antidepressants will experience some side effect(s) initially.**
  Identify an accessible health professional who can answer your questions.
- **Antidepressants should be taken at the same time daily.**
  This will make it easier for you to remember to take the medication and may also minimize side effects.
- **The response to antidepressants is delayed.**
  Several weeks may pass before you begin to feel better and it may take 4 to 6 weeks before maximal benefits are evident.
- **Antidepressants must be taken for at least 6 to 9 months.**
  Even if you are feeling completely better, studies have shown that people who stop their medication during the first 6 months are much more likely to become depressed again.
- **Antidepressants are NOT addictive substances.**
  Antidepressants may elevate the moods of depressed individuals but they do not act as stimulants and are not associated with craving or other abuse patterns. However, if certain antidepressants are discontinued abruptly, mild withdrawal reactions may occur.

The reader is referred to Chapter 77: Mood Disorders I: Major Depressive Disorders, written by *Patrick R. Finley, Pharm.D., Lyle K. Laird, Pharm.D.,* and *William H. Benefield, Jr., Pharm.D.,* in the seventh edition of **Applied Therapeutics: The Clinical Use of Drugs** for a more in-depth discussion. All notations to reference numbers are based on the reference list at the end of that chapter. The editors of this handbook express their thanks to Drs. Finley, Laird, and Benefield and acknowledge that this chapter is based upon their work.

Notes:

Chapter 76

Mood Disorders II: Bipolar Disorders

Definition. *Bipolar disorder* also is known as *manic-depressive disease* and is used for a person who has had at least 2 years of cycling mood characterized by numerous periods of hypomanic symptoms (see Table 76.1) and separate periods with depressive symptoms that do not meet the criteria for a major depressive episode (see Chapter 75: Mood Disorders I: Major Depressive Disorders).

Classification of Mood Disorders. Discrete episodes of mood disturbances are examined and classified as *major depressive* episodes, *manic* episodes (episodes of elevated mood), *mixed* episodes (with features of both depression and mania), or *hypomanic* episodes (elevated mood less severe than mania and insufficient to impair functioning).

♦ A history of manic, mixed, or hypomanic episodes precludes the diagnosis of major depressive disorder. See Chapter 75.

♦ An individual who has experienced manic *or* mixed episodes has a *Bipolar I Disorder.* An individual who has experienced both hypomania and depression (without a history of manic or mixed episodes) has a *Bipolar II Disorder.*

Signs and Symptoms. The diagnostic criteria for mania are described in Table 76.1. DSM-IV "specifiers" further characterize the course and pattern of illness, severity, presence of psychotic features, recovery between episodes, and whether rapid cycling (>4/year) is involved. A manic episode typically begins with a change in sleep patterns, and symptoms gradually develop over several days in three stages.

♦ *Stage I* is characterized by euphoria, labile affect, grandiosity, overconfidence, racing thoughts, increased psychomotor activity, and an increased rate and amount of speech. This stage corresponds to an episode of hypomania.

♦ *Stage II* features increased irritability, dysphoria, hostility, anger, delusions, and cognitive disorganization. Many patients progress no further than this stage.

♦ *Stage III* features progression of the mania to an undifferentiated psychotic state. Individuals in this stage experience terror, panic, and hallucination. Their behavior is bizarre and psychomotor activity is frenzied.

Course of Illness. Usually is characterized by variations in episode length, length of euthymic intervals, frequency of relapse, severity of episode, and predominant syndrome (i.e., mania, hypomania, or depression).

♦ The first attack usually begins before the age of 33, but after age 15, as a manic episode.

♦ An untreated episode can last for several months.

♦ Most have multiple episodes of mania, hypomania, or depression separated by periods of euthymia throughout their lives. Often the euthymic interval and cycle length decrease with additional episodes.

♦ Individuals who experience shorter cycle lengths and suffer from >4 episodes/year of depression, hypomania, or mania are identified as rapid cyclers. Women comprise

80%-95% of patients with *rapid-cycling* bipolar disorder. Individuals with rapid-cycling bipolar disorder often are refractory to conventional treatment and suffer significant morbidity and mortality due to rapid mood changes.

♦ Manic episodes can be precipitated by drugs listed in Table 76.2.

Treatment is comprised of 1) acute treatment of manic episodes, 2) acute treatment of depressive episodes, and 3) maintenance pharmacotherapy. See Table 76.3.

♦ *Clinical Pharmacology of Mood Stabilizing Agents.* See Table 76.4.
♦ *Prelithium Wakeup.* See Table 76.5.
♦ *Side Effects of Lithium.* See Table 76.6.
♦ *Lithium Drug Interactions.* See Table 76.7.

Table 76.1 • DSM-IV Criteria for a Manic Episode[a]

1. A distinct period of abnormally and persistently elevated, expansive, or irritable mood, lasting at least 1 week (or of any duration if hospitalization is necessary).
2. During the period of mood disturbance, ≥3 of the following symptoms have persisted (4 if the mood is only irritable) and have been present to a significant degree:
   - Inflated self-esteem or grandiosity
   - Decreased need for sleep (e.g., feels rested after only 3 hours of sleep)
   - More talkative than usual or pressure to keep talking
   - Flight of ideas or subjective experience that thoughts are racing
   - Distractibility (i.e., attention too easily drawn to unimportant or irrelevant external stimuli)
   - Increase in goal-directed activity (either social, at work, at school, or sexually) or psychomotor agitation
   - Excessive involvement in pleasurable activities that have a high potential for painful consequences (e.g., the person engages in unrestrained buying sprees, sexual indiscretions, or foolish business investing)
3. The symptoms do not meet the criteria for a Mixed Episode.
4. The mood disturbance is sufficiently severe to cause marked impairment in occupational functioning or in usual social activities or relationships with others, or to necessitate hospitalization to prevent harm to self or others, or there are psychotic features.
5. The symptoms are not due to the direct physiologic effects of a substance (e.g., a drug of abuse, a medication, or other treatment) or a general medical condition (e.g., hyperthyroidism).

[a]A "manic syndrome" is defined as including criteria 1, 2, and 3. A "hypomanic syndrome" is defined as including criteria 1 and 2, but not 3 (i.e., no marked impairment). Maniclike episodes that are clearly caused by somatic antidepressant treatment (e.g., medication, electroconvulsive therapy, light therapy) should not count toward a diagnosis of bipolar I disorder.
Reprinted with permission from reference 2.

Notes:

Table 76.2 • Drugs Reported to Induce Mania

Antidepressants
  Monoamine oxidase inhibitors[19,22,23]
  Tricyclic antidepressants[21,23,24]
  Bupropion[25-27]
  Fluoxetine[28,29]
  Fluvoxamine[30]
  Sertraline[23,24]
  Paroxetine[23,24]
  Nefazodone[31]
  Mirtazapine[32]
  Venlafaxine[33]

Antipsychotics
  Olanzapine[34,35]
  Risperidone[36-38]

Anxiolytics/Hypnotics
  Buspirone[39]
  Alprazolam[40]
  Triazolam[41]

Miscellaneous
  Levodopa[42]
  Amantadine[43]
  Cimetidine[44]
  Tolmetin[45]
  Folate[46]
  Pindolol[47]
  Interferon-α[48]
  Donepezil[49]
  Clarithromycin[50]
  Tramadol[51]
  Guanfacine[52]

Herbals
  St. John's Wort[53]
  Ginseng[54]
  Ma-huang[55]
  Chromium piccolinate[55]

Stimulants
  Cocaine[42]
  Methylphenidate[56]
  Dexfenfluramine[57]
  Phentermine[58]

Anticonvulsants
  Felbamate[59]
  Gabapentin[60]

Endocrine
  Corticosteroids[61]
  Thyroid[42]
  Androgens[62]
  Dehydroepiandrosterone (DHEA)[63]
  Testosterone patch[64]
  Leuprolide[65]

Notes:

Table 76.3 • Bipolar Disorders—Treatment Overview

Disease Stage	Recommended Treatment
Acute Manic Episode	
• First-line[c] (see Table 76.4)	
• Mania with psychosis	• Divalproex[a] *or* lithium
• Dysphoric mania or true mixed mania	• Divalproex[a] *or* lithium
• Euphoric mania	• Lithium[a] *or* divalproex (carbamazepine is an alternative)
• Hypomania	• Lithium *or* divalproex
• Rapid cycling	• Divalproex or carbamazepine
• Partial or poor responders after 1–2 weeks	Divalproex (or carbamazepine) *plus* Lithium
• Adjunctive agents	
• For agitation, hyperactivity, and sleep disorders	Benzodiazepines (e.g. lorazepam 2 mg PO or IM, Q 2–8 hr PRN; taper as patient responds to mood stabilizer)
• For pyschosis	SSRIs[a,b] (e.g. risperidone 2 mg/day initially; <6 mg/day as maintenance to avoid extrapyramidal symptoms and mania; discontinue when mania resolves, usually within 2 weeks. Bupropion[b] is an alternative.
Acute Depressive Episode	Lithium alone *or combined with* bupropion or an SSRI[b]
Maintenance (prophylactic) therapy	Lithium or divalproex

[a]Drug of choice
[b]Antidepressants have the potential to switch a depressed patient into a manic episode. Bupropion and serotonin reuptake inhibitors (SSRIs) may be less likely to do so.
[c]Adapted from Sachs GS et al, eds. The expert consensus guideline series: medication treatment of bipolar disorder 2000. Postgrad Med 2000;Special: 1.

Notes:

Table 76.4 • Mood Stabilizing Agents

	Valproic Acid Divalproex Sodium	Lithium	Carbamazepine
Brand name	Generic, Depakene Depakote	Generic, Eskalith Capsules, Eskalith CR Controlled Release Tablets, Lithobid Slow-Release Tablets	Generic, Tegretol, Tegretol XR
Dosage form	250 mg capsules 125, 250 mg delayed release tablets	300 mg capsules 450 mg CR tablets 300 mg Slow-Release tablets	100 mg chewable tablets, 100 mg/mL suspension, 200 mg tablet, 100, 200, 400 mg extended release tablets.
Dose	250 mg TID initially. Increase by 250 mg Q 2 days to target serum levels. Mean dose is 1250–1500 mg daily.	300 mg TID (extended release dosage forms are given BID initially). Titrate over a few days as tolerated. Typical dose for acute mania is 1800 mg/day; for maintenance, it is 900–1200 mg/day in divided doses, or a single dose of the long-acting form.	100–200 mg BID initially. Increase by 200 mg/day every 3–4 days to target serum levels.
Target levels	45–125 μg/mL	0.5–1.2 mEq/L for acute episodes; 0.5–0.8 for maintenance. Draw levels just before next dose.	8–12 mg/mL. Toxicity associated with >12 mg/mL.
Onset	5–7 days	1–2 weeks	1–2 weeks
Side effects	GI (nausea, diarrhea, dyspepsia, anorexia), sedation, ataxia, tremor, alopecia, weight gain. Transient liver enzyme elevations, thrombocytopenia (rare).	See Table 76.6 and Table 76.7 Toxicity can occur at levels >1.5 mEq/L (tremor, slurred speech, unsteady gait, drowsiness, confusion, muscle twitches, blurred vision.) At levels >2.5 mEq/L, seizures, stupor, coma, and cardiovascular collapse can occur.	Hematologic (transient leukopenia, agranulocytosis, thrombocytopenia, aplastic anemia), hyponatremia, ataxia, lethargy, skin rash, increased LFTs, GI complaints.

(continued)

Table 76.4 • Mood Stabilizing Agents (continued)

	Valproic Acid Divalproex Sodium	Lithium	Carbamazepine
Predrug work-up	CBC with differential, weight, neurological status, pregnancy test, drug history for interacting drugs (e.g. ASA, warfarin, rifampin, anticonvulsants).	See Table 76.5	CBC with differential and platelets, LFTs, electrolytes, neurologic status, BP, skin rashes, pregnancy test. Drug history of interacting drugs (e.g., oral contraceptives, warfarin, valproic acid, haloperidol, tricylic antidepressants).
Monitoring	Target symptoms, LFTs, valproic serum levels, CBC with differential monthly for 3 months, then Q 3–6 months.	Target symptoms; lithium levels every several days until stable, than Q 3 months; thyroid and renal function tests Q 6–12 months.	Target symptoms, carbamazepine levels, CBC with differential and platelets Q 3 weeks for 3 months, then Q 6 months. Petechiae, bleeding, rashes, infection, mental status changes indicative of hyponatremia.
Notes	Divalproex is enteric-coated form of valproic acid with fewer GI effects initially. Once stabilized, many patients can be switched to less expensive valproic acid.	Adjunctive therapy is needed due to long onset of action. As patients recover from acute mania, clearance may decrease leading to higher levels and side effects. Sustained release products have been used to enhance compliance and reduce side effects. BID administration lowers peak levels and higher trough levels which can lead to polyuria.	Can induce its own metabolism causing levels to decrease for up to 1 month after any dose adjustment is made.

Table 76.5 • Prelithium Workup[a]

Baseline Determination[18,85]	Rationale
SrCr, BUN	Lithium is excreted renally.
Urine-specific gravity	Lithium may cause polyuria.
Electrolytes	Hyponatremia and dehydration lead to ↑ renal reabsorption of lithium and subsequent lithium toxicity; hypokalemia may ↑ the risk of lithium-induced cardiac toxicity.
ECG[b]	Lithium may worsen severe cardiac disease.
CBC with differential	Lithium may cause a 15–45% ↑ in the numbers of all WBC lines except basophils; lithium also may cause an ↑ in platelet counts.[86,87]
T$_4$, TSH	Lithium may induce hypothyroidism.[88–90]
Glucose	Lithium may induce weight gain and complicate the presentation of diabetes mellitus.[91]
Weight	Lithium may induce weight gain.[92]
Lithium level	Manic patients may at times be poor historians.
Pregnancy test	Lithium is a potential teratogen.[93,94]

[a]BUN = Blood urea nitrogen; CBC = Complete blood count; ECG = Electrocardiograph; SrCr = Serum creatinine; TSH = Thyroid-stimulating hormone; WBC = White blood cell.
[b]In those patients with a history or at risk for cardiac disease.

Table 76.6 • Side Effects of Lithium[a]

Lithium Side Effect	Occurrence	Treatment Strategy
Cognitive effects[17,96]	9%	Ensure that patient is not depressed; consider supportive therapy; differentiate from manic hyperacuity; lower dosage.
Fine tremor[86,97]	15% but ↓ with time	May resolve with time; lower dosage; reduce caffeine intake; avoid tricyclic antidepressants, sympathomimetics; consider β-adrenergic blocking agents such as propranolol 40–160 mg/day.
GI upset[17]	33% in first 2 wk	May resolve or improve with time; may be related to speed of rise of serum levels; consider divided doses or sustained-release preparations.
Diarrhea[17,92]	6–20%	May be related to serum levels; reduce dosage.
Hypothyroidism[16,17]	5–8%	Discontinue lithium or treat with levothyroxine.
Polyuria, polydipsia[98,99]	36%	May be related to serum levels; reduce dosage; consider reducing frequency of administration; consider amiloride.
Weight gain[92]	50–75%; average ↑ of 4 kg	Try to avoid polyuria and polydipsia and discourage use of high-calorie drinks; regular exercise; dietary consultation.
Worsening of dermatologic conditions[100]	Follicular eruptions 33%	Consider reduction in dosage or discontinuation depending on severity of reaction; provide symptomatic treatment.

[a]GI = Gastrointestinal.

Table 76.7 • Lithium Drug Interactions of Clinical Significance[115,a]

Drugs That May Increase Lithium Levels

NSAIDs[113]

Many NSAIDs have been reported to ↑ lithium levels as much as 50–60%. This probably is due to an enhanced reabsorption of sodium and lithium secondary to inhibition of prostaglandin synthesis.

Diuretics

All diuretics can contribute to sodium depletion. Sodium depletion can result in an ↑ proximal tubular reabsorption of sodium and lithium. Thiazide-like diuretics cause the greatest ↑ in lithium levels, whereas loop diuretics and potassium-sparing diuretics appear somewhat safer.

ACE inhibitors

ACE inhibitors and lithium both result in volume depletion and a reduction in glomerular filtration rate. This results in reduced lithium excretion.

Drugs That May Decrease Lithium Levels

Theophylline, caffeine

Theophylline and caffeine may ↑ renal clearance of lithium and result in a ↓ in levels in the range of 20%.

Acetazolamide

Acetazolamide may impair proximal tubular reabsorption of lithium ions.

Sodium

High dietary sodium intake promotes the renal clearance of lithium.

Drugs That Increase Lithium Toxicity

Methyldopa

Cases of sedation, dysphoria, and confusion due to the combined use of lithium and methyldopa have been reported.

Carbamazepine

Cases of neurotoxicity involving the combined use of lithium and carbamazepine have been reported in patients with normal lithium levels.

Calcium channel antagonists

Cases of neurotoxicity involving the combined use of lithium and the calcium channel blockers verapamil and diltiazem have been reported. Lithium does interfere with calcium transport across cells.

Antipsychotics

Cases of neurotoxicity (encephalopathic syndrome, extrapyramidal effects, cerebellar effect, EEG abnormalities) have been reported due to the combined use of lithium and various antipsychotics. The interaction may be related to ↑ in phenothiazine levels, changes in tissue uptake of lithium, and/or dopamine-blocking effects of lithium. Studies attempting to demonstrate this effect have yielded differing results.

Serotonin-specific reuptake inhibitors

Fluvoxamines and fluoxetine have been reported to result in an ↑ of toxicity when added to lithium. Sertraline has been reported to ↑ nausea and tremor in lithium recipients.[116]

[a]ACE = Angiotensin-converting enzyme; EEG = Electroencephalogram; NSAIDs = Nonsteroidal anti-inflammatory drugs.

The reader is referred to Chapter 77: Mood Disorders II: Bipolar Affective Disorders, written by *Raymond C. Love, Pharm.D.*, and *Mary C. Borovicka, Pharm.D.*, in the seventh edition of **Applied Therapeutics: The Clinical Use of Drugs** for a more in-depth discussion. All notations to reference numbers are based on the reference list at the end of that chapter. The editors of this handbook express their thanks to Drs. Love and Borovicka and acknowledge that this chapter is based upon their work.

Notes:

Chapter 77

Psychiatric Disorders in Children, Adolescents, and People with Developmental Disabilities

Attention-Deficit Hyperactivity Disorder (ADHD)
Clinical Features
♦ Most common psychiatric disorder in children, with male to female ratio of 4:1.
♦ A developmentally inappropriate ability to maintain attention
♦ Hyperactivity; impulsivity (e.g., acts before thinking) for >6 months
♦ Social and academic function significantly impaired
♦ Onset before age 7 years; can persist into adulthood

Treatment. Use one of the stimulants below or antidepressants if there are symptoms of anxiety, mood lability, or depression. All stimulants are equally effective in normalizing behavior and improving academic performance and peer interactions; 15–20% are unresponsive.

♦ *Methylphenidate (Ritalin)*
  • Dose: 5 mg in the morning, additional dose at noon and at 4 p.m. if needed. Gradually increase dose to 0.3–0.6 mg/kg/day (maximum 60 mg/day).
  • Maximum benefits occur 2–3 hours after the dose.
  • Side effects: insomnia, anorexia, and growth retardation. Latter can be avoided by use of drug holidays on weekends and during the summer months.
  • Sustained release form (Ritalin SR, 20 mg) may be less effective.
♦ *Dextroamphetamine (Dexedrine)*
  • Dose: 2.5 mg in the morning, with an additional dose at noon if needed.
  • Peak benefit: 1–2 hours after dosing
  • Side effects: Similar to methylphenidate, but tachycardia, anorexia, and compulsivity more common.
♦ *Magnesium Pemoline (Cylert)*.
  • Dose: Initially, 18.75 mg once daily. Gradually increase to 112.5 mg/day max. Twice daily dosing may be required.
  • Onset is 1–2 hours; duration 8–12 hours.
  • Side effects: Similar to other stimulants, except for rare, but serious liver toxicity. LFTs required every 2 weeks. Discontinue if ALT is >2 times normal.

♦ *Antidepressants*
  • SSRIs ineffective in ADHD
  • Tricyclic antidepressants (TCAs) are best studied and may be more efficacious in patients with comorbid depression.
    —Desipramine (Norpramin) 5 mg/kg/day
    —No relationship between serum level and response
    —Side effects: no growth suppression but sudden cardiac death a concern. Get baseline vitals and ECG during dose titration and maintenance. Watch for prolongation of the PR and QTc intervals and QRS widening.

Depressive Disorders
Clinical Features
♦ Common, affecting 2% of all children and 4–8% of adolescents. Cumulative prevalence is 20% by age 18.
♦ Often chronic and associated with other disorders (e.g., anxiety)
♦ Symptoms vary with child's age:
  • *Ages 3–4.* "Acting out" (hyperactivity, aggression, temper tantrums, social withdrawal, separation problems, eating or sleeping difficulties).
  • *Ages 5–8.* Low self-esteem, sadness, self-blame, feelings of guilt, social withdrawal, accident-prone, somatic symptoms, lying, stealing, aggression, and underachievement academically.
  • *Ages 9–12.* Sadness, apathy, sense of helplessness, anhedonia, anxiety, irritability, somatic symptoms, academic problems, and suicidal ideation.
  • *Ages 13–18.* Symptoms similar to adults (see Chapter 72: Anxiety Disorders). Sleep and appetite disturbance, anhedonia, somatic symptoms, social withdrawal, antisocial behavior, drug or alcohol abuse. Risk of youth suicide highest in this age group. See Table 77.1.

Treatment
♦ *SSRIs* are considered first-line therapy but are not FDA-approved for this use.
  • Fluoxetine (Prozac) and sertraline (Zoloft) have been studied. Citalopram (Celexa) has not been studied but may be considered due to mild side effect profile.
  • Dose: For children 6 years or older, start with half adult doses (5–10 mg/day fluoxetine; 12.5–25 mg sertraline). Adolescents may start paroxetine (Paxil) at 20 mg/day but seldom used in children. Increase to tolerable dose in a week and maintain for at least 4 weeks. If no response at 4 weeks, increase the dose. Full response can take 10 weeks. Typical adequate daily doses are fluoxetine 10–20 mg, sertraline 25–200 mg, and paroxetine 20–50 mg (lower in preadolescents).
♦ *TCAs*
  • Use in children who do not respond to or are intolerant of SSRIs or who have relevant comorbid conditions such as ADHD.
  • Obtain baseline ECG, pulse, blood pressure, and weight. Follow as dose is escalated and within several days of achieving final dose.
  • Dose. Initially 1–2 mg/kg/day of imipramine (best studied) or desipramine or 1 mg/kg/day nortriptyline in 2 or more divided doses. Increase by 10–25 mg/day once or twice weekly based on side effects. Usual daily dose is 2–5 mg/kg/day for imipramine and desipramine or 1–3 mg/kg/day for nortriptyline.
  • Response correlates with serum levels of 125–225 ng/mL; higher levels associated with tachycardia and slowed cardiac conduction. Nortriptyline levels of 60–100

ng/mL are considered safe but are not correlated with efficacy. Lower levels than that required for adults may be related to lower protein binding and more lean body mass.

- Full response takes 4–10 weeks.
- Side effects similar to adults. See Chapter 72. Do not prescribe amounts that can be fatal. Lowest fatal dose is 8 mg/kg.

Bipolar Disorder

Clinical Features

♦ Silly, excited, hyperactive, irritable, paranoid, withdrawn, angry, or explosive behavior and affective lability

♦ Adolescents may have several depressive episodes before the first manic episode, which has a greater likelihood of presenting as psychosis than in adults

♦ Can be misdiagnosed as schizophrenia or ADHD

Treatment

♦ *Lithium*

- Dose: 30 mg (or 0.8 mEq/kg) per day in 3 divided doses with food. Increase to serum concentration of 0.6–1.2 mEq/L.
- Side Effects. Similar to adults (see Chapter 76: Mood Disorders II: Bipolar Disorders), but watch for situations that could lead to dehydration, especially over the summer; watch for hypothyroidism, which can impair growth; and acne.

♦ *Valproic Acid (Depakote)*

- Approved for bipolar disorder in adults but no placebo-controlled studies in children
- Dose: Initially 15 mg/kg/day. Clinical benefit has been seen at 10–60 mg/kg/day for children and 1000–3000 mg/day in adolescents. Anticonvulsant levels of 50–100 mcg/mL have been used.
- Side Effects. See Chapter 76. Severe liver toxicity a problem in children younger than 2 years old or in those taking other anticonvulsants. Long-term therapy may cause polycystic ovaries and weight gain.

Anxiety Disorders

Clinical Features

♦ Symptoms similar to adults. See Chapter 72: Anxiety Disorders

♦ Separation Anxiety Disorder (SAD) is only anxiety disorder specific to children: excessive or unrealistic worry about harm to self or parents, refusal to attend school, reluctance to sleep alone, go away from home, or to be alone. Physical symptoms include stomachaches, headaches, palpitations, and dizziness.

♦ Prevalence: Social phobia 1.1%, SAD 3.5%, obsessive-compulsive disorder 1–3.6%, generalized anxiety 4.6%, all anxiety disorders 8.7%.

♦ Diagnosis is confounded by developmental level, difficulty getting accurate information, and comorbid psychiatric disorders.

Treatment

♦ Behavioral treatment, psychotherapy, and family therapy are primary modes of treatment.

♦ Drugs should only be used as an adjunct to behavioral therapy. SSRIs have become first-line agents over TCAs. Benzodiazepines are recommended for short-term use only.

Schizophrenia

Clinical Features

♦ Early-onset schizophrenia (EOS), occurring between 13 and 18 years of age, and very-early-onset schizophrenia (VEOS), occurring before 13 years of age, are very rare (<0.04%).

♦ Must be differentiated from autism, bipolar disorder, schizoaffective disorder, and organic brain disorder.

♦ Symptoms include social withdrawal, odd personality, and delays in cognitive, motor, sensory, and social functioning.

Treatment

♦ Similar to adults. See Chapter 74: Schizophrenia.

♦ Atypical antipsychotics, or serotonin-dopamine antagonists—SDAs (e.g., risperidone, olanzapine, quetiapine), which are preferred over conventional agents (e.g., haloperidol, chlorpromazine, thiothixene) because they have a more tolerable side effect profile

♦ Baseline assessment for antipsychotic medications is recommended. See Table 77.2.

♦ Dose: Risperidone (Risperdal), 0.05–0.17 mg/kg/day, olanzapine (Zyprexa), 0.15–0.41 mg/kg/day.

Tourette's Syndrome

Clinical Features

♦ A familial disorder with an autosomal dominant pattern of inheritance

♦ Onset is 2–15 years of age, with a mean of 7 years for motor tics and 11 years for vocal tics.

♦ Sudden involuntary movements or sounds (grunts, foul language) wax and wane and are difficult to suppress.

♦ Behavioral symptoms common: OCD present in 55–74%. ADHD present in 50%

Treatment

Many drugs have been used to suppress tics

♦ *Clonidine* (generic, Catapres) is effective in 40–60% of patients, is well tolerated in patients with coexisting ADHD. Initial dose is 0.05 mg once or twice daily, with initial dose at bedtime to avoid daytime sedation. Increase by 0.05 mg Q 3 days until sedation or dizziness is noted. Usual dose is 5.5 mcg/kg/day. Effect may require several weeks.

♦ *Guanfacine* (Tenex) may have less hypotensive and sedative effects than clonidine. Dose is 0.5–4 mg/day

♦ *Haloperidol* (Haldol) is a mainstay, but 14% discontinue drug due to extrapyramidal effects (EPSs). Dose is 2–6 mg/day.

♦ *Pimozide* (Orap) may be better tolerated than haldol and may be more efficacious but is associated with cardiac effects. Periodic ECGs are recommended.

Autistic Disorder

Clinical Features

♦ A rare developmental disorder (1 in 10,000) characterized by qualitative impairment in social interaction (they do not "connect"), verbal and nonverbal communication skills (inability to use and interpret body language or speech for communication), a restricted set of activities and interests (e.g., repetitive movements and insistence on an unchanging environment).

♦ About 75% are developmentally delayed, and 25% have a seizure disorder.

♦ Diagnosis is typically at less than 36 months of age but can be detected as early as 18 months.

Treatment

♦ Highly individualized behavioral therapy and special education

♦ Many drugs have been used, including naltrexone, clonidine, clomipramine, and SSRIs.

♦ SDAs such as *risperidone* can reduce repetitive behavior, aggression, anxiety, depression, and irritability. Start with 0.5 mg once daily and increase slowly because autistic children seem to respond to low doses. Dose used in one trial was 2 to 4 mg/day. Onset 1–2 weeks. Monitor for weight gain, EPSs, and sedation.

♦ *Haloperidol* in low doses (0.25 to 4.0 mg/day) reduces repetitive movements and withdrawal but carries the risk of EFSs and tardive dyskinesia.

Disorders Associated with Developmental Disabilities

See Table 77.3.

Table 77.1 • Risk Factors for Adolescent Suicide[45]

Psychiatric Diagnosis	Genetic Predisposition
Mood disorders	Family history of mood disorders
Schizophrenia	Family history of suicide attempts
Conduct disorders	Family history of alcohol abuse
Substance abuse	**Other Factors**
Personality disorders (especially borderline and antisocial)	Biologic factors (serotonin and dopamine)
	"Contagion" effect (suicide clusters)
Personality Traits	Dysphoria regarding sexual orientation
Aggression	
Impulsiveness	
Hopelessness	
Psychosocial stressors	
Family dysfunction	
Parental loss	
Medical illness	
Lack of social supports	

Data from reference 45.

Table 77.2 • Recommended Baseline Assessment for Antipsychotic Medications

Medical history (including seizures, liver and cardiac disease)
Weight, height, BP, pulse rate
Sleep and eating patterns
CBC, LFTs
Glucose
ECG (for pimozide)
Abnormal movement assessment (using an established rating scale)

BP, blood pressure; CBC, complete blood count; ECG, electrocardiogram; LFTs, liver function tests.

Notes:

Table 77.3 • Developmental Syndromes and Associated Behavioral and Psychiatric Disorders

Developmental Syndrome	Associated Behavioral Disorder
Down syndrome	Alzheimer's dementia
Fragile X syndrome	Autism, hyperactivity, inattention, temper tantrums, anxiety
Prader-Willi syndrome	Compulsive eating, hoarding
Lesch-Nyhan syndrome	Severe self-injury (self-biting)
Cornelia de Lange syndrome	Self-injury
Rett's syndrome	Stereotypic hand movements (hand clasping, washing)
Fetal alcohol syndrome	Hyperactivity

The reader is referred to Chapter 79: Psychiatric Disorders in Children, Adolescents, and People with Developmental Disabilities, written by *Judy L. Curtis, Pharm.D.*, and *Jay D. Sherr, Pharm.D.*, in the seventh edition of **Applied Therapeutics: The Clinical Use of Drugs** for a more in-depth discussion, and in particular, the treatment of behavioral disorders associated with developmental disabilities (schizophrenia, depression, self-injurious behavior, and aggression). All notations to reference numbers are based on the reference list at the end of that chapter. The editors of this handbook express their thanks to Drs. Curtis and Sherr and acknowledge that this chapter is based upon their work.

Notes:

Chapter 78

Secondary Neuropsychiatric Disorders

Definition
Secondary neuropsychiatric disorders include emotional, behavioral, or cognitive syndromes triggered by another medical condition affecting the brain. See Table 78.1.

Clinical Presentation
Symptoms closely resemble those characteristic of primary psychiatric disorders (e.g., impulsivity, mood instability, irritability, agitation, aggression, sleep disorders, lack of interest, depression, anxiety, mania, crying, and psychosis). Different pathologies may lead to similar clinical symptoms, and conversely, the same underlying medical condition can produce a variety of neuropsychiatric presentations. This chapter focuses on treatment of aggression and apathy.

Diagnoses
 ♦ Diagnostic criteria. See Table 78.2.
 ♦ Use detailed physical examination and history along with tests and procedures used by clinical neurologists (e.g., EEG, neuroimaging)

Treatment
 ♦ Diagnose and treat underlying medical condition
 ♦ No medications are approved specifically for treatment of secondary neuropsychiatric disorders. Treatment is largely empirical due to general lack of evidence.
 ♦ Identification of target symptoms and intense clinical monitoring for response are pivotal to successfully treat these behaviors
 ♦ Drug therapy alone is seldom efficacious and must be combined with environmental and behavioral interventions

Disinhibition and Aggression
 ♦ Patients with disinhibited behavior require constant supervision. Symptoms are hard to eliminate, making it difficult for patients to integrate back into the community. See Table 78.3.
 ♦ Aggressive behavior that is explosive or impulsive in nature may be more responsive to therapy than that which is premeditated and predatory.
 ♦ Dysregulation of several neurotransmitters may underlie aggressive behavior. See Table 78.4.
 ♦ *Typical antipsychotic agents* have been the preferred drugs of choice to control acutely aggressive and violent patients (e.g., haloperidol 5 mg IM with 1 to 2 mg lorazepam IM if needed).
 ♦ *Atypical antipsychotics* (e.g., risperidone, olanzapine, quetiapine) are used to manage chronic aggressive behaviors, but their use should be limited to patients that exhibit behavior clearly related to psychotic symptoms because they can worsen pre-existing cognitive dysfunction.

♦ Other agents that have been used are listed in Table 78.5

♦ Combination therapy (e.g., risperidone and valproic acid) is used in patients who only partially respond to a single drug.

Apathy

♦ Defined as a state of reduced emotion and motivation or the inability to feel emotion, interest, or concern.

♦ Commonly associated with neurodegenerative disorders (e.g., Alzheimer's or Parkinson's disease) and acute neurologic insults (e.g., strokes)

♦ Antidepressant therapy is generally ineffective

♦ *Dopamine agonists* (e.g., bromcriptine, amantadine) have been used successfully, but tolerance may occur. Bromocriptine may be particularly useful in apathy associated with stroke

♦ *Methylphenidate,* a psychostimulant may be useful in apathy associated with AIDS, stroke, or traumatic brain injury.

Table 78.1 • Medical Conditions Triggering Neuropsychiatric Disorders (Examples)

Alzheimer's disease	Endocrine disorders (e.g., thyroid abnormalities)
Brain tumors	Neurotoxins
CNS infections and inflammation (e.g., AIDS)	Parkinson's disease
CNS degenerative disorders (e.g., multiple	Seizures disorders
sclerosis, Huntington's)	Stroke
Developmental disorders	Traumatic brain injury

Table 78.2 • DSM-IV Diagnostic Criteria for Personality Change Due to a General Medical Condition[a]

• A persistent personality disturbance that represents a change from the individual's previous characteristic personality pattern. (In children, the disturbance involves a marked deviation from normal development or a significant change in the child's usual behavior patterns, lasting at least 1 year.)
• There is evidence from the history, physical examination, or laboratory findings that the disturbance is the direct physiologic consequence of a general medical condition.
• The disturbance is not better accounted for by another mental disorder (including other mental disorders due to a general medical condition).
• The disturbance does not occur exclusively during the course of a delirium and does not meet the criteria for a dementia.
• The disturbance causes clinically significant distress or impairment in social, occupational, or other important areas of functioning.

Specify Type
Labile Type: if the predominant feature is affective lability
Disinhibited Type: if the predominant feature is poor impulse control (e.g., sexual indiscretions)
Aggressive Type: if the predominant feature is aggressive behavior
Apathetic Type: if the predominant feature is marked apathy and indifference
Paranoid Type: if the predominant feature is suspiciousness or paranoid ideation
Other Type: if the predominant feature is not one of the above (e.g., personality change associated with a seizure disorder)
Combined Type: if more than one feature predominates in the clinical picture
Unspecified Type

[a]The name of the general medical condition always is included with the diagnosis.
Adapted from reference 11.

Table 78.3 • Types of Disinhibited Behaviors

Motor disinhibition	Hyperactivity Pressured speech Decreased need for sleep
Instinctive disinhibition	Hypersexuality Hyperphagia Aggressive outbursts
Emotional disinhibition	Euphoria Elation Irritability
Intellectual disinhibition	Grandiose delusions Paranoid delusions Flight of ideas
Sensory disinhibition	Visual hallucinations Auditory hallucinations

Adapted from reference 10.

Table 78.4 • Proposed Neurotransmitter Activity and Aggression[a]

Increased Aggression	Decreased Aggression
↓ 5HT	↑ 5HT
↓ GABA	↑ GABA
↑ NE	↓ NE
↑ DA	↓ DA

[a] 5HT = Serotonin; DA = Dopamine; GABA = Gamma-aminobutyric acid; NE = Norepinephrine.

Table 78.5 • Agents Used in the Chronic Management of Aggressive and Disinhibited Behaviors

Drug	Dosage
β-Blockers	
Propranolol (Inderal)	100–600 mg/day in divided doses
Pindolol (Visken)	20–60 mg/day in divided doses
Nadolol (Corgard)	80–320 mg/day in divided doses
Metoprolol (Lopressor)	100–400 mg/day in divided doses
Serotonin Agonists	
Buspirone (BuSpar)	30–120 mg/day in 3 or 4 divided doses
Fluoxetine (Prozac)	10–60 mg/day
Paroxetine (Paxil)	10–60 mg/day
Sertraline (Zoloft)	50–200 mg/day
Citalopram (Celexa)	10–40 mg/day
Mood Stabilizers/Anticonvulsants	
Lithium	600–1,200 mg/day in 2 or 3 divided doses (0.6–1.2 mEq/mL)
Carbamazepine (Tegretol)	600–1,400 mg/day in 2 or 3 divided doses (8–12 μg/mL)
Valproate (Depakene, Depakote)	1,000–3,000 mg/day in 2 or 3 divided doses (50–120 μg/mL)
Gabapentin (Neurontin)	200–2,400 mg/day in 2 or 3 divided doses

Notes:

The reader is referred to Chapter 80: Secondary Neuropsychiatric Disorders, written by *Deborah A. Stanley, Pharm.D.*, and *Steven W. Stanislav, Pharm.D.*, in the seventh edition of **Applied Therapeutics: The Clinical Use of Drugs** for a more in-depth discussion. All notations to reference numbers are based on the reference list at the end of that chapter. The editors of this handbook express their thanks to Drs. Stanley and Stanislav and acknowledge that this chapter is based upon their work.

Notes:

Chapter 79

Eating Disorders

Definitions

♦ *Anorexia Nervosa.* A condition characterized by a focus on weight loss and thinness to the extent that it becomes detrimental to health. See Tables 79.1, 79.2, and 79.3.

♦ *Bulimia Nervosa.* A condition characterized by binge eating along with inappropriate compensatory behaviors and methods to prevent weight gain that occur, on average, at least twice weekly for 3 months. See Tables 79.2 and 79.4.

♦ *Eating Disorder Not Otherwise Specified.* Also called *atypical eating disorder.* Characterized by an abuse of weight reduction medications, use of excessive exercise to lose weight, or binge eating behaviors that do not meet the strict diagnostic criteria for anorexia nervosa or bulimia nervosa.

♦ *Binge Eating Disorder.* Recurrent binge eating episodes unaccompanied by behaviors to prevent weight gain. Often triggered by anxiety or depression.

♦ *Obesity.* A chronic metabolic disorder defined as a body mass index (BMI) ≥ 30 kg/m^2 or a waist circumference of 102 cm or 40 inches in men and ≥ 89 cm or 35 inches in women. See Table 79.1.

♦ *Body Dysmorphic Disorder.* Characterized by a preoccupation with a defect in appearance or body shame that results in significant distress or impaired function. Associated with depression, anxiety, phobias, frequent checking of the "defect" in a mirror, excessive grooming, skin picking, compulsive exercising, cosmetic surgery.

Medical Complications of Eating Disorders. See Table 79.5

Anorexia Nervosa—Treatment

♦ *Criteria for hospitalization:* rapid weight loss of >15% of body weight, hypotension with a systolic BP <90 mm Hg, bradycardia (heart rate ≤ 50 beat/minute), core body temperature <97°F, suicide ideation, medical complications, nonresponsiveness to outpatient treatment after 3 to 4 months.

♦ *Therapeutic Goal:* 90% of ideal body weight. A healthy weight is that at which normal ovulation and menstruation occur. Inpatient weight restoration programs can add 2 to 3 pounds/week. Outpatient programs can add 0.5 to 1 pound/week.

♦ Responds to a variety of psychotherapeutic approaches

♦ *Pharmacotherapy.* See Table 79.6
  • No pharmacological agents are more effective than placebo
  • Malnourished patients may be prone to side effects of medications.
  • Tricyclic antidepressants can increase the risk of dehydration, hypotension, arrhythmias, and seizures.
  • The pharmacokinetics of drugs may be altered due to changes in body fat and protein. Always start with low doses of any drug.
  • Selective serotonin reuptake inhibitors (SSRIs) are considered safest antidepressant for comorbid anxiety, obsessive-compulsive behaviors, social phobia, and depression.

Bulimia Nervosa—Treatment

♦ Behavioral and cognitive techniques help individuals modify their binge eating and purging behavior
♦ *Antidepressants* are drugs of choice.
  • Beneficial even in the absence of clinical depression
  • All agents are effective, but SSRIs are most prescribed due to favorable side effect profile.
  • Fluoxetine (up to 60 mg/day) is only agent that is FDA-approved for bulimia. Reduced number of binge eating and vomiting episodes by about 70%, with complete recovery in 25%.
  • Patients treated for at least 6 months have better long-term outcomes

Obesity—Treatment

♦ Moderate caloric reduction to obtain a weight loss of 5 to 10% body weight over a year: 1,000 to 1,200 kcal/day for women and 1,200 to 1,500 kcal/day for men.
♦ Increased physical activity to facilitate weight loss and prevent weight gain: 30 minutes of moderate-intensity exercise/day
♦ Behavioral modification through nutritional education, cognitive restructuring, and self-monitoring
♦ Pharmacotherapy. See Table 79.7.
  • *Amphetamines* are not routinely used because of their euphoric properties and risks of drug abuse
  • Over-the-counter weight loss products include sympathomimetics, including ephedrine (ma huang). *Phenylpropanolamine* was withdrawn from the market due to increased incidence of stroke in young women
  • *Sibutramine* (Meridia) is a serotonin/norepinephrine reuptake inhibitor, which promotes satiety and decreases appetite. Produced a weight loss of 4.8 to 6.1 kg over 12 months (versus 1.8 mg for placebo). Takes several weeks to have a clinical effect. Common adverse effects include headache, dry mouth, constipation and insomnia, increased BP (1 to 3 mm Hg) and heart rate (4 to 5 beats/minute). Use cautiously in patients with hypertension; not recommended in heart disease. Combined use with other CNS medications that increase levels of norepinephrine and serotonin (e.g., other antidepressants), lithium, antimigraine agents (e.g., sumatriptan, dihydroergotamine), some opioid analgesics (e.g., tramadol, dextromethorphan), and other centrally acting appetite suppressant agents or sympathomimetics are contraindicated. Drugs that inhibit liver enzymes (cytochrome P450 [CYP]3A4), such as ketoconazole and erythromycin, can increase serum concentrations of sibutramine.
  • *Orlistat (Xenical)* reduces dietary fat absorption by inhibiting GI (stomach and pancreas) lipase activity. About 30% of ingested fat are excreted in the feces. Onset is 24–48 hours after dosing. Most effective if combined with low-fat diet; patients lost 9% of body weight in 12 months vs. 5.8% for placebo. Common adverse effects include loose stools, oily spotting, flatus with discharge, fecal urgency, fecal incontinence, bloating, and cramping. Side effects persist for 1 to 4 weeks but occasionally last >6 months. Take multivitamin that includes vitamins K, A, D, and E daily. Dose is 120 g TID during or up to 1 hour after each main meal.

Notes:

Table 79.1 • Body Mass Index (BMI) and Guidelines for Weight Classes

Metric Conversion Formula Using Kilograms and Meters

$$BMI = \frac{Weight\ in\ kilograms}{Height\ in\ meters^2}$$

Nonmetric Conversion Formula Using Pounds and Inches

$$BMI = \frac{Weight\ in\ pounds}{Height\ in\ inches^2} \times 703$$

Weight Status	BMI	Obesity Class
Anorexia nervosa	≤17.5	
Underweight	<18.5	
Normal	18.5–24.9	
Overweight	25.0–29.9	
Obesity	30.0–34.9	I
	35.0–39.9	II
Extreme obesity	≥40	III

Adapted from reference 20.

Table 79.2 • Comparison of Eating Disorders

	Anorexia Nervosa	Bulimia Nervosa	Binge Eating Disorder
Lifetime prevalence	0.5–1% females	1–3% females	Unknown
Prevalence rates			0.7–4% (community) 15–50% (weight control programs)
Female:male	10:1	10:1	1.5:1
Onset	Mid- to late adolescence (14–18 years)	Late adolescence or early adulthood	Late adolescence or early 20s
Dietary restriction	++	+	+
Bingeing	+	+++	++
Purging	++	+++	—

Adapted from references 5, 6, and 113.

Table 79.3 • DSM-IV-TR Diagnostic Criteria for Anorexia Nervosa[6]

A. Refusal to maintain body weight at or above a minimally normal weight for age and height (e.g., weight loss leading to maintenance of body weight <85% of that expected; or failure to make expected weight gain during period of growth, leading to body weight <85% of that expected).
B. Intense fear of gaining weight or becoming fat, even though underweight.
C. Disturbances in the way that one's body weight or shape is experienced, undue influence of body weight or shape on self-evaluation, or denial of the seriousness of the current low body weight.
D. In postmenarchal females, amenorrhea (i.e., the absence of at least three consecutive menstrual cycles). (A woman is considered to have amenorrhea if her periods occur only following hormone [e.g., estrogen] administration.)

Specify Type:
Restricting Type: During the current episode of anorexia nervosa, the person has not regularly engaged in binge eating or purging behavior (i.e., self-induced vomiting or the misuse of laxatives, diuretics, or enemas).
Binge Eating/Purging Type: During the current episode of anorexia nervosa, the person has regularly engaged in binge eating or purging behavior (i.e., self-induced vomiting or the misuse of laxatives, diuretics, or enemas).

Reprinted with permission from the Diagnostic and Statistical Manual of Mental Disorders, Fourth Edition, Text Revision. Copyright 2000 American Psychiatric Association.

Table 79.4 • DSM-IV-TR Diagnostic Criteria for Bulimia Nervosa[6]

A. Recurrent episodes of binge eating. An episode of binge eating is characterized by both of the following:
- (1) eating, in a discrete period of time (e.g., within any 2-hour period), an amount of food that is definitely larger than most people would eat during a similar period of time and under similar circumstances
- (2) a sense of lack of control over eating during the episode (e.g., a feeling that one cannot stop eating or control what or how much one is eating)

B. Recurrent inappropriate compensatory behavior to prevent weight gain, such as self-induced vomiting; misuse of laxatives, diuretics, enemas, or other medications; fasting; or excessive exercise

C. The binge eating and inappropriate compensatory behaviors both occur, on average, at least twice a week for 3 months

D. Self-evaluation is unduly influenced by body shape and weight

E. The disturbance does not occur exclusively during episodes of anorexia nervosa

Specify Type:

Purging Type: During the current episode of bulimia nervosa, the person has regularly engaged in self-induced vomiting or the misuse of laxatives, diuretics, or enemas

Nonpurging Type: During the current episode of bulimia nervosa, the person has used other inappropriate compensatory behaviors, such as fasting or excessive exercise, but has not regularly engaged in self-induced vomiting or the misuse of laxatives, diuretics, or enemas

Notes:

Table 79.5 • Medical Complications of Eating Disorders[a]

Related to Weight Loss and Starvation:

- Cardiac
  Acrocyanosis (circulatory disorder in which hands and feet are cold, blue, and sweaty)
  Arrhythmias (supraventricular premature beats or ventricular tachycardia)
  Bradycardia
  Dizziness or lightheadedness (from dehydration)
  Electrocardiogram changes
    QT_c prolongation
    ST-segment depression
    T-wave inversion
  Left ventricular changes (decreased mass and cavity size)
  Mitral valve prolapse
  Orthostatic hypotension (from dehydration)
  Peripheral edema
  Syncope
  Tachycardia
- Central Nervous System
  Anxiety symptoms
  Brain imaging changes
    Cortical atrophy
    Decreased gray and white matter (MRI)
    Increased ventricular:brain ratio
    Ventricular enlargement
  Cognitive impairment
  Decreased attention and concentration
  Depressed, irritable mood with suicidal thoughts
  Electroencephalogram changes
    Diffuse abnormalities secondary to fluid and electrolyte changes
    Metabolic encephalopathy
  Headache
  Lethargy
  Obsessional thinking about food, weight, metabolism, body image
  Peripheral neuropathy
  Seizures
- Dermatologic
  Alopecia
  Brittle nails
  Dry skin and hair
  Hair thinning
  Lanugo (fine body hair)
  Petechiae
  Yellow skin (hypercarotenemia)
- Endocrine/Metabolic
  Carbohydrate intolerance
  Cold intolerance
  Hyperamylasemia
  Hypercortisolism
  Hypoglycemia
  Hypothermia
  Hypothyroidism
    Serum thyroxine (T_4)—in low-normal range
    Triiodothyronine (T_3)—low
  Impaired temperature regulation
  Lipid abnormalities
  Low basal metabolic rate

- Fluid/Electrolyte/Renal
  Decreased glomerular filtration rate
  Dehydration
  Diuresis
  Hypokalemia
  Hypomagnesemia
  Hyponatremia
  Hypophosphatemia (especially on refeeding)
  Hypozincemia
  Ketonuria
  Peripheral edema
  Polyuria (from decreased renal concentration ability)
  Renal dysfunction (dehydration and hypokalemia)
- Gastrointestinal
  Abdominal pain
  Abnormal bowel sounds
  Abnormal taste sensation (zinc deficiency)
  Bloating (abdominal distension with meals)
  Constipation
  Delayed gastric emptying
  Gastric dilation (rapid refeeding)
  Parotitis
- Genitourinary
  Elevated blood urea nitrogen
  Hypovolemic nephropathy
  Impaired renal function (associated with chronic dehydration and hypokalemia)
  Low glomerular filtration rate
  Pitting edema
  Renal calculi
- Hematologic
  Anemia (normochromic normocytic)
  Hypercholesterolemia
  Leukopenia
  Neutropenia
  Thrombocytopenia
- Hypoalbuminemia
- Increased liver enzymes
- Musculoskeletal
  Bone pain with exercise
  Delayed linear growth
  Fractures (from bone loss)
  Muscle wasting, weakness, and aches
  Myopathy
  Osteopenia or osteoporosis (decreased bone density)
  Short stature (arrested skeletal growth)
  Stress fractures
- Reproductive
  Amenorrhea
  Arrested sexual development
    Atrophy of the breasts
    Delayed puberty
    Ovarian and uterine regression
    Regression in secondary sexual characteristics
  Estrogen deficiency
  Follicle-stimulating hormone (prepubertal levels)

Table 79.5 • Medical Complications of Eating Disorders[a] (continued)

Related to Weight Loss and Starvation (continued):
- Reproductive (continued)
  Hypogonadism (men)
  Infertility
  Luteinizing hormone (prepubertal patterns)
  Loss of libido
  Oligomenorrhea
  Pregnancy (low weight gain and low-birth-weight infant)
  Testosterone deficiency (men)

- Vitamin and Mineral Deficiencies
  Calcium
  Iron
  Zinc

Related to Purging (Vomiting and Laxative Abuse):
- Cardiac
  Cardiomyopathy (from emetine toxicity from ipecac)
  Mild ST changes
- Dental
  Calluses on the dorsum of the hand (from hand-induced vomiting)
  Dental caries (from acidic vomitus)
  Dental enamel erosion (from acidic vomitus)
- Digestive/Gastrointestinal
  Abdominal pain and discomfort
  Barrett esophagus
  Constipation and decreased intestinal motility (from chronic laxative abuse)
  Dehydration
  Delayed gastric emptying and motility
  Diarrhea (from laxative abuse and excessive hydration)
  Esophageal or gastric erosion and rupture (from vomiting)
  Esophagitis
  Gallstones
  Gastric dilation and rupture (from binge eating)

  Hyperamylasemia
  Hypertrophy of salivary and parotid glands
  Mallory-Weiss tears
  Pancreatic inflammation and enlargement (increase in serum amylase)
  Rectal prolapse
- Fluid/Electrolyte
  Hypochloremia
  Hypokalemia
  Hypomagnesemia
  Hyponatremia
  Metabolic acidosis (laxative abuse)
  Metabolic alkalosis (vomiting)
    Elevated serum bicarbonate
    Hypochloremic alkalosis
  Peripheral edema (cessation of laxative and diuretic abuse)
- Neuropsychiatric
  Fatigue and weakness
  Mild cognitive disorder
  Neuropathies
  Seizures (related to large fluid shifts and electrolyte disturbances)

[a]MRI = Magnetic resonance imaging.
Adapted from references 2–4, 6, 10, 11, and 95.

Notes:

Table 79.6 • Pharmacologic Treatment Approaches for Anorexia and Bulimia Nervosa

Severe constipation	Hydration, stool softeners, and bulk-forming laxatives
Decreased gastric motility	Metoclopramide (Reglan)
Amenorrhea	Estrogen and progesterone combination therapy
Bone loss	Calcium 1,500 mg/day Multivitamin Vitamin D 400 IU/day Estrogen therapy (controversial; not always recommended because of negative studies in reversing bone loss) Exercise (nonstrenuous, aerobic, weight bearing)
Electrolyte depletion	Potassium supplements
Anxiety	Benzodiazepine (low dose before meals) Buspirone (BuSpar)

Bulimia nervosa, binge eating, depression, and obsessive-compulsive disorder	Serotonin-augmenting antidepressant:
	    Citalopram (Celexa)
	    Clomipramine (Anafranil)
	    Fluoxetine (Prozac)
	    Fluvoxamine (Luvox)
	    Paroxetine (Paxil)
	    Sertraline (Zoloft)

Stimulation of appetite	Cyproheptadine (Periactin)

Notes:

Table 79.7 • Medications Marketed or Used for the Treatment of Obesity

Generic Name	Trade Name	Dosage	DEA Schedule or Class
Amphetamine/dextroamphetamine	Adderall	5–30 mg/day	II[a]
	Biphetamine	12.5–20 mg/day	II[a]
Benzphetamine hydrochloride	Didrex	25–50 mg one to three times daily	III
Dextroamphetamine			
Immediate release	Dexedrine	5–10 mg before meals	II[a]
Extended release	Dexedrine	10–30 mg AM	II[a]
Diethylpropion hydrochloride			
Immediate release	Tenuate	25 mg TID; 75 mg AM	IV
Controlled release	Tenuate Dospan	75 mg AM	IV
Ephedrine	Various products	20–60 mg/day	Over-the-counter
Fluoxetine	Prozac	20–60 mg AM	Prescription
Mazindol	Sanorex	1 mg TID; 2 mg AM	IV
Methamphetamine hydrochloride			
Immediate release	Desoxyn	2.5–5 mg before meals	II[a]
Extended release	Desoxyn	10–15 mg AM	II[a]
Orlistat	Xenical	120 mg TID	Prescription
Phendimetrazine tartrate	Bontril, Plegine, Prelu-2, X-Trozine	35 mg TID; 105 mg AM	III
Phenmetrazine	Preludin	25 mg BID–TID	II[a]
Phenylpropanolamine	Dexatrim, Acutrim	25 mg TID; 75 mg AM	Over-the-counter
Phentermine			
Hydrochloride	Adipex-P, Fastin, Oby-Cap, Phentride	8 mg TID; 30–37.5 mg AM	IV
Resin	Ionamin	15–30 mg AM	IV
Sibutramine	Meridia	5–15 mg/day	IV

[a]High abuse potential, not recommended for routine or long-term use.
Adapted from references 11 and 54.

The reader is referred to Chapter 81: Eating Disorders, written by *Martha P. Fankhauser, Pharm.D.*, in the seventh edition of **Applied Therapeutics: The Clinical Use of Drugs** for a more in-depth discussion of the pathophysiology, clinical presentation, and treatment of eating disorders. All notations to reference numbers are based on the reference list at the end of that chapter. The editors of this handbook express their thanks to Dr. Fankhauser and acknowledge that this chapter is based upon her work.

Notes:

Notes:

Chapter 80

Psychoactive Substance Abuse Disorders

Definition of terms as recommended by the American Society of Addiction Medicine

♦ *Abstinence:* Nonuse of a specific substance. In recovery, nonuse of any addictive psychoactive substance. May also denote cessation of addictive behavior (e.g., gambling, overeating).

♦ *Abuse:* Harmful use of a specific psychoactive substance. The term also applies to one category of psychoactive substance use disorder. Although recognizing that "abuse" is part of present diagnostic terminology, ASAM recommends that an alternative term be found for this purpose because of the pejorative connotations of the word "abuse."

♦ *Addiction:* A disease process characterized by the continued use of a specific psychoactive substance despite physical, psychologic, or social harm.

♦ *Addictionist:* A physician who specializes in addiction medicine.

♦ *Blackout:* Acute antegrade amnesia with no formation of long-term memory, resulting from the ingestion of alcohol or other drugs (i.e., a period of memory loss for which there is no recall of activities).

♦ *Chemical dependency:* A generic term relating to psychologic or physical dependency, or both, on one or more psychoactive substances.

♦ *Dependence:* Used in three different ways: (1) physical dependence, a physiologic state of adaptation to a specific psychoactive substance, characterized by the emergence of a withdrawal syndrome during abstinence, which may be relieved in total or in part by readministration of the substance, (2) psychologic dependence, a subjective sense of need for a specific psychoactive substance, either for its positive effects or to avoid negative effects associated with its absence; and (3) one category of psychoactive substance use disorder.

♦ *Detoxification:* A process of withdrawing a person from a specific psychoactive substance in a safe and effective manner.

♦ *Enabling:* Any action by another person or an institution that intentionally or unintentionally has the effect of facilitating the continuation of an individual's addictive process.

♦ *Impairment:* A dysfunctional state resulting from use of psychoactive substances.

♦ *Intervention:* A planned intervention with an individual who may be dependent on one or more psychoactive substances, with the aim of making a full assessment, overcoming denial, interrupting drug-taking behavior, or inducing the individual to initiate treatment. The preferred technique is to present facts regarding psychoactive substance use in a caring, believable, and understandable manner.

♦ *Loss of control:* The inability to consistently limit the self-administration of psychoactive substances.

♦ *Misuse:* Any use of a prescription drug that varies from accepted medical practice.

♦ *Problem drinking:* An informal term describing a pattern of drinking associated with life problems before establishing a definitive diagnosis of alcoholism. Also, an umbrella term for any harmful use of alcohol, including alcoholism. ASAM recommends that the term not be used in the latter sense.

♦ *Recovery:* A process of overcoming both physical and psychologic dependence on a psychoactive substance, with a commitment to sobriety.

♦ *Relapse:* Recurrence of psychoactive substance–dependent behavior in an individual who has previously achieved and maintained abstinence for a significant period beyond withdrawal.

♦ *Sobriety:* A state of complete abstinence from psychoactive substances by an addicted individual, in conjunction with a satisfactory quality of life.

♦ *Tolerance:* State in which an increased dosage of a pychoactive substance is needed to produce a desired effect.

♦ *Withdrawal syndrome:* The onset of a predictable constellation of signs and symptoms after the abrupt discontinuation of, or rapid decrease in, dosage of a psychoactive substance.

Diagnostic Classification

♦ Psychoactive substance–use disorders define the specific patterns of behavior related to drug use. These are divided into psychoactive substance *abuse* and psychoactive substance *dependence.*

♦ Diagnostic criteria for *psychoactive substance abuse* is most applicable to people who only recently have started taking psychoactive substances and who are using substances least likely to cause marked physiologic signs of withdrawal (e.g., cannabis cocaine hallucinogens). See Table 80.1.

♦ Diagnostic criteria for *psychoactive substance dependence* are the same for each of the individual psychoactive drugs or drug classes. See Table 80.2.

♦ *Polysubstance dependence* exists when there is repeated use of at least three categories of substances (except nicotine and caffeine), but no single agent predominates.

♦ A category for *"other " (or unknown) substance-related disorders* is used to classify disorders associated with use of substances without their own *Diagnostic and Statistical Manual of Mental Disorders,* fourth edition (DSM-IV) category. Examples include anabolic steroids, nitrate inhalants, nitrous oxide, OTC medications, and antihistamines.

♦ *Dual Diagnosis* is used to describe patients who have comorbid diagnoses for a psychiatric disorder and a psychoactive substance use disorder, but it is an imprecise term that is used in other contexts. Other psychiatric diagnoses coexist in about 50% of substance abusers and about 50 to 75% of patients with a primary psychiatric diagnosis have a coexisting substance abuse diagnosis.

Diagnosis

♦ Alcohol and substance abuse is often unrecognized

♦ Patterns of behavior commonly observed across addictions:
  • Mood swings
  • Changes in social behaviors and contacts, often with increasing isolation
  • Family and financial problems
  • Dishonesty
  • Neglect of physical appearance and diet
  • Uncharacteristic deterioration of health

- Traumatic injuries
- Memory lapses
- Poor job performance or behavior

♦ Denial is a major impediment in diagnosis. Alcoholics or other drug addicts often truly believe they do not have a problem (delusional). Formal confrontation by family and friends may be needed to convince patients that they need treatment

♦ Diagnosis of "dual diagnosis" may require several weeks to assess the patient's baseline because symptoms of substance intoxication and withdrawal may resemble mania or depression.

Treatment

♦ Treatment that focuses only on the symptoms of addictive disease has little or no impact on the progression of the disease. Current approaches safely withdraw patients from the substance, treat continuing symptoms, and provide continual recovery through education in the disease process and involvement with long-term, self-help groups.

♦ *Acute Intervention* treatment goals (inpatient):
  - Abstinence is the initial and primary goal
  - Detoxification
  - Medical evaluation
  - Stabilization of life-threatening emotional issues
  - Education
  - Identification of barriers to recovery
  - Readjustment of behavior toward recovery
  - Orientation and membership in a self-help or mutual help 12-step program. See Table 80.3. The basic principles of recovery are available at the Alcoholics Anonymous website: http://www.alcoholics-anonymous.org.
  - Family members also may need treatment to address their physical, emotional, and spiritual distress

♦ *Continuing care* maintains the link between the patient and the professional recovery community after discharge

♦ *Extended care* allows for structured support of sobriety

♦ *Multidisciplinary, integrated* treatment approaches are needed for people with dual diagnosis, who have a higher rate of relapse

Populations at Risk for Chemical Dependency

Fetuses and neonates born to mothers who abuse alcohol, nicotine, marijuana, amphetamines, cocaine, opiates, and other substances.

Adolescents. Alcohol is the drug of choice (75%), then marijuana (29 to 42%), cocaine (4 to 6%), LSD (5 to 8%), and heroin (0.4 to 1.2%)

Women with a history of depression, abuse of tranquilizers, physical and sexual abuse and whose spouse is chemically dependent.

Elderly, especially medical and psychiatric inpatients, are prone to alcoholism (44%).

Gay and lesbian populations (30%)

Health Care Professionals. Incidence similar to population, but drug of choice and route of administration vary among professions: nurses and doctors more likely to use injections than pharmacists, who abuse multiple oral drugs and stimulants. Drug of choice for dentists is nitrous oxide; fentanyl or its analogs is used by anesthesiologists and nurse anesthetists

Table 80.1 • Diagnostic Criteria for Psychoactive Substance Abuse[a]

A) A maladaptive pattern of psychoactive substance use leading to clinically significant impairment or distress, as manifested by one or more of the following, occurring within a 12-month period:
  1) Recurrent substance use resulting in a failure to fulfill major role obligations at work, school, or home (e.g., repeated absences or poor work performance related to substance used; substance-related absences, suspensions, or expulsions from school; neglect of children or household)
  2) Recurrent substance use in situations in which it is physically hazardous (e.g., driving an automobile or operating a machine when one is impaired by substance use)
  3) Recurrent substance-related legal problems (e.g., arrests for substance-related disorderly conduct)
  4) Continued substance use despite having persistent or recurrent social or interpersonal problems caused by or exacerbated by the effects of the substance (e.g., arguments with spouse about consequences of intoxication, physical fights)
B) The symptoms have never met the criteria for psychoactive Substance Dependence for this class of substance

[a]Reprinted with permission from American Psychiatric Association. Diagnostic and Statistical Manual of Mental Disorders. 4th ed. Washington, DC: American Psychiatric Association; 1994.

Table 80.2 • Diagnostic Criteria for Psychoactive Substance Dependence[a]

A maladaptive pattern of substance use, leading to clinically significant impairment or distress, as manifested by three (or more) of the following, occurring at any time in the same 12-month period:

1) Tolerance, as defined by either of the following:
   a) A need for markedly increased amounts of the substance to achieve intoxication or desired effect
   b) Markedly diminished effect with continued use of the same amount of the substance

2) Withdrawal, as manifested by either of the following:
   a) The characteristic withdrawal syndrome for the substance
   b) The same (or closely related) substance is taken to relieve or avoid withdrawal symptoms

3) The substance is often taken in larger amounts or over a longer period than was intended

4) There is persistent desire or unsuccessful efforts to cut down or control substance use

5) A great deal of time is spent in activities to obtain the substance (e.g., visiting multiple doctors or driving long distances), use the substance (e.g., chain smoking), or recover from its effects

6) Important social, occupational, or recreational activities are given up or reduced because of substance use

7) The substance use is continued despite knowledge of having a persistent or recurrent physical or psychological problem that is likely to have been caused or exacerbated by the substance (e.g., current cocaine use despite recognition of cocaine-induced depression or continued drinking despite recognition that an ulcer was made worse by alcohol consumption)

[a]Reprinted with permission from American Psychiatric Association. Diagnostic and Statistical Manual of Mental Disorders. 4th ed. Washington, DC: American Psychiatric Association; 1994.

Notes:

Table 80.3 • Twelve-Step Group Directory

Adult Children of Alcoholics
ACA WSO
P.O. Box 3216
Torrance, CA 90510
(310) 534-1815
http://www.adultchildren.org

Al-Anon (or Alateen)
Al-Anon Family Group Headquarters, Inc.
1600 Corporate Landing Parkway
Virginia Beach, VA 23454-5617
(757) 563-1600
http://www.Al-Anon-Alateen.org

Alcoholics Anonymous
A.A. World Services, Inc.
P.O. Box 459
New York, NY 10163
(212) 870-3400
http://www.alcoholics-anonymous.org

Cocaine Anonymous
CAWSO, Inc.
P.O. Box 2000
Los Angeles, CA 90049-8000
(310) 559-5833
800-347-8998
http://www.ca.org

Co-Dependents Anonymous, Inc. (CoDA)
P.O. Box 33577
Phoenix, AZ 85067-3577
(602) 277-7991
http://www.codependents.org

Drugs Anonymous
P.O. Box 473
Ansonia Station
New York, NY 10023
(212) 484-9095

International Doctors in Alcoholics Anonymous
C. Richard McKinley, M.D., Listkeeper
P.O. Box 199
Augusta, MO 63332
(314) 482-4548
http://www.members.aol.com/aadocs/

International Nurses Anonymous
Pat Green, R.N., M.S.W., Listkeeper
1020 Sunset Drive
Lawrence, KS 66044
(913) 842-3893

International Pharmacists Anonymous
IPA Listkeeper
11 Dewey Lane
Glen Gardner, NJ 08826-3102
(908) 537-4295
http://members.home.com/mitchfields/ipa/ipapage.htm

Marijuana Anonymous World Services
P.O. Box 2912
Van Nuys, CA 91404
(800) 766-6779
http://www.marijuana-anonymous.org

Nar-Anon World Service Office
P.O. Box 2562
Palos Verdes Peninsula, CA 90274
(310) 547-5800

Narcotics Anonymous
P.O. Box 9999
Van Nuys, CA 91409
(818) 773-9999
http://www.na.org

Pill Addicts Anonymous
P.O. Box 278
Reading, PA 19603
(215) 372-1128

The reader is referred to Chapter 82: Psychoactive Substance Use Disorders, written by *Jeffrey N. Baldwin, Pharm.D.*, and *Teri L. Gabel, Pharm.D.*, in the seventh edition of **Applied Therapeutics: The Clinical Use of Drugs** for a more in-depth discussion of patient assessment and treatment, populations at risk, drugs in the workplace, and drug testing. The editors of this handbook express their thanks to Drs. Baldwin and Gabel and acknowledge that this chapter is based upon their work.

Notes:

Chapter 81

Alcohol Abuse

Alcohol Content and Definitions

♦ *"Proof"* is a term used to describe the alcohol content of distilled beverages and is twice the percent of ethanol by volume (e.g., 80 proof = 40% ethanol).

♦ *Ethanol content* varies widely among beverages. See Table 81.1

♦ *Denatured alcohol* is ethanol rendered unsuitable for human consumption by addition of toxic contaminants and is identified as SD alcohol or SDA (special denatured alcohol). Examples include rubbing alcohols, colognes, and aftershave lotions.

♦ *Drunkenness* in most of the United States is a blood alcohol concentration of 0.1% or 100 mg/dL (2.7 mmol/L). Some states have lowered the legal limit to 0.08% or 80 mg/dL

Pharmacokinetics

♦ *Absorption* from the stomach, intestine, and colon is complete, but the rate is variable. Peak concentrations under fasting conditions are reached in 30 to 75 minutes. Alcohol is most rapidly absorbed from carbonated drinks containing 10 to 30% ethanol (e.g., champagne). Food and other factors that slow gastric emptying slow ethanol absorption because it is most rapidly absorbed from the small intestine.

♦ *Volume of distribution* is 0.65 L/kg on average (0.58–0.70 L/kg).

♦ *Metabolism*

• Primarily (90–96%) oxidized in the liver via the alcohol dehydrogenase pathway, resulting in a reduction of NAD+ to NADH. Some first-pass metabolism occurs by gastric alcohol dehydrogenase. In chronic alcoholics, all metabolic reactions that convert NADH back to NAD+ are favored (e.g., pyruvate is reduced to lactate).

• When large amounts of alcohol (>200 mg/dL) deplete NAD+, the alcohol dehydrogenase system becomes saturated and metabolism tends to become nonlinear. Cytochrome P-4502E is stimulated, which produces metabolic tolerance to ethanol in chronic users.

• The average rate of oxidation varies widely but is reported as 15 mg/dL/hr for men and 18 mg/dL/hr for women. Chronic heavy drinkers oxidize ethanol at twice this rate. Patients with end-state liver disease may have no metabolic capacity

Acute Intoxication

♦ *Symptoms:* Blood alcohol concentrations generally correlate with the clinical presentation. See Table 81.2. Symptoms include acute central nervous system depression through all stages of anesthesia, respiratory depression (primary cause of death), respiratory acidosis, and vomiting with aspiration. Other symptoms, their causes and management are described in Table 81.3.

Alcohol Withdrawal

♦ *Symptoms.* See Table 81.4.

♦ *Diagnosis.* Patients must have at least two of the following symptoms after reduction or cessation of prolonged or heavy alcohol ingestion:

- Autonomic hyperactivity
- Increased hand tremor
- Insomnia
- Nausea or vomiting
- Transient visual, tactile, or auditory hallucinations or illusions
- Psychomotor agitation
- Anxiety
- Grand mal seizures

♦ Therapy

- Supportive care: fluids, electrolytes, thiamine
- Benzodiazepines are drugs of choice to manage symptoms and to prevent agitation and seizures. Most can be managed with oral therapy, but parenteral therapy may be required for acutely agitated patients (e.g., diazepam 10 mg IV repeated every 5 minutes until calm). See Table 81.5.

Chronic Alcoholism

♦ *Diagnosis.* Must fulfill three of seven criteria for psychoactive substance dependence. See Chapter 80, Table 80.3.

♦ *Treatment*

- After treatment for withdrawal, refer to a treatment program. See Chapter 80, Table 80.3.
- *Disulfiram*

    —Aversion therapy will most benefit those who want to remain abstinent but have had periodic binge relapses.

    —Blocks aldehyde dehydrogenase, resulting in a 5- to 10-fold increase in acetaldehyde concentrations within 15 minutes

    —Disulfiram-ethanol reaction: flushing, tachycardia, dyspnea, palpitations, headache, nausea, vomiting, thirst, diaphoresis, chest pain, postural hypotension.

    —Typical dose: 500 mg/day for 2 weeks; then 250 mg/day after at least 12 hours of abstinence. After discontinuation, the disulfiram reaction can persist for 14 days.

Medical Complications of Chronic Alcoholism. See Table 81.6

Notes:

Table 81.1 • Alcohol Content

Product	Ethanol Content (%)
Light beer	2%–4%
Beer	4%–6%
Ales and special beers	≤12%
Wines	10%–20%
Distilled spirits (whiskey, rum, cognac)	35%–55% (some as high as 95%)
Colognes, aftershave	70%–90%

Table 81.2 • Blood Alcohol Relationship to Clinical Status

Blood Ethanol Concentration	Clinical Presentation[a]
50 mg/dL (0.05 mg%)	Motor function impairment observable
80 mg/dL (0.08 mg%)	Moderate impairment[b]
100 mg/dL (0.1 mg%)	Legal definition of intoxication[b]
450 mg/dL	Respiratory depression
500 mg/dL	LD_{50} for ethanol

[a] Tolerance to alcohol varies among individuals.
[b] Some states define legal intoxication as 80 mg/dL (0.08 mg%).

Table 81.3 • Acute Alcohol Intoxication: Symptoms and Treatment

Symptom	Cause	Treatment
Respiratory Acidosis	Alcohol-induced respiratory depression; blunted response to hypercapnia and hypoxia	Endotracheal intubation for respiratory support
Coma	Alcohol-induced CNS depression; ingestion of other drugs	Gastric lavage, naloxone (Narcan) 1 mg; repeat every 2 to 3 minutes up to 10 doses, depending on response and suspicion of ingestion. Dialysis possible
Hypotension	Hypovolemia	IV fluid replacement
Hypoglycemia	Most often occurs in malnourished patients. Pyruvate is converted to lactate, rather than glucose, through gluconeogenesis.	50 mL 50% glucose by IV push

Notes:

Table 81.4 • Stages of Ethanol Withdrawal

Stage	Onset After ↓ in Ethanol Blood Level	Clinical Features
I	≈6–8 hr	Moderate autonomic hyperactivity (anxiety, tremulousness, tachycardia, insomnia, nausea, vomiting, diaphoresis) and a craving for alcohol
II	≈24 hr	Autonomic hyperactivity with auditory and visual hallucinations lasting for 1–3 days. Most remain lucid and oriented
III	≈1–2 days	About 4% of untreated patients develop grand mal seizures about 7–48 hr after ↓ in blood alcohol concentration
IV	3–5 days	Delirium tremens (DTs) in ≈5% patients (confusion, illusions, hallucinations, agitation, tachycardia, hyperthermia). Mortality as high as 25% attributed to arrhythmias, shock, infection, trauma, or aspiration

Table 81.5 • Summary of the Oral Dosing Considerations for Benzodiazepines in the Management of Acute Alcohol Withdrawal[92]

Drug	Dose: Day 1	Dose: Taper
Diazepam[93]	20 mg, then 20 mg Q 2 hr until calm	Day 2: 10 mg, 5 mg, 10 mg Day 3: 5 mg TID Day 4: 5 mg BID
Chlordiazepoxide[94]	50–100 mg Q 6–8 hr until calm	Day 2: 50–100 mg Q 8 hr Day 3: 50–100 mg Q 12 hr Day 4: 50–100 mg HS
Lorazepam[95,96]	2 mg Q 6–8 hr until calm	Day 2: 2 mg Q 8 hr Day 3: 1 mg Q 8 hr Day 4: 1 mg Q 12 hr

Notes:

Table 81.6 • Medical Complications of Chronic Alcoholism: Presentation and Treatment

Complication	Presentation	Treatment
Liver Disease • Progressive: fatty liver, steatosis, hepatitis, then cirrhosis. • Hepatitis occurs in all who drink 20–40 g daily.	Varies from asymptomatic to fulminant. Anorexia, weight loss, abdominal pain, chills, fevers, vomiting, jaundice, GI bleeding, elevated AST and ALT, cholestatic changes, low albumin, high prothrombin time. Also see Chapter 27.	Abstinence to prevent progression. Supportive care: bed rest, hydration, nutrition
Hematologic Complications • Megaloblastic anemia due to folate deficiency • Sideroblastic anemia and hemosiderosis due to deranged iron metabolism • Iron deficiency anemia due to poor diet and GI blood loss • Thrombocytopenia due to interference with platelet function and formation	See Chapter 83.	Oral multiple vitamins, folic acid, iron sulfate (326 mg/day)
Gastrointestinal Effects • Diarrhea • Acute hemorrhagic, chronic and atrophic gastritis, may be due to *H. pylori* • Gastroesophageal reflux disease (GERD)	Acute abdominal pain, nausea, esophageal reflux, vomiting	Gastritis typically resolves a few days after discontinuing alcohol. Antacids and H2-receptor antagonists may provide pain relief and speed healing
Pancreatitis • Heavy alcohol consumption is second most common cause (35% of cases) • Typically occurs after binge drinking	Severe abdominal pain radiating from the upper abdomen through to the back and flanks, nausea, vomiting, elevated lipase to amylase levels.	Supportive care: NPO, parenteral analgesia, hydration and nutrition.
Wernicke-Korsakoff Syndrome • A neurologic disorder caused by thiamine deficiency • Wernicke's encephalopathy can be precipitated by large glucose load • Korsakoff's psychosis develops in 80% who survive but fail to recover in 48–72 hours • A medical emergency	• Wernicke's: CNS depression (mental sluggishness, restlessness, confusion, coma), ambulatory problems (wide-based, ataxic gait), ocular problems, hypothermia, hypotension, polyneuropathy • Korsakoff's: retrograde amnesia, anterograde amnesia, confabulation	Thiamine 100 mg by slow IV push before or concurrently with dextrose-containing fluids, then oral thiamine 50 to 100 mg/day.

(continued)

Table 81.6 • Medical Complications of Chronic Alcoholism: Presentation and Treatment (continued)

Complication	Presentation	Treatment
Cardiovascular Effects • Alcoholic cardiomyopathy after 10+ years of excessive alcohol leads to decreased contractile function • Hypertension associated with >3 standard drinks/day • Arrhythmias can occur after heavy alcohol consumption	Cardiomyopathy occurs between 30–60 years of age as low output failure	See appropriate cardiovascular chapters.
Endocrine Effects Hypogonadism due to reduced synthesis and increased metabolism of testosterone.	• Women: amenorrhea, anovulation, hyperprolactinemia leading to infertility, spontaneous abortion, and impaired fetal growth and development • Men: loss of facial hair, gynecomastia, decreased muscle and bone mass, testicular atrophy, decreased libido, and sexual impotence	No treatment except discontinuation of alcohol
Myopathy A syndrome of muscle necrosis perhaps caused by direct toxicity of alcohol on muscle tissue	Ranges from asymptomatic to weakness, pain and swelling of muscles to frank rhabdomyolysis. Myoglobinuria and elevated MM fraction of creatine kinase	Correct electrolyte abnormalities, maintain urine output, and use sodium bicarbonate to alkalinize the urine if myoglobin is present to prevent precipitation

The reader is referred to Chapter 83: Alcohol Abuse, written by *Paul W. Jungnickel, Pharm.D.*, in the seventh edition of **Applied Therapeutics: The Clinical Use of Drugs** for a more in-depth discussion of diagnosis and medical management of conditions related to alcohol abuse. All notations to reference numbers are based on the reference list at the end of that chapter. The editors of this handbook express their thanks to Dr. Jungnickel and acknowledge that this chapter is based upon his work.

Notes:

Notes:

Chapter 82

Anemias

ANEMIA

- **Definition.** A decrease in the number of red blood cells (RBCs)/mm^3 or hemoglobin concentration in blood. Associated with nutritional deficiencies and acute and chronic diseases; it also may be drug induced. Diagnostic terminology for anemia requires inclusion of the RBC morphology and pathogenesis (e.g., megaloblastic anemia secondary to folate deficiency). See Table 82.1.
- **Pathophysiology**
  - Caused by decreased RBC production, increased RBC loss (e.g., bleeding), or increased RBC destruction (e.g., hemolysis).
  - Normally, RBC mass is maintained by a feedback mechanism (e.g., hypoxia) that regulates levels of erythropoietin, a hormone that stimulates proliferation and differentiation of erythroid precursors in bone marrow. The kidney produces 90% of erythropoietin.
- **Signs and Symptoms**
  - Related to tissue hypoxia: pallor (skin, mucous membranes, nailbeds, conjunctivae); exertional dyspnea; increased angina, fatigue, or malaise; tachycardia.
  - Can be asymptomatic or mild if anemia develops gradually.
  - Some symptoms are specific to the etiology (e.g., neurological symptoms related to vitamin B_{12} deficiency).
- **Diagnosis**
  - Physical examination, including history and signs and symptoms
  - Laboratory evaluation is critical
    - —Morphologic appearance of the RBC provides useful information about the nature of the anemia. Microscopic evaluation of the peripheral blood smear can detect the presence of large (macrocytic), small (microcytic), or normal-size (normocytic) RBCs.
    - —*Routine Laboratory Evaluation for Anemia Workup.* See Table 82.2.
    - —*Normal Hematology Values.* See Table 82.3.
    - —*Laboratory Diagnosis of Anemia.* See Figure 82.1.

IRON DEFICIENCY (MICROCYTIC) ANEMIA

- A state of negative iron balance in which the daily iron intake and stores cannot meet the RBC and other body tissue needs. The body contains 3.5 g of iron; 2.5 g is in Hgb.
- Iron metabolism, pathophysiology, symptoms, treatment. See Table 82.4.
- **Iron Products**
  - *Iron Content of Liquid Iron Preparations.* See Table 82.5.
  - *Comparisons of Iron Preparations.* See Table 82.6.
  - *Combination Iron Products.* See Table 82.7.

- Dispense in childproof container and store away from children; accidental ingestion of only 3 to 4 tablets can cause serious toxicity in small children.
- Parenteral iron therapy
  —Indications: Failure to respond to oral iron therapy due to noncompliance or malabsorption; intolerance to oral therapy; significant blood loss in patients refusing transfusion.
  —Iron-dextran is FDA approved for IM injection at a maximum dose of 100 mg/day in the gluteus muscle using a Z-track technique to avoid skin staining. Although not approved for IV administration, infusions of "total doses" over 2 to 6 hours (no >50 mg/minute) are used in clinical practice.
  —The total dose of iron dextran can be determined using the following equation.

$$\text{Iron (mg)} = [\text{Weight (pounds)} \times 0.3]\left[100 - \frac{100(\text{Hgb})}{14.8}\right]$$

MEGALOBLASTIC ANEMIA

♦ **Causes.** Deficiencies of folic acid or vitamin B_{12} or by metabolic or inherited defects resulting in the inability to use these vitamins.
♦ **Morphology and Labs:** Large, oval, well-hemoglobinized RBCs; low reticulocyte count; thrombocytopenia with large platelets; leukopenia; hyperbilirubinemia.
♦ *Vitamin B_{12} Deficiency Anemia*
  - Vitamin B_{12} is essential for hematopoiesis, maintenance of myelin, and production of epithelial cells.
  - Humans cannot synthesize B_{12} and must obtain it primarily through ingestion of animal proteins.
  - A typical Western diet contains 5 to 15 µg/day, an amount sufficient to replace the 1 µg/day lost.
  - Total body stores are 2000–5000 µg; thus 3 to 4 years elapse before deficiency develops.
  - Intrinsic factor in the stomach is essential for absorption. Pernicious anemia develops from lack of intrinsic factor production. Normal levels of intrinsic factor permit oral B_{12} therapy.
  - Serum B_{12} concentration reliably reflects B_{12} tissue stores. Shilling test evaluates B_{12} absorption from the GI track.
  - Clinical presentation, treatment, and monitoring. See Table 82.8.
♦ *Folic Acid Deficiency*
  - The minimum adult requirement of folate is 50 µg/day, but an intake of 200 µg/day is recommended because absorption from food sources is incomplete.
  - Estimates of folate requirements based on age and growth needs:
    —Children 3.3 µg/kg/day
    —Infants 16 µg/day
    —Pregnancy 100 µg/day plus 3 µg/kg/day
    —Lactating women 300 µg/day
  - Folate stores are small (5 to 10 mg); thus, deficiency and anemia may occur within 3 to 4 months of decreased folate intake.
  - Folate deficiency absolutely must be differentiated from vitamin B_{12} deficiency before folate therapy is initiated because folate can reverse the hematological, but not the neurological, damage caused by B_{12} deficiency.
  - Clinical presentation, treatment, and monitoring. See Table 82.8

SICKLE CELL ANEMIA

♦ An inherited hemoglobin disorder characterized by a more negatively charged hemoglobin A that favors hemoglobin aggregation and polymerization resulting in sickle-shaped RBCs. Sickled RBCs are more rigid and may become lodged when passing through microvasculature, resulting in vascular occlusions.

♦ There are several inheritance patterns. Patients with sickle cell anemia are homozygous, whereas patients with sickle cell trait are heterozygous.

♦ **Clinical course** is variable and difficult to predict. Kidneys, retina, spleen, and bones are frequent sites of vaso-occlusive events. Pain anemia infections and cardiac, pulmonary, neurological, hepatobiliary, obstetrical, gynecological, ocular, dermatological, and orthopedic complications occur.

♦ **Management** is organ specific and aimed at supportive measures.

- *Hemolytic anemia* is caused by splenic sequestration of abnormal RBCs, reducing the life span from 120 to 15 to 25 days. It is usually self limiting. Treat with blood transfusions or splenectomy.

- *Infections* (e.g., pneumonia, osteomyelitis) are more common. Hypoxia from pneumonia can cause progression to vaso-occlusion, acute chest syndrome, and right heart failure. Prophylactic treatment with penicillin and pneumococcal vaccine, as well as early treatment of infections, is essential.

- *Vascular occlusion episodes* ("sickle cell crises") cause severe pain and organ damage. Pain typically lasts 2 to 6 days and should be managed with narcotic analgesics. Hydroxyurea (15 to 35 mg/kg/day) has been used to increase hemoglobin F synthesis, which may reduce the frequency of crises. Many toxicities, including bone marrow suppression, GI effects, rash, and secondary neoplasms.

- *Neurologic complications* include strokes in the first decade of life and cerebral hemorrhage in adulthood. Maintain hemoglobin S level below 30%.

- *Renal and genital complications* include reduced potassium excretion, hyperuricemia, hematuria, renal failure with decreased erythropoietin production, and priapism. Manage with IV fluids, pain control, transfusions, and surgery.

ANEMIA OF CHRONIC DISEASE

♦ **Definition.** Mild-to-moderate anemia that accompanies diseases that last >1 to 2 months, including:

- Chronic infections (e.g., endocarditis, osteomyelitis, UTIs, TB, HIV)
- Chronic inflammatory conditions (e.g., SLE, rheumatoid arthritis)
- Malignancies and chemotherapy
- Renal insufficiency

♦ **Pathogenesis**

- Impaired iron release from reticuloendothelial stores
- Decreased erythrocyte life span
- Inadequate bone marrow response to decreased erythrocyte life span
- Decreased erythropoietin is rarely important, except in the case of renal failure

♦ **Symptoms and Clinical Course**

- Symptoms are nonspecific and vary greatly with underlying disease
- Usually not progressive or life-threatening but can affect quality of life

♦ **Treatment**

- Blood transfusions for symptomatic anemia
- Vitamins are of no value unless a concurrent deficiency exists

- *Human recombinant erythropoietin (rhEPO)* may be indicated for anemia associated with end-stage renal disease, AIDS, cancer, and drug-induced anemia (chemotherapy and zidovudine therapy); in patients with low endogenous EPO levels; and with autologous blood transfusions for elective surgery.
  —Response is dose dependent and variable; often depends on underlying cause of anemia
  —Dose in cancer patients often higher than renal failure patients
  —Patients who have received intensive chemotherapy or radiotherapy are less responsive
  —Lack of response is most commonly associated with iron deficiency
  —Current therapeutic uses. See Table 82.9

Table 82.1 • Classifications of Anemia[a]

Pathophysiologic (Classifies Anemias Based on Pathophysiologic Presentation)

Blood Loss
Acute: Trauma, ulcer, hemorrhoids
Chronic: Ulcer, vaginal bleeding, aspirin ingestion

Inadequate Red Blood Cell Production
Nutritional deficiency: B_{12}, folic acid, iron
Erythroblast deficiency: Bone marrow failure (aplastic anemia, irradiation, chemotherapy, folic acid antagonists) or bone marrow infiltration (leukemia, lymphoma, myeloma, metastatic solid tumors, myelofibrosis)
Endocrine deficiency: Pituitary, adrenal, thyroid, testicular
Chronic disease: Renal, liver, infection, granulomatous, collagen vascular

Excessive Red Blood Cell Destruction
Intrinsic factors: Hereditary (G6PD), abnormal hemoglobin synthesis
Extrinsic factors: Autoimmune reactions, drug reactions, infection (endotoxin)

Morphologic (Classifies Anemias by Red Blood Cell Size [Microcytic, Normocytic, Macrocytic] and Hemoglobin Content [Hypochromic, Normochromic, Hyperchromic])

Macrocytic
Defective maturation with decreased production
Megaloblastic: Pernicious (B_{12} deficiency), folic acid deficiency

Normochromic, normocytic
Recent blood loss
Hemolysis
Chronic disease
Renal failure
Autoimmune
Endocrine

Microcytic, hyperchromic
Iron deficiency
Genetic abnormalities: Sickle cell, thalassemia

[a]G6PD = Glucose-6-phosphate dehydrogenase.

Notes:

Table 82.2 • Routine Laboratory Evaluation for Anemia Workup[a]

Complete blood count (CBC): Hgb, Hct, RBC count, red cell indices (MCV, MCH, MCHC),
    WBC count (and differential)
Platelet count
Red cell morphology
Reticulocyte count
Bilirubin and LDH
Serum iron, TIBC, serum ferritin, transferrin saturation
Peripheral blood smear examination
Stool examination for occult blood
Bone marrow aspiration and biopsy[b]

[a]Hct = Hematocrit; Hgb = Hemoglobin; LDH = Lactic dehydrogenase; MCV = Mean corpuscular volume;
MCH = Mean corpuscular hemoglobin; MCHC = Mean corpuscular hemoglobin concentration; RBC = Red blood cell;
TIBC = Total iron-binding capacity; WBC = White blood cell.
[b]Performed in patients with abnormal peripheral blood smears.

Table 82.3 • Normal Hematology Values[a]

Laboratory Test	Pediatric			Adult	
	1 wk	6 mo	1–15 yr	Male	Female
RBC (mm³)	5.3 ± 7	4.5 ± 6	4.7 ± 6	5.4 ± 0.7	4.8 ± 6
Hgb (g/dL)	18 ± 4	12.5 ± 1.5	13 ± 2	16 ± 2	14 ± 2
Hct (%)	53 ± 9	37 ± 4	40 ± 5	47 ± 5	42 ± 2
MCV (mm³)	101 ± 5	78 ± 5	80 ± 5	87 ± 7	90 ± 9
MCH (pg/cell)	37 ± 2	34 ± 2	33.5 ± 2	29 ± 2	34 ± 2
MCHC (g/dL)	33–37	31–36	31–36	31–36	31–36
Erythropoietin (mU/mL)	6–7	10–13	4–26	4–26	4–26
Reticulocyte count (%)	0.5–1.5	0.5–1.5	0.5–1.5	0.5–1.5	0.5–1.5
TIBC (mg/dL)	100–400	250–400	250–400	250–400	250–400
Fe (mg/dL)	100–250	100–400	50–120	50–160	40–150
Folate (ng/mL)	7–25	7–25	7–25	7–25	7–25
RBC Folate (ng/mL)	None found			140–960	140–960
Fe/TIBC (%)	62.5–100		20–30	20–40	16–38
Vitamin B$_{12}$ (pg/mL)	>200	>200	>200	>200	>200
Ferritin (ng/mL)	25–200	50–200	7–140	15–200	12–150

[a]Fe = Iron; Hgb = Hemoglobin; Hct = Hematocrit; MCH = Mean corpuscular hemoglobin; MCV = Mean corpuscular
volume; RBC = Red blood cell; TIBC = Total iron-binding capacity.

Notes:

Table 82.4 • Iron Deficiency Anemia

Iron Metabolism	Pathogenesis	Symptoms and Labs	Prevention and Treatment
• Iron stores are 600–1,200 mg for males and 100–400 mg for females • Only 0.5–1 mg/day is lost; another 0.5 to 1 mg is lost daily during menstruation; more lost during pregnancy and lactation • Average American diet contains 6 mg elemental iron/1000 Kcal or 10 to 12 mg/day. • Ferric iron converted to more easily absorbed ferrous iron in acid environment of stomach; 10% dietary iron absorbed in the duodenum and upper jejunum; 20 to 30% absorbed in iron deficiency states	• Blood loss (menstruation, GI, trauma) • Decreased absorption (e.g. drugs—tetracycline, gastrectomy, regional enteritis) • Increased requirement (infancy, pregnant/lactating females) • Impaired utilization (hereditary, decreased iron use)	• Symptoms of generic anemia (see text) • Low serum iron • Serum ferritin, an iron storage compound, <12 ng/mL • High total iron binding capacity (TIBC) • Low reticulocyte count indicating poor RBC production • 10% of patients also have neutropenia and thrombocytosis or thrombocytopenia	*Prevention.* Use Fe supplements to prevent anemia in high-risk populations: • Pregnant and nursing women. See Chapter 43. • Premature infants: 10 to 15 mg/day • Infants and children: 1 to 2 mg/kg/day (not to exceed 20 mg) *Treatment* • Correct underlying cause and modify diet • Fe SO$_4$ 325 mg TID between meals. Start slowly with 1 tablet to minimize GI irritation and diarrhea. Increase by 1 tablet every 2 to 3 days • Goals: Normalize Hgb and Hct and replete iron stores. Reticulocyte count should increased by 3rd or 4th day and peak by 7th to 10th day. In 3 weeks, Hgb increases 2 g/dL and Hct increases by 6%. Symptoms resolve in 1 to 2 months. Continue therapy 3 to 6 months after normalization.

Table 82.5 • Iron Content of Liquid Iron Preparations[a-c]

Preparation	Trade Name	Iron Content (mg Fe++/mL)
Ferrous Sulfate		
Elixir (44 mg/mL)	Feosol	8.8
Drops (125 mg/mL)	Fer-in-Sol	25.0
Syrup (18 mg/mL)	Fer-in-Sol	3.6
Ferrous Gluconate		
Elixir (60 mg/mL)	Fergon	7

[a]Fe = Iron.
[b]There are other iron preparations that may be equally efficacious, and generic equivalents may be available.
[c]The listed preparations are not being endorsed.

Table 82.6 • Comparisons of Iron Preparations[a]

Preparation	Dose (mg)	Fe++ Content (mg)	% Fe	AWP[b] ($/100)
Ferrous sulfate	325	65	20	0.85
Ferrous sulfate (enteric coated)	325	65	20	1.91
Ferrous fumarate	300	99	33	1.87
Ferrous gluconate	300	35	11	1.75
Feosol tablets	200	60	20	8.04
Fero-Gradumet (slow-release)	525	105	20	27.65

[a]AWP = Average wholesale price; Fe = Iron.
[b]This price does not include a prescription fee. Prescription fees will vary among pharmacies. AWP is based on the 1999 Red Book.

Table 82.7 • Combination Iron Products[a]

Drug	DOSS (mg)	Vitamin C (mg)	Fe++ Content (mg)	AWP[b] ($/100)
Ferrous sulfate	0	0	65	0.85
Ferro-Grad 500 (Filmtabs)	0	500	105	30.83
Feostat chew tabs	0	0	33	18.73
Vitron C	0	125	66	8.76
Vitron C-Plus	0	250	132	16.80
Ferro DSS	100	0	50	7.95
Slow Fe	0	0	50	19.25

[a]AWP = Average wholesale price; DOSS = Dioctyl sodium sulfosuccinate; docusate sodium; Fe = Iron.
[b]This price does not include a prescription fee. Prescription fees will vary among pharmacies. AWP is based on the 1999 Red Book.

Notes:

Table 82.8 • Megaloblastic Anemias

Type of Deficiency	Etiology	Signs and Symptoms	Treatment	Monitoring
Folic acid	Alcoholism, hemodialysis, impaired GI absorption,[a] pregnancy,[b] rapid cell turnover states,[c] drug induced[d]	Diarrhea, cheilosis, glossitis with hematologic abnormalities similar to B_{12} deficiency, thrombocytopenia. Neurologic abnormalities do not occur	1 mg/day for 2–3 weeks to replace storage pool. Must rule out B_{12} deficiency before beginning folate[g]	Reticulocytosis should begin in 3–5 days and peak in 5–10 days. Constitutional symptoms should improve within 2 weeks[h]
B_{12}	Rarely dietary deficiency; usually impaired GI absorption (lack of intrinsic factor, achlorhydria, bacterial overgrowth, blind loop strictures, diverticuli)	Onset gradual and insidious. Classic triad of weakness, sore tongue, and tingling of extremities; other neurologic deficits,[e] mental changes, anorexia, pallor, and dyspnea on exertion	30–100 µg/day IM × 2–3 weeks; then 100 µg IM Q 2–4 weeks[f]	Patient feels better within 24 hr and bone marrow normoblastic within 48 hr. Reticulocytosis within 5 days. Check CBC Q 3–6 months. Neurologic changes are reversible with early treatment

[a]From jejunal resection, regional enteritis.
[b]Usually 3rd trimester because of marginal diet and rapid metabolism by fetus.
[c]Hemolytic anemias, leukemias, lymphomas, multiple myeloma.
[d]Barbiturates, oral contraceptives, ethanol, phenytoin, sulfasalazine, trimethoprim.
[e]Loss of vibratory sense, ↑ deep tendon reflexes, ataxia, motor weakness.
[f]Single dose >100 µg are rapidly excreted renally. Oral supplementation, 25 to 250 µg/day, can be used if bacterial overgrowth is the cause after appropriate antibiotic therapy.
[g]Folate doses >0.5 mg/day can reverse hematological but not neurological damage caused by B_{12} deficiency.
[h]Serum chemistries and hematocrit begin to normalize within 10 days. RBC morphology begins to revert back to normal within 1–2 days of initiation of therapy.

Table 82.9 • Therapeutic Uses and Regimens for Recombinant Human Erythropoietin (rhEPO)[a,b]

Anemia Pathogenesis[c]	Dose (U/kg)	Frequency	Maximum Dose Escalation[d]	Time to Respond (wk)	Overall Response Rate (%)
AIDS	100	3 times/wk	200	8–12	17–35
Chemotherapy-induced	150 or 40,000 units	3 times/wk or once a week, respectively	300	2–8	32–61
MDS	40	3 times/wk	570	4–6	20–30
Malignancy	150 or 40,000 U	3 times/wk once a week	150	4–5	47–85
Renal insufficiency	50	3 times/wk	500	2–8	90–97

[a] MDS = Myelodysplastic syndrome.
[b] Twelve- to sixteen-week course of rhEPO therapy.
[c] AIDS patients with endogenous erythropoietin levels <500 U/L.
[d] Moderate dose escalation is indicated if a partial response is observed after 4–8 weeks of therapy.

Notes:

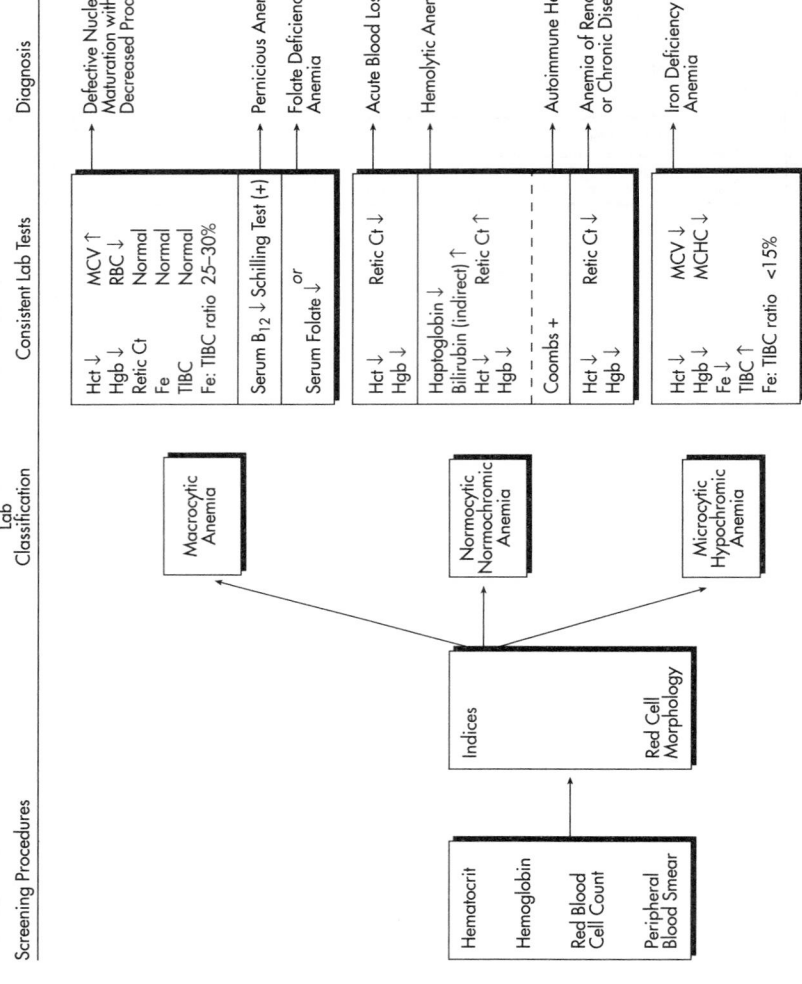

Fig. 82.1 Laboratory Diagnosis of Anemia.

The reader is referred to Chapter 84: Hematopoietic Disorders, written by *Carla Van Den Berg, Pharm.D.,* and *Cindy O'Bryant, Pharm.D.,* in the seventh edition of **Applied Therapeutics: The Clinical Use of Drugs** for a more in-depth discussion of the pathogenesis and treatment of the anemias described briefly above, particularly anemias of chronic disease responsive to RhEPO. All notations to reference numbers are based on the reference list at the end of that chapter. The editors of this handbook express their thanks to Drs. Van Den Berg and O'Bryant and acknowledge that this chapter is based upon their work.

Notes:

Notes:

Chapter 83

Drug-Induced Blood Disorders

Blood Dyscrasias. Drug-induced injuries to the blood that are unpredictable, are not a direct extension of a drug's pharmacological action, and occur in a small number of persons exposed to the agent. Accurate estimates of incidence are unobtainable.

Drug-induced Hemolytic Anemia

♦ Refers to an increased rate of red blood cell (RBC) destruction caused directly or indirectly by a drug. It can occur either within the blood vessels (intravascular hemolysis) or outside the vascular space (extravascular hemolysis). Anemia develops when the rate of hemolysis exceeds the rate of bone marrow RBC production

♦ *Mechanisms and Presentation.* See Table 83.1

♦ *G6PD Deficiency*
   • *Pathophysiology.* RBCs deficient in G6PD are susceptible to hemolysis when exposed to certain oxidant drugs. The hexose monophosphate shunt in RBCs is responsible for maintaining glutathione in the reduced state. Glutathione is an antioxidant that prevents oxidation of hemoglobin to methemoglobin. NADPH is required to keep glutathione in the reduced state and G6PD is needed to reduce NADP to NADPH. NADPH is inadequate to keep glutathione in a reduced state in RBCs deficient in G6PD; methemoglobin is produced; Heinz bodies (condensations of precipitated, denatured Hgb) appear in RBCs. The fragile cells are removed (lysed) prematurely by the spleen.

   • The degree of hemolysis induced by drugs is related to the oxidant potential of the drug, its dose, and the extent of G6PD deficiency. See Table 83.2.

♦ *Immune Hemolytic Anemia*
   • *Mechanisms and Common Drugs.* Drugs or their metabolites can serve as haptens and be immunogenic when combined with cell membranes or circulating proteins. See Table 83.3
   • *Coombs Test (Antiglobulin Test).* Detects both antibody coating of RBCs and circulating immunoglobulins against RBCs. The direct antiglobulin test (DAT) is the most important laboratory test consistent with immune hemolysis and will direct further investigation. It detects IgG class immunoglobulin and complement or both on RBCs but does not indicate whether hemolysis is occurring.

Drug-induced Thrombocytopenia, Neutropenia, and Aplastic Anemia

♦ *Definition and Mechanisms.* See Table 83.4.

♦ *Heparin* is the most common cause of drug-induced thrombocytopenia. Type I HIT occurs early in therapy and may resolve with continued therapy. Caused by a direct, reversible platelet-aggregating effect that leads to undercounting. Type II HIT is less common but can be severe with devastating thromboembolic sequelae. See Table 83.5.

Table 83.1 • Mechanisms and Metabolic Effects of Drug-induced Hemolytic Anemia[a]

Mechanism	Explanation	Site of Destruction & Metabolic Effects	Presentation
Hereditary RBC Defects • G6PD deficiency • Defects in glutathione metabolism • Unstable hemoglobins	Hereditary enzymopathies or hemoglobinopathies predispose RBCs to lysis when exposed to certain drugs or chemicals.	Intravascular. Free Hgb binds to haptoglobin. The complex is removed by the liver where heme is converted to bilirubin; iron is conserved; and haptoglobin levels fall. Excess free Hgb spills into urine. Hyperbilirubinemia and urobilinogenuria can be observed.	Fatigue, jaundice, dark urine, decreased hematocrit and hemoglobin (Hgb), reticulocytosis, hyperbilirubinemia, urobilinogenuria. Positive test for "blood" or hemoglobin in the urine.
Immunologic Destruction • Immune • Autoimmune	Some drugs elicit an idiosyncratic immune response that results in destruction of normal RBCs.	Extravascular in most cases. Reticuloendothelial cells phagocytize RBCs. The heme portion is metabolized to unconjugated (indirect) bilirubin, which can be elevated, causing jaundice. Urobilogen can be excreted into the urine.	As above. Elevated indirect (unconjugated bilirubin), positive Coomb's (antiglobulin) test.

[a]G6PD = Glucose 6-phosphate dehydrogenase; Hgb = Hemoglobin; RBC = Red blood cell

Notes:

Table 83.2 • Drugs and Chemicals Associated with Hemolysis in G6PD Deficiency[a]

Acetanilid	Phenazopyridine	Sulfanilamide
Furazolidone	Phenylhydrazine	Thiazolsulfone
Isobutyl nitrate	Primaquine	Toluidine
Methylene blue	Sulfapyridine	Trinitrotoluene
Naphthalene	Sulfacetamide	Urate oxidase
Nitrofurantoin	Sulfamethoxazole	

[a]G6PD = Glucose 6-phosphate dehydrogenase.
From reference 7.

Table 83.3 • Drug-induced Immunologic Hemolytic Anemia[a]

Mechanism	Process	Common Drugs	Comment
High-affinity hapten-type reaction	Drug binds tightly to RBC membrane surface; immunoglobulins then form against the drug-membrane complex	Cephalosporins, penicillin, tetracycline	Penicillin is the classic prototype of this dose-related reaction
Low-affinity hapten-type reaction or Immune complex formation	Drug binds to either (1) low-affinity specific antigenic loci on the cell membrane or (2) to circulating proteins to form an immune complex that adheres loosely to RBCs. Lysis via complement activation ensues	Acetaminophen, ASA, chlorpromazine, chlorpropamide, hydrochlorothiazide, INH, PAS, phenacetin, probenecid, quinidine, quinine, rifampin, sulfonamides	Subsequent to hemolysis, the drug or immune complex dissociates from RBC fragments, adheres to another RBC, and repeats the process. Small doses can cause large scale hemolysis. Quinidine is the prototype drug
Autoimmune reaction	Drug stimulates production of anti-RBC antibodies. Autoantibodies coat RBCs and extravascular lysis occurs	Levodopa, mefenamic acid, methyldopa, procainamide	Methyldopa is the prototype drug for autoimmune hemolysis

[a]ASA = Acetylsalicylic acid; INH = Isoniazid; PAS = Para-aminosalicylate sodium; RBC = Red blood cell.

Notes:

Table 83.4 • Drug-Induced Blood Disorders[a]

Type	Definition	Mechanism (Drug)	Comment
Thrombocytopenia	↓ platelets <100,000/mm³	1) ↓ platelet formation (thiazides) 2) Immune suppression or destruction of platelets (gold, quinine, quinidine) 3) Nonimmune, dose-related destruction of platelets (heparin)	>100 implicated drugs but most are anecdotal reports or based on circumstantial evidence. Heparin is most common drug-induced cause
Neutropenia[c,d]	Leukopenia = WBC <3000/mm³; granulocytopenia = granulocytes (including eosinophils and basophils) <1500/mm³; neutropenia = neutrophils (PMNs and bands) <1500/mm³; agranulocytosis = total granulocyte count <500/mm³	1) Immunological suppression or destruction of marrow precursors (nafcillin) 2) Direct toxicity to marrow precursors (chlorpromazine; clozapine)	>100 implicated drugs, but case reports do not provide enough data to establish mechanisms[b]
Aplastic anemia[e]	Severe marrow aplasia and pancytopenia (↓ or absent RBCs, WBCs, and platelets) or bicytopenia as any 2 of the 3 abnormalities present in pancytopenia	1) Toxicity to the pluripotential stem cell before process of differentiation to committed stem cells (chloramphenicol, felbamate, phenylbutazone)	Rarest, least understood, most serious (50% mortality) of blood dyscrasias

[a]Other than drug-induced hemolytic anemia.
[b]The incidence of agranulocytosis with clozapine is <1%. The WBC ↓s steadily over a period of at least 4 weeks with clozapine-induced agranulocytosis. Clozapine apparently causes immune suppression of myeloid precursors independent of a dose-relationship.
[c]Agranulocytosis implies a total or near absence of granulocytes but generally used when total granulocyte count <100/mm³.
[d]Colony-stimulating factors (G-CSF, GM-CSF) should be used in supporting patients with symptomatic drug-induced neutropenic; however, use for this indication is not FDA-approved.
[e]Bone-marrow transplantation from an HLA-identical sibling donor is treatment of choice for younger patients (i.e., <45 yr). Immune suppression is alternative for older patients and for those without a suitable bone-marrow donor.

Table 83.5 • Characteristics of Type I and II Heparin-induced Thrombocytopenia (HIT)

	Type I	Type II
Frequency	10–20%	2–30%
Timing of onset	1–4 days	5–10 days
Nadir platelet count	100,000/µL	30,000–55,000/µL
Antibody-mediated	No	Yes
Thromboembolic sequelae	None	30–80%
Hemorrhagic sequelae	None	Rarely
Management	Observe	Cessation of heparin, alternative anticoagulation, additional therapy

From reference 66.

The reader is referred to Chapter 85: Drug-induced Blood Disorders, written by *Larry D. Sasich, Pharm.D.,* and *Sana R. Sukkari, Pharm.D.,* in the seventh edition of **Applied Therapeutics: The Clinical Use of Drugs** for a more in-depth discussion of pathogenesis and clinical presentation of drug-induced thrombocytopenia, neutropenia, and aplastic anemia. All notations to reference numbers are based on the reference list at the end of that chapter. The editors of this handbook express their thanks to Drs. Sasisch and Sukkari and acknowledge that this chapter is based upon their work.

Notes:

Notes:

Chapter 84

Neoplastic Disorders and Their Treatment: General Principles

CAUTION: *Cancer chemotherapy is a rapidly changing field. Doses provided in this chapter may not correspond to the latest protocols. For definitive treatment guidelines always use approved protocols.*

Inside . . .

Inside . . .

Etiology and Prevention

♦ Cancer is a group of diseases characterized by uncontrolled growth and spread of abnormal cells.

♦ About 1 in 2 American men and 1 in 3 American women will eventually develop cancer. See Figure 84.1 for the most *common cancers.*

♦ Some initial "event" causes damage or mutation to the cell's DNA, causing it to multiply. *Carcinogenic factors* are listed in Table 84.1.

♦ Two gene classes, *oncogenes and tumor-suppressor genes* may play a major role in the origin of cancer. Oncogenes cause overproduction of proteins that stimulate cell proliferation. Tumor-suppressor genes encode for proteins that control inappropriate cell division or growth. Loss or mutation of these genes can lead to malignant transformation. See Table 84.2

♦ Cancer chemoprevention focuses on reversing carcinogenesis in the early phases and preventing malignancies. It includes preventing the formation of carcinogens; blocking the carcinogen from reacting with critical target sites; or suppressing the promotion of an epidermal neoplasia. Clinical trials and their outcomes are described in Table 84.3.

Tumor Growth and Spread

♦ **Growth.** Cancer cells and normal cells proceed through a specific and orderly set of events during cellular replication. The cell cycle contains four phases (S, M, G1, and G2) of activity, each responsible for a different task in cell division. In a normal cell, a "cell-cycle clock" regulates cell division by interpreting the inhibitory and stimulatory signals it receives from surrounding cells. Altered inhibitory (e.g., pRB, p53) and stimulatory signals (e.g., cyclins, cyclin-dependent kinases -cdks) can lead to malignant transformation. See Figure 84.2.

♦ **Spread.** The ability of cancer cells to disseminate and form metastases is their most malignant characteristic because metastases are associated with the majority of cancer-related deaths. Cancer cells must develop new blood cells to supply nutrients and spread to distant sites. To do this they secrete growth factors to stimulate growth of new blood vessels (angiogenesis) and other chemicals involved in invasion and spread into surrounding tissue. These substances have become molecular targets. See Tables 84.4 and 84.5.

Screening and Early Detection

♦ Standardized screening tests can help identify disease in asymptomatic people or help diagnose a disease in symptomatic individuals.

♦ Screening tests must meet four requirements: there must be good evidence that the test is effective in reducing morbidity or mortality; the benefits should outweigh the risks; it should be cost-beneficial; it should be practical and feasible. See Table 84.6.

Diagnosis and Screening

♦ A tumor's histologic diagnosis determines its natural history, pattern of progression, and responsiveness to treatment.

♦ Staging is the process that determines the extent or spread of the disease and significantly influences its treatment and prognosis. Schema have been developed for all major types of cancer, and many incorporate the TNM system, which incorporates the size of the primary rumor (T), the extent of regional lymph node spread (N), and the presence of metastatic spread to distant organs (M). See Table 86.7.

Clinical Presentation

♦ The initial signs and symptoms of malignant disease are variable and predominantly depend on the histologic diagnosis, the location, and the size of the tumor.

♦ Pain due to compression and obstruction and destruction of adjacent tissues and organs is the most common presenting symptom. Others include anorexia, weight loss, and fatigue. See Table 84.8.

♦ Substances secreted by the tumor produce *paraneoplastic* signs or symptoms. See Table 84.9.

Treatment Principles

♦ The choice of therapy depends not only on the histology and stage but also on the patient's predicted tolerance of the side effects and complications.

♦ The goal of therapy should always be to cure the patient, and the likelihood of this is greatest when the tumor burden is low.

♦ Surgery or radiation is the initial choice of therapy for localized tumors. See Table 84.10.

Chemotherapy

♦ Cytotoxic chemotherapy kills cancer cells by damaging DNA or interfering with DNA synthesis or other steps during cell division. They are most cytotoxic to tumor cells with a high-growth fraction.

♦ *Phase-specific or schedule-dependent agents* affect the cell only during a specific phase of the cell cycle. *Phase-nonspecific or dose-dependent agents* affect the cell during any phase of the cell cycle. See Figure 84.2.

♦ **Pharmacology.** See Table 84.11.

♦ **Cell-kill Hypothesis.** The number of tumor cells killed by chemotherapy is proportional to the dose when the growth fraction is 100% (i.e., all cells are dividing). Tumor cells do not decrease predictably because the growth fraction is not 100%, and some cells are resistant. When the growth of large tumors has plateaued, the fraction of cells killed with each treatment is low. Drugs are administered every 3 to 4 weeks to allow normal cells to recover from the toxic effects. See Figure 84.3.

♦ Factors Influencing Response to Therapy

- *Dose intensity* equals the amount of chemotherapy administered per unit of time. There is a direct relationship between dose intensity and response rate, but this is limited by toxicity.
- *Schedule dependency.* The schedule of chemotherapy administration can reduce toxicity and allow greater dose intensity. Rates of administration are also determined by the pharmacokinetic properties of an agent.
- *Drug resistance.* Biochemical resistance to chemotherapy is a major impediment to successful treatment. It can occur de novo or develop during cell division by several mechanisms. Resistant cell lines may also be resistant to structurally unrelated cytotoxic compounds (pleiotropic drug resistance or multidrug resistance). See Table 84.12.
- *Tumor site.* The cytotoxic effects of chemotherapy agents are related to the time the tumor is exposed to an effective concentration. This is determined by the dose, route, and lipophilicity of the drug, as well as by the tumor size and location.

♦ Combination chemotherapy provides broader coverage against resistant cell lines within a heterogeneous tumor. See Table 84.13. Agents used together:

- Should have activity against the tumor as a single agent
- Should have different mechanisms of action
- Should not have overlapping toxicities
- Should be used in their optimal dose and schedule

♦ Tumors That Respond to Chemotherapy. See Table 84.14.

♦ Phases of Chemotherapy. See Figure 84.4.

- *Primary chemotherapy* is the primary treatment modality used for leukemias as well as solid tumors that have metastasized at the time of diagnosis or have recurred at metastatic sites following initial therapy. Can be curative or palliative.
- *Induction chemotherapy* is additional therapy given after a patient fails primary chemotherapy in an attempt to eradicate the tumor. Can also refer to the initial treatment of patients who present with leukemias.
- *Postremission therapy* is given after induction therapy to improve chances of long-term survival. It includes consolidation, intensification, and maintenance treatment phases.
- Other additional therapy is referred to as secondary chemotherapy, second-line chemotherapy, or salvage chemotherapy.
- *Adjuvant chemotherapy* is given after primary therapy to eradicate any undetectable tumor after initial curative surgery or radiation therapy. Because the tumor burden is relatively low, chemotherapy should immediately follow the primary therapy.
- *Neoadjuvant chemotherapy* is initial treatment for patients who present with locally advanced tumors that are unlikely to be cured with primary surgery or radiation therapy. The objective is to reduce the tumor mass to increase the likelihood of eradication by surgery or radiation.

♦ Administration

- *Systemic* chemotherapy is most commonly administered by the intravenous route by IV bolus (<15 minutes), short infusion (15 minutes to several hours), or continuous infusion (24 hrs to several weeks). Some can be administered orally.
- *Regional* chemotherapy is that administered locally to specific sites of the body affected by the tumor. See Table 84.15.

+ **Assessing Response to Therapy**
  • *Standard criteria* are used. See Table 84.16.
  • *Tumor markers* are biochemical indicators commonly found in abnormally high concentrations with cancer. They should be produced and released primarily by the cancer cells at levels proportional to the tumor mass and should be detectable at low levels. See Table 84.17.

Other Therapies

+ **Endocrine therapy** Can be used to treat several cancers that arise from hormone-sensitive tissues: breast, prostate, and endometrial cancers. See Table 84.18

+ **Gene therapy** represents a potential treatment modality in which a functioning gene is inserted into a cell to correct a metabolic abnormality or to introduce a new function. In cancer the goal is to inactivate an oncogene or replace a missing or mutant tumor suppressor gene. Not technically feasible.

+ **Biologic response modifiers** target molecular changes associated with carcinogenesis. They include organic substances such as proteins, antibodies, cells, and genes. They are used to kill cancer cells or to bolster the host's defense mechanism.

  • *Interferon-Alpha* is a recombinant cytokine that has a direct antiproliferative effect; an immunomodulatory effect on natural killer cells, T cells, B cells, and macrophages; an induction of tumor cell antigens; and a differentiating effect on tumor cells. Causes many side effects, including a flu-like effect, profound fatigue, anorexia, weight loss, and disordered mentation.

  • *Interleukin-2* is a lymphokine with many immunoregulatory functions. Lymphoid cells incubated with IL-2 develop the capacity to lyse tumor cells. There is significant dose-related toxicity caused by diffuse capillary leaks (hypotension, pulmonary edema, oliguria, hyperbilirubinemia).

Notes:

Table 84.1 • Carcinogens Associated with an Increased Risk of Cancer

Carcinogenic Risk Factor	Associated Cancer(s)
Environmental	
Ionizing radiation (radon gas emitted from soil containing uranium deposits)	Leukemia, breast, thyroid, lung
Ultraviolet radiation	Skin melanoma
Viruses[a]	Leukemia, lymphoma, nasopharyngeal
Occupational	
Asbestos	Lung, mesothelioma
Chromium, nickel	Lung
Vinyl chloride	Liver
Aniline dye	Bladder
Benzene	Leukemia
Lifestyle	
Alcohol	Esophagus, liver, stomach, oropharynx, larynx
Dietary factors	Colon, breast, gallbladder
Tobacco	Lung, oropharynx, pharynx, larynx, esophagus, bladder
Medical Drugs	
Diethylstilbestrol	Vaginal in offspring, breast, testes, ovary
Alkylating agents	Leukemia, bladder
Azathioprine	Lymphoma
Phenacetin	Bladder
Estrogens, tamoxifen	Endometrial
Cyclophosphamide	Bladder

[a]Casual relationship credible but not firmly established.

Notes:

Table 84.2 • Some Genes Involved in Human Cancers[13]

Oncogenes

Genes for Growth Factors or Their Receptors
PDGF	Codes for platelet-derived growth factor; involved in glioma (a brain cancer)
erb-B	Codes for the receptor for epidermal growth factor; involved in glioblastoma (a brain cancer and breast cancer)
erb-B2	Also called *Her-2* or *neu;* codes for a growth factor receptor; involved in breast, salivary gland, and ovarian cancers
RET	Codes for a growth factor receptor; involved in thyroid cancer

Genes for Cytoplasmic Relays in Stimulatory Signaling Pathways
Ki-ras	Involved in lung, ovarian, colon, and pancreatic cancers
N-ras	Involved in leukemias

Genes for Transcription Factors That Activate Growth-Promoting Genes
c-myc	Involved in leukemias and breast, stomach, and lung cancers
N-myc	Involved in neuroblastoma (a nerve cell cancer) and glioblastoma
L-myc	Involved in lung cancer

Genes for Other Kinds of Molecules
Bcl-2	Codes for a protein that normally blocks cell suicide; involved in follicular B-cell lymphoma
Bcl-1	Also called *PRAD1;* codes for cyclin D1, a stimulatory component of the cell-cycle clock; involved in breast, head, and neck cancers
MDM2	Codes for an antagonist of the p53 tumor-suppressor protein; involved in sarcomas (connective tissue cancers) and others cancers

Tumor-Suppressor Genes

Genes for Proteins in the Cytoplasm
APC	Involved in colon and stomach cancers
DPC-4	Codes for a relay molecule in a signaling pathway that inhibits cell division; involved in pancreatic cancer
NF-1	Codes for a protein that inhibits a stimulatory (Ras) protein; involved in neuro-fibroma and pheochromocytoma (cancers of the peripheral nervous system) and myeloid leukemia
NF-2	Involved in meningioma and ependymoma (brain cancers) and schwannoma (affecting the wrapping around peripheral nerves)

Genes for Proteins in the Nucleus
MTS1	Codes for the p16 protein, a braking component of the cell-cycle clock; involved in a wide range of cancers
RB	Codes for the pRB protein, a master brake of the cell cycle; involved in retino-blastoma and bone, bladder, and small cell lung and breast cancer
p53	Codes for the p53 protein, which can halt cell division and induce abnormal cells to kill themselves; involved in a wide range of cancers
WT1	Involved in Wilms' tumor of the kidney

Genes for Proteins Whose Cellular Location Is Not Yet Clear
BRCA1	Involved in breast and ovarian cancers
BRCA2	Involved in breast cancer
VHL	Involved in renal cell cancer

Notes:

Table 84.3 • Large, Randomized Chemoprevention Trials

Trial	Agents	Population	Duration of Intervention (yr)	End Points	Outcomes
Nutrients					
ATBC[16]	Vitamin E β-Carotene	Men with a history of smoking or a current smoker (n = 29,133)	6	Lung cancer	Negative: β-carotene showed no chemoprotective benefit with an increase in incidence and mortality; vitamin A showed no effect
CARET[17,18]	Vitamin A β-Carotene	Individuals with a history of smoking or a current smoker (n = 18,344)	4	Lung cancer	Negative: showed no chemoprotective benefit with an increase in incidence and mortality
Physician's Health Study[19]	β-Carotene	Male physicians with no significant medical history (n = 22,071)	12	Lung cancer	Negative: showed no chemoprotective benefit
Antiestrogens					
BCPT[20]	Tamoxifen	Women of higher-than-average risk of breast cancer (n = 13,000)	5.7	Breast cancer	Positive: reduced the risk of invasive and noninvasive cancers and the occurrence of estrogen receptor–positive tumors; tamoxifen received an indication for chemoprevention from the U.S. Food and Drug Administration
MORE[21]	Raloxifene	Postmenopausal women with osteoporosis (n = 7705)	3	Breast cancer	Positive: reduced the risk of invasive cancers
STAR[22]	Tamoxifen Raloxifene	Postmenopausal women at high risk of breast cancer (n = 22,000)	Ongoing	Breast cancer	
α-Reductase Inhibitors					
PCPT[23,24]	Finasteride	Men with no significant medical history	Ongoing	Prostate cancer	

Table 84.4 • Molecular Approaches in Cancer Therapy[36]

Cancer Feature	Molecular Targets	Therapeutics
Oncogene activation leading to excessive Ras protein or kinase activity	Ras proteins	Farnesyl transferase inhibitors: L-744,832; SCH 44352; BZA-5B
	Abl, EGF receptor, Erb-B2, and Src kinases	Tyrosine kinase inhibitors: tyrphostins (RG 13 022); lavendustins (AG 957); quinazolines (PD 153 035) Antisense inhibitors
	PKC-α, Raf, and cyclin-dependent kinases	Serine/threonine kinase inhibitors: olomoucine; staurosporine; butryolactone Antisense inhibitors
Loss of tumor-suppressor genes	APC, AT, DCC, RB, and p53 genes	Gene therapy to restore normal suppressor gene function Antisense agents to block E2F synthesis
Abnormal DNA repair mechanisms	DNA mismatch repair enzymes: MSH2; MLH1; PMS1; PMS2	Gene therapy to restore normal enzyme activity Checkpoint inhibitors to promote susceptibility to DNA-damaging agents
Lack of senescence (cell aging) in tumor cells	Telomerase	Telomerase inhibitors
Angiogenesis	FGF, FCF, VEGF growth factors	TNP-470, suramin
	Integrin receptors	$\alpha_v\beta_3$, $\alpha_v\beta_5$ antagonists
Metastases	Metalloproteases Collagenases	Protease inhibitors Collagenase inhibitors

Table 84.5 • Common Cancers and Sites of Metastases[a]

Cancer	Most Common Sites of Metastases
Breast	
Premenopausal	Lymph nodes, skin, lung, liver, bone, brain
Postmenopausal	Lymph nodes, bone, soft tissue
Prostate	Lymph nodes, bone, liver
Lung	
Non–small cell	Lymph nodes, liver, bone, brain
Small cell	Lymph nodes, bone, liver, bone marrow, brain
Colon	Lymph nodes, liver, lung, adrenals, ovary, bone
Lymphomas	
Hodgkin's disease	Liver, spleen, stomach, bone marrow, lung
Non-Hodgkin's lymphoma	GI tract, bone marrow, liver, lung, CNS
Ovary	Peritoneum, lung
Bladder	Pelvis, lymph nodes

[a]CNS = Central nervous system; GI = Gastrointestinal.

Notes:

Table 84.6 • Guidelines for Screening Cancer

	U.S. Preventative Task Force	American Cancer Society	National Cancer Society
Self-Examination			
Breast self-examination	Not recommended	≥20 yr: monthly	Not recommended
Testicular self-examination	Not recommended (unless high risk)	Not recommended	With periodic examination
Skin	High risk	Not recommended	With periodic examination
Clinician Examination			
Clinical breast examination	20–40 yr: not recommended[a]; 50–60 yr: annually with mammogram	20–40 yr: every 3 yr; ≥40 yr: annually	40–48 yr: periodicity unspecified; ≥50 yr: with mammogram
Digital rectal examination	Not recommended	Colon: not recommended; Prostate: ≥50 yr: annually	Not recommended
Pelvic examination	Not recommended	20–40 yr: every 1–3 yr; ≥40 yr: annually	Annually
Sigmoidoscopy	Recommended: periodicity unspecified	≥50 yr: every 5 yr	≥50 yr: periodicity unspecified
Colonoscopy	Not recommended	≥50 yr: every 10 yr	
Laboratory Tests			
Stool guaiac	≥50 yr: annually	≥50 yr: annually	≥50 yr: annually
Prostate-specific antigen	Not recommended	≥50 yr: annually	Not recommended
Pap smear	When sexually active: every 3 yr	18 yr or sexually active[b]: annually	18 yr or sexually active: annually
Mammogram	40–49 yr: not recommended; 50–69 yr: every 1–2 yr; ≥70 yr: not recommended	≥40 yr: annually; ≥50 yr: every 1–2 yr; ≥50 yr: based on health and patient's choice	40–49 yr: patient's choice

[a]For high-risk women, start clinical breast examination at age 35.
[b]If Pap smear is normal for 3 consecutive years, then less frequently.

Table 84.7 • Staging of Breast Carcinoma[a]

TNM Classification[a]

Primary Tumor (T)

T1	Tumor ≤2 cm in greatest dimension
T2	Tumor >2 cm but not >5 cm in greatest dimension
T3	Tumor >5 cm in greatest dimension
T4	Tumor of any size with direct extension to chest wall or skin

Regional Lymph Nodes (N)

N0	No regional lymph node metastasis
N1	Metastasis to movable ipsilateral axillary lymph node(s)
N2	Metastasis to ipsilateral axillary lymph node(s) fixed to one another or other structures
N3	Metastasis to ipsilateral internal mammary lymph node(s)

Distant Metastasis (M)

M0	No distant metastasis
M1	Distant metastasis (includes metastasis to ipsilateral supraclavicular lymph nodes)

Stage Grouping

Stage I	T1	N0	M0
Stage II$_A$	T0	N1	M0
	T1	N1	M0
	T2	N0	M0
Stage II$_B$	T2	N1	M0
	T3	N0	M0
Stage III$_A$	T0	N2	M0
	T1	N2	M0
	T2	N2	M0
	T3	N1, N2	M0
Stage III$_B$	T4	Any N	M0
	Any T	N3	M0
Stage IV	Any T	Any N	M1

[a]TNM = Tumor-node-metastasis.
[b]See text for full explanation of TNM system of classification.

Notes:

Table 84.8 • Signs and Symptoms Associated with Common Cancers[a]

Cancer	Local	Distant[b]
Breast	Breast lumps; nipple retraction, dimpling, discharge; skin changes; axillary lymphadenopathy	Bone pain; elevated LFTs; hypercalcemia
Prostate	Urinary hesitancy: nocturia; poor urine stream; dribbling; terminal hematuria	Bone pain; elevated acid phosphatase, PSA, and alkaline phosphatase
Lung	New cough; hoarseness hemoptysis, dyspnea; unresolving pneumonias; chest wall pain; pain; dysphagia; effusion; tracheal obstruction	Anorexia; weight loss; elevated LFTs; bone pain, hypercalcemia; jaundice; lymphadenopathy; osteoarthropathy; neurologic (brain metastases and neuromuscular disorders)
Colorectal	Change in bowel habits; ↓ in stool caliber; occult bleeding; constipation	Elevated LFTs, CEA, and alkaline, phosphatase; obstruction hepatomegaly; perforation
Ovarian	Abdominal pain, discomfort, or enlargement; postprandial flatulence; vaginal bleeding; abdominal mass; urinary frequency; constipation, nausea; dyspepsia; early satiety	Peripheral neuropathies; pleural effusion; thrombophlebitis; elevated LFTs; abdominal distention or pain; Addison's or Cushing's syndrome
Testicular	Painless enlargement; epididymitis; gynecomastia; back pain; infertility/erectile dysfunction	Elevated HCG, α-fetoprotein, LD
Bladder	Hematuria; bladder irritability; urinary hesitancy, frequency or urgency; dysuria; flank or pelvic pain	Edema of lower extremities and genitalia
Melanoma	Change in size, color, or shape of a pre-existing nevus	Lymphadenopathy; elevated LFTs
Lymphomas	Painless lymphadenopathy	Fever; night sweats; weight loss; bone or retroperitoneal pain; hepatomegaly; splenomegaly: abnormal CBC

[a]CBC = Complete blood count; CEA = Carcinoembryonic antigen; HCG = β-human chorionic gonadotropin; LD = Lactate dehydrogenase; LFTs = Liver function tests; PSA = Prostate-specific antigen; SIADH = Syndrome of inappropriate antidiuretic hormone secretion.
[b]Local effects include those produced by the primary tumor, and distant effects include those associated with metastatic spread and paraneoplastic syndromes. Many cancers may not produce symptoms in the early stages, and diagnosis at that time is depend on early detection and screening efforts.

Table 84.9 • Paraneoplastic Syndromes Associated with Cancers

Syndrome	Cancer
Dermatologic	
Sweet's syndrome	Hematologic malignancies and various carcinomas
Endocrine	
Addison's syndrome[a]	Adrenal carcinoma, lymphomas, and ovarian cancer
Cushing's syndrome[a]	Lung, thyroid, testicular, adrenal, and ovarian cancers
Hypercalcemia (not associated with bone metastases)[a]	Lung cancer
Syndrome of inappropriate antidiuretic hormone secretion	Lung and head and neck cancers
Hematologic/Coagulation	
Anemia[a]	Various cancers
Autoimmune hemolytic anemia[a]	Chronic lymphocytic leukemia, lymphomas, ovarian cancer
Disseminated intravascular coagulation[a]	Acute progranulocytic leukemia, lung and prostate cancers
Thrombophlebitis	Lung, breast, ovarian, prostate, and pancreatic cancers
Neuromuscular	
Dermatomyositis and polymyositis	Lung and breast cancers
Myasthenic syndrome (Eaton-Lambert syndrome)	Small cell lung, gastric, and ovarian cancers
Sensory neuropathies	Small cell lung and ovarian cancers

[a]This syndrome is discussed in more detail in other sections of this text. See the index.

Table 84.10 • Radiation Sensitivity of Common Tumors[39,40]

Radiosensitive	Intermediate	Radioresistant
Acute lymphocytic leukemia	Squamous cell carcinoma of the head and neck	Gliomas
Testicular, seminoma	Cervix cancer	Melanomas
Neuroblastoma	Breast cancer	Soft-tissue sarcomas
Hodgkin's disease	Ovarian cancer	Thyroid cancer
Basal cell and squamous cell skin cancer	Bladder cancer	

Notes:

Table 84.11 • Clinical Pharmacology of Chemotherapy Agents[a]

Agents	Mechanism of Action	Pharmacokinetic Characteristics	Dosage Adjustment for Organ Dysfunction	Major Toxicities
Altretamine (Hexalen)[43–46] Cap: 50 mg	Nonclassic alkylating agent. Metabolites generate reactive intermediates that cross-link DNA.	Bioavailability variable, probably due to extensive metabolism $t_{1/2\alpha}$ = 30 min; $t_{1/2\beta}$ = 4.7–13 hr.		Anorexia; nausea, vomiting; diarrhea; neurologic toxicity; myelosuppression
Asparaginase (Elspar)[39,40,47] Inj: 10,000 IU/vial	Enzyme; depletes essential amino acids and inhibits protein synthesis.	$t_{1/2}$ = 14–22 hr; plasma clearance greatly accelerated in patients who develop hypersensitivity.		Hypersensitivity; hypoalbuminemia; hyperglycemia; ↓ clotting factors (↑ PT, ↑ PTT); ↓ LFT; nausea/ vomiting; chills
Bleomycin (Blenoxane)[48–52] Inj: 15 mg/vial	Antitumor antibiotic; causes single- and double-strand breaks in DNA by generating free radicals.	$t_{1/2\alpha}$ = 24 min; $t_{1/2\beta}$ = 2–4 hr; longer $t_{1/2}$ reported in patients with renal insufficiency; 45–70% excreted in urine in 24 hr.	↓ if Cl_{CR} <25 mL/min/m² in proportion with ↓.	Pulmonary toxicity; fever; skin changes: erythema, induration, hyperkeratosis, hyperpigmentation, peeling, and nail changes
Busulfan (Myleran)[53–56] Tab: 2 mg	Alkylating agent; forms reactive intermediates that cross-link DNA.	Well absorbed orally; metabolized extensively; no intact drug recovered in urine, but metabolites are excreted renally; 90% of dose cleared from plasma in 3 min.		Myelosuppression; pulmonary fibrosis; hyperpigmentation; suppression of testicular, ovarian, and adrenal function
Capecitabine (Xeloda)[57]	Antimetabolite; prodrug metabolized to fluorouracil; incorporates into RNA and interferes with RNA function; inhibits thymidylate synthase and causes inhibition of DNA synthesis.	$t_{1/2}$ = 0.75 hr; 35% protein bound; C_{max} and AUC varies >85%.		Nausea/vomiting; stomatitis; hand-foot syndrome; bone marrow suppression; anorexia
Carboplatin (Paraplatin)[58–62] Inj: 50, 150, 450 mg/vial	Nonclassic alkylating agent; binds to DNA to form interstrand cross-links and adducts.	$t_{1/2\alpha}$ = 12–24 min; $t_{1/2\beta}$ = 22–40 hr; ≤90% excreted in urine.	↓ if Cl_{CR} <60 mL/min or use methods described by Egorin or Calvert.[70,71]	Myelosuppression (especially thrombocytopenia); nausea/ vomiting
Carmustine (BiCNU)[63–65] Inj: 100 mg/vial	Alkylating agent; metabolites generate, reactive intermediates that cross-link DNA.	>30% metabolite excreted in urine; $t_{1/2}$ = 5 min; good CSF penetration.	↓ may be necessary if a patient has ↓ bone marrow reserve.	Delayed myelosuppression; nausea/ vomiting; pulmonary fibrosis; hepatotoxicity; renal toxicity

Chlorambucil (Leukeran)[66–69] Tab: 2 mg	Alkylating agent; forms reactive intermediates that cross-link DNA.	Oral bioavailability 70–80%, reduced by 10–20% if ingested with food; rapidly metabolized to inactive metabolites and active phenylacetic acid mustard; $t_{1/2}$ = 1.5–2 hr (parent), 2.5 hr (active metabolite); <1% excreted unchanged in urine in 24 hr.		Myelosuppression; pulmonary fibrosis
Cladribine (Leustatin)[70–72] Inj: 10 mg/vial	Antimetabolite; following intracellular phosphorylation, causes inhibition of enzymes that impair DNA synthesis; impairs DNA repair.	$t_{1/2\alpha}$ = 35 min; $t_{1/2\beta}$ = 6.7 hr.	?; effect of renal or hepatic disease is unknown.	Myelosuppression; fever; immunosuppresion (B and T cells); acute tubular necrosis; neurotoxicity (paraparesis, quadriplegia); rash
Cisplatin (Platinol)[73–77] Inj: 10, 50 mg/vial	Nonclassic alkylating agents; binds to DNA to form interstrand cross-links and adducts.	$t_{1/2\alpha}$ = 20–30 min; $t_{1/2\beta}$ = 60 min; $t_{1/2\gamma}$ = 24 hr; >90% excreted in urine.	↓ or discontinue for renal dysfunction.	Nephrotoxicity; nausea/vomiting; peripheral neuropathy; ototoxicity; hypomagnesemia; visual disturbances (rare)
Cyclophosphamide (Cytoxan)[78–82] Inj: 100, 200, 500, 1,000, 2,000 mg/vial	Alkylating agent; metabolite generates reactive intermediates that cross-link DNA.	Oral bioavailability ≈100%; must be activated in liver by microsomal enzymes to active compounds and toxic metabolites; 22% of parent and 60% of metabolites excreted in urine; $t_{1/2}$ = 3–10 hr; 6.5–≥8 hr (alkylating activity).		Myelosuppression; hemorrhagic cystitis; nausea/vomiting; alopecia; cardiomyopathy (rare); "allergic" interstitial pneumonitis; SIADH
Cytarabine (Cytosar)[83–86] Inj: 100, 500, 1,000, 2,000 mg/vial	Antimetabolite; incorporates into DNA and causes termination of DNA chain elongation and inhibition of DNA polymerase.	Metabolized by deamination primarily in liver, 8% parent and 72% as metabolite excreted unchanged; in urine; $t_{1/2\alpha}$ = 1.6–20 min; $t_{1/2\beta}$ = 9–111 min.		Myelosuppression; nausea/vomiting; stomatitis; fever; rash; intrahepatic cholestasis, ↑ LFT and bilirubin (rare)
Dacarbazine (DTIC-Dome)[87–92] Inj: 50 μg/vial	Nonclassic alkylating agent; metabolite causes methylation of nucleic acids; causes direct DNA damage and inhibits purine synthesis.	Extensively metabolized to active compound; 50% parent and 9–18% major metabolite excreted in urine; some hepatobiliary excretion; $t_{1/2\alpha}$ = 3 min; $t_{1/2\beta}$ = 41 min.	↓ may be required for moderate-to-severe hepatic or renal dysfunction.	Myelosuppression; nausea/vomiting; myalgias; fever; malaise; headache; pain at injection site; photosensitivity; fatal hepatic vein occlusion (rare)

(continued)

Table 84.11 • Clinical Pharmacology of Chemotherapy Agents[a] (continued)

Agents	Mechanism of Action	Pharmacokinetic Characteristics	Dosage Adjustment for Organ Dysfunction	Major Toxicities
Dactinomycin (Cosmegen)[93–95] Inj: 500 µg/vial	Antitumor antibiotic; intercalates into DNA and inhibits RNA and protein synthesis.	Urinary excretion 20% fecal excretion 14%; $t_{1/2\beta} \geq 36$ hr.		Myelosuppression, nausea, vomiting, diarrhea; mucositis; alopecia; hepatotoxicity; vesicant if extravasated
Daunorubicin (Cerubidine)[96–99] Inj: 20 mg/vial	Antitumor antibiotic, intercalates to DNA double helix; topoisomerase II–mediated DNA damage; produces oxygen-free radicals.	Extensive binding to tissues; know routes of elimination account for only 50–60% of dose; extensively metabolized by liver; $t_{1/2\alpha} = 40$ min; $t_{1/2\beta} = 45$–55 hr; 20–30% biliary excretion; 14–23% excreted in urine as parent and metabolites.	↓ if very severe hepatic dysfunction; 75% if severe renal dysfunction.	Myelosuppression, mucositis; alopecia cumulative cardiac toxicity; dose-related acute ECG changes; severe tissue damage if extravasated
Daunorubicin, liposomal (Daunoxome)[100] Inj: 50 mg/vial	Antitumor antibiotic: intercalates into DNA double helix; topoisomerase II–mediated DNA damage; produces oxygen-free radicals.		↓ with hepatic dysfunction: 75% if bilirubin 1.2–3.0; 50% if bilirubin >3.0.	
Docetaxal (Taxotere)[101] Inj: 40 mg/mL	Taxane; promotes microtubule assembly and arrests cell cycle in G_2 and M phases.	$t_{1/2\alpha} = 4$ min; $t_{1/2\beta} = 36$ min; $t_{1/2\gamma} = 11$ hr; Cl 21 L/hr/m²; Vd = 113 L.	Discontinue treatment if bilirubin > ULN; SGOT/ SGPT >1.5 × ULN or alkaline phosphatase >2.5 × ULN.	Peripheral edema; bone marrow suppression; hypersensitivity reaction
Doxorubicin (Adriamycin, Rubex)[102–104] Inj: 10, 20, 50, 100, 150, 200 mg/vial	Antitumor antibiotic; intercalates into DNA double helix; topoisomerase II–mediated DNA damage; produces oxygen-free radicals.	Extensive binding to tissues; known routes of elimination only account for 50–60% of dose; extensively metabolized by liver; $t_{1/2\alpha} = 40$ min; $t_{1/2\beta} = 45$–55 hr; 20–30% biliary excretion; 14–23% excreted in urine as parent and metabolites.	↓ if hepatic dysfunction: 100% if bilirubin ≤1.2; 50% if bilirubin 1.2–3.0; 25% if bilirubin >3.0.	Myelosuppression; mucositis; nausea/vomiting; alopecia; cumulative cardiac toxicity; dose-related acute ECG changes; severe tissue damage (extravasated)
Doxorubicin, liposomal (Doxil)[105] Inj: 20 mg SDV	Antitumor antibiotic; intercalates into DNA double helix; topoisomerase II–mediated DNA damage; produces oxygen-free radicals.		↓ if hepatic dysfunction 50% if bilirubin 2.0–3.0; 25% if bilirubin ≥3.	

Drug	Mechanism	Pharmacokinetics	Dose Adjustment	Toxicity
Estramustine (Emcyt)[106,107] Cap: 140 mg	Endocrine therapy and alkylating agent; probably impairs mitotic spindle formation.	Milk ↓ absorption; readily dephosphorylated absorption to estradiol and estrone congeners.		Estrogenic effects; cardiovascular (edema, thrombophlebitis, pulmonary embolus); nausea/vomiting; diarrhea; gynecomastia; mild ↑ LFT
Etoposide (VePesid)[108–114] Inj: 100 mg/5 mL Cap: 50 mg	Epipodophyllotoxin; produces DNA strand breaks by inhibiting topoisomerase II; arrests cells in late S or early G_2 phase.	Oral bioavailability 37–67% (average 50%); 30–40% excreted rapidly in the urine (70% of excreted drug is unchanged); terminal $t_{1/2}$ = 6–8 hr; <2% excreted in bile; <2% excreted in feces.		Myelosuppression; nausea/vomiting; alopecia; mucositis; hypotension (related to rapid-infusion); hypersensitivity reactions; fever; bronchospasm
Floxuridine (FUDR)[115–117] Inj: 500 mg/vial	Antimetabolite; incorporates into RNA and interferes with RNA function; inhibits thymidylate synthase and inhibits DNA synthesis.	$t_{1/2}$ = 20 min; >90% hepatically metabolized.	Adjustments are made depending on clinical hematologic and GI toxicity.	Mucositis; myelosuppression; nausea/vomiting; diarrhea; skin changes
Fludarabine (Fludara IV)[118–121] Inj: 50 mg/vial	Antimetabolite; inhibits ribonucleotide reductase and DNA polymerase causing inhibition DNA synthesis.	Undergoes rapid dephosphorylation to F-ara-A; terminal $t_{1/2}$ F-ara-A 8 hr; terminal $t_{1/2}$ F-ara-ATP 15 hr.	↓ if renal dysfunction in proportion to ↓ in CL_{Cr}.	Myelosuppression; neurotoxicity; peripheral neuropathy; pulmonary toxicity; nausea/vomiting
Fluorouracil[122,123] Inj: 500 mg/vial	Antimetabolite; incorporates into RNA interferes with RNA function.	$t_{1/2}$ = 6–20 min; ≥90% hepatically metabolized.		Mucositis; myelosuppression; nausea/vomiting; diarrhea; dermatologic
Gemcitabine (Gemzar)[124] Inj: 200 mg/vial or 1,000 mg/10 mL	Antimetabolite; inhibits ribonucleotide synthesis reductase and inhibits DNA synthesis.	Parameters dependent on infusion; $t_{1/2}$ = 32–94 min or 245–638 min; V = 50 L/m² or 370 L/m².	Adjustments are made depending on clinical, hematologic, and GI toxicity.	Bone marrow suppression; elevated LFT; protein or blood in urine, diarrhea; alopecia
Hydroxyurea (Hydrea)[125] Cap: 500 mg	Antimetabolite; inhibits ribonucleotide reductase and inhibits DNA synthesis.	T_{max} = 2 hr; 80% excreted in urine in 12 hr.		Bone marrow suppression; stomatitis; nausea/vomiting; diarrhea; rash
Idarubicin (Idamycin)[126–130] Inj: 5, 10 mg/vial	Antitumor antibiotic; intercalates into DNA double helix; topoisomerase II–mediated DNA damage; produces oxygen-free radicals.	Terminal $t_{1/2}$ = 15–18 hr.		Myelosuppression; mucositis; anorexia; nausea/vomiting; diarrhea; fever; alopecia

(continued)

Table 84.11 • Clinical Pharmacology of Chemotherapy Agents ^{a} **(continued)**

Agents	Mechanism of Action	Pharmacokinetic Characteristics	Dosage Adjustment for Organ Dysfunction	Major Toxicities
Irinotecan (Camptostar)[131] Inj: 20 mg/mL	Campthothecin; inhibits DNA-strand religation by binding topoisomerase I-DNA complex.	$t_{1/2}$ = 6 hr, 36–68% protein bound.		Diarrhea; cholinergic syndrome
Isofamide (Ifex)[132–135] Inj: 1, 3 g/vial	Alkylating agent; metabolites generate reactive intermediates that cross-link DNA.	Parameters are dose and schedule dependent; 60–80% excreted in urine as unchanged drug or metabolite within 72 hr.	Adjustments may be necessary based on clinical response.	Myelopsuppression; hemorrhagic cystitis (should be administered with MESNA); nephrotoxicity; neurotoxicity; anorexia; nausea/vomiting; alopecia
Lomustine (CeeNu)[136–138] Cap: 10, 40, 100 mg	Nonclassic alkylating agent; metabolites generate reactive intermediates that cross-link DNA.	Well absorbed orally; $t_{1/2}$ of metabolites = 16–48 hr; 50% metabolites excreted in urine within 24 hr.	↓ may be required for patients with ↓ bone marrow reserves.	Myelosuppression; nausea/vomiting; nephrotoxicity; pulmonary infiltrates/fibrosis; hepatotoxicity
Mechlorethamine (Mustargen)[139,140]	Alkylating agent; forms reactive intermediates that cross-link DNA.	Rapid metabolism; <0.01% unchanged drug excreted in urine; 50% of metabolites excreted in urine within 24 hr.		Myelosuppression; nausea/vomiting; sterility, menstrual irregularities; local irritant/vesicant (if extravasated)
Melphalan (Alkeran)[141–144] Tab: 2 mg Inj: 50 mg/vial	Alkylating agent; forms intermediates that cross-link DNA.	Oral absorption erratic and incomplete (≈30%); not actively metabolized but spontaneous chemical degradation; $t_{1/2}$ = 90 min; 10–15% excreted in urine within 24 hr.	↓ if renal dysfunction: 50% dose for BUN >30 mg/dL or creatinine >1.5 mg/dL.	Myelosuppression; pulmonary fibrosis
Mercaptopurine (Purinethol)[145,146] Tab: 50 mg	Antimetabolite; metabolites incorporate into DNA or RNA and inhibit purine synthesis.	Oral absorption highly variable; $t_{1/2}$ = 20–60 min; elimination primarily hepatic.	↓ if hepatic or renal dysfunction.	Myelosuppression; anorexia, nausea, vomiting; hepatic toxicity (biliary stasis)
Methotrexate[147–152] Tab: 2.5 mg Inj: 25, 50, 100, 200, 250, 1,000 mg/vial	Antifolate; inhibits dihydrofolate reductase and depletes reduced folates and inhibits DNA synthesis.	Oral absorption appears to be better with smaller doses; exhibits interpatient bioavailability; "third space" collections of fluid may provide a reservoir for drug accumulation; $t_{1/2\alpha}$ = 1.5–3.5 hr; $t_{1/2\beta}$ = 8–15 hr; 90% dose excreted in urine within 24 hr.	↓ or discontinue if renal dysfunction; monitor serum methotrexate levels with ↓ renal function or fluid accumulation.	Myelosuppression; nephrotoxicity; hepatotoxicity; mucositis, pulmonary toxicity; neurotoxicity

Drug	Mechanism	Pharmacokinetics	Dosage adjustment	Toxicity
Mitoxantrone (Novatrone)[153–159] Inj: 20, 25, 30 mg/vial	Antitumor antibiotic; intercalates into DNA double helix; topoisomerase II–mediated DNA damage; produces oxygen-free radicals.	$t_{1/2\alpha} = 10$ min, $t_{1/2\beta} = 6$ hr; $t_{1/2\gamma} = 2$ days; <10% excreted in the urine.		Myelosuppression; cumulative cardiac toxicity (total dose >100 mg); ↑ risk with prior anthracycline therapy; nausea/vomiting; mild stomatitis
Paclitaxel (Taxol)[160–164] Inj: 30 mg/vial	Taxane; promotes microtubule assembly and arrests cell cycle in G_2 and M phases.	<10% excreted in urine; liver and biliary primary routes of elimination; $t_{1/2\alpha} = 0.3$ hr; $t_{1/2\beta} = 1.3$–8.6 hr.	↓ for severe neutropenia (following prior therapy), severe peripheral neuropathy or hepatic dysfunction.	Hypersensitivity reactions (premedications recommended); cardiac disturbances; sensory neuropathy; myalgia; arthralgia
Pentostatin (Nipent)[165–167] Inj: 10 mg/vial	Antimetabolite; inhibits adenosine deaminase and subsequent DNA and RNA synthesis.	90% excreted in urine; $t_{1/2\alpha} = 11$–85 min; $t_{1/2\beta} = 5$–15 hr (longer in patients with ↓ renal function).	↓ for renal dysfunction: $Cl_{CR} < 60$ mL/min.	Myelosuppression; immunosuppression; lethargy; seizures; conjunctivitis; rash; nausea/vomiting; renal dysfunction (rare)
Procarbazine (Matulane)[168–170] Cap: 50 mg	Nonclassic alkylating agent; prodrug metabolite causes methylation of nucleic acids; causes direct DNA damage and inhibits purine synthesis.	Oral dose well absorbed; 70% excreted in urine as active metabolite.	↓ for renal dysfunction: SrCr >2.0 or bilirubin >3.0.	Myelosuppression; nausea/vomiting; neurotoxicity; sterility; pulmonary hypersensitivity; ↑ with drugs metabolized by phase I enzymes, sympathomimetic drugs, and tyramine-rich foods; disulfiram-like reaction with alcohol
Rituximab (Rituxan)[171] Inj: 10 mg/mL 100 mg, 500 mg	Monoclonal antibody; lyses B cells by recruiting immune effectors.	$t_{1/2}$ variable.		Tumor lysis; hypersensitivity reactions
Streptozocin (Zanosar)[172–174] Inj: 1,000 mg/vial	Alkylating agent; forms reactive intermediate that cross-links DNA.	$t_{1/2\alpha} = 5$–15 min; $t_{1/2\beta} = 35$ min; 60–72% excreted in urine within 4 hr.	↓ may be required in patients with renal dysfunction.	Renal toxicity-dose related; nausea/vomiting; myelosuppression; abnormal glucose tolerance; hepatotoxicity
Teniposide (Vumon)[175–177] Inj: 50 mg/ampule	Epipodophyllotoxin; produces DNA strand breaks by inhibiting topoisomerase II; arrests cells in late S or early G_2 phases.	4–12% excreted in urine; terminal $t_{1/2} = 6$–10 hr; ↑ hepatic enzymes correlate with ↓ clearance.	Adjustments may be necessary for hepatic dysfunction.	Myelosuppression; hypotension; nausea, vomiting; secondary leukemia

(continued)

Table 84.11 • Clinical Pharmacology of Chemotherapy Agents^a *(continued)*

Agents	Mechanism of Action	Pharmacokinetic Characteristics	Dosage Adjustment for Organ Dysfunction	Major Toxicities
Thioguanine[145,178] Tab: 40 mg	Antimetabolite; interrupts purine synthesis and inhibits RNA and DNA synthesis.	Oral absorption incomplete and ↓ with food; clearance is mainly hepatic with methylation of parent drug to inactive metabolites; $t_{1/2\alpha}$ = 15 min; $t_{1/2\beta}$ = 11 hr.	No adjustment necessary.	Myelosuppression; stomatitis; hepatotoxicity (↑ alkaline phosphatase and ↑ direct bilirubin); nausea/vomiting
Thiotepa[54,66,179] Inj: 15 mg/vial	Alkylating agent; forms reactive intermediates that cross-link DNA.	Metabolized to TEPA; 15% of TEPA excreted in urine within 24 hr; $t_{1/2\alpha}$ = 7.5 min; $t_{1/2\beta}$ = 109 min.	↓ may be required for patients with ↓ bone marrow reserve.	Myelosuppression; nausea/vomiting
Topotecan (Hycamtin)[180] Inj: 10 mg/mL	Camptothecin; inhibits DNA-strand religation by binding topoisomerase I-DNA complex.	$t_{1/2}$ = 2–3 hr; 35% protein bound; 30% excreted in urine.	↓ renal dysfunction: 0.75 mg/m^2 if Cl$_{CR}$ 20–39 mL/min.	Bone marrow suppression; nausea/vomiting; diarrhea; alopecia
Trastuzamab (Herceptin)[181] Inj: 440 mg/30 mL	Monoclonal antibody; inhibits proliferation of human tumor cells that express HER2 proto-oncogene.	$t_{1/2}$ = 5.8 hr; Vd = 44 mL/kg.		Cardiomyopathy; diarrhea; nausea/vomiting hypersensitivity reaction
Vinblastine (Velban)[54,182–185] Inj: 10 mg/vial	Vinca alkaloid; reversibly inhibits mitosis; binds to microtubule protein and tubulin and ultimately inhibits formation.	Primarily metabolized and excreted in bile; 10% excreted in feces; $t_{1/2\alpha}$ = 4.5 min.	↓ if hepatic dysfunction: >50% if bilirubin >3.0.	Myelosuppression; neurotoxicity (rare); vesicant (if extravasated)
Vincristine (Oncovin)[54,184–187] Inj: 1, 2, 5 mg/vial; 2-mg prefilled syringe	Vinca alkaloid; reversibly inhibits mitosis; binds to microtubule protein and tubulin and ultimately inhibiting formation of mitotic spindles.	$t_{1/2\alpha}$ = <1 min; $t_{1/2\beta}$ = 7.4 min; $t_{1/2\gamma}$ = 164 min.		Neurotoxicity (primarily distal neuropathy that affects sensory and motor abilities); autonomic neuropathies (high dosages); SIADH; vesicant (if extravasated)
Vinorelbine (Navelbine)[188–191]	Vinca alkaloid; reversibly inhibits mitosis; binds to microtubule protein and tubulin and ultimately inhibits formation of mitotic spindles.	<20% excreted in urine; $t_{1/2\alpha}$ = 2–6 min; $t_{1/2\beta}$ = 1.9 hr.		Leukopenia; neurotoxicity; ↓ DTR; vesicant (if extravasated)

^{a}BUN = Blood urea nitrogen; Cl$_{CR}$ = Creatinine clearance; CSF = Cerebrospinal fluid; DTR = Deep tendon reflexes; GI = Gastrointestinal; LFT = Liver function tests; PT = Prothrombin time; PPT = Partial thromboplastin time; SIADH = Syndrome of inappropriate antidiuretic hormone secretion; SrCr = Serum creatinine; $t_{1/2\alpha}$ = α half-life; $t_{1/2\beta}$ = β half-life; $t_{1/2\gamma}$ = γ half-life.

Table 84.12 • Possible Mechanisms of Anticancer Drug Resistance

Mechanism	Chemotherapy Agents
Improved proficiency in repair of DNA	Cisplatin, cyclophosphamide, melphalan, mitomycin, mechlorethamine
↓ in drug activation	Cytarabine, doxorubicin, fluorouracil mercaptopurine, methotrexate, thioguanine
↑ in drug inactivation	Cytarabine, mercaptopurine
↓ in cellular uptake of drug	Methotrexate, melphalan
↑ in efflux of drug (multidrug resistance)	Doxorubicin, daunorubicin, etoposide, vincristine, vinblastine, teniposide, docetaxel, paclitaxel, vinorelbine
Alternative biochemical pathways	Cytarabine, fluorouracil, methotrexate
Alterations in target enzymes (DHFR, topoisomerase II)	Fluorouracil, hydroxyurea, mercaptopurine, methotrexate, thioguanine, etoposide, teniposide, doxorubicin, daunorubicin, idarubicin

Notes:

Table 84.13 • Commonly Used Chemotherapy Regimens[a,b]

Acronym	Agents	Dose/Schedule	Cycle
Breast Cancer			
CMF	Cyclophosphamide[211]	100 mg/m^2 PO days 1–14	Q 28 days
	Methotrexate	40–60 mg/m^2 IV days 1 and 8	
	Fluorouracil	600 mg/m^2 IV days 1 and 8	
Herceptin-tax	Herceptin[212]	4 mg/kg IV week 1, then 2 mg/kg IV Q wk	Q 21 days
	Paclitaxel	175 mg/m^2 IV over 3 hr day 1	
CAF	Cyclophosphamide[213]	100 mg/m^2 PO days 1–14	Q 28 days
	Doxorubicin (Adriamycin)	30–50 mg/m^2 IV days 1 and 8	
	Fluorouracil	500 mg/m^2 IV days 1 and 8	
	or		
	Cyclophosphamide[214]	400 mg/m^2 IV day 1	Q 21 days
	Doxorubicin (Adriamycin)	40 mg/m^2 IV day 1	
	Fluorouracil	400 mg/m^2 IV day 1	
	or		
	Cyclophosphamide[215]	500 mg/m^2 IV day 1	Q 21 days
	Doxorubicin (Adriamycin)	50 mg/m^2 IV day 1	
	Fluorouracil	500 mg/m^2 IV day 1	
AC	Doxorubicin (Adriamycin)[216,217]	60 mg/m^2 day 1	Q 21 days
	Cyclophosphamide	400–600 mg/m^2 day 1	
Colorectal Cancer			
5-FU	Fluorouracil[218]	500 mg/m^2/day IVP days 1–5	Q 5 wk
FU/leucovorin	Fluorouracil[218]	370 mg/m^2/day IVP days 1–5	Q 28 days × 2, then Q 35 days
	Leucovorin	20 mg/m^2/days 1–5 immediately following by FU	
	or		
	Fluorouracil[219]	600 mg/m^2 IVP at 1 hr after starting leucovorin infusion	Q wk × 6 wk
	Leucovorin	500 mg/m^2 IV over 2 hr	
	or		
	Fluorouracil[220]	435 mg/m^2 IVP days 1–5	Q 4–5 wk
	Leucovorin	20 mg/m^2 IVP days 1–5	
FU/levamisole	Fluorouracil[221]	450 mg/m^2/day IVP days 1–5; then beginning day 29, 450 mg/m^2 Q wk for 1 yr	Q 4–5 wk
	Levamisole	50 mg/m^2 PO Q 8 hr × 3 days Q 2 wk for 1 yr	

Gastric Cancer

FAM
- Fluorouracil[222] — 600 mg/m² IV days 1, 8, 29, and 36
- Doxorubicin (Adriamycin) — 30 mg/m² IV days 1 and 29
- Mitomycin — 10 mg/m² IV day 1
— Q 8 wk

EAP
- Etoposide[223] — 120 mg/m² IV days 4, 5, and 6
- Doxorubicin (Adriamycin) — 20 mg/m² IV days 1 and 7
- Cisplatin — 40 mg/m² IV days 2 and 8
— Q 21–28 days

Pancreatic Cancer

FAM
- Fluorouracil[222] — 600 mg/m² IV days 1, 8, 29, and 36
- Doxorubicin (Adriamycin) — 30 mg/m² IV days 1 and 29
- Methotrexate — 10 mg/m² IV day 1
— Q 8 wk

CF
- Fluorouracil[224] — 300 mg/m² CIV for 10 wk
- Cisplatin — 20 mg/m² IV Q wk for 10 wk
— Q 12 wk

Ovarian Cancer

CP
- Cyclophosphamide[225] — 1000 mg/m² IV day 1
- Cisplatin — 50 mg/m² IV day 1
— Q 21 days

CT
- Paclitaxel[226] — 135 mg/m² IV over 3 or 24 hr day 1
- Cisplatin — 75 mg/m² IV
— Q 21 days

Carbo-tax
- Paclitaxel[227] — 135 mg/m² IV over 24 hr or 175 mg/m² over 3 hr, day 1
- Carboplatin — Targeted by Calvert equation to AUC 7.5 IV
— Q 21 days

Testicular Cancer

BEP
- Bleomycin[228] — 30 units IV days 2, 9, and 16
- Etoposide — 100 mg/m² IV days 1–5 IV
- Cisplatin — 20 mg/m² IV days 1–5
— Q 21 days

EP
- Etoposide[229] — 100 mg/m² IV day 1–5
- Cisplatin — 20 mg/m² IV days 1–5
— Q 21 days

Bladder Cancer

M-VAC
- Methotrexate[230] — 30 mg/m² IV days 1, 15, and 22
- Vinblastine — 3 mg/m² IV days 2, 15, and 22
- Adriamycin (Doxorubicin) — 30 mg/m² IV day 2
— Q 28 days

PC
- Paclitaxel[231] — 200 mg/m² over 3 hr day 1
- Carboplatin — Targeted by Calvert equation to AUC 5.0 after paclitaxel day 1
— Q 21 days

(continued)

Table 84.13 • Commonly Used Chemotherapy Regimens[a,b] (continued)

Acronym	Agents	Dose/Schedule	Cycle
Small Cell Lung Cancer			
EP or PE	Cisplatin[232]	25 mg/m^2/day IV days 1–3	Q 21–28 days
	Etoposide	100 mg/m^2/day IV days 1–3 + radiation therapy	
Non-Small Cell Lung Cancer			
EP or PE	Cisplatin[233]	100 mg/m^2 IV day 1	Q 21 days
	Etoposide	80 mg/m^2 IV days 1–3	
	or		
	Cisplatin[234]	60 mg/m^2 IV day 1	Q 21–28 days
	Etoposide	120 mg/m^2 IV days 4, 6, and 8	
Carbo-tax	Paclitaxel[232]	135 mg/m^2 IV over 24 hr or 175 mg/m^2 over 3 hr, day 1	Q 21 days
	Carboplatin	Targeted by Calvert equation to AUC 7.5 IV	
EC	Etoposide[235,236]	100–120 mg/m^2 IV days 1–3	Q 21–28 days
	Carboplatin	300–325 mg/m^2 IV day 1	
Gemcitabine-Cis	Gemcitabine[237,238]	1,000 mg/m^2 IV days 1, 8, and 15	Q 28 days
	Cisplatin	100 mg/m^2 IV days 2 or 15	
Head and Neck Cancer			
CF	Cisplatin[239]	100 mg/m^2 IV day 1	Q 21–28 days
	Fluorouracil	1,000 mg/m^2/day CI days 1–5	
Lymphomas			
Non-Hodgkin's Lymphomas			
CHOP	Cyclophosphamide[240]	750 mg/m^2 IV day 1	Q 21 days
	Doxorubicin (Hydroxyl Daunorubicin)	50 mg/m^2 IV day 1	
	Vincristine (Oncovin)	2 mg IV days 1 and 5	
	Prednisone	100 mg/m^2/day PO days 1–5	
m-BACOD	Methotrexate[241]	200 mg/m^2 IV with leucovorin rescue days 8 and 15	Q 21 days
	Bleomycin	4 mg/m^2 IV day 1	
	Doxorubicin (Adriamycin)	45 mg/m^2 IV day 1	
	Cyclophosphamide	600 mg/m^2 IV day 1	
	Vincristine (Oncovin)	1 mg/m^2 IV day 1	
	Dexamethasone	6 mg/m^2 PO days 1–5	

Non-Hodgkin's Lymphomas

MACOP-B	Methotrexate[242]	400 mg/m² IV weeks 2, 6, and 10	Only 1 cycle
	Doxorubicin (Adriamycin)	50 mg/m² IV weeks 1, 3, 5, 7, 9, and 11	
	Cyclophosphamide	350 mg/m² IV weeks 1, 3, 5, 7, 9, and 11	
	Vincristine (Oncovin)	1.4 mg/m² IV weeks 2, 4, 6, 8, 10, and 12	
	Prednisone	75 mg/m² PO daily, tapered over the last 15 days	
	Bleomycin	10 U/m² IV weeks 4, 8, and 12	
ESHAP	Etoposide[243,244]	60 mg/m² IV days 1–4	Q 21–28 days
	Methylprednisolone	500 mg IV days 1–4	
	Cisplatin	25 mg/m²/day CI days 1–4	
	Cytarabine	2,000 mg/m² IV day 5 immediately following completion of etoposide and cisplatin	

Hodgkin's Disease

MOPP	Mechlorethamine[245]	6 mg/m² IV days 1 and 8	Q 28 days
	Vincristine (Oncovin)	1.4 mg/m² IV days 1 and 8	
	Prednisone	40 mg/m² PO days 1–14, cycles 1 and 4	
	Procarbazine	100 mg/m² PO days 1–14	
ABVD	Doxorubicin (Adriamycin)[246]	25 mg/m² IV days 1 and 15	Q 28 days
	Bleomycin	10 mg/m² IV days 1 and 15	
	Vinblastine	6 mg/m² IV days 1 and 15	
	Dacarbazine	375 mg/m² IV days 1 and 15	

Multiple Myeloma

VAD	Vincristine[247]	0.4 mg/m²/day CIV days 1–4	Q 28 days
	Doxorubicin (Adriamycin)	9 mg/m²/day CIV days 1–4	
	Dexamethasone	40 mg/m² PO days 1–4, 9–12, and 17–20	
MP	Melphalan[248]	0.25 mg/kg/day PO days 1–4	Q 42 days
	Prednisone	2 mg/kg/day PO days 1–4	

aCIV = Continuous intravenous infusion; IV = Intravenous; IVP = Intravenous push; PO = Oral.
bOriginal citations should be consulted for dosage adjustments due to toxicity.

Table 84.14 • Tumors That Respond to Chemotherapy

Advanced Tumors That Can Be Cured with Chemotherapy

Choriocarcinoma	Wilms' tumor
Acute lymphocytic leukemia	Embryonal rhabdomyosarcoma
Testicular cancer	Peripheral neuroepithelioma
Acute myelogenous leukemia	Neuroblastoma
Hodgkin's disease	Small cell lung cancer (limited stage)
Non-Hodgkin's lymphoma (especially high-grade lymphomas)	Hairy cell leukemia

Chemotherapy Used as Adjuvant Therapy with Curative Intent

Breast cancer (stages I and II)	Wilms' tumor
Colorectal cancer (stages III and IV)	Osteosarcoma
Ewing's sarcoma	Ovarian cancer

Chemotherapy Used as Neoadjuvant Therapy with Potential Curative Intent

Soft-tissue sarcoma	Head and neck cancer
Anal cancer	Non–small cell lung cancer (stage III$_A$)
Breast cancer (locally advanced)	Osteosarcoma
Esophageal cancer	Bladder cancer
Cervical cancer	Cervical cancer

Advanced Tumors in Which Chemotherapy May Prolong Survival or Palliate Symptoms

Bladder cancer	Endometrial cancer
Chronic myelogenous leukemia	Adrenocortical carcinoma
Multiple myeloma	Medulloblastoma
Gastric carcinoma	Prostate cancer
Cervical carcinoma	Insulinoma
Soft-tissue sarcoma	Breast cancer
Head and neck cancer	Colorectal cancer
Osteogenic sarcoma	Non–small cell cancer
Pancreatic cancer	Melanoma

Table 84.15 • Local/Regional Routes of Administration of Cancer Chemotherapy

Route of Administration	Cancer Managed with Alternative Route
Intrathecal/intraventricular	Leukemia, lymphoma
Intravesicular	Bladder cancer
Intraperitoneal	Ovarian cancer
Intrapleural	Malignant pleural effusions
Intra-arterial	
hepatic artery	Liver metastases
Chemoembolization (intra-arterial or intravenous)	Colon cancer, rectal cancer, carcinoid, liver metastases

Notes:

Table 84.16 • Response Criteria Used for Evaluating Effects of Chemotherapy

Complete Response
Disappearance of all clinical evidence of active disease for at least 4 weeks. No new lesions may appear during this period.

Partial Response
>50% reduction in the sum of the products of two perpendicular diameters of all measured tumors for at least 4 weeks. No tumor or metastasis may show progression and no new lesions may appear.

Stable Disease
<50% reduction or 25% ↑ in the sum of the product of two perpendicular diameters of all measured lesions; no appearance of new lesions; and no deterioration of the performance status for a minimum of 4 weeks.

Disease Progression
Reappearance of a lesion after complete response, appearance of any new lesions or an ↑ of ≥25% in the product of the two perpendicular diameters of any measurable lesion.

Disease-Free Survival
Time from documentation of complete response until disease relapse or death.

Overall Survival
Time from treatment until time of death.

Table 84.17 • Clinically Useful Tumor Markers

Tumor Marker	Cancers Commonly Associated with Increased Markers
CA-19-9	Colon, rectal
CA-15-3	Breast
CA-27-29	Breast
Neuron-specific enolase	Neuroblastoma, small cell lung cancer
α-Fetoprotein	Liver
CA-125	Ovarian, testicular—nonseminoma
Carcinoembryonic antigen	Colon, lung
Human chorionic gonadotropin	Trophoblastic, testicular
β_2-Microglobulin	Multiple myeloma
Prostate-specific antigen	Prostate

Notes:

Table 84.18 • Endocrine Therapy Used for Hormone-Sensitive Tumors

Class	Drug	Dosage	Side Effects	Indication
Antiestrogens	Tamoxifen Toremifene	10–20 mg PO BID 60 mg PO QD	Disease flare, hot flashes, nausea, vomiting, edema, thromboembolism, endometrial cancer	Breast
LHRH analogs	Leuprolide Goserelin	7.5 mg SC Q 28 days 3.6 mg SC Q 28 days	Amenorrhea, hot flashes, occasional nausea	Breast, prostate
Progestins	Medroxyprogesterone acetate Megestrol acetate	400–1,000 mg IM Q wk	Weight gain, hot flashes, vaginal bleeding, edema, thromboembolism	Breast, prostate, anorexia
Aromatase inhibitors	Anastrazole Letrozole Aminoglutethimide	1 mg PO QD 2.5 mg PO QD 250 mg PO QID with hydrocortisone 40 mg PO QD	Lethargy, rash, postural dizziness, ataxia, nystagmus, nausea	Breast, prostate
Estrogens	Ethynylestradiol Conjugated estrogens	1 mg PO TID 2.5 mg PO TID	Nausea/vomiting, fluid retention, hot flashes, anorexia, thromboembolism, hepatic dysfunction	Breast, prostate
Androgens	Fluoxymesterone	10 mg PO BID	Deepening voice, alopecia, hirsutism, facial/truncal acne, fluid retention, menstrual irregularities, cholestatic jaundice	Breast
Antiandrogens	Bicalutamide Flutamide Nilutamide	50 mg PO QD 750 mg PO QD 300 mg PO QD × 1 mo, then 150 mg PO QD	Gynecomastia, hot flashes, diarrhea, breast tenderness, hepatic dysfunction	Prostate

Table 84.19 • Factors That May Increase the Risk of Medication Errors Involving Chemotherapy

Contributing Factor	Recommendation
Verbal orders	Do not accept; accept only written signed orders. If not possible have two health professionals accept verbal orders, have written policy regarding verbal orders.
Multiple-day drug courses (e.g., etoposide 50 mg/m² × 5)	Use standardized order forms or format. Order should clearly state total dose to be administered each day and actual dates of administration (e.g., etoposide 50 mg/m²/day = 100 mg per day on 3/1, 3/2, 3/3, 3/4, and 3/5/00). Orders should also explicitly state infusion guidelines, other specific instructions (e.g., administer 30 min after antiemetic), and other pertinent patient information such as body surface area, weight, height, and age.
Trailing zeros following decimal points (example, 50.0 mg) or the decimal point may be lost or overlooked on carbon or fax copies	Do not permit trailing zeros. Leading zeros before decimal points should be required (example, 0.5 mg) so that the decimal point will not be overlooked.
Orders written by prescribers unfamiliar with chemotherapy	Require orders to be written by appropriately credentialed practitioners.
Use of abbreviations	Only approved generic names should be used when ordering chemotherapy or documenting regimens in patient records
Wide variability in chemotherapy doses that may be appropriate for different disease states or combinations	Educate all practitioners involved in the chemotherapy use process (physicians, nurses, pharmacists) regarding commonly used regimens and make printed or electronic resources to verify doses and regimens readily available. Institutional dosing guidelines are recommended.
Inappropriate interpretation of orders	Two pharmacists should verify orders at the point of entry and nurses should reverify prior to administration. All practitioners should be instructed to resolve all questions prior to dispensing or administration.
Labeling errors	Labels should be double-checked and include all pertinent information including route of administration. Syringe labels should be directly attached to the syringe.
Poor communication or confusion regarding chemotherapy	Written institutional policies and procedures should address every aspect of the chemotherapy use process, including ordering, preparing, dispensing, administration, and documentation.

Notes:

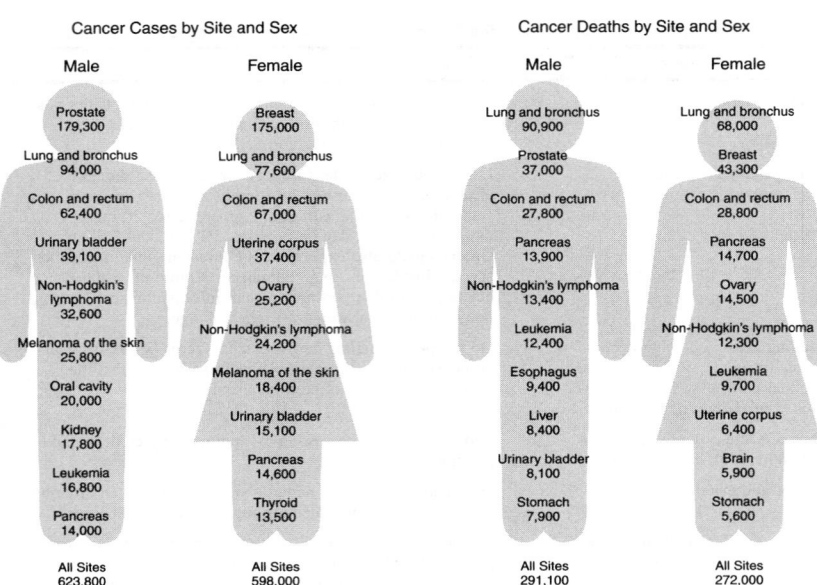

Fig. 84.1 Leading Sites of New Cancer Cases and Deaths. (Data from reference 1.)

Notes:

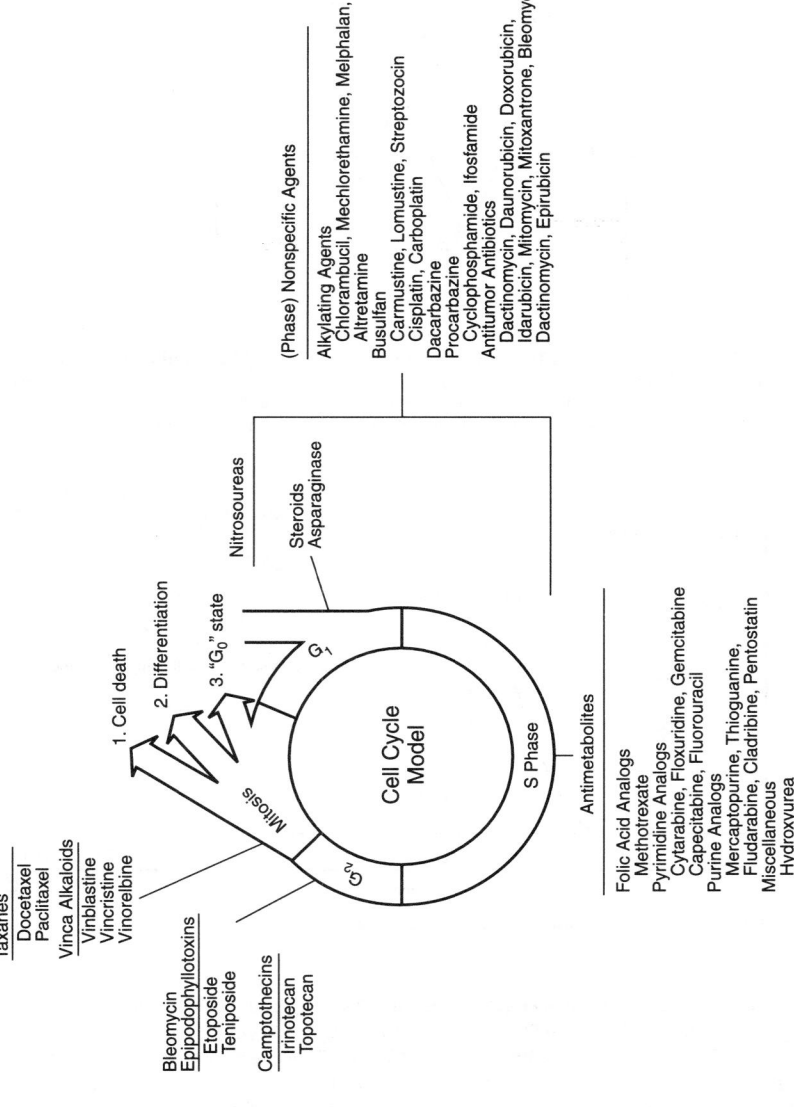

Fig. 84.2 Effect of Cytotoxic Chemotherapeutic Drugs on the Cell Cycle.

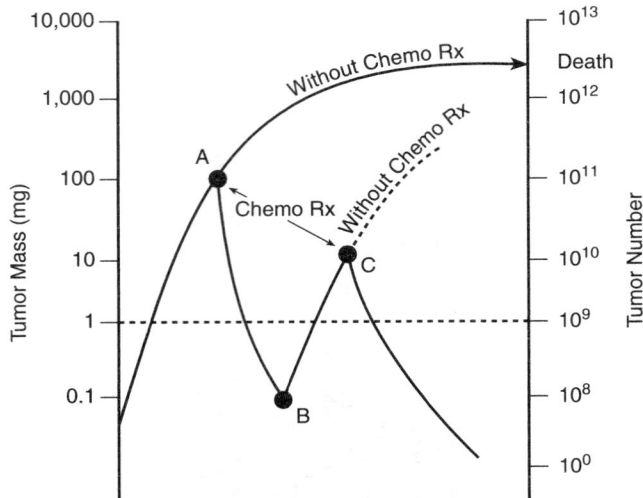

Fig. 84.3 The Growth Rate of a Tumor is Initially Very Rapid and Eventually Slows as It Approaches 10^{11} Cells. Two trillion (2×10^{12}) cells or 2 kg of tumor is lethal to humans. An effective chemotherapy treatment given at point A will decrease the tumor number to point B. Regrowth of the tumor will occur during the recovery period until further chemotherapy is given at point C.

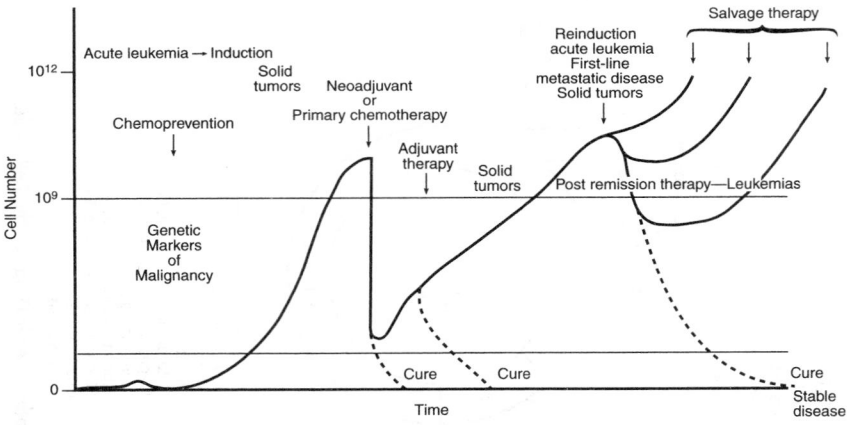

Fig. 84.4 Chemotherapy During Various Phases of Malignancy.

The reader is referred to Chapter 86: Neoplastic Disorders and Their Treatment: General Principles, written by *Celeste Lindley, Pharm.D., Stacy Shifflett Shord, Pharm. D.,* and *Rebecca S. Finley, Pharm.D.*, in the seventh edition of **Applied Therapeutics: The Clinical Use of Drugs** for a more in-depth discussion of the principles underlying chemotherapy, combination chemotherapy, the use of biologic response modifiers, and the handling of cytotoxic agents. All notations to reference numbers are based on the reference list at the end of that chapter. The editors of this handbook express their thanks to Drs. Lindley, Shifflett Shord, and Finley and acknowledge that this chapter is based upon their work.

Chapter 85

Adverse Effects of Chemotherapy

Inside . . .

Common and Acute Toxicities

♦ **Hematologic.** Bone marrow suppression used to be a dose-limiting toxicity of chemotherapy, but can now be ameliorated or prevented by colony-stimulating factors (CSFs). Factors that influence the degree of cytopenia include the chemotherapy agent used, dose intensity, schedule of administration, concurrent chemotherapy, patient age (older patients are more susceptible), bone marrow reserve, the patient's nutritional status, kidney function, and liver function. Cell-cycle phase-specific agents, such as the antimitotics and antimetabolites, produce fairly rapid cytopenia with faster recovery than agents that are cell-cycle phase-nonspecific, such as the alkylating agents and antitumor antibiotics. Also see Table 85.10.

- *Time Course.* The survival time of granulocytes in the periphery is 6 to 8 hours and that for platelets is about 10 days. Thus, granulocytopenia generally is more severe and occurs before thrombocytopenia. Both may be observed following a single course of chemotherapy. WBC and platelet counts begin to fall in 5 to 7 days; the nadir occurs in 7 to 10 days; and recovery is observed in 14 to 26 days. For unknown reasons, nitrosureas, mitomycin, and mechlorethamine produce a second delayed nadir at 4 to 6 weeks. Since RBCs survive 120 days in the periphery, brief impairment of RBC production does not cause significant anemia; it is observed after several courses of therapy. Time frames vary widely, and combination therapy can intensify effects.

- *Neutropenia.* Neutrophil counts <500–1000/mm^3 place patients at risk for life-threatening infections. The prophylactic administration of CSFs can protect against the myelosuppressive effects of chemotherapy. The American Society of Clinical Oncology (ASCO) recommends primary prophylaxis for all patients receiving chemotherapy regimens that have a ≥40% incidence of febrile neutropenia. G-CSF 5 µg/kg/day or GM-CSF 6 µg/kg/day rounded to the nearest vial size can be initiated the day after the last dose of chemotherapy and continued until the neutrophil count exceeds 2000 to 4000/mm^3 after the expected nadir. Whether CSFs are cost-beneficial in patients with established febrile neutropenia remains unsettled

- *Thrombocytopenia.* Platelet counts <20,000 can lead to bleeding, usually from the GI and GU tract. Oprelvekin (Neumega) is indicated to prevent severe thrombocytopenia and reduce the need for platelet transfusions following chemotherapy in patients with nonmyeloid malignancies. The dose is 50 mg/kg per day until the postnadir platelet count is >50,000/mm^3 or up to 21 days following chemotherapy. The cost benefit of oprelvekin versus platelet transfusions has not been demonstrated, since only 20% respond. Vaginal bleeding can be suppressed with uninterrupted birth control therapy.

- *Anemia.* Anemia is not the dose-limiting toxicity of chemotherapy, and chemotherapy is not the sole cause of anemia in a cancer patient. Because of its high cost, erythropoietin generally is reserved for patients who require blood transfusions to alleviate symptoms. The starting dose is 150 U/kg or a standard dose of 10,000 U (equivalent to the vial size) three times a week *or* 40,000 U once weekly. Continue for 4 weeks and increase the dose if the Hgb increases <1 gm/dL (300 U/kg three times weekly or 60,000 U once weekly). Up to 8 weeks of therapy may be required to see a response, and only 50% of patients respond. Discontinue if no response is seen in 8 to 12 weeks.

♦ **Gastrointestinal Toxicities**

- *Nausea and vomiting* are common. Emesis most commonly occurs on the first day of chemotherapy and often persists for several days thereafter. Most patients require antiemetics before chemotherapy and after for several days. See Chapter 5 and Table 85.10.

- *Complications of the oral cavity* occur in ≈40% of patients treated with chemotherapy and all patients who receive radiation. These include mucositis and stomatitis, xerostomia (dry mouth), infection (from neutropenia), and bleeding (from thrombocytopenia). See Tables 85.1 and 85.2.

- *Xerostomia.* In addition to dry mouth, patients lose ability to differentiate between sweet and salty foods and are at increased risk for caries. Amifostine (Ethyol), an organic thiophosphate chemoprotectant agent, is approved to reduce the incidence of moderate to severe xerostomia in patients undergoing postoperative radiation treatment for head and neck cancer. Xerostomia was reduced by about 30% in patients receiving 200 mg/m^2 as a 3-minute IV infusion 15 to 30 minutes before each fraction of radiation.

- *Mucositis and stomatitis* present as pain and burning of the buccal, labial, and soft palate mucosa along with the ventral surface of the tongue and floor of the mouth. Discrete lesions may be present initially but often progress to large areas of ulceration. Pain occurs in 5 to 7 days. Antimetabolites and antitumor antibiotics are directly toxic to the mucosa. It is difficult to prevent mucositis; treatment is palliative. See Table 85.2.

- *Esophagitis* is caused by damage to the mucosal lining and commonly presents as dysphagia. Follow treatment guidelines for mucositis, assure there is adequate fluid and nutritional intake, avoid acidic fluids, and consider proton pump inhibitors. Generally resolves I to 2 weeks after bone marrow recovery.

- *Lower GI complications* include malabsorption, diarrhea (irinotecan, high-dose cytarabine and 5-FU), and constipation (vinca alkaloids). Changes in small-bowel integrity may decrease drug absorption (e.g., phenytoin, verapamil, digoxin). Diarrhea should be treated promptly with loperamide and fluid and electrolyte replacement. Octreotide (Sandostatin) may be used for resistant cases.

♦ **Dermatologic Toxicities.** Inhibition of epidermal mitotic activity causes alopecia, nail changes, dry skin, and blistering. Other reactions result from altered epidermal response to UV light or radiation and vesicant properties. Several agents cause rashes. See Table 85.3.

- *Alopecia.* Hair loss begins 7 to 10 days after a single treatment and is prominent within 1 to 2 months. Beards, eyebrows, eyelashes, axillary and pubic hair are also affected. Regeneration begins 1 to 2 months after therapy is discontinued, but color and texture may be altered. Resources are available to help patients look and feel more comfortable with changes in appearance caused by chemotherapy. See Table 85.4.

- *Nail changes* are cosmetic in nature and resolve 6 to 12 months after therapy is completed. Nail growth is arrested causing pale horizontal lines (Beau's lines). Some agents cause brown or blue horizontal or vertical bands in the nails, especially in dark-skinned patients.

- *Pigment changes* are common, but poorly understood. Although hypopigmentation can occur, generalized hyperpigmentation is most common. Pigmentation localized to the mucous membrane, hair, or nails also can occur. This is primarily a cosmetic concern

- *Hand-foot syndrome* presents as tender, burning, tingling erythematous skin on the palms and soles. These symptoms may resolve or progress to bullous lesions.

- *Dry skin* may be caused by the cytostatic effect of chemotherapy on sebaceous and sweat glands. Treatment is with emollient creams.

- *Chemotherapy Interactions with Radiation and UV light.* Chemotherapy can interact with radiation or UV light to cause radiation enhancement reactions, radiation recall reactions, and photosensitivity reactions. See Table 85.5. Patients should be advised to wear protective clothing and sunscreens.

- *Local hypersensitivity reactions* are characterized by immediate local burning, itching, and erythema. Some patients also experience a "flare" reaction along the length of the vein used for treatment. Pretreatment with antihistamines may be needed.

- *Local irritant reactions and vesicant extravasations* may be difficult to differentiate initially and must always be treated as a potential extravasation. Infiltration of a vesicant can produce severe burning that lasts for several days or an asymptomatic period of days to weeks followed by redness and firmness that progresses to ulceration and necrosis. See Tables 85.6 to 85.9.

♦ **Hypersensitivity Reactions.** See Tables 85.11 and 85.12.

- Reactions often occur after the first dose, and most are mild (transient rash) or moderate (mild bronchospasm).

- Premedication with corticosteroids and antihistamines together with modified administration rates often allow safe readministration in most patients.

- Humanized monoclonal antibodies contain foreign proteins and cause more hypersensitivity reactions than traditional chemotherapy.

♦ **Grading Toxicities.** See Table 85.10.

Specific Organ Toxicities

♦ *Neurotoxicity*

- Chemotherapeutic agents associated with neurotoxicity are summarized in Table 85.13. Some are dose, route, and schedule-related, and symptoms can occur early or late. For each agent, symptoms are characteristic, and there may be associated risk factors.

♦ *Cardiac Toxicities*

- All anthracyclines (doxorubicin, daunorubicin, idarubicin, epirubicin, mitoxantrone) cause total dose-related *cardiomyopathy* that presents as congestive heart failure.

- Risk factors include total cumulative dose, mediastinal radiation therapy, preexisting cardiac disease, hypertension, and age (young children and older adults).

- The risk of CHF rises rapidly when the total dose of doxorubicin exceeds 550 mg/m^2 (0.1% to 50% probability).

- Prevention measures include lower total doses for patients at high risk, lower doses administered weekly or by prolonged continuous IV infusions (48 to 96 hours), careful monitoring using radionuclide ventriculography (RNV) and endomyocardial biopsy, and use of dexrazoxane.

- Dexrazoxane (Zinecard) is indicated to reduce the incidence and severity of cardiomyopathy associated with doxorubicin in women with metastatic breast cancer who have received a cumulative dose of 300 mg/m^2.

- *Electrocardiographic changes and non-life-threatening arrhythmias* also can be caused by anthracyclines and several other agents.

- Fluorouracil has been associated with angina pectoris and myocardial infarction; alkylating agents in high doses rarely cause myocardial necrosis; trastuzumab (Herceptin) can cause CHF, which is more likely when patients concurrently receive paclitaxel, cyclophosphamide, or doxorubicin.

♦ *Nephrotoxicity*

- *Cisplatin.* Nephrotoxicity is a major dose-limiting toxicity. Acute renal failure is now uncommon with the use of vigorous hydration, mannitol, and prophylactic magnesium; however, tubular dysfunction (which primarily presents as hypomagnesemia) and chronic renal toxicity (decreased GFR) remain problems. *Amiphostine* (Ethyol), an organic thiophosphate, is a chemoprotectant indicated to reduce the cumulative renal toxicity associated with repeated administration of cisplatin in patients with advanced ovarian cancer.

- *Proximal tubule dysfunction* also is caused by streptozocin, lomustine (CCNU), carmustine (BCNU), plicamycin, and ifosfamide. Changes in serum creatinine as well as acid and electrolyte imbalances suggest toxicity.

- *Hemolytic uremic syndrome* is often fatal and has been associated with several courses of mitomycin, carboplatin, and combination chemotherapy (bleomycin, cisplatin, and vincristine or bleomycin, cisplatin, and methotrexate). There is an abrupt onset of hemolytic anemia, elevated creatinine, increased fibrin degradation products, thrombocytopenia, and hypertension.

- *Acute tubular obstruction* has been associated with high-dose methotrexate if appropriate precautions (hydration and urine alkalinization) are not taken.

- *Hemorrhagic cystitis* is associated with ifosfamide and, to a lesser extent, cyclophosphamide. This can be prevented with forced hydration to wash out toxic metabolites and *mesna,* a uroprotective agent.

- *Dose adjustment* of chemotherapy in patients with decreased renal function is described in Table 85.14.

◆ Pulmonary Toxicities

- Several agents cause pulmonary toxicity, especially in patients with risk factors. Symptoms are often specific to the agent but include nonproductive cough, fever, dyspnea, tachypnea, and interstitial infiltrates on chest x-ray. Other treatable causes of pulmonary infiltrates (e.g., infection or disease progression) should be ruled out. See Tables 85.15 and 85.16.

◆ Hepatotoxicity

- Several drugs cause hepatocellular damage, but elevated LFTs are common in cancer patients and these must be considered. Routinely monitor serum transaminases, alkaline phosphatase, bilirubin, and serum levels of protein produced by the liver. If hepatotoxicity is suspected, withhold the drug until LFTs are within normal limits or substitute another drug that is not hepatotoxic. Drugs cleared predominantly by the liver may require dose adjustments. See Tables 85.17 to 85.19.

Long-Term Complications

◆ Secondary Malignancies

- *Acute nonlymphocytic leukemia* has been associated with chemotherapy used to treat hematological malignancies, solid tumors, and nonmalignant disease. The onset is about 3–4 years after therapy. Alkylating agents—especially melphalan—carry the greatest risk. Risk increases with large doses, continuous daily dosing, prolonged treatment, age >40 years, and concomitant radiation therapy. Regimens that include teniposide and etoposide also produce ANLL, but the onset is sooner.

- *Non-Hodgkins lymphoma* also is associated with chemotherapy.

◆ Fertility

- *Oogenesis.* Gonadal toxicity is most prominently caused by cyclophosphamide and other alkylating agents, doxorubicin, vinblastine, etoposide, and cisplatin. Permanent amenorrhea is both dose- and age-related. Prepubertal girls can sustain substantial doses without apparent effect.

- *Spermatogenesis.* The alkylating agents, in particular, can cause progressive dose-related reduction in the testicular volume and azoospermia. Recovery can occur in 2 to 3 years. Libido and sexual activity may decline during treatment but return to pretreatment levels.

- Cryopreservation of oocytes and sperm should be considered.

♦ *Teratogenicity*

- Men and women should be explicitly discouraged from conception during chemotherapy, and survivors should wait two or more years after completion of therapy before attempting to conceive. There is no evidence that spontaneous abortion, genetic disease, or congenital anomalies occur more frequently in the progeny of cancer survivors, nor is there increased risk of malignancy in offspring.

Notes:

Table 85.1 • Topical Medications for Oral Complications of Chemotherapy and/or Radiation Therapy

Problem	Products	Use
Xerostomia	Pilocarpine 5-mg tablet + Saliva substitutes and/or	1–2 tablets TID to QID Rinse or spray PRN
Mucositis	Sugar-free hard candy; sugar-free gum; ice chips	PRN
Generalized	Dyclonine HCL 0.5% or 1% solution or	Swish and expectorate 5–15 mL Q 2–3 hr PRN
	Viscous lidocaine 2% solution or	Swish and expectorate 5–15 mL Q 2–3 hr PRN
	Diphenhydramine capsules (125 mg) Dyclonine 1% 30 mL Nystatin 1 mL and ≤120 mL Maalox or	Swish and expectorate 5–15 mL Q 2–3 hr PRN
	Diphenhydramine + nystatin + hydrocortisone (various formulations) or	Swish and expectorate 5–15 mL Q 2–3 hr PRN
	Sucralfate suspension (8 tablets in 40 mL sterile water plus 40 mL 70% sorbitol; shake well and add water to 120 mL)	Swish and expectorate 5–15 mL Q 2–3 hr PRN
	Capsaicin candy[31]: Combine sugar, corn syrup, water, cornstarch, butter, and salt in 2-quart saucepan; cook over medium heat, stirring constantly to 256° on candy thermometer; remove from heat; stir in vanilla and cayenne pepper; pull taffy until light in color and stiff; pull into ½-inch long strip; cut with scissors into 1-inch pieces	Dissolve candy in mouth PRN
Localized	Benzocaine in orabase	Apply to affected dried area Q 2–3 hr; not to be used in the presence of an infection

(continued)

Table 85.1 • Topical Medications for Oral Complications of Chemotherapy and/or Radiation Therapy (continued)

Problem	Products	Use
Local bleeding (gingival)	Topical thrombin solution	Apply to affected area with gauze sponge and hold in place with pressure for 30 min; do not remove formed clots
	Aminocaproic acid	Swish and spit 250 mg Q 4 hr for up to 12 hr
Mucosal surface bleeding	Aminocaproic acid	Swish and spit 250 mg Q 4 hr for up to 12 hr
General infection	Chlorhexidine gluconate 0.12% oral rinse	Rinse BID after breakfast and at HS for 30 sec; do not swallow
Prevention and treatment of oral candidiasis	Nystatin oral suspension	Rinse and swallow (if tolerated) 500,000–1,000,000 units TID to QID
	or	
	Clotrimazole troche 10 mg	Dissolve 1 tablet 5 times/day
Prevention of caries	Acidulated fluoride rinse	Rinse daily for 1 min with 5–10 mL; do not swallow; switch to neutral fluoride if mucositis is present
	or	
	Neutral fluoride rinse	Rinse daily for 1 min with 5 mL; do not swallow; switch back to acidulated fluoride rinse when mucositis resolves
	or	
	Stannous fluoride gel 0.4%	Brush daily at HS; swish for 30 sec; spit out and rinse
	or	
	Sodium fluoride gel 1.1%	Brush daily at HS; swish for 30 sec; spit out and rinse

Table 85.2 • Guidelines for the Management of Stomatitis

1. Remove dentures to prevent further irritation and tissue damage.
2. Maintain gentle brushing of teeth with a soft toothbrush.
3. Avoid mouthwashes or rinses that contain alcohol because they may be painful and cause drying of the mucosa. Consider normal saline or sodium bicarbonate.
4. Lubricants, such as artificial saliva, may loosen mucus and prevent membranes from sticking together. Avoid mineral oil and petroleum jelly because they can be aspirated.
5. Apply local anesthetics for localized pain control, especially before meals (may add an antacid or an antihistamine). Systemic analgesics may be required to control pain associated with severe mucositis.
6. Ensure that adequate hydration and nutrition are maintained:
   - Eat a bland diet, avoiding spiced, acidic, and salted foods.
   - Avoid rough food; process in a blender if necessary.
   - Use sugar-free gum or sugar-free hard candy to stimulate salivation and facilitate mastication.
   - If necessary, provide intravenous support.
   - Avoid extremely hot or cold foods.
   - Use shakes with nutritional supplements or ice cream.

Table 85.3 • Single Agents Associated with Alopecia, Pigmentation Changes, and Nail Disorders

	Frequent	Occasional
Alopecia[a]	Cyclophosphamide	Mechlorethamine
	Ifosfamide	Thiotepa
	Fluorouracil	Methotrexate
	Dactinomycin	Vinblastine
	Daunorubicin	Vincristine
	Doxorubicin	Etoposide
	Bleomycin	Carmustine
	Vindesine	Hydroxyurea
	Paclitaxel	Cytarabine
	Irinotecan	Topotecan
	Epirubicin	Gemcitabine
	Docetaxel	
Pigmentation	Busulfan	Cyclophosphamide
	Fluorouracil	Methotrexate
	Doxorubicin	Dactinomycin
	Bleomycin	Daunorubicin
	Epirubicin	Hydroxyurea
		Ifosfamide
		Thiotepa
Nail		Cyclophosphamide
		Fluorouracil
		Daunorubicin
		Doxorubicin
		Bleomycin
		Hydroxyurea
		Epirubicin
		Docetaxel
		Paclitaxel

[a]Degree and onset of alopecia depend on dose, schedule of administration, rate and route of delivery, and various combinations of agents.

Notes:

Table 85.4 • Information and Toll-Free Hotlines for Cancer Support

Toll-Free Hotlines
- The American Cancer Society's (ACS) National Toll-Free Hotline: 800-ACS-2345
- The American College of Radiology (ACR): 800-648-8900
- The American Society of Plastic and Reconstructive Surgeons: 800-635-0635
- Breast Settlement Information Line: 800-887-6828
- The FDA Breast Implant Hotline: 800-532-4440
- National Bone Marrow Transplant Link: 800-546-5268
- The National Cancer Institute (NCI): 800-4-CANCER
- The National Cancer Information Service (NCI): 800-4-CANCER
- The National Consumer Insurance Helpline (HIAA): 800-942-4242
- The National Council Against Health Fraud: 800-821-6671
- The National Lymphedema Network: 800-541-3259
- PDQ (Physicians Data Query): 800-4-CANCER
- The Susan Komen Alliance Treatment and Information Line: 800-462-9273 [800-I'M AWARE]
- The Susan G. Komen Breast Cancer Foundation: 800-462-9273 [800-I'M AWARE]
- The Y-ME National Organization for Breast Cancer Information and Support's National Toll-free Hotline: 800-221-2141[a]

Organizations for Information and Support
- Cancer Care, Inc., and the National Cancer Care Foundation: 212-221-3300
- Cancer Research Council: 301-654-7933
- The Chemotherapy Foundation: 212-213-9292
- The Health Insurance Association of America (HIAA): 202-866-6244
- The National Alliance of Breast Cancer Organizations (NABCO): 212-719-0154
- The National Breast Cancer Coalition: 202-296-7477
- The National Coalition for Cancer Survivorship: 505-764-9956

[a]A support line for husbands.

Table 85.5 • Chemotherapy and Radiation Reactions

Radiation Enhancement Reactions

Bleomycin	Doxorubicin	Hydroxyurea
Dactinomycin	Fluorouracil	Methotrexate
Etoposide		

Radiation Recall Reactions
All of the above *plus*

Vinblastine	Epirubicin	Capecitabine
Etoposide	Paclitaxel	

Reactions with Ultraviolet Light
Phototoxic reactions

Dacarbazine	Thioguanine	Methotrexate
Fluorouracil	Vinblastine	Mitomycin

Reactivation of sunburn
Methotrexate

Notes:

Table 85.6 • Chemotherapeutic Drugs Reported to Produce Local Toxicities

Potential Vesicants

Dactinomycin	Plicamycin
Daunorubicin	Streptozocin
Doxorubicin	Vinblastine
Idarubicin	Vincristine
Mechlorethamine	Paclitaxel
Mitomycin	

Potential Irritants

Carmustine	Etoposide
Cisplatin	Mitoxantrone
Dacarbazine	Melphalan
Vinorelabine	Vindesine

Drugs That Produce Local Hypersensitivity Reactions

Daunorubicin	Mechlorethamine
Doxorubicin	Docetaxel
Idarubicin	

Table 85.7 • Guidelines for Administration of Cytotoxic Agents[89,90,92]

- Administration of chemotherapy should be performed only by persons familiar with its toxic effects.
- The site of infusion is selected with consideration of visualization of the vessel, its size, and potential damage if extravasation occurs in the following order of preference: forearm > dorsum of the hand > wrist > antecubital fossa.
  - Limbs with compromised circulation (e.g., invading neoplasm, axillary dissection, severe bruising) should not be used.
  - The lower extremities should not be used.
  - Pre-existing IV lines should not be used because the site may already have occult vein or tissue irritation or phlebitis.
- A 23- or 25-gauge scalp vein ("butterfly") needle is inserted into the vein. Only 1 venipuncture should be performed on a vein to avoid leakage.
- The wings of the needle should be lightly taped in place with care not to obscure the injection site so that it may be visualized during injection.
- Test the integrity of the IV line by injecting a small volume of saline solution and withdrawing a small amount of blood. If extravasation of the saline is obvious, select another vein or a site proximal on the same vein to avoid upstream leakage.
- Administer the drug at the recommended rate (preferably through the tubing of an IV running by gravity to assess for back pressure).
- During the administration, question the patient about discomfort, check for blood return by aspirating the syringe gently, observe the continuous flow of the running IV, and visualize the IV site frequently. If the patency of the line is in doubt at any time, the injection should be stopped and an alternate site selected.
- After administration, the IV line should be flushed with at least 10 mL of saline or other IV fluid to flush the needle and tubing of all drug.
- If multiple drugs are to be given, the IV should be flushed between each drug.
- Apply pressure with sterile gauze for 3–4 minutes after the needle is removed. Inspect the site before applying a bandage.

IV, intravenous.

Notes:

Table 85.8 • Suggested Procedures for Management of Suspected Extravasation of Vesicant Drugs[89,90,92]

1. Stop the injection immediately, but do not remove the needle. Any drug remaining in the tubing or needle, as well as the infiltrated area, should be aspirated.
2. Contact a physician as soon as possible.
3. If deemed appropriate, instill an antidote in the infiltrated areas (via the extravasated IV needle if possible).
4. Remove the needle.
5. Apply ice to the site and elevate the extremity for the first 24 to 48 hr (if vinca or podophyllotoxin, use warm compresses).
6. Document the drug, suspected volume extravasated, and the treatment in the patient's medical record.
7. Check the site frequently for 5–7 days.
8. Consult a surgeon familiar with extravasations early so that he or she can periodically review the site, and if ulceration begins, the surgeon can rapidly assess if surgical debridement or excision is necessary.

Table 85.9 • Recommended Extravasation Antidotes[a]

Class/Specific Agents	Local Antidote Recommended	Specific Procedure
Alkylating agents Cisplatin[a] Mechlorethamine	⅙ or ⅓ M solution sodium thiosulfate	Mix 4–8 mL 10% sodium thiosulfate USP with 6 mL of sterile water for injection, USP for a ⅙ or ⅓ M solution. Into site, inject 2 mL for each mg of mechlorethamine or 100 mg of cisplatin extravasated.
Mitomycin-C	Dimethylsulfoxide 50–99% (w/v)	Apply 1–2 mL to the site Q 6 hr for 14 days. Allow to air-dry; do not cover.
DNA intercalators Doxorubicin Daunorubicin	Cold compresses Dimethylsulfoxicle 50–99% (w/v)	Apply immediately for 30–60 min for 1 day. Apply 1–2 mL to the site Q 6 hr for 14 days. Allow to air dry; do not cover.
Vinca alkaloids Vinblastine Vincristine	Warm compresses Hyaluronidase	Apply immediately for 30–60 min, then alternate off/on every 15 min for 1 day. Inject 150 U into site.
Epipodophyllotoxins[a] Etoposide Teniposide	Warm compresses Hyaluronidase	Apply immediately for 30–60 min, then alternate off/on every 15 min for 1 day. Inject 150 U into site.
Paclitaxel	Hyaluronidase	Dilute 150 U in 3 mL NS; inject locally into site.

[a]Treatment indicated only for large extravasations (e.g., doses one-half or more of the planned total dose for the course of therapy). NS = Normal saline; W/V = Weight per volume.
Reprinted with permission from Dorr RT. Pharmacologic management of vesicant chemotherapy reactions. In: Dorr RT, von Hoff DD, eds. Cancer Chemotherapy Handbook. 2nd ed. East Norwalk: Appleton and Lange, 1993.

Notes:

Table 85.10 • National Cancer Institute Common Toxicity Criteria[a]

Toxicity[a]	Grade 0	Grade 1	Grade 2	Grade 3	Grade 4
Hematologic					
WBC	≥4.0	3.0–3.9	2.0–2.9	1.0–1.9	<1.0
Platelets	WNL	75.0–normal	50.0–74.9	25.0–49.9	<25.0
Hgb g/100 mL	WNL	10.0–normal	8.0–10.0	6.5–7.9	<6.5
g/L	WNL	100–normal	80–100	65–79	<65
mmol/L	WNL	6.2–normal	4.95–6.2	4.0–4.9	<4.0
Granulocytes/bands	≥2.0	1.5–1.9	1.0–1.4	0.5–0.9	<0.5
Lymphocytes	≥2.0	1.5–1.9	1.0–1.4	0.5–0.9	<0.5
Hematologic (other)	None	Mild	Moderate	Severe	Life-threatening
Hemorrhage (Clinical)	None	Mild, no transfusion	Gross, 1–2 units transfusion per episode	Gross, 3–4 units transfusion per episode	Massive, >4 units transfusion per episode
Infection	None	Mild, no active treatment	Moderate, PO antibiotic	Severe, IV antibiotic, anti-fungal, or hospitalization	Life-threatening
Gastrointestinal					
Nausea	None	Can eat reasonable intake	Intake significantly ↓ but can eat	No significant intake	—
Vomiting	None	1 episode in 24 hr	2–5 episodes in 24 hr	6–10 episodes in 24 hr	>10 episodes in 24 hr or requiring parenteral support
Diarrhea	None	↑ of 2–3 stools/day over pretreatment	↑ of 4–6 stools/day or noc-turnal stools, or moderate cramping	↑ of 7–9 stools/day or incon-tinence, or severe cramping	↑ of ≥10 stools/day or grossly bloody diarrhea, or need for parenteral support

[a]IV = Intravenous; PO = Orally; WBC = White blood cell; WNL = Within normal limits.

Table 85.11 • Cancer Chemotherapeutic Agents Commonly Causing Hypersensitivity[a]

Drug	Frequency	Risk Factors	Manifestations	Mechanism	Comments
L-Asparaginase[101–104]	10–20%	Increasing doses; interval (weeks to months) between doses; IV administration; history of atopy/allergy; use without prednisone 6-MP and/or vincristine	Pruritus, dyspnea, agitation, urticaria, angioedema, laryngeal spasm	Type I	Substitute PEG-L-asparaginase, but up to 32% may demonstrate mild hypersensitivity
Paclitaxel[105,106]	Up to 10% first or second dose	None known	Rashes, dyspnea, bronchospasm, hypotension	Nonspecific release of mediators; ? Cremophor	Premedicate with diphenhydramine corticosteroids, and H_2-receptor antagonists
Teniposide[107–112]	6–40%; can occur with first dose	Increasing doses or number of doses; young age/ leukemia	Dyspnea, wheezing, hypotension, rash, facial flushing	Type I versus nonspecific; ? Cremophor	Etoposide may be substituted in some cases; decrease rate of infusion
Cisplatin[113–118]	Up to 20% intravesicular 5–10% systemic; case reports of hemolytic anemia	Increasing number of doses Anemia: None known	Rash, urticaria, bronchospasm Anemia: Hemolytic anemia	Type I Anemia: Type III	Carboplatin may be substituted in some cases, but cross-reactivity has been reported
Procarbazine[119–124]	Up to 15% case reports	None known	Urticaria Pneumonitis	Type I Type III	All patients rechallenged have prompt return of symptoms
Anthracyclines[125–131]	1–15% depending on anthracycline	None known	Dyspnea, bronchospasm, angioedema	Unknown; ? nonspecific release	Cross-reactivity documented, but incidence and likelihood unknown

Drug	Incidence	Risk Factors	Signs/Symptoms	Mechanism	Management
Bleomycin[132–134]	Common	Lymphoma	Fever (up to 42°C) tachypnea	Endogenous pyrogen release	Not technically classified as HSR; premedicate with acetaminophen and diphenhydramine
Rituximab[135]	First treatment 80%; subsequent treatments 40%	Female gender; pulmonary infiltrates, CLL or mantle cell lymphoma	Fevers, chills; occasional nausea, urticaria, fatigue, headache, pain, pruritis, bronchospasm, SOB, angioedema, rhinitis, vomiting, ↓ BP, flushing	Unknown; ? related to manufacturing process	Stop or ↓ infusion rate by 50%; provide supportive care with IV fluids, acetaminophen, diphenhydramine, vasodepressors PRN
Trastuzamab[136]	First treatment 40%; subsequent treatments rare	None known	Chills, fever; occasional nausea/vomiting; pain rigors, headaches, dizziness, SOB, ↓ BP, rash, asthenia	Unknown, ?, related to manufacturing process	Manage with acetaminophen, diphenhydramine, meperidine
Docetaxel[137]	0.9% with premedication	None known	↓ BP, bronchospasm, rash, flushing, pruritus, SOB, pain, fever, chills	Unknown	Premedicate with acetaminophen, dexamethasone, and diphenhydramine
Doxorubicin[138] liposomal	6.8%	None known	Flushing, SOB, angioedema, HA, chills, ↓ BP	Unknown, ?, related liposomal components	Stop infusion; restart at a lower rate
Daunorubicin[139] liposomal	13.8%	None known	Back pain, flushing, chest tightness	Unknown, ?, related liposomal components	Stop infusion; restart at a lower rate

Type I: Antigen interaction with IgE bound to mast cell membrane causes degranulation. Drug binding to mast cell surface causes degranulation. Neurogenic release of vasoactive substances. Type III: Antigen–antibody complexes form intravascularly and deposit in or on tissues. Activation of classic or alternative complement pathways produces anaphylatoxins.

aBP = Blood pressure; CLL = Chronic lymphocytic leukemia; HA = Headache; HSR = Hypersensitivity reaction; 6-MP = 6-mercaptopurine; PEG-L-asparaginase = Pegaspargase; SOB = Shortness of breath.

Table 85.12 • Prophylaxis and Treatment of Hypersensitivity Reactions from Antitumor Drugs[a]

Prophylaxis

IV access must be established.

BP monitoring must be available.

Premedication

- Dexamethasone 20 mg PO and diphenhydramine 50 mg PO 12 and 6 hr before treatment, then the same dose IV immediately before treatment
- Consider addition of H_2-antagonist with similar schedule

Have epinephrine and diphenhydramine readily available for use in case of a reaction.

Observe the patient up to 2 hr after discontinuing treatment.

Treatment

Discontinue the drug (immediately if being administered IV).

Administer epinephrine 0.35–0.5 mL IV Q 15–20 min until reaction subsides or a total of 6 doses is administered.

Administer diphenhydramine 50 mg IV.

If hypotension is present that does not respond to epinephrine, administer IV fluids.

If wheezing is present that does not respond to epinephrine, administer nebulized albuterol solution 0.35 mL.

Although corticosteroids have no effect on the initial reaction, they can block late allergic symptoms. Thus, administer methylprednisolone 125 mg (or its equivalent) IV to prevent recurrent allergic manifestations.

[a]BP = Blood pressure; IV = Intravenous; PO = Orally.

Notes:

Table 87.13 • Neurotoxicity of Selected Chemotherapeutic Agents[a]

	Acute Encephalopathy	Chronic Syndrome	Cerebellar Neuropathy	Peripheral Neuropathy	Cranial Neuropathy	Autonomic (IT Dose)	Arachnoiditis Syndrome	Strokelike	SIADH
Alkylating Agents									
Cyclophosphamide									+
Ifosfamide	+			+	+				
Thiotepa		+	+	+			+		
Cisplatin	+			++	++				
Oxaliplatin				++					
Altretamine	+		+						
Procarbazine	++		+	+					
Antimetabolites									
Fluorouracil	+		++	+	+				
Fludarabine	+		+						
Cytarabine	+	+					+		
Methotrexate	+	+					+	+	
Plant Alkaloids									
Vinca alkaloids				++					
Vincristine						++			+
Vinblastine									
Vinorelabine				+					
Taxanes				+					
Paclitaxel									
Docetaxel									
Miscellaneous									
Asparginase	++								

+, reported but appears rare; ++, common in some cases and may present a clinical problem; +++, common and/or dose-limiting.
[a]SIADH = Syndrome of inappropriate secretion of antidiuretic hormone.

Table 85.14 • Chemotherapeutics Requiring Dosage Modification in Renal Failure[a]

Drug	>60 mL/min	30–60 mL/min	10–30 mL/min
Bleomycin	NC	75%	75%
Cisplatin	NC	50%	Omit
Cyclophosphamide	NC	NC	NC
Methotrexate	NC	50%	Omit
Mitomycin	NC	75%	75%
Nitrosureas	NC	Omit	Omit
Topotecan	NC	NC	25%

Carboplatin Dosing Recommendation
Calvert equation

$$\text{Dose (mg)} = \text{Target AUC (mg/mL} \times \text{min)} \times [\text{GFR (mL/min)} + 25]$$

Suggested Target AUC for Adults

Single agent, untreated	7 mg/mL/min
Single agent, previously treated	5 mg/mL/min
Combination chemotherapy	4.5 mg/mL/min

[a]NC = No change.

Notes:

Table 85.15 • Chemotherapy-Induced Pulmonary Toxicity[a]

Drug	Histopathology	Clinical Features	Treatment/Outcome
Aldesleukin[246]	Capillary leak, pulmonary edema	*Clinical presentation:* ↓ BP, fever, SOB, anorexia, rash, mucositis	Stop infusion; provide supportive care to cause a quick resolution of symptoms.
Bleomycin[247–255]	Interstitial edema and hyaline membrane formation; mononuclear cell infiltration pneumonitis with progression to fibrosis; eosinophilic infiltrations seen in patients with suspected hypersensitivity-type reactions	Cumulative dose-related toxicity with risk increasing substantially with total dose >450 mg or 200 mg/m²; may occur during or after treatment. *Clinical presentation:* cough, fever, dyspnea, tachypnea, rales, hypoxemia, bilateral infiltrates, dose-related ↓ in diffusing capacity	Recovery if bleomycin is discontinued while symptoms and radiologic changes still minimal; progressive and usually fatal if symptoms severe. Avoid cumulative doses >200 mg/m²; monitor serial pulmonary function tests. Discontinue therapy if diffusing capacity ≤40% of baseline, FVC <25% of baseline, or if any signs or symptoms suggestive of pulmonary toxicity occur. Steroids may be helpful if toxicity is result of hypersensitivity.
Busulfan[254]	Pneumocyte dysplasia; mononuclear cell infiltrations; fibrosis	Does not appear to be dose-related, but no cases reported with total doses <500 mg. *Clinical presentation:* insidious onset of dyspnea, dry cough, fever, tachypnea, rales, hypoxemia diffuse linear infiltrate, ↓ in diffusing capacity	Fatal in most patients; progressive despite discontinuation of busulfan. High-dose steroids (50–100 mg prednisone daily) have been helpful in a few cases.
Carmustine[255–259]		Dose-related; usually occurs with doses >1,400 mg/m² *Clinical presentation:* dyspnea, tachypnea, dry hacking cough, bibasilar rales, hypoxemia, interstitial infiltrates; spontaneous pneumothorax has been reported	May continue to progress after carmustine discontinued. No evidence that steroids improve or alter incidence. High mortality rate if symptoms severe. Serial pulmonary function studies recommended. Total cumulative dose should not exceed 1,400 mg/m².
Chlorambucil[260]	Pneumocyte dysplasia; fibrosis	Usually occurs after at least 6 months of treatment with total cumulative doses of >2 g *Clinical presentation:* dyspnea, dry cough, anorexia, fatigue, fever, hypoxemia, bibasilar rales, localized infiltrates progressing to diffusing involvement of both lung fields	Fatal in most cases despite discontinuation of chlorambucil and treatment with high-dose steroids.

(continued)

Table 85.15 • Chemotherapy-Induced Pulmonary Toxicity[a] (continued)

Drug	Histopathology	Clinical Features	Treatment/Outcome
Cyclophosphamide[257,260]	Endothelial swelling, pneumocyte dysplasia, lymphocyte infiltration fibrosis	Does not appear to be schedule- or dose-related and may occur after discontinuation. *Clinical presentation:* progressive dyspnea, fever, dry cough, tachypnea, fine rales, ↓ diffusing capacity and restrictive ventilatory defect, bilateral interstitial infiltrates	Clinical recovery reported in about 50% of patients within 1–8 wk if therapy stopped. Some of these patients received steroid therapy; however, others have died despite steroid therapy. Occasionally, therapy has been restarted without recurrence.
Cytarabine[261]	Pulmonary edema	*Clinical presentation:* tachypnea, hypoxemia, interstitial/alveolar infiltrates	Not always fatal.
Gemcitabine[262]	Pulmonary edema	Dyspnea was reported in 23% of patients; severe dyspnea in 3%; dyspnea occasionally accompanied by bronchospasm (<2% of patients); rare reports of parenchymal lung toxicity consistent with drug-induced pneumonitis	Treatment is support care measures. Symptoms resolve and are usually not seen with rechallenge.
Fludarabine[263]	Interstitial infiltrates, alveolitis, centrilobular emphysema	*Clinical presentation:* fever, dyspnea, cough, hypoxia; onset 3–28 days after third or fourth course; bilateral infiltrates and effusions	Resolves spontaneously over several weeks with or without corticosteroids.
Melphalan[260]	Pneumocyte dysplasia	Not dose-related. *Clinical presentation:* dyspnea, dry cough, fever, tachypnea, rales, pleuritic chest pain, hypoxemia. Usually progresses rapidly	Most patients die because of progressive pulmonary disease. Most reported cases occurred while patients were receiving concomitant prednisone therapy.
Methotrexate[260,264–267] *Delayed*	Nonspecific changes; occasional fibrosis	No evidence that dose related; daily or weekly schedules more likely to cause toxicity than monthly dosing. *Clinical presentation:* headache, malaise prodrome, dyspnea, dry cough, fever, hypoxemia, tachypnea, rales, eosinophilia, cyanosis in up to 50% of patients, interstitial infiltrates, ↓ diffusing capacity, restrictive ventilatory defect	Most patients recover within 1–6 wk (some may have persistent infiltrates or ↓ pulmonary function parameters). Steroids may produce more rapid resolution. May resolve despite continuation of methotrexate, but discontinuation may speed resolution. Rarely fatal.

Noncardiac pulmonary edema *Pleuritic chest pain*	Acute pulmonary edema	Occurs very rarely 6–12 hr after PO or IT methotrexate Not related to other methotrexate toxicities or serum levels; may not occur with each course of therapy *Clinical presentation*: right-sided chest pain, occasional pleural effusion or collapse of lung, thickened pleural densities	Fatal in 2 of 3 reported cases. Resolved within 3 days in 1 case. Usually resolves within 3–5 days.
Mitomycin[260,268]	Similar to bleomycin	*Clinical presentation*: dyspnea, dry cough, basilar rales, hypoxemia, bilateral interstitial or finely nodular infiltrates, ↓ diffusing capacity	Fatal in ≈50% of cases. Complete resolution reported in some patients, including some who received steroid therapy.
Procarbazine[269,270]	Hypersensitivity pneumonitis with eosinophilia and interstitial fibrosis	*Clinical presentation*: nausea, fever, dry cough, dyspnea within a few hours of ingestion, bilateral interstitial infiltrates, and pleural effusion	Rapid resolution after discontinuation.
Vinblastine[271]	Hyperplasia, dysplasia, interstitial edema, and fibrosis	Associated with concomitant treatment with mitomycin *Clinical presentation*: acute respiratory distress, bilateral infiltrates	Initial improvement with subsequent progression.

aBP = Blood pressure; FVC = Forced vital capacity; IT = Intrathecal; SOB = Shortness of breath.

Table 85.16 • Factors Associated with Increased Risk of Chemotherapy-induced Pulmonary Toxicity

Risk Factor	Drug(s)
Total cumulative dose	Bleomycin,[247,248,260,268,272] carmustine[260]
Age	Bleomycin[248]
Oxygen therapy	Bleomycin,[251–253] cyclophosphamide,[252] mitomycin[260]
Irradiation to lungs	Bleomycin,[251,273] busulfan,[274] carmustine,[255] mitomycin[254]
Concurrent therapy with other drugs	Bleomycin,[257,273] carmustine,[255,256] cyclophosphamide,[257,273] methotrexate,[275] mitomycin,[276,277] vinblastine[278]
Pre-existing pulmonary disease	Carmustine[277]
Tobacco use	Carmustine[277]

Adapted from reference 272.

Table 85.17 • Common Causes of Elevated LFTs in Patients with Cancer[a]

Primary or metastatic tumor involvement of the liver
Hepatotoxic drugs (e.g., cytotoxics, hormones [estrogens, androgens], antiemetics [phenothiazines], antimicrobials [rifampin, isoniazid])
Infections (e.g., hepatic candidiasis, viral hepatitis)
Parenteral nutrition
Allopurinol
Portal vein thrombosis
Paraneoplastic syndrome
History of liver disease

[a]LFTs = Liver function tests.

Notes:

Table 85.18 • Hepatotoxicity from Antineoplastic Drugs

Drug/Schedule	Prevalence	Type
Asparaginase[279–281]		
Daily	Frequent	Hepatocellular fatty metamorphosis
Carmustine[282,283]		
Weekly bolus	Common	Hepatocellular
Daily × 3	Common	
Bolus	Infrequent	
Cytarbine[284]		
Daily	Common	Cholestatic
Decarbazine[285,286]		
Daily × 5	Infrequent	Hepatocellular
Bolus		
Etoposide[287]		
High dose	Common with high dose	Hepatocellular
Lomustine[288,289]	Infrequent	
Mercaptopurine[290,291]		
Daily	Common	Cholestatic
High dose		Hepatocellular
Methotrexate[292,293]		
Daily	Common	Hepatocellular
Weekly bolus	Rare	Hepatocellular
High dose	Uncommon	Hepatocellular
Mitomycin[294]		
High dose	Infrequent	Veno-occlusive disease
Plicamycin[295,296]		
Daily × 5	Common	Hepatocellular
Streptozocin[297]		
Bolus	Common	Hepatocellular
Thioguanine[298]		
Daily	Rare	Veno-occlusive disease
Epirubicin	Infrequent	Hepatocellular

Notes:

Table 85.19 • Chemotherapeutics Requiring Dose Modification in Hepatic Dysfunction[a]

Bilirubin	AST	Adriamycin	Daunorubicin	Vincristine Vinblastine Etoposide	Methotrexate	5-Fluorouracil
<1.5	<60	100%	100%	100%	100%	100%
1.5–3.0	60–80	50%	75%	50%	100%	100%
3.1–5.0	>180	25%	50%	Omit	75%	100%
5.0		Omit	Omit	Omit	Omit	Omit

Paclitaxel-CALGB Recommendations for Dosing in Patients with Liver Dysfunction

AST >2 × ULN
Bilirubin ≤1.5   <135 mg/m²
Bilirubin = 1.6–3.0   ≤75 mg/m²
Bilirubin ≥3.1   50 mg/m²

Epirubicin

Bilirubin 1.2–3.0
AST 2–4 × ULN   ↓ dosage by 50%
Bilirubin ≥3 or
AST ≥4 × ULN   ↓ dosage by 75%

[a]AST = Aspartate aminotransferase; CALGB = Cancer and leukemia group B; ULN = Upper limit of normal.

The reader is referred to Chapter 87: Adverse Effects of Chemotherapy, written by *Celeste Lindley, Pharm.D., Rebecca S. Finley, Pharm.D.*, and *Stacy L. Shifflett, Pharm.D.*, in the seventh edition of **Applied Therapeutics: The Clinical Use of Drugs** for a more in-depth discussion of common and acute toxicities, specific organ toxicities, and long-term complications of chemotherapy, their presentations, and their management. All notations to reference numbers are based on the reference list at the end of that chapter. The editors of this handbook express their thanks to Drs. Lindley, Finley, and Shifflett and acknowledge that this chapter is based upon their work.

Notes:

Notes:

Chapter 86

Hematological Malignancies

CAUTION: Several errors related to overdoses of chemotherapy recently have caught the public's eye. The authors and editors have tried very hard to carefully check doses; however, we strongly urge clinicians to check two to three sources to minimize errors. Occasionally, total doses that are to be divided over the course of a day or several-day period are given repeatedly as single doses. Thus, it is extremely important to study the details of the dosage regimen.

Topics covered in this chapter include cancers arising from the bone marrow and lymphoreticular system. Major categories include the leukemias, lymphomas, and plasma cell disorders.

Definition and Classification

♦ *Leukemias.* A progressive proliferation of leukocytes that are either lymphocytic or nonlymphocytic or myeloid (granulocytes, monocytes, RBCs, or platelets).

  • *Acute leukemia* results from proliferation of immature hematopoietic cells (blasts) that appear in the bone marrow and periphery. If immature cells have lymphoid features, the condition is called acute lymphocytic leukemia (ALL); if they are myeloid in nature, the condition is referred to as acute nonlymphocytic leukemia (ANLL) or acute myelogenous leukemia (AML). See Table 86.1 for distinctive characteristics of these two leukemias. Acute leukemias appear suddenly and progress to death within weeks or months if the patient is not effectively treated.

  • *Chronic leukemias* follow a more insidious onset and course and are associated with proliferation of mature cells which can be lymphocytes (CLL) or granulocytes (CGL or CML). Cells accumulate in various organs as well as the periphery and the bone marrow; decreased RBC and platelet production results. Patients may survive for years with suppressive therapies, but chronic leukemias are not curable.

♦ *Lymphomas* are a heterogeneous group of neoplasms originating from lymphoid cells. Can arise in the lymph nodes or from lymphoid tissue in the GI tract, CNS, and bone. There are two major types: Hodgkin's disease (HD) and non-Hodgkin's lymphoma (NHL), which is 3 times more common. Table 86.2 compares the characteristics of each.

♦ *Plasma cell disorders* arise from antibody-secreting cells that overproduce immunoglobulins (Ig). In Waldenström's macroglobulinemia, the malignant cells are plasmacytoid lymphocytes, and excess IgM is produced. In multiple myeloma, plasma cells produce high levels of IgG, IgA, IgD, or IgE. Clinical manifestations include osteoporosis, hypercalcemia, renal disease, anemia, and thrombocytopenia.

Acute Nonlymphocytic Leukemia (ANLL, also referred to as Acute Myelocytic Leukemia, or AML)

+ **Signs and symptoms** are consistent with rapid reduction of RBCs, neutrophils, and platelets in the periphery due to rapid proliferation of malignant cells.

  • Fatigue (anemia), fever, night sweats, infection, bleeding, or bruising. (*Note:* Lymphadenopathy and hepatosplenomegaly are common if leukemia is lymphoid in origin).

  • Decreased Hct and platelet counts. High WBC count with abnormal differential and presence of leukemic blast cells (e.g., WBC 120,000 with 90% blasts).

  • Bone marrow biopsy reveals >30% of all nucleated bone marrow cells are immature blast cells of myeloid origin. Eight French-American-British (FAB) subtypes are based on morphologic and cytochemical characteristics. See Table 86.3.

+ **Goals of Therapy.** Initial goal is to clear bone marrow and peripheral blood of all leukemic blast cells so that normal blood cell components can regenerate.

+ **Induction Therapy**

  • *Standard therapy* for all FAB subtypes (except M3 or promyelocytic leukemia) includes an anthracycline (daunorubicin or idarubicin) and cytarabine, an antimetabolite. Complete response rates of 60%–80% have been reported. Continuous infusions of cytarabine produce higher response rates than bolus injections.

  • *Promyelocytic leukemia (FAB M3)* is characterized by disseminated intravascular coagulation and associated bleeding complications. Heparin is used to correct coagulation abnormalities. *Tretinoin or all-transretinoic acid (ATRA)* is used to induce promyelocyte differentiation and maturation. After 2 days, patients receive standard induction therapy as above. Toxicities include hyperleukocytosis and retinoic acid syndrome: fever, pulmonary infiltrates, pulmonary capillary leak, and acute renal failure. Also causes dryness of skin and mucous membranes, rash, hair loss, muscle weakness, depression, and elevated liver enzymes.

  • *Tumor lysis syndrome (TLS)* is a complication of induction therapy in patients with a high tumor burden and results from rapid lysis of leukemic cells. Occurs 12–24 hr after chemotherapy. Symptoms include hypocalcemia, hyperkalemia, hyperphosphatemia, hyperuricemia, acidosis, renal failure, and ECG changes. Leukophoresis or hydroxyurea can decrease tumor burden, but the most common approach is prevention:

    —*IV Hydration (2–3 L/day).* Begin 24–48 hr before chemotherapy to maintain renal perfusion, solubilize tumor lysis products (e.g., uric acid), and replace lost fluids from fever and vomiting.

    —*Allopurinol.* Initiate 300–600 mg/day before chemotherapy and monitor uric acid 3 to 4 times daily for 24 to 48 hours. Can be discontinued after chemotherapy completed and WBC <500/mm^3. Watch for rash and adjust dose if renal function deteriorates.

    —*Dialysis.* Use in extreme circumstances to correct metabolic abnormalities.

  • *Myelosuppression* is a common and dose-limiting effect of chemotherapy. (See Chapter 85: Adverse Effects of Chemotherapy.)

+ **Postremission therapy** (previously called consolidation therapy) is indicated to lengthen remissions since median duration is only 12–18 months, and only 20%–40% have a disease-free survival of >5 yr. Strategies vary from low-dose chronic maintenance therapy for years to 2 to 4 cycles of high-dose chemotherapy. The latter has best results. Regimens usually include high-dose cytarabine alone or in combination with other agents. Elderly or very ill may not receive therapy. Allogeneic bone marrow transplant also has been studied (see Chapter 88: Hematopoietic Cell Transplantation).

- *High-dose cytarabine adverse effects* include myelosuppression, moderate nausea and vomiting, fever, and skin rashes. (See Chapters 84: Neoplastic Disorders and Their Treatment: General Principles and 85: Adverse Effects of Chemotherapy.)

  —*Ocular toxicity* includes conjunctivitis, lacrimation, burning, photophobia, and blurred vision. Artificial tears or two drops in each eye Q 6 hr before initiating high-dose cytarabine can prevent it. Corticosteroid eyedrops can be used in the case of conjunctivitis.

  —*Rash* may present as total body or plantar-palmar eythema, which can progress to desquamation.

Chronic Myelogenous Leukemia (CML)

- ◆ **Signs and Symptoms.** Characterized by unregulated granulocyte proliferation in the bone marrow and an increase in mature granulocytes in the peripheral blood. *Leukocytosis* increases blood viscosity, which causes *headaches* and *stroke*. Histamines cause *pruritus*. Increased cell turnover leads to *hyperuricemia, gouty arthritis,* and *nephrolithiasis*. *Splenomegaly* is due to increased activity of reticuloendothelial system. Low-grade *fever* results from release of granulocyte lysozymes. Normochromic, normocytic *anemia* is due to suppression of RBC precursors. Increased megakaryocytes lead to *thrombocytosis*, thrombotic episodes, and hemorrhagic complications due to impaired platelet function. *Fatigue* and *weight loss* are common.

- ◆ **Staging.** There are 3 distinct phases.
  - *Chronic phase* as described above may last from weeks to years (mean: 3 yr).
  - *Accelerated Phase.* In this phase, immature leukocytes or blasts appear in the peripheral blood. Symptoms are more problematic. Lasts <6 weeks.
  - *Acute phase or "blast crisis"* is characterized by many blasts in the periphery, bone pain, fatigue, worsening anemia, infections, and bleeding complications. Indistinguishable from ANLL. Final phase is refractory to treatment, and survival is <3 months.

- ◆ **Treatment** of chronic phase is aimed at reducing leukocytosis and related symptoms. Hydroxyurea and interferon-alfa are most widely used.
  - *Hydroxyurea.* Typical dose is 2 gm/day PO, and the dosage is titrated to a WBC count of <20,000/mm^3. Remarkably free of side effects.
  - *Interferon-alfa* has a direct antiproliferative effect on leukemic cells and platelets. Dose is 5 million units/m^2/day IM or SQ. 30%–60% of patients respond, but it may take weeks to months for maximum effect. Side effects include fever, chills, myalgias, malaise, headache, chronic fatigue, impaired cognition, and depression. When used with hydroxyurea, improves survival.
  - *Bone marrow transplants* from HLA identical donors before the blast phase are successful in 50%–60% of patients who are alive and disease free at 5 yr. (See Chapter 88: Hematopoietic Cell Transplantation.)

Chronic Lymphocytic Leukemia (CLL)

- ◆ A monoclonal neoplasm of slowly proliferating, long-lived lymphocytes that are immunologically incompetent. Most common type of leukemia; occurs 2 times more often in men than women; age typically >55 yr. Median survival for patients with early disease is >10 yr.

- ◆ **Signs and Symptoms.** 25% of patients are asymptomatic with lymphocytosis (5000/mm^3). Many other causes of lymphocytosis must be ruled out (e.g., mononucleosis, acute infection). Bone marrow biopsy and cell surface markers are required for definitive diagnosis. As disease progresses, one sees enlarged lymph nodes, hepatosplenomegaly, and progressive lymphocytosis. Anemia and thrombocytopenia also can occur.

♦ **Treatment.** Asymptomatic patients in early-stage disease are not treated. Initial treatment when the disease progresses usually consists of chlorambucil with or without corticosteroids or fludarabine.

- *Chlorambucil* is given daily or intermittently. Approximately 70% respond. Doses are 6–14 mg/day until signs and symptoms diminish; then lower doses for 6 months. Intermittent therapy: 0.7 mg/kg PO *over* 2–4 days; repeat Q 3 weeks until disease stabilizes. Watch for myelosuppression.

- *Corticosteroids* are reserved for the 15% of patients who have immune complications (e.g., hemolytic anemia or thrombocytopenia). Prednisone is given 20–60 mg/m^2/day for 5–7 days each month.

- *Fludarabine* has been reserved for patients failing chlorambucil. A dose of 20–25 mg/m^2 IV daily for 5 days produced responses in about 50% of patients. Courses repeated every 4 weeks; acute toxicities are mild, but profound lymphopenia can occur.

Non-Hodgkin's Lymphoma (NHL)

♦ **Classification.** The Working Formulation (WF) is used to classify this diverse group of malignancies based on morphology and clinical course (see below). The Revised European-American Lymphoma (REAL) classification incorporates morphology, immunophenotype, genetics, and clinical information. See Tables 86.4 and 86.5

- *Low-grade lymphomas* have an indolent history. They are not curable, but patients have a prolonged survival (7 to 10 years) with minimal symptoms. Comprised of small cleaved cells.

- *High-grade lymphomas* spread rapidly to other organs and result in death within weeks to months if untreated. However, they are very responsive to chemotherapy (60 to 70% cure). Composed of large cells with diffuse growth patterns.

- *Intermediate-grade lymphomas* have an intermediate grade and prognosis.

♦ **Staging and Prognosis.** See Tables 86.6 and 86.7.

♦ **Clinical Presentation.** The most common presentation is painless enlargement of one or more lymph nodes with fever, night sweats, and weight loss.

♦ **Treatment.** See Chapter 84, Table 84.13

- *Aggressive Lymphomas.* Prompt treatment is required. The CHOP regimen is considered the gold standard. See Table 86.8 and Chapter 84: Neoplastic Disorders and Their Treatment.

- *Highly Aggressive Lymphomas.* Treatment is more similar to that of ALL, because they provide continuous exposures to chemotherapy. CNS prophylaxis with intermittent intrathecal methotrexate or cytarabine also is used.

- *Indolent Lymphomas.* Most experts treat only after patients become symptomatic. Patients with bulky disease or systemic symptoms should be treated immediately. Treatment is usually initiated with an oral alkylating agent because it is safe, convenient, and inexpensive (e.g., chlorambucil). Response lasts about 18 to 24 months. Rituximab, a chimeric anti-CD20 antibody, is used for progressive (relapsed or refractory) low-grade, CD20-positive B-cell NHL (40 to 50% response).

Hodgkin's Disease

♦ **Clinical Presentation and Prognosis.** Presentation is similar to NHL. See Table 86.4 for staging. Hodgkin's Disease represents <1% or all cancers in the United States, but it is typically curable even in the advanced stages.

♦ **Treatment.** The ABVD regimen is the preferred regimen. Cycles are given every 28 days and continued for two cycles beyond documentation of complete remission for a total of six to eight cycles. See Chapter 84, Table 84.13.

Multiple Myeloma

♦ **Clinical Presentation.** Manifestations are caused by proliferation and accumulation of plasma cells in bone and other organs and the overproduction and deposition of immunoglobulin. Bone pain and compression fractures, hypercalcemia, and anemia are common. Hyperviscosity syndrome can cause cardiac and CNS symptoms. Infectious complications are due to depressed production of other immunoglobulin classes.

♦ **Diagnosis.** See Table 86.9.

♦ **Staging and Prognosis.** Median survival ranges from 5 years for patients with stage I to 2 years for patients with Stage III. See Table 86.10.

♦ **Treatment.** Patient receive two to six cycles of conventional therapy (e.g., VAD—vincristine, adriamcin, and dexamethasone) followed by high-dose chemotherapy with stem cell support. See Chapter 84, Table 84.13.

♦ **Pamidronate.** Monthly pamidronate (90 mg IV over 2 to 3 hours) for MM patients with evidence of osteolytic lesions is standard care, because it significantly reduces bone pain and skeletal events and improves quality of life.

CHILDHOOD HEMATOLOGICAL MALIGNANCIES
Acute Lymphoplastic Leukemia (ALL)

♦ **Epidemiology.** The most common childhood leukemia (75% of cases) and the most common childhood cancer (30% of cases). Peak incidence occurs at ages 2 to 3 years, predominantly in white children. More than 80% will achieve prolonged survival, and the majority will be cured.

♦ **Clinical Presentation.** Normal bone marrow is replaced with immature lymphoid cells. The signs and symptoms are nonspecific, and many are similar to other childhood diseases such as juvenile rheumatoid arthritis. Frequent symptoms include fever (61%), bleeding (48%), and bone pain (23%). On physical examination many patients have lymphadenopathy (50%), splenomegaly (63%), and hepatosplenomegaly (68%). The WBC count will be normal or low with marked lymphocytosis; lymphoblasts may be present in the periphery. Normochromic, normocytic anemia, along with thrombocytopenia, is present in most cases. A bone marrow biopsy is necessary to confirm the diagnosis.

♦ **Prognostic Variables.**

  • *Clinical Variables.* The two most important prognostic factors are WBC count and age at diagnosis. Generally, a WBC count >50,000/mm^3 and age younger than 1 year or older than 9 years carry poor prognoses. Higher relapse rates also are seen in males and black children.

  • *Immunological Variables.* ALL is classified into different immunologic subsets based on cell surface markers and/or antigens present on the leukemic lymphoblasts at diagnosis. These can be categorized as cells of B-cell (80%) and T-cell (20%) origin. About 1 to 2% of children have mature B-cell disease. Patients with T-cell disease have a poorer prognosis.

  • *Cytogenic Variables.* Abnormalities in chromosome number (ploidy) is found in 60 to 75% of ALL cases. Ploidy is represented by the DNA index: A value of 1.0 is normal, whereas a value >1.0 represents an increased number. An index >1.16 has a better prognosis than <1.16. Translocations also are common in ALL, and certain ones (e.g., Philadelphia chromosome) are associated with treatment failure and relapse.

- *Early Response,* as measured by clearance of blasts from the peripheral blood or morphologic bone marrow remission on days 7 or 14 of therapy, is predictive of long-term, disease-free survival.

- *Minimum Residual Disease (MRD)* can be detected in bone marrow samples using PCR-based assays. Persistence of MRD beyond 4 to 6 months or re-emergence almost always is predictive of future relapse. Monitoring MRD is not yet standard practice.

♦ **Treatment**

- *Remission Induction Therapy.* The goal is complete remission (i.e., no detectable leukemic cells in the peripheral blood or bone marrow). Agents most commonly used are prednisone, vincristine, asparaginase, and daunorubicin. A 3-drug regimen is standard for children with low-to-medium risk of relapse. Four drugs are used when children are at high risk. See Table 86.11

  —*Vincristine toxicity.* Constipation with colicky abdominal pain appears in 3 to 10 days and is caused by autonomic neuropathy. Prophylactic use of a stool softener or laxative may lessen the severity.

  —*Asparaginase toxicity* includes severe, sometimes fatal pancreatitis (abdominal pain, elevated serum amylase, hyperglycemia) and frequent (20 to 35%) hypersensitivity reactions, ranging from urticarial eruptions to anaphylaxis. Asparaginase must be discontinued permanently if pancreatitis occurs. An investigational form derived from *Erwinia* may be useful in the case of hypersensitivity, although there are cross reactions in 17 to 26% of patients. Coagulopathies, which occasionally lead to cerebral hemorrhage or infarction, can occur.

- *CNS Preventive Therapy.* Because many chemotherapeutic agents do not reach the CNS, it is a common site for leukemic relapse. The purpose of CNS or intrathecal (IT) preventive therapy is to decrease the chance of relapse within the CNS and increase the chance of long-term survival. Low- or intermediate-risk patients are treated with triple intrathecal chemotherapy or IT methotrexate. High-risk patients also receive cranial radiation (1,200 cGY).

  —*IT doses* are based on the CSF volume, which correlates best with age. See Table 86.12

  —*IT vincristine* given in error is uniformly fatal. Institutional precautions must be taken to avoid this error

  —*Acute adverse effects* include acute arachnoiditis 12 to 24 hours after injection; headache, nausea, and vomiting. It generally is self limiting. Severe nausea and vomiting can be minimized with the addition of ondansetron. See Chapter 5: Nausea and Vomiting.

- *Consolidation (Early Intensification) Therapy* is intensive chemotherapy following induction therapy. It is vital to prevent relapse of ALL and has produced event-free survival of about 80% in low-risk children. The ideal regimen, which always includes methotrexate, is yet to be determined. See Table 86.13

  —*Methotrexate Concentration Monitoring* is crucial to establish the dose of leucovorin and duration of hydration and alkalinization needed to prevent systemic MTX toxicity. Measure about 24 hours after completion of the infusion and repeat daily until the concentration falls below the toxic threshold of 0.05 μmol/L.

  —*Allopurinol-MTX Interaction.* Allopurinol can markedly increase the plasma concentrations of mercaptopurine by inhibiting first-pass metabolism which can lead to toxicity. Usually the interaction is irrelevant because allopurinol is employed early in the first week of induction therapy.

- *Maintenance or Continuation Therapy.* The purpose is to sustain the complete remission, since without it, the majority of patients will relapse in 1 to 2 months. This is because patients who have responded to induction and consolidation therapy still have a high, though undetectable, leukemic cell burden.

  —Two of the most effective and least toxic agents are oral, IV, or IM methotrexate (20 mg/m^2/week) plus mercaptopurine (50 to 75 g/m^2/day). This is given along with periodic pulse therapy with vincristine 1.5 mg/m^2 for 1 day, and prednisone 40 mg/m^2 orally for 7 days every 4 weeks. IT chemotherapy should be repeated every 8 to 12 weeks.

  —Doses are adjusted to achieve an absolute neutrophil count of 300 to 2000/mm^3, and treatment is continued for 2.5 to 3 years, including the length of induction therapy.

  —*Teniposide and Etoposide Adverse Effects. Hypersensitivity* reactions (flushing, chills, bronchospasm, and hypotension) occur in 50% of children receiving these drugs repeatedly. Risk increases with total cumulative dose and happens at the end of infusion. Manage by switching from teniposide to etoposide. If on etoposide, pretreat with antihistamines with or without corticosteroids. *Secondary AML* unresponsive to standard therapy is another risk of long-term therapy with these agents.

- *Salvage Therapy for Relapsed ALL.* About 80 to 85% will attain a second remission, but long-term survival is poor; only 6 to 29% are disease free for 2 years. Allogeneic bone marrow transplantation after a 2nd remission has been achieved and can produce 5-year, disease-free survivals in 40 to 64%. See Chapter 88: Hematopoietic Cell Transplantation

Pediatric Non-Hodgkin's Lymphoma

- ♦ Lymphomas account for about 10% of all childhood malignancies, but they are less common in children than in adults. Children younger than 16 years of age account for only 3% of all lymphoma cases.

- ♦ **Classification.** Pediatric NHLs are best classified using histopathology, which divides them into three different categories: lymphoblastic, small noncleaved, and large-cell lymphomas. See Table 86.14.

- ♦ **Clinical Presentation.** In contrast to adults, pediatric NHL is extranodal in origin; thus, symptoms relate to the organ of origin. See Table 86.14.

- ♦ **Staging.** Most systems include four or more stages, with stage I being a single tumor and higher stages involving one or more anatomic sites. The highest stage includes patients with bone marrow or CNS involvement. The main predictor of outcome is tumor burden at presentation.

- ♦ **Treatment**

  - *Lymphoblastic Lymphoma (T-Cell).* The primary treatment for all stages and histologic types is combination chemotherapy because the disease is generalized at the time of diagnosis. The Memorial Sloan-Kettering LSA2L2 protocol is one of the most effective (60 to 80% long-term disease-free survival). See Table 86.15.

    —*CNS prophylaxis* should be given to all patients with lymphoblastic lymphoma. See ALL above.

    —*Toxicity* associated with treatment includes neuropathy from vincristine; myelosuppression from daunorubicin and cyclophosphamide; hemorrhagic cystitis from cyclophosphamide; and nausea and vomiting induced by both doxorubicin and cyclophosphamide.

    —*Hematopoietic recovery* is monitored weekly throughout the continuation phase before the next treatment is given. Adequate recovery is considered an ANC of

$\geq 500/mm^3$ (some use $1000/mm^3$) and platelets of $100,000/mm^3$. Use of a colony-stimulating factor may speed recovery when it is delayed.

- *Small Noncleaved (B Cell)*. The main difference in treatment is the less frequent use of anthracyclines, shorter treatment duration, and more frequent use of methotrexate. The trend is to use short-duration, intensive therapy using alkylating agents in conjunction with high-dose antimetabolite therapy. Chemotherapy is administered in rapid succession with limited recovery from neutropenia for 2 to 3 cycles in children with limited stage disease and for 4 to 6 cycles in children with advanced-stage disease. Survival rates are about 80%. See Table 86.16.
- *Large cell lymphoma* responds to both regimens; therefore, the shorter COMP regimen is appropriate.

Table 86.1 • Distinction of Acute Myelogenous from Acute Lymphocytic Leukemia[a]

	AML	ALL
Clinical Features		
Age	Commonly adults	Commonly children
Lymphadenopathy	Rare	Common
CNS involvement	Unusual	5%
Cytochemical Stains		
Myeloperoxidase	Positive	Negative
Periodic acid (Schiff)	Negative (except M_6)	Positive
Other Studies		
Surface markers	Myeloid	Lymphoid
CALLA	No	In early pre-B lineage ALL
Tdt	Absent	Present
Gene Arrangement Studies		
T-cell receptor	Absent	Present in T-cell ALL
Immunoglobulin	Absent	Present in B-cell ALL
Common Cytogenic Abnormalities	t(9,22)	t(9,22)
	t(8,21)	t(4,11) null cell ALL
	t(15,17) in AML-M_3	t(8,14) B-cell Burkitt's type
	5q-, 7q-	t(11,14) B-cell
	Inv 16 in AML-M_4Eo	t(1,19) B-cell

[a]ALL = Acute lymphocytic leukemia; AML = Acute myelogenous leukemia; CALLA = Common ALL antigen; CNS = Central nervous system.

Notes:

Table 86.2 • Comparison of Hodgkin's Disease and Non-Hodgkin's Lymphomas[a]

Characteristic	Hodgkin's Disease	Non-Hodgkin's Lymphomas	
		Low-Grade	Intermediate-High Grade
Site(s) of origin	Nodal	Extranodal (≈10%)	Extranodal (≈35%)
Nodal distribution	Axial (centripetal)	Centrifugal	Centrifugal
Nodal spread	Contiguous	Noncontiguous	Noncontiguous
CNS involvement	Rare (<1%)	Rare (<1%)	Uncommon (<10%)
Hepatic involvement	Uncommon	Common (>50%)	Uncommon
Bone marrow involvement	Uncommon (<10%)	Common (>50%)	Uncommon (<20%)
Marrow involvement adversely affects prognosis	Yes	No	Yes
Curable by chemotherapy	Yes	No	Yes

[a]CNS = Central nervous system.

Notes:

Table 86.3 • Classification of Acute Nonlymphocytic Leukemia (ANLL) and Acute Myeloid Leukemia (AML)[a]

Designation	ANLL Name	Predominant Cell Type	Cytogenetics	Frequency (%)	AML Morphology
M_0	Undifferentiated myeloblastic				No maturation of myeloblasts
M_1	Undifferentiated myelocytic	Myeloblasts	t(9;22) + 8 del(5), del(7)	2–3	Minimal maturation of myeloblasts
M_2	Myelocytic	Myeloblasts, promyelocytes, myelocytes	t(8;21) + 8 del(5), del(7)	20	Prominent maturation of myeloblasts
M_3	Promyelocytic	Hypergranular promyelocytes	t(15;17)	25–30	Promyelocytic
M_3 variant					Promyelocytic in marrow; atypical monocytes in blood
M_4	Myelomonocytic	Promyelocytes, myelocytes, promonocytes, monocytes	t(4;11), t(9;11) + 8 del(5), del(7)	8–15	Myelomonocytic
M_4Eo			inv(16)		With atypical eosinophils
M_{5a}	Monoblastic	Monoblasts	t(9;11) + 8 del(5), del(7)		Monoblastic
M_{5b}	Differentiated monocytic	Monoblasts, promonocytes, monocytes		20–25	Promonocytic
M_6	Erythroleukemia	Erythroblasts	+ 8 del(5), del(7)	5	Erythroblastic
M_7	Megakaryocytic	Megakaryocytes		1–2	Megakaryoblastic

[a] French-American-British (FAB) classification system.

Table 86.4 • Comparison of the Working Formulation with the REAL Classification[a]

Working Formulation	Revised European-American Classification	
	B-Cell Neoplasms	T-Cell Neoplasms
Low-Grade		
Small lymphocytic consistent with CLL	B-cell CLL/PLL/SLL Marginal zone/MALT Mantle cell	T-cell CLL/PLL LGL ATL/L (chronic and smoldering)
Plasmacytoid	Lymphoplasmacytic-immunocytoma Marginal zone/MALT B-cell CLL/PLL/SLL	
Follicular, predominately small cleaved cell	Follicle center, follicular, grade I Mantle cell Marginal zone/MALT	
Follicular, mixed small cleaved and large cell	Follicle center, follicular, grade II Marginal zone/MALT	
Intermediate Grade		
Follicular, large cell	Follicle center, follicular, grade III	
Diffuse, small cleaved cell	Mantle cell Follicle center, diffuse small cell Marginal zone/MALT	T-cell CLL/PLL LGL ATL/L Angioimmunoblastic Angiocentric
Diffuse, mixed small and large cell	Large B-cell lymphoma (rich in T cells) Follicle center, diffuse small cell Lymphoplasmacytoid Marginal zone/MALT Mantle cell	Peripheral T-cell, unspecified ATL/L Angioimmunoblastic Angiocentric Intestinal T-cell lymphoma
Diffuse, large cell	Diffuse large B-cell lymphoma	Peripheral T-cell, unspecified ATL/L Angioimmunoblastic Angiocentric Intestinal T-cell lymphoma
High Grade		
Large-cell immunoblastic	Diffuse large B-cell lymphoma	Peripheral T-cell, unspecified ATL/L Angioimmunoblastic Angiocentric Intestinal T-cell Anaplastic large cell
Lymphoblastic	Precursor B-lymphoblastic	Precursor T-lymphoblastic
Small noncleaved cell		
Burkitt's	Burkitt's	
Non-Burkitt's	High-grade B-cell Burkitt-like diffuse large B-cell	Peripheral T-cell, unspecified

[a]ATL/L = Adult T-cell lymphoma; CLL = Chronic lymphocytic leukemia; LGL = Large granular lymphocyte leukemia; MALT = Mucosa-associated lymphoid tissue; PLL = Prolymphocytic leukemia; SLL = Small lymphocytic lymphoma.
Adapted from reference 70.

Notes:

Table 86.5 • Clinical Grouping of Currently Recognized Non-Hodgkin's Lymphomas[a]

B-Cell Neoplasms	TNK Cell Neoplasms

Indolent Lymphomas (Untreated Survival Measured in Years)

Indolent Disseminated Lymphomas/Leukemias

B-cell CLL/SLL/PLL	T-cell CLL/PLL
Lymphoplasmacytic lymphoma/immunocytoma	Large granular lymphocyte leukemia
Splenic marginal zone lymphoma/SLVL	
Hairy cell leukemia	
Plasmacytoma/myeloma	

Indolent Extranodal Lymphomas

Extranodal marginal zone/MALT lymphomas	Mycosis fungoides

Indolent Nodal Lymphomas

Nodal marginal zone B-cell lymphoma	
Follicle center lymphoma, follicular	
Mantle cell lymphoma	

Aggressive Lymphomas (Untreated Survival Measured in Months)

Diffuse large B-cell lymphoma	Anaplastic large-cell lymphoma
	Peripheral T-cell lymphomas

Highly Aggressive Acute Lymphomas/Leukemias (Untreated Survival Measures in Weeks)

Precursor B-lymphoblastic leukemia/lymphoma	Precursor T-lymphoblastic lymphoma/leukemia
Burkitt's lymphoma	Adult T-cell lymphoma/leukemia (HTLVI+)

[a]CLL = Chronic lymphocytic leukemia; HTLVI = Human T-cell leukemia virus type I; MALT = Mucosa-associated lymphoid tissue; PLL = Prolymphocytic leukemia; SLL = Small lymphocytic lymphoma; SLVL = Splenic lymphoma with villous lymphocytes.
Adapted from reference 70.

Table 86.6 • Cotswold (Ann Arbor) Classification for the Staging of Non-Hodgkin's Lymphoma and Hodgkin's Lymphoma

Stage I:	Disease involvement of a single lymph node region (I) or lymphoid structure (e.g., spleen, thymus) or a single localized extranodal organ or site (I_E)
Stage II:	Disease involvement of two or more lymph node regions on the same side of the diaphragm (II); localized contiguous involvement of one extranodal organ or site and lymph node region on the same side of the diaphragm (II_E); the number of anatomic sites is indicated by a subscript (e.g., II_3)
Stage III:	Disease involvement of lymph node regions on both sides of the diaphragm (III); may also be accompanied by localized involvement of an extralymphatic organ or site (III_E) or by involvement of the spleen (III_S), or both (III_{SE})
	III_1: indicates with or without involvement of splenic, hilar, celiac, or portal nodes
	III_2: indicates involvement of para-aortic, iliac, or mesenteric nodes
Stage IV:	Diffuse or disseminated disease involvement of one or more extranodal organs or tissues, with or without associated lymph node enlargement

Designations Applicable to Any Stage Disease

A	Asymptomatic
B	Symptomatic: weight loss >10% of body weight, unexplained fever with temperature >39°C (100.4°F), and night sweats
X	Designates bulky disease as >⅓ widening of the mediastinum or >10 cm maximum dimension of nodal mass
E	Involvement of a single extranodal site that is contiguous or proximal to the known nodal site.

Staging should be identified as clinical stage (CS) or pathologic stage (PS).

Adapted from reference 33.

Table 86.7 • Risk Factors and Survival According to the International Non-Hodgkin's Lymphoma Prognostic Factors Project[a]

All Patients	Patients <60 Years of Age
Age ≥60 years of age LDH > normal Performance status ≥2 Ann Arbor stage III or IV Extranodal involvement > 1 site	LDH > normal Performance status ≥2 Ann Arbor stage III or IV

Risk Group	# of Risk Factors	5-Year Survival Rate (%)
Patients of All Ages		
Low	0, 1	73
Low-intermediate	2	51
High-intermediate	3	43
High	4, 5	26
Patients ≤60 Years of Age		
Low	0	83
Low-intermediate	1	69
High-intermediate	2	46
High	3	32

[a]LDH = Lactate dehydrogenase.
Adapted from reference 94.

Table 86.8 • Comparison of a Standard CHOP with Three Intensive Chemotherapy Regimens for Advanced Non-Hodgkin's Lymphoma

Regimen	6-Year Overall Survival (%)	Fatal Toxicities (%)
CHOP	33	1
m-BACOD	36	5
ProMACE-CytaBOM	34	3
MACOP-B	32	6

Adapted from reference 100.

Notes:

Table 86.9 • Diagnostic Criteria for Plasma Cell Disorders

Multiple Myeloma (MM)
Major criteria:
  1. Plasmacytoma on tissues biopsy
  2. Bone marrow plasmacytosis with >30% plasma cells
  3. Monoclonal globulin spike on serum electrophoresis: IgG >35 g/L, IgA >20 g/L, light chain excretion on urine electrophoresis >1.0 g/24 hr in the absence of amyloidosis
Minor criteria:
  1. Bone marrow plasmacytosis with 10–30% plasma cells
  2. Monoclonal globulin spike present but less than levels defined above
  3. Lytic bone lesions
  4. Normal IgM <500 mg/L, IgA <1 g/L, or IgG <6 g/L
The diagnosis of myeloma generally requires a minimum of one major and one minor criterion (1 + 1 not considered sufficient) or three minor criteria that must include 1 + 2

Indolent Myeloma (IMM)
Criteria as for myeloma with the following limitations:
  1. Absent or only limited bone lesions (≤3 lytic lesions), no compression fractures
  2. Paraprotein levels IgG <70 g/L, IgA <50 g/L
  3. No symptoms or associated disease features: Karnofsky performance status >70%, hemoglobin >6.8 mmol/L (100 g/L), serum calcium normal, serum creatinine <175 μmol/L (<3.0 mg/dL) no infections

Smoldering Myeloma (SMM)
Criteria as for indolent myeloma with additional constraints:
  1. No demonstrable bone lesions
  2. Bone marrow plasma cells 10–30%

Monoclonal Gammopathy of Undetermined Significance (MGUS)
  1. Paraprotein levels IgG ≤35 g/L, IgA ≤20 g/L, Bence Jones protein ≤1.0 g/24 hr
  2. Bone marrow plasma cells <10%
  3. No bone lesions
  4. No symptoms

Adapted from reference 33.

Notes:

Table 86.10 • Myeloma Staging System

Stage	Criteria	Measured Myeloma Cell Mass (Cells × 10^{12}/m^2)

I	All of the following:
	1. Hemoglobin value >100 g/L
	2. Serum calcium value normal (≤12 mg/dL)
	3. On radiograph, normal bone structure (scale 0) or solitary bone plasmacytoma only
	4. Low M-component production rates
	   A. IgG value <50 g/L
	   B. IgA value <30 g/L
	   C. Urine light chain M-component on electrophoresis <4 g/24 hr
		<0.6
		(low)

II	Fitting neither stage I nor stage II	0.6–1.2 (intermediate)

III	One or more of the following:
	1. Hemoglobin value <85 g/L
	2. Serum calcium value >12 mg/dL
	3. Advanced lytic bone lesions (scale 3)
	4. High M-component production rates
	   A. IgG value >70 g/L
	   B. IgA value >50 g/L
	   C. Urine light chain M-component on electrophoresis >12 g/24 hr
		>1.2 (high)

Subclassification
A = Relatively normal renal function (serum creatinine value <2.0 mg/dL).
B = Abnormal renal function (serum creatinine value ≥2.0 mg/dL).

Examples
Stage IA = Low cell mass with normal renal function.
Stage IIIB = High cell mass with abnormal renal function.

Adapted from reference 33.

Table 86.11 • Induction Regimens for Childhood Acute Lymphocytic Leukemia[a]

Agent	Route	Dose/Schedule
Prednisone	PO	40 mg/m^2/day × 28 days
Vincristine with:	IV	1.5 mg/m^2/week (*max*: 2 mg) × 4
Asparaginase	IM	10,000 units/m^2 3 × week × 9 doses
and/or		
Daunorubicin	IV	25 mg/m^2 on days 2, 8, ±15
and/or		
Methotrexate	IV	4 g/m^2 on day 1

[a]IM = Intramuscularly; IV = Intravenously; PO = Orally.
Adapted from references 214–220, 238, 261–264, and 400–404.

Notes:

Table 86.12 • Dosage Regimen for IT Methotrexate Based On Patient Age[a]

Patient Age	Methotrexate	Hydrocortisone	Cytarabine
<1 yr	6 mg	6 mg	12 mg
1 yr	8 mg	8 mg	16 mg
2 yr	10 mg	10 mg	20 mg
3 yr	12 mg	12 mg	24 mg
≥9 yr	15 mg	15 mg	30 mg

[a]IT = Intrathecal.
Adapted from reference 259.

Table 86.13 • Consolidation Regimens[a]

	Reference
Week 1: Methotrexate 1 g/m^2 IV over 24 hours Mercaptopurine 1 g/m^2 IV over 6 hours	
Week 2: Methotrexate 20 mg/m^2 IM × 1 dose Mercaptopurine 50 mg/m^2 PO daily × 7 days Triple intrathecal therapy on weeks 1, 2, 3, 7, 13, 19, and 25 Repeat 2-week cycles for a total of 12 courses	276
Cyclophosphamide 1 g/m^2 IV on days 0 and 14 Cytarabine 75 mg/m^2 SC or IV on days 1–4, 8–11, 15–18, and 22–25 Mercaptopurine 60 mg/m^2 PO daily × 28 days Methotrexate IT weekly × 4 weeks	228
Mercaptopurine 25 mg/m^2 PO daily on days 1–56 Methotrexate 5 g/m^2 IV over 24 hours on days 8, 22, 36, and 50 Methotrexate IT on days 8, 22, 36, and 50	223
Methotrexate 1 g/m^2 IV over 24 hours, every 3 weeks × 6 doses Vincristine 1.5 mg/m^2 IV on weeks 8, 9, 17, and 18 Prednisone 40 mg/m^2 PO daily × 7 days on weeks 8 and 17	229

[a]IM = Intramuscularly; IT = Intrathecally; IV = Intravenously; PO = Orally; SC = Subcutaneously.

Table 86.14 • Classification and Clinical Presentation of Pediatric NHL

Name	% of Cases	Cell Type	Symptoms
Lymphoblastic	30%	Immature T-cells similar to ALL	Mediastinal mass, pleural effusion, pain, dyspnea, swelling of face and upper arms; lympadenopathy is above diaphragm. Usually in bone marrow and CNS
Small Noncleaved	50%	B-cells: Burkitt's and non-Burkitt's	Abdominal tumor and pain, altered bowel function, occasional N/V. Bone marrow involved. Lymphadenopathy below the diaphragm: inguinal and ileac area
Large Cell	20%	B- or T-cells	Involves gut, lung, face, or CNS

Table 86.15 • LSA₂L₂ Regimen for Lymphoblastic Lymphomas^a

Induction
Cyclophosphamide	1 g/m² IV on day 1
Vincristine	1.5 mg/m² IV (max, 2 mg) IV on days 1 and 4
Methotrexate	12 mg^a IT on days 5, 31, and 34
Daunorubicin	60 mg/m² IV on days 12 and 13
Prednisone	60 mg/m² (max, 60 mg) PO daily in 3 divided doses on days 3–30, with doses decreasing to 0 on days 31–37

Consolidation
Cytarabine	100 mg/m² daily × 5 days × 4 wk
Thioguanine	50 mg/m² PO 8–12 hr after each cytarabine dose
Asparaginase	6,000 U/m² IM daily × 14 days following completion of cytarabine
Methotrexate	12 mg IT twice (3 days apart), beginning 3 days after last asparaginase dose
Carmustine	60 mg/m² IV × 1, given 2–3 days after completion of methotrexate

Maintenance (Cycles Separated by 1–2 Weeks and Repeated for ≈15 Months)
1. Thioguanine	300 mg/m² PO on days 1–4
Cyclophosphamide	600 mg/m² IV on day 5
2. Hydroxyurea	2.4 gm/m² PO on days 1–4
Daunorubicin	45 mg/m² IV on day 5
3. Methotrexate	10 mg/m² PO on days 1–4
Carmustine	60 mg/m² IV on day 5
4. Cytarabine	150 mg/m² IV on days 1–4
Vincristine	2 mg/m² (max, 2 mg) IV on day 5
5. Methotrexate	12 mg IT × 2 (3 days apart)

^{a}IM = Intramuscular; IT = Intrathecal; IV = Intravenous; PO = Oral.
^{b}Dosage based on patient's age.
Adapted from reference 371.

Table 86.16 • COMP Protocol for Localized Small Noncleaved Lymphoma

Induction
Cyclophosphamide	1.2 g/m² IV on day 1
Vincristine	2 mg/m² (max, 2 mg) IV on days 3, 10, 17, and 24
Methotrexate	12 mg^a IT on days 5, 31, and 34
Methotrexate	300 mg/m² IV on day 12
Prednisone	60 mg/m² (max, 60 mg) PO daily in 3 divided doses on days 3–30, with doses decreasing to 0 on days 31–37

Maintenance (Repeated Q 28 days × 5)
Cyclophosphamide	1 g/m² IV on day 1
Vincristine	1.5 mg/m² (max, 2 mg) IV on days 1 and 15
Methotrexate	12 mg IT on day 1
Methotrexate	300 mg/m² IV on day 15
Prednisone	60 mg/m² (max, 60 mg) on days 1–5 (excluded from 1st maintenance cycle)

^{a}Dosage based upon patient age.
Adapted from references 371 and 374.

Notes:

The reader is referred to Chapter 88: Hematologic Malignancies, written by *Rebecca S. Finley, Pharm.D., Imad M. Treish, Pharm.D., Celeste M. Lindley, Pharm.D.,* and *Mark T. Holdsworth, Pharm.D.,* in the seventh edition of **Applied Therapeutics: The Clinical Use of Drugs** for a more in-depth discussion of the pathophysiology and medical management of adult and childhood hematologic malignancies. All notations to reference numbers are based on the reference list at the end of that chapter. The editors of this handbook express their thanks to Drs. Finley, Treish, Lindley, and Holdsworth and acknowledge that this chapter is based upon their work.

Notes:

Chapter 87

Solid Tumors

Solid tumors include malignancies that present as discrete masses. They arise from malignant transformation of cells within virtually any organ system, except the hematopoietic system. Solid tumors are the major cause of cancer-related morbidity and mortality. For additional details on the pharmacology of drugs used to treat solid tumors and treatment regimens, see Chapter 84, and in particular, Tables 84.11 and 84.13.

ADULT SOLID TUMORS
Breast Cancer

♦ *Epidemiology.* Most common cancer in women accounting for 29% of cases. About 1 in 8 women develop breast cancer with the greatest risk occurring after age 65.

♦ *Risk Factors.* See Table 87.1.

♦ *Screening* for breast cancer is described in Chapter 84: Neoplastic Disorders and Their Treatment. See Table 84.6. Since nearly 75% of cases occur in women >50 years old, annual mammography is recommended in this age group.

♦ *Prognosis* is related to the likelihood of disease recurrence, which is determined by the size of the primary tumor; number of involved axillary lymph nodes; nuclear or histologic grade; and the presence of estrogen and/or progesterone receptors. Other factors include tumor growth fraction, HER-2/new oncogen amplification, and perhaps ploidy (DNA content)

♦ *Surgery.* There is no difference in survival between patients undergoing conservative surgery (e.g., partial mastectomy) followed by local radiation therapy and those treated with radical mastectomy. Women with negative lymph nodes have a 90% chance of cure with surgery alone; this is reduced to 40 to 60% in women with positive nodes.

♦ *Adjuvant Therapy.* Chemotherapy following surgery reduces the risk of death by 30 to 40% in patients with Stage I and Stage II (positive nodes) disease. Combination chemotherapy is typically used for premenopausal women who are usually hormone receptor negative. Tamoxifen benefits hormone receptor positive breast cancers, which typically occur in postmenopausal women. Treatment for node-negative patients is based on three risk categories. See Table 87.2

• *Combination Chemotherapy.* Response is 80 to 90% in patients who have not received prior chemotherapy. This drops to 20 to 30% in patients who have been previously exposed. See Chapter 84, Table 84.13 for several combination regimens that have been used to treat breast cancer.

• *Hormonal Therapy. Tamoxifen* consists of 20 mg daily or 10 mg BID for 5 years. It is started after chemotherapy because its cytostatic effects may interfere with the cytocidal effects of chemotherapy.

♦ *Metastatic Disease*

• *Metastatic Sites.* Common sites of metastatic spread of breast cancer are described in Chapter 84, Table 84.5.

• *Prognosis.* Metastatic disease is rarely curable. Median duration of survival is about 2 years. Poor prognostic factors include short disease-free interval (<l year); liver

involvement; negative estrogen and progesterone receptors at the time of diagnosis, and premenopausal status.

- *Combination Chemotherapy.* See above.

- *Paclitaxel (Taxol) and docetaxel* are approved for breast cancer after failure of combination chemotherapy for metastatic disease or relapse within 6 months of adjuvant chemotherapy. A 60% response rate has been reported in patients who have developed metastases >12 months after adjuvant therapy.

- *Capecitabine* is used in patients unresponsive to the above and has a response rate of about 18 to 20%.

- *Transtuzumab (Herceptin)* produces responses in about 14% of heavily pretreated patients whose tumors are HER-2/neu positive.

- *High-Dose Chemotherapy With Autologous Bone Marrow Transplant* does not appear to offer an advantage over conventional combination chemotherapy.

- *Spinal Cord Compression* by expansion of the tumor or fracture of the vertebrae can result in paralysis and anal sphincter dysfunction. Impending compression is treated with high-dose steroids (e.g., dexamethasone 10 mg every 6 hours PO or IV titrated for maximum response) followed by radiation therapy.

- *Hormonal therapy* is used to treat metastatic disease in women whose tumors are hormone receptor positive. Hormone-positive patients have a longer survival after metastases. See Chapter 84, Table 84.18.

  —*Response* is highest (70%) in patients who are both estrogen and progestogen receptor-positive (ER+, PR+); 30% in patients who are ER+ and PR−; 10% in patients who are both ER- and PR-negative.

  —*Antiestrogens (tamoxifen, toremifene), progesterone (e.g., megestrol acetate), and aromatase inhibitors* are equally effective, but antiestrogens are considered first-line therapy because they have a low toxicity profile. Aromatase inhibitors are second line and progesterones are third line if disease progresses. See Chapter 84, Table 84.16.

  —*Therapeutic response* to tamoxifen usually takes 4 to 6 weeks (less bone pain, no new sites of metastases); steady-state levels are not achieved for 16 weeks.

  —*Flare reactions* (transient worsening of symptoms within hours or days after therapy is started) are common. Symptoms generally subside within a month. Continue therapy unless hypercalcemia is severe.

Colon Cancer

- ♦ **Epidemiology and Prognosis.** Colon cancer is the second leading cause of cancer death in the adult U.S. population, but it is curable with surgical intervention if detected early; >90% survive 5 years. This drops to 40 to 50% if it is diagnosed at later stages.

- ♦ **Risk Factors** include family history; age >50 years; high-fat, low fiber diet; obesity; chronic inflammatory bowel disease; and history or colorectal polyps or cancer. Continuous aspirin or other NSAIDs may prevent colorectal cancer.

- ♦ **Screening** is by fecal occult blood testing, which decreases mortality. The guaiac test is commonly used. Foods, other substances, and medical conditions that contain or produce peroxidase activity may yield false readings. See Table 87.3.

- ♦ **Clinical Presentation.** See Chapter 84, Table 84.8.

- ♦ **Staging.** Stage A indicates penetration into but not through the bower wall. Stage B indicates penetration through the bowel wall. Stage C indicates lymph node involvement. CEA or CA-19–9 levels are elevated in relation to the extent of disease, the degree of tumor differentiation, and the site of metastases.

♦ **Adjuvant Therapy**

- Indicated for Stage C and high-risk Stage B because up to 60% of surgically treated patients will develop local recurrence.

- Current favored regimen is fluorouracil (FU) 425 mg/m^2 per day plus leucovorin 20 mg/m^2 for 5 consecutive days repeated every 4 weeks for 6 months, beginning 3 weeks after surgery. Toxicities include leukopenia, severe diarrhea, and stomatitis.

- Follow-up care includes evaluation (including CEA levels) every 3 months for 3 years, then every 6 months for 2 more years.

♦ **Recurrent Disease**

- *Rising CEA levels* may be first indication; >50% of patients with recurrent local or metastatic disease have elevated levels. The liver is the most common metastatic site.

- *FU plus leucovorin* (a reduced folate that augments the cytotoxicity of FU) is the most promising systemic regimen. It is given as a high-dose weekly regimen or as a 5-day low-dose regimen. Both are equally effective, but the 5-day regimen has substantially less toxicity and is less costly.

- *Irinotecan* (a topoisomerase I inhibitor) or oxaliplatin (a third-generation cisplatin analog) have activity against colorectal cancer if FU regimen fails. Several manufacturers are pursuing the development of orally administered fluoropyrimidines.

- *Hepatic Intra-Arterial Chemotherapy* is indicated for hepatic metastases. It produces a higher response rate than systemic chemotherapy (40 to 60% versus 10 to 20%), but survival is not improved. *Floxuridine* is used because the liver extracts 95% of the dose, and it has a half-life of only 20 minutes when it does reach the systemic circulation. Biliary sclerosis and liver failure is related to the total dose and duration of therapy. Interrupt treatment or lower the dose if alkaline phosphatase rises.

Lung Cancer

♦ **Epidemiology.** Cigarette smoking causes 75 to 80% of lung cancer cases, especially SCLC. Four major types of lung carcinomas account for 95% of all lung cancers.

- *Small cell lung cancer (SCLC)* comprises 25% of cases. It progresses rapidly and is responsive to many chemotherapeutic agents. Surgery is almost never indicated because of spread.

- *Nonsmall cell lung cancers (NSCLC)* is comprised of the other three types because they have similar prognoses and responses to therapy. These include epidermoid or squamous cell (30%), adenocarcinoma (25%), and large cell carcinoma (15%). NSCLC is slower growing and less likely to metastasize, but it is less sensitive to chemotherapy than SCLC.

♦ **Prevention and Screening.** The most important intervention to prevent lung cancer is not to smoke and to avoid secondary smoke. No screening measures affect overall mortality.

♦ **Staging.** Complex staging schemes do not correlate with survival. Therefore, a simple two-stage system is used for SCLC. "Limited" disease is defined as that confined to one hemithorax and the regional lymph nodes. "Extensive" disease extends beyond the thorax.

♦ **Clinical Presentation.** Signs and symptoms depend on the size and location and degree of spread. Most common are cough, wheezing, chest pain, hemoptysis, and dyspnea. These may be overlooked in heavy smokers. Obstruction from a large tumor can lead to pneumonia and fever. Spread to other structures in the thorax can cause dysphagia, hoarseness, and pleural effusion. Paraneoplastic symptoms include cancer cachexia in 33%, clubbing, pulmonary osteoarthropathy, Cushing's, and SIADH. See Chapter 84, Tables 84.8 and 84.9.

♦ **Treatment of NSCLC** includes surgery, which is curative only in the early stages. Radiation is used for large tumors or when there is extensive lymph node involvement. In advanced stages, response to combination chemotherapy is 25 to 40%, but <5% achieve complete response. The best response is to 2 to 8 cycles of high-dose cisplatin or carboplatin combined with etoposide, paclitaxel, docetaxel, vinorelbine, and gemcitabine. See Chapter 84, Table 84.13.

♦ **Treatment of SCLC.** When disease is "limited," 85 to 95% respond, with 50 to 60% achieving complete response. Nevertheless, median survival is 12 to 16 months, and the 2-year disease-free survival (DFS) rate is 15 to 20%. When disease is "extensive," median survival is 7 to 11 months, and 2-year DFS is <2%.

- SCLC responds to many drugs. See Chapter 84, Table 84.13. There is not evidence to support the use of more than 3 to 4 drugs. Current first-line regimens include cisplatin or carboplatin in combination with etoposide. After nausea and vomiting from cisplatin are alleviated, etoposide can be administered orally by doubling the IV dose and rounding up to the next 50 mg to offset poor bioavailability (50%). Duration of therapy is 4 to 6 months. Other active agents include topotecan, paclitaxel, docetaxel, ifosfamide, cyclophosphamide, teniposide, doxorubicin, vincristine, and methotrexate.

- Prophylactic cranial irradiation after remission can decrease brain metastases, which occur in 20 to 25%.

Ovarian Cancer

♦ **Epidemiology.** Ovarian cancer is one of the leading causes of cancer deaths in women. Carcinoma is more common in postmenopausal women 40 to 70+ years of age, whereas germ cell neoplasms are more common in younger women.

♦ **Risk factors** include endocrine disorders, nulliparity or a low number of pregnancies, positive family history, and a history of previous malignancies, especially breast cancer.

♦ **Screening.** Unfortunately, there are no effective screening methods for ovarian cancer.

♦ **Clinical Presentation.** Because the ovaries are suspended in the pelvis, early disease is typically asymptomatic or accompanied by mild vague abdominal pain. Pain, abdominal distention, and vaginal bleeding are common symptoms of advanced disease. Others include weight loss, nausea, or change in bowel or bladder habits if the tumor compresses adjacent structures. See Chapter 84, Table 84.8.

♦ **Treatment** includes surgery followed by combination chemotherapy and, perhaps, intraperitoneal chemotherapy.

- *Combination Chemotherapy* currently includes carboplatin plus paclitaxel, which has a response rate of 73%. Overall survival is 38 months. See Chapter 84, Table 84.13.

- *Intraperitoneal cisplatin* has been widely studied and compared to high-dose IV cisplatin. Median survival was significantly longer, and moderate-to-severe toxicities were fewer in the IP group. Toxicities include chemical peritonitis, fibrosis, and pain.

- *Recurrent Disease.* Treatment for recurrence within 6 months of treatment should be with drugs that have a different mechanism of action. Topotecan produces response rates of 14 to 25%. The dose is 1.5 mg/m^2 daily as a 30-minute infusion for 5 consecutive days; this course is repeated every 21 days. The major toxicity is myelosuppression.

Bladder Cancer

+ **Risk factors** include age >60 years, male gender, occupational exposure to chemical carcinogens (aryl amines found in dye, rubber, and paint industries), cigarette smoking, drugs (cyclophosphamide and phenacetin), and chronic urinary tract infections

+ **Clinical Presentation.** Bladder irritation may be the only symptom. Microscopic or gross hematuria often prompts medical intervention. Flank pain, constipation, or lower extremity edema are symptoms of advanced disease. See Chapter 84, Table 84.8.

+ **Treatment**

  • *Surgical resection* effectively eradicates existing lesions, but 30 to 85% eventually develop new lesions.

  • *Adjuvant intravesical therapy* (instillation into the urinary bladder) is recommended to reduce the risk of recurrence. Limited systemic absorption minimizes the risk of serious systemic toxicities. BCG (Bacille-Calmette-Guerin), 120 mg in sterile saline weekly for 6 weeks, then monthly for up to 12 months is standard therapy. Some patients experience a dose-limiting local irritation (dysuria, hematuria, increased urinary frequency), and 6% experience fever, chills, and joint pain. Other drugs that are used include thiotepa, doxorubicin, and mitomycin C.

  • *Metastatic disease.* About 40% develop metastases to the lymph nodes, liver, lung, and bone. Since the prognosis is poor in these cases, the focus of therapy is to reduce symptoms and prolong survival. Many experimental combinations are under investigation, including carboplatin plus paclitaxel (50% response) and gemcitabine as a single agent.

Melanoma

+ **Epidemiology.** Melanoma accounts for only 3% of cancers but is expected to increase due to sun exposure. It occurs in adults of all ages but predominantly Caucasians. Cutaneous melanoma can arise on any surface of the skin. It occasionally develops in noncutaneous tissues, such as the retina.

+ **Clinical Presentation.** See Table 87.4. See Chapter 84, Table 84.8.

+ **Treatment**

  • *Surgical excision* is the first line of treatment for localized melanoma lesions. The prognosis is determined by vertical extension of the lesion into the skin and subcutaneous tissue. Extension into the subcutaneous fat is associated with a high rate of tumor recurrence and a grave prognosis.

  • *Chemotherapy* has been disappointing. Alkylating agents have demonstrated modest (20%) activity.

  • *Immunotherapy* has been studied extensively because melanoma cells express surface antigens and may produce their own growth factors. Interleukin-2 (IL-2) has been used alone or in combination with LAK cells. The overall response rate is 10 to 20%, but 5% have responded completely for many years. Also see Chapter 84: Biologic Response Modifiers.

Prostate Cancer

+ **Epidemiology.** The most common malignancy in adult males. The highest incidence is in black men, which is 1.7 times that of white men in the United States.

+ **Risk factors** include male gender and increasing age. Other possible risk factors include high meat and saturated fat diets, exposure to cadmium, high testosterone levels, and perhaps a family history of the disease or prior venereal disease.

◆ **Screening.** There is no evidence that widespread screening and early detection improve survival, but routine evaluation of PSA in men >50 years old is standard.

◆ **Staging** is based on location of the cancer. Stage B is confined to the prostate, and Stage D is spread to the lymph nodes and other tissues (e.g., bone)

◆ **Clinical Presentation.** Almost all patients are asymptomatic unless there are metastases, which can lead to pain and neurologic dysfunction. See Chapter 84, Table 84.8.

◆ **Treatment**

- *Stage B* is treated with surgery (radical prostatectomy) or radiation therapy
- *Stage D.* Hormonal therapy is associated with a survival advantage, even when started before symptoms develop. Hormonal manipulation reduces testosterone to levels consistent with castration because the growth of both normal and malignant prostate tissue depends on testosterone. See Chapter 84, Table 84.18. Options include:

    —*Bilateral orchiectomy* is considered by many to be the therapy of choice because it permanently removes the primary source of testosterone production. Causes impotence but avoids need for long-term administration of drugs.

    —*LHRH analogs (leuprolide—Leupron; goserelin—Zoladex)* decrease testosterone production. Initially, they stimulate the release of FSH and LH by the pituitary, which increases testosterone production, but over several weeks, the LHRH receptors are down regulated. The initial testosterone surge may transiently worsen symptoms such as pain. These are long-acting parenteral preparations that are administered monthly (leuprolide 7.5 mg IM or goserelin 1.6 mg SQ). Response rates equivalent to diethylstilbesterol but with less toxicity.

    —*Antiandrogens (flutamide, bicalutamide, nilutamide)* prevent the action of testosterone at the prostate. Response rates are 50 to 87% for flutamide, but a compensatory increase in LH ultimately reverses the blockade. Side effects include gynecomastia, hot flashes, GI disturbances, breast tenderness, and liver function abnormalities. Patients can often maintain sexual potency.

    —*Combination androgen blockade* (e.g., leuprolide plus flutamide or orchiectomy plus flutamide) is often used in patients with minimal disease.

    —*Monitor* serial PSA levels as well as control of symptoms.

◆ **Second-line Therapy for Disease Progression**

- For patients receiving combination therapy, withdraw the antiandrogen, which may have converted to an agonist due to a change in the receptor. Up to 35% of patients respond.

- *Aromatase inhibitors,* which interfere with adrenal steroidgenesis can be added. Concurrent replacement of glucocorticoids is essential, and mineralocorticoids may be needed.

    —*Aminoglutethimide* is initiated with 250 mg BID and gradually increased to QID. Onset may take 4 to 6 weeks. Adverse effects are common (50%) and include lethargy, ataxia, dizziness, and a rash that resolves in 5 to 8 days.

    —*Ketoconazole* interferes with testicular steroidgenesis as well. Doses are 400 mg Q 8 hours, and response is rapid. Adverse effects include GI intolerance, weakness, lethargy, and skin pigmentation. There may be transient increases in liver and kidney function tests.

- *Cytotoxic Chemotherapy.* Estramustine combined with vinblastine and itoxantrone combined with prednisone are active against refractory prostate cancer. Partial response rates are 30%.

Testicular Cancer

- **Epidemiology.** The most common malignancy in men between ages 15 to 25 years.
- **Risk factors** include crytorchidism, race (lower in black males), and family history.
- **Staging and Histology.** Germinal neoplasms are divided into seminomas (arising from spermatocytes) and nonseminomas (arising from germ cells of placental origin). Stage I is limited to the testes; Stage II involves the lymph nodes; Stage III includes all metastatic tumors.
- **Clinical Presentation.** Typical presentation is painless swelling in one gonad. Alpha fetoprotein and beta human chorionic gonadotropin are typically elevated and are monitored as tumor markers. See Chapter 84, Table 84.8.
- **Treatment**
  - Treatment of seminoma and advanced disease is similar, but seminoma is exquisitely sensitive to radiation.
  - *Initial treatment* is surgical resection (orchiectomy), but 20 to 30% ultimately relapse. Adjuvant therapy with two cycles of a platinum-based regimen dramatically reduces this risk.
  - *Metastatic disease.* Combination cisplastin, etoposide, and bleomycin therapy (up to four courses) has produced responses in almost all men and complete responses in 60 to 80%. See Chapter 84, Table 84.13. The most significant toxicities include myelosuppression, nephrotoxicity, and neurotoxicity associated with cisplatin. If tumor markers plateau, additional cycles with the same regimen are not likely to produce further regression, and salvage therapy with other agents should be initiated. See Chapter 84, Table 84–13. The response and long-term survival for both first-line and salvage chemotherapy are considerably higher for testicular cancer than for most solid tumors.

PEDIATRIC SOLID TUMORS
Epidemiology

- In the U.S., more children between 1 and 14 years old die of cancer than any other disease.
- Nevertheless, many common pediatric cancers now have 5-year survivals >65%.
- Acute leukemias are the most common malignancies of childhood, whereas the solid tumors represent only 3 to 7% of all childhood malignancies. See Table 87.5.

Neuroblastoma

- **Epidemiology.** Neuroblastoma develops in immature cells of sympathetic nervous system origin; 65% are abdominal (half of these adrenal) and 20% thoracic. It is the most common extracranial tumor of childhood. The median age at diagnosis is 22 months; 36% occur in children younger than 1 year of age and 79% before 4 years of age.
- **Screening.** Urine is screened for VMA and HVA (see below) in infants who have a better prognosis than older children do.
- **Staging and Prognosis.** See Tables 87.6, 87.7, and 87.8. The 2-year disease-free survival (DFS) is 75 to 90% for stage 1 or 2 disease and 10 to 30% for stage 3 to 4 disease. At diagnosis, children are more likely to present with stage 3 or 4 disease than infants (78% versus 43%) are.
- **Clinical Presentation.** Often presents as a fixed, hard abdominal mass without other signs or symptoms, except those that may depend on the location of the tumor and

metastases. The most common metastatic sites are the bone marrow, bone, liver, and skin. The catecholamine metabolites vanillylmandelic acid (VMA) and homovanillic acid (HVA) are elevated in the urine in 90% of patients.

+ **Treatment**

  • *Low-risk disease* is treated with surgery. Recurrence is treated with surgery again. Two to four courses of chemotherapy are used if organ or life-threatening symptoms are present. (See Table 87.8.)

  • *Intermediate-risk disease* is treated with surgery and four or eight courses of chemotherapy, which avoids cisplatin to reduce nephrotoxicity and ototoxicity; limits the total dose of doxorubicin to avoid cardiac toxicity; and limits the total dose of etoposide to reduce the risk of secondary AML. See Table 87.9.

  • *High-risk disease* is treated with surgery for biopsy, aggressive chemotherapy, second surgery for tumor resection, additional chemotherapy or high-dose chemotherapy with progenitor cell rescue, and then radiation. High-dose chemotherapy with progenitor cell rescue has raised survival from 10 to 20% to 49%. 13-cis-retinoic acid may also improve survival.

Wilms' Tumor (Nephroblastoma)

+ **Epidemiology.** Wilms' tumor is a kidney tumor composed of various kidney cell types at different stages of maturation. Comprises about 6% of all childhood cancers and is the most common intraabdominal tumor of childhood. The peak incidence occurs at 3 years of age.

+ **Staging and Prognosis.** Overall prognosis is good (90% for stage I, 75% for stage IV with favorable histology, 55% for stage IV with unfavorable histology). Stage I is confined to the kidneys; Stage II extends beyond the kidney but can be excised; Stage II is residual tumor confined to the abdomen; stage IV is distant metastases; and stage V is bilateral disease.

+ **Clinical Presentation.** Typically presents as an asymptomatic abdominal mass, although malaise and pain may be reported. Hematuria and high-renin hypertension are present in 25%. Metastases most commonly involve the lung and liver.

+ **Treatment**

  • Many national studies have tried to minimize toxicities from radiation and chemotherapy while maintaining the excellent cure rate.

  • Table 87.10 outlines the current protocol for Wilms' tumor.

  • The following lessons were learned from the previous studies:

    —Intermittent, higher doses of dactinomycin allowed higher dose intensity with less myelosuppression.

    —With greater dose intensity and density, 6 months therapy was as effective as 15 months of therapy.

    —Chemotherapy doses reduced by 50% in infants decreased the number of severe hematologic toxicity, toxic deaths, and pulmonary and hepatic complications without a decrease in efficacy.

    —Dactinomycin and doxorubicin doses should be reduced by 50% or withheld in patients receiving concurrent radiation because they enhance radiation effects and cause recurrence of radiation effects on skin and mucous membranes up to several weeks later.

    —Dactinomycin hepatotoxicity remains higher than with previous regimens. If ALT rises to 2 to 5 times normal or the total bilirubin is 3 to 5 mg/dL, doses of all chemotherapy should be reduced by 50% or discontinued if LFTs continue to rise.

Osteosarcoma

♦ **Epidemiology.** Osteosarcoma is a bone tumor that most commonly occurs in children in the second decade of life. It occurs most frequently in the metaphyseal ends of the distal femur, proximal tibia, or proximal humerus.

♦ **Prognosis.** When chemotherapy is used with surgery, 2- to 5-year DFS is 50 to 75%. Clinically apparent metastases or a location that does not allow complete surgical removal of the primary tumor are associated with a poor prognosis.

♦ **Clinical Presentation.** Most common presentation is pain at the site for weeks to months. Metastases are clinically detectable in 15 to 20%, usually in the lungs, but micrometastases are likely present in all patients.

♦ **Treatment** includes surgery and chemotherapy to prevent metastases. Frequently used drugs include high-dose methotrexate, cisplatin, doxorubicin, ifosfamide, carboplatin, and etoposide. The tumor is relatively resistant to radiation therapy.

♦ **High-Dose Methotrexate—Leucovorin Rescue.** Cytotoxic effects of methotrexate depend on concentration and duration of exposure. Many high-dose MTX protocols continue leucovorin rescue until serum MTX concentrations are 0.1 μmol/L. However, some patients have delayed clearance with persistence of low MTX levels past 72 hours. Prevention of GI and bone marrow toxicity may require continuation of leucovorin rescue until MTX concentrations are <0.01 to 0.05 μmol/L. Figure 87.1 helps identify patients who are at high risk of MTX toxicity if given the usual low doses of leucovorin rescue.

Rhabdomyosarcoma

♦ **Epidemiology.** The most common soft tissue sarcoma of childhood, comprising 3.4% of all childhood cancers. Two types are most common. Embryonal cells resemble striated muscle and occur most frequently in young children with involvement in the head and neck or genitourinary tract. Alveolar cells resemble the lung parenchymal cells and occur more frequently in older children or adolescents with involvement of the trunk or extremities.

♦ **Staging and Prognosis.** The embryonal classification has a better prognosis than the alveolar one. Complete surgical removal and lack of metastases both correlate with good prognosis. A TNM staging system is used. See Chapter 84, Table 84.7.

♦ **Clinical presentation** is determined by the tumor location (e.g., periparotid mass).

♦ **Treatment** combines surgery, irradiation, and chemotherapy. Complete surgical removal is often difficult; irradiation is used to gain further local control; combination chemotherapy is needed because the 5-year survival with local control alone is 10 to 30%. Vincristine, dactinomycin, and cyclophosphamide (VAC regimen) have been used extensively. The 3-year survival is 67 to 76% for nonmetastatic patients.

• *Low-risk disease* (patients with embryonal cells at favorable sites or at unfavorable sites with no more than microscopic residual tumor) are treated with vincristine and dactinomycin.

• *Intermediate-risk disease* (embryonal subtype with gross residual or with metastatic disease if they are younger than 10 years old) are treated with vincristine, dactinomycin, and high-dose cyclophosphamide.

• *High-risk disease* (metastatic alveolar disease or metastatic embryonal disease in patients >10 years old) are treated with newer drugs such as irinotecan. They are candidates for treatment trials.

• *TMP-SMX* is used for 6 months after chemotherapy as prophylaxis against *Pneumocystis carinii*. Filgrastim is used to minimize neutropenia while maintaining dose intensity.

Table 87.1 • Risk Factors Associated with Development of Breast Cancer

Strong Risk Factors
- History of breast cancer in the contralateral breast
- Family history of breast cancer, especially in first-degree relatives[a]
- Benign breast "cancer" (i.e., atypical hyperplasia)
- Early menarche, late menopause
- Late first pregnancy greater than no pregnancy
- Advancing age

Possible Risk Factors
- Obesity
- High-fat diet
- Long-term use of exogenous estrogens
- Alcohol

[a]Some cases of familial breast cancer, especially those in premenopausal women, have been linked to specific breast cancer susceptibility genes, BRCA-1 and BRCA-2.

Notes:

Table 87.2 • Adjuvant Treatment for Patients with Node-Negative (A) and Node-Positive (B) Breast Cancer^{a,b}

Patient Group	Node Negative		
	Minimal/Low Risk[c]	Intermediate Risk[d]	High Risk[e]
Premenopausal, ER- or PR-positive	**None or tamoxifen**	**Tamoxifen ± chemotherapy**[f] Ovarian ablation[g] Gn-RH analog[g]	**Chemotherapy ± tamoxifen**[f] Ovarian ablation[g] Gn-RH analog[g]
Premenopausal, ER- and PR-negative	Not applicable	Not applicable	**Chemotherapy**[h]
Postmenopausal, ER- or PR-positive	**None or tamoxifen**	**Tamoxifen ± chemotherapy**[f]	**Tamoxifen + chemotherapy**[f]
Postmenopausal, ER- and PR-negative	Not applicable	Not applicable	**Chemotherapy**[h]
Elderly	**None or tamoxifen**	**Tamoxifen ± chemotherapy**	**Tamoxifen** If no ER and PR expression: chemotherapy

Patient Group	Node Positive
	Treatments
Premenopausal, ER- or PR-positive	**Chemotherapy ± tamoxifen** **Ovarian ablation (or Gn-RH analog) ± tamoxifen**[g] Chemotherapy ± ovarian ablation or (Gn-RH analog) ± tamoxifen[f]
Premenopausal, ER- and PR-negative	**Chemotherapy**[h]
Postmenopausal, ER- or PR-positive	**Tamoxifen ± chemotherapy**[f]
Postmenopausal, ER- and PR-negative	**Chemotherapy**[h]
Elderly	**Tamoxifen** If no ER and PR expression: **chemotherapy**

[a]ER = Estrogen receptor; Gn-RH = Gonadotropin releasing hormone; PR = Progesterone receptor.
[b]Bold entries are treatments accepted for routine use or baseline in clinical trials.
[c]Minimal/low risk includes patients with negative lymph nodes, tumors ≤1 cm in diameter estrogen receptor-positive, histologic grade 1, and age 35 years or older
[d]Intermediate risk includes all patients who fall outside these criteria.
[e]High-risk, node-negative patients have one of the following: tumor >2 cm, estrogen receptor negative, histologic grade 2 or 3, and age younger than 35 years. All node-positive patients are high risk
[f]The addition of chemotherapy is considered an acceptable option based on evidence from clinical trials. Considerations about a low relative risk of relapse, age, toxic effects, socioeconomic implications, and information on patient's preference might justify the use of **tamoxifen alone.**
[g]Indicates treatments still being tested in randomized clinical trials.
[h]The addition of tamoxifen following chemotherapy might be considered for patients whose tumors are classified as ER and PR negative but that exhibit minimal/trace levels of either ER or PR.
Adapted with permission from Dipiro JT et al. Pharmacotherapy: a pathophysiological approach, 4th ed. Stamford, CT: Appleton & Lange, 1999:2028.

Table 87.3 • Causes of Positive Fecal Guaiac Test[a]

Foods with Peroxidase Activity	Medications That Interfere with Fecal Blood Testing	Common Causes of Blood in the Stool
Broccoli	Steroids	Colorectal cancer
Cauliflower	NSAIDs	Colorectal polyps
Turnips	Reserpine	Diverticulitis
Horseradish		Hemorrhoids
Cabbage		Fissures
Potatoes		Proctitis
Cucumbers		Inflammatory bowel disease
Mushrooms		
Artichokes		

[a]NSAIDs = Nonsteroidal anti-inflammatory drugs.

Table 87.4 • Danger Signs of Malignant Melanoma

Examine Skin Lesions for:

Change in Color
Especially multiple shades of dark brown or black; red, white, and blue; spread of color from the edge of the lesion into surrounding skin

Change in Size
Especially sudden or continuous enlargement

Change in Shape
Especially development of irregular margins

Change in Elevation
Especially sudden elevation of a previously macular pigmented lesion

Change in Surface
Especially scaliness, erosion, oozing, crusting, ulceration, bleeding

Change in Surrounding Skin
Especially redness, swelling, satellite pigmentations

Change in Sensation
Especially itching, tenderness, pain

Change in Consistency
Especially softening or friability

Notes:

Table 87.5 • Relative Incidence of Malignancies in Children 0 to 14 Years of Age

Malignancy	Relative Incidence (%)
Acute lymphoblastic leukemia	23.2
Central nervous system	20.7
Neuroblastoma	7.3
Non-Hodgkin's lymphoma	6.3
Wilms' tumor	6.1
Hodgkin's lymphoma	5.0
Acute myeloid leukemia	4.2
Rhabdomyosarcoma	3.4
Retinoblastoma	2.9
Osteosarcoma	2.6
Ewing's sarcoma	2.1
Other histologic types	16.4

Adapted from Gurney JG et al. Incidence of cancer in children in the United States. Cancer 1995;75(8):2186. Copyright 1995 American Cancer Society. Reprinted by permission of Wiley-Liss, Inc., a subsidiary of John Wiley & Sons, Inc. Based on National Cancer Institute Surveillance, Epidemiology, and End Results data from 1974–1989. Total Incidence = 133.3 per million children.

Table 87.6 • International Neuroblastoma Staging System (Abbreviated)

Stage 1	Local tumor with complete gross excision
Stage 2A	Unilateral localized tumor with incomplete gross excision
Stage 2B	Unilateral localized tumor, complete or incomplete excision, with ipsilateral nonadherent lymph node spread
Stage 3	Involves both sides of the midline
Stage 4	Distant lymph node or organ involvement
Stage 4S	Infants less than 1 year of age with localized primary tumor (stage 1 or 2) with dissemination limited to liver, skin, and/or <10% of bone marrow

Adapted from reference 215.

Table 87.7 • Factors Associated with a Poor Prognosis in Neuroblastoma

Stages 3 or 4 disease
Age older than 1 year
N-myc oncogene amplification
DNA index = 1 (diploid)
Shimada unfavorable histology
Ferritin >142 ng/mL
Neuron-specific enolase >100 ng/mL
Lactate dehydrogenase >1,500 units/mL in infants
Deletions of the short arm of chromosome 1

Adapted from references 216–228.

Notes:

Table 87.8 • National Comprehensive Cancer Network Neuroblastoma Risk Groups

Low-Risk
All stage 1 patients
Infants younger than 1 year with stages 2, 3, or 4S and hyperdiploidy

Intermediate-Risk
Patients more than 1 year old at diagnosis with stage 2 or 3 and N-myc not amplified
Infants with stages 2, 3, or 4S and diploidy
Infants with stage 4 and hyperdiploidy

High-Risk
Infants with stage 4 and diploidy
Patients with stage 2A and N-myc amplification

Very High-Risk
Patients more than 1 year old at diagnosis with stage 4
Patients with stages 2B, 3, or 4S and N-myc amplification
Infants with stage 4 and N-myc amplification

Adapted from reference 229.

Table 87.9 • Sequence of Chemotherapy Combinations Used in U.S. Intergroup Low- and Intermediate-Risk Neuroblastoma Clinical Trials[a]

1. Carboplatin, etoposide
2. Carboplatin, cyclophosphamide, doxorubicin
3. Cyclophosphamide, etoposide
4. Carboplatin, doxorubicin, etoposide
5. Cyclophosphamide, etoposide
6. Carboplatin, cyclophosphamide, doxorubicin
7. Carboplatin, etoposide
8. Cyclophosphamide, doxorubicin

[a]Generally the first four courses are used in patients with favorable histology disease and all eight for patients with unfavorable histology.

Table 87.10 • National Wilms' Tumor Study V Treatment Regimens by Stage and Histology

Stages I and II, Favorable Histology; Stage I, Focal or Diffuse Unfavorable Histology:
1. Surgery followed by 18 weeks of vincristine and dactinomycin

Stage III, Favorable Histology; Stages II and III, Focal Anaplasia:
2. Surgery followed by 24 weeks of vincristine, dactinomycin, and doxorubicin, with abdominal radiation. *Stage IV, Favorable Histology or Focal Anaplasia:* Add pulmonary radiation if chest radiograph shows metastases

Stage II or III, Diffuse Anaplasia; Stages I to III Clear Cell Sarcoma of the Kidney (Unfavorable Histology):
3. Surgery followed by 24 weeks of vincristine, doxorubicin, etoposide, and cyclophosphamide with mesna, abdominal radiation. *Stage IV, Diffuse Anaplasia or Clear Cell Sarcoma of the Kidney:* Add pulmonary radiation if chest radiograph is positive for metastases

Stage V:
4. Biopsy followed by neoadjuvant vincristine, dactinomycin, and doxorubicin, then complete resection or debulking followed by more chemotherapy and if a poor response, radiation therapy; more aggressive treatment if unfavorable histology (10%)

Stages I–IV, Rhabdoid Tumor (Unfavorable Histology):
5. Surgery followed by 24 weeks of carboplatin, etoposide, and cyclophosphamide with mesna, abdominal radiation

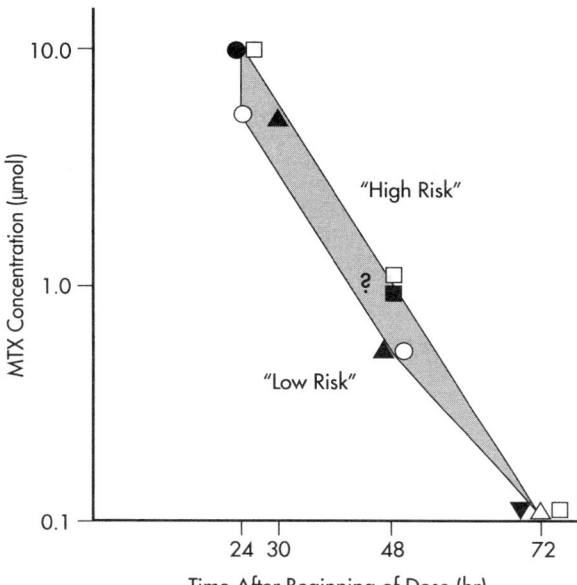

Time After Beginning of Dose (hr)

Fig. 87.1 Composite Semilogarithmic Plot of Serum Methotrexate (MTX) Concentrations That Have Been Proposed to Identify Patients at "High Risk" to Develop Toxicity from High-Dose MTX if Conventional Low-Dose Leucovorin is Administered. Data obtained from reports of (▲) Evans,[294] (△)Tattersal,[295] (●) Isacoff,[296] (○) Isacoff,[297] (□)Nirenberg,[298] (■) Stoller,[299] (▼) Rechnitzer.[300] (Reprinted from Evans WE et al. *Applied Pharmacokinetics: Principles of Therapeutic Drug Monitoring.* 3rd Ed. Vancouver, WA: Applied Therapeutics Inc., 1992.)

The reader is referred to Chapter 89: Solid Tumors, written by *Celeste M. Lindley, Pharm.D., Rebecca S. Finley, Pharm.D.,* and *David W. Henry, Pharm.D.,* in the seventh edition of **Applied Therapeutics: The Clinical Use of Drugs** for a more in-depth discussion of the pathophysiology and treatment of adult and childhood solid tumors. All notations to reference numbers are based on the reference list at the end of that chapter. The editors of this handbook express their thanks to Drs. Lindley, Finley, and Henry and acknowledge that this chapter is based upon their work.

Notes:

Notes:

Chapter 88

Hematopoietic Cell Transplantation

Definitions

♦ *Hematopoietic cell transplantation (HCT)* is broadly defined as the infusion of hematopoietic stem cells (HSCs) into a patient to treat disease and/or restore normal hematopoiesis and lymphopoiesis. Previously called bone marrow transplant, HCT is a more appropriate term because cells are obtained from the donor's bone marrow, peripheral blood, or umbilical cord.

♦ *Allogeneic HCT* involves "transplantation" of bone marrow from one individual to another and is potentially curative for diseases involving the bone marrow or immune system. The procedure has also allowed dose-intensive chemotherapy in the treatment of malignancy. (See Chapter 84: Neoplastic Disorders and Their Treatment.) Histocompatibility is a major consideration because there is potential for bidirectional graft rejection. Human leukocyte antigen (HLA) typing is used to test for compatibility; rejection reactions are least likely if the donor is fully matched with the patient at HLA-A, HLA-B, and HLA-DR. Intensive pre- and posttransplant immunosuppression is needed to prevent rejection or graft-versus-host disease (GVHD). See Tables 88.1 and 88.2.

♦ *Syngeneic HCT* is infusion of HSCs from an identical twin.

♦ *Autologous HCT* is the use of the patient's own hematopoietic stem cells to allow the use of escalating doses of chemotherapy, radiation, or both. More aptly called hematopoietic cell rescue, the procedure permits use of doses of chemotherapy otherwise limited by hematopoietic toxicity. See Tables 88.1 and 88.2.

♦ *Cord blood stem cell transplantation (CBT),* a form of allogeneic HCT, is restricted to children and adults weighing <60 kg because of the limited number of stem cells that can be obtained from this source.

♦ *Peripheral blood stem cell transplantation (PBSCT)* has replaced BMT for autologous rescue after high-dose chemotherapy and is being used increasingly in the allogeneic setting.

Allogeneic HCT

♦ *Basic Schema.* See Figure 88.1. A 1- to 2-day rest and then infusion of stem cells generally follow administration of near-lethal doses of chemotherapy and/or radiation. A period of pancytopenia (2 to 6 weeks) follows until engraftment or the re-establishment of functional hematopoiesis by the infused stem cells occurs. This is defined as an absolute neutrophil count (ANC) of 500 cells/mm^3 for 2 to 3 consecutive days. Time to engraftment is determined by several factors. See Figure 88.2.

♦ *Preparative or conditioning regimens* are used in recipients who have functioning immune systems and are designed to eradicate immunologically active host tissues (to prevent host-versus-graft reactions), to destroy residual malignant cells, or both. Table 88.3 describes common preparative regimens, but most contain cyclophosphamide, total body irradiation (TBI) or both if used to treat hematologic malignancies. Antithymocyte globulin (ATG) may be added in the case of a mismatched allogeneic HCT. Preparative conditioning regimens are not needed for patients with poor immune systems.

♦ **Post-transplant immunosuppressive therapy** is used for 6 months to 1 year to prevent or minimize GVHD. Common regimens include cyclosporine or tacrolimus with a short course of low-dose methotrexate. Therapy is not needed in the case of a syngeneic HCT or a T-cell-depleted histocompatible HCT for the treatment of severe combined immunodeficiency disease.

♦ **Acute leukemia** is the most common indication for allogeneic BMT, accounting for 40% of procedures. HCT improves disease-free survival for patients with AML in first remission compared to intensive chemotherapy. However, higher early mortality in the HCT arms and a higher incidence of relapse in the chemotherapy-treated patients equalizes overall survival. See Chapter 86.

♦ **Supportive care** is directed toward maintaining an adequate complete blood count (CBC), preventing or treating infection, and providing adequate nutrition. It includes placement of a central venous catheter, transfusions of packed RBCs when the hematocrit is <25% and platelets when the counts are <10,000 to 20,000/mm^3, strict isolation in rooms equipped with laminar air flow, prophylactic antibacterial and antifungal therapy, good oral hygiene, low microbial diets, antiemetics, analgesics, and total parenteral nutrition as necessary. The use of hematopoietic growth factors is yet unsettled due to concern that they may enhance GVHD.

Autologous HCT

♦ **Basic Schema.** Since the donor and patient are the same, pre- and posttransplant immunotherapy are unnecessary. However, since the HSCs must be harvested before chemotherapy, they must be cryopreserved and stored for future use. Once harvested, they may be purged to minimize tumor contamination or to enrich the hematopoietic cell composition.

♦ **PBSCs** are preferred to bone marrow and are obtained by daily apheresis, a procedure similar to dialysis, until an adequate number of hematopoietic progenitor cells have been obtained. Chemotherapy (e.g., a single dose of cyclophosphamide 4 gm/m^2 by IV infusion) and hematopoietic growth factors (e.g., filgrastim 5 to 15 μg/kg per day or sargramostim 250 to 500 μg/m^2 per day) are used as priming agents for PBSC collection. PBSC HCT rescue is associated with more rapid engraftment and decreased health care resource use relative to BMT. See Table 88.4.

♦ **Indications** primarily include chemotherapy-sensitive malignancies, such as intermediate or high-grade non-Hodgkin's lymphoma, since patients who do not respond to chemotherapy are unlikely to respond to autologous HCT. See Table 88.2.

♦ **Supportive Therapy.** Profound aplasia lasting 20 to 30 days occurs after high-dose chemotherapy and autologous BMT, but only for 7 to 14 days after PBSC infusion. Both sargramostim (250 μg/m^2 per day IV over 2 hours beginning on the day of infusion for 21 days) and filgrastim accelerate the time to engraftment following BMT and, perhaps, after PBSC infusion. Growth factor-treated BMT patients also had fewer days of antibiotics, fewer documented bacterial infections, and a shorter initial hospital stay. However, platelet production is not enhanced. There is no established role for erythropoietin or interleukin-2. Other supportive measures include use of central venous catheters, blood product support, and medical management of nausea, vomiting, mucositis, and pain. Autologous HCT patients are not subject to extended immunosuppressive therapy and are less susceptible to infection; thus, the use of isolation is unnecessary, and outpatient care often can be incorporated into the initial recovery.

Complications Associated with HCT

Regimen-Related Toxicities. HCT patients experience toxicities commonly associated with chemotherapy (see Chapter 85: Adverse Effects of Chemotherapy); however, these are often magnified. Mucositis, for example, is often severe enough to warrant airway protection, preclude oral intake, and require IV narcotics for pain control. Table 88.5 lists extramedullary (nonhematopoietic) toxicities that become dose-limiting in HCT patients. Table 88.6 depicts the range of toxicities that can occur following HCT, and Figure 88.3 depicts the time course for complications following HCT.

   ♦ **Overdosing Obese Patients.** Doses of immunosuppressants used for preparatory therapy should not be based on actual body weight (ABW) in obese patients because this may expose them to severe toxicity. Instead ideal body weight (IBW) or an adjusted ideal body weight = IBW + 0.25 (ABW − IBW) should be used.

   ♦ **Busulfan seizures** occurred in up to 7.5% of children in one series. They are characterized by a single seizure that occurs after at least 6 or 7 of the 16 total doses and usually do not result in permanent neurologic deficits. Prophylactic oral phenytoin to achieve concentrations of 10 to 20 ng/mL is used before, during, and for 24 to 48 hours after the last dose. Seizures may, nevertheless, occur.

   ♦ **Cyclophosphamide hemorrhagic cystitis** occurs in 12 to 73% of HCT patients. Prophylaxis includes forced hydration with normal saline (NS) or dextrose 5% in NS, 3000 mL/m^2 per day; continuous bladder irrigation with NS 200 to 1000 mL/hr via a 3-way Foley catheter; and/or use of the uroprotectant, mesna. To date, there have been no randomized comparative trials evaluating the most effective prophylactic method.

   ♦ **Veno-occlusive disease (VOD) of the liver** is a life-threatening (50% mortality) complication of high-dose chemotherapy or radiation that has a prevalence of 4 to 54%. It is defined as a fibrous narrowing or obliteration of the small hepatic venules that presents as hepatic failure. The signs and symptoms are listed in Table 88.7, but the first manifestation is weight gain exceeding 5% of baseline within 3 to 6 days of marrow infusion. A diagnosis is made if any two of the following occur in the first 30 days after HCT: hyperbilirubinemia, hepatomegaly and RUQ pain, or ascites and/or unexplained weight gain. Treatment is supportive and aimed at increasing intravascular volume (colloids; albumin), decreasing extracellular fluid accumulation (spironolactone), and minimizing encephalopathy (low-protein diet; lactulose). Recombinant tissue plasminogen activator and heparin have been used experimentally in severe cases.

Graft failure is a lack of functional hematopoiesis after HCT and is classified as primary graft failure (failure to engraft) or graft rejection.

   ♦ *Primary failure* most often occurs following autologous HCT. Contributing factors include intensive chemotherapy, which reduces the inoculum or viability of progenitor cells, residual malignancy, and ex vivo purging. In allogeneic HCT, primary graft failure is uncommon because the donor marrow in unmanipulated and is free from the toxic effects of prior chemotherapy.

   ♦ *Graft rejection* is more common in allogeneic HCTs. However, it is rare when histocompatible donors are used to treat leukemia. The incidence is higher in patients with aplastic anemia and in those who have received a histoincompatible or T-cell-depleted marrow.

   ♦ *Treatment* options are limited but include antithymocyte globulin and hematopoietic growth factors.

Graft-Versus-Host Disease (GVHD) is one of the most serious complications after allogeneic HCT, occurring in about 45% of patients; the overall mortality is 48% but increases to 90% with grade IV GVHD. The pathogenesis is complex but involves immunocompetent donor T-cells that recognize host histocompatibility antigens as foreign. Destruction of tissues disrupts the integrity of protective mucosal barriers, which leads to opportunistic infections. GVHD is classified as acute or chronic based on clinical manifestations and an arbitrarily designated time relative to day 0 of HCT.

♦ *Acute GVHD* primarily affects the skin, liver, and GI tract and usually occurs within the first 100 days after HCT. The single most important risk factor is the degree of histocompatibility between the donor and recipient. See Figure 88.4.

  • *Symptoms* include a diffuse maculopapular rash that starts on the palms, soles, or behind the ears, which can progress to a generalized erythrodermal bullae and desquamation; severe bloody diarrhea; and hyperbilirubinemia that can progress to hepatic failure.

  • A *staging system* first evaluates the severity of organ involvement (Table 88.8) and then establishes an overall grade based on the number and extent of involved organs (Table 88.9).

  • *Posttransplant immunosuppressive therapy* or infusion of T-cell-depleted hemato-poietic cells are two methods used to prevent or minimize GVHD. Combination therapy is superior to single-agent therapy, except in acute leukemia when a single agent allows for the development of low-grade GVHD, which has a beneficial graft-versus-leukemia effect. Table 88.10 describes regimens that have been used. There is no consensus on the best regimen. Methotrexate, cyclosporine or tacroli-mus, and corticosteroids are the agents most commonly incorporated into these regimens. Table 88.11 describes characteristics of regimens containing these drugs. Trough cyclosporine levels of 200 to 400 ng/mL may enhance effectiveness while minimizing nephrotoxicity.

  • *Treatment* of established acute GVHD consists of high-dose corticosteroids: methylprednisolone 2 mg/kg per day IV or PO in four divided doses for a minimum of 14 days, followed by a tapering schedule over at least 1 month as determined by patient response. About 40% respond. ATG, OKT3, or investigational drugs are used as salvage therapy for those who do not respond.

♦ *Chronic GVHD* can affect almost any organ system and closely resembles several autoimmune diseases. It occurs in about 45% of patients who have undergone allogeneic HCT and is unrelated to the regimen used for prophylaxis of acute GVHD. Risk factors include increasing age, history, and acuity of acute GVHD.

  • *Signs and symptoms* are multifaceted because any organ system can be involved. See Table 88.12.

  • *Time Course.* There are three patterns: progressive, quiescent, or de novo. The progressive form evolves directly from acute GVHD and has the worst prognosis. The quiescent form appears slowly after a period of complete resolution of acute GVHD. De novo chronic GVHD occurs spontaneously in the absence of a history of acute GVHD.

  • *Severity* is described as "limited" or "extensive" based on the extent of involve-ment. Limited GVHD is localized to the skin or liver. Extensive GVHD is characterized by extensive skin or hepatic involvement, mucosal changes, and/or involvement of other organ systems.

  • *Treatment* is with immunosuppressive agents. Prednisone, azathioprine, and cyclo-sporine have the best efficacy and toxicity profiles and are most commonly used. Single-agent therapy with prednisone is the treatment of choice for lim-ited involvement, quiescent, or de novo chronic GVHD. The dose of prednisone is 1 mg/kg per day in divided doses for 30 days; then convert slowly to 2 mg/kg per day every other day (QOD); then taper slowly to 1 mg/kg QOD. Onset of improvement is in 1 to 2 months; therapy is continued for 9 to 12 months. The dose of azathioprine alone or in combination is 1.5 mg/kg per day. For progressive GVHD, cyclosporine plus prednisone or thalidomide are used.

- *Adjuvant therapy* includes trimethoprim-sulfamethoxazole for prophylaxis of *P. carinii;* sunscreens, artificial tears and saliva to prevent fissures and cracking of the mucous membranes, and nutritional supplements as needed.

Infectious Complications

♦ *Periods of Infectious Risk.* There are 3 periods depicted in Figure 88.3.

- In the early period when neutropenia and mucositis are present, the primary pathogens are aerobic bacteria (*Staphylococcus, S. viridans,* vancomycin-resistant enterococci), herpes simplex virus (now rare with the use of antiviral prophylaxis), respiratory viruses, and candida (oral and systemic)

- The second period spans from marrow engraftment to posttransplant day +100. CMV, adenovirus, *P. carinii,* and aspergillosis are common pathogens, and interstitial pneumonia is a common clinical manifestation.

- During the late period (after day +100), the predominant organisms are encapsulated bacteria (e.g., *S. pneumoniae, H. influenzae, N. meningitides), fungi,* and varicella-zoster virus. The encapsulated organisms commonly cause sinopulmonary infections.

♦ *Prevention of Herpes Simplex Virus (HSV).* Reactivation occurs in 43 to 70% of patients who are HSV antibody seropositive before allogeneic or autologous HCT. Acyclovir reduces the occurrence to 0 to 45%. HSV seronegative patients rarely develop HSV so acyclovir is not warranted. IV acyclovir is given from the day of admission until the patient can tolerate and reliably absorb oral medication. Dose: 250 mg/m^2 or 5 mg/kg IV every 12 hours; convert to oral acyclovir 400 mg TID for patients >7 years old and 200 mg TID if <7 years old. Duration of therapy is +30 to +180 days. Patients on ganciclovir prophylaxis for CMV do not require acyclovir for HSV.

♦ *Prevention of CMV.* CMV is common in allogeneic, but not autologous HCTs. Primary CMV can be prevented by avoiding exposure to the virus (CMV-negative donor, blood products), but this is difficult. Other strategies include the use of filtered blood products, immune globulin, prophylactic antiviral therapy, or a combination of these.

- *Antivirals.* To prevent secondary CMV, high-dose acyclovir or ganciclovir (most common) are used from the time of engraftment to day +100. Ganciclovir also is used as pre-emptive therapy at the time of CMV reactivation following HCT. The goal is to prevent progression to CMV disease while the patient is symptomatic. Table 88.13 presents doses of ganciclovir commonly used as prophylactic and pre-emptive therapy. Reversible neutropenia occurs in 30 to 58% of patients within a median of 36 days. If ganciclovir is discontinued, the ANC recovers to >1000/mm^3 at which time ganciclovir can be reinstituted on an every other day schedule. Sargramostim (250 μg/m^2 per day) or filgrastim (5 μg/kg per day) IV or SC may be used to speed recovery and titrated to maintain the ANC >1000 cells/mL. Thrombocytopenia also can occur.

- *Immunoglobulin (IVIG).* Humoral immunity is depressed for 3 to 4 months following HCT. IVIG prophylaxis reduces CMV infection, interstitial pneumonia, septicemia, and GVHD. Most centers use unselected IVIG prophylactically, while others use IVIG when IgG levels are <650 mg/dL. The optimal dose and schedule are not known.

♦ *CMV infection* is one of the most serious infectious complications following HCT. The usual onset is between days +30 to +90 after an allogeneic HCT and is most often due to reactivation of a latent virus. Diagnosis is difficult, but the infection most often manifests as interstitial pneumonitis (CMV IP) or enteritis (epigastric pain, nausea, vomiting, diarrhea, anorexia, weight loss, or GI hemorrhage).

- CMV-IP following HCT best responds to combined therapy with ganciclovir and unselected IVIG. Induction therapy should be administered for 3 weeks, and maintenance therapy should be given for an additional 2 to 3 weeks or longer if pulmonary symptoms persist. See Table 88.14 for doses and outcomes.

- GI-CMV often is self-limited but can be progressive in HCT patients. Although the benefit of ganciclovir has not been demonstrated, it is used because the condition is so debilitating. Induction doses are 2.5 mg/kg every 8 hours or 5 mg/kg every 12 hours IV for 2 to 3 weeks. Maintenance therapy similar to that given for CMV-IP may prevent or delay recurrences. Foscarnet can be used for patients who cannot tolerate ganciclovir (60 mg/kg every 8 hours IV for 2 to 3 weeks followed by a maintenance dose of 60 mg/kg IV daily). Although it does not have hematologic effects, it is nephrotoxic.

♦ *Pneumocystis carinii Pneumonia (PCP) Prevention.* PCP is a common cause of infection after allogeneic HCT. Most centers administer co-trimoxazole after engraftment (ANC >1000/mm^3) and pentamidine or dapsone in those allergic to sulfas. See Table 88.15. Although some administer co-trimoxazole during the neutropenic period, it has myelosuppressive effects and should be used cautiously. Prophylaxis should be continued for 6 to 12 months. Routine prophylaxis following autologous HCTs is controversial.

Table 88.1 • Comparison of Allogeneic and Autologous HCT

	Allogeneic	Autologous
Risk of[a]:		
Relapse after HCT	+	+++
Rejection	+	—
Delayed engraftment	+	++
GVHD	+	—
Infection	++−+++[b]	+
Transplant-related morbidity	+++	+
Transplant-related mortality	++	+
Cost of procedure	+++	++

[a]Risk will vary depending on underlying disease, patient characteristics, and previous medical history.
[b]Risk of infection increases with presence of prolonged immunosuppression and/or chronic graft-versus-host disease.

Notes:

Table 88.2 • Indications for BMT[a,b,1,5a,16]

	Established Role	Promising/ Experimental
Allogeneic		
Nonmalignant	Aplastic anemia Homozygous β-thalassemia Severe combined immunodeficiency disease Wiskott-Aldrich syndrome Fanconi's anemia Infantile osteopetrosis Chediak-Higashi syndrome	Sickle cell anemia Severe leukocyte adhesion deficiency X-linked agammaglobulinemia Common variable immunodeficiency
Malignant	AML ALL CML (Intermediate- and high-grade NHL)	CLL (young patients only) Multiple myeloma Myelodysplastic syndrome
Autologous		
Nonmalignant	—	Genetic disorders with gene therapy
Malignant	Intermediate and high-grade NHL AML (patients who lack suitable allogeneic donors) Relapsed or refractory HD Testicular cancer	Breast cancer (high-risk adjuvant or metastatic) Multiple myeloma Neuroblastoma Small-cell lung cancer Ovarian cancer Low-grade lymphomas Rhabdomyosarcoma

[a]AML = Acute myelogenous leukemia; BMT = Bone marrow transplantation; CLL = Chronic lymphocytic leukemia; CML = Chronic myelogenous leukemia; HD = Hodgkin's disease; NHL = Non-Hodgkin's lymphoma.
[b]Timing relative to diagnosis and other therapies may vary.

Notes:

Table 88.3 • Representative Preparative Regimens Used in BMT[a]

Type of BMT	Disease State	Regimen[a]	Dose/Schedule
Allogeneic[2,18]	Hematologic malignancies[a]	Cy + TBI	Cy 60 mg/kg/day IV on 2 consecutive days before TBI + 1,000–1,575 rads TBI fractionated over 1–7 days
Allogeneic[19]	Aplastic anemia	Cy	Cy 60 mg/kg/day IV on 4 consecutive days (–5, –4, –3, –2)
Allogeneic, Autologous[20–22]	Acute and chronic leukemias	Bu + Cy	Bu (adult): 1 mg/kg/dose PO Q 6 hr × 16 doses Age <7 yr: 37.5 mg/m² PO Q 6 hr × 16 doses + Cy 50 mg/kg/day IV QD × 4 days following Bu or 60 mg/kg/day IV QD × 2 days following Bu
Allogeneic[23]	Hematologic malignancies	TBI + VP-16	1320 rads TBI over 4 consecutive days (–7, –6, –5, –4) + VP-16 60 mg/kg/day IV on day –3
Allogeneic Autologous, PBSC[24,25]	Hematologic malignancies	Cy + BCNU + VP-16	Cy 1,500 mg/m²/day IV on 4 consecutive days (–6, –5, –4, –3) + BCNU 300 mg/m²/day IV × 1, day –6 + VP-16 100 mg/m²/dose IV Q 12 hr for 6 doses (–6, –5, –4)
Autologous, PBSC[26]	HD, NHL	BCNU + VP-16 + Ara-C + melphalan	BCNU 300 mg/m²/day IV × 1, day –6 + VP-16 100–200 mg/m²/day IV QD × 4 (days –5, –4, –3, –2) + Ara-C 200–400 mg/m²/day IV QD × 4 (days –5, –4, –3, –2) + melphalan 140 mg/m²/day IV, day –1
Autologous, PBSC[27]	Breast	Cy + Cisplatin + BCNU	Cy 1875 mg/m²/day IV QD × 3 (–6, –5, –4) + CDDP 55 mg/m²/day as a 72 hr IV continuous infusion (–6, –5, –4) + BCNU 600 mg/m²/day IV × 1, day –6
Autologous, PBSC[29]	Testicular	Carbo + VP-16	Carbo 500 mg/m²/day IV QD × 3 (days –7, –5, –3) + VP-16 400 mg/m²/day IV QD × 3 (days –7, –5, –3)

[a]Ara-C = Cytarabine; BCNU = Carmustine; BMT = Bone marrow transplantation; Carbo = Carboplatin; CDDP = Cisplatin; Cy = Cyclophosphamide; HD = Hodgkin's disease; NHL = Non-Hodgkin's lymphoma; TBI = Total body irradiation; VP-16 = Etoposide. [a]Ara-C = Cytarabine; BCNU = Carmustine; BMT = Bone marrow transplantation; Carbo = Carboplatin; CDDP = Cisplatin; Cy = Cyclophosphamide; HD = Hodgkin's disease; NHL = Non-Hodgkin's lymphoma; TBI = Total body irradiation; VP-16 = Etoposide.
[b]Includes acute myelogenous leukemia, acute lymphocytic leukemia, chronic myelogenous leukemia, non-Hodgkin's lymphoma, and Hodgkin's disease.

Table 88.4 • Comparison of Source of Hematopoietic Cells in Autologous HCT Bone Marrow Versus Peripheral Blood

	Bone Marrow	Peripheral Blood
Duration of neutropenia	++	+
Duration of thrombocytopenia	++	+
Transfusion support needs	++	+
Number of hematopoietic cells collected/infused	+	++
Duration of hospitalization	++	+
Early complications	++	+
Late complications[a]	= ?	= ?
Tumor contamination of hematopoietic cell product[b]	++	+
Cost of procedure	+++	++

[a]Limited comparative data on long-term complications.
[b]Clinical relevance of differences in tumor contamination for certain diseases under evaluation.

Table 88.5 • Single-Agent Dose Escalation[95,96]

Agent	Usual Dose (mg/m^2)	Maximum Dose with Stem Cell Rescue (mg/m^2)	Extramedullary Toxicity
Total body irradiation	—	1,300–1,500 rads[a]	Hepatic, pulmonary
Cyclophosphamide	500–1,000	7,500 (200 mg/kg)	Cardiac, bladder
Busulfan	2–8 mg/day	16 mg/kg	Hepatic (VOD)
Carmustine	200	1,200	Pulmonary, hepatic
Melphalan	40	200	Mucositis[b]
Thiotepa	50	1,135	Mucositis,[b] central nervous system
Etoposide	200	2,400 (60 mg/kg)	Mucositis[d]
Carboplatin	400	2,000	Renal, hepatic
Cisplatin	100	200	Renal

[a]Administered in fractionated doses.
[b]Mucositis requiring airway protection, parenteral nutrition, and intravenous narcotic analgesics.

Notes:

Table 88.6 • Common Toxicities Associated with BMT[a]

Early	Late
Nausea, vomiting, diarrhea	Cardiotoxicity
Mucositis	Cataracts
Infectious complications	Sterility
Hemorrhagic cystitis	Delayed puberty
Renal dysfunction	Growth retardation
VOD	Second malignancies
Acute GVHD	Chronic GVHD
Cardiotoxicity	
Idiopathic pneumonitis	
Viral pneumonitis	
Graft failure, graft rejection	

[a]BMT = Bone marrow transplantation; GVHD = Graft-versus-host disease; VOD = Veno-occlusive disease.

Table 88.7 • Signs and Symptoms of VOD of the Liver[a,116]

Hyperbilirubinemia	Elevated alkaline phosphatase
Weight gain (>5% above baseline)	Ascites
Hepatomegaly	Elevated AST
Azotemia	Encephalopathy

[a]AST = Aspartate aminotransferase; VOD = Veno-occlusive disease.

Table 88.8 • Proposed Clinical Stage of GVHD According to Organ System[a]

Stage	Skin	Liver	GI Tract
+	Maculopapular rash 25% of BSA	Bilirubin 2–3 mg/dL	>500 mL/day diarrhea
++	Maculopapular rash 25–50% of BSA	Bilirubin 3–6 mg/dL	>1,000 mL/day diarrhea
+++	Generalized erythroderma	Bilirubin 6–15 mg/dL	>1,500 mL/day diarrhea
++++	Generalized erythroderma with bullous formation and desquamation	Bilirubin >15 mg/dL	Severe abdominal pain with or without ileus

[a]BSA = Body surface area; GI = Gastrointestinal; GVHD = Graft-versus-host disease.
Reprinted with permission from Thomas ED et al. Bone-marrow transplantation. N Engl J Med 1975;292:895. Copyright © 2001 Massachusetts Medical Society. All rights reserved.

Notes:

Table 88.9 • Overall Clinical Grading of Severity of GVHD[a]

Grade	Degree of Organ Involvement
I	+ to ++ skin rash; no gut involvement; no liver involvement; no ↓ in clinical performance
II	+ to +++ skin rash; + gut involvement or + liver involvement (or both); mild ↓ in performance status
III	++ to +++ skin rash; ++ to +++ gut involvement or ++ to ++++ liver involvement (or both); marked ↓ in performance status
IV	Similar to grade III with ++ to ++++ organ involvement and extreme ↓ in clinical performance

[a]GVHD = Graft-versus-host disease.
Reprinted with permission from Thomas ED et al. Bone-marrow transplantation. N Engl J Med 1975;292:895. Copyright © 2001 Massachusetts Medical Society. All rights reserved.

Table 88.10 • Regimens of Prophylaxis of Acute GVHD[a]

Drug	Regimen
Single Agent	
MTX "long course"[2]	15 mg/m² IV, day +1
	10 mg/m² IV, day +3, +6, +11; then Q wk until day 100
MTX "short course"	Same dose but no doses after day +11
CTX[147]	7.5 mg/kg IV, day +1, +3, +5, +7, +9; then Q wk until day +10
ATG[148]	7 mg/kg IV over 6 hr QOD × 6 doses, days +8 to +29
CSA[144,149,150]	1.5 mg/kg IV or 6.25 mg/kg PO Q 12 hr, days −1 to +50; then taper 5% per week and discontinue by day +180
Combination Therapy	
MTX "short course"[146,151,152]	15 mg/m² IV, day +1; 10 mg/m², days +3, +6, +11
+	
CSA	1.5 mg/kg IV Q 12 hr (or 6.25 mg/kg PO Q 12 hr), days −1 to +50; then taper by 5% per week and discontinue by day +180
MTX[160]	15 mg/m² IV, days +1, +3, +6
+	
CSA	5 mg/kg/day IV continuous infusion, day −2 to +3, then 3–3.75 mg/kg IV until day +35; then switch to 10 mg/kg/day PO and taper by 20% Q 2 wk; then discontinue by day +180 (dosage adjusted to maintain serum concentration between 200–600 ng/mL)
+	
Pred	0.5 mg/kg/day IV for 1 wk beginning day +7; then 1.0 mg/kg/day IV for 2 wk beginning day +14 or +15; then taper slowly and discontinue by day +180
CSA[161]	5 mg/kg/day IV continuous infusion days 0 to +3; then 3.75 mg/kg/day IV days +4 to +14; then 10 mg/kg/day PO days +15 to +42; then 7.5 mg/kg/day PO days +43 to +180; then discontinue
+	
MP	0.5 mg/kg/day IV day +8 to +14; 1.0 mg/kg/day IV days +15 to +28; then taper slowly and discontinue by day +72
CTX[161]	7.5 mg/kg IV, days +1, +3, +5, +7, +9; then Q wk until day +100
+	
MP	0.5 mg/kg/day IV day +8 to +14; 1.0 mg/kg/day IV, day +15 to day +28; then taper slowly and discontinue by day +72

[a]ATG = Antithymocyte globulin; CSA = Cyclosporine; CTX = Cyclophosphamide; GVHD = Graft-versus-host disease; MP = Methylprednisolone; MTX = Methotrexate; Pred = Prednisone or prednisolone.

Table 88.11 • Characteristics of Combination Regimens for Prophylaxis of Acute GVHD[a]

Regimens Containing	Characteristic
MTX	Delayed engraftment ↑ time to platelet independence ↑ incidence and severity of mucositis Elevations in LFTs
CSA	Marrow sparing ↑ incidence of nephrotoxicity ↑ incidence of neurotoxicity ↑ incidence of hypertension ↓ clearance of MTX if nephrotoxicity develops
Corticosteroids	↑ infectious complications ↑ incidence of hypertension in combination with CSA Hyperglycemia

[a]CSA = Cyclosporine; GVHD = Graft-versus-host disease; LFTs = Liver function tests; MTX = Methotrexate.

Table 88.12 • Signs and Symptoms of Chronic GVHD[a,207,208]

Affected Organ	Clinical Manifestations
Skin	Rash, hypopigmentation or hyperpigmentation, erythema, alopecia, sclerosis, or scleroderma with joint contractures if severe lichen planus lesions
Eyes	↓ tear formation, dry eyes, burning, photophobia
GI tract	↓ saliva production, dry mouth leading to cracking or fissure formation, change in taste sensation, diarrhea and abdominal pain, fat malabsorption, chronic malnutrition, web formation
Liver	Increased LFTs, histologic changes consistent with combined hepatocellular injury and cholestasis
Lungs	Nonproductive cough, wheezing, bronchospasm, diffuse interstitial pneumonitis, restrictive or obstructive abnormalities on PFTs
Bone marrow	Eosinophilia, thrombocytopenia, ↓ antibody formation and subclass distribution
Musculoskeletal	Myalgias, arthralgias, clinical picture resembling systemic lupus erythematosus or rheumatoid arthritis
Miscellaneous	Circulating autoantibodies (antinuclear antibody, rheumatoid factor, positive direct Coombs' test)

[a]GI = Gastrointestinal; GVHD = Graft-versus-host disease; LFTs = Liver function tests; PFTs = Pulmonary function tests.

Notes:

Table 88.13 • Strategies to Prevent CMV Infection and Disease in CMV-Seropositive Patients Undergoing Allogeneic Hematopoietic Cell Transplantation[a]

Strategy/Drug	Regimen
Prophylaxis	
Ganciclovir	5 mg/kg IV Q12 hr × 5 days, then 5 mg/kg/day until day +100 (beginning after engraftment)[227]
	or
	2.5 mg/kg IV Q 8 hr (admission to day −1); then 6 mg/kg/day Mon–Fri only until day +120 (beginning after engraftment)[230]
Foscarnet	40 mg/kg IV Q 8 hr (day −7 to +30), then 60 mg/kg QD until day +75[232]
Pre-Emptive	
Ganciclovir	If BAL positive for CMV at day +35, then 5 mg/kg IV 12 hr × 14 days, then 5 mg/kg Mon–Fri until day +120[228]
	or
	If weekly surveillance blood culture positive for CMV, then 5 mg/kg IV Q 12 hr × 7 days, then 5 mg/kg QD until day +100[229]
	or
	If weekly surveillance blood sample positive for CMV by PCR, 5 mg/kg IV Q 12 hr × 14 days, then 5 mg/kg QD until PCR negative[231]

[a]BAL = Bronchoalveolar lavage; CMV = Cytomegalovirus; PCR = Polymerase chain reaction.

Table 88-14 • Treatment of CMV-IP[a]

Induction	Maintenance	Outcome
Ganciclovir 5 mg/kg Q 12 hr IV (range, 10–59 days)	Ganciclovir 5 mg/kg/dose 5 days/wk	11/13 (85%) responded 9/13 (69%) alive at median of 211 days[260]
+	+	
IVIG (Gammagard) 500 mg/kg QOD (range, 10–59 days)	IVIG 500 mg/kg Q week	
Ganciclovir 2.5 mg/kg Q 8 hr IV × 20 days	Ganciclovir 5 mg/kg/dose 3–5 days/wk × 20 doses	10/10 (100%) responded 7/10 (70%) alive at median of 10 months[261]
+	+	
IVIG (Gammagard) 500 mg/kg QOD × 10 doses	IVIG (Gammagard) 500 mg/kg 2×/wk × 8 doses	
Ganciclovir 2.5 mg/kg Q 8 hr IV × 14 days	Ganciclovir 5 mg/kg/day × 14 days	13/25 (52%) survived initial episode 8/25 (32%) long-term survival[262]
+	+	
CMV-IVIG 400 mg/kg on days 1, 2, 7; 200 mg/kg on day 14	CMV-IVIG 200 mg/kg on day 21 (only received maintenance if symptomatic after completion of induction)	
Ganciclovir 2.5 mg/kg Q 8 hr IV	None	4/6 died[263]
+		
CMV-IVIG 20 g QOD until signs and symptoms resolved		

[a]CMV-IP = Cytomegalovirus interstitial pneumonitis; CMV-IVIG = Cytomegalovirus hyperimmune globulin; IVIG = Intravenous immune globulin.

Table 88.15 • Common PCP Prophylactic Regimens[a]

Co-trimoxazole	5 mg/kg QD divided in 2 doses on 2 or 3 consecutive days of the week or Mon-Wed-Fri
Pentamidine aerosolized	4 mg/kg or 300 mg Q mo
Pentamidine IV	4 mg/kg or 300 mg Q 2–4 wk

[a]PCP = *Pneumocystis carinii* pneumonia.

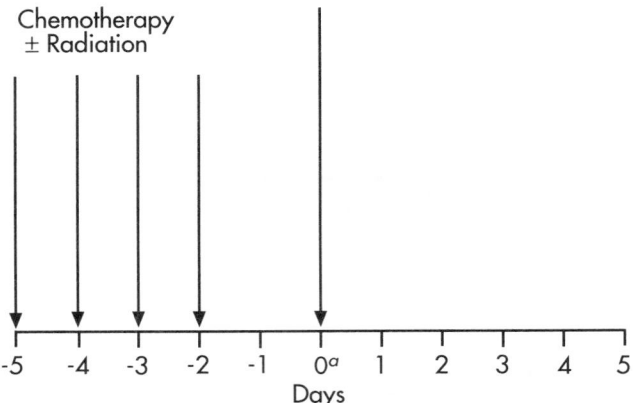

Fig. 88.1 Basic Schema for Bone Marrow Transplantation. [a]Day 0 = bone marrow or stem cell infusion.

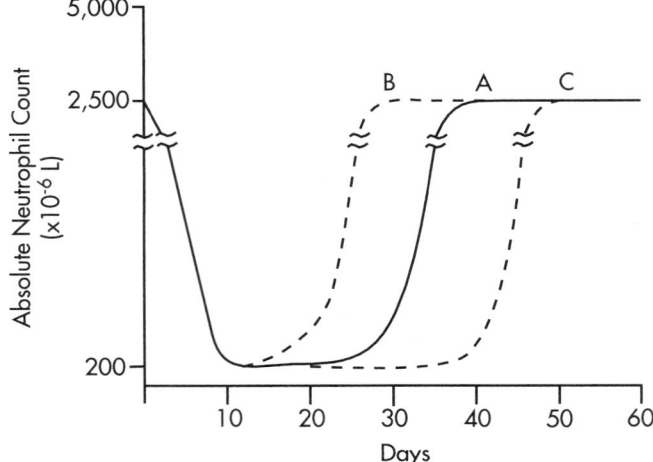

Fig. 88.2 Time to Engraftment. *A,* Bone marrow infusion without complications or hematopoietic growth factors. *B,* Accelerated engraftment with hematopoietic growth factors, peripheral blood stem cells (PBSCs), and/or combination of bone marrow, PBSCs, and hematopoietic growth factors. *C,* Delayed engraftment caused by infection, purged bone marrow, and/or inadequate inoculum.

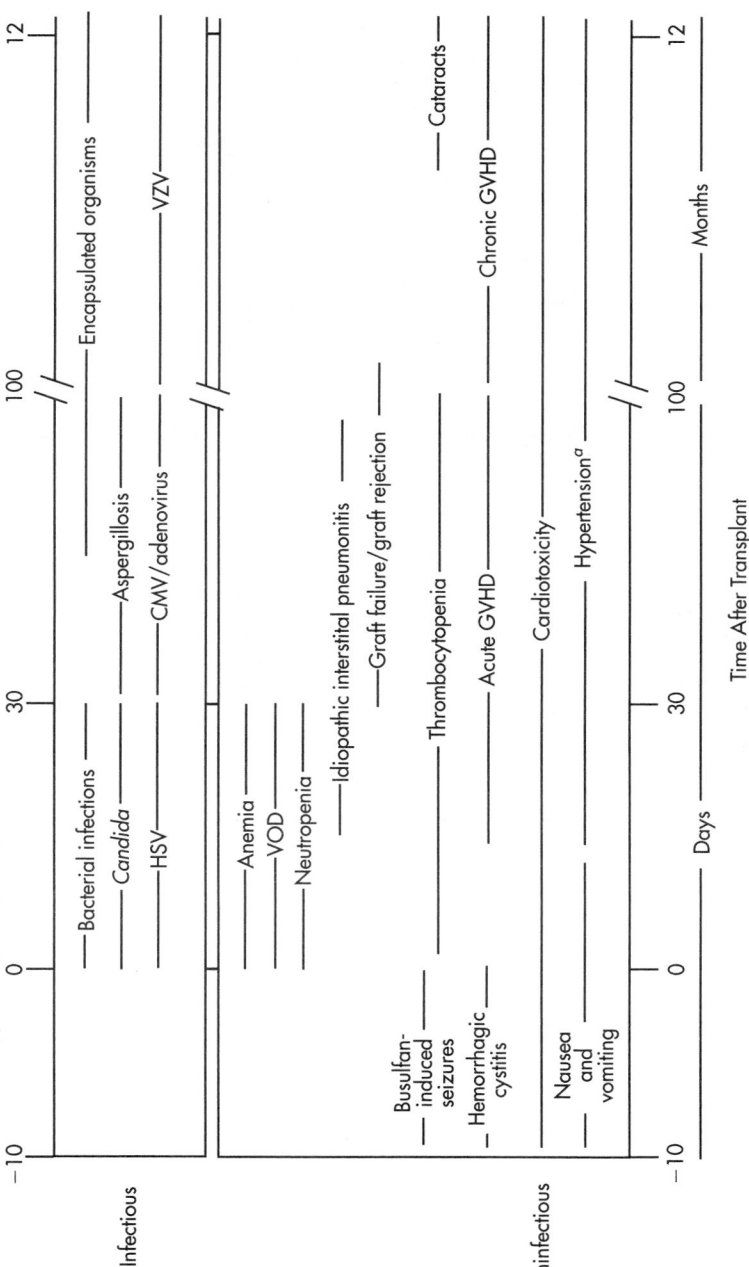

Fig. 88.3 Complications After Bone Marrow Transplantation by Time. [a]Patients undergoing allogeneic bone marrow transplantation only. CMV, cytomegalovirus; GVHD, graft-versus-host disease; HSV, herpes simplex virus; VOD, veno-occlusive disease; VZV, varicella-zoster virus.

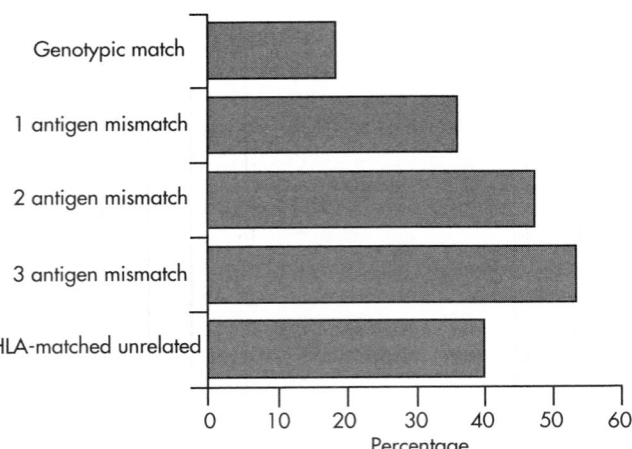

Fig. 88.4 Probability of Developing Severe Acute (Grade III or IV) Graft-Versus-Host Disease (GVHD) by Degree of Histocompatibility. This graph assumes all combination therapy with methotrexate and cyclosporine for prevention of acute GVHD. (Reprinted with permission from reference 14.)

The reader is referred to Chapter 90: Hematopoietic Cell Transplantation, written by *Suzanne P. Dix, Pharm.D.,* and *Dayna L. McCauley, Pharm.D.,* in the seventh edition of **Applied Therapeutics: The Clinical Use of Drugs** for a more in-depth discussion of supportive care, guidelines for use of post-transplant immunosuppressive therapy, pharmacokinetic monitoring of cyclosporine or tacrolimus, treatment of high-risk chronic GVHD, and other details of drug therapy. All notations to reference numbers are based on the reference list at the end of that chapter. The editors of this handbook express their thanks to Drs. Dix and McCauley and acknowledge that this chapter is based upon their work.

Notes:

Chapter 89

Pediatric Considerations

General Pediatric Therapy

The reader is also referred to other chapters in this handbook that further address the treatment of pediatric patients.

Teething

- ◆ Eruption of primary or deciduous teeth occurs at 4–5 months and is complete by 30 months. A significant number of children erupt no teeth until the end of the 1st yr.
- ◆ Symptoms of teething include drooling, restlessness, thumbsucking, and gum-rubbing.
- ◆ Manage by allowing the child to chew on blunt, formed objects (e.g., teething ring) or on cracked ice to hasten eruption and relieve pain. Occasional topical anesthetics can be used such as benzocaine 7.5%. Lidocaine should be avoided. Ibuprofen and acetaminophen can be used to relieve pain.

Diaper Rash

- ◆ Irritants (e.g., urine, stool, detergents), occlusion, and fungal or bacterial overgrowth can cause diaper rash.
- ◆ Candidal rash is typically a beefy red rash with satellite vesicular lesions that persists longer than 3 days with diffuse involvement of genitalia and inguinal folds.
- ◆ Treat by rinsing the area gently with plain water and apply a drying agent like cornstarch. Avoid talcum powder (aspiration can occur). Change diapers frequently and avoid plastic pants. Hydrocortisone ointment, 0.5%–1% BID for up to 1 week, also can be used. For rash due to *Candida albicans,* apply nystatin powder or ointment QID or clotrimazole cream to area BID until resolved.

Fever

- ◆ Defined as oral temperature of 37.8°C or higher (37.2° axillary, 38.8° rectal)
- ◆ Fever in children younger than 2 months of age is not predictive of the degree of illness
- ◆ Children 6–24 months with temperature >38.9°C and WBC count <5,000/mm^3 or >15,000 mm^3 are at increased risk for bacteremia
- ◆ Temperature >41°C commonly is associated with bacterial disease, including meningitis
- ◆ Febrile seizures occur in 4% of children 6 months → 6 years with temperature >38°C
- ◆ Antipyretic therapy
  - • Acetaminophen 10–15 mg/kg/dose Q 4–6 H (maximum 65 mg/kg/day)
  - • Ibuprofen 5–10 mg/kg/dose Q 6–8 H (maximum 40 mg/kg/day)
  - • Aspirin should be avoided in patients with viral infections

Diarrhea

♦ Most cases are self-limited, but severe cases can cause serious complications.

♦ Dehydration is a major risk in infants and children because percent of total body water is higher in children and renal capacity to compensate for fluid and electrolyte losses is limited.

♦ Symptoms of dehydration include depressed fontanel (useful up to 6 months of age), sunken eyes, dry mucus membranes around the mouth and eyes, crying without tears, decreased urine output, fever without perspiration, thirst, and weight loss (5%-mild; 10%-moderate; >10%-severe).

♦ Acute diarrhea is usually abrupt in onset, lasts a few days, and usually is of viral etiology.

♦ Chronic diarrhea can be caused by malabsorption and milk or protein intolerance.

♦ Mild-to-moderate diarrhea without dehydration can be managed at home with elimination of solids and addition of oral *electrolyte solutions* (see Table 89.5). Avoid giving milk and bouillon. Decarbonated beverages, diluted flavored gelatin, and juices may be used.

♦ IV replacement is indicated if the infant is in shock, unable to drink, vomiting, or has stool losses ≥100 mL/kg/hr.

♦ In situations of mild dehydration caused by diarrhea, oral electrolyte solutions containing 75–90 mEq/L of sodium should be given in a volume equal to the estimated fluid deficit (usually 40–50 mL/kg) over ≈4 hr. See Table 89.1.

♦ Maintenance hydration should replace ongoing losses. For each diarrhea stool, 10 mL/kg of oral electrolyte solution usually is needed.

♦ Maintenance fluid requirements are increased 10% for every degree (Celsius) body temperature increases above normal.

♦ Reinstitute breast-feeding 6–8 hr after oral replacement of fluid losses. Restart formulas at 1/2 strength for 1–2 days. Institute solids gradually.

♦ Medications play a minor role in treatment. Avoid anticholinergic agents in all children. Avoid other drugs that decrease motility in children with high fever, toxemia, or bloody mucoid stool.

Vomiting

♦ The most common cause of vomiting beyond the neonatal period is infection. See Table 89.2.

♦ Antiemetic drugs should be avoided in children. Sucking lollipops or popsicles with a sweet aroma and taste may decrease the urge to vomit. Prevention and treatment of dehydration and electrolyte loss are critical components of therapy.

♦ A pediatrician should be called if a child appears toxic or has signs of abdominal pain or distention, red or black vomitus, ear infection, or suspicion of head trauma or ingestion of a toxic substance.

♦ No food or drink should be given for the first 2–4 hr after vomiting begins. Clear liquids should be given for 24 hr, followed by soft foods such as cereal, crackers, rice, and cooked fruit.

♦ Milk, other dairy products, fatty meats, and fried food may decrease gastric emptying and make vomiting worse.

♦ For infants and young children, an oral electrolyte solution is recommended.

♦ Jello water, apple juice, and carbonated beverages supply fluid and carbohydrate but lack essential electrolytes.

♦ Estimate maintenance and replacement fluid requirements. Infants should be given 15 mL of liquid Q 20 min for 1–2 hr. Two times that amount is given to children >1 yr.

Gastroesophageal Reflux (GER)

♦ Most common symptom of GER in infants is vomiting or regurgitation.

♦ Failure to thrive, recurrent pneumonia, apnea, dysphagia, hematemesis, and anemia also might be indicative of GER.

♦ GER often resolves spontaneously by 18–24 months of age.

♦ Therapy is aimed at preventing complications to avoid the need for surgery.

♦ *Initial treatment* is to thicken foods with cereal, feed smaller volumes more frequently, and maintain the infant in a semiupright position 24 hr/day. Prop infant upright 1 hr after feedings.

♦ *More severe* GER can be treated with drugs that increase GI motility or neutralize/decrease acid secretion. Continue therapy for 3–4 months. See Table 89.3.

Hemolytic uremic syndrome (HUS) is characterized by microangiopathic hemolytic anemia, thrombocytopenia, and nephropathy. It is an acute illness that primarily affects children <4 yr.

♦ Onset is typically days to 2 weeks following an episode of gastroenteritis, upper respiratory infection, or flu-like illness.

♦ Patients usually present with hemolysis (decreased Hct, decreased Hgb, increased reticulocytes, dark urine, and lethargy); nephropathy (anuria, increased BUN, increased creatinine, hyperkalemia, and hypertension); thrombocytopenia (bruising and bleeding); and normal coagulation studies.

♦ Packed RBCs, platelets, dialysis, antihypertensives, and supportive care should be initiated as necessary.

♦ Antiplatelet agents are used to decrease platelet thrombi on damaged endothelium and to limit renal damage. ASA 1–60 mg/kg/day alone or with dipyridamole 3–10 mg/kg/day in 2 doses.

♦ Plasmapheresis is thought to enhance prostacyclin production and, thereby, to decrease platelet aggregation in renal capillaries.

Short Stature

♦ Short stature is height 3–4 standard deviations below the mean for age and sex. Three children in 100 are short.

♦ Growth hormone deficiency (GHD) is a relatively rare cause of short stature. Most children are intrinsically short or are experiencing delayed growth.

♦ Children with delayed bone age are most likely to respond to therapy.

♦ *Growth hormone* (GH) is the treatment of choice for children with GHD who have open epiphyses (bone age <12–13 yr).

♦ The optimal GH dose is unknown. Doses higher than those currently recommended may be more effective.

♦ Although GH is given IM, SQ may be less painful and as effective.

♦ GH is administered at night to mimic physiologic GH secretion. Response is enhanced by coadministration of androgens or GH withdrawal for several months.

♦ Adverse effects to GH include occasional local tenderness at injection site; hyothyroidism and hypertension are uncommon. Supraphysiologic doses lead to glucose intolerance and acromegaly.

Idiopathic Thrombocytopenic Purpura (ITP)

♦ *Disease Characteristics.* Generally an acute, self-limited, benign disease with spontaneous remission in 80%-90% within 6 months of diagnosis.

♦ Mortality rates are low (0.2%-2.1%), and most are attributed to intracranial hemorrhage within weeks of diagnosis.

♦ Social and psychological effects secondary to restriction of normal childhood activity constitute the primary morbidity.

♦ Chronic ITP evolves from the acute form in <20% of patients.

♦ Etiology is unknown. Pathogenesis of acute and chronic ITP is probably different.

♦ Acute ITP is thought to be triggered by a viral infection that induces antigen-antibody complexes which adhere to platelets, resulting in increased platelet consumption.

♦ *Clinical presentation of acute ITP* is characterized by: sudden onset of purpura or petechiae within a month after onset of a viral infection; about 25% have nosebleeds; 5% have hematuria; <4% have massive purpura or retinal hemorrhages; platelet count <50,000 cells/mm^3 with a normal CBC; eosinophilia in 15%-20%; bone marrow usually shows a normocellular marrow with increased megakaryocytes.

♦ *Treatment of Acute ITP.* Splenectomy is the only therapeutic modality with undisputed efficacy and is only performed in children with catastrophic hemorrhage.

♦ Plasmapheresis, steroids, and intravenous gamma globulin therapies are controversial because mortality rate is low, rate of spontaneous remission is high, and data for these therapies are inconsistent.

♦ Medications with antiplatelet effects (e.g., ASA, dipyridamole, NSAIDs) should be avoided.

Enuresis

♦ Enuresis is involuntary voiding of urine in the absence of any organic lesion after 5–6 yr. Most children become dry at night between 18 months and 4 yrs. This benign condition is most common in males and more common in children with positive family histories (77% if both parents enuretic; 44% if 1 parent enuretic; 15% if neither parent enuretic).

♦ A physical and neurological evaluation should rule out urologic abnormality or spinal lesion.

♦ *Conditioning Therapy.* Alarms, bladder training, and motivational counseling are used in addition to drugs.

♦ Drug Therapy
  • Desmopressin (DDAVP) used when conditioning therapy has failed
  • DDAVP dose is 40 µg intranasal at HS
  • Imipramine alternatively can be used in patients refractory to DDAVP; dose ranges from 1–1.5 mg/kg/day and titratable to a maximum of 2.5 mg/kg/day

Conscious Sedation. See Table 89.4.

Analgesia. See Table 89.5.

Notes:

Table 89.1 • Oral Electrolyte Solutions[37,39,40]

Solution	Compositions			
	Sodium (mEq/L)	Potassium (mEq/L)	Carbohydrate (g/L)	Osmolality
Rehydration				
Rehydralyte	75	20	25	305
WHO formula	90	20	25	310
Maintenance				
Infalyte	50	25	20	290
Pedialyte	45	20	25	250
Resol	50	20	20	270
Rice-Lyte	50	25	30	200
Home Remedies				
Jell-O	15–27	0.1–20	100–150	570–640
Apple juice	0.1–3.5	24–32	120	650–734
Gatorade	20	3	46	330
Ginger ale	0.8–5.5	0.1–1.5	53	520–560
Chicken broth	140–251	1.5–8.2	—	380–500

Table 89.2 • Causes of Vomiting in Infants and Children[a,29]

Causes	Other Signs and Symptoms
Drug-induced	
Cancer chemotherapy	Nausea
Narcotics	
Theophylline/aminophylline	
Antibiotics	
Alcohol	
Anesthetics	
Metabolic or Endocrine Disorders	Alteration in behavior
Infectious Diseases	Fever
Otitis media	Symptoms of otitis media
Meningitis	Stiff neck, toxic appearance
Appendicitis	Abdominal pain
Urinary tract infection/pyelonephritis	Dysuria, frequency, and urgency in older children
Viral or bacterial gastroenteritis	Diarrhea
Mechanical Obstruction	
Bowel obstruction	Abdominal distention, green emesis
Pyloric stenosis	Projectile nonbilious vomiting
Inflammatory	Abdominal pain
Pancreatitis	
Inflammatory bowel	Diarrhea
PUD	Black or red vomitus
Psychologic	
Chemotherapy	
Bulimia	
Miscellaneous	
Gastroesophageal reflux	Usually self-limited; indications for evaluation include recurrent pneumonia, poor growth, GI blood loss, dysphagia, or heartburn
↑ Intracranial pressure	Mental status alternation
Head injury/trauma	History of trauma, mental status changes
Food or milk intolerance or allergy	Irritability, loose stool, blood in stool

[a]GI = Gastrointestinal; PUD = Peptic ulcer disease.

Table 89.3 • Oral Drugs Used to Treat GER in Infants[a,46-50]

Agent	Mode of Action	Oral Dosage
Antacids (aluminum/ magnesium hydroxide)	Neutralizes acid; ↑ LES pressure	0.5–1.0 mL/kg/dose before and after feeding (max: 15 mL/dose)
Bethanechol	↑ LES pressure; augments esophageal clearance; corrects delayed gastric emptying	0.1–0.2 mg/kg/dose QID given 30–60 min before feeding and HS
Cimetidine	Blocks H_2-receptors; ↓ acid secretion	5–10 mg/kg/dose QID
Metoclopramide	Prokinetic agent; corrects delayed gastric emptying; ↑ LES pressure; augments esophageal clearance	0.1–0.2 mg/kg/dose QID given 30 min before feeding and HS
Omeprazole	Inhibits gastric secretion via inhibition of gastric hydrogen-potassium adenosine triphosphatase	0.7–3.5 mg/kg/day Q AM; used for resistant GER
Ranitidine	Blocks H_2-receptors; ↓ acid secretion	1.25–2.5 mg/kg/dose BID

[a]GER = Gastroesophageal reflux; LES = Lower esophageal sphincter.

Notes:

Table 89.4 • Drugs Commonly Used for Conscious Sedation[48]

Drug	Dosage[a]	Onset of Action	Duration	Comments
Chloral hydrate	*Adults:* 500–1000 mg *Children:* 25–100 mg/kg (max: 1 g/dose to a total of 2 g) *Route:* PO, PR	20–30 min	Unpredictable	Rapidly metabolized to active metabolite trichloroethanol; paradoxical excitation may occur; hyperbilirubinemia has been associated with chloral hydrate (repeated doses) in premature infants and neonates
Diazepam (Valium)	*Adults:* *PO:* 5–10 mg *IV:* 5–7.5 mg *Children:* *IV:* 0.05–0.2 mg/kg (max: 10 mg) *PO:* 0.1–0.5 mg/kg (max: 10 mg)	*IV:* 2–3 min *PO:* 30–45 min	2–6 hr	May burn when given IV (lipid soluble); do not use small veins; infuse IV over 3 min and at most 5 mg/min; potentiates the effect of narcotics and barbiturates
Fentanyl (Sublimaze)	*Adults:* *IV:* 0.5–1.0 µg/kg *Children:* *IV:* 1–2 µg/kg (up to 100 µg/dose) *PO:* 5–15 µg/kg (max: 400 µg)	*IV:* 1–1.5 min *IM:* 7–8 min *PO:* 5–15 min	*IV:* 30–60 min *IM:* 1–2 hr *PO:* 1–2 hr	Infuse IV over 3–5 min; effects potentiated by benzodiazepines; Oralet available in 200-, 300-, and 400-µg doses
Lorazepam (Ativan)	*Adults:* *IV:* 2 mg/dose *PO:* 2–4 mg/dose *Children:* *IV:* 0.05 mg/kg *PO:* 0.05–0.1 mg/kg	*IV:* 2–5 min *IM:* 15–30 min *PO:* 30–60 min	6–24 hr	Infuse IV over 2–3 min, not to exceed 2 mg/min; potentiates the effect of narcotics and barbiturates
Meperidine (Demerol)	*Adults:* *IV/IM:* 50–100 mg *Children:* *IV:* 0.5–1.0 mg/kg *SC/IM:* 1–2 mg/kg (max: 100 mg/dose) See Combination Drugs below for Meperidine/ Promethazine/Chlorpromazine dosage	*IV:* 1–5 min *SC/IM:* 10 min	*IV:* 1–2 hr *SC/IM:* 2–4 hr	Metabolite (normeperidine) has neurotoxic effect; accumulation of normeperidine may result in central nervous system manifestation; caution in patients with renal impairment after high or repeated doses; infuse IV dose over 3–5 min

(continued)

Table 89.4 • Drugs Commonly Used for Conscious Sedation[48] (continued)

Drug	Dosage[a]	Onset of Action	Duration	Comments
Midazolam (Versed)	*Adults:* IV: 0.5–2 mg/dose; may repeat to total dose of 2.5–5 mg *Children:* IV: 0.05–0.1 mg/kg Intranasal: 0.2–0.3 mg/kg PO: 0.2–0.4 mg/kg (max: 15 mg)	*IV:* 1–3 min *IM:* 10–15 min *Intranasal:* 5 min *PO:* 5–10 min	*IV:* 30–60 min *IM:* 2–6 hr *Intranasal:* 40–75 min *PO:* 30–90 min	3–4 times potency of diazepam; potentiates the effect of narcotics; infuse IV dose over 1–2 min
Morphine	*Adults:* IV: 2–15 mg/dose *Children:* IV: 0.05–0.1 mg/kg	*IV:* 1.0–2.5 min	1–2 hr	Maximal respiratory depression occurs within 7 min; effect potentiated by benzodiazepines; infuse IV dose over 3–5 min
Pentobarbital (Nembutal)	*Adults:* PO/IV: 100 mg *Children:* PO/PR/IM: 2–6 mg/kg (max: 100 mg/dose) IV: 1–3 mg/kg in increments of 1 mg/kg (max: 100 mg/dose)	*PO/PR:* 15–60 min *IM:* 10–25 min *IV:* 1–2 min	*PO/PR:* 1–4 hr *IM:* 30–60 min *IV:* 15–20 min	IV administration over at least 1 min or not to exceed 50 mg/min
Propofol (Diprivan)	*Adults:* <55 yr 2 mg/kg × 1, 6–12 mg/kg/hr *Children:* 2.5 mg/kg × 1 6–18 mg/kg/hr	*IV:* 30 sec after bolus	3–10 min, longer with prolonged use	Titrate to desired effect; lower dosages required when used with narcotics
Combination drugs Meperidine/ Promethazine/ Chlorpromazine	*IM:* *Demerol:* 2 mg/kg (up to 50 mg) *Phenergan:* 1 mg/kg (up to 12.5 mg) *Thorazine:* 1 mg/kg (up to 12.5 mg) *IV:* ½ of IM dose	*IM:* 10–15 min *IV:* 5–10 min	2–5 hr	Infuse IV dose over 5 min; hypotension can occur with rapid IV infusion; may be mixed in the same syringe

[a]Use low end of the dose if combined with another agent(s).

Table 89.5 • Analgesic Agents Used in Children[a,48]

Product	Initial Dose	Comments
Nonopioid		
Acetaminophen	10–15 mg/kg/dose Q 4–6 hr	No anti-inflammatory effect
Salicylates	10–15 mg/kg/dose Q 4–6 hr	Associated with Reye's syndrome; has anti-inflammatory effect
NSAIDs		
Ibuprofen	5–10 mg/kg/dose Q 6–8 hr	Gastritis with prolonged use
Naprosyn	5–7 mg/kg/dose Q 8–12 hr	Gastritis with prolonged use
Ketorolac	*Adults*: 15–30 mg IM/IV Q 6 hr *Children*: Not well established; 0.25–5 mg/kg IM/IV Q 6 hr; do not exceed adult dose	Increased risk of bleeding if high doses are used for >5 days
Opioids		
Codeine	0.5–1.0 mg/kg/dose Q 4–6 hr (*Adults*: 30–60 mg/dose)	Frequently combined with acetaminophen
Fentanyl	1–2 µg/kg/dose IV/IM (*Adults*: 50–100 µg/dose) *Infusion*: 3–10 µg/kg/hr	Chest wall rigidity, especially after rapid IV administration
Meperidine	*IV/IM*: 1.0–1.5 mg/kg Q 2–4 hr *PO*: 1–2 mg/kg Q 3–4 hr (*Adults*: 50–100 mg/dose)	Active metabolite has neurotoxic effect; avoid in renal failure
Morphine	*IV*: 0.1 mg/kg/dose Q 2–4 hr *IM*: 0.1–0.2 mg/kg Q 3–4 hr *PO*: 0.3–0.6 mg/kg Q 3–4 hr *IV infusion*: 0.05–0.1 mg/kg/hr	When changing to sustained release formulation, give daily dose as 2–3 divided doses

[a] IM = Intramuscular; IV = Intravenous; NSAID = Nonsteroidal anti-inflammatory drug; PO = Oral.

Notes:

The reader is referred to Chapter 91: Pediatric Considerations, written by *Ann M. Bolinger, Pharm.D., C.Y. Jennifer Chan, Pharm.D.,* and *Abby B. Zangwill, Pharm.D.,* in the seventh edition of **Applied Therapeutics: The Clinical Use of Drugs** for a more in-depth discussion. All notations to reference numbers are based on the reference list at the end of that chapter. The editors of this handbook express their thanks to Drs. Bolinger, Chan, and Zangwill and acknowledge that this chapter is based upon their work.

Notes:

Chapter 90

Neonatal Therapy

Terminology. Every newborn is evaluated and classified at birth according to birth weight, gestational age, and intrauterine growth status. Some common neonatal terminology for these evaluations and classifications can be found in Table 90.1.

Neonatal Pharmacokinetics (Table 90.2)
Absorption
- ♦ *Gastrointestinal Absorption.* Gastric acidity is lower during the neonatal period and for the first 2 yrs of age. The relatively alkaline gastric pH in neonates can decrease bioavailability of acidic drugs (e.g., phenobarbital, phenytoin) and increase bioavailability of weakly basic or acid-labile drugs (e.g., penicillin, erythromycin).
  - • Gastric emptying is affected by numerous variables and can offset bioavailability alterations.
  - • During the neonatal period, phenobarbital, digoxin, and sulfonamides are absorbed at a slower rate, but total amount absorbed is not decreased. Total amount absorbed of phenytoin, acetaminophen, carbamazepine, and rifampin is decreased in neonates.
- ♦ *Intramuscular absorption* is variable and unpredictable because of relative decrease in muscle blood flow, increased percentage of water in muscle mass, decreased strength of muscle contractions, and varying degrees of muscle activity.
- ♦ *Percutaneous absorption* increases in neonates (especially in preterm newborns) because of decreased thickness of stratum corneum, increased skin hydration, and increased ratio of skin surface area/kg of body weight.
  - • Toxicities have occurred after topical application of iodine, hexachlorophene, boric acid, salicylic acid, alcohol, epinephrine, and corticosteroids.

Distribution
- ♦ Distribution differs from adults because of differences in extracellular fluid volume, adipose tissue, protein binding, and other factors.
- ♦ *Water Compartments.* Total body water of a preterm 1 kg newborn is 80%, a term newborn 75%, a three-month-old 60%, and an adult 55%.
  - • More total body water and extracellular water mean >Vd for water-soluble drugs.
  - • Dosing on a mg/kg basis decreases with increasing age because of changes in body water and clearance.
- ♦ *Adipose Tissue.* Neonates have much less adipose tissue than adults.
  - • Preterm newborns have decreased fat (1%-2%) compared to term neonates (15% fat).
  - • Decreased Vd for fat-soluble or lipophilic drugs results in smaller mg/kg/doses.
  - • Some drugs (digoxin, theophylline) penetrate into the CNS and RBCs of newborns more readily, and larger mg/kg doses sometimes are needed.

♦ *Protein-Binding.* Binding of drugs to proteins (albumin, lipoproteins. α_1-acid glyco-protein, beta globulin) is decreased.

• Fetal albumin has decreased affinity for drugs.

• Total plasma-protein concentration and affinity of albumin for acidic drugs increases with age (adult values at 10–12 months of age).

Hepatic Metabolism

♦ Hepatic metabolism is decreased because of decreases in hepatic blood flow, cellular uptake of drugs, hepatic enzyme capacity, and biliary excretion.

♦ Hepatic oxidation, reduction, hydrolysis, and demethylation are significantly decreased but increase with gestational and postnatal age.

♦ Phase I biotransformation reactions include the cytochrome P450 enzymes (Table 90.3).

♦ Phase II reactions (conjugation with sulfate, glucuronide, glycine, glutathione, and hippurate; acetylation; and methylation) can be decreased (Table 90.4).

Renal Elimination

♦ Glomerular filtration, tubular secretion, and tubular reabsorption are decreased, and clearance of drugs eliminated by more than one of these mechanisms is difficult to predict.

♦ Digoxin, vancomycin, and gentamicin are eliminated primarily by glomerular filtration, and doses need to be adjusted for immature glomerular filtration. Gentamicin dosing guidelines are listed in Table 90.5.

Respiratory Distress Syndrome (RDS)

♦ RDS is a major cause of morbidity and mortality in preterm neonates, resulting from decreased production of surfactant in the lungs.

♦ Pulmonary surfactant decreases surface tension at the air:fluid interface in the alveoli, facilitates clearance of pulmonary fluid, prevents pulmonary edema, and prevents alveolar collapse.

Clinical Presentation

♦ *Tachypnea* is the first sign of respiratory distress. It attempts to compensate for inadequate ventilation, hypercapnia, and acidosis.

♦ *Retracting respirations* (i.e., use of intercostal, subcostal, suprasternal, or sternal accessory muscles) reflect the increased work of breathing needed to maintain ventilation.

♦ *Nasal flaring* decreases resistance during inspiration and increases oxygenation.

♦ *Grunting* is the result of forceful exhalation against a partially closed glottis in an effort to prolong expiration and maximize oxygenation.

♦ *Cyanosis, hypoxemia, hypercapnia, and acidosis* are other consequences of inadequate oxygenation and poor ventilation.

Prevention

♦ Prolong pregnancy by suppressing premature labor with drugs that inhibit uterine contractions (*tocolytics* such as ritodrine or terbutaline) to allow time for fetal lungs to mature. Chapter 41: Obstetrics describes the use of these tocolytic agents.

♦ Accelerate production of pulmonary surfactant *in utero* by maternal administration of *corticosteroids* (e.g., betamethasone 12 mg IM Q 12–24 hr times 2 doses, dexamethasone 6 IM/IV Q 12 hr times 4 doses when preterm labor occurs at 24–36 weeks of gestation.

Treatment

♦ *Surfactant therapy*

- Three types of exogenous surfactants have been evaluated: natural, modified natural, and synthetic
- Four surfactant products are commercially available in the U.S.: Exosurf (colfosceril palmitate) is synthetic; Survanta (beractant) is a modified natural; and Infasurf (calfactant) and Curosurf (poractant alfa) and natural surfactants

Bronchopulmonary Dysplasia (BPD)

♦ Most common form of chronic pulmonary disease in infants. Develops in newborns requiring supplemental oxygen and positive pressure ventilation for respiratory distress syndrome or other primary disorders.

♦ Defined as chronic lung disease associated with supplemental oxygen dependency at 28 days of life and/or at 36 weeks postconceptional age; clinical signs of respiratory distress; abnormal chest radiograph; and a history of oxygen requirement in the first week of life for a minimum of 3 days.

♦ Surfactant deficiency, barotrauma due to positive-pressure ventilation, inflammation, infection, and nutrient deficiency all play a role in the pathogenesis of BPD.

♦ Management

- Nonpharmacologic—oxygen, fluid restriction, nutrition.
- Pharmacologic

Patent Ductus Arteriosus (PDA)

♦ When the ductus arteriosus (a blood vessel connecting the left pulmonary artery to the aorta) remains open after birth, unoxygenated blood from the right ventricle is shunted to the systemic circulation through the patent ductus arteriosus. Normally, the ductus arteriosus closes rapidly within 12–24 hr after birth in full-term neonates.

♦ Major *risk factors* for PDA are premature delivery and respiratory distress syndrome.

Clinical Presentation

♦ Shunting of left ventricular cardiac output through an open ductus arteriosus into the lungs increases left ventricular volume, increases pulmonary blood flow, and decreases oxygenation of organ systems.

♦ Tachycardia, hyperactive precordium, and a continuous murmur, although not always present, are results of left-to-right shunting through ductus arteriosus during systole.

♦ Increased pulmonary blood flow and resultant pulmonary edema worsen respiratory disease and increases the need for ventilatory support. Higher ventilatory settings can increase the risk of development of bronchopulmonary dysplasia.

♦ If PDA is left untreated, CHF can develop secondary to increased left ventricular end-diastolic volume. Intraventricular hemorrhage and necrotizing enterocolitis are other complications.

Treatment

♦ *Indomethacin* in an initial dose of 0.2 mg/kg IV for all neonates with PDA. Subsequent 2nd and 3rd indomethacin doses given at 12–24 hr intervals are determined by postnatal age.

- Indomethacin 0.1 mg/kg/dose if neonates <2 postnatal days in age.
- Indomethacin 0.2 mg/kg/dose if neonates 2–7 days postnatal age.
- Indomethacin 0.25 mg/kg/dose if neonates >7 days postnatal age.

♦ *Surgical ligation* of open ductus arteriosus.

Necrotizing Enterocolitis (NEC)

♦ NEC is a type of acute intestinal necrosis.

♦ It is the most common life-threatening nonrespiratory condition affecting newborns.

♦ It primarily affects preterm neonates, but up to 20% of cases occur in full-term infants.

♦ **Pathogenesis** is unknown but most likely results from effects of intestinal bacteria in combination with other multiple factors on injured intestinal mucosa (Fig. 90.1).

♦ **Clinical Presentation.** Patients present with a wide range of manifestations from benign GI disturbance to a rapidly fulminant course that could include intestinal gangrene, perforation, sepsis, and shock.

  • *Stage I* refers to infants or neonates with suspected NEC and mild GI problems (e.g., emesis, ileus).

  • *Stage II* NEC with systemic and abdominal signs (abdominal distention, bloody stools) can be confirmed by presence of pneumatosis intestinalis on x-ray.

  • *Stage III* is advanced NEC with peritonitis, shock, and possible intestinal perforation.

♦ **Treatment** is based on managing the disparate symptoms and is dependent upon the severity of the illness.

  • *Stage I* illness generally can be managed with supportive therapy, bowel rest (NPO), and empiric antibiotics for 72 hr, pending culture and sensitivity results.

  • *Stage II* usually requires 7–14 days of bowel rest, total parenteral nutrition, and parenteral antibiotics.

  • *Stage III* usually requires fluid resuscitation, inotropic agents (e.g., dopamine, dobutamine), and surgical intervention.

Neonatal Sepsis

♦ Neonates, especially preterm newborns, are at increased risk for infections because of decreased immune function.

♦ Risk factors include prematurity, low birthweight, predisposing maternal conditions (e.g., prolonged rupture of membranes, maternal infection), and prolonged hospital stay.

Pathogens

♦ *Early onset sepsis* (during first 5–7 days of life): Pathogens usually are acquired from maternal genital tract (group *B Streptococcus, Escherichia coli, Klebsiella pneumoniae, Proteus* sp., *Listeria monocytogenes,* and *Enterococcus* sp.).

♦ *Late onset sepsis* (>5–7 days postnatal life): Pathogens are usually nosocomial pathogens (*Staphylococcus epidermidis, Staphylococcus aureus, Pseudomonas* sp., *Candida* sp., and anaerobes).

Clinical Presentation

♦ Sepsis can present with nonspecific or subtle signs (poor feeding, temperature instability, lethargy, apnea).

♦ Hypothermia is more common than fever, especially in preterm newborns. Fever, if present, is strongly associated with bacterial infection.

♦ Neutropenia, shift to the left, tachypnea, vomiting, and diarrhea can be other early signs of neonatal sepsis.

♦ Late signs can include jaundice, hepatosplenomegaly, and petechiae.

♦ Bulging fontanelle, posturing, or seizures suggest meningitis (see Chapter 53: Central Nervous System Infections).

Treatment

♦ Initiate *empiric antibiotics* IV immediately after collecting blood, CSF, and urine for C&S. Use doses as recommended for meningitis until CNS infection is excluded. Modify therapy based upon C&S results.

♦ *Early-Onset Sepsis and Meningitis.* Ampicillin plus either an aminoglycoside or a 3rd-generation cephalosporin in doses listed below (Table 90.8). Cephalosporins are insufficient alone for *Listeria.*

♦ *Late-Onset Sepsis.* Consider nosocomial pathogens, early-onset sepsis pathogens, and coverage for staphylococci (e.g., nafcillin or vancomycin).

Congenital Infections

Pathogens can be categorized into the acronym TORCH.

T = Toxoplasmosis
O = Other (syphilis, gonorrhea, hepatitis B, listeria)
R = Rubella
C = Cytomegaloviris
H = Herpes simplex

Selected congenital infections, manifestations, and treatment are described below. (See Table 90.9.)

Apnea

♦ Is defined as a cessation of breathing for >15 seconds, or less if accompanied by bradycardia (rate <100 beats/min), hypoxemia, cyanosis, pallor, or hypotonia.

♦ Apnea can be caused by prematurity or by severe underlying diseases as shown below.

♦ It is important to rule out sepsis before apnea of prematurity is presumed.

♦ In apnea of prematurity, about 40% of apneic episodes are of central origin (i.e., no respiratory effort), 10% to obstruction, and 50% to both (i.e., mixed events).

♦ Heart rate and respiratory rate should be monitored continuously.

♦ Time, duration, and severity of episodes and activity of infant should be documented.

Treatment includes:

♦ Treat underlying cause (e.g., RDS, PDA, infection, metabolic disorders);
♦ Supplemental oxygen;
♦ Gentle tactile stimulation;
♦ Environmental temperature control;
♦ Oscillation water beds;
♦ Nasal continuous positive airway pressure; and
♦ Positive pressure ventilation.
♦ *Methylxanthines* (e.g., caffeine, theophylline) are widely accepted as initial pharmacologic therapy of choice.

• The goal of methylxanthines is to decrease the number of episodes of apnea and bradycardia.

• Initiate methylxanthines when:

Apneic episodes are >3 episodes;

Duration >20 seconds;

Severe (accompanied by cyanosis, bradycardia);

Nonpharmacological interventions (tactile stimulation, environmental temperature control) have been ineffective.

- It acts by stimulating the medullary respiratory center and increasing receptor responsiveness to CO_2.
- The most common adverse effect of tachycardia responds to a decrease in dose but may persist for 1–3 days because of slow elimination of theophylline-derived caffeine.

Periventricular-Intraventricular Hemorrhage (PV-IVH)

- ♦ PV-IVH occurs in 40%-50% of premature newborns <1500 gm birth weight or <35 weeks of gestation.
- ♦ The most common site of hemorrhage is the periventricular germinal matrix, a highly vascularized network of neuronal precursor cells supported by blood vessels that are fragile and vulnerable to injury.
- ♦ *Clinical presentation* includes hypotension, hypotonia, decreased hematocrit, decreased responsiveness, apnea, areflexia, tonic posturing, and seizures.
- ♦ *Prognosis* for normal neurological development in survivors depends upon the location and severity of hemorrhage.
- ♦ *Preventive therapy* with phenobarbital, indomethacin, vitamin E, and pancuronium requires further investigations. Indomethacin appears to be the most promising.

Neonatal Seizures

- ♦ Seizures rarely are generalized tonic-clonic but can be tonic, clonic, myoclonic, or subtle.
- ♦ It often is a common manifestation of life-threatening underlying neurological processes such as those listed.
- ♦ Definitive treatment is directed toward specific etiologies.
- ♦ Acute *evaluation* includes assessment of infant's airway, breathing, circulation, and a review of history, physical examination, and laboratory determinations of serum electrolytes, BUN, glucose, Ca^{++}, Mg^{++}, blood gases, and bilirubin. An infectious disease work-up consisting of CBC with platelets, blood culture, urine culture, and lumbar puncture with CSF analysis may be necessary.
- ♦ *Pharmacotherapy*

Neonatal Abstinence Syndrome

- ♦ Occurs in 55%-95% of infants born to narcotic-dependent mothers.
- ♦ *Symptoms*
  - Onset, severity, and duration of neonatal abstinence syndrome are dependent upon specific drug(s) abused, time and amount of mother's last dose before delivery, elimination of drug by infant, and gestational age of infant at birth.
- ♦ *Initial treatment* should include nonpharmacologic supportive measures after excluding other serious neonatal disorders (e.g., sepsis, meningitis, hypoglycemia, hypocalcemia, adrenal insufficiency, CNS hemorrhage, or anoxia).
- ♦ *Pharmacologic treatment* is indicated in the presence of seizures, excessive weight loss or dehydration due to diarrhea or vomiting, severe hyperactivity or tachypnea that interferes with feeding, inability to sleep, and significant hypo- or hyperthermia.
  - *Phenobarbital* (loading dose of 15–20 mg/kg over 24–48 hr and maintenance dose of 4.5 mg/kg/day); *diluted tincture of opium* (0.08–0.2 mg morphine PO Q 3–4 hr) or *diazepam* (0.3 to 0.5 mg/kg Q 8 hr PO) are the most common drugs used to treat neonatal narcotic or CNS depressant withdrawal.

Table 90.1 • Common Neonatal Terminology[6,8]

Term	Definition
Gestational age	*By Dates*: The number of weeks from the onset of the mother's last menstrual period until birth *By Examination*: Assessment of gestational maturity by physical and neuromuscular examination; gestational age estimates the time from conception until birth
Postnatal age	Chronologic age after birth
Postconceptional age	Gestational age plus postnatal age
Corrected age	Postconceptional age in weeks minus 40; represents postnatal age if neonate had been born at term (40 weeks' gestational age)
Preterm	<38 weeks' gestational age at birth
Term	38–42 weeks' gestational age at birth
Postterm	≥43 weeks' gestational age at birth
Extremely-low birth weight	Birth weight <1 kg
Very low birth weight	Birth weight <1.5 kg
Low birth weight	Birth weight <2.5 kg
Small for gestational age	Birth weight below 10th percentile for gestational age
Appropriate for gestational age	Birth weight between 10th and 90th percentiles for gestational age
Large for gestational age	Birth weight above 90th percentile for gestational age

Notes:

Table 90.2 • Pharmacokinetics of Selected Drugs in Neonates and Adults[a,8,12,21,22]

Drug	Plasma $t_{1/2}$ (hr)		Vd (L/kg)		% Protein Bound	
	Neonates	Adults	Neonates	Adults	Neonates	Adults
Caffeine	40–230	3–7	1.0	0.5–0.6	N/A	30–40
Diazepam	25–100	20–30	1.8–2.1	1.6–3.2	84–86	94–98
Digoxin	20–80	25–50	4–10	7	14–26	23–40
Gentamicin	3–12	1.5–3	0.4–0.7	0.2–0.3	<10	<10
Indomethacin	15–30	4–10	0.35–0.53	0.15–0.26	95–98	90–95
Morphine	5–14	2–4	1.7–4.5	2.4–4.2	18–22	33–37
Phenobarbital	40–400	50–180	1.0	0.6–0.7	28–43	45–50
Phenytoin	15–105	15–30	1.0	0.6–0.7	70–90	89–93
Theophylline	20–60	6–12	1.0	0.45	36–50	50–65
Vancomycin	6–12	5–8	0.48–0.97	0.3–0.7	N/A	30–55

[a]N/A = Not available; $t_{1/2}$ = Half-life; Vd = Volume of distribution.

Table 90.3 • Important Neonatal Phase I Drug-Metabolizing Enzymes, Substrates, and Known Developmental Patterns

Enzyme	Neonatal Substrates	Known Developmental Pattern
CYP1A2	Acetaminophen, caffeine, theophylline, warfarin	Not present to an appreciable extent in human fetal liver. Adult levels reached by 4 months of age and may be exceeded in children 1 to 2 years of age. Activity slowly declines to adult levels, which are attained at the conclusion of puberty. Gender differences in activity are possible during puberty.
CYP2C9 CYP2C19	S-warfarin; diazepam, phenytoin, propranolol	Not apparent in fetal liver. Inferential data using phenytoin disposition as a nonspecific pharmacologic probe suggest low activity in first week of life, with adult activity reached by 6 months of age. Peak activity (as reflected by average values for V_{max}, which are 1.5- to 1.8-fold adult values) may be reached at 3 to 4 years of age and declines to adult values at the conclusion of puberty.
CYP2D6	Captopril, codeine, propranolol	Low to absent in fetal liver but uniformly present at 1 week of postnatal age. Poor activity (approximately 20% of that in adults) at 1 month of postnatal age. Adult competence attained by approximately 3 to 5 years of age.
CYP3A4	Acetaminophen, alfentanil, carbamazepine, cisapride, diazepam, erythromycin, lidocaine, midazolam, theophylline, verapamil, R-warfarin	Low activity in the first month of life, with approach toward adult levels by 6 to 12 months of postnatal age. Pharmacokinetic data for CYP3A4 substrates suggest that adult activity may be exceeded between 1 and 4 years of age. Activity then progressively declines, reaching adult levels at the conclusion of puberty.
CYP3A7	Dehydroepiandrosterone sulfate, ethinylestradiol, triazolam	Functional activity in fetus is approximately 30 to 75% of adult levels of CYP3A4.

Modified with permission from Leeder JS, Kearns GL. Pharmacogenetics in pediatrics: implications for practice. Pediatr Clin North Am 1997;44:55.

Notes:

Table 90.4 • Important Neonatal Phase II Drug-Metabolizing Enzymes, Substrates, and Known Developmental Patterns

Enzyme	Neonatal Substrates	Known Developmental Pattern
N-acetyltransferase-2 (NAT2)	Caffeine, clonazepam, hydralazine, procainamide, sulfamethoxazole	Some fetal activity present by 16 weeks. Virtually 100% of infants between birth and 2 months of age exhibit the slow metabolizer phenotype. Adult phenotype distribution reached by 4 to 6 months of postnatal age, with adult activity present by approximately 1 to 3 years of age.
Thiopurine methyltransferase	Azathioprine, mercaptopurine, thioguanine	Levels in fetal liver are approximately 30% of those in adult liver. In newborn infants, activity is approximately 50% higher than in adults, with a phenotype distribution that parallels that in adults. In Korean children, adult activity appears at approximately 7 to 9 years of age.
Glucuronosyltransferase (UGT)	Acetaminophen, chloramphenicol, morphine, valproic acid	Ontogeny is isoform specific, as reflected by pharmacokinetic data for certain pharmacologic substrates (e.g., acetaminophen or chloramphenicol). In general, adult activity as reflected from pharmacokinetic data seems to be achieved by 6 to 18 months of age.
Sulfotransferase	Acetaminophen, bile acids, chloramphenicol, cholesterol, dopamine, polyethylene glycols	Ontogeny (based on pharmacokinetic studies) seems to be more rapid than that for UGT; however, it is substrate specific. Activity for some isoforms (e.g., that are responsible for acetaminophen metabolism) may exceed adult levels during infancy and early childhood.

Modified with permission from Leeder JS, Kearns GL. Pharmacogenetics in pediatrics: implications for practice. Pediatr Clin North Am 1997;44:55.

Table 90.5 • Gentamicin Dosing Guidelines for Neonates and Infants

Postconceptional Age (wk)	Postnatal Age (days)	Dose (mg/kg/dose)	Interval (hr)
≤29 or significant asphyxia	0–28	2.5	24
	>28	3.0	24
30–36	0–14	3.0	24
	>14	2.5	12[a]
≥37	0–7	2.5	12
	>7	2.5	8

[a]Use 18 to 24 hours if birth weight ≤1,200 g and postnatal age <28 days.[52]
Adapted with permission from Young TE, Mangum OB. Neofax '96: A Manual of Drugs Used in Neonatal Care. 9th ed. Raleigh, NC: Acorn Publishing, Inc., 1996:30. A more recent version of this table appears in the 2000 edition of Neofax. The 2000 version recommends extended-interval dosing of gentamicin.

Notes:

Table 90.6 • Comparison of Currently Marketed Surfactant Products[a,68-71]		
Variable	Calfactant (Infasurf)	Poractant (Curosurf)
Type and source	Natural surfactant, calf lung wash	Natural surfactant, porcine lung mince extract
Phospholipids	Natural DPPC with mixed phospholipids	Natural and DPPC and mixed phospholipids
Proteins	Calf proteins SP-B and SP-C	Porcine proteins SP-B and SP-C
Dispersing and adsorption agents	Proteins SP-B and SP-C	Proteins SP-B and SP-C
Recommended dose	3 mL/kg (phospholipids 105 mg/kg)	Initial dose: 2.5 mL/kg (phospholipids 200 mg/kg); Repeat dose: 1.25 mL/kg (phospholipids 100 mg/kg)
Indications	Prophylaxis and rescue therapy	Rescue therapy
Criteria for prophylaxis	Premature infants <29 weeks' gestational age at high risk for RDS	Not approved
Recommended regimen for prophylaxis	Give first dose ASAP after birth, preferably within 30 minutes; repeat every 12 hours up to a total of three doses if infant still remains intubated or repeat as early as 6 hours up to a total of four doses if infant still remains intubated and requires $Fio_2 \geq 0.3$ with $Pao_2 \leq 80$ mm Hg	Not approved
Criterion for rescue therapy	Infants ≤72 hours of age with confirmed RDS who require endotracheal intubation	Infants with confirmed RDS who require endotracheal intubation
Recommended regimen for rescue therapy	Give first dose ASAP after RDS diagnosed, repeat every 12 hours up to a total of three doses if infant still remains intubated or repeat as early as 6 hours up to a total of four doses if infant still remains intubated and requires $Fio_2 \geq 0.3$ with $Pao_2 \leq 80$ mm Hg	Give first dose ASAP after RDS diagnosed, repeat every 12 hours up to a total of three doses if infant still remains intubated and requires mechanical ventilation with supplemental oxygen
Recommended administration technique	Administer through side-port of ETT adapter via ventilator, divide dose into 2 aliquots with position change OR through disconnected ETT via 5-French catheter, divide dose into 4 aliquots with position change	Administer through disconnected ETT via 5-French catheter, divide dose into 2 aliquots with position change
Formulation	Suspension	Suspension
Storage	Refrigerate 2 to 8°C; protect from light	Refrigerate 2 to 8°C; protect from light
Volume/vial	6 mL	1.5 mL, 3 mL

(continued)

Table 90.6 • Comparison of Currently Marketed Surfactant Products[a,68-71] (continued)

Variable	Calfactant (Infasurf)	Poractant (Curosurf)
Special instructions	Gentle swirling of the vial may be necessary for redispersion; warming to room temperature is *not* necessary; do not shake	Warm to room temperature before use; do not shake
Stability	If warmed to room temperature <24 hours, unopened, unused vials may be returned once to refrigerator; single-use vial contains no preservative; discard unused portion	If warmed to room temperature for <24 hours, unopened, unused vials may be returned only once to refrigerator; single-use vial contains no preservative; discard unused portion
Cost per vial[a]	$732	$440 (1.5 mL), $762 (3 mL)
Type and source	Synthetic	Modified natural surfactant, bovine lung mince extract
Phospholipids	Synthetic DPPC (hexadecanol and DPPC)	Natural and supplemented DPPC and mixed phospholipids
Proteins	None	Bovine proteins SP-B and SP-C
Dispersing and adsorption agents	Cetyl alcohol, tyloxapol	Proteins SP-B and SP-C
Recommended dose	5 mL/kg (DPPC 67.5 mg/kg)	4 mL/kg (phospholipids 100 mg/kg)
Indications	Prophylaxis or rescue therapy	Prophylaxis or rescue therapy
Criteria for prophylaxis	Birth weight <1350 g with risk for RDS; birth weight >1,350 g with evidence of lung immaturity	Birth weight <1,250 g or evidence of surfactant deficiency
Recommended regimen for prophylaxis	Give first dose ASAP after birth; give second and third doses 12 and 24 hours later to all who remain on ventilator	Give first dose ASAP after birth, preferably within 15 min; repeat as early as 6 hours up to a total of four doses if infant still remains intubated and requires Fio_2 ≥0.3 with Pao_2 ≤80 mm Hg

Criterion for rescue therapy	Infants with confirmed RDS who require endotracheal intubation	Infants with confirmed RDS who require endotracheal intubation
Recommended regimen for rescue therapy	Give first dose ASAP after RDS diagnosed; give second dose 12 hours later to all who remain on ventilator	Give first dose ASAP after RDS diagnosed, preferably by 8 hours postnatal age; repeat as early as 6 hours up to a total of four doses if infant still remains intubated and requires FiO_2 ≥0.3 with PaO_2 ≤80 mm Hg
Recommended administration technique	Administer through side port of ETT adapter via ventilator, divide dose into 2 aliquots with position change	Administer through disconnected ETT via 5-French catheter, divide dose into 4 aliquots with position change
Formulation	Lyophilized powder	Suspension
Storage	Room temperature	Refrigerate 2 to 8°C; protect from light
Volume/vial	8 mL (after reconstitution)	4 mL, 8 mL
Special instructions	Reconstitute with 8 mL of preservative-free Sterile Water for Injection, follow mixing procedures carefully; do not shake vigorously; use gentle shaking or swirling	Warm to room temperature before use; do not shake
Stability	Stable up to 12 hours after reconstitution; single-use vial contains no preservative; discard unused portion	If warmed to room temperature for <8 hours, unopened, unused vials may be returned only once to refrigerator; single-use vial contains no preservative; discard unused portion
Cost per vial[a]	$719	$455 (4 mL), $807 (8 mL)

[a]ASAP = As soon as possible; DPPC = Dipalmitoylphosphatidylcholine; ETT = Endotracheal tube; FiO_2 = Fractional inspired oxygen; PaO_2 = Partial pressure of oxygen; RDS = Respiratory distress syndrome.
[b]Average wholesale price 1999 Red Book.

Table 90.7 • Pharmacologic Management of Bronchopulmonary Dysplasia[a,8,84,86,88]

Drug Therapy	Dosage Regimen
Diuretics	
Chlorothiazide	*Neonates and infants <6 months*: PO: 20–40 mg/kg/day in two divided doses; maximum dose: 375 mg/day *Infants >6 months*: PO: 20 mg/kg/day in two divided doses; maximum dose: 1 g/day
Furosemide	PO: 1–4 mg/kg/dose 1–2 times/day IV: 1–2 mg/kg/dose Q 12–24 hr Nebulized: 1 mg/kg/dose diluted to a final volume of 2 mL with NS (use IV form)
Hydrochlorothiazide/ Spironolactone	PO: 1–2 mg/kg/dose Q 12 hr (dose based on hydrochlorothiazide)
Systemic Bronchodilators	
Caffeine citrate	*Loading dose*: 20 mg/kg (10 mg/kg as caffeine base) IV over 30 min *Maintenance dose*: 5 mg/kg/dose (2.5 mg/kg/dose as caffeine base) Q 24 hr; start 24 hr after loading dose; may administer IV (over 10 min) or PO (use IV form)
Theophylline	*Loading dose*: 5 mg/kg IV or PO *Maintenance dose*: 2–3 mg/kg/dose Q 8–12 hr IV or PO
Inhaled Bronchodilators	
Albuterol	0.02–0.04 mL/kg/dose of 0.5% solution (0.1–0.2 mg/kg/dose) diluted to 1–2 mL NS; give via nebulization Q 4–6 hr or PRN; minimum dose: 0.1 mL (0.5 mg); maximum dose: 1 mL (5 mg)
Cromolyn sodium	20 mg (2 mL) via nebulization Q 6–8 hr; may need up to 2–4 weeks for response to occur
Ipratropium bromide	0.13–0.4 mL/kg/dose of 0.02% solution (0.026–0.08 mg/kg/dose) diluted to 2–2.5 mL NS; give via nebulization Q 6–8 hr; do not exceed 0.9 mL (0.18 mg) per dose
Metaproterenol	0.01–0.02 mL/kg/dose of 5% solution (0.5–1 mg/kg) diluted to 1.5–2 mL NS; give via nebulization Q 6 hr or PRN; minimum dose: 0.1 mL (5 mg); maximum dose: 0.3 mL (15 mg)

[a]IV = Intravenous; NS = Normal saline; PO = Oral; PRN = As needed.

Notes:

Table 90.8 • Antibiotic Dosage Regimens for Neonates: Dosages and Intervals of Administration

Drug	Weight <1,200 g[52] 0–4 Weeks[a] (mg/kg)	Weight 1,200–2,000 g 0–7 Days[a] (mg/kg)	Weight 1,200–2,000 g >7 Days[a] (mg/kg)	Weight >2,000 g 0–7 Days[a] (mg/kg)	Weight >2,000 g >7 Days[a] (mg/kg)
Ampicillin					
Meningitis	50 Q 12 hr	50 Q 12 hr	50 Q 8 hr	50 Q 8 hr	50 Q 6 hr
Other diseases	25 Q 12 hr	25 Q 12 hr	25 Q 8 hr	25 Q 8 hr	25 Q 6 hr
Cefazolin	20 Q 12 hr	20 Q 12 hr	20 Q 12 hr	20 Q 12 hr	20 Q 8 hr
Cefotaxime	50 Q 12 hr	50 Q 12 hr	50 Q 8 hr	50 Q 12 hr	50 Q 8 hr
Ceftazidime	50 Q 12 hr	50 Q 12 hr	50 Q 8 hr	50 Q 12 hr	50 Q 8 hr
Ceftriaxone	50 Q 24 hr	50 Q 24 hr	50 Q 24 hr	50 Q 24 hr	75 Q 24 hr
Chloramphenicol	22 Q 24 hr	25 Q 24 hr	25 Q 24 hr	25 Q 24 hr	25 Q 12 hr
Clindamycin	5 Q 12 hr	5 Q 12 hr	5 Q 8 hr	5 Q 8 hr	5 Q 6 hr
Erythromycin	10 Q 12 hr	10 Q 12 hr	10 Q 8 hr	10 Q 12 hr	13.3 Q 8 hr
Methicillin					
Meningitis	50 Q 12 hr	50 Q 12 hr	50 Q 8 hr	50 Q 8 hr	50 Q 6 hr
Other diseases	25 Q 12 hr	25 Q 12 hr	25 Q 8 hr	25 Q 8 hr	25 Q 6 hr
Metronidazole	7.5 Q 48 hr	7.5 Q 24 hr	7.5 Q 12 hr	7.5 Q 12 hr	15 Q 12 hr
Mezlocillin	75 Q 12 hr	75 Q 12 hr	75 Q 8 hr	75 Q 12 hr	75 Q 8 hr
Oxacillin	25 Q 12 hr	25 Q 12 hr	25 Q 8 hr	25 Q 8 hr	37.5 Q 6 hr
Nafcillin	25 Q 12 hr	25 Q 12 hr	25 Q 8 hr	25 Q 8 hr	37.5 Q 6 hr
Penicillin G					
Meningitis	50,000 units Q 12 hr	50,000 units Q 12 hr	75,000 units Q 8 hr	50,000 units Q 8 hr	50,000 units Q 6 hr
Other diseases	25,000 units Q 12 hr	25,000 units Q 12 hr	25,000 units Q 8 hr	25,000 units Q 8 hr	25,000 units Q 6 hr
Piperacillin	75 Q 12 hr	75 Q 12 hr	75 Q 8 hr	75 Q 8 hr	75 Q 6 hr
Ticarcillin	75 Q 12 hr	75 Q 12 hr	75 Q 8 hr	75 Q 8 hr	75 Q 6 hr
Vancomycin	15 Q 24 hr[b]	20 Q 24 hr	15 Q 12 hr	15 Q 12 hr	15 Q 8 hr

[a]Postnatal age.
[b]If weight <750 g and postnatal age <14 days, use 10.0 to 12.5 mg/kg every 24 hours.
Adapted with permission from Nelson JD, Bradley JS. Nelson's Pocket Book of Pediatric Antimicrobial Therapy. 14th ed. Philadelphia: Lippincott Williams & Wilkins, 2000:16; incorporating references 8,145.

Notes:

Table 90.9 • Selected Congenital and Perinatal Infections in the Neonate[a,8,156–161]

Organism	Primary Clinical Manifestations	Treatment of Proven or Highly Probable Disease
Herpes simplex	Cutaneous vesicles, keratoconjunctivitis, microcephaly, CNS infection, hepatitis, pneumonitis, prematurity, respiratory distress, sepsis, convulsion, chorioretinitis	*Acyclovir:* Term neonate: 10 mg/kg Q 8 hr IV × 14–21 days; Preterm: 10 mg/kg Q 12 hr IV × 14–21 days *Ocular Involvement:* Acyclovir IV plus topical therapy: 1–2% trifluridine, 1% iododeoxyuridine, or 3% vidarabine
Toxoplasmosis	Chorioretinitis, ventriculomegaly, microcephaly, hydrocephaly, intracranial calcifications, ascites, hepatosplenomegaly, lymphadenopathy, jaundice, anemia, mental retardation	Sulfadiazine 100 mg/kg/day in two divided doses PO for 1 year *AND* pyrimethamine 1 mg/kg/day for 2–6 months followed by 1 mg/kg QOD to complete 1-year therapy *AND* folinic acid (leucovorin) 5–10 mg three times/week
Treponema pallidum	*Early:* Osteochondritis/periostitis, hepatosplenomegaly, skin rash (maculopapular or vesiculobullous), rhinitis, meningitis, IUGR, jaundice, hepatitis, anemia, thrombocytopenia, chorioretinitis *Late:* Hutchinson's triad (interstitial keratitis, eighth-nerve deafness, Hutchinson's teeth), mental retardation, hydrocephalus, saddle nose, mulberry molars	Aqueous crystalline penicillin G × 10–14 days IV (preferred) or IM: ≤7 days postnatal age: 50,000 units/kg Q 12 hr >7 days postnatal age: 50,000 units/kg Q 8 hr *OR* Procaine penicillin G 50,000 units/kg/day IM Q 24 hr × 10–14 days
Hepatitis B	Prematurity; usually asymptomatic; long-term effects include chronic hepatitis, cirrhosis, liver failure, hepatocellular carcinoma	*Perinatal Exposure (maternal HBsAg-positive):* HBIG 0.5 mL IM and hepatitis B vaccine IM (different IM sites) within 12 hours after birth; repeat hepatitis B vaccine at 1 and 6 months

Rubella	*Early:* IUGR, retinopathy, hypotonia, hepatosplenomegaly, thrombocytopenic purpura, bone lesions, cardiac effects *Late:* Hearing loss, mental retardation, diabetes *Rare:* Myocarditis, glaucoma, microcephaly, hepatitis, anemia	Supportive care
Cytomegalovirus	Petechiae, hepatosplenomegaly, jaundice, prematurity, IUGR, increased liver enzymes, hyperbilirubinemia, anemia, thrombocytopenia, interstitial pneumonitis, microcephaly, chorioretinitis, intracranial calcifications *Late:* Hearing loss, mental retardation, learning and motor abnormalities, visual disturbances	IV ganciclovir (under investigation)
Neisseria gonorrhea	Ophthalmia neonatorum, scalp abscess, sepsis, arthritis, meningitis, endocarditis	*Nondisseminated (including ophthalmia neonatorum):* Ceftriaxone 25–50 mg/kg IV or IM × 1 (maximum dose: 125 mg); alternative for ophthalmic neonatorum: cefotaxime 100 mg/kg IM or IV × 1; use saline eye irrigations for ophthalmia neonatorum *Disseminated:* Ceftriaxone 25–50 mg/kg IV or IM Q 24 hr; cefotaxime 25–50 mg/kg IV or IM Q 12 hr Duration of therapy: • Arthritis or septicemia: 7 days • Meningitis: 10–14 days Use cefotaxime if hyperbilirubinemic

^aCNS = Central nervous system; HBIG = Hepatitis B immune globulin; HBsAg = Hepatitis B surface antigen; IM = Intramuscular; IUGR = Intrauterine growth retardation; IV = Intravenous; QOD = Every other day.

Table 90.10 • Causes of Neonatal Seizures

Metabolic
Hypoxic-ischemia (i.e., asphyxia)
  Hypoxia
  Hypoglycemia
  Hypocalcemia
Hypoglycemia
  Intrauterine growth retardation
  Infant of a diabetic mother
  Glycogen storage disease
  Galactosemia
  Idiopathic
Hypocalcemia
  Hypomagnesemia
  Infant of a diabetic mother
  Neonatal hypoparathyroidism
  Maternal hyperparathyroidism
  High phosphate load
Other electrolyte imbalances
  Hypernatremia
  Hyponatremia

Cerebrovascular Lesions (Other Than Trauma)
Cerebral infarction (thrombotic versus embolic)
  ischemic versus hemorrhagic
Cortical vein thrombosis

Trauma
Subarachnoid hemorrhage
Intracranial hemorrhage
Subdural/epidural hematoma
Intraventricular hemorrhage

Infections
Bacterial meningitis
Viral-induced encephalitis

Congenital infections
  Herpes
  Cytomegalovirus
  Toxoplasmosis
  Syphilis
  Coxsackie meningoencephalitis
  AIDS
Brain abscess

Brain Anomalies (i.e., Cerebral Dysgenesis from Either Congenital or Acquired Causes)
Drug Withdrawal or Toxins
Prenatal substance: methadone, heroin, barbiturate, cocaine, etc.
Prescribed medications: propoxyphene, isoniazid
Local anesthetics
Bilirubin

Hypertensive Encephalopathy
Amino-Acid Metabolism
Branched-chain amino acidopathies
Urea-cycle abnormalities
Nonketotic hyperglycinemia
Ketotic hyperglycinemia

Pyridoxine Dependency
Familial Seizures
Neurocutaneous syndromes
Tuberous sclerosis
Incontinentia pigmenti
Autosomal-dominant neonatal seizures

Selected Genetic Syndrome
Zellweger syndrome
Neonatal adrenal leukodystrophy
Smith-Lemli-Opitz syndrome

Adapted with permission from Scher MS. Seizures in the newborn infant: diagnosis, treatment, and outcome. Clin Perinatol 1997;24:735.

Notes:

Table 90.11 • Pharmacotherapy of Neonatal Seizures [a,b]

Drug	Loading Dose	Maintenance Dose	Therapeutic Concentration
Phenobarbital	*IV:* Initial: 20 mg/kg, then 5–10 mg/kg Q 15–20 min if needed until total load of 40 mg/kg	*IV PO:* Initial: Premature: 3 mg/kg/day Term: 4 mg/kg/day May need to ↑ to 4–5 mg/kg/day by 2–4 weeks of therapy	20–40 µg/mL
Phenytoin	*IV:* 15–20 mg/kg	*IV:* Initial: 5 mg/kg/day May need to ↑ to ≥10 mg/kg/day by 2–4 weeks of therapy	8–15 µg/mL
Lorazepam	*IV:* 0.05–0.1 mg/kg	May repeat doses if needed Q 10–15 min	—
Diazepam	*IV:* 0.1–0.3 mg/kg	May repeat doses if needed Q 10–15 min	—
Pyridoxine	*IV:* 50–100 mg	*IV PO:* 20–50 mg/day; ↑ dose PRN with age	—
Paraldehyde	*Rectal:* 0.3 mL/kg; dilute 2:1 with mineral oil	May repeat dose if needed in 4–6 hours	—
Valproic acid	*PO:* 20 mg/kg	*PO:* 10 mg/kg/dose Q 12 hr	40–50 µg/mL

[a]IV = Intravenous; PO = Oral.
[b]See text for comments on appropriate IV administration and monitoring.

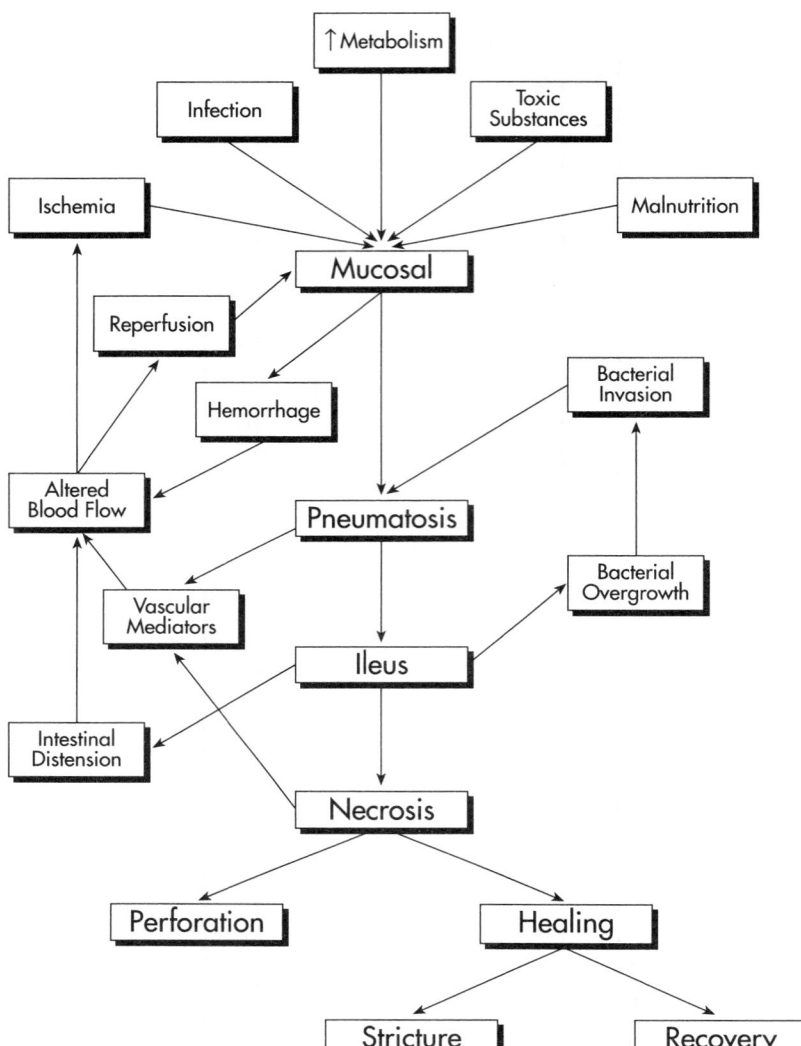

Fig. 90.1 Necrotizing Enterocolitis (NEC). This schematic is a composite of the theories about factors believed to be involved in the pathogenesis of NEC. The progression of this disease is denoted in large type. The factors believed to initiate or propagate the disease process are in smaller type. (Reproduced with permission from Crouse DT. Necrotizing enterocolitis. In: Pomerance JJ, Richardson CJ, eds. Neonatology for the Clinician. Norwalk, CT: Appleton & Lange, 1993:364.)

Notes:

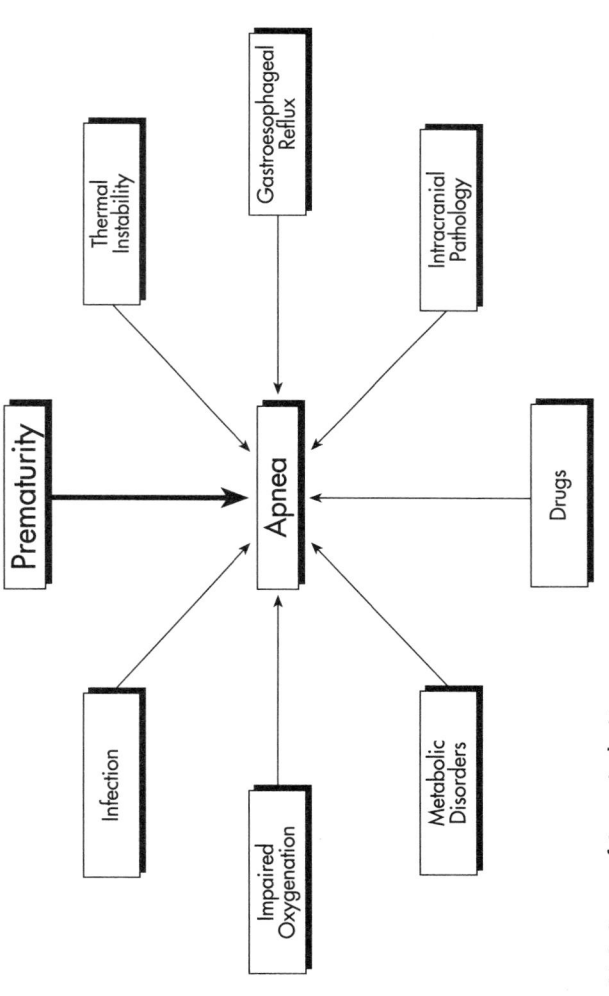

Fig. 90.2 Causes of Apnea in the Neonate. (Reproduced with permission from Martin RJ et al. Pathogenesis of apnea in preterm infants. J Pediatr 1986;109:738.)

The reader is referred to Chapter 92: Neonatal Therapy, written by *Donna M. Kraus, Pharm.D.,* and *Jennifer Tran Pham, Pharm.D.,* in the seventh edition of **Applied Therapeutics: The Clinical Use of Drugs** for a more in-depth discussion. All notations to reference numbers are based on the reference list at the end of that chapter. The editors of this handbook express their thanks to Drs. Kraus and Pham and acknowledge that this chapter is based upon their work.

Notes:

Chapter 91

Immunizations

Common Childhood Diseases See Table 91.1.

Immunization Schedule See Figure 91.1.

Tetanus Prophylaxis in Routine Wound Management See Table 91.2.

Notes:

Table 91.1 • Common Childhood Diseases[a,9,18,102]

Disease	Organism	Incubation Period	Communicability	Treatment	Immunization
Chickenpox	Varicella-zoster virus	10–21 days	1–2 days before and 5–6 days after rash	*Patient:* Acyclovir *Contact:* VZIG	*Active:* Vaccine *Passive:* VZIG
Diphtheria	C. diphtheria	2–6 days	2–4 wk untreated; 1–2 days after antibiotics initiated	*Patient:* Diphtheria antitoxin combined with penicillin or erythromycin *Contact:* (1) Oral erythromycin or IM benzathine penicillin; (2) diphtheria toxoid immunization	*Active:* Diphtheria toxoids *Passive:* Diphtheria/toxoid antitoxin
Hepatitis	Hepatitis B	120 days	Transmission via contaminated blood, sexual intimacy, and perinatal transmission from a HBsAg-positive mother to her child	*Patient:* HBIG *Contact:* HBIG and Hepatitis B vaccine series	*Active:* Hepatitis B vaccine series *Passive:* HBIG
Invasive bacteremic disease	H. influenzae type b (Hib)			*Patient:* Ampicillin combined with chloramphenicol or third-generation cephalosporin *Contact:* Rifampin 20 mg/kg/day QD × 4 days	*Active:* HbCV vaccine
Measles (Rubeola)	Measles virus	10–12 days	Beginning fifth day of incubation through first few days of rash	*Patient:* None *Contact:* As under immunizations	*Active:* Measles virus vaccine *Passive:* Unvaccinated normal children with severe systemic infection: IVIG 500 mg/kg. Non-vaccinated immunosuppressed children: IVIG 500 mg/kg

Mumps	Mumps virus	14–21 days	7 days before and 9 days after parotid swelling	*Patient:* None *Contact:* Mumps immune serum globulin	*Active:* Mumps virus vaccine *Passive:* Mumps immunoglobulin
Pertussis	*B. pertussis*	5–21 days	Greatest during disease; ranges include 4 wk; lessened with antibiotics	*Patient:* Erythromycin *Contact:* Erythromycin or ampicillin for 10 days after contact or for duration of cough in contacted patient	*Active:* Pertussis vaccine *Passive:* None
Polio	Polio viruses types 1, 2, and 3	7–14 days	Virus persists in throat 1 wk after onset of symptoms, also may be excreted in feces 46 weeks	*Patient:* None *Contact:* TOPV	*Active:* TOPV or IPV *Passive:* None
Rubella (German measles)	Rubella virus	14–21 days	7 days before and 5 days after appearance of rash	*Patient:* None *Contact:* See text	*Active:* Rubella virus vaccine *Passive:* ISG
Tetanus (lockjaw)	*C. tetani*	3 days–3 wk	None	*Patient:* Tetanus immunoglobulin (human), penicillin G, or tetracycline *Contact:* None required	*Active:* Tetanus toxoid *Passive:* Tetanus immunoglobulin (human)

[a]HbCV = *H. influenzae* type b conjugate vaccine; HBIG = Hepatitis B immunoglobulin; IPV = Inactive polio vaccine; ISG = Immune serum globulin; IVIG = Intravenous immunoglobulin; TOPV = Trivalent oral polio vaccine; VZIG = Varicella-zoster immunoglobulin.

Table 91.2 • Tetanus Prophylaxis in Routine Wound Management[a,b]

Tetanus Toxoid Adsorbed History	Clean, Minor Wounds		All Other Wounds[c]	
	Td	TIG	Td	TIG
Not known or <3 doses	Yes	No	Yes	Yes
≥3 doses[d]	No[e]	No	No[f]	No

[a]Adapted from reference 103.
[b]Td, Adult tetanus and diphtheria toxoids, adsorbed; for children <7 years old, use DTP or DT; TIG, tetanus immunoglobulin.
[c]Including, but not limited to, wounds contaminated with saliva, soil, feces, dirt; puncture wounds; avulsions; and wounds from crushing, burns, or frostbite.
[d]If only three doses of tetanus toxoid have been received, a fourth dose (using tetanus toxoid adsorbed) should be given.
[e]Yes, if >10 years since last dose.
[f]Yes, if >5 years since last dose.

Notes:

Notes:

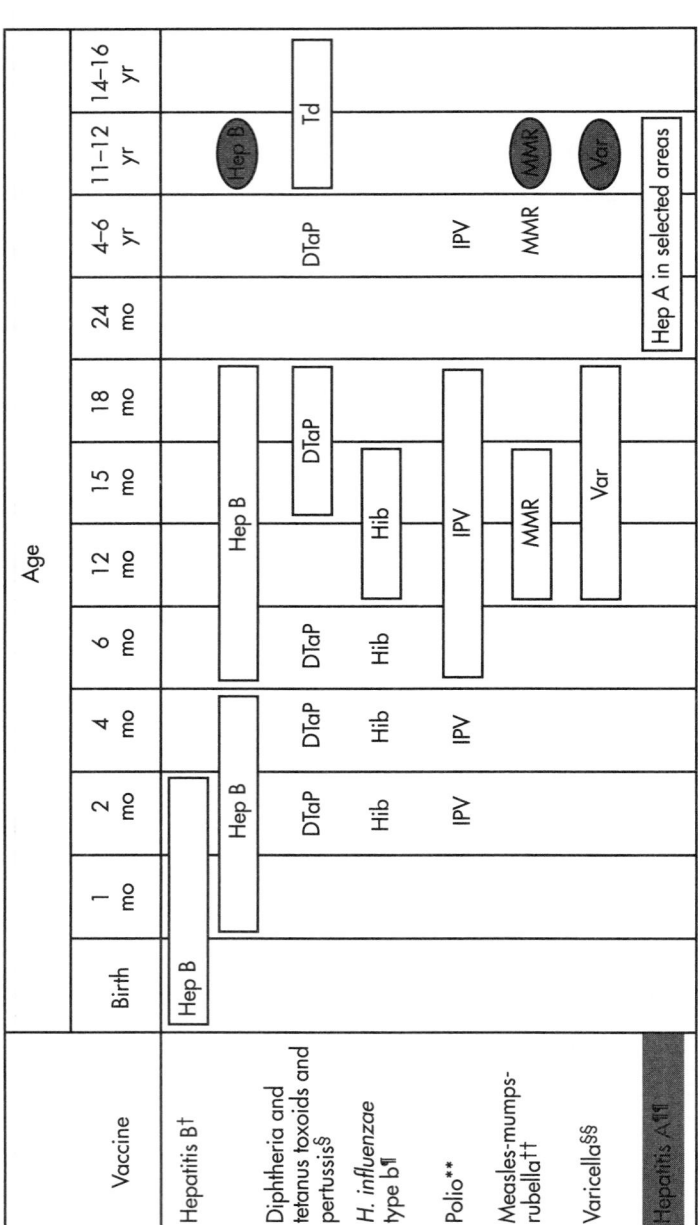

Age

Vaccine	Birth	1 mo	2 mo	4 mo	6 mo	12 mo	15 mo	18 mo	24 mo	4–6 yr	11–12 yr	14–16 yr
Hepatitis B[†]	Hep B	Hep B	Hep B		Hep B						Hep B	
Diphtheria and tetanus toxoids and pertussis[§]			DTaP	DTaP	DTaP		DTaP	DTaP		DTaP	Td	Td
H. influenzae type b[¶]			Hib	Hib	Hib	Hib	Hib					
Polio**			IPV	IPV	IPV	IPV	IPV			IPV		
Measles-mumps-rubella[††]						MMR	MMR			MMR	MMR	
Varicella[§§]						Var	Var				Var	
Hepatitis A[¶¶]									Hep A in selected areas			

☐ Range of recommended ages for vaccination.

⬭ Vaccines to be given if previously recommended doses were missed or were given earlier than the recommended minimum age.

▨ Recommended in selected states and/or regions.

On October 22, 1999, the Advisory Committee on Immunization Practices (ACIP) recommended that Rotashield (rhesus rotavirus vaccine-tetravalent [RRV-TV]), the only U.S.-licensed rotavirus vaccine, no longer be used in the United States (MMWR, 1999;48:[43]). Parents should be reassured that children who received rotavirus vaccine before July 1999 are not now at increased risk for intussusception.

*This schedule indicates the recommended ages for routine administration of licensed childhood vaccines as of November 1, 1999. Any dose not given at the recommended age should be given as a "catch-up" vaccination at any subsequent visit when indicated and feasible. Additional vaccines may be licensed and recommended during the year. Licensed combination vaccines may be used whenever any components of the combination are indicated, and the vaccine's other components are not contraindicated. Providers should consult the manufacturers' package inserts for detailed recommendations.

†Infants born to hepatitis B surface antigen (HBsAg)-negative mothers should receive the first dose of hepatitis B vaccine (Hep B) by age 2 months. The second dose should be administered at least 1 month after the first dose. The third dose should be administered at least 4 months after the first dose and at least 2 months after the second dose but not before age 6 months. Infants born to HBsAg-positive mothers should receive Hep B and 0.5 mL hepatitis B immunoglobulin (HBIG) within 12 hours of birth at separate sites. The second dose is recommended at age 1 to 2 months and the third dose at age 6 months. Infants born to mothers whose HBsAg status is unknown should receive Hep B within 12 hours of birth. Maternal blood should be drawn at delivery to determine the mother's HBsAg status; if the HBsAg test is positive, the infant should receive HBIG as soon as possible (no later than age 1 week). All children and adolescents (through age 18 years) who have not been vaccinated against hepatitis B may begin the series during any visit. Providers should make special efforts to vaccinate children who were born in or whose parents were born in areas of the world where hepatitis B virus infection is moderately or highly endemic.

§The fourth dose of diphtheria and tetanus toxoids and acellular pertussis vaccine (DTaP) can be administered as early as age 12 months, provided 6 months have elapsed since the third dose and the child is unlikely to return at age 15 to 18 months. Tetanus and diphtheria toxoids (Td) are recommended at age 11 to 12 years if at least 5 years have elapsed since the last dose of diphtheria and tetanus toxoids and pertussis vaccine (DTP), DTaP, or diphtheria and tetanus toxoids (DT). Subsequent routine Td boosters are recommended every 10 years.

¶Three Haemophilus influenzae type b (Hib) conjugate vaccines are licensed for infant use. If Hib conjugate vaccine (PRP-OMP) [PedvaxHIB or ComVax [Merck]) is administered at ages 2 months and 4 months, a dose at age 6 months is not required. Because clinical studies in infants have demonstrated that using some combination products may induce a lower immune response to the Hib vaccine component, DTaP/Hib combination products should not be used for primary vaccination in infants at ages 2, 4, or 6 months unless approved by the Food and Drug Administration for these ages.

**To eliminate the risk for vaccine-associated paralytic poliomyelitis (VAPP), an all-inactivated poliovirus vaccine (IPV) schedule is now recommended for routine childhood polio vaccination in the United States. All children should receive four doses of IPV: at age 2 months, age 4 months, between ages 6 and 18 months, and between ages 4 and 6 years. Oral poliovirus vaccine (OPV) (if available) may be used only for the following special circumstances: 1) mass vaccination campaigns to control outbreaks of paralytic polio; 2) unvaccinated children who will be traveling in <4 weeks to areas where polio is endemic or epidemic; and 3) children of parents who do not accept the recommended number of vaccine injections. Children of parents who do not accept the recommended number of vaccine injections may receive OPV only for the third or fourth dose or both; in this situation, health-care providers should administer OPV only after discussing the risk for VAPP with parents or caregivers. During the transition to an all-IPV schedule, recommendations for the use of remaining OPV supplies in physicians' offices and clinics have been issued by the American Academy of Pediatrics (Pediatrics 1999;104(6)).

††The second dose of measles, mumps, and rubella vaccine (MMR) is recommended routinely at age 4 to 6 years but may be administered during any visit, provided at least 4 weeks have elapsed since receipt of the first dose and that both doses are administered beginning at or after age 12 months. Those who previously have not received the second dose should complete the schedule no later than the routine visit to a health-care provider at age 11 to 12 years.

§§Varicella (Var) vaccine is recommended at any visit on or after the first birthday for susceptible children (i.e., those who lack a reliable history of chickenpox as judged by a health-care provider) and who have not been vaccinated. Susceptible persons aged ≥13 years should receive two doses given at least 4 weeks apart.

¶¶Hepatitis A vaccine (Hep A) is recommended for use in selected states and regions. Information is available from local public health authorities and MMWR, 1999;48:RR-12).

Use of trade names and commercial sources is for identification only and does not constitute or imply endorsement by CDC or the U.S. Department of Health and Human Services.

Fig. 91.1 Recommended Childhood Immunization Schedule*—United States, January–December 2000. (From Advisory Committee on Immunization Practices [ACIP], American Academy of Family Physicians [AAFP], and American Academy of Pediatrics [AAP].)

The reader is referred to Chapter 93: Immunizations, written by *Ann M. Bolinger, Pharm.D.,* and *C.Y. Jennifer Chan, Pharm.D.,* in the seventh edition of **Applied Therapeutics: The Clinical Use of Drugs** for a more in-depth discussion. All notations to reference numbers are based on the reference list at the end of that chapter. The editors of this handbook express their thanks to Drs. Bolinger and Chan and acknowledge that this chapter is based upon their work.

Notes:

Chapter 92

Pediatric Infectious Diseases

Pathogenesis

♦ Humoral and cellular immunity are not fully developed in the immediate newborn period and in the first years of life. Serum concentrations of immunoglobulins at various early ages are listed in Table 92.1.

♦ Maternal immunity transferred to the newborn dissipates during the first year of life.

♦ Imperfect complement and C-reactive proteins decrease opsonization. Phagocytosis and intracellular cidal function of neutrophils and macrophages are depressed.

♦ Incomplete development of a full complement of normal bacterial flora permit colonization of potential pathogens. Common pathogens associated with specific infectious diseases are listed in Table 92.2.

♦ Inadequate exposure to antigens decreases immunity.

Antibiotics for Common Pediatric Infectious Diseases (Table 92.3)

Otitis Media

Otitis media is an inflammation of the middle ear caused by viral or bacterial pathogens. Clinical presentation, common pathogens, and treatment are presented in Chapter 55: Respiratory Tract Infections.

Sinusitis

Clinical presentation includes a preceding history of an upper respiratory infection;

♦ excessive nasal discharge that changes in color (e.g., greenish-yellow), but nasal discharge also can be clear and nonpurulent;

♦ fever and decreased appetite; and

♦ an increased WBC count with a predominance of neutrophils.

♦ Headaches are rare; although they are common in adults.

Microbiology

♦ Acute sinusitis is most commonly caused by *S. pneumoniae, H. influenzae,* and *M. catarrhalis.*

♦ Chronic sinusitis is caused by more atypical organisms such as *S. aureus, S. pyogenes,* anaerobes, or penicillin-resistant strains of *S. pneumoniae, M. catarrhalis,* and *H. influenzae.*

♦ Treatment can be discontinued after 10–14 days, but if residual signs or symptoms (e.g., fever, cough, nasal discharge) remain, 7–10 additional days of antibiotics are needed.

♦ Decongestants and antihistamines reduce congestion and the risk of secondary bacterial sinusitis only in patients with significant allergic history and nasal congestion.

Pharyngitis

Clinical presentation includes rapid onset of symptoms, high fever, exudative patches in the throat, and painful "sore throats."

♦ Differentiation between viral and bacterial pharyngitis is difficult because of considerable overlap of common signs and symptoms.

♦ It is often a self-limiting infection that generally resolves in a few days without treatment.

Complications. A few patients with group A beta-hemolytic streptococci (GABHS) pharyngitis develop peritonsillar abscess, cervical lymphadenitis, otitis media, mastoiditis, sinusitis, or other toxin-mediated complications (e.g., scarlet fever, toxic-shock syndrome). Only 10%–20% of *toxic-shock syndrome* results from GABHS pharyngitis, but severe multisystem organ failure can occur. Antibiotic treatment of GABHS infection can prevent the immunological complication of *rheumatic heart disease* but does not appear to directly prevent GABHS *poststreptococcal glomerulonephritis*. Antibiotics can indirectly reduce the incidence of GABHS poststreptococcal glomerulonephritis by decreasing the transmission of this infection to others.

Microbiology

♦ Common viral and bacterial pathogens associated with pharyngitis are listed in Table 92.2.

♦ Group A beta hemolytic streptococci (GABHS), also known as *Streptococcus pyogenes,* accounts for the vast majority of bacterial pharyngitis.

Treatment

♦ GABHS are exquisitely sensitive to all beta-lactam antibiotics. Penicillin is the treatment of choice. Erythromycin is the alternative of choice in patients allergic to penicillin.

♦ Despite improvement of pharyngitis symptoms after 24–48 hr, penicillin should be continued for 10 days to reduce the risk of subsequent rheumatic fever.

Rheumatic Fever

Clinical Presentation See Table 92.4.

Treatment

♦ Penicillin G IV 100,000 units/kg/day divided Q 6 hr is the antimicrobial therapy of choice.

♦ Parenteral vancomycin or erythromycin are alternatives in penicillin-allergic patients.

Prophylactic Antibiotics

♦ There is recurrence of rheumatic fever in 75% without long-term antibiotic prophylaxis.

♦ Prophylactic antibiotic regimens for acute rheumatic fever and recommendations for penicillin-allergic patients are summarized below. See Table 92.5.

♦ Respiratory difficulty classified based upon signs and symptoms is listed in Table 92.4.

Bronchiolitis

Pathogenesis

♦ Differentiation between bronchiolitis and acute exacerbation of reactive airway disease is difficult and the two can occur concurrently.

♦ A positive swab for RSV *(respiratory syncytial virus)* is suggestive of bronchiolitis infection.

Treatment

♦ Inhaled *beta-agonists* in infants can provide subjective improvement in clinical symptoms and can be justified despite controversy as to efficacy in infants <18 months of age. Albuterol (or another similar beta-agonist) can be initiated at 0.10–0.15 mg/kg/dose as often as Q 30 minutes if needed. If a response is not observed within 6 hr, therapy should be re-evaluated.

♦ *Ribavirin* should be reserved for infants with the highest risk of complications from RSV infection (e.g., those with congenital heart disease, chronic pulmonary disease, immunodeficiency of prematurity). It also is indicated when respiratory distress is severe (e.g., pCO2 is >60 mm Hg venous, pH <7.32 venous, O_2 <90% saturation). Aerosol therapy is initiated with a standard regimen of 6 gm ribavirin diluted in 300 mL of sterile water delivered by a small-particle aerosol generator over 18–20 hr daily for 3–5 days.

Croup Syndrome

♦ A spectrum of upper respiratory tract infections that affect the larynx, trachea, and upper bronchial airways (e.g., epiglottitis, laryngotracheobronchitis). See Table 92.6.

Pertussis

Pathogenesis

♦ Pertussis is a rare respiratory infection caused by *Bordetella pertussis*. A resurgence of the disease because of inadequate immunization with DPT (diphtheria, pertussis, tetanus toxoid) intermittently has been reported.

Clinical Presentation

♦ The first phase of disease with symptoms of coryza, congestion, low-grade fever, and irritability is difficult to differentiate from a viral upper respiratory tract infection.

♦ A subsequent whooping cough develops and lasts up to 2 weeks.

♦ Cough may persist for up to 3 months during the convalescent phase.

Treatment

♦ Erythromycin is the drug of choice. Treat for at least 14 days to ensure eradication of the organism.

Prophylaxis

♦ Erythromycin is indicated for household members and close contacts even if previously vaccinated because immunity from pertussis vaccine wanes over time.

Measles

♦ Measles is a relatively self-limiting disease.

♦ Mild cases are usually without complications but secondary bacterial infections (primarily otitis media and bacterial pneumonia) occur in 5%–15%.

♦ *Vitamin A* reduces pulmonary complications, fever, hospital stay, and mortality. Infants <6 months of age should receive a single dose of 100,000 units. Vitamin A 200,000 units is recommended for infants >6 months of age. Doses can be repeated at 24 hr and 4 weeks later for malnourished or vitamin A-deficient patients.

Kawasaki Disease

Clinical Presentation

♦ Kawasaki is a systemic vasculitis presenting as a mucocutaneous lymph node syndrome in children 6 months to 5 yr of age.

♦ The etiology is unknown, and no test can confirm the diagnosis. It must be a diagnosis of exclusion after ruling out scarlet fever, JRA, toxic-shock syndrome, and other likely diagnoses.

♦ A constellation of symptoms including fever of >5 days with at least 4 of the following:

• Mucous membrane changes such as swollen "strawberry" tongue or perioral fissures.

• Cervical lymphadenopathy.

• Bilateral conjunctivitis.

• Rash.

• Swollen feet or hands with desquamation.

♦ Other nondiagnostic characteristics include arthritis, irritability, lack of response to antibiotics, and urethritis.

♦ *Acute phase* of 1–2 weeks is followed by a *subacute phase* in which coronary aneurysms tend to form. In the final *convalescent phase,* the patient may be asymptomatic, and the risk of aneurysms diminishes

♦ Risk factors for development of coronary aneurysms include:

• Asian descent.

• <5 yr of age.

• Fever >14 days.

• Platelet count >900,000/mm^3.

• ESR >100 mm/hr.

Treatment

♦ *Aspirin* 50–100 mg/kg/day is recommended as an anti-inflammatory during acute phase to reduce risk of coronary aneurysm and to modify arthritic component. Oral absorption of aspirin can be decreased by as much as 50% in these patients, and higher doses may be needed. Serum trough salicylate concentrations of 20–30 mg/dL are recommended. During the subacute and convalescent phase, aspirin can be decreased to 3–10 mg/kg/day for an antithrombotic effect.

♦ Administration of *IV immunoglobulin (IVIG)* within 10 days of fever onset decreases the incidence of coronary aneurysms from about 20% to 5%. Most respond to IVIG with resolution of fever, rash, and decreased ESR within 72 hr. Dosage regimens of 400 mg/kg/day for 4 days, 1 gm/kg or 2 gm/kg as single doses have been successful. The single daily dose regimens might be more effective. IVIG is usually well tolerated, but hypo- or hypertension, tachycardia, and tachypnea can arise during infusion of IVIG.

Notes:

Table 92.1 • Immunologic Parameters in Infants, Children, and Adults

	Birth	1 Month	1 Year	5 Years	Adult
Average white blood cell count (cells/mm^3)	18,100	10,800	10,600	8,500	7,400
Average neutrophil count (cells/mm^3)	8,500	2,700	2,900	3,200	3,700
Average lymphocyte count (cells/mm^3)	4,300	6,000	6,400	3,200	2,500
Average serum immunoglobulin G concentration (mg/dL)	1,100	650	800	900	1,000
Average serum immunoglobulin M concentration (mg/dL)	15	80	140	150	200
Average serum immunoglobulin A concentration (mg/dL)	3	35	140	120	230
Average complement C^3 concentration (mg/dL)	—	110	130	140	130
Average complement C^4 concentration (mg/dL)	—	25	25	25	30

Compiled from reference 1.

Notes:

Table 92.2 • Common Viral and Bacterial Pathogens Associated with Specific Pediatric Infectious Diseases[a]

	Otitis Media	Sinusitis	Pharyngitis	Bronchiolitis	Croup Syndrome[b]
Viral					
Parainfluenza	+	+	++	++	+++
Influenza	++	+	++		++
Adenovirus	+	+	+++	+	+
Rhinovirus		++	+		+
RSV	+++	+	+	+++	+
Coronavirus		++			+
Enterovirus	+	+	+++		+
EBV			++		
Bacterial					
S. pneumoniae	+++	+++	+		
S. pyogenes	+	+	+++		
S. aureus		+[b]	+		+[d]
H. influenzae	++	++	++		+[d]
M. catarrhalis	++	++			
C. diphtheria			+		+
Oral anaerobes		+[c]	+		
M. pneumoniae	+	+	+	+	+

[a] +++ = Most common pathogens; ++ = Common pathogens; + = Occasional pathogens; EBV = Epstein-Barr virus; RSV = Respiratory syncytial virus.
[b] See Table 92.6 for specific bacterial pathogens for croup syndrome.
[c] Mostly isolated to chronic infections.
[d] Most common bacterial pathogens but are rare overall. S. aureus is more common than H. influenzae as a cause of bacterial tracheitis, but H. influenzae is more common as cause for supraglottitis.
Adapted with permission from the University of Kentucky College of Pharmacy Office of Continuing Education Independent Study Program entitled Pediatric Pharmacotherapy.

Notes:

Table 92.3 • Oral Antibiotics for the Treatment of Common Pediatric Infectious Diseases

Antibiotic	Dose	S. aureus	S. pneumoniae	H. influenzae	M. catarrhalis	Group B β-Hemolytic Strep	Compliance Factor Rating[c]	Side Effects/Comments	Refrigeration Required
Penicillins									
Penicillin VK,[d] Penicillin V	250 mg = 400,000 units of Penicillin G. 25–50 mg/kg/day divided Q 6 hr (max, 3 g/day)	+	+++	—	—	+++	1	Allergy, drug fever, eosinophilia, interstitial nephritis, CNS toxicity; ↓ dose in renal failure	
Penicillinase-resistant Penicillins									
Dicloxacillin[e]	25–50 mg/kg/day divided Q 6 hr	+++	+++	—	—	+++	1	Mild GI symptoms, diarrhea	
Cloxacillin[f]	50–100 mg/kg/day divided Q 6 hr	+++	+++	—	—	+++	1	Mild GI symptoms, diarrhea	
Broad-Spectrum Penicillins									
Amoxicillin[g]	Standard dose: 20–40 mg/kg/day divided BID to TID High dose: 80–90 mg/kg/day divided BID	+	+++	++	+	+++	2	↓ dose in renal failure; good activity against Salmonella; poor activity against Shigella	Preferred
Amoxicillin-clavulanate[h]	25–45 mg/kg/day divided BID	+++	+++	+++	+++	+++	2	Nausea, vomiting, diarrhea, abdominal cramps; take with food; do not give two of the 250 mg amoxicillin/125 mg clavulanate at one time; may result in GI toxicity	Yes
Ampicillin[i]	50–100 mg/kg/day divided Q 6 hr	+	+++	++	+	+++	1	Useful in treatment of Shigella; fair-to-good activity against Salmonella	

(continued)

Table 92.3 • Oral Antibiotics for the Treatment of Common Pediatric Infectious Diseases (continued)

Antibiotic	Dose	Spectrum[a]					Compliance Factor Rating[c]	Side Effects/Comments	Refrigeration Required
		S. aureus	S. pneumoniae	H. influenzae	M. catarrhalis	Group B β-Hemolytic Strep			
Cephalosporins (All Adjusted in Renal Failure)									
1st Generation									
Cephalexin (Keflex)[j]	25–50 mg/kg/day divided Q 6 hr	+++	+++	+	+	+++	2	GI distress, dizziness, fatigue, headache, neutropenia, rash, ↑AST, false-positive test for urinary reducing substances	Yes
Cephradine (Velosef, Anspor)[k]	25–50 mg/kg/day divided Q 6 hr	+++	+++	+	+	+++	2	GI distress, diarrhea, pseudomembranous colitis, rash, joint pains, transient leukopenia or neutropenia, ↑ hepatic enzymes or bili	
Cefadroxil (Duricef)[l]	30 mg/kg/day divided Q 12 hr	+++	+++	+	+	+++	3	Allergy, GI distress, transient neutropenia, pruritus	
2nd Generation									
Cefaclor (Ceclor)[m]	20–40 mg/kg/day divided Q 8–12 hr	+	+++	++	+	+++	3	GI distress, eosinophilia, pruritus, positive Coombs, false-positive test for urinary glucose, serum sickness	Yes
Loracarbef (Lorabid)[n]	15 mg/kg/day divided Q 12 hr	++	+++	+++	++	+++	3	GI distress, eosinophilia, pruritus, positive Coombs, false-positive test for urinary glucose	Preferred
Cefuroxime axetil (Ceftin)[o]	30 mg/kg/day divided Q 12 hr (40 mg/kg/day for otitis)	+++	+++	+++	+++	+++	1	Minor GI complaints	Preferred
3rd Generation									
Cefixime (Suprax)[p]	8 mg/kg/day divided Q 12–24 hr	+	++	+++	+++	+++	3	GI distress	Yes

3rd Generation

Drug	Dose					Comments	
Cefpodoxime (Vantin)[g]	10 mg/kg/day divided Q 12 hr	++	+++	+++	3	Not approved in infants less than 6 months of age; suspension contains phenylalanine; side effects include GI distress, ↑ liver enzymes, allergy, dizziness, ↓ leukocytes, eosinophilia; suspension does not contain phenylalanine	Yes
Cefprozil (Cefzil)[r]	30 mg/kg/day divided Q 12 hr	+++	+++	++	3	Not approved in infants less than 6 months of age; suspension contains phenylalanine; side effects include GI distress, ↑ liver enzymes allergy, dizziness, ↓ leukoctes, eosinophilia	Yes

Macrolides

Drug	Dose					Comments	
Erythromycin[s]	30–50 mg/kg/day divided Q 6 hr. Infants less than 4 months of age: 20–40 mg/kg/day divided Q 6 hr	+	++	+++	1	In pediatrics, estolate has greater bioavailability than ethylsuccinate; absorption not affected by food; no adjustment in renal failure; avoid in hepatic failure; GI: epigastric distress, diarrhea; drug interactions with theophylline, carbamazepine, digoxin, cyclosporine	
Clarithromycin (Biaxin)[t]	15 mg/kg/day divided BID	+	+++	+++	2	GI side effects less than erythromycin; drug interactions include ↑ theophylline and carbamazepine concentrations, failure of oral contraceptives	No

(continued)

Table 92.3 • Oral Antibiotics for the Treatment of Common Pediatric Infectious Diseases (continued)

Antibiotic	Dose	Spectrum[a] S. aureus	S. pneumoniae	H. influenzae	M. catarrhalis	Group B β-Hemolytic Strep	Compliance Factor Rating[c]	Side Effects/Comments	Refrigeration Required
Macrolides (continued)									
Azithromycin (Zithromax)	10 mg/kg on day 1, followed by 5 mg/kg on days 2–5	+	++	++	++	+++	1	GI side effects less than erythromycin; drug interactions include ↑ theophylline and carbamazepine concentrations, failure of oral contraceptives	Yes
Others									
TMP-SMX[u]	6–12 mg TMP/ 30–60 mg SMX/ kg/day divided Q 12 hr	+	+++	+++	+++	—	3	Not in patients less than 2 months (kernicterus); mild GI symptoms, skin rash, thrombocytopenia (rare), neutropenia (rare); ↑ half-life of phenytoin	No
Erythromycin-sulfisoxazole[v] (Pediazole)	40 mg/kg/day of erythromycin divided Q 6–8 hr	++	+++	+++	+++	+++	1	Same as erythromycin; also, neutropenia, agranulocytosis, thrombocytopenia, aplastic anemia, allergy, GI distress, crystalluria	Yes
Metronidazole[w]	15–35 mg/kg/day divided Q 6 hr	—	—	—	—	—	1	Anaerobic infections, C. difficile colitis, alcohol intolerance, GI distress, metallic or unpleasant taste	No
Tetracycline[x]	25–50 mg/kg/day divided Q 6 hr. **Use only in patients older than 9 years.**	++	++	+	+	+++	1	Depress bone growth, discolor teeth, enamel hypoplasia, photosensitivy, nausea, vomiting, epigastric distress, esophageal ulceration	No
Doxycycline[y]	2–4 mg/kg/day divided Q 12 hr on day 1, then half dose Q 24 hr. **Use only in patients older than 9 years.**	++	++	+	+	+++	2	Depress bone growth, discolor teeth, enamel hypoplasia, photosensitivity, nausea, vomiting, epigastric distress, esophageal ulceration	

Drug	Dose					FR[b]	Adverse Effects/Comments
Clindamycin[z]	20–30 mg/kg/day divided Q 6–8 hr	++	++	—	+	2	C. difficile diarrhea, allergy, minor ↑ in hepatocellular enzymes, neutropenia, thrombocytopenia
Rifampin[aa]	H. influenzae: 20 mg/kg/day QD × 4 days; N. meningitis: 20 mg/kg/day divided BID × 2 days	++	++	+++	++	2	Resistance develops rapidly; drug interactions with theophylline, cyclosporine, ketoconazole, β-blockers, digoxin, verapamil, phenytoin; diverse effects include allergies, ↑ cortisol metabolism, flu-like syndrome, hepatotoxicity, exudative conjunctivitis

[a] +++, good; ++, average; +, minimal; —, none.
[b] FR, factor ratings; 1, less favorable; 2, average; 3, more favorable.
[c] Penicillin VK available as 125, 250, 500 mg tablets; 125, 250 mg/5 mL suspension; Penicillin V available as 250, 500 mg tablets; 125, 250 mg/5 mL suspension.
[d] Dicloxacillin available as 250, 500 mg capsules; 62.5 mg/5 mL suspension.
[e] Cloxacillin available as 250, 500 mg capsules; 125 mg/5 mL suspension.
[f] Amoxicillin available as 250, 500 mg capsules; 125, 250 mg chewable tablets; 125, 250 mg/5 mL suspension.
[g] Amoxicillin-clavulanate available as 250 mg amoxicillin/125 mg clavulanate chewable tablets; 500 mg amoxicillin/125 mg clavulanate chewable tablets; 250 mg amoxicillin/62.5 mg clavulanate/5 mL suspension.
[h] Ampicillin available as 250, 500 mg capsules; 125, 250 mg/5 mL suspension.
[i] Cepholexin available as 250, 500 mg capsules; 125, 250 mg/5 mL suspension.
[j] Cephradine available as 250, 500 mg capsules; 125, 250 mg/15 mL suspension.
[k] Cefadroxil available as 50 mg, 1 g capsules; 125, 250, 500 mg/5 mL suspension.
[l] Cefaclor available as 250, 500 mg capsules; 125, 187, 250, 375 mg/5 mL suspension.
[m] Loracarbef available as 200 mg pulvules; 100 mg/5 mL suspension.
[n] Cefuroxime axetil available as 125, 250, 500 mg tablets; 125 mg/5 mL suspension.
[o] Cefixime available as 200, 400 mg tablets; 100 mg/5 mL suspension.
[p] Cefpodoxime available as 100, 200 mg capsules; 50, 100 mg/5 mL suspension.
[q] Cefprozil available as 250, 500 mg tablets; 125, 250 mg/mL suspension.
[r] Erythromycin available as Estolate: 125, 250 mg/5 mL suspension; ethylsuccinate available as 200, 400 mg/5 mL suspension; base available as 400 mg/5 mL tablets; stearate available as 250, 500 mg tablets.
[s] Clarithromycin available as 250, 500 mg tablets; 125, 250 mg/5 mL suspension.
[t] TMP-SMX, trimethoprim-sulfamethoxazole. Regular strength tablets: 80 mg TMP/400 mg SMX; double-strength tablets: 160 mg TMP/800 mg SMX; suspension: 40 mg TMP/200 mg SMX/5 mL.
[u] Erythromycin-sulfisoxazole available as 200 mg erythromycin + 600 mg sulfisoxazole/5 mL.
[v] Metronidazole available as 250, 500 mg tablets.
[w] Tetracycline available as 250, 500 mg capsules.
[x] Doxycycline available as 50, 100 mg capsules and tablets; 25 mg/5 mL suspension; 50 mg/5 mL syrup.
[y] Clindamycin available as 75, 150, 300 mg capsules; 75 mg/5 mL suspension.
[z] Rifampin available as 150, 300 mg capsules; suspension can be compounded.
AST, aspartate transaminase; BUN, blood urea nitrogen; CNS, central nervous system; GI, gastrointestinal.

Table 92.4 • The Modified Jones Criteria for the Diagnosis of Acute Rheumatic Fever

Clinical Findings	Description
Major Manifestations	
Carditis	Carditis usually manifests as a valvulitis and is associated with a systolic or diastolic murmur; myocarditis and pericarditis in the absence of a murmur are not likely
Polyarthritis	Frequently in the larger joints and migratory in nature; classically responds to salicylates within 48 hours
Chorea	Involuntary movements of the trunk or extremities that tend to have a delayed appearance
Erythema marginatum	The rash is a rare occurrence and is transitory and migrant; the lesions are nonpruritic, round with a pale center, and occur mostly on the trunk
Subcutaneous nodules	Firm, painless nodules develop over bony surfaces such as the elbows and knees; they move freely and are not inflamed; most often seen in patients with carditis
Minor Manifestations	
Arthralgia	Arthralgia is a joint pain without evidence of inflammation, which would be arthritis
Fever	A temperature of at least 39°C that usually occurs early in the course of the disease
Elevated erythrocyte sedimentation rate (ESR)	↑ acute-phase reactant that is relatively nonspecific
Elevated C-reactive protein	↑ acute-phase reactant that is more specific than ESR
Prolonged PR interval	Nonspecific finding suggestive of carditis; does not predict development of chronic heart disease
Evidence of Antecedent Group A Streptococcal Infection	
(+) Throat culture	Does not differentiate between acute infection and carrier state; only positive in approximately 25% of acute rheumatic fever patients
(+) Rapid streptococcal antigen screen	Does not differentiate between acute infection and carrier state; relatively specific but lacks sensitivity; negative results need to be confirmed with culture
Elevated or rising antibody titers	A ≥2 dilution ↑ in titers is suggestive of recent infection; Antistreptolysin O and Anti-DNase B are the most common; Antistreptolysin O titers >320 Todd units and Anti-DNase titers >240 Todd units generally are considered elevated in children

Notes:

Table 92.5 • Prophylactic Antibiotic Regimens for Acute Rheumatic Fever Patients

Long-Term Antibiotic Prophylaxis for the Prevention of Secondary Rheumatic Fever or Heart Disease

Benzathine penicillin G 1.2 million units IM Q 3–4 wk

or

Penicillin V 125–250 mg PO Q 12 hr (125 mg <60 lb >250 mg)

or

Sulfadiazine or sulfisoxazole 500–1,000 mg QD (500 mg <60 lb >1,000 mg)

or

Erythromycin 250 mg Q 12 hr

Prophylaxis for Endocarditis in Patients with Rheumatic Fever or Heart Disease Already Receiving Long-Term Secondary Prophylaxis

Dental, Oral, and Upper Respiratory Procedures

Azithromycin or clarithromycin 15 mg/kg PO 1 hr before procedure (max dose, 500 mg)

or

Clindamycin PO or IV, 20 mg/kg 1 hr before procedure (max dose, 300 mg)

or

Cephalexin or cefadroxil 50 mg/kg PO 1 hr before procedure (max dose, 2 g)

Genitourinary and Gastrointestinal Procedures

Vancomycin IV, 20 mg/kg (max dose, 1 g) *and* gentamicin IV 1.5 mg/kg (max dose, 120 mg) are both given within 30 min of starting procedure

Notes:

Table 92.6 • Characteristics of the Different Classifications of Croup Syndrome[a]

	Spasmodic Croup	Viral Croup	Bacterial Tracheitis	Supraglottitis
Synonyms	Subglottic allergic edema	Laryngotracheitis, laryngitis, LTB	Pseudomembranous croup, LTB	Epiglottitis
Frequency	Common	Most common	Less common	Rare
Age group	3 mo–3 yr	3 mo–3 yr	3 mo–3 yr	2–8 yr
Common pathogens	None (parainfluenza), (influenza)	Parainfluenza, adenovirus, influenza	S. aureus, S. pyogenes, S. pneumoniae	H. influenzae, S. pyogenes, S. pneumoniae
Clinical Presentation				
Onset	Rapid, nocturnal	Gradual, preceding URI	Gradual, preceding URI	Rapid
Signs and symptoms	Afebrile, cough, stridor	Fever, cough, stridor	Fever, cough, stridor, "toxic" appearance	Fever, dysphagia, drooling, stridor, "toxic" appearance
Neck radiography	Normal	Subglottic narrowing (steeple sign)	Subglottic narrowing (steeple sign)	Swollen epiglottis (thumb sign)
Laboratory	Normal	↑ WBC count, no shift	↑ WBC count, left shift, ↑ CRP	↑ WBC count, left shift, ↑ CRP

[a]CRP = C-reactive protein; LTB = Laryngotracheobronchitis; URI = Upper respiratory tract infection; WBC = White blood cell.
Adapted with permission from the University of Kentucky, College of Pharmacy, Office of Continuing Education, Independent Study Program, Pediatric Pharmacotherapy.

The reader is referred to Chapter 94: Pediatric Infectious Diseases, written by *Nicholas Blanchard, Pharm.D.*, in the seventh edition of **Applied Therapeutics: The Clinical Use of Drugs** for a more in-depth discussion. All notations to reference numbers are based on the reference list at the end of that chapter. The editors of this handbook express their thanks to Dr. Blanchard and acknowledge that this chapter is based upon his work.

Notes:

Notes:

Chapter 93

Pediatric Nutrition

Fluid and Electrolyte Requirements

♦ Dehydration. See Tables 93.1, 93.2 and 93.3.

♦ Electrolyte replacement. See Tables 93.4 and 93.5.

♦ Human milk feeding

• Human milk is the ideal food for an infant

• 3 phases of human milk production:

—colostrum: viscous, yellow fluid produced during first 5 days of lactation

—transitional: 5th → 10th day lactation

—mature: has sufficient protein, minerals, and calories, regardless of mother's nutritional status

• Mature milk: provides 70 kcal/100 mL with fat accounting for >50% of caloric content. Iron, vitamin D, and fluoride content are inadequate; thus supplementation is necessary.

♦ Infant formula. See Table 93.6.

♦ Parenteral nutrition

• Indications. See Table 93.7.

• Monitoring. See Table 93.8.

• Pediatric amino acid solutions. See Table 93.9.

Notes:

Table 93.1 • Parenteral Nutrient Requirements in Children[2-5]

Nutrient	Requirement
Fluid[1]	<1–1.5 kg 150 mL/kg 1.5–2.5 kg 120 mL/kg 2.5–10 kg 100 mL/kg 10–20 kg 1,000 mL + 50 mL/kg for each kg >10 kg >20 kg 1,500 mL + 20 mL/kg for each kg >20 kg
Calories	<10 kg 100 kcal/kg 10–20 kg 1,000 kcal + 50 kcal/kg for each kg >10 kg >20 kg 1,500 kcal + 20 kcal/kg for each kg >20 kg
Protein[a]	*Infants:* 2–3 g/kg *Older children:* 1.5–2.0 g/kg *Adolescents and beyond:* 1.0–1.5 g/kg
Fat[b]	Initially: 0.5–1 g/kg/day then increase by 0.5–1 g/kg/day (max, 3 g/kg/day) (≥4% of calories as linoleic acid)
Sodium	2–4 mEq/kg (max, 100–120 mEq/day)
Potassium	2–3 mEq/kg (max, 100–120 mEq/day)
Chloride	2–4 mEq/kg (max, 100–120 mEq/day)
Magnesium	0.25–0.5 mEq/kg
Calcium	0.5–3.0 mEq/kg
Phosphorus	1.0–1.5 mmol/kg
Zinc	<3 kg: 300 µg/kg >3 kg: 100 µg/kg (max, 4 mg/day)
Copper	20 µg/kg (max, 1 mg/day)
Manganese	2–10 µg/kg (max, 400 µg/day)
Chromium	0.1–0.5 µg/kg (max, 10–15 µg/day)
Selenium	2–3 µg/kg (max, 80 µg/day)
Vitamin A	230 U/kg (max, 2,300 units)
Vitamin D	40 U/kg (max, 400 units)
Vitamin E	0.7 U/kg (max, 7 units)
Vitamin K	20 mg/kg (max, 200 µg)
Thiamine	0.12 mg/kg (max, 1.2 mg)
Niacin	1.7 mg/kg (max, 17 mg)
Riboflavin	0.14 mg/kg (max, 1.4 mg)
Pyridoxine	0.1 mg/kg (max, 1 mg)
Vitamin B$_{12}$	0.1 µg/kg (max, 1 µg)
Biotin	2 µg/kg (max, 20 µg)
Vitamin C	8 mg/kg (max, 80 mg)
Folic acid	14 µg/kg (max, 140 µg)

[a]"Infant" amino acids contain histidine, taurine, tyrosine, and cysteine, which are essential in infants but not older patients.
[b]Because linoleic acid represents 54% of the fatty acid in soy bean oil and 77% in safflower oil, 7–10% of calories must be provided as fat emulsion. This can be given daily over 24 hours (preferred in patients predisposed to sepsis and preterm infants) or 2–3 times weekly.

Notes:

Table 93.2 • Clinical Signs of Dehydration

Severity	% Dehydration	Psyche	Thirst	Mucous Membranes	Tears	Anterior Fontanel	Skin	Urine-Specific Gravity
Mild	<5	Normal	Slight	Normal to dry	Present	Flat	Normal	Slight change
Moderate	6–10	Irritable	Moderate	Dry	+/−	+/−	+/−	↑
Severe	10–15	Hyperirritable to lethargic	Intense	Parched	Absent	Sunken	Tenting	Greatly ↑

Notes:

Table 93.3 • Situations That Alter Maintenance Fluid Requirements[a]

Situation	Mechanism	Extent of Change
Extreme prematurity	↑ skin losses	Varies
Radiant warmer use	↑ insensible water loss	20–40%
Croup tent	↓ evaporative water loss	20–50%
Diarrhea or vomiting	↑ GI loss	Varies
Fever	↑ insensible water loss	10–15% per °C
Renal dysfunction	↑ or ↓ renal loss	Varies
Hyperventilation	↑ pulmonary evaporative loss	Varies
Phototherapy for hyperbilirubinemia	↑ insensible water loss	10–20%
GI tract suction or ostomy	↑ GI loss	Varies
Mechanical ventilation	↓ insensible water loss	20–30%

[a]GI = Gastrointestinal.

Table 93.4 • Body Fluid Volumes and Electrolyte Content

Source	Volume (L/day)	Na^+ (mEq/L)	K^+ (mEq/L)	Cl^- (mEq/L)	HCO_3^- (mEq/L)
Salivary glands	1.5 (0.5–2)	10 (2–10)	26 (20–30)	10 (8–18)	30
Stomach	1.5 (0.1–4)	60 (9–116)	10 (0–32)	130 (8–154)	—
Duodenum	(0.1–2)	140	5	80	—
Ileum	3 (0.1–9)	140 (80–150)	5 (2–8)	104 (43–137)	30
Colon	—	60	30	40	—
Pancreas	(0.1–0.8)	140 (113–185)	5 (3–7)	75 (54–95)	115
Bile	(0.05–0.8)	145 (131–164)	5 (3–12)	100 (89–180)	35

Table 93.5 • Composition of Oral Rehydration Products[a]

Product	Na^+ (mEq/L)	K^+ (mEq/L)	Cl (mEq/L)	Bicarbonate Source (mEq/L)	Carbohydrate (%)
Gastrolyte	90	20	80	30 citrate	2
Rehydrate	75	20	65	30 citrate	2.5
Lytren	50	25	45	30 citrate	2
Pedialyte	45	20	35	30 citrate	2.5
WHO salts	90	20	80	30 bicarbonate	2

[a]WHO = World Health Organization.

Notes:

Table 93.6 • Examples of Infant Formulas and Their Individual Components[a]

Product	Calories per 100 mL	Carbo-hydrate g/100 mL	Caloric Source	Protein g/100 mL	Protein Source	Fat g/100 mL	Fat Source	Osmolality mOsm/L	Sodium mEq/L	Potassium mEq/L	Chloride mEq/L	Calcium mEq (mg)/L	Phosphorus mEq/L	Iron mg/L
Human Milk–Based, Milk-Based, and Soy-Based Formulas														
Human milk	72 ± 5	7.2 ± 0.25	Lactose	1.05 ± 0.2	Whey 55% Casein 45%	3.9 ± 0.4	Human milk fat	290 ± 5	7.8 ± 1.7	13.4 ± 0.9	11.8 ± 1.7	14 ± 1.3 (280 ± 26)	9.0 ± 1.4	0.3 ± 0.1
Enfamil with iron	67	6.9	Lactose	1.5	Whey 50% Casein 50%	3.8	Soy and coconut oils	300	7.9	18.4	11.9	23	17.4	12.6
Similac with iron	68	7.23	Lactose	1.5	Casein (nonfat milk)	3.63	Soy and coconut oils	290	10	21	15	25	25.2	12
SMA	68	7.2	Lactose	1.5	Whey 60% Casein 40% L-methionine	3.6	Oleo, saf-flower oleic, soy, and coconut oils	300	6.4	14	10.6	21.9	20.9	12
Isomil	68	6.83	Corn syrup solids, sucrose	1.8	Soy protein isolate, L-methionine	3.69	Soy and coconut oils	250	14	24	12	35	32.9	12
Nursoy	68	6.9	Sucrose	2.1	Soy protein isolate, L-methionine	3.6	Oleo, saf-flower oleic, soy, and coconut oils	296	8.7	17.9	10.6	29.9	27.1	11.5
ProSobee	68	6.7	Corn syrup solids	2.0	Soybean solids, L-methioninic	3.5	Olein, soy, coconut, oleic, and sunflower oil	200	11	21	15	35	26	12
Soyalac	69	6.8	Corn syrup, sucrose, soy	2.1	Soybean solids, L-methionine	3.7	Soy oil	240	13	20	13	32	12	12.8
Casein Hydrolysate, Modified Fat, and Premature LBW Formulas														
Nutramigen	67	9.1	Corn syrup solids, modified corn starch	1.9	Hydrolyzed casein	2.6	Corn oil	320	14.0	18.9	16.4	31.3	24.0	12.7
Pregestimil	67	9.1	Corn syrup solids, modified corn starch	2.4	Hydrolyzed casein	2.7	MCT oil 42%, corn oil 57%, lecithin 1%	350	14.0	19.0	16.0	31.3	24.0	12.7

(continued)

Table 93.6 • Examples of Infant Formulas and Their Individual Components[a] (continued)

Product	Calories per 100 mL	Carbo-hydrate g/100 mL	Caloric Source	Protein g/100 mL	Protein Source	Fat g/100 mL	Fat Source	Osmolality mOsm/L	Sodium mEq/L	Potassium mEq/L	Chloride mEq/L	Calcium mEq (mg)/L	Phosphorus mEq/L	Iron mg/L
Casein Hydrolysate, Modified Fat, and Premature LBW Formulas *(continued)*														
Portagen 20	67	7.8	Corn syrup, sucrose	2.4	Sodium caseinate	3.4	MCT oil 86%, corn oil 12%, soy lecithin 2%	220	13.9	22.0	16.4	31.3	27.0	12.7
NeoCare	73	7.7	Corn syrup solids, lactose	1.9	Nonfat milk, whey	4.1	Soy and coconut oil, 25% MCT oil	250	11	27	16	16		13
NeoCate	67	7.1	Corn syrup solids	1.9	Free amino acids	2.8	Vegetable, safflower, coconut	342	9	24	14	37		12
Enfamil Premature Formula	67	7.4	Corn syrup solids, lactose	2.0	Whey 50% Casein 50%	3.4	MCT oil 39%, soy 39%, coco-nut 20%, lecithin 2%	244	11.3	19.2	16.1	39.0	22.0	1.7
Enfamil Premature Formula 24	81	8.9	Corn syrup solids, lactose	2.4	Whey 50% Casein 50%	4.1	MCT oil 39%, soy 39%, coco-nut 20%, lecithin 2%	300	13.9	23.0	19.5	47.0	27.0	2.0
Similac Special Care	68	7.17	Lactose, glucose polymers	1.83	Whey 60% Casein 40%	3.67	MCT, soy, and coconut oils	250	15	24	17	61	35.5	2.5

Similac Special Care 24	81	8.61	Lactose, glucose polymers	2.2	Whey 60% Casein 40%	4.41	MCT, soy, and coconut oils	300	18	29	21	73	42.4	3.0
Similac 24 LBW	81	8.53	Lactose, glucose polymers	2.2	Nonfat milk	4.49	MCT, soy, and coconut oils	290	16	31	25	36	33.1	3.0
Hypercaloric and Low-Electrolyte Formulas														
Similac 27	91	9.59	Lactose	2.47	Casein (nonfat milk)	4.81	Soy and coconut oils	410	17	32	23	41	41.3	2.0
Similac PM 60:40	68	6.9	Lactose	1.58	Whey 60% Casein 40%	3.76	Soy and coconut oils	260	7	15	11	19	11	1.5
SMA 24	81	8.6	Lactose	1.8	Whey 60% Casein 40%	4.3	Oleo, safflower, oleic, soy, and coconut oils	364	7.8	17	12.7	25.1	21.7	14.4
SMA 27	91.3	9.7	Lactose	2.0	Whey 60% Casein 40%	4.9	Oleo, safflower oleic, soy, and coconut oils	416	8.8	19.3	14.3	28.2	24.4	16.2

Adapted from information provided by the American Academy of Pediatrics.

a LBW = Low body weight; MCT = Medium-chain triglyceride.

Table 93.7 • Indications for Parenteral Nutrition Support [a]

Extreme prematurity
Respiratory distress
Congenital GI anomalies
   Duodenal atresia
     Jejunal atresia
     Esophageal atresia
     Tracheoesophageal fistula
   Pyloric stenosis
   Congenital webs
   Hirschsprung's disease
   Malrotation
   Volvulus
Abdominal wall defects
   Omphalocele (herniation of viscera into the umbilical cord base)
   Gastroschisis (defect of abdominal wall, any location except umbilical cord)
   Congenital diaphragmatic hernia
Necrotizing enterocolitis
Chronic diarrhea
Inflammatory bowel disease
Chylothorax
Pseudo-obstruction
Megacystic microcolon
Abdominal trauma involving viscera
Adverse effects of treating neoplastic disease
   Radiation enteritis
   Nausea and vomiting
   Stomatitis, glossitis, and esophagitis
Anorexia nervosa
Cystic fibrosis
Chronic renal failure
Hepatic failure
Metabolic errors

[a] GI = Gastrointestinal.

Table 93.8 • Routine Laboratory Monitoring of Pediatric and Neonatal Parenteral Nutrition [a,b]

Test	Frequency
Electrolytes, glucose, BUN, SrCr	Daily until stable, then 2–3 times/wk
Calcium	1–2 times/wk
Phosphorus	1–2 times/wk
Magnesium	1–2 times/wk
Triglycerides	QOD until stable on maximum fat dose, then weekly
PA or RBP	Weekly
Total protein, albumin	Weekly if PA, RBP not available
Alkaline phosphatase	Weekly
Bilirubin (total, direct) [a]	Weekly
Hgb, WBC count	Weekly
AST, ALT	Monthly

[a] ALT = Alanine aminotransferase; AST = Aspartate aminotransferase; BUN = Blood urea nitrogen; Hgb = Hemoglobin; PA = Prealbumin; RBP = Retinol binding protein; SrCr = Serum creatinine; WBC = White blood cell.
[b] Bilirubin [indirect] daily in the newborn, until normal.

Table 93.9 • Pediatric Amino Acid Solutions

	TrophAmine 6%	Aminosyn-PF 7%
Essential Amino Acids (EEA) (mg/1 g total amino acids)		
Isoleucine	81.7	76.3
Leucine	140.0	118.7
Lysine	81.7	67.9
Methionine	33.3	17.9
Phenylalanine	48.3	42.9
Threonine	41.7	51.4
Tryptophan	20.0	17.9
Valine	78.3	64.6
Cysteine HCl[a]	3.3	0
Histidine	48.3	31.4
Tyrosine	23.3	6.3
Taurine	2.5	7.1
Nonessential Amino Acids (mg/1 g total amino acids)		
Alanine	53.3	70.0
Arginine	121.7	123.0
Proline	68.3	81.4
Serine	38.3	49.6
Glycine	36.7	38.6
L-aspartic acid	31.7	52.9
L-glutamic acid	50.0	82.3
Sodium (mEq/L)	5.0	3.4
Acetate (mEq/L)	56.0	32.5
Chloride (mEq/L)	<3.0	0
% essential amino acid	60.1	50.2
% branched chain amino acid (g amino acid/1 g nitrogen)	30.0	26.0

[a] 40 g of cysteine syringe available.

Notes:

The reader is referred to Chapter 95: Pediatric Nutrition, written by *Michael F. Chicella, Pharm.D.,* and *Emily B. Hak, Pharm.D.,* in the seventh edition of **Applied Therapeutics: The Clinical Use of Drugs** for a more in-depth discussion. All notations to reference numbers are based on the reference list at the end of that chapter. The editors of this handbook express their thanks to Drs. Chicella and Hak and acknowledge that this chapter is based upon their work.

Notes:

Chapter 94

Cystic Fibrosis (CF)

♦ CF is inherited as an autosomal recessive trait.

♦ The gene product is known as cystic fibrosis transmembrane regulator (CFTR), which functions as a chloride channel throughout the body. In sweat glands it reabsorbs chloride, while in the lung it excretes chloride.

♦ *Pathophysiology:*

Lungs: chronic infection and inflammation leading to destruction of lung tissue

Pancreas: insufficiency and maldigestion limit nutrition and ability to gain weight

♦ *Clinical Manifestations.* See Table 94.1.

♦ *Treatment of Respiratory Tract Infection in CF*

• Selection of therapy: exclude antibiotics to which the patient's organism are resistant; monotherapy is beneficial but associated with increased bacterial resistance. See Table 94.2. Optimal therapy is 2-drug coverage of *Pseudomonas aeruginosa.*

♦ *Pharmacokinetic Differences*

Absorption: CF patients manifest gastric hyperacidity, a decreased bicarbonate secretion along with pancreatic insufficiency, and a prolonged small intestinal transit time. These changes will affect the solubility, rate, and extent of absorption of some oral drugs (e.g., ciprofloxacin).

Distribution: The apparent volume of distribution (Vd) for some drugs (e.g., aminoglycosides, β-lactams) is increased in CF patients, which may necessitate using higher doses to achieve therapeutic serum concentrations.

Elimination: Individuals with CF manifest a higher total clearance of many drugs. This increased clearance is not limited to one particular route of elimination and can affect drugs eliminated by the kidneys without significant metabolism (e.g., aminoglycosides), those eliminated mostly by metabolism (e.g., theophylline), and those with a combination of renal and metabolic elimination (e.g., cloxacillin). Increased glomerular filtration rate (GFR), increased tubular secretion, and decreased tubular reabsorption all have been proposed as the mechanism for the increased renal clearance, but the actual mechanism is unknown. Metabolism of drugs takes place in a number of organs in the body, but the majority occur in the liver. The increases in nonrenal clearance (i.e., hepatic biotransformation) of drugs can be explained in part by the following: (1) an increase in hepatic blood flow, which has been observed in CF patients and which would increase metabolism of restrictively cleared drugs (i.e., those drugs whose clearance is dependent on liver blood flow) and (2) the induction of various hepatic enzymes (e.g., cytochrome P450).[34] The result of these differences is that antibiotics need to be given more frequently and in larger doses.

♦ *Pancreatic Enzyme Replacement.* See Table 94.3.

• With the malabsorption of fats, deficiencies in the fat-soluble vitamins take place. Thus, CF patients require supplementation with the fat-soluble vitamins. See Table 94.4.

♦ *Other Therapies*

DNase (Pulmozyme)

- Recombinant human DNase, when administered via aerosol into the lungs, breaks down intrapulmonary free DNA, reducing the viscosity of the sputum.

Chloride Channel Modifiers

- Amiloride, duramycin, and isobutylmethylxanthine inhibit reabsorption of sodium and water into the lung epithelium and have been associated with increased mucociliary clearance and decreased sputum viscosity.

Table 94.1 • Clinical Manifestations of Cystic Fibrosis

Manifestation	Approximate Incidence (%)		
	Infants	Children	Adults
Pancreatic			
Insufficiency	80–85	85	90
Pancreatitis	—	1–2	2–4
Abnormal glucose tolerance	—	5/yr[a]	30
Diabetes mellitus	—	2–4	8–15
Hepatobiliary			
Biliary cirrhosis	—	10–20	>20
Cholelithiasis	—	5	5–10
Biliary obstruction	—	1–2	5
Intestinal			
Meconium ileus	10–15	—	—
Meconium ileus equivalent	—	1–5	10–20
Rectal prolapse	—	10–15	1–2
Intussusception	—	1–5	1–2
Gastroesophageal reflux	—	1–5	>10
Appendiceal abscess	—	0–1	1–2
Respiratory			
Upper			
Nasal polyps	<1	4–10	15–20
Pansinusitis	—	—	90–100
Lower			
Bronchiectasis	—	30–50	>90
Pneumothorax	—	1–2	10–15
Hemoptysis[b]	—	5–15	50–60
Genitourinary			
Delayed puberty	—	—	85
Infertility			
Males	—	—	98
Females	—	—	70–80

[a] ↑ in glucose intolerance of approximately 5% per year.
[b] Percentage includes both major and minor hemoptysis.
Reprinted with permission from Wilson J. Adenoviruses as gene-delivery vehicles. N Engl J Med 1996;334:1185.

Notes:

Table 94.2 • Beginning Antibiotic Dosing in Cystic Fibrosis

Drug	Dose	Interval	Notes
Intravenous Antibiotic Dosages for the Treatment of Pulmonary Exacerbations in Cystic Fibrosis			
Amikacin[a]	7.5 mg/kg	6–8	Max 500 mg/dose; *monitor levels to adjust*
Ampicillin/sulbactam[b]	50 mg/kg	6	Max 2,000 mg/dose; 8 g/day
Aztreonam	50 mg/kg	6	Max 2,000 mg/dose; 8 g/day
Ceftazidime[c]	50 mg/kg	(6)–8	Max 2,000 mg/dose (Q 8 hr); 6 g/day
Ceftriaxone	75 mg/kg	24	Max 2,000 mg/dose; meningitis dosage higher
Cefuroxime	50 mg/kg	8	Max 1,500 mg/dose; 4.5 g/day
Chloramphenicol	20 mg/kg	6	Max 1,000 mg/dose; *monitor levels to adjust*
Ciprofloxacin	10 mg/kg	8	Max 400 mg/dose; 1.2 g/day
Gentamicin[a]	2.5 mg/kg	6–8	Max 180 mg/dose; *monitor levels to adjust*
Imipenem/cilistatin[b]	25 mg/kg	6	Max 1,000 mg/dose; 4 g/day
Mezlocillin	100 mg/kg	4–6	Max 4,000 mg/dose; 24 g/day
Meropenem	40 mg/kg	8	Max 2,000 mg/dose; 6 g/day
Piperacillin	100 mg/kg	4–6	Max 4,000 mg/dose; 24 g/day
Piperacillin/tazobactam[b]	100 mg/kg	6	Max 3,000 mg/dose; 12 g/day
Ticarcillin	100 mg/kg	4–6	Max 3,000 mg/dose; 18 g/day
Ticarcillin/clavulanate[b]	100 mg/kg	6	Max 3,000 mg/dose; 12 g/day
Trimethoprim-sulfamethoxazole[b]	5 mg/kg	6	Dosed on TMP; serious infection dosing
Tobramycin[a]	2.5 mg/kg	6–8	Max 180 mg/dose; *monitor levels to adjust*

(continued)

Table 94.2 • Beginning Antibiotic Dosing in Cystic Fibrosis (continued)

Drug	Dose	Interval	Notes
Inhaled Antibiotic Dosages in Cystic Fibrosis			
Amikacin	7.5 mg/kg/dose	BID–TID	Traditional outpatient dosing
Gentamicin	2.5 mg/kg/dose	BID–TID	Traditional outpatient dosing
TOBI	300 mg	BID	Proprietary formulation for aerosol: 30 days on, 30 days off
Colistin (Coly-Mycin-S)	37.5–75 mg	BID–QID	Used for changing resistance patterns of *P. aeruginosa*

[a]Levels:	Peak (µg/mL)	Trough (µg/mL)
Amikacin	25–30	2–5
Gentamicin	8–12	<2
Tobramycin	8–12	<2
Chloramphenicol	10–20	5–10

[b]**Combination medications** are written in terms of only one of their components:

- Ampicillin/sulbactam: dosed on ampicillin; standard adult dose is 3 g Unasyn IV Q 6 hr (equals 2 g ampicillin).
- Trimethoprim-sulfamethoxazole: dosed on trimethoprim.
- Imipenem/cilastatin: dosed on imipenem; standard adult dose is 1 g imipenem IV Q 6 hr.
- Piperacillin/tazobactam: dosed on piperacillin; standard adult dose is 3.375 g IV Q 6 hr (equals 3 g piperacillin).
- Ticarcillin/clavulanate: dosed on ticarcillin; standard adult dose is 3.1 g IV Q 6 hr (equals for 3 g ticarcillin).

[c]Ceftazidime: if using Q 6 hr dosing, 150 mg/kg/day ÷ 4 for Q 6 hr dose (max, 1.5 g/dose for Q 6 hr).

Table 94.3 • Pancreatic Enzymes

| Product[a] | Microencapsulated Enzymes | | |
	Lipase	Protease	Amylase
Cotazym-S	5,000	20,000	20,000
Creon 5	5,000	18,750	16,600
Creon 10	10,000	37,500	33,200
Creon 20	20,000	75,000	66,400
Pancrease	4,500	25,000	20,000
Pancrease MT 4	4,500	12,000	12,000
Pancrease MT 10	10,000	30,000	30,000
Pancrease MT 16	16,000	48,000	48,000
Pancrease MT 20	20,000	44,000	56,000
Pancrecarb	8,000	45,000	40,000
Ultrase	4,500	25,000	20,000
Ultrase MT 12	12,000	39,000	39,000
Ultrase MT 18	18,000	58,500	58,500
Ultrase MT 20	20,000	65,000	65,000
Zymase	12,000	24,000	24,000

[a]Dosing and comparison of products based on lipase content.
Adapted from Drug Facts and Comparisons, Inc., 2000.

Table 94.4 • Guidelines for Fat-Soluble Vitamins in Cystic Fibrosis[72]

Vitamin	Age	Dose
A and D	<2 yr	A: 1,500 international units D: 400 international units
	2–8 yr	A: 5,000 international units D: 400 international units
E	0–6 mo	25 international units
	6–12 mo	50 international units
	1–4 yr	100 international units
	4–10 yr	100–200 international units
	>10 yr	200–400 international units
K[a]	0–12 mo	2.5 mg/wk
		2.5 mg twice a week
	>1 yr	5 mg twice a week
Multi	Adolescent/adult	1–2 multivitamins QD

[a]Vitamin K is supplemented in cholestatic liver disease; prolonged antibiotics dosing in active hemoptysis is higher.

Notes:

The reader is referred to Chapter 96: Cystic Fibrosis, written by *James W. Jones, Pharm.D.*, and *Richard Shell, Pharm.D.*, in the seventh edition of **Applied Therapeutics: The Clinical Use of Drugs** for a more in-depth discussion. All notations to reference numbers are based on the reference list at the end of that chapter. The editors of this handbook express their thanks to Drs. Jones and Shell and acknowledge that this chapter is based upon their work.

Notes:

Chapter 95

Geriatric Drug Use

Demographics and Epidemiology of Drugs in the Elderly

♦ An increasing number of adults are living longer with multiple health problems. See Table 95.1.
♦ *Facts About Drug Use in the Older Population.* See Table 95.2.

Pharmacokinetic Changes in the Elderly

♦ Physiologic aging, or a progressive decrease in the ability of each organ system to maintain homeostasis in the face of challenge, increases vulnerability to disease symptoms or medication-adverse events. Functional age is affected by many factors and does not necessarily correlate with chronological age. See Table 95.3.
♦ Physiologic changes associated with aging, diseases, and pharmacological factors can affect pharmacokinetic parameters. These changes can alter drug response. See Table 95.4.
♦ The age-related changes in renal function are probably the single most important physiologic factors resulting in adverse drug reactions. Thus, drugs primarily eliminated by the kidneys require dose adjustment. See Table 95.5.

Pharmacodynamic Changes in the Elderly

♦ Defined as alterations in concentration-response relationships due to inefficient homeostatic adjustments or receptor sensitivity.
♦ *Homeostasis:* Orthostasis or postural hypotension occurs as a result of impaired baroreceptor function and a failure of cerebral blood flow autoregulation. Can be aggravated by sympatholytics, volume-depleting drugs, and vasodilating agents. These can contribute to falls. See Table 95.6.
♦ *Receptor sensitivity* changes can lead to exaggerated response (e.g., nitrazepam, heparin in females, warfarin). A decline in the dopamine system increases sensitivity to dopamine-blocking agents (e.g., neuroleptics, metoclopramide). Cholinergic deficits in the CNS can increase susceptibility to confusion caused by anticholinergic agents. See Table 95.7.

Effects of Drugs on Functional Ability

♦ Many medicines can induce functional impairments, especially in the elderly. This must be considered when assessing the patient's functional status. See Table 95.8.

Principles of Clinical Care and Prescribing in the Elderly

♦ *Geriatric Clinical Care Principles.* See Table 95.9.
♦ *Strategies for Healthy Prescribing in the Older Patient.* See Table 95.10.

♦ Adverse drug reactions can be difficult to detect in older patients because they often exhibit an atypical response and present with nonspecific symptoms such as lethargy, confusion, lightheadedness, or falls. Nevertheless, most adverse reactions are predictable extensions of a drug's pharmacologic effects and can be predicted and prevented. See Table 95.11.

♦ The ability of older persons to take medications is important to assess. Several conditions or skills have been identified as possible indicators. See Table 95.12.

♦ *Noncompliance* with medications regimens can be a source of drug misadventures and is important to assess. Over 50% of medications are taken incorrectly, and 30 to 50% of prescribed medications fail to produce their intended results. Several factors contribute to noncompliance in the older patient. See Table 95.13.

Table 95.1 • Profile of Older Americans[1]

Current Status of the Older Population
- The older population, persons ≥65 years of age, numbered 34 million in 1997, representing 13% of the U.S. population. This means since 1900, the percentage of Americans aged ≥65 tripled (4.1% in 1900 to 13% in 1997), and their numbers have increased 11-fold (from 3.1 million to 34 million in 1997).
- There are more women than men among the older population. Among persons ≥65 years old in 1997, 59% were women. In the oldest group, 71% of persons ≥85 years were women.
- The older population is getting older. In 1997 the ≥85 age group (4 million) was 31 times larger than in 1900.
- The expected number of years of life increased by approximately 60% since 1900. In 1997, life expectancy was 79.4 years for women and 73.6 years for men.
- In 1995, among noninstitutionalized elderly ≥70 years of age, 79% had at least one of the seven chronic conditions common among the elderly (arthritis, hypertension, respiratory illnesses, heart disease, diabetes, stroke, cancer).
- Among all persons ≥65 years of age, the five leading causes of death are heart disease, cancer, stroke, chronic obstructive pulmonary diseases, and pneumonia and influenza.

Future Growth of the Older Population
- Although the rate of growth slowed during the 1990s because of the relatively small number of births during the Great Depression of the 1930s, the most rapid increase is expected between the years 2010 and 2030, when the "baby boom" generation reaches age 65.
- By 2030, there will be about 70 million older persons, 2.7 times their number in 1980. If current fertility and immigration levels remain stable, the only age groups to grow significantly will be those >55 years of age.
- By the year 2030, persons aged ≥65 are expected to represent 20% of the population; the population ≥85 years of age will more than double to approximately 8.5 million persons.

Notes:

Table 95.2 • Facts About Drug Use in the Older Population[75]

Approximately 90% of Americans (35.5 million) >60 years of age are taking ≥1 prescription drugs.
The average older outpatient uses 2–4 different prescription drugs at the same time.
Among people aged 65–84 who live in the community, 61% receive ≥3 different drugs in a year, 37% receive ≥5, and 19% receive ≥7.
Each year, >9 million adverse drug reactions occur in older Americans.
Unwanted side effects of drugs are 7 times more common in older patients than in younger adults.
Nearly one-fourth of all nursing home admissions result from the inability of older adults to take their medications properly.

Table 95.3 • Factors That May Influence Functional Age

Poor versus good or adequate nutrition
Smoking versus quit smoking versus never a smoker
Acute or chronic diseases versus good health
Acute or chronic drug therapy versus no drug use
"Couch potato" versus lifelong habit of exercise
Institutionalized versus living independently at home

Notes:

Table 95.4 • Changes Affecting Pharmacokinetic Parameters[a]

Parameter	Physiologic Changes	Disease States	Pharmacologic Factors
Absorption (bioavailability, first-pass metabolism)	↑ Gastric pH ↓ Absorptive surface ↓ Splanchnic blood flow ↑ GI motility ↓ Gastric emptying rate	Achlorhydria, diarrhea, gastrectomy, malabsorptive syndromes, pancreatitis	Drug interactions, antacids, anticholinergics, cholestyramine, food
Distribution	↓ Cardiac output ↓ TBW ↓ Lean body mass ↓ Serum albumin ↑ α_1-Acid glycoprotein ↑ Body fat ↓ Altered relative tissue perfusion	CHF; dehydration; edema, ascites; hepatic failure; malnutrition; renal failure	Drug interactions, protein-binding displacement
Metabolism	↓ Hepatic mass ↓ Enzyme activity ↓ Hepatic blood flow	CHF, fever, hepatic failure, malignancy, malnutrition, thyroid disease, viral infection, or immunization	Dietary makeup, drug interactions, insecticides, alcohol, smoking, induction of metabolism, inhibition of metabolism
Excretion	↓ Renal blood flow ↓ GFR ↓ Tubular secretion ↓ Renal mass	Hypovolemia, renal insufficiency	Drug interactions

[a]CHF = Congestive heart failure; GFR = Glomerular filtration rate; GI = Gastrointestinal; TBW = Total body water.

Table 95.5 • Drugs Highly Dependent on Renal Function for Elimination^a

Acetazolamide	Diflunisal	Nadolol
Acyclovir	Digoxin	Nitrosourea
Allopurinol	Enalapril	Penicillamine
Amantadine	Ethambutol	Pentamidine
Amiloride	Fluconazole	Phenazopyridine
Aminoglycosides	Flucytosine	Plicamycin
Amphotericin B	Fluoroquinolones (most)	Probenecid
Atenolol	Furosemide	Procainamide
Aztreonam	Gallamine	Pyridostigmine
Bleomycin	Gold sodium thiomalate	Spironolactone
Bretylium	H$_2$ blockers (most)	Sulfamethoxazole
Captopril	Imipenem	Sulfinpyrazone
Cephalosporins (most)	Lisinopril	Thiazides
Chlorpropamide	Lithium	Ticarcillin
Cisplatin	Methenamine	Trimethoprim
Clonidine	Methotrexate	Vancomycin
Colistimethate	Metoclopramide	

^aThis list is not comprehensive; see references 159 and 160 for additional details.

Table 95.6 • Adverse Drug Reactions That May Affect Mobility of the Older Patient^a

Medication Class	Adverse Drug Reaction
TCAs	Orthostatic hypotension, tremor, cardiac arrhythmias, sedation
Benzodiazepines and sedative hypnotics	Sedation, weakness, ↓ coordination, confusion
Narcotic analgesics	Sedation, ↓ coordination, confusion
Antipsychotics	Orthostatic hypotension, sedation, extrapyramidal effects
Antihypertensives	Orthostatic hypotension
β-Adrenergic blockers	↓ Ability to respond to work load

^aTCAs = Tricyclic antidepressants.

Notes:

Table 95.7 • Categories of Anticholinergic Drugs That Can Induce Confusion in Older Patients[a]

Therapeutic Class	Examples (Brand Name)
Antispasmodic	Belladonna (generic) Dicyclomine (Bentyl) Propantheline (Probanthine)
Antiparkinson	Benztropine (Cogentin) Trihexyphenidyl (Artane)
Antihistamine	Diphenhydramine (Benadryl) Chlorpheniramine (Chlor-Trimeton)
Antidepressant	Amitriptyline (Elavil) Imipramine (Tofranil)
Antiarrhythmic	Quinidine Disopyramide (Norpace)
Neuroleptic	Thioridazine (Mellaril) Chlorpromazine (Thorazine)
Hypnotic	Hydroxyzine (Vistaril)
OTC agents	Antidiarrheals Doxylamine Cold remedies

[a]OTC = Over-the-counter.

Notes:

Table 95.8 • Drug Effects on Other Assessments[a]

Assessments	Drug Effects	Drug Examples
Functional	Movement disorders (extrapyramidal, tardive dyskinesia)	Neuroleptics, metoclopramide, amoxapine, methyldopa
	Balance (neuritis, neuropathies, tinnitus, dizziness; hypotension)	Metronidazole, phenytoin, aspirin, aminoglycosides, furosemide, ethacrynic acid, β-blockers, calcium channel blockers, neuroleptics, antidepressants, diuretics, vasodilators, benzodiazepines, levodopa, metoclopramide
Physical	Supporting structures (arthralgias, myopathies, osteoporosis, osteomalacia)	Corticosteroids, lithium, phenytoin, heparin
	Incontinence (urinary retention; secondary oversedation)	Anticholinergic agents, TCAs, neuroleptics, antihistamines, smooth muscle relaxants, nifedipine, phenylpropanolamine, prazosin; benzodiazepines, sedatives, hypnotics
	Sexual dysfunction	Hypotensive agents, CNS depressants, SSRI antidepressants
Social	Malnutrition	Drugs affecting appetite
	Poor dental health	Anticholinergic agents, glucose-containing oral liquid/chewable dosage forms
Psychologic	Cognitive impairment (metabolic alterations; memory loss, dementia)	β-Blockers, corticosteroids, diuretics, sulfonylureas, methyldopa, propranolol, hydrochlorothiazide, reserpine, neuroleptics, opiates, cimetidine, amantadine, benzodiazepines, anticonvulsants
	Behavioral toxicity (insomnia, nightmares, sedation, agitation, delirium, psychosis, hallucinations)	Anticholinergics, cimetidine, ranitidine, famotidine, digoxin, bromocriptine, amantadine, baclofen, levodopa, opiates, sympathomimetics, corticosteroids
	Depression	Reserpine, methyldopa, β-blockers, metoclopramide, corticosteroids, CNS depressants

Adapted from reference 60.
[a]CNS = Central nervous system; SSRI = Selective serotonin reuptake inhibitors; TCA = Tricyclic antidepressant.

Notes:

Table 95.9 • Geriatric Clinical Care Principles[11,a]

Care Principle	Outcome/Example
Because of impaired physiologic reserve in older patients, disease often presents at an earlier stage.	• Mild disease may tip the "balance." • Drug side effects may occur with agents and doses unlikely to be toxic in younger people. • Stoic elderly may be less likely to seek help for dysfunction until symptoms are advanced.
Presentation of a new disease depends on the organ system made most vulnerable by previous changes, and this "weak link" often differs from the organ newly diseased.	• Presentation is often atypical, with the "weakest link" being the brain (confusion), lower urinary tract (incontinence), musculoskeletal system (falling), or cardiovascular system (fainting).
Clinical findings abnormal in younger patients are common in older people and may not be responsible for a particular symptom.	• An elderly patient with syncope due to medications and dehydration, but with ventricular ectopy on a cardiac monitor, may be harmed by misdirected antiarrhythmic therapy.
Because comorbid disease and drug use are common, symptoms are often due to multiple causes.	• Incontinence may involve a combination of fecal impaction, drugs inducing confusion, and impaired mobility due to arthritis.
Because many homeostatic mechanisms may be compromised concurrently, multiple abnormalities can be amenable to treatment, and small improvements in several areas may yield dramatic benefits to overall function.	• Falls associated with diabetic polyneuropathy are exacerbated by concomitant drug use, arthritis, and orthostatic hypotension, which are more easily treated than the underlying disease.
Because older patients are more likely to suffer adverse consequences of disease, treatment and prevention may be equally or more effective.	• Thrombolytics for AMI. • β-Blockers after MI. • Hypertension treatment. • Immunization (influenza, pneumococcal pneumonia). • Fall prevention (modify drugs that induce orthostasis or confusion, remove environmental hazards, address balance, peripheral edema, nocturia).

[a]AMI = Acute myocardial infarction; MI = Myocardial infarction.

Notes:

Table 95.10 • Strategies for Healthy Prescribing in the Older Patient[57,67,84,85,95,a]

Ensure that a proper indication is established; do not just treat symptoms.

Put the problem in context. Is it affecting the patient's quality of life or causing functional decline? Balance the risks of the medication with its potential benefits.

Know the patient. What is his or her overall health status? Is there known hepatic or renal impairment?

What drugs, including nonprescription drugs, social drugs, and other self-medication, is the patient taking? Who else is prescribing?

Consider nondrug alternatives to therapy (e.g., physical exercise, physical therapy, counseling, and relaxation techniques).

If drug treatment is necessary, know the drug well, including its mechanism of action, route of metabolism and excretion, side effect profile in the elderly, and clinically significant drug interactions.

Dose carefully. The well-known adage "start low and go slow" is appropriate. Adjust the dosage according to the patient's response.

Simplify the regimen as much as possible by minimizing dose frequency, using monotherapy or at least a minimum number of drugs possible, avoiding "PRN" orders, and reviewing the need for all prescribed medications periodically with the intent to eliminate unnecessary drugs.

Try to anticipate and minimize adverse drug reactions by considering side effect profiles in selecting a specific drug group.

In general, if an older patient receives a new drug and develops new symptoms (e.g., confusion, instability, orthostatic hypotension, or falls), seriously consider that the symptoms may be drug induced.

Beware of enforced compliance and its potential for ADEs when an elder is moving from an ambulatory to a LTCF or hospital setting.

Minimize use of potentially inappropriate medications in the frail elderly with diseases that may be exacerbated (e.g., disopyramide in heart failure, diet pills in hypertension, β-blockers in asthma or severe peripheral vascular disease, ASA or NSAIDs with ulcers and cautiously with anticoagulants, anticholinergic agents in benign prostatic hypertrophy, dementia or confusional states).

Determine whether the patient needs help using the medication. Pharmacists, nurses, and caregivers all can serve as resources for older patients who are living alone or are functionally or cognitively impaired. Written instruction, information leaflets, calendars, special containers, special packaging, and a variety of other reminder devices can enhance the appropriate use of medication.

Educate the patient (and caregiver/family when needed) about intended therapeutic effects, possible adverse drug reactions, and signs of toxicity.

Be sure to schedule regular follow-ups, constantly re-evaluate the older patient's medication regimen, and document the outcomes of your interventions based on predetermined therapeutic goals.

[a]ADE = Adverse drug effects; ASA = Aspirin; LTCF = Long-term care facility; NSAIDs = Nonsteroidal anti-inflammatory drugs.

Table 95.11 • Predictors of Adverse Drug Events[95,96]

- >4 prescription medications
- Length of stay in hospital >14 days
- >4 active medical problems
- Admission to a general medical unit versus a specialized geriatric ward
- History of alcohol use
- Lower mean Mini-Mental Status Examination score (confusion, dementia)
- 2–4 new medications added to medication regimen during hospitalization

Table 95.12 • Indicators of the Inability to Self-Medicate[161,162]

Cognitive impairments
>5 prescription medications
Inability to read prescription and auxiliary labels
Difficulty opening nonchildproof containers
Problems removing small tablets from containers
Inability to discriminate between medication colors and shapes

Table 95.13 • Factors Influencing the Inability to Comply with a Medication Regimen

≥3 chronic conditions
>5 prescription medications
≥12 medication dosages per day
Medication regimen changed ≥4 times during the past 12 months
≥3 prescribers involved
Significant cognitive or physical impairments (e.g., memory, hearing, vision, color discrimination,
    child-resistant containers)
Living alone in the community
Recently discharged from the hospital
Reliance on a caregiver
Low literacy
Medication cost
Demonstrated poor compliance history

Adapted from reference 151.

The reader is referred to Chapter 97: Geriatric Drug Use, written by *Robin H. Fuerst, Pharm.D.,* in the seventh edition of **Applied Therapeutics: The Clinical Use of Drugs** for a more in-depth discussion of the specific nature of drug problems encountered in the elderly, their assessment, and the specific role of rehabilitation. All notations to reference numbers are based on the reference list at the end of that chapter. The editors of this handbook express their thanks to Dr. Fuerst and acknowledge that this chapter is based upon her work.

Notes:

Chapter 96

Geriatric Dementias

Types of Dementias

♦ Dementia is a syndrome, the most prominent feature of which is impaired short-term and long-term memory.

♦ The majority of individuals with dementias suffer from primary degenerative dementia (i.e., Alzheimer's).

♦ *Alzheimer's disease* accounts for ≅ 50% of all diagnosed cases of dementia

♦ *Vascular dementias* (including multi-infarct dementias and Binswanger's disease) are second most common.

♦ *Parkinson's dementia, pseudodementia, Pick's disease,* and others occur less frequently.

Diagnosis

♦ Multiple cognitive deficits sufficiently severe to compromise normal social or occupational function must be present before dementia can be diagnosed. See Table 96.1.

♦ Family members or others may note several symptoms that should prompt a medical evaluation. See Table 96.2.

♦ Memory loss often accompanies several diseases or disorders in the elderly, and these must be ruled out. See Table 96.3.

♦ Laboratory and other tests are used to assist in differentiating dementia disorders. See Table 96.4.

Alzheimer's Disease (AD)

♦ A definitive cause has not been determined, but genetic factors play a significant role.

♦ Risk factors include aluminum toxicity, young or old maternal age, head trauma, small head circumference and brain size, low intelligence, and family history of Alzheimer's disease or Down syndrome.

♦ Criteria for definite, probable, and possible dementia of the Alzheimer's type have been established. See Table 96.5.

♦ AD progresses over 10 years or more. See Table 96.6.

♦ Treatment

  • Goal is to maintain independence as long as possible by keeping patient in familiar surroundings and supporting the family. A good resource is the Alzheimer's Disease and Related Disorders Association, 360 N. Michigan Avenue, Chicago, IL 60601.

  • No drugs are available that can halt or reverse the progression of AD. Two cholinesterase inhibitors are FDA-approved to treat memory deficits. Other cholinergic agents, estrogens, and NSAIDs are examples of drugs under investigation. See Table 96.7.

Vascular Dementias

◆ The most common cause is occlusion of cerebral blood vessels by a thrombus or embolus, leading to ischemic brain injury. See Table 96.8.

◆ *Multi-infarct dementia (MID)* refers specifically to the cognitive decline that follows multiple small or large cerebrovascular occlusions.

◆ *Presentation.* Typically presents suddenly after a cerebrovascular insult. This is followed by a period of stability and further declines after additional episodes in a stepwise pattern. Cognitive impairments are variable and depend on the area of the brain affected.

◆ *Diagnosis.* Because criteria are vague, diagnosis is difficult. See Tables 96.9 and 96.10.

◆ Treatment includes smoking cessation, treatment of underlying hypertension and dyslipidemias, and antiplatelet therapy such as aspirin.

Behavior Disturbances in Dementia

◆ Several behavioral disturbances may develop during the course of dementia, particularly during the later stages. Rule out unrecognized medical problems and medication adverse effects first.

◆ *Psychological behavior* includes anxiety, depression, withdrawal, psychotic behaviors, and aggression. These respond reasonably well to nonpharmacologic and pharmacologic intervention.

◆ *Nonpsychologic behaviors* such as wandering, inappropriate motor activity, shouting, and incontinence respond better to environmental modification.

Table 96.1 • Diagnostic Criteria for Alzheimer-Type Dementia[a]

1. The presence of multiple cognitive deficits manifested by both:
   • Impaired memory (↓ ability to learn new information or to retrieve information previously learned), and
   • At least one of the following:
      Aphasia (language difficulties)
      Apraxia (diminished ability to perform motor activities in the presence of intact motor function)
      Agnosia (inability to recognize or name objects despite intact sensory function)
      Disruption of executive function (diminished ability to plan, organize)
2. The deficits above significantly interfere with normal work or social activities and represent a decline from previous ability to function.
3. The deficits above cannot be attributed to any of the following:
   • CNS conditions that cause progressive cognitive or memory impairment (e.g., cerebrovascular disease)
   • Systemic conditions known to cause dementia (e.g., hypothyroidism, neurosyphilis, HIV infection)
   • Substance-induced conditions (e.g., drug toxicity)
4. The deficits do not occur exclusively during the course of a delirium.
5. The disturbance is not better accounted for by another Axis I disorder (schizophrenia, major depressive disorder).

[a]CNS = Central nervous system; HIV = Human immunodeficiency virus.
Adapted from reference 19.

Notes:

Table 96.2 • Symptoms Suggesting Dementia

Symptom	Evidence
Difficulty learning or retaining new information	Repeats questions; difficulty remembering recent conversations, events, etc.; loses items
Unable to handle complex tasks	Cannot complete tasks that require multiple steps (e.g., difficulty following a shopping list)
Impaired reasoning	Difficulty solving everyday problems; inappropriate social behavior
Impaired spatial orientation and abilities	Gets lost in familiar places; difficulty with driving
Language deficits	Problems finding appropriate words (e.g., difficulty with naming common objects)
Behavior changes	Changes in personality; suspiciousness

Adapted from reference 20.

Table 96.3 • Causes of Dementia Symptoms

CNS Disorders	Systemic Illness	Medications
Adjustment disorder (e.g., inability to adjust to retirement)	Cardiovascular disease	Anticholinergic agents
	Arrhythmia	Anticonvulsants
Amnestic syndrome (e.g., isolated memory impairment)	Heart failure	Antidepressants
	Vascular occlusion	Antihistamines
Delirium	Deficiency states	Anti-infectives
Depression	Vitamin B_{12}	Antineoplastic agents
Intracranial causes	Folate	Antipsychotic agents
Brain abscess	Iron	Cardiovascular agents
Normal pressure Hydrocephalus	Infections	Antiarrhythmics
	Metabolic disorders	Antihypertensives
Stroke	Adrenal	Corticosteroids
Subdural hematoma	Glucose	H_2-receptor antagonists
Tumor	Renal failure	Immunosuppressants
	Thyroid	Narcotic analgesics
		Nonsteroidal anti-inflammatory agents
		Sedative hypnotics and anxiolytics
		Skeletal muscle relaxants

Notes:

Table 96.4 • Dementia Screening Tests[a]

Test	Rationale for Testing
CBC with sedimentation rate	Anemic anoxia, infection, neoplasms
Metabolic screen	
Serum electrolytes	Hypernatremia, hyponatremia; renal function
BUN, creatinine	Renal function
Bilirubin	Hepatic dysfunction (e.g., portal systemic encephalopathy, hepato-cerebral degeneration)
Thyroid function	Hypothyroidism, apathetic hyperthyroidism
Iron, B_{12}, folate	Deficiency states (B_{12}, folate neuropathies), anemias
Stool occult blood	Blood loss, anemia
Syphilis serology	Neurosyphilis
UA	Infection, proteinuria
Chest roentgenogram	Neoplasms, infection, airway disease (anoxia)
ECG	Cardiac disease (stagnant anoxia)
Brain scan	Cerebral tumors, cerebrovascular disease
Mental status testing	General cognitive screen
Depression testing	Depression, pseudodementia

[a]BUN = Blood urea nitrogen; CBC = Complete blood cell count; ECG = Electrocardiogram; UA = Urinalysis.

Table 96.5 • NINCDS-ADRDA Criteria for Dementia of the Alzheimer Type[a,87]

Definite DAT
Clinical criteria for probable DAT
Histopathologic evidence for DAT (autopsy or biopsy confirmed)

Probable DAT
Dementia established by clinical examination and documented by mental status testing (e.g., history and physical examination, Folstein Mini-Mental)
Confirmation of dementia by neuropsychologic tests (e.g., Blessed Dementia Screen and other tests)
Deficits in at least 2 areas of cognitive function (e.g., language and memory)
Progressive deterioration of memory and other cognitive function
Undisturbed consciousness
Onset between the ages of 40 and 90
Absence of systemic or other brain disease capable of producing dementia

Possible DAT
Atypical onset, presentation, or progression of dementia with an unknown etiology
Presence of a systemic or other brain disease capable of producing dementia but not thought to be the cause of the dementia
Gradually progressive decline in one intellectual function in the absence of another identifiable cause

Unlikely DAT
Sudden onset
Focal neurologic findings (e.g., ↑ DTRs, hemiparesis)

[a]DAT = Dementia of the Alzheimer type; DTRs = Deep tendon reflexes; NINCDS-ADRDA = National Institute of Neurological and Communicative Disorders–Alzheimer's Disease and Related Disorders Association.

Notes:

Table 96.6 • Stages of Dementia of the Alzheimer Type

Stage of Cognitive Decline	Features
No cognitive decline	Normal cognitive state
Very mild cognitive decline	Forgetfulness, subjective complaints only; no objective decline
Mild cognitive decline	Objective decline through psychiatric testing; work and social impairment; mild anxiety and denial
Moderate cognitive decline	Concentration, complex skills decline; flat affect and withdrawal
Moderately severe cognitive decline	Early dementia; difficulty in interactions; unable to recall or recognize people or places
Severe cognitive decline	Requires assistance with bathing, toileting; behavioral symptoms present (agitation, delusions, aggressive behavior)
Very severe cognitive decline	Loss of psychomotor skills and verbal abilities; incontinence; total dependence

Adapted from reference 92.

Table 96.7 • Drugs FDA-Approved For Alzheimer's Disease

Drug (Brand) Mechanism	Dosage	Indication and Effect	Adverse Effects	Other
Donepezil HCl (Aricept) 5, 10 mg tablets Reversibly inhibits acetylcholinesterase. More specific than tacrine.	5 mg daily. 10 mg daily does not provide greater benefit, but if used, do not increase dose for 4 to 6 weeks.	Symptomatic treatment of mild-to-moderate AD. All patients experience cognitive improvement over a 12- to 24-week period.	Cholinergic effects (see below) are milder. Dropout rates at 5 mg were similar to placebo.	Completely bioavailable and can be given as a single daily dose due to long half-life (70 hr).
Tacrine HCl (Cognex) 10, 20, 30, 40 mg capsules Reversibly inhibits acetylcholinesterase and butyrylcholinesterase	Titrate slowly to minimize side effects. Initially 10 mg QID between meals for 4 weeks. Increase by 10 mg/dose Q 4 weeks to 120 to 160 mg per day in divided doses.	Symptomatic treatment of mild-to-moderate AD. Cognitive improvement noted in 33% to 50% of subjects over 30 weeks.	Cholinergic effects may cause withdrawal of 17%: nausea, vomiting, diarrhea, and abdominal pain. ALT elevations in 49%.	Poor bioavailability made worse by meals. Multiple daily doses required due to short half-life (5–7 hr).

Notes:

Table 96.8 • Vascular Dementia Etiologies

Thrombotic Causes	Embolic Causes
Atherosclerosis	Atherosclerotic Stenosis
Arteriosclerosis	Atherosclerotic Ulcerative Plaques
Diabetes Mellitus	Cardiac Disease
	Atrial fibrillation
Hematologic Disorders	Cardiac surgery
Hyperlipidemia	Cardiomyopathy
Leukemia	Mitral valve prolapse
Sickle cell disease	MI with mural thrombus
	Prosthetic valves
Inflammatory Vascular Disorders	Rheumatic heart disease
Giant cell arteritis	Rheumatic valve disease
Polyarteritis nodosa	
Rheumatoid arthritis with arteritis	Metastatic Deposits
Scleroderma	
Systemic lupus erythematosus	Parasites and Ova
	Septic Emboli

Table 96.9 • DSM-IV Criteria for Vascular Dementia[a]

1. The presence of multiple cognitive deficits manifested by both:
   - Impaired memory ($\downarrow$ ability to learn new information or to retrieve information previously learned)
   - At least one of the following:
     Aphasia (language difficulties)
     Apraxia (diminished ability to perform motor activities in the presence of intact motor function)
     Agnosia (inability to recognize or name objects despite intact sensory function)
     Disruption of executive function (diminished ability to plan, organize)
2. The deficits above significantly interfere with normal work or social activities and represent a decline from previous ability to function.
3. Focal neurologic deficits (e.g., hyperactive DTRs, gait disturbances, weak extremities) or laboratory evidence indicating cerebrovascular disease (e.g., multiple infarctions of the cortex or white matter) judged to be etiologically linked to the disorder.
4. The deficits do not occur exclusively during the course of a delirium.

Adapted from reference 19.
[a]DSM-IV = Diagnostic and Statistical Manual of Mental Disorders, 4th ed; DTRs = Deep tendon reflexes.

Notes:

Table 96.10 • Proposed Diagnostic Criteria for Ischemic Vascular Dementia[a]

Definite IVD (Requires Histopathologic Examination of the Brain)
Clinical evidence of dementia
Pathologic confirmation of multiple infarcts, some extracerebellar

Probable IVD
Dementia
Evidence of at least two ischemic strokes by history, neurologic signs, or neuroimaging or by a
   single stroke with clearly documented temporal relationship to the dementia onset
Supporting evidence of multiple infarcts in regions affecting cognition, history of TIAs or vascular
   risk factors, elevated Hachinski score

Possible IVD
Dementia, plus one or more of the following:
• History or evidence of a single stroke (but not multiple strokes) without clearly documented tem-
   poral relationship to dementia onset
• Binswanger's disease (without multiple strokes), including all of the following:
      Early-onset urinary incontinence unexplained by urologic disease or gait disturbance not
         explained by peripheral cause
      Vascular risk factors
      Extensive white matter change on neuroimaging

Adapted from reference 140.
[a]IVD = Ischemic vascular dementia; TIAs = Transient ischemic attacks.

The reader is referred to Chapter 98: Geriatric Dementias, written by *Bradley R. Williams, Pharm.D.,* in the seventh edition of **Applied Therapeutics: The Clinical Use of Drugs** for a more in-depth discussion of the etiology, neuropathology, diagnosis, and treatment of dementias and their associated behavioral disturbances. All notations to reference numbers are based on the reference list at the end of that chapter. The editors of this handbook express their thanks to Dr. Williams and acknowledge that this chapter is based upon his work.

Notes:

Notes:

Chapter 97

Geriatric Urological Disorders

Sexual Dysfunction

- ◆ Highly prevalent in both sexes: 10 to 25% in men and 25–63% in women.
- ◆ Erectile dysfunction exists in 52% of elderly males.
  - • 80% of all cases are thought to be related to organic disease. See Table 97.1.
  - • Severe atherosclerosis is most common cause.
  - • Hypertension, smoking, and diabetes are commonly associated with erectile dysfunction.
- ◆ Drugs can induce sexual dysfunction. See Table 97.2.
- ◆ Treatment includes eliminating drugs that might be contributing to sexual dysfunction and drugs directed primarily toward erectile dysfunction. See Table 97.3.

Benign Prostatic Hyperplasia (BPH)

- ◆ Prevalence is age dependent; 75% of men who live to age 70 will develop signs and symptoms of BPH.
- ◆ *Clinical Presentation*
  - • Symptoms are both obstructive (difficulty initiating urination, a decrease in urinary force, midstream stoppage, postvoiding dribbling, a feeling of incomplete bladder emptying) and irritative (nocturia and daytime frequency) in nature. Incontinence and acute urinary retention can occur.
  - • Alcohol, anticholinergic agents, α-adrenergic agents, and neuroleptics can cause and exacerbate acute urinary retention in men with BPH.
  - • The Boyarsky Index is a symptom scoring system that is used to assess BPH and the effectiveness of treatment in an individual. See Table 97.4.
  - • The American Urologic Association's Urinary Symptom Index for Prostatism is a validated instrument that can be used to assess the baseline severity of prostatism, disease progression, and the effectiveness of different therapies. It is the preferred patient questionnaire. See Table 97.5.
- ◆ Examination should include urinalysis to rule out urinary tract infection and a serum PSA before the rectal digital examination. The latter is used to determine the size, shape, consistency, and nodularity of the prostate.
- ◆ PSA or prostate-specific antigen is thought to be specific for prostate origin. PSA correlates well with prostate weight, but prostate cancer produces about 10 times the amount of PSA on a tissue volume basis than does BPH. PSA values also increase with age. See Table 97.6.
- ◆ *Transurethral Resection of the Prostate (TURP)* is the gold standard for treatment of BPH and is used in 90% of patients with symptoms of residual urine or acute urinary retention. Erectile dysfunction, urinary incontinence, and bladder neck contractures are late complications of the procedure.

◆ *Drug therapy* is used to reduce the tension of the bladder neck and prostatic capsule and to induce atrophy of the prostate gland for patients awaiting TURP or for those who will not undergo surgery.

- α-Adrenergic antagonists and drugs that suppress androgens are used. See Table 97.7. Phenoxybenzamine (Dibenzyline), flutamide (Eulexin), and leuprolide should not be used because they carry more risk than benefit.

Urinary Incontinence

◆ Affects about 50% of institutionalized elderly and 20% of community-dwelling elderly

◆ Neurologic impairment, immobility, female gender, and hysterectomy are independent risk factors for urinary incontinence, but advanced age or chronic bacteriuria do not seem to be.

◆ *Drug-induced urinary incontinence.* Occasionally, α_1-antagonists (e.g., prazosin) have been associated with female stress incontinence; they have a relaxant effect on smooth muscle. Other drugs include diuretics, α-adrenergic agonists (e.g. pseudoephedrine), anticholinergics, and neuroleptics.

◆ *Acute incontinence* is urinary incontinence that is of relatively recent onset or associated with an acute medical problem (e.g., cystitis, atrophic vaginitis, urethritis, CHF, diabetes, delirium, and immobility). First treat reversible conditions. Women with urethritis and atrophic vaginitis can benefit from intravaginal estrogen cream administered nightly for 7 days followed by at least once weekly application thereafter or oral conjugated estrogen 0.625 mg/day.

◆ *Persistent urinary incontinence* occurs in three forms.

- *Urge incontinence* is the most common form affecting the elderly and occurs when involuntary voiding is preceded by a warning of a few seconds to a few minutes. It is characterized by precipitous urine leakage. It is most often associated with involuntary contraction of the bladder or detrusor motor instability caused by a neurologic disorder. Treatment is with anticholinergic antispasmodic agents.

- *Stress incontinence* is the involuntary leakage that occurs only when there is an abrupt increase in intra-abdominal pressure (coughing, sneezing, laughing, lifting) that overcomes urethral resistance. Primarily occurs in elderly women and is due to weakness and laxity of the pelvic floor musculature. Estrogen deficiency and a genetic defect in the connective tissue may contribute. Obesity or TURP can predispose men to stress incontinence. Treatment is with phenylpropanolamine, pseudoephedrine, impramine, or estrogens.

- *Overflow incontinence* occurs when the weight of urine in a distended bladder overcomes outlet resistance. Typically there is leakage of small amounts throughout the day. Patients complain of hesitancy, diminished and interrupted flow, a need to strain to void, and a sense of incomplete emptying. It usually results from an anatomic outlet obstruction. Treatment is with prazosin (0.5 to 1.0 mg QD at bedtime) or bethanechol 10 mg TID.

- *Functional incontinence* occurs when a continent individual is unable or unwilling to reach the toilet to urinate.

- *Drug therapy* is aimed at modifying bladder contractility (anticholinergic agents, since the major neurohormonal stimulus for bladder muscle contraction is acetylcholine)) and increasing bladder outlet resistance (imipramine, sympathomimetics, estrogens). See Table 97.8.

Notes:

Table 97.1 • Causes of Impotence

Vascular
Atherosclerosis
Penile Raynaud's phenomenon

Neurologic
Cerebrovascular accident
Spinal cord damage
Autonomic neuropathy
Peripheral neuropathy

Endocrine
Diabetes mellitus
Hypogonadism
Prolactinomas
Hyperthyroidism
Hypothyroidism

Iatrogenic
Pelvic radiation
Lumbar sympathectomy
Prostatectomy
Renal transplantation
Spinal cord resection

Psychogenic
Performance anxiety
Depression
Widower's syndrome

Adapted with permission from reference 74.

Table 97.2 • Common Drug-induced Alterations in Sexual Response[a]

Drug Categories	Clinical Considerations
Antihypertensives	
Diuretics	
Thiazides	Temporal association with sexual dysfunction. Reported incidence varies between 0 and 32%[283–287]; however, impotence generally is not considered common. Mechanism believed to be a "steal syndrome" whereby blood is routed from erectile tissues to skeletal muscle.[84]
Spironolactone	Associated with ↓ libido, impotence, and gynecomastia. Mechanism may be hormone related. Incidence is dose related and reported to be 5–67%[84,288,289] and much more commonly encountered than with the thiazides. May be due to antiandrogen effects of drug.
Sympatholytics	
Methyldopa	Central action mediated causing vasodilation resulting in erectile dysfunction. Reported incidence: 10%.[84,88] Also ↓ libido.
Clonidine	Induces erectile dysfunction. Mechanism similar to methyldopa and other central α_2-agonists. Incidence reported to be 4–70% and dose related.[290–292] Also ↓ libido.
Guanabenz, guanfacine	Incidence and mechanism believed to be similar to other central α_2-agonists.
Nonselective β-Blockers	
Propranolol	Associated with erectile dysfunction and ↓ libido. Mechanism believed to be due to ↓ vascular resistance and central effects. Erectile dysfunction reported to begin at doses of 120 mg/day. Incidence may be as high as 100% at higher dosages.[81,88,293]
Selective β-Blockers	
Atenolol, metoprolol, pindolol, timolol (drops)	Incidence of erectile dysfunction is significantly less than nonselective β-blockers.[294]
α-Blockers	
Doxazosin, prazosin, terazosin	Associated with erectile dysfunction and priapism.[88,295] Reported incidence: 0.6–4%.[296] Mechanism is local α_1-blockade resulting in vasodilation. Erectile dysfunction and priapism appear to be unique to the nonspecific α_1-antagonists.
Phenoxybenzamine	Associated with priapism, retrograde ejaculation, and inhibited emissions during erection. Effects are dose related.[297,298]

(continued)

Table 97.2 • Common Drug-induced Alterations in Sexual Response[a] (continued)

Drug Categories	Clinical Considerations
Direct Vasodilators Hydralazine	Associated with erectile dysfunction. Mechanism is vascular smooth muscle relaxation. Incidence not reported.[297]
Calcium Channel Blockers Nifedipine	Associated with erectile dysfunction. Mechanism believed to be vasodilation and possibly muscle relaxation. Reported incidence: <2%.[74]
Diltiazem, verapamil	Similar to nifedipine. Reported incidence: <1%.
Antiarrhythmics Class IA disopyramide	Associated with erectile dysfunction in patients treated for ventricular arrhythmias. Incidence not reported. Mechanism believed to be due to strong anticholinergic effect.[84,297]
Anticonvulsants Carbamazepine, phenytoin	May be associated with sexual dysfunction through decreasing DHEA, which is a precursor to testosterone, estrogen, and pheromones.[248]
Antidepressants SSRIs	Drugs with prominent serotonin agonist effects commonly cause delayed ejaculation and anorgasmia. The reported incidence for delayed ejaculation among men is 2–12%; for anorgasmia among women users, the incidence appears to be <3%. This adverse effect is directly dose related.[248]
Tricyclic antidepressants, monoamine oxidase inhibitors	Associated with impairment of sexual performance in both male and female: ↓ libido, anorgasmia, retrograde ejaculation, erectile dysfunction. Mechanism believed to be due to anticholinergic and serotonergic effects. Incidence not reported; several case studies in the literature.[21]
Trazodone	Associated with priapism in men and ↑ libido in women. Mechanism similar to TCAs. Incidence not reported but believed to be dose related.[21] (*Note:* The literature reports that overall there is less sexual dysfunction with desipramine than with other antidepressants.)
Antipsychotics Phenothiazines	Frequently associated with sexual dysfunction. Commonly, ↓ libido is reported. Mechanism is due to hyperprolactinemia secondary to central dopamine antagonism. Thioridazine is the most often reported offender. Erectile and ejaculatory pain are very common with this drug class; the α-antagonism and anticholinergic effects are responsible. Priapism is common with this drug group, owing to the peripheral α-blockade property. Incidence for all sexual dysfunction with this drug class: approximately 50% of users.[21]
Anxiolytics Short-acting barbiturates	Biphasic effect. At low doses, libido ↑, similar to ethanol, and at higher doses, CNS depression causes ↓ libido and performance.[21]
Benzodiazepines	Biphasic effect. At low doses, libido ↑, whereas at higher dosages, CNS depression causes performance failure. Some reports of anorgasmia (men and women) and ejaculatory failure.[21]
Substances of Abuse Alcohol	Alcohol is thought to impair sexual function through its chronic effects on the nervous system. Short-term use of alcohol can induce erectile dysfunction through its sedative effects. More than 600 mL alcohol per week increases the probability of erectile dysfunction.[212]

(continued)

Table 97.2 • Common Drug-induced Alterations in Sexual Response[a] (continued)

Drug Categories	Clinical Considerations
Substances of Abuse (continued)	
Cocaine	Biphasic effect. At low doses, there is enhanced sexual desire (similar to amphetamines) and possibly performance. At higher dosages, there may be arousal dysfunction, ejaculatory dysfunction, anorgasmia. Freebasing has been associated with spontaneous orgasm. Continued use ("on a run") causes significant loss of sexual interest and performance ability. Chronic use associated with hyperprolactinemia resulting in ↓ libido.[21]
Ethanol	At low doses actually may enhance libido. Sexual dysfunction is dose related and due to CNS depressant effects.[84,88,295]
Hallucinogens	Biphasic effect for majority of drugs in this category. At low doses, libido is enhanced; at higher doses, libido is severely ↓. No reports on chronic use.[21]
Marijuana	Biphasic effect similar to ethanol. With chronic use there is a ↓ in libido. Mechanism may be due to ↓ testosterone. Incidence not reported.[21]
Opioids	Associated with sexual dysfunction: erection lubrication, orgasm, and ejaculation. Chronic use associated with ↓ libido. Mechanism may be due to α-antagonism, alterations in testosterone, and the intoxicating effects. Incidence not reported.[83,88,295,299]
Miscellaneous	
Amyl nitrite	Associated with intense and prolonged orgasms in both male and female. Impotence has been reported in some cases due to vasodilation.[21]
Cimetidine, ranitidine	Associated with ↓ libido and erectile dysfunction. Mechanism due to antiandrogen qualities and drug-induced elevation of prolactin. May be dose related.[88,300]
Metoclopramide	Associated with ↓ libido and erectile dysfunction. Mechanism is through CNS dopamine antagonism, resulting in hyperprolactinemia. Incidence not reported.[88]

[a]CNS = Central nervous system; DHEA = Dehydroepiandrosterone; TCAs = Tricyclic antidepressants.

Notes:

Table 97.3. • Treatment of Erectile Dysfunction

Drug (Brand)	Indication and Mechanism of Action	Dosage	Precautions and Adverse Effects	Other
Alprostadil or prostaglandin E₁ (Caverject, MUSE urethral suppository)	Erectile dysfunction unresponsive to oral therapy. Blocks α-membrane receptors thereby relaxing the cavernous and arteriolar smooth muscle while restricting venous outflow.	IC injection and suppositories require careful titration in the physician's office. Consult package insert. Onset is 5 to 10 minutes. Duration is 30 to 60 minutes.	Urethral pain (11% for suppository users), hypotension, leg swelling, and perineal pain	Users had successful intercourse 65% to 80% of the time.
Bromocriptine (Parlodel, generic) 2.5 mg tablets	Hyperprolactinemia with secondary hypogonadism. Dopamine agonist, which suppresses prolactin.	1.25 mg BID with meals	Dizziness, drowsiness, hypotension, cerebral vascular accidents, dyskinesia, hallucinations, dystonia, confusion	Even with normalization of prolactin only 50% of elderly males achieved erectile function and desire.
Papaverine-phentolamine (extemporaneously compounded for intracavernous injections) 30 mg/mL papaverine and 1 mg/mL phentolamine	Erectile dysfunction of various etiologies that have failed to respond to oral therapy. Papaverine is a phosphodiesterase inhibitor that relaxes penile arteriolar and corporal sinusoidal smooth muscle. Phentolamine blocks both α₁ and α₂ receptors.	0.5 mL for mild to 1.0 mL for severe dysfunction.* Initial test dose administered in physician office. Papaverine 25 to 60 mg can be used as a single drug as well.	Priapism, penile induration, corporeal fibrosis, bradycardia, hypertension, dizziness, flushing	IC epinephrine is used to counteract priapism; atropine is used to counteract other effects.
Pergolide (Permax) 0.05, 0.25, 1 mg tablets	Hyperprolactinemia with secondary hypogonadism. Dopamine agonist, which suppresses prolactin.	0.05 mg daily for 2 days initially. Every 3rd day increase by 0.1 to 0.15 mg for 12 days. Thereafter, increase by 0.25 mg every 3rd day until average dose of 1.0 mg TID is achieved.	Nausea, hypotension, cerebral vascular accidents, dyskinesia, hallucinations, dystonia, confusion	As with bromocriptine, response rate is 50%.

Sildenafil (Viagra) 25, 50, 100 mg tablets	Erectile dysfunction of various etiologies. Enhances the nitric oxide-induced relaxation of corpus cavernosal smooth muscle.	50 mg 1 hour before sexual activity (range is 4 hours to 30 minutes before intercourse). Use 25 mg in patients >65 years old, those with severe liver or renal impairment, and those taking potent P450 (CYP) 3A4 inhibitors.	Headache and facial flushing are most frequent. Contraindicated in patients using nitrates. Use cautiously in patients with retinitis pigmentosa (causes transient visual anomalies).	Significantly improves erectile function and the rate of successful sexual intercourse approaching normal men of same age.
Testosterone enanthate (Delatestryl injection) or *testosterone cypionate* (Virilon IM) or *testosterone transdermal system* (Testoderm Transdermal Systems)	Primary hypogonadism with severely deficient serum testosterone levels is only indication.	• 50 to 400 mg IM every 2 to 4 weeks *or* • One patch to skin on the back, abdomen, upper arms, or thighs applied nightly. Rotate sites.	Gynecomastia, edema, acne, dermatologic reactions, ? increased risk of prostate cancer	Baseline assessment of the prostate, including PSA, digital palpation, and fine needle biopsy
Yohimbine (Generic) 5.4 mg tablets	Psychogenic erectile dysfunction, diabetes mellitus. An α-adrenergic antagonist that decreases outward blood flow from the penile corporal tissue	5.4 mg orally QID. Beneficial effects usually occur in 2 to 3 weeks.	Nausea, tachycardia, slight elevations in blood pressure, anxiety, panic attacks	Only modestly effective, but relatively safe and easy to take. Worth trying before intracorporeal injections.

*Inject within a 1- to 2-minute period into the right side of the penis (lateral aspect), approximately 4 cm from the glans. If pain occurs extend injection time to 3 or 4 minutes. Compress puncture site and massage penis for about 3 minutes to distribute drug throughout the shaft.

Table 97.4 • BPH Symptom Scoring System (Boyarsky Index)[a,b]

Nocturia

0	Absence of symptoms
1	Urinates 1 time/night
2	Urinates 2–3 times/night
3	Urinates ≥4 times/night

Daytime Frequency

0	Urinates 1–4 times/day
1	Urinates 5–7 times/day
2	Urinates 8–12 times/day
3	Urinates ≥13 times/day

Hesitance (Lasts ≥1 min)

0	Occasional (≤20% of the time)
1	Moderate (20–50% of the time)
2	Frequent (≥50% of the time)
3	Always present

Intermittency (Lasts ≥1 min)

0	Occasional (≤20% of the time)
1	Moderate (20–50% of the time)
2	Frequent (≥50% of the time)
3	Always present

Terminal Dribbling (At end of voiding)

0	Occasional (≤20% of the time)
1	Moderate (20–50% of the time)
2	Frequent (≥50% of the time)
3	Always present (may wet clothes)

Urgency

0	Absence
1	Occasionally difficult to postpone urination
2	Frequently difficult to postpone urination
3	Always difficult to postpone urination

Impairment of Size and Force of Urinary Stream

0	Absence
1	Impaired trajectory
2	Most of the time size and force are restricted
3	Urinates with great effort and stream is interrupted

Dysuria

0	Absence
1	Occasional burning sensation during urination
2	Frequent (>50% of the time) burning sensation
3	Frequent and painful burning sensation during urination

Sensation of Incomplete Voiding

0	Absence
1	Occasional sensation
2	Frequent (>50% of the time) sensation
3	Constant and urgent sensation, no relief on voiding

[a] Symptom scoring provides the clinician with a tool to measure the relative need for, and efficacy of, different interventions. No specific score is associated with the need for a specific intervention. A low symptom score in the absence of significant urine retention generally indicates that medical management can be attempted before considering surgical intervention.[158]

[b] BPH = Benign prostatic hyperplasia.

Notes:

Table 97.5 • American Urological Association (AUA) Urinary Symptom Index for Prostatism

Symptom				Score			
	Not at All	<1 in 5 Times	<½ the Time	≈½ the Time	>½ the Time	Almost Always
1. Over the past month or so, how often have you had a sensation of not emptying your bladder completely after you finished urinating?	0	1	2	3	4	5
2. Over the past month or so, how often have you had to urinate again <2 hr after you finished urinating?	0	1	2	3	4	5
3. Over the past month or so, how often have you found you stopped and started several times when you urinated?	0	1	2	3	4	5
4. Over the past month or so, how often have you found it difficult to postpone urination?	0	1	2	3	4	5
5. Over the past month or so, how often have you had a weak urinary stream?	0	1	2	3	4	5
6. Over the past month or so, how often have you had to push or strain to begin urination?	0	1	2	3	4	5
7. Over the past month or so, how many times did you most typically get up to urinate from the time you went to bed at night until the time you got up in the morning?	0 times	1 time	2 times	3 times	4 times	5 times

AUA Symptom Score = Sum of questions 1–7 = _____

Interpretation of AUA Symptom Index
Mild prostatism ≤7
Moderate prostatism 8–18
Severe prostatism >18
Highest possible score 35

Reprinted with permission from reference 301.

Table 97.6 • Age-Adjusted PSA Values[a]

Age Range (yrs)	PSA Upper Limit (ng/mL)	PSA Density
40–49	2.5	0.08
50–59	3.5	0.10
60–69	4.5	0.11
70–79	6.5	0.13

[a]PSA = Prostate-specific antigen.

Notes:

Table 97.7 • Drug Treatment of BPH

Drug	Indication/Effect	Dose	Adverse Effects	Comments
α-Adrenergic Antagonists	Reduce smooth muscle tone of the prostatic urethra thereby decreasing the functional component of urethral constriction and obstruction, leading to increased urinary flow			
Prazosin (Minipress, Generic) 1 mg capsule	More specific α-adrenergic blocker (α_{1A})	1 mg at bedtime initially. Increase slowly to 2 to 4 mg daily in 2 to 3 divided doses.	First-dose syncope (1 to 2% in patients receiving ≥2 mg). Dizziness, headache, drowsiness, fatigue, palpitations (5 to 10%).	Give first dose and any increase in dose at night to minimize syncope.
Terazosin (Hytrin) 1, 2, 5, 10 mg capsule.	Long-acting, selective α_{1A}-blocker significantly improves urinary flow rates.	1 mg at bedtime initially. Gradually increase dose in 2 mg increments to 5 to 10 mg once daily. Trial of 4 to 6 weeks needed to assess effects.	Similar to prazosin above.	Commonly prescribed with finasteride to control progression and symptoms. Lower doses of terazosin can be used (1 to 5 mg/day).
Doxazosin (Cardura) 1, 2, 4, 8 mg tablets	Long-acting, selective α_{1A}-blocker. Improves urinary flow rates in about 70% of subjects within weeks	1 mg daily at bedtime initially. After 1 to 2 weeks, increase dose over several weeks to 4 to 8 mg daily.	Similar to prazosin above. Doses >4 mg are most often associated with dizziness and syncope.	Give first dose at night.

(continued)

Table 97.7 • Drug Treatment of BPH (continued)

Drug	Indication/Effect	Dose	Adverse Effects	Comments
Androgen Suppression	Testosterone is converted to dihydrotestosterone (DHT), which stimulates prostatic growth. The conversion is facilitated by 5-α-reductase. All agents that suppress androgen action, therefore, will induce prostatic atrophy.			
Finasteride (Proscar) 5 mg tablet	Inhibits 5-α-reductase thereby decreasing DHT production. Halts disease progression and decreases the size of an enlarged prostate. Urine flow increases in most patients. Reduces risk for acute urinary retention and surgery.	5 mg/day	Generally well tolerated. Inhibition of DHT does not affect testosterone-mediated functions on muscle mass, libido, or spermatogenesis.	Drug must be taken indefinitely.

Notes:

Table 97.8 • Drugs Most Commonly Used for Persistent Urinary Incontinence

Drug	Indication/Effect	Dose	Comments
Anticholinergic, Local Anesthetic, Antispasmodic Agents	Indicated for urge incontinence. Inhibit detrusor contractions in patients with or without neurogenic bladder. Improve bladder capacity, number of voids, and incontinent episodes per day.	See below. Several must be given in multiple daily doses. Evaluate after 2 weeks and consider switching to another agent if there is no response to maximum recommended doses.	Vary with regard to efficacy, propensity for anticholinergic side effects (dry mouth, CNS, urinary hesitancy, urinary retention), and dosing frequency.
Oxybutynin chloride (Ditropan, Ditropan XL, generic) 5 mg tablets; 5 mg/5 mL syrup; 5, 10, 15 mg XL tablets	Strong independent effect on smooth muscle with local anesthetic and minor anticholinergic effects. Inhibits detrusor contractions in patients with and without neurogenic bladder dysfunction.	2.5 (elderly) daily up to 5 mg TID. Increase by 2.5 mg. Or, once daily doses of controlled-release form (5 to 30 mg)	Oral agent most commonly used for neurogenic urinary incontinence. Has fewer anticholinergic effects and more prominent detrusor relaxant effects than any antispasmodic except tolterodine. Potential for CNS toxicity increases with dose. Maximum benefit at week 4.
Tolterodine tartrate (Detrol) 1, 2 mg tablets	Competitive muscarinic receptor antagonist and antispasmodic indicated for urinary frequency and urge incontinence. Decreases number of voids and episodes of incontinence and increases volume per void.	1 to 2 mg BID. Onset is <1 hour and effect is sustained as long as drug is taken.	More selective for bladder than salivary glands. Better tolerated, but more expensive than oxybutynin. Reserve for patients who cannot tolerate oxybutynin.
Propantheline bromide (Pro-Banthine, generic) 15 mg tablets	Quaternary amine anticholinergic agent that does not cross blood-brain barrier	15 to 30 mg every 4 to 6 hours. Higher doses sometimes necessary	Effect approximates that of oxybutynin. Multiple daily doses required.
Dicyclomine hydrochloride (Bentyl, generic) 10 mg capsules, 20 mg tablets	Smooth muscle relaxant with anticholinergic properties; a tertiary amine	10 to 20 mg TID for elderly; up to 30 mg TID	Anticholinergic side effects, including CNS effects, become prominent as dose increases.
Flavoxate hydrochloride (Urispas) 100 mg tablets	Smooth muscle relaxant with anticholinergic properties	100 to 200 mg TID to QID	Conflicting efficacy results

(continued)

Table 97.8 • Drugs Most Commonly Used for Persistent Urinary Incontinence (continued)

Drug	Indication/Effect	Dose	Comments
Imipramine Hydrochloride (Tofranil, generic) 10, 25, 50 mg tablets	Indicated for stress incontinence. Relaxes detrusor muscle unrelated to anticholinergic and adrenergic effects. Increases bladder outlet resistance via enhanced α-adrenergic effects in smooth muscle of bladder base and proximal urethra.	25 mg at bedtime. Increase by 25 mg every 3rd day until continent, side effects occur, or a dose of 150 mg/day is reached. Usual dose is 25 mg BID for elderly and 25 mg QID for others.	Imipramine 75 mg/day produced continence in 68% in 4 weeks. Most become continent in 7 to 10 days. Weakness, fatigue, and postural hypotension are significant problems.
Estrogens	α-adrenergic stimulation of the urethra is estrogen dependent. Increases urethral outlet resistance in postmenopausal females.	Vaginal suppositories 1 mg/day	Can be additive with α-adrenergic agents, but additional study is needed.

Notes:

The reader is referred to Chapter 99: Geriatric Urologic Disorders, written by *John F. Thompson, Pharm.D.*, in the seventh edition of **Applied Therapeutics: The Clinical Use of Drugs** for a more in-depth discussion of the pathophysiology and pharmacotherapy of erectile dysfunction, benign prostatic hyperplasia, and urinary incontinence. All notations to reference numbers are to those listed in the original chapter noted above. The editors of this handbook express their thanks to Dr. Thompson and acknowledge that this chapter is based upon his work.

Notes:

Notes:

Index

Page numbers in *italics* denote figures; those followed by a "t" denote tables.